Getting Ready and Finishing Up

Getting Ready

Pre-procedure actions ("Getting Ready" steps) are taken before every patient or resident care procedure. These actions promote efficiency, safety, and respect of the patient's or resident's rights. You can remember the steps by thinking of the word **"WEAVERS"**

WASH – Hand hygiene

EQUIPMENT – Assemble needed supplies

ANNOUNCE – Knock and introduce yourself

VERIFY – Identify the person and check the person's care plan

EXPLAIN – Explain the procedure

RESPECT – Respect the person's privacy

SAFETY – See to safety

Finishing Up

Post-procedure actions ("Finishing Up" steps) are taken after every patient or resident care procedure. These actions promote comfort, safety, and communication among members of the health care team. You can remember the steps by thinking of the term **"ALSO Wash & Document."**

ALIGNMENT – Confirm comfort and body alignment

LIGHT – Leave the call light within the person's reach

SAFETY – See to safety

OPEN – Open the curtain and door

WASH – Hand hygiene

&

DOCUMENT – Report and record

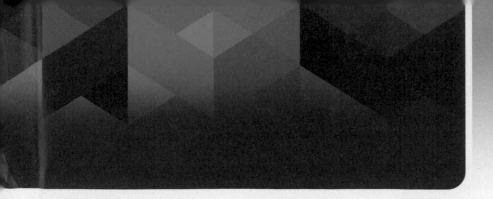

Contents in Brief

Lippincott Textbook for

Nursing

SIXTH EDITION

Assistants

A Humanistic Approach to Caregiving

Pamela J. Carter, RN, BSN, MEd, CNOR

Davis Hospital and Medical Center
Layton, Utah

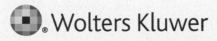 **Wolters Kluwer**

Philadelphia • Baltimore • New York • London
Buenos Aires • Hong Kong • Sydney • Tokyo

Vice President and Publisher: Julie K. Stegman
Senior Acquisitions Editor: Jonathan Joyce
Director of Nursing Education and Practice Content: Jamie Blum
Development Editor: Chelsea Neve
Editorial Coordinator: Anthony Gonzalez
Marketing Manager: Brittany Riney
Editorial Assistant: Devika Kishore
Design Coordinator: Stephen Druding
Art Director, Illustration: Jennifer Clements
Production Project Manager: Bridgett Dougherty
Manufacturing Coordinator: Margie Orzech-Zeranko
Prepress Vendor: Aptara, Inc.

Sixth edition

9 8 7 6 5 4 3 2 1

Printed in Mexico

Library of Congress Cataloging-in-Publication Data available upon request.
978-1-9751-9890-9

shop.lww.com

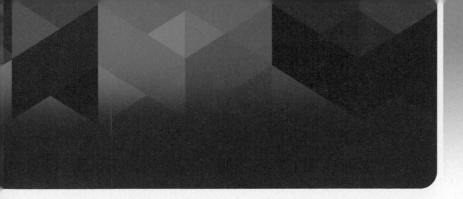

About the Author

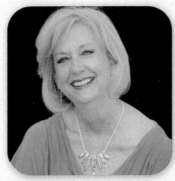

Pamela J. Carter is a registered nurse and an award-winning teacher. After receiving her bachelor's degree in nursing from the University of Alabama in Huntsville, Pamela immediately began a career as a perioperative nurse. Over the course of her nursing career, she also worked in a physician's office and as a staff nurse in an intensive care unit.

Pamela started teaching informally while serving as an officer in the United States Air Force Nurse Corps. She formally entered the field of health care education by accepting a position at the Athens Area Technical Institute in Athens, Georgia, where she taught surgical technology. After obtaining a master's degree in adult vocational education from the University of Georgia, Pamela moved to Florida and took a position teaching nursing assisting students. She continued teaching nursing assisting after accepting a position at Davis Technical College in Kaysville, Utah. During her first year at Davis Tech, Pamela piloted a new "open-entry/open-exit" method of curriculum delivery for the nursing assistant program at the college

and was awarded the Superintendent's Award for Outstanding Faculty for her work. She then opened a surgical technology program at the college and has obtained national accreditation from the Commission on Accreditation of Allied Health Education Programs (CAAHEP) for delivery of this program using the "open-entry/open-exit" method. In 2002, and again in 2014, 2015, 2016, and 2017, Pamela received a National Merit Award for having her program rank in the top 10% in the nation for students passing their national certification exam. After enjoying over 26 years teaching and preparing students to become health care professionals, Pamela has decided to return to her love of providing patient care to finish out her nursing career.

In addition to authoring this textbook, Pamela has also authored "Lippincott Essentials for Nursing Assistants," "Lippincott Advanced Skills for Nursing Assistants," and "Lippincott Textbook for Long-Term Care Nursing Assistants."

Pamela's writing style reflects her love of teaching, and of nursing. She is grateful for the opportunity teaching and writing have afforded her to share her experience and knowledge with those just entering the health care profession, and to help those who are new to the profession to see how they can have a profound effect on the lives of others.

DEDICATION

This book is dedicated to my colleagues, both past and present, who have worked with me and who share my passion for providing compassionate, humanistic care for all our patients. These past few years have taken a toll, both physically and emotionally, on all health care personnel. I applaud you all for continuing to care for those in need and for being such a positive influence for those entering the profession.

Pam

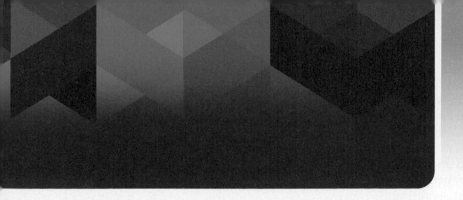

Preface

Nursing assistant education is changing. Indeed, it must change if we are to keep pace with the needs of the health care industry. Today, the need for competent nursing assistants by hospitals, acute and extended-care facilities, hospice agencies, and home health care agencies is growing rapidly. In addition, the composition of the long-term care population (the population most frequently cared for by nursing assistants) is changing. Shorter hospital stays and advances in medicine and technology mean that today's long-term care resident tends to be older, sicker, and in need of more assistance with activities of daily living than the resident of 15 years ago. As educators, we must seek to provide our students with the skills and knowledge that they will need to meet the changing needs of their patients, residents, and clients, and to advance in their own careers. In the past, the focus of nursing assistant education was on skill competency. However, that focus is shifting now toward graduating nursing assistants who not only possess the technical skills they need to provide competent care, but also the compassion and the communication and critical thinking skills they need to function effectively in the health care setting. It is no longer enough for nursing assistants to be competent at changing bed linens and measuring vital signs. Today's nursing assistants must also be able to recognize the person within the patient, resident, or client, and to understand that each person they are responsible for providing care for is unique and special, with individual needs that are very different from those of the person in the next bed. This textbook, *Lippincott Textbook for Nursing Assistants, 6th edition*, has been written not only to help students develop the skills they need to become nursing assistants, but also to introduce them to a very humanistic approach to caregiving. Because so many students use a Nursing Assisting course as the starting point for other endeavors in the health care profession, developing that sense of humanistic care early on assures its use throughout a person's career.

THEMES

Three key beliefs informed the writing of this textbook:

1. Students need a textbook that captures their interest and increases their desire to learn.
2. Graduates of nursing assistant training programs must be able to provide competent, skilled care in a compassionate way.
3. The nursing assistant is a vital member of the health care team.

These beliefs form the basis for the textbook you hold in your hands.

Lippincott Textbook for Nursing Assistants, 6e, Is Written With the Student in Mind

One of the primary goals in writing this textbook was to make the information it contains interesting and accessible to the student. Great care has been taken to present the student with a textbook that is easy and enjoyable to read, with a well-developed art program and proven learning aids.

A Student-Focused Writing Style

Educators know that a student can easily understand complex information if it is explained in a way that the student can understand. *Lippincott Textbook for Nursing Assistants* uses a conversational, yet professional, writing style that respects the student's intelligence. Concepts are presented in a straightforward, accessible way, and the text is enlivened through the frequent use of examples and anecdotes from the author's own experience with patients and residents. Recognizing that many students entering nursing assistant training programs speak English as a second language or are resource students, each chapter has been thoroughly reviewed by a special needs consultant to ensure an appropriate reading level.

An Art Program Developed Alongside the Text

The purpose of an art program is to reinforce and expand on concepts discussed in the text. To do this effectively, the art must be planned and developed alongside the manuscript. Numerous photographs, both alone and in combination with line art that has been created specifically for this textbook, help students to visualize and remember important concepts.

Proven Learning Aids in Every Chapter

Learning and remembering new information is challenging for many students. To help them meet the challenge of mastering the information in the textbook, we have developed features to assist students with studying and internalizing information:

- **What Will You Learn?** Each chapter begins with a *What Will You Learn?* section, which previews the chapter and helps to focus the student's reading. Each *What Will You Learn?* section begins with a paragraph that introduces the topic of the chapter to the student and explains why the topic is important. This introductory paragraph is then followed by a list of learning objectives and vocabulary words.
- **Summary.** Each chapter ends with a summary in a unique narrative outline format. This summary helps students to review the key, "take home" concepts of the chapter.
- **What Did You Learn?** Multiple-choice and matching exercises at the end of each chapter provide students with the opportunity to evaluate their understanding of the material they have just studied. Answers to these exercises are given in Appendix A.
- **Highlighted figure, table, and box call-outs.** The references to figures, tables, and boxes are highlighted with color in the narrative, helping students to quickly find their place in the text after stopping to look at a figure, table, or box.

New to This Edition!

Health care is always evolving with new discoveries and advances in treatment occurring constantly. It seems that the more we learn, the more there is to know. We strive to ensure that the material found in our textbook is based on the latest information and is current at the time of publication.

A primary focus of this new edition has been to streamline current information by focusing more on the "need to know" content that students need to succeed. Art and images have been reviewed and updated for relevancy and currency. Unit 7, which covers information on anatomy, physiology, normal aging, and system-specific diseases, has been reviewed and updated by a contributor with expertise in this field.

With this sixth edition, we wish to bring into focus the impact that the COVID-19 pandemic has had on how health care is provided. Changes in how we respond to communicable diseases have affected not only how health care workers provide care, but also how patients, residents, and clients live their daily lives. The infection control chapters in this book have been thoroughly updated and revised to improve their organization and make this important information easier for students to understand.

Recent years have shone a greater spotlight on many social justice issues in the United States, which have impacted us all on both personal and professional levels. With these ongoing challenges in mind, we are introducing a new feature, *Respect*, at the end of each unit. This feature focuses on inclusion and respect of all people, and includes short stories illustrating how nursing assistants learn more about caring for others simply by listening to their patients and residents share their unique backgrounds and experiences. These lessons remind us all that respect for the individual is central to humanistic care.

Other updates specific to this edition are summarized as follows:

- Terminology has been updated where needed throughout the text, including for inclusivity.
- Updated information related to nutrition and new dietary recommendations from the *2020–2025 Dietary Guidelines for Americans* has been included, along with the related art and descriptions of MyPlate and MyPlate for Older Adults.

Lippincott Textbook for Nursing Assistants, 6e, is Designed to Prepare Students for Clinical Practice

It is the author's desire to help prepare students to enter the health care profession with the knowledge, skills, and confidence that education and training can provide. Several of the textbook's features were designed specifically to help prepare the student for clinical practice:

■ **Procedures.** Certainly, a major objective of any nursing assistant training course is to ensure that graduates are able to provide care in a safe and correct manner. Each procedure in this text has been revised and updated in accordance with new infection control standards, current practice, and the current National Nurse Aide Assessment Program (NNAAP) Skills List. Those particular skills can be found in the following chapters:

■ **Hand Hygiene (Handwashing):** Chapter 12
■ **Applied One Knee-High Elastic Stocking:** Chapter 32
■ **Assists to Ambulate Using Transfer Belt:** Chapter 15
■ **Assists With Use of Bedpan:** Chapter 25
■ **Cleans Upper or Lower Denture:** Chapter 22
■ **Counts and records Radial Pulse/Respiration/Blood Pressure:** Chapter 20
■ **Donning and Removing PPE (Gown and Gloves):** Chapter 12
■ **Dresses Clients With Affected (Weak) Right Arm:** Chapter 23
■ **Feeds Client Who Cannot Feed Self:** Chapter 24
■ **Gives Modified Bed Bath:** Chapter 22
■ **Measures and Records Urinary Output:** Chapter 25
■ **Measures and Records Weight of Ambulatory Client:** Chapter 20
■ **Performs Modified PROM for Knee and Ankle/Shoulder:** Chapter 30
■ **Positions on Side:** Chapter 15
■ **Provides Catheter Care for Female:** Chapter 25
■ **Provides Foot Care:** Chapter 23
■ **Provides Mouth Care:** Chapter 22
■ **Provides Perineal Care for Female:** Chapter 22
■ **Transfers From Bed to Wheelchair Using Transfer Belt:** Chapter 15

Seventy-nine core procedures are presented in this text. The procedures for each chapter are grouped at the end of the chapter, to avoid breaking up the text with lengthy boxes. Each procedure box begins with a "Why You Do It" statement, to help students understand the "why behind the what," an understanding that is the foundation for the development of critical thinking skills. The concepts of privacy, safety, infection control, comfort, and communication are emphasized consistently in every procedure. *"Getting Ready"* and *"Finishing Up"* steps are included in every procedure box to help students remember these very important pre- and postprocedure actions. Easy-to-remember

mnemonics for the pre- and postprocedure actions help students remember. The steps of the procedure are given using clear and concise language, and photographs and illustrations are provided as necessary. A "What You Document" section at the end of each procedure reminds the student to document the care given and what important observations should be noted. An icon ▶ identifies procedures that are demonstrated in *Lippincott Video Series for Nursing Assistants*.

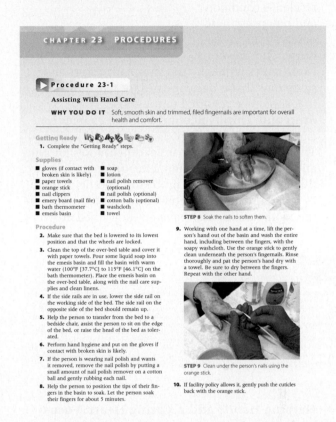

■ **Guidelines Boxes.** These boxes summarize general guidelines for various aspects of the nursing assistant's job. The unique "What You Do/Why You Do It" format helps students to understand why things are done a certain way. Rather than just presenting students with an endless list of guidelines to memorize, these boxes help them to remember why these guidelines are important to follow.

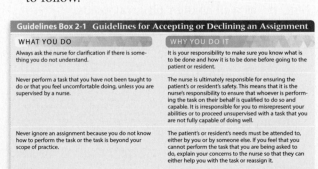

■ **Tell the Nurse! Notes.** A recurrent theme throughout the book is the important role the nursing assistant plays in making observations about a patient's or resident's condition and reporting these observations to the nurse. The *Tell the Nurse!* notes highlight and summarize signs and symptoms that a nursing assistant may observe that should be reported to the nurse.

Tell the Nurse!

As a nursing assistant, you may be the first to notice changes in a resident's behavior that may suggest delirium. If you notice any of the following in a person who is normally alert and oriented, report your observations to a nurse immediately:

● The person is hallucinating (seeing or hearing something that you know cannot possibly be true, such as mice crawling all over the bed)

● The person does not recognize someone familiar, or mistakes a stranger for a family member or close friend

● The person is very restless, especially at night

● The person seems confused

● The person talks frequently about events from the past, but cannot remember events that occurred recently (such as a meal eaten 2 hours ago)

● The person gets lost and wanders the halls aimlessly, even though the person knows their way around the facility

■ **Stop and Think! Scenarios.** Each chapter concludes with one or more *Stop and Think!* scenarios. These scenarios, which are excellent tools for initiating classroom discussion, encourage students to think critically to solve problems, and help them to see that many situations they will encounter in the workplace do not have cut-and-dried answers.

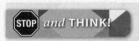

Imagine that you have just completed your nursing assistant training and taken the state test. While you are waiting for your test results, you decide to begin searching job postings to see what opportunities are available. At this point, you are considering several options. You are excited about beginning your career in the health care field, and you are anxious to get into the workforce and put your new skills to use. However, you think that you might also want to continue your education and become either a licensed practical nurse (LPN) or a registered nurse (RN) someday. What sorts of organizations may be looking for nursing assistants in your community? How could working as a nursing assistant now help you to further define your career goals?

You are a nursing assistant student completing your training in a local health care facility. Do you think that the nurses and nursing assistants view you as a potential employee? What actions can you take as a student to make a good impression?

■ **Helping Hands and a Caring Heart: Focus on Humanistic Health Care Boxes.** These boxes, found throughout the text, encourage students to empathize with those in their care, and emphasize the importance of meeting patients' and residents' emotional and spiritual needs, as well as their physical needs.

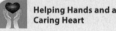 **Helping Hands and a Caring Heart**

Focus on Humanistic Health Care

Physically and emotionally, restraints have a very negative impact on a person's quality of life. Imagine how you would feel if you had to be "tied down." You might feel embarrassed, frightened, or humiliated. As a nursing assistant, there are many things you can do that may eliminate or reduce the need for restraints. These things require planning and effort, but the effort is considered part of the quality, individualized care that should be given to each person.

■ **Concerns for Long-Term Care.** This feature is found throughout the textbook and focuses on specific information that is important to remember when providing care for older residents in the long-term care setting.

Concerns for Long-Term Care

The majority of your residents in the long-term care setting are older adults and may experience difficulty with communication due to hearing loss, aphasia, or dementia. Unfortunately, many people think of older adults as people who are "going through their second childhood" and speak to them accordingly. When speaking with your older adult residents, avoid the use of "baby talk" or calling them all "sweetie" or "honey." These residents, like all people needing health care services, deserve to be spoken to with respect and as the adults they are. If a resident has a specific communication difficulty, learn about why the person has the difficulty and use communication techniques specific for that problem.

■ **Taking It to the Next Level: Advanced Skills.** This feature is found throughout the textbook where related information on advanced skills that nursing assistants may be providing in an advanced care setting can be accessed through the new ebook.

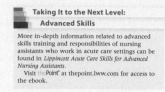 **Taking It to the Next Level: Advanced Skills**

More in-depth information related to advanced skills training and responsibilities of nursing assistants who work in acute care settings can be found in *Lippincott Acute Care Skills for Advanced Nursing Assistants*.

Visit *the*Point* at thepoint.lww.com for access to the ebook.

Lippincott Textbook for Nursing Assistants, 6e, Seeks to Instill in Students Pride in Themselves and Their Chosen Profession

It is important to impress upon students entering the health care profession that no one is "just" a nursing assistant. Nursing assistants are often the members of the health care team with the most day-to-day contact with patients, residents, and clients. As such, they bear a large part of the responsibility for the well-being of those in their care. To highlight the contributions that nursing assistants make, on *the*Point* can be found first-person accounts of how a nursing assistant had a positive impact on the lives of patients, residents, and clients or the lives of their loved ones. The goal of these *Nursing Assistants Make a Difference!* stories is to help students to see that nursing assistants are vital members of the health care team. Nursing assistants who feel that they can and do make a difference in the lives of others will go the "extra mile" to ensure that the care they provide is humanistic.

AN OVERVIEW OF LIPPINCOTT TEXTBOOK FOR NURSING ASSISTANTS

Lippincott Textbook for Nursing Assistants is a comprehensive textbook, designed to prepare students to work as nursing assistants in any health care setting, as well as to open their eyes to the many career opportunities that exist within the health care field and to entice them to further their learning. The United States is in the midst of a health care crisis—profound demographic changes have led to an ever-widening gap between the number of people who need care and the number of people who are qualified to provide that care. Educators of future health care professionals are charged with providing the community with competent, dedicated, and compassionate caregivers. In recognition of this need, this textbook has been designed to be in accordance with standards for curriculum development established by organizations such as the National Consortium on Health Science and Technology Education (NCHSTE) and Health Occupations Students of America (HOSA). Each instructional objective for approved nursing assistant training, as mandated by the Omnibus Budget Reconciliation Act (OBRA), is covered in-depth.

A lifelong interest in learning new information is an important quality for any health care professional to have, as the body of information related to medicine and health care is constantly evolving. A lifelong interest in learning benefits the recipients of care as well as the caregivers themselves. Awareness of career pathways allows those just entering the health care profession to set goals for career advancement and reach them, over time receiving higher levels of compensation for higher levels of experience, skills, and responsibilities.

This textbook consists of 10 units. The following is a brief survey of these units and the information they contain.

Unit 1: Introduction to Health Care

The six chapters that make up Unit 1 provide the student with basic background knowledge. Chapter 1 begins with an overview of how health care has evolved, and continues to evolve, in the United States. It then provides the student with a basic understanding of how the governmental regulations that control health care standards and payment came into existence. The nursing home survey process is introduced so that students become better informed of how regulatory organizations determine a facility's ability to provide quality care to the residents. Chapter 1 also provides an overview of the many different types of health care facilities, and introduces the idea of holistic, humanistic health care and the "health care team." Chapter 2 focuses on the nursing assistant's roles and responsibilities as a member of the health care team, and on the concept of delegation. Professionalism, the concept of work ethic, and job-seeking skills are thoroughly discussed in Chapter 3, introducing students to the idea that a professional attitude promotes respect and is necessary for career advancement. Legal and ethical issues, including patient and resident rights and the Health Insurance Portability and Accountability Act (HIPAA), are covered in Chapter 4. Information specific to abuse and defining "vulnerable adults" who are often victims of abuse, is included. Communication, one of the most essential responsibilities of the nursing assistant, is discussed in Chapter 5. This unit concludes with Chapter 6, which focuses on the central member of the health care team—the patient, resident, or client. Information has been included to stress the importance of the person's family members and how

they should be included in the health care plan of care. This final chapter introduces the concept of human needs and explains how the person being cared for in a health care setting has many needs other than those specifically associated with illness or disability.

Unit 2: Long-Term Care

This unit is comprised of three chapters that focus on the long-term care setting and the care of residents. Chapter 7, Overview of Long-Term Care, introduces the student to the long-term care setting and includes a discussion about the past, present, and future of long-term care. Chapter 8, The Long-Term Care Resident, helps students understand the factors that can lead to admission to a long-term care facility, and the special needs that residents of long-term care facilities, and their families, may have. Chapter 9 continues the discussion by providing information about dementia, a condition that affects many long-term care residents.

Unit 3: Infection Control

Unit 3 is a new unit in this edition and contains current information about communicable disease, how it is transmitted, and the measures that health care workers take to protect their patients and residents as well as themselves from contracting these illnesses. Chapter 10 introduces students to communicable disease and how our bodies can either fight off an infection or become infected. Chapter 11 continues with a discussion of common communicable diseases and how they can be transmitted within a health care setting. Chapter 12 concludes this unit with measures that health care workers use to help prevent the spread of infection in the health care setting. Updated recommendations by the CDC and management of epidemics and pandemics are also included.

Unit 4: Safety

The four chapters that compose Unit 4 are concerned with the measures taken to ensure safety. Chapter 13 deals with workplace safety, and includes an extensive discussion about the importance of using proper body mechanics and ergonomics to prevent work-related injuries. Also in Chapter 13, the student is introduced to the "Getting Ready" and "Finishing Up" steps that are taken before and after each procedure. Colorful and descriptive mnemonics help students to easily remember each of these important pre- and post-procedure steps. Chapter 14 explores some of the conditions that put patients, residents, or clients at risk for injury, followed by a discussion about methods used to prevent accidents from occurring. Restraints, with a focus on methods that can be used as an alternative to a restraint, are discussed in-depth. In Chapter 15, the techniques used to safely assist patients, residents, and clients with repositioning and transferring are covered. This unit concludes with Chapter 16, which contains information related to recognizing emergencies and responding to them. Included in Chapter 16 are the current AHA BLS guidelines.

Unit 5: Basic Patient and Resident Care

The nine chapters in this unit focus on the skills and equipment used to provide basic daily care to patients, residents, and clients. Chapters 17 and 18 introduce the student to the health care environment and explain the processes for admitting, transferring, or discharging patients, residents, and clients. Chapter 19 covers bed-making. Chapter 20 covers vital signs, with an emphasis on exactly what function of the body is being measured and situations that may alter these measurements. Also included are practical tips to take the mystery out of taking vital sign measurements, procedures that many students find intimidating and difficult to master at first. Chapter 21 discusses the importance of rest and sleep and how the nursing assistant can help to promote a person's comfort in the health care setting. Pain, and information on pain relief measures are also included here. Chapters 22 and 23 cover bathing and grooming, with a focus on empathizing with the person receiving the care. In Chapter 24, current dietary recommendations from the *2020–2025 Dietary Guidelines for Americans* discusses MyPlate and MyPlate for Older Adults, along with basic information about nutrition and the nursing assistant's role in assisting patients or residents with meeting their nutritional needs. We conclude Unit 5 with Chapter 25, a discussion about assisting with elimination. Again, much emphasis is placed on empathizing with the patient, resident, or client who requires assistance with this most intimate of activities.

Unit 6: Death and Dying

This unit has been written as two separate chapters to emphasize that a person may cope with a terminal illness and the stages of grief for a long period of time before the actual physical process of dying takes place. Chapter 26 introduces the student to the stages of grief within the context of a discussion about terminal illness. Important concepts such as advance directives, wills, and palliative care are also discussed in this chapter. Chapter 27 focuses on the care a nursing assistant provides to the dying person and their family members in the hours immediately leading up to, and following, death. Both chapters in this unit include discussions about the grief a nursing assistant can

expect to feel when a patient, resident, or client dies or receives a diagnosis of a terminal illness.

Unit 7: Body Systems: Normal Function and the Effects of Aging and Disease

Unit 7 has been reviewed and revised by an expert in the field of anatomy and physiology to provide the most current information related to the body systems. Having a basic understanding of how each of the body's organ systems functions in health is essential to understanding how failure of an organ system to work properly leads to disease and disability. This unit begins with Chapter 28, which provides an overview of the body's organization and introduces the student to different types of disease processes that can affect each body system. Chapters 29 through 38 each cover one of the organ systems. A basic explanation of the normal structure and function of the organ system is given, with an emphasis on homeostasis. Next, the normal effects of aging are discussed and differentiated from the effects of disease and disability. Key disorders specific to that particular body system are then discussed. Diagnostic tests and treatments are also covered. Throughout these chapters, the nursing assistant's role in recognizing problems and providing care is emphasized.

Unit 8: Special Care Concerns

This unit, which consists of four chapters, introduces the student to the special needs of certain groups of people. Chapter 39 introduces the student to the different phases of the rehabilitation process and discusses rehabilitation measures specific for different types of disability. In Chapter 40, some of the major types of developmental disabilities are reviewed, along with updated information related to each disability. Chapter 41 is dedicated to a discussion about mental disorders, including the importance of recognizing depression in older adult patients, residents, and clients. Information that discusses posttraumatic stress disorder and substance use disorder is also included. The final chapter in this unit, Chapter 42, discusses the diagnosis and treatment of cancer, as well as the special needs of people with cancer.

Unit 9: Acute Care

Nursing assistants provide care in many different types of health care settings. Many work in hospitals and clinics and assist nurses in caring for patients with acute conditions. The focus of the three chapters in Unit 9 is on special populations of patients that the nursing assistant may encounter in the acute care setting. Chapter 43 is dedicated to the surgical patient, Chapter 44 to obstetrical patients and newborns, and Chapter 45 to the pediatric patient.

Unit 10: Home Health Care

The two chapters in this final unit introduce the student to the home health care setting. These two chapters have been revised in accordance to suggestions and recommendations from experts who currently work in the home health care field. Building on the basic knowledge and skills presented in previous units, this unit explores some of the concerns and issues that are unique to the home health care setting. Chapter 46 provides the student with an overview of what home health care is, who might require it, and how it is paid for, and explores some of the qualities that a person must have to succeed as a home health care aide. Chapter 47 covers specific issues related to safety and infection control within the home.

Appendices and Glossary

The textbook concludes with two appendices and a comprehensive glossary. Appendix A contains the answers to the *What Did You Learn?* exercises that appear at the end of each chapter. Appendix B introduces the student to the language of health care. We chose to include this discussion about medical terminology as an appendix so that it could be introduced at any point during the training course, and referred to frequently. The tables containing common roots, prefixes, suffixes, and updated abbreviations are in close physical proximity to the glossary for easy and quick reference. The glossary is the most comprehensive found in any nursing assistant textbook. A precise definition of each vocabulary word is given. The number in parentheses at the end of each entry indicates the chapter where the term is introduced as a vocabulary word. Extensive cross-references remind students of synonyms and antonyms, and help them to differentiate related words.

A NOTE ABOUT THE LANGUAGE USED IN THIS BOOK

Wolters Kluwer recognizes that people have a diverse range of identities, and we are committed to using inclusive and nonbiased language in our content. In line with the principles of nursing, we strive not to define people by their diagnoses, but to recognize their personhood first and foremost, using as much as possible the language diverse groups use to define themselves, and including only information that is relevant to nursing care.

We strive to better address the unique perspectives, complex challenges, and lived experiences of diverse populations traditionally underrepresented in health literature. When describing or referencing populations discussed in research studies, we will adhere to the identities presented in those studies to maintain fidelity to the evidence presented by the study investigators. We follow best practices of language set forth by the Publication Manual of the American Psychological Association, 7th edition, but acknowledge that language evolves rapidly, and we will update the language used in future editions of this book as necessary.

A COMPREHENSIVE PACKAGE FOR TEACHING AND LEARNING

To further facilitate teaching and learning, a carefully designed ancillary package is available. In addition to the usual print resources, we are pleased to present multimedia tools that have been developed in conjunction with the text.

Resources for Instructors

- ***Lippincott Acute Care Skills for Advanced Nursing Assistants* first edition ebook.** Depending on the needs of the different types of facilities that hire nursing assistants, the skills required and the daily duties of the nursing assistant varies greatly. As a nursing assistant advances within their career, the need for additional training increases.

  Because of this, we are providing an ebook addition, titled *Lippincott Acute Care Skills for Advanced Nursing Assistants*, as a companion to this textbook. We feel that the ebook companion will be a useful tool for nursing assisting instructors who teach advanced skills in their programs. It has also been developed for use by nursing assistants who have completed their basic nursing assisting training and have obtained employment in an acute care setting where they are required to perform advanced skills.

- ***Lippincott® CoursePoint.*** This integrated, digital curriculum solution for nursing education provides other course knowledge and prepares students for practice. The time-tested, easy-to-use and trusted solution includes engaging learning tools and in-depth reporting to meet students where they are in their learning, combined with the most trusted nursing education content on the market to help prepare students for practice. This easy-to-use digital learning solution of *Lippincott® CoursePoint*, combined with unmatched support, gives instructors and students everything they need for course and curriculum success!

- *Lippincott® CoursePoint* includes:
  - Engaging course content provides a variety of learning tools to engage students of all learning styles.
  - Adaptive and personalized learning helps students learn the critical thinking and clinical judgment skills needed to help them become practice-ready nurses.
  - Unparalleled reporting provides in-depth dashboards with several data points to track student progress and help identify strengths and weaknesses.
  - Unmatched support includes training coaches, product trainers, and nursing education consultants to help educators and students implement CoursePoint with ease.
- *Lippincott Video Series for Nursing Assistants.* Procedure-based modules provide step-by-step demonstrations of the core skills that form the basis of the daily care the nursing assistant provides. As in the textbook, all procedures have been reviewed and updated in accordance with current practice, infection control, and the current NNAAP skills. *Getting Ready and Finishing Up* actions are reviewed on every procedure-based module, and the concepts of privacy, safety, infection control, comfort, and communication are emphasized throughout. Four non–procedure-based modules, on the topics of preparing for entry into the workforce, caring for people with dementia, death and dying, and communication and patient and resident rights, are also available.

Tools to assist you with teaching your course are available upon adoption of this text on thePoint® at https://thePoint.lww.com/Carter6e.

- **Stop and Think! Scenario Discussion Points** outline the main concepts of the text's *Stop and Think!* feature.
- A **Test Generator** lets you put together exclusive new tests from a bank containing hundreds of questions to help you in assessing your students' understanding of the material. Test questions link to chapter learning objectives.
- **PowerPoint Presentations** provide an easy way for you to integrate the textbook with your students' classroom experience, either via slideshows or handouts. Multiple-choice and true/false questions are integrated into the presentations to promote class participation and allow you to use i-clicker technology.
- An **Image Bank** lets you use the photographs and illustrations from this textbook in your PowerPoint slides or as you see fit in your course.

- **Guided Lecture Notes** include Learning Objectives and references to PowerPoint presentation slides.
- **Sample Syllabi** for long and short courses.
- **Answers and Rationales to** *Workbook for Lippincott Textbook for Nursing Assistants*, Assignments, Pre-Lecture Quizzes, and Discussion Topics.
- Plus **Strategies for Effective Teaching, Discussion Topics, Assignments**, and **Pre-Lecture Quizzes**.

Resources for Students

An exciting set of free resources is available on thePoint® to help students review material and become even more familiar with vital concepts. Students can access all these resources at https://thePoint.lww.com/Carter6e using the codes printed in the front of their textbooks.

- *Watch and Learn!,* a series of video clips that support information given in the text.
- **Audio Clips for** *Nursing Assistants Make a Difference!* allow the student to listen to first-person accounts of how nursing assistants have made a difference in the lives of patients, residents, clients, and family members.
- **Certification-Style Review Questions** for each chapter help students review important concepts and practice for certification exams.
- Plus downloadable **Procedures** checklists from the text.

Workbook to Accompany *Lippincott Textbook for Nursing Assistants, 6e.* Developed by an instructional design team, this workbook provides the student with a fun and engaging way of reviewing important concepts and vocabulary. Each part of the student workbook has been updated and revised alongside the changes made in the sixth edition of the textbook. Multiple-choice questions, matching exercises, true/false exercises, word finds, crossword puzzles, labeling exercises, and other types of active learning tools are provided to appeal to many different learning styles. The workbook also contains procedure checklists for each procedure in the textbook.

It is with great pleasure that the author and publisher introduce these resources—the textbook, the ancillary package, the videos, and the companion ebook—to you. One of my primary goals in creating these resources has been to share with those just entering the health care field my sense of excitement about the health care profession, and my commitment to the idea that being a nursing assistant involves much more than just "bedpans and blood pressures." I hope I have succeeded in that goal, and I welcome your feedback.

Pamela J. Carter

To the Students

Welcome! By enrolling in this nursing assistant training course, you have taken a big first step. You may be taking this course for any number of different reasons. For example, you may be taking this course to "test the waters"—to see if working in health care is something you really want to do. Or, you may already know that you want to work in health care, and you are taking this course because it is the first step toward reaching your goal. Health care is an exciting, yet demanding, field. During your training course, you will be expected to learn and apply a lot of new information. You will even have to learn a new language, the language of health care! My name is Pam Carter, and I am the author of this book. It is my pleasure and my honor to assist you on your journey toward becoming a health care professional.

HOW TO USE THE BOOK TO PREPARE FOR CLASS AND STUDY

Learning is an active process. You need to read, make notes, and ask questions about anything you are having trouble understanding. Most students who are successful learners take a three-step approach to learning:

Preview

During the *preview* stage of learning, you focus on preparing yourself for class. Most likely, your instructor will give you reading and possibly video assignments that must be completed before each class. The course *syllabus* that you will receive at the beginning of the course will tell you when each reading assignment must be completed. The reading assignments give you the chance to get a general idea of what is going to be discussed in the next class.

To prepare for class, just read the assignment as if you were reading a novel, magazine, or news story for enjoyment. During the preview, you do not need to take notes or try to memorize facts—just read through the material to get the "big picture" of the information you are about to learn. Some people find it helpful to read the chapter out loud to themselves (or into an audio recorder, so that they can listen to the chapter again later). Others like to highlight parts of the chapter using a highlighting pen, or make notes in the margin. Learning becomes much easier when you discover what methods work best for you. To assist you with previewing, each chapter in the book begins with a *What Will You Learn?* section. This section contains a list of specific goals for the chapter, called *learning objectives*. Learning objectives tell you what you will be expected to know or be able to do to demonstrate complete understanding of the material in the chapter. During the preview stage, the learning objectives are useful for giving you an overview of the key goals of the chapter. The *What Will You Learn?* section also contains a list of the new vocabulary words you will need to learn. The vocabulary words, which appear in

---

WHAT WILL YOU LEARN?

As a health care professional, you will be part of the health care system. In this chapter, you will learn about the many different types of organizations that make up the health care system. You will also learn about some of the government regulations that affect the health care system. Finally, we will discuss some of the ways that health care is paid for in the United States. When you are finished with this chapter, you will be able to:

1. Identify changes that have occurred in how health care is delivered.
2. Describe the different types of health care organizations.
3. Briefly explain the structure of a health care organization.
4. List some of the government and private agencies that provide oversight of the health care system.
5. Describe how the survey process is used to monitor the quality of care given by health care organizations.
6. Discuss how health care is paid for.

bold type throughout the chapter, are listed in the order that they appear. You can also look each word up in the glossary at the back of the book to find a complete definition. Familiarizing yourself with the chapter's vocabulary words before class puts you one step ahead, because when you hear those words in class, they will not sound strange to you, and you may already know what they mean.

If you are a nursing assistant who is working or planning to work in an acute care setting, look for the *Taking It to the Next Level: Advanced Skills* feature. The feature calls out information that is further explained in the updated companion ebook, *Lippincott Acute Care Skills for Advanced Nursing Assistants*. This ebook is available on thePoint® and is written in mind for the nursing assistant who is already progressing to the next level in their nursing assistant careers.

View

The *viewing* stage is when you get down to business and really work to understand the material. During the classroom lecture or discussion, highlight important points and take notes as you need to. Ask questions about any of the material that you do not fully understand. Remember, there are no "stupid" questions! If you do not fully understand something, you need to speak up so that the instructor can help you. This is your instructor's job.

Review

After class, go back over the notes you took in class, and review the chapter in your book. Some students like to read the entire chapter over again. Others just skim the chapter, paying close attention to the topics they still have questions about. Read the chapter summary, which reviews the key concepts of the chapter. If you are using the student workbook in your class, complete the exercises by looking the answers up in the textbook chapter. Looking for the answers is another way of reviewing the information in the chapter, and many students find that the act of writing the answers down helps them to remember the information. When you feel comfortable with your understanding of the material, test yourself! Go back to the learning objectives in the *What Will You Learn?* section at the beginning of the chapter and pretend they are questions. Try to answer them. If you have trouble answering them, then you know that you need to review certain parts of the chapter again. You can also test yourself using the *What Did You Learn?* section, at the end of each chapter. The answers to the questions in the *What Did You Learn?* section are in Appendix A in the back of the book so that you can

see how well you understood the material you just studied. Again, if you have trouble answering these questions, then you will know that your studying is not quite finished! You may need to read certain parts of the chapter again, or ask your instructor for help. Try to set aside short periods of time for studying each day. For example, you might study for 30 to 45 minutes, take a break to attend to other activities or chores, and then come back and study for another 30 to 45 minutes. After 30 to 45 minutes of studying, most people become tired and lose their ability to concentrate. Studying in short bursts will help keep you focused on the material you are trying to learn.

SUMMARY

- No matter what the setting, nursing assistants are an integral part of the nursing team, a subset of the health care team.
- Like all of the members of the nursing team, nursing assistants undergo training that authorizes them to perform certain tasks.
- Nursing assistants assist the nurse by performing basic nursing functions, such as those related to hygiene, safety, comfort, nutrition, exercise, and elimination.
- To ensure that the nursing team operates smoothly and efficiently, a "chain of command" exists. This means that licensed nurses (RNs or LPNs) are able to assign (delegate) certain tasks to nursing assistants.
- The delegation of tasks cannot be taken lightly by either the delegator (the licensed nurse) or the delegatee (the nursing assistant). Both share the responsibility of ensuring that the procedure is carried out without harm to the patient or resident.
- The nursing assistant must know which tasks are within their scope of practice and which tasks are not.

WHAT DID YOU LEARN?

Multiple Choice

Select the single best answer for each of the following questions.

1. Nursing assistants who work in the long-term care setting must complete a course of training and undergo a competency evaluation. These requirements are set by the:
   a. Centers for Disease Control (CDC)
   b. Food and Drug Administration (FDA)
   c. Omnibus Budget Reconciliation Act of 1987 (OBRA)
   d. Occupational Safety and Health Administration (OSHA)

2. As a nursing assistant, it is your responsibility to:
   a. Plan the patient's or resident's care
   b. Perform the tasks your supervisor assigns to you
   c. Do the best you can without asking for help
   d. Compare assignments with your coworkers

3. If you do not know how to do an assigned task, you should:
   a. Call another nursing assistant for help
   b. Ask the patient or resident how they prefer to have it done
   c. Call the charge nurse and ask for help
   d. Follow the instructions in the procedure manual

4. Nursing assistants work under the supervision of:
   a. A doctor
   b. A registered nurse (RN) or licensed practical nurse (LPN)
   c. Other nursing assistants
   d. The long-term care facility administrator

5. To "delegate" means to:
   a. Do what you are told to do
   b. Give another person permission to perform a task on your behalf
   c. Transfer your duties to another assistant
   d. Have the charge nurse take your assignment

6. What information is included in the registry?
   a. The nursing assistant's full name
   b. The nursing assistant's registry number and date of expiration
   c. Any reported incidents of abuse or theft
   d. All of the above

HOW TO PREPARE FOR TESTS

Did you learn the material or not? This is what instructors want to know when they give tests, quizzes, and exams. Not doing well on a test does not mean that you are a failure. It just means that you need to figure out what went wrong, and make an effort to improve the next time. Perhaps you did not study as well as you could have for the test. Or maybe you got so nervous, you forgot everything you learned when it came time to take the test!

The course syllabus will tell you when a test is scheduled to be given, and what material it will cover. Mark these dates on your calendar, so you are not surprised! Preparing for a test should not be a major event. If you use the preview–view–review approach and study each day, when it comes time to prepare for the test, you will be very well prepared. In the days leading up to the test, all you will need to do is review the material that will be covered on the test one more time, by skimming the chapters in the book and reviewing the notes you took in class. When it comes time to actually take the test, remember the following tips:

- Relax! You have prepared for this test, and you know the answers to these questions!

- Take a deep breath and make sure you read the directions carefully. The directions will tell you whether there is only one correct answer for each question, or whether it is possible for a question to have more than one correct answer.

- Read each question completely and carefully. Many students answer questions incorrectly simply because they are in a hurry and miss important words, like "except" or "not."

- If the question is a multiple-choice question, try to state the answer in your head before looking at the answer choices. Then read each answer choice before choosing the one that best matches the answer you have in your head. This will increase your confidence that the answer you have selected is the correct one.

- After selecting an answer, avoid second-guessing yourself. Research has shown that your first choice is most likely to be correct, if you studied the material well. Sometimes, however, you will come across a question later in the test that makes you realize that you answered an earlier question incorrectly. In this case, when you are sure that you have made a mistake, it is all right to go back and change your answer. But if you do not have a clear idea of what the correct answer is, doubting your first choice will most likely result in changing a correct answer to an incorrect one!

- If you cannot answer a question, go on to the next. Often, another question on the test will jog your memory and help you to remember the answer to the question you skipped earlier. Just remember to go back over your answer sheet before you hand in your test to make sure you have answered all of the questions.

Many people think that the goal of studying is to pass a test. It is true that as you work through your training course, you will have to pass many tests. And most states require people who want to be nursing assistants to pass a certification exam at the end of the training course. But passing the test is a short-term goal. It is more important for you to be able to remember and use the information that you learned during your training course long after you complete the course and pass the certification exam. The people you will be caring for are depending on you to be knowledgeable and good at what you do. They are trusting you with their health and well-being. Study hard, ask questions, and remember that each and every person you care for throughout your career deserves the same type of competent, compassionate care that you would expect to be given to your own parents, spouse, partner, sibling, or child. As a nursing assistant, you will have the chance to have a positive effect on the lives of many people. Caring for those in need is very important work. Let me be among the first to thank you for your interest in pursuing a career in health care, and to wish you luck on your journey.

Sincerely,
PAM

Acknowledgments

Health care has undergone some unique and challenging changes since our last edition! These changes have affected our society and how we interact with other people and have increased our need to practice tolerance and respect for everyone. The pandemic has not only changed how we provide health care, but how we live our daily lives. It has also stressed the providers of health care to the breaking point. As we work to regroup and move forward, new challenges will face us, and it is our responsibility to teach and support the next generation of health care workers as they enter this field. Thank you all for your hard work as you strive to mentor and nurture the future of health care.

I wish to extend my sincere thanks to Chelsea Neve, Development Editor, for her exceptional assistance in making this edition more streamlined, inclusive, and sensitive in content. She is such a pleasure to work with! Also to Anthony Gonzalez, Editorial Coordinator, who has worked so hard to keep this project on track, even when my eyes would not work. And finally, to Jonathon Joyce, Senior Acquisitions Editor, for continuing to believe in me and what I write. You are all exceptional and I am truly honored to be able to work with such a great crew!

I would also like to personally thank the OR crew at Davis Hospital and Medical Center for their care and concern during my surgeries this year. And a special thanks to Dr. Mark Rush, Dr. Jason Rupp. Dr. Claron Alldredge, and Trish Perkins for your care and expertise to help save my eyesight. Without you all, completing this book would not have been possible.

Contents

UNIT 5

UNIT 6

Death and Dying 497
CHAPTER 26
Caring for People Who Are Terminally Ill 498

UNIT 8

Special Care Concerns   721

UNIT 10

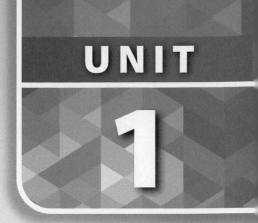

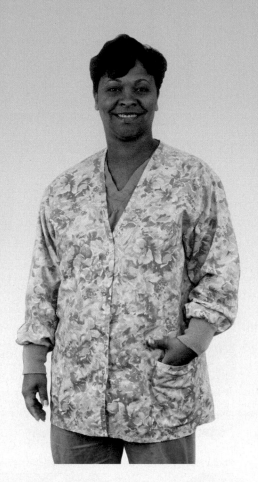

Introduction to Health Care

WELCOME TO THE HEALTH CARE FIELD! TODAY IN THE UNITED STATES, the health care field is one of the largest fields and is expected to grow on average by about one million new jobs per year. In 2020, over 1.4 million of those employed by the health care industry were nursing assistants, with the number of job openings expected to increase by 8% through 2030.* The health care field is the focus of Unit 1.

*Bureau of Labor Statistics, U.S. Department of Labor, Occupational Outlook Handbook 2020–21 edition.

Photo: Welcome to the health care field! Nursing assistants are key members of the health care team.

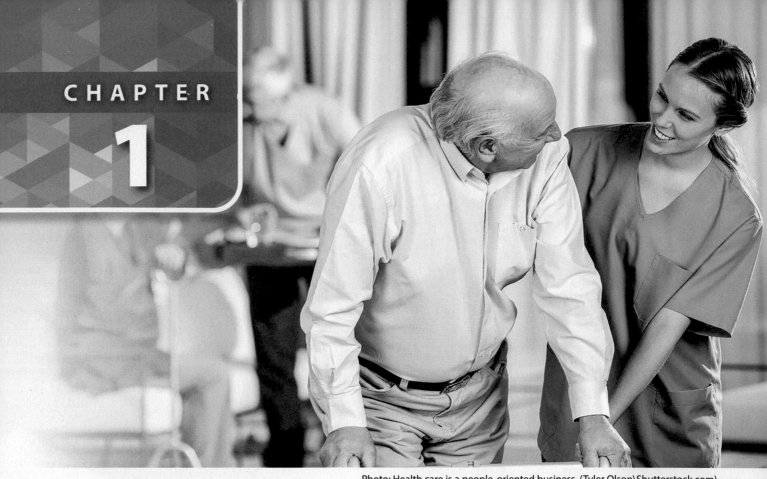

Photo: Health care is a people-oriented business. (Tyler Olson\Shutterstock.com)

The Health Care System

 WHAT WILL YOU LEARN?

As a health care professional, you will be part of the health care system. In this chapter, you will learn about the many different types of organizations that make up the health care system. You will also learn about some of the government regulations that affect the health care system. Finally, we will discuss some of the ways that health care is paid for in the United States. When you are finished with this chapter, you will be able to:

1. Identify changes that have occurred in how health care is delivered.
2. Describe the different types of health care organizations.
3. Briefly explain the structure of a health care organization.
4. List some of the government and private agencies that provide oversight of the health care system.
5. Describe how the survey process is used to monitor the quality of care given by health care organizations.
6. Discuss how health care is paid for.

Vocabulary

Holistic
Mission
Hospital
Acute care setting
Patients
Subacute care unit
    (skilled nursing unit,
    skilled nursing facility)

Long-term care facility
    (nursing home)
Residents
Assisted-living facility
Home health care agency
Clients
Hospice organizations
Health care team

United States
    Department of Health
    and Human Services
    (DHHS)
Omnibus Budget
    Reconciliation Act
    (OBRA) of 1987
Accreditation

Survey
Occupational Safety and
    Health Administration
    (OSHA)
Managed care system
Medicare
Minimum Data Set (MDS)
Medicaid

HEALTH CARE DELIVERY, PAST AND PRESENT

In the United States during the 18th, 19th, and early part of the 20th centuries, health care delivery focused mainly around the home and family. The health care provider was trained in general health care skills. The provider delivered babies, attended to wounds and broken bones, and provided comfort to both the dying person and the family (Fig. 1-1).

Present-day delivery of health care has changed dramatically. More intensive educational preparation for health care providers has become the standard and, in the United States, is required for those who want to care for those in need. Large facilities dedicated to providing on-site patient care have been established, replacing the home as the primary site for patient care. Doctors treat people in doctor's offices, clinics, work areas, schools, and other types of health care settings. A variety of medications and other treatments allow us to treat and cure many diseases that in the past would have been fatal, increasing the average person's life span. The family doctor who attended a person from birth to death is now called a "general practitioner" or "family physician," and in many cases, they are supported by a team of specialists.

Although in the recent past the trend was to *replace* the family doctor with a team of specialists, today we are seeing a return to a more **holistic** approach to health care. A holistic approach focuses on the care of the whole person, not just the person's physical condition or disease. When a holistic approach to care is taken, the person's physical *and* emotional needs are met. The best aspect of the care provided by the old-fashioned "family doctor"—the doctor's familiarity with the person as an individual—is combined with modern-day availability of specialized care when needed.

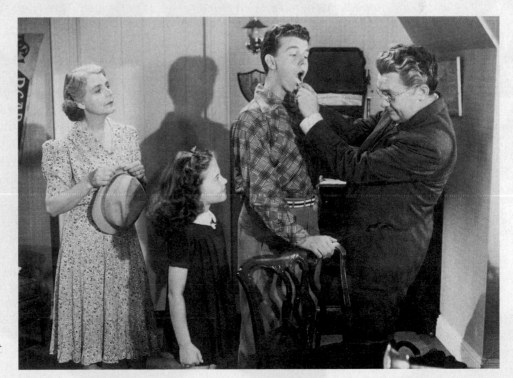

Figure 1-1 In the past, health care was delivered in the home, usually by a "family doctor." (*Everett Collection\Shutterstock.com*)

Helping Hands and a Caring Heart

Focus on Humanistic Health Care

A "humanistic" approach to health care is one that focuses on the person receiving the care. When we take a humanistic approach to health care, we:

- Consider the qualities that make the person unique and use that knowledge to guide the care that we provide.
- Imagine how it would feel to be in the person's situation and act with empathy and compassion.
- Consider the person's emotional, social, and spiritual needs, as well as their physical needs.

A humanistic approach to health care is the basis for providing quality care. Here is a true story that will help you understand how a humanistic approach can make a real difference in the lives of your patients or residents and their family members:

"Nell was a woman I visited in her home and later in a nursing home. She came from a Catholic background. Although I am a Methodist pastor, I told Nell I would be glad to get a rosary and pray it with her. I was willing to do anything that would help her feel closer to God. She said she was fine and didn't need anything from her background. Instead, I began the ritual of closing our visits with prayer and ending with the two of us saying the Lord's Prayer together. Visit after visit over the course of a couple of years, we prayed together. We were creating our own ritual.

Eventually, Nell became very ill and was dying. She was in the hospital. I went to visit and found her son and daughter-in-law with her in the hospital room. She had been unconscious that day and the day before. I visited with them for a while. As I prepared to leave, I asked them if they would like to pray together. They said they would appreciate a prayer. So, we circled around Nell's bed and prayed. As usual, I began to end the time of prayer with the Lord's Prayer as Nell and I had done so often in the past. At that point, Nell began to pray aloud with us. The ritual we had created together stirred within her and spoke through her unconsciousness. The time I shared with Nell and her family that day was so special. The time was healing because Nell's son and daughter-in-law heard Nell speak one more time. She did not come out of her unconscious state, but she responded from deep within to join us in the words of the Lord's Prayer."

—Reverend Diane M. Bell

Many of the things Reverend Bell did to help Nell are things you can do too in your work as a nursing assistant. Spend time with your patients or residents and get to know them as individuals. Using that knowledge, think about things you can do that will help them feel more comfortable, both physically and emotionally. Act with compassion. Everyone will benefit! You will have the satisfaction of knowing that you are providing the best care possible, and your patients or residents will feel well cared for and valued as individuals. That is what a humanistic approach to health care is all about.

HEALTH CARE ORGANIZATIONS

As the health care system has developed and changed over the years, we have seen more and more variety in the organizations that provide health care to people in need. As a nursing assistant, you will be employed by a health care organization. All health care organizations have a purpose, or **mission**. Some health care organizations, such as university hospitals, are associated directly with schools. The primary mission of a university hospital may be to train people in the field of health care. Other health care organizations are associated with a religious group. Some health care organizations are owned by corporations and use the health care industry as a financial investment in order to turn a profit. Although some health care organizations have very specific missions, others combine many of the following:

- To prevent disease by providing immunizations, teaching people how to control chronic health problems, and identifying factors that could place a person at risk for a disease
- To detect and treat disease
- To promote health by teaching people about ways to achieve and maintain both physical and mental fitness
- To offer rehabilitation (restorative care) services in order to help people return to their highest possible level of physical or emotional function
- To provide emergency care to people with life-threatening illnesses or injuries
- To educate health care professionals by providing work-based training for medical students, student nurses, and many other types of students training for a career in the health care field

Types of Health Care Organizations

There are many different types of health care organizations. Depending on where you live, you may be able to work as a nursing assistant in all of these organizations, or just some. For example, in some states, nursing assistants are only employed in long-term care facilities (nursing homes), but in others, nursing assistants can work in hospitals.

Hospitals

A person who has a severe illness or whose condition is unstable and who requires a great deal of care and close monitoring is usually treated in a **hospital**, which is a type of **acute care setting**. The services provided by a hospital differ according to the hospital's mission and location. Some hospitals, such as children's hospitals, women's centers, cancer centers, or orthopedic hospitals, have very specific missions, either in terms of the type of people they serve or the services that they offer. Other hospitals, sometimes called "general hospitals," provide a variety of services, such as:

- Delivering babies
- Diagnosing diseases
- Treating diseases with drugs, surgery, or both
- Providing emergency and intensive care services
- Providing mental health services
- Providing rehabilitation and physical therapy

People who receive the services of a hospital are typically referred to as **patients**. A hospital may admit a patient for care (have the patient stay for one or more nights). This is called *inpatient care*. Or a hospital may provide its services on an outpatient basis (the patient goes home the same day). For example, a patient with cancer who returns to the hospital every day for a period of time to receive radiation therapy would be receiving *outpatient care*.

Subacute Care Units (Skilled Nursing Units)

The care provided in a hospital is costly, and the number of beds in the hospital is limited. Therefore, once a patient has recovered enough to be out of danger, they are usually moved from the acute care setting. Often, these patients still need some care from a skilled health care professional. This care may be provided in a **subacute care unit** (also called a **skilled nursing unit** or a **skilled nursing facility**). A subacute care unit may be a unit within a hospital or a long-term care facility, or it may be a separate facility.

Patients in subacute care units may require intravenous drugs, physical therapy, respiratory care or

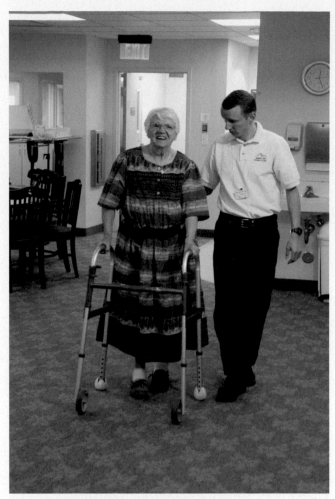

Figure 1-2 The care provided in subacute care units, also called skilled nursing units or skilled nursing facilities, often focuses on rehabilitation. Here, a physical therapist teaches a patient how to use a walker.

ventilator services, or wound management. The care given in these units focuses on rehabilitation and helping the patient to move from hospital care to home care (Fig. 1-2). Some patients in subacute care units recover fully, but others may need to move to a long-term care facility or arrange for continued care from home health care services after they return home.

Long-Term Care Facilities (Nursing Homes)

A **long-term care facility (nursing home)** is for people who are unable to care for themselves at home but who do not need to be hospitalized (Fig. 1-3). Because the long-term care facility becomes the person's home, either temporarily or permanently, people being cared for in long-term care facilities are referred to as **residents**, rather than patients. Some residents will stay in the facility for a short period of time, until they are well enough to return home. Others will

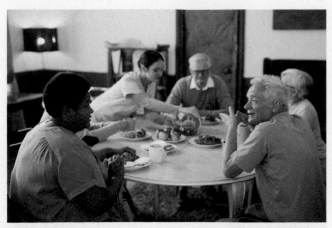

Figure 1-3 Residents of long-term care facilities (nursing homes) are unable to care for themselves at home yet do not need to be hospitalized. (*Photographee.eu\Shutterstock.com*)

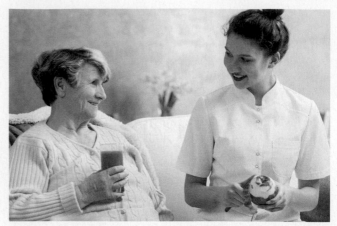

Figure 1-5 Nursing assistants who work for home health care agencies provide health care to people in their homes. A home health care aide's responsibilities might also include preparing and serving light meals and light housekeeping, depending on the client's needs and agency policy. (*Photographee.eu\Shutterstock.com*)

remain in the long-term care facility for the rest of their lives.

Assisted-Living Facilities

An **assisted-living facility** is a type of long-term care facility. People who live in an assisted-living facility are able to provide most of their own care, but they may need some limited help with medications, transportation, meals, and housekeeping. The residents of an assisted-living facility usually live in private apartments and can feel safe and secure knowing that if they need help, someone is nearby to provide it, 24 hours a day (Fig. 1-4). Many retirement communities offer both assisted-living services and long-term care services. If the resident's needs

change, they can move to the long-term care facility to receive more advanced care.

Home Health Care Agencies

Home health care agencies provide skilled care in a person's home (Fig. 1-5). In the home health care setting, people who receive care are typically called **clients**, rather than patients or residents. Home health care services are available for people of all ages with any number of different medical needs. For example, a new parent and their baby may need home care, especially if the baby was born too early.

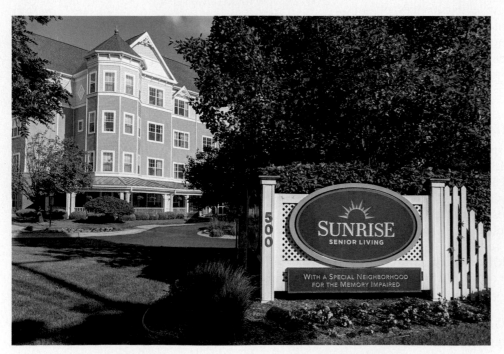

Figure 1-4 Residents of assisted-living communities often live in individual apartments. These residents are able to provide most of their own care but need help with certain things, such as medications, transportation, meals, or housekeeping. (*Shutterstock (2039551112).*)

A person recovering from an accident, a stroke, or surgery may also need home care.

Hospice Organizations

Hospice organizations provide care for people who are dying and their families. People are able to receive the services of a hospice organization when they have been diagnosed with an illness or condition from which they will not recover. The focus of hospice care is on relieving pain and providing emotional and spiritual support for both the dying person and the family. Hospice care can be provided in the home, hospital, or long-term care facility, or in a facility devoted exclusively to providing care to the dying.

Structure of Health Care Organizations

Most health care organizations are set up in a way similar to that shown in Figure 1-6. Most are governed by a board of trustees (also called a board of directors), and most have divisions (groups in charge of certain aspects of the organization's function). An administrator or chief executive officer (CEO) usually manages the organization and is the link between the board and the organization.

The board is made up of community members. The board sets policies to ensure that the care offered by the organization is safe and of good quality. The board also makes sure that the organization meets the needs of the community. Each division within a health care organization is responsible for one key aspect of the organization's function. Each division is managed by a division director or division manager. The medical services division is led by a medical director and is responsible for the doctors on staff. Nursing services division is headed by a director of nursing (DON) or chief nursing officer (CNO) and is responsible for all aspects of the organization that have to do with patient or resident care. Business services division is led by a business director and usually oversees admissions, billing, and payroll. The business division may also oversee maintenance and housekeeping. The ancillary services division typically contains the departments in the organization that provide patient or resident services, such as lab, pharmacy, and dietary services.

Within each facility, care of patients or residents is provided by a **health care team**, made up of many people with different types of knowledge and skill levels (Fig. 1-7). The patient or resident is always the focus of the health care team's efforts. The goal of the health care team is to provide holistic care (care of the whole person, physically and emotionally). Each member of the health care team's job is as important as any other member's. Think of the members of the health care team as links in the chain of care provided for the patient or resident. Because a chain is only as strong as its weakest link, each member of the health care team must provide care to the best of their ability. For example, the maintenance staff keeps the facility running smoothly by keeping equipment in good working order. The housekeeping staff keeps the facility clean. The people who work in the lab must be precise when performing laboratory studies and writing reports. In short, everyone must provide competent care in order for the health care team to function properly.

OVERSIGHT OF THE HEALTH CARE SYSTEM

Today in the United States, many agencies exist to protect both the recipients and the providers of health care.

Ensuring Quality Health Care

Agencies involved with making sure that the health care provided in the United States is safe and of high quality may be associated with the government, or they may be independent nonprofit organizations. These agencies may have one or more of the following objectives:

- To ensure that providers of health care are properly trained and competent
- To ensure that health care facilities meet standards of cleanliness and quality

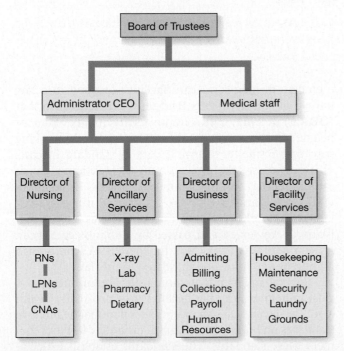

Figure 1-6 Most health care organizations are organized in similar ways. Each division within a health care organization is responsible for one key aspect of the organization's function.

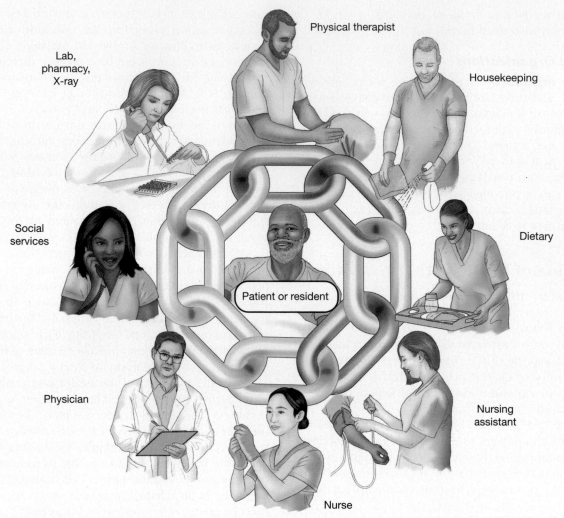

Lab,
pharmacy,
X-ray

Physical therapist

Housekeeping

Social
services

Patient or resident

Dietary

Physician

Nursing
assistant

Nurse

Figure 1-7 Care is provided by the health care team. The patient or resident is the primary focus of the health care team's efforts. Because a chain is only as strong as its weakest link, each member of the health care team must provide care to the best of their ability.

- To ensure that all products used in the delivery of health care are safe
- To ensure that quality health care is available to everyone

The **United States Department of Health and Human Services (DHHS)** is the primary government agency responsible for protecting this nation's health. Under the umbrella of the DHHS, there are multiple agencies involved in overseeing many different aspects of the health care system in the United States (Fig. 1-8). Some of these agencies are involved with inspecting health care organizations regularly to make sure that the standards set by the government are being followed. Any problems are addressed and, if the problems are serious, the organization faces being fined or closed, or the loss of government funding.

An in-depth investigation of long-term care facilities initiated by the DHHS in response to complaints of neglect and abuse from people who had family members in long-term care facilities resulted in a law known as the **Omnibus Budget Reconciliation Act (OBRA) of 1987**. OBRA improves the quality of life for people who live in long-term care facilities by making sure that residents receive a certain standard of care. This care must take into account the resident's physical, emotional, spiritual, and social needs. In addition, OBRA sets standards for the training of nursing assistants who work in long-term care facilities. OBRA legislation is reviewed and passed by Congress each year. As you read this book, look for the OBRA icon, which highlights key information related to this law.

Several independent, nonprofit organizations also exist to help ensure that facilities provide quality health care. These various organizations set national health care standards and officially recognize (accredit) facilities that meet these standards. The standards establish expectations for how to carry out certain activities, especially those that affect patient and resident safety and the quality of patient and resident care. For example, one

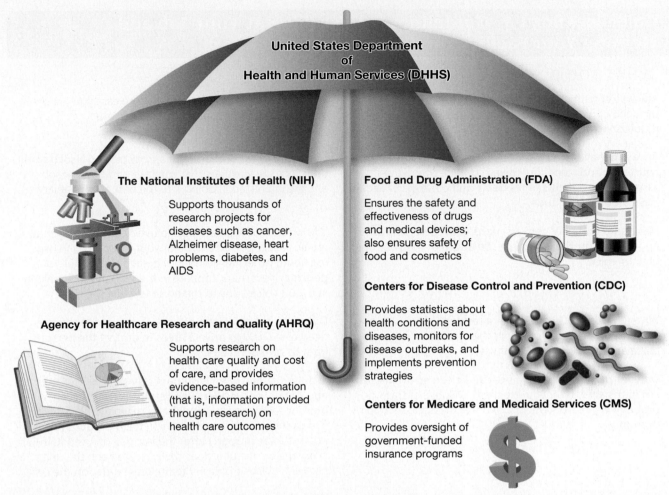

The National Institutes of Health (NIH)

Supports thousands of research projects for diseases such as cancer, Alzheimer disease, heart problems, diabetes, and AIDS

Agency for Healthcare Research and Quality (AHRQ)

Supports research on health care quality and cost of care, and provides evidence-based information (that is, information provided through research) on health care outcomes

Food and Drug Administration (FDA)

Ensures the safety and effectiveness of drugs and medical devices; also ensures safety of food and cosmetics

Centers for Disease Control and Prevention (CDC)

Provides statistics about health conditions and diseases, monitors for disease outbreaks, and implements prevention strategies

Centers for Medicare and Medicaid Services (CMS)

Provides oversight of government-funded insurance programs

Figure 1-8 The United States Department of Health and Human Services (DHHS) oversees many different agencies that are responsible for protecting the health of the people in this country. Some of the key agencies that you may hear about are shown in the figure.

such organization, *The Joint Commission,* has established standards for safe medication administration, infection control, the use of abbreviations in documentation, staffing levels and staff education, and responding to emergencies.

Like the government agencies, these independent organizations also inspect health care facilities regularly to make sure that standards are being followed. However, unlike the government inspections, inspections by independent organizations are voluntary. Health care organizations request and pay for these inspections to be done to receive **accreditation** (official recognition that the organization meets certain standards of quality). After receiving accreditation status, a health care organization must continue to provide proof that it meets the standards of quality and demonstrate a commitment to continuously improving its performance.

The Survey Process

To ensure that a health care organization is meeting the established regulations, standards, or requirements

set by the government agency or private organization that accredits or approves it, a survey process is utilized. A **survey** is an actual inspection and evaluation of a health care organization or facility. A *survey team,* comprised of a specific group of officials from the accrediting organization, visits the facility and works together to complete specified survey tasks.

During the survey, the surveyors directly observe the care and services provided in the facility. They look at the overall appearance and condition of the building. They review patient and resident services, such as the laundry, housekeeping, food service, and activities programming departments, and of course, they review the nursing care that is provided.

At the end of the survey, the survey team presents a written report of their findings. If the facility is found to be out of compliance, the report will include *deficiency citations* (statements that identify the standards that were not met, as well as the survey team's findings that indicate how the facility failed to meet the standards).

Guidelines Box 1-1 Guidelines for Excelling at Your Job and Helping Your Facility Do Well During a Survey

WHAT YOU DO	WHY YOU DO IT
Always act within your scope of practice, as defined by facility policy, your job description, and your state's regulations.	This is the best way to ensure that the care you are providing is within the legal limits of your job.
Always behave like the professional that you are. Be courteous and respectful toward others. Offer your assistance to patients or residents and coworkers readily. Have a positive attitude.	Having a professional attitude and displaying a solid work ethic indicate to others that you take pride in your job and are interested in doing it to the best of your ability.
Make sure that your conversations with coworkers are appropriate for the workplace. Be aware of the volume of your voice.	You would not want anyone to overhear anything that would reflect poorly on you or your work ethic. Gossiping about others or going into great detail about your personal life is inappropriate in the workplace. Speaking in a loud voice adds to the noise level on the unit.
When discussing a patient's or a resident's care with a coworker, be mindful of where the discussion is taking place and the volume of your voice.	Discussions that involve a patient's or a resident's care need to be held in private areas to protect the person's right to confidentiality.
Do your part to maintain a neat and clean environment. Put items away after you use them. Dispose of trash properly. If you notice a spill or other mess, clean it up promptly.	A cluttered, messy environment is unpleasant for everyone, patients or residents and staff alike. It may even present safety issues. It is difficult to work efficiently if you cannot locate something you need because it was not put away properly after the last person used it. If everyone on the unit does their part to keep the unit neat and clean, it is easier to maintain order on the unit.
Always put your patient's or resident's needs first. Strive to provide humanistic, holistic care.	When you are at work, your first priority must be helping your patients or residents to meet their physical, emotional, social, and spiritual needs. A humanistic, holistic approach to health care is the basis for providing quality care.
Answer questions honestly and to the best of your ability. If you do not know the answer to a question, simply say that you do not know and offer your help in getting the person the answer they need.	Most people are quick to recognize bluffing. Admitting that you do not know the answer to a question conveys to the other person that you are honest. Offering to find out the answer for the person or directing the person to someone who is better able to answer the person's question indicates that you are helpful and conscientious.

The facility must respond to the deficiency citations by submitting and carrying out a formal plan of correction that outlines specific actions that the facility will take to fix the problems and achieve compliance. Depending on the seriousness of the deficiency, the survey team may return to the facility at a future date to make sure that the plan of correction has worked and the facility is back in compliance. A facility that does not regain compliance status may face serious penalties, such as:

- Loss of accreditation status
- Substantial fines
- An inability to qualify for Medicare or Medicaid payments
- An admission ban (a long-term care facility may not be allowed to admit new residents)
- Closure

People who work in a health care facility may actually fear the survey process. However, if you are providing the type of quality care that you have been trained to do and are following the policies and procedures that have been established by your facility, you have nothing to be nervous about. Guidelines Box 1-1 lists ways that you can both excel at your job and help your facility do well during a survey, regardless of the type of facility you work at. Health care organizations are being trusted to care for those who are unable to care for themselves, which is a very serious business!

Protecting Health Care Workers

The **Occupational Safety and Health Administration (OSHA)** is a government agency that is responsible for protecting the health and safety of American workers by enforcing standards and providing education to improve conditions in the workplace. OSHA, which is part of the U.S. Department of Labor, seeks to protect workers across all industries, not just the health care industry. OSHA was formed after a key piece of legislation (the Occupational Safety and Health Act of 1970) was passed in response to public concern over increasing numbers of on-the-job injuries and deaths. You will see OSHA standards referenced frequently throughout this text. These standards protect you while you care for others.

PAYING FOR HEALTH CARE

If you have ever received a bill for health care in the United States, you know that health care can be expensive. Insurance can help to lessen these costs to the individual. Having a basic understanding of the ways health care is paid for is an important part of your job. In many cases, proper documentation of the care you give to your patients or residents is required to ensure that your facility is paid for the services it provides.

Private and Group Insurance

Although people can pay for health insurance privately, using their own funds, most people are covered by *group insurance* (insurance that is purchased at group rates by an employer or corporation). The employee may be covered in full as a benefit of employment, or they may pay a certain percentage of their coverage. The insurance company then pays for health care according to the individual policy.

As a result of *the Patient Protection and Affordable Care Act* of 2010, health insurance is available for people who do not qualify for group insurance, Medicare, or Medicaid. Insurance is available for purchase at affordable rates through the federal or state government.

Due to the increasing costs of medical care, the insurance industry has taken measures to control costs. Some insurance companies have a *precertification (preapproval) process*. This means that in order to be paid, the health care provider must prove that a person's medical condition meets certain criteria and obtain the insurance company's go-ahead for the proposed treatment before starting treatment.

Other insurance companies use a **managed care system**. Managed care systems assist in delivering health care to people who need it by arranging contracts with various health care providers (doctors' offices, hospitals, ambulance services, pharmacies). In addition, they help to reduce unnecessary costs associated with medical and surgical procedures by authorizing treatments before they are carried out. One form of managed care system is the *Preferred Provider Organization (PPO)*, in which health care providers contract with an insurance company to accept a standard payment as total payment for services rendered. In return for seeking care only from health care providers who are part of the PPO network, the insured person usually receives that care at a reduced cost. A *Health Maintenance Organization (HMO)* is another type of managed care system. Like PPOs, HMOs contract with health care providers to provide health care services for a prepaid fee, and people seeking care agree to see only health care providers who are part of the HMO network. An underlying principle of HMOs is that it costs less to keep a person healthy than it does to treat an illness. Therefore, these organizations typically promote regular physical examinations and screening to detect and prevent illnesses.

Medicare

Medicare is a type of insurance plan that is federally funded by Social Security, under the administration of the Center for Medicare and Medicaid Services (CMS). People who are 65 years or older are eligible for Medicare, regardless of their financial situation. Some younger people with a disability also qualify for Medicare. Health care facilities that are eligible to receive Medicare reimbursements must follow strict rules and guidelines to receive payment. For example, to receive Medicare reimbursements, long-term care facilities must complete a **Minimum Data Set (MDS)** report for each resident in their care (Fig. 1-9). This report focuses on the degree of assistance or skilled care that the resident needs. Information, such as the person's weight, bowel and bladder habits, and ability to care for themselves, is recorded regularly as part of the MDS report. Changes in these areas could indicate that a higher level of care is needed or that the person is not receiving the necessary care and as a result, their condition is getting worse. Nursing assistants who work in long-term care settings play a very important role in providing care and documenting that care for the MDS report.

Like insurance companies that insure the general public, the Medicare program is faced with the problem of controlling ever-increasing health care costs. In

Section G Functional Status

G1. Activities of Daily Living (ADL) Assistance

Code for most dependent episode in last 5 days:

Coding:

0. **Independent**—resident completes activity with no help or oversight

1. **Set up assistance**

2. **Supervision**—oversight, encouragement or cueing provided throughout the activity

3. **Limited assistance**—guided maneuvering of limbs or other non-weight bearing assistance provided at least once

4. **Extensive assistance, 1 person assist**—resident performed part of the activity while one staff member provided weight-bearing support or completed part of the activity at least once

5. **Extensive assistance, 2 + person assist**—resident performed part of the activity while two or more staff members provided weight-bearing support or completed part of the activity at least once

6. **Total dependence, 1 person assist**—full staff performance of activity (requiring only 1 person assistance) at least once. The resident must be unable or unwilling to perform any part of the activity.

7. **Total dependence, 2 + person assist**—full staff performance of activity (requiring 2 or more person assistance) at least once. The resident must be unable or unwilling to perform any part of the activity.

8. **Activity did not occur** during entire period

→ **Enter Codes in Boxes** →

Enter Code		
☐	**a.**	**Bed mobility**—moving to and from lying position, turning side to side and positioning body while in bed.
☐	**b.**	**Transfer**—moving between surfaces including to or from: bed, chair, wheelchair, standing position (**excludes** to/from bath/toilet).
☐	**c.**	**Toilet transfer**—how resident gets to and moves on and off toilet or commode.
☐	**d.**	**Toileting**—using the toilet room (or commode, bedpan, urinal); cleaning self after toileting or incontinent episode(s); changing pad, managing ostomy or catheter, adjusting clothes (**excludes** toilet transfer).
☐	**e.**	**Walk in room**—walking between locations in his/her room.
☐	**f.**	**Walk in facility**—walking in corridor or other places in facility.
☐	**g.**	**Locomotion**—moving about facility, with wheelchair if used.
☐	**h.**	**Dressing upper body**—dressing and undressing above the waist, includes prostheses, orthotics, fasteners, pullovers.
☐	**i.**	**Dressing lower body**—dressing and undressing from the waist down, includes prostheses, orthotics, fasteners, pullovers.
☐	**j.**	**Eating**—includes eating, drinking (regardless of skill) or intake of nourishment by other means (for example, tube feeding, total parenteral nutrition, IV fluids for hydration).
☐	**k.**	**Grooming/personal hygiene**—includes combing hair, brushing teeth, shaving, applying makeup, washing/drying face and hands (**excludes** bath and shower).
☐	**l.**	**Bathing**—how resident takes full-body bath/shower, sponge bath and transfers in/out of tub/shower (**excludes** washing of back and hair).

G2. Mobility Prior to Admission—complete only on admission assessment (A10a = 01)

Enter Code		
☐	**a.**	Did resident have a **hip fracture, hip replacement, or knee replacement** in the 30 days prior to this admission? 0. **No** ➜ Skip to G3, Balance During Transitions and Walking 1. **Yes** ➜ Continue to G2b

Check all that apply.

b. If yes, check all that apply for tasks in which the resident was independent prior to fracture/replacement.

☐ 1. **Transfer**

☐ 2. **Walk across room**

☐ 3. **Walk 1 block on a level surface**

☐ 4. **Resident was not independent in any of these activities**

☐ 9. **Unable to determine**

Recommended MDS 3.0   14

Figure 1-9 Nurses in long-term care facilities that receive Medicare funding must complete a Minimum Data Set (MDS) report for each resident in their care. This report is used to assess the degree of assistance that each resident needs. The form is broken down into Sections A–T and addresses all aspects related to a resident's care needs. The MDS report helps to ensure that the resident receives quality care that is directed toward their specific needs by requiring the nursing staff to evaluate these needs at regular intervals.

Section G Functional Status

G3.   Balance During Transitions and Walking

After observing the resident, **code the following walking and transition items for most dependent** over the last 5 days:

Coding:

0.   **Steady at all times**
1.   **Not steady, but <u>able</u> to stabilize without human assistance**
2.   **Not steady, <u>only able</u> to stabilize with human assistance**
8.   **Activity did not occur**

Enter Codes in Boxes

→ *Enter Code* [ ] **a.   Moving from seated to standing position**

Enter Code [ ] **b.   Walking** (with assistive device if used)

Enter Code [ ] **c.   Turning around** and facing the opposite direction while walking

Enter Code [ ] **d.   Moving on and off toilet**

→ *Enter Code* [ ] **e.   Surface-to-surface transfer** (transfer between bed and chair or wheelchair)

G4.   Functional Limitation in Range of Motion

Code for limitation during last 5 days that interfered with daily functions or placed resident at risk of injury.

Coding:

0.   **No impairment**
1.   **Impairment on one side**
2.   **Impairment on both sides**

Enter Codes in Boxes

→ *Enter Code* [ ] **a.   Upper extremity** (shoulder, elbow, wrist, hand)

Enter Code [ ] **b.   Lower extremity** (hip, knee, ankle, foot)

G5.   Mobility Devices

Check all that were normally used in the past 5 days:

Check all that apply.

- [ ] **a.   Cane/crutch**
- [ ] **b.   Walker**
- [ ] **c.   Wheelchair (manual or electric)**
- [ ] **d.   Lower extremity limb prosthesis**
- [ ] **e.   None of the above** were used

G6.   Bedfast

Enter Code [ ] **Has the resident been in bed or in recliner in room** for more than 22 hours on at least three of the past 5 days?

   0.   **No**
   1.   **Yes**

G7.   Functional Rehabilitation Potential—complete only on full assessment (A10a = 01)

Enter Code [ ] **a.   Resident believes he or she is capable of increased independence** in at least some ADL's.
   0.   **No**
   1.   **Yes**
   9.   **Unable to determine**

Enter Code [ ] **b.   Direct care staff believe resident is capable of increased independence** in at least some ADL's.
   0.   **No**
   1.   **Yes**

Recommended MDS 3.0   15

Figure 1-9 (*Continued*)

an effort to control these costs, Medicare uses a system known as a *Prospective Payment System (PPS)*. Under this system, payment for hospitalization, surgery, or other treatment is fixed. Lengths of hospital stays are also determined by the PPS and are typically short. Adjustments may be made based on the severity of the person's related condition. As a result of the PPS system, patients are discharged sooner and sicker than in the past, a situation that has created an increased need for extended care and home health care.

Medicaid

Medicaid is a federally funded and state-regulated plan designed to help people with low incomes to pay for health care. Older adults, as well as people with a disability, may also be eligible, especially if they have limited incomes. To receive Medicaid reimbursement, a facility must be approved by the state agency. Not all facilities or health care providers choose to participate in the Medicaid plan.

SUMMARY

- Society has historically sought to care for the sick and injured.
    - In the United States during the 1700s, 1800s, and early part of the 1900s, most people who needed health care received it in their homes. Most care was provided by family members and a "family doctor."
    - Today, health care is delivered in the home through home health care agencies and hospice organizations. In addition, people can receive care at facilities such as hospitals, subacute care units, long-term care facilities ("nursing homes"), and assisted-living facilities.
- Today, we strive to take a holistic approach to health care, taking into consideration the person's emotional, as well as physical, needs.
    - Health care is provided by a team of people, each with different areas of expertise and job responsibilities.
    - As a nursing assistant, you are a critical part of the health care team.
- Numerous agencies monitor health care organizations to protect both the recipients and the providers of health care.
    - The DHHS is the primary government agency responsible for protecting this nation's health and oversees government agencies such as the Centers for Disease Control and Prevention (CDC), the National Institutes of Health (NIH), and the Centers for Medicare and Medicaid Services (CMS).
    - Independent, nonprofit organizations offer accreditation to health care facilities that meet their quality standards.
    - The survey is an inspection of a health care organization or facility done to ensure that care is being provided according to standards and regulations.
    - OSHA is a government agency responsible for protecting the health and safety of American workers by enforcing standards and providing education to improve conditions in the workplace.
- As the health care system has become more complex, the cost of health care has increased, and the way health care is paid for has changed.
    - Private and group insurance policies are one way that individuals pay for health care.
    - Medicare is insurance that is funded by the US government.
        - All people who are 65 years or older are eligible for Medicare.
        - Health care facilities must meet government regulations to receive Medicare reimbursement for services provided. For example, long-term care facilities must complete an MDS report for each person in their care.
- Medicaid is also funded by the US government and is designed to help people with low incomes pay for health care.

WHAT DID YOU LEARN?

Matching

Match each type of health care facility with its appropriate description.

_____ **1.** Assisted-living facility

_____ **2.** Long-term care facility (nursing home)

_____ **3.** Hospice

_____ **4.** Home health care agency

_____ **5.** Subacute care unit (skilled nursing unit, skilled nursing facility)

a. Place where people who can provide for most of their own care but who need limited assistance can live

b. Provides skilled care in a person's home

c. Provides care for people who cannot care for themselves yet are not ill enough to be hospitalized

d. Care devoted exclusively to the dying

e. Provides care that is focused on rehabilitation; assists patients in making the transition from hospital care to home care

Match each insurance term with its appropriate description.

_____ **6.** Medicaid

_____ **7.** Patient Protection and Affordable Care Act of 2010

_____ **8.** Prospective Payment Systems

_____ **9.** Medicare

_____ **10.** Minimum Data Set (MDS)

f. Low-cost insurance available for purchase through the federal or state government

g. Federally funded and state-regulated plan to help people with low income

h. Report that focuses on the degree of assistance or care a resident requires

i. Used to regulate the payment for health services

j. Federally funded by Social Security

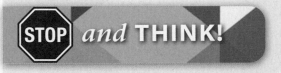

Think about what health care was like in the United States 100 years ago. How has health care delivery changed in the United States since the early 1900s?

What aspects of the "old-fashioned" way of delivering health care were good? Not so good? What aspects of modern health care delivery are good? Not so good?

CHAPTER 2

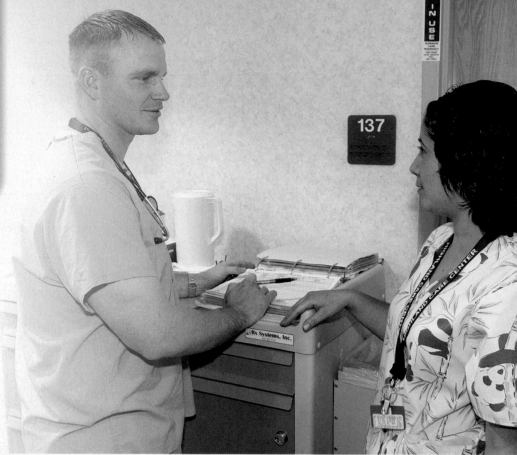

Photo: Nurses and nursing assistants work together to provide patient or resident care.

The Nursing Assistant

 WHAT WILL YOU LEARN?

In the previous chapter, you were introduced to the idea of a "health care team," a group of employees with varying types of knowledge and skill levels who provide holistic care to a patient or resident. If you think of the members of the health care team as "links" in the chain of care, then as a nursing assistant, you are a very critical "link." What contributions does the nursing assistant make to the health care team, and what education is needed to become a nursing assistant? In this chapter, we will answer those questions, as well as describe ways in which nursing care can be delivered. We will also discuss how the nursing assistant and nurse interact to achieve the goal of safe, efficient patient or resident care. When you are finished with this chapter, you will be able to:

1. Discuss the *Omnibus Budget Reconciliation Act of 1987* (OBRA) requirements for nursing assistant training.
2. Describe the contents of the registry.
3. Discuss the responsibilities of the nursing assistant.
4. List the members of the nursing team and describe the role of each team member.
5. Discuss the delegation process as it relates to the nursing assistant.
6. List the five rights of delegation.

Vocabulary

Competency evaluation	Registered nurse (RN)	Certified registered nurse	Delegate
Registry	Charge nurse	practitioner (CRNP)	Scope of practice
Reciprocity	Unit manager	Team nursing	Five rights of delegation
Licensed practical nurse (LPN) or licensed vocational nurse (LVN)	Director of nursing (DON)	Patient-centered or patient-focused care	

NURSING, PAST AND PRESENT

Very simply stated, the field of nursing involves caring for others. People who enter the field of nursing, such as nurses and nursing assistants, provide physical and emotional care for people who are sick, disabled, or injured. Many nurses also work to keep people healthy, by teaching them about ways to maintain health and prevent illness.

Perhaps you have heard of Florence Nightingale. Florence Nightingale (1820–1910) was a British nurse who is credited with making nursing into the profession that it is today (Fig. 2-1). Ms. Nightingale started training programs for nurses and set up practices for hospital cleanliness and patient care that are followed to this day. By establishing educational standards for nursing professionals, Ms. Nightingale improved conditions for both the people receiving health care and those providing it. For the first time, those in the nursing field were regarded as professionals in their own right, with specialized knowledge, skills, and responsibilities.

The knowledge, skills, and responsibilities of the nursing assistant have grown over the years too. Early nursing assistants, often referred to as "aides" or "orderlies," were employed in long-term care facilities and hospitals to help the nurses care for residents and patients. These nursing assistants usually did not have training in the health care field, which led to poor care in many cases. Today's nursing assistants, however, are well-trained members of the health care team with many important responsibilities.

EDUCATION OF THE NURSING ASSISTANT

Omnibus Budget Reconciliation Act of 1987 Requirements for Certification

As you learned in Chapter 1, a major goal of the *Omnibus Budget Reconciliation Act of 1987* (OBRA) was to

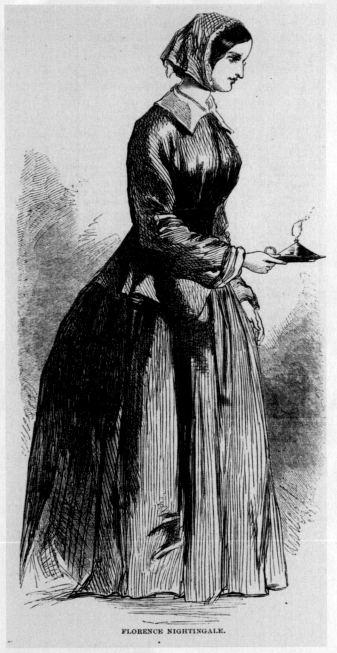

Figure 2-1 Florence Nightingale was a British nurse who established educational standards for nursing professionals. (*Florence Nightingale, National Library of Medicine.*)

improve the quality of care given to residents of long-term care facilities. To ensure that nursing assistants have the necessary knowledge and skills to give care, OBRA requires all nursing assistants who want to be employed in long-term care facilities to complete a training program and to pass a test that evaluates their knowledge and skills.

Training can be offered in vocational schools, community colleges, and private training academies. In addition, many long-term care facilities have their own nursing assistant training programs. Although the minimum training and competency evaluation requirements for nursing assistant training programs are set by OBRA, each state must create and regulate its own training programs following the education and certification requirements specified by OBRA. To be approved by the state's authorizing agency, all state training programs, known as nursing assistant training and competency evaluation programs (NATCEPs), must submit proof that they meet the federal standards as well as any state-specific standards. Any nursing assistant who is employed by a long-term care facility or home care agency that receives Medicare funds must have successfully completed an approved NATCEP.

OBRA mandates a *minimum* of 75 hours of training. States must meet that minimum, but many require more hours. This training must include classroom lectures and hands-on practice of skills, as well as at least 16 hours of supervised practical training. Although most state NATCEPs require that this practical training occurs in a long-term care facility, it can be accomplished in a lab setting. Since nursing assistants often are employed in home care and acute care settings, some states add clinical experience in those health care settings as part of their NATCEP.

As you complete your nursing assistant training program, you will study communication skills, infection control, safety and emergency procedures, residents' rights, basic nursing skills, personal care skills, feeding techniques, and skin care. You will also learn how to help residents move from place to place, change positions, dress, and perform range-of-motion exercises. In addition, you will learn the signs and symptoms of common diseases and how to care for people who have problems with thinking and memory. During the practical experience portion of the course, you will have the opportunity to practice what you have learned by performing skills on other people in a lab setting or caring for patients or residents in a health care facility (Fig. 2-2).

The training ends with a **competency evaluation**, which involves a written test (consisting of approximately 75 multiple-choice questions) and a skills test (during which you will be asked to perform selected nursing skills learned in the training

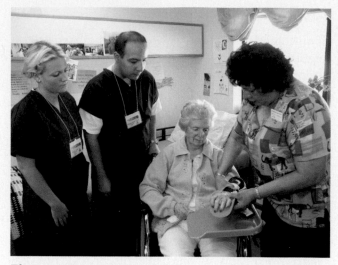

Figure 2-2 Part of a nursing assistant's training involves working with patients or residents in an actual health care setting.

program). The actual number of test questions that you must answer and skills that you must demonstrate is determined by each state. You will have three opportunities to complete the evaluation successfully. This is mandated by OBRA. The pass rate (or score that you must attain in order to pass the evaluation) varies from state to state.

Some states allow a person who has on-the-job experience as a health care worker or one who has been trained in a related field to take the competency evaluation without completing the training course. However, the person must pass both the written and skills portions of the test on the first try. If the person does not, then they must complete the course before taking the competency evaluation again.

When you complete your training program and pass the competency evaluation, you will be certified to work as a nursing assistant in the state where you completed your training and passed your competency evaluation. To remain certified, you must work as a nursing assistant providing direct care for residents or patients for a minimum number of hours (determined by the state) to keep your knowledge and skills current. You may also need to provide proof of your employment status to renew your certificate. OBRA requires nursing assistants who have not met the minimum requirement for 2 years in a row to undergo retraining and pass a competency evaluation. It is your professional responsibility to maintain your certification and to renew when you are required.

Registry

OBRA requires every state to maintain a **registry**, an official record of the people who have successfully completed the nursing assistant training program. The registry contains the following information about each nursing assistant:

- Full name, including maiden name and any married names
- Last known home address
- Registry number and the date of expiration
- Date of birth
- Date the competency evaluation was passed
- Last known employer and dates of employment
- Reported incidents of resident abuse or neglect, or theft of resident property

Long-term care employers check this registry to verify certifications as part of the hiring process. Information about performance concerns, such as resident abuse, must remain in the registry for at least 5 years. It is important that you notify the nurse aide registry in the state that issued your most recent certification of any changes in the information contained in your registry record, especially address changes. Notification that it is time to renew your certification will be sent to the address that the registry has on file for you. Many states notify you via email. If you do not receive this notification and as a result fail to renew your certification, your certification could lapse, making you ineligible to work as a nursing assistant.

Reciprocity

Some states practice the principle of **reciprocity**. This means that in many cases, your certification will be valid in states other than where you originally trained. However, before working in another state, you must go through the official process of getting your certification approved by that state. Usually, this involves contacting the state's nurse aide registry and completing an application. In addition to submitting the application, you may also be required to demonstrate competency in the new state. If you want to work in a state that requires more hours of training than you have, additional training can be obtained.

Continuing Education

Regular in-service education and performance reviews are also mandated by OBRA. Once you are certified, you must complete a *minimum* of 12 hours of continuing education per year (some states require more). Most health care facilities provide for this requirement through their in-service training programs. During in-service training, new knowledge and skills may be taught or existing ones reviewed, depending on the needs of the facility. Although it is the facility's responsibility to provide in-service training, it is your responsibility to attend the training to complete the required hours.

RESPONSIBILITIES OF THE NURSING ASSISTANT

The duties of the nursing assistant vary according to the setting, but all nursing assistants assist nurses in giving care to patients or residents by performing simple, basic nursing functions. As a nursing assistant, most of your responsibilities will relate to meeting the basic physical needs of patients and residents, which include hygiene, safety, comfort, nutrition, exercise, and elimination (Fig. 2-3). In addition to taking care of patients' or residents' physical needs, you will play an important role in meeting patients' or residents' emotional needs. A kind word, a gentle touch, and a willingness to listen let your residents or patients know that they are important to you and that you care for them as individuals. Finally, you will play an important role as "observer and communicator." As the member of the health care team with the most opportunity to interact with the patients or residents, you will be in a unique position to observe changes in the patient's or resident's physical or mental status and report these observations to the nurse.

Many nursing assistants are now being hired to work in acute care settings and are receiving additional training so that they can perform advanced care skills that have previously only been the responsibility of licensed nurses. See the following "Taking It to the Next Level: Advanced Skills" box for information about additional resources. At relevant points throughout this book, this feature box will also provide additional information about many of the skills that nursing assistants may be trained to perform in these care settings.

Taking It to the Next Level: Advanced Skills

More in-depth information related to advanced skills training and responsibilities of nursing assistants who work in acute care settings can be found in *Lippincott Acute Care Skills for Advanced Nursing Assistants.*

Visit thePoint® at thepoint.lww.com for access to the ebook.

THE NURSING TEAM

The nursing team, a subset of the health care team, is responsible for all aspects of the nursing care provided to patients and residents. In a health care facility, the nursing team is made up of licensed nurses in a variety of different roles, as well as nursing assistants

JOB DESCRIPTION

JOB TITLE: Certified Nursing Assistant (Class 1)   (Non-Exempt Employee)

DEPARTMENT NAME: Nursing Services

OVERALL RESPONSIBILITIES

Responsible for the hands on delivery of care and assistance with activities of daily living for all residents. Provides care in a manner that meets or exceeds Western States Senior Communities expectations.

WORKING RELATIONSHIPS

Reports to: Assistant Living Administrator

Supervises: None

Interfaces with: Resident Care Coordinator Residents, Families, Visitors, and Associates

PRIMARY JOB DUTIES

Provide assistance to residents with activities of daily living (ADL).

Maintain the dignity and privacy of all residents. Protect all resident rights.

Assist residents with personal needs as requested, while helping to maintain the resident's independence and well-being.

Document appropriately services delivered to residents and any significant changes in condition.

Report any concerns with the health and well-being to the Assistant Living Administrator.

Maintain and protect the confidentiality of resident information at all times.

Meet or exceed, Western States Senior Communities standards of appearance; comply with Western States Senior Communities sanitation, hygiene, and health standards of community personnel.

Serve meals in a fine and gracious manner, ensuring the dignity and nutritional needs of the resident.

Perform other reasonable tasks as assigned by supervisor.

JOB QUALIFICATIONS

Completion of state of Utah approved Certified Nursing Assistants Course.

Must possess a current Nursing Assistant certificate or be able to obtain one within four months of employment.

Must possess a current Food Handlers permit.

Ability to effectively communicate with residents, families, supervisor, and employees.

Willingness to work with the elderly.

OSHA OCCUPATIONAL EXPOSURE CATEGORY

After careful analysis, it has been determined that this position falls into the OSHA Occupational Exposure Category _____ and requires the following protective equipment to be worn by anyone filling this position: Gloves and eye protection.

I have read and agree that the contents of this job description accurately reflect what is expected of me in my current position.

_____   _____
Associate's Signature   *Date*

_____
Associate's Printed Name

_____   _____
Immediate Supervisor's Signature   *Date*

Figure 2-3 It is always a good idea to be very familiar with your formal job description at each facility where you work. Here is an example of a typical job description for a nursing assistant. *(Courtesy of Legacy Village of Layton—A Continuing Care Senior Living Community, Layton, Utah.)*

TABLE 2-1   The Nursing Team

TEAM MEMBER	REQUIREMENTS TO PRACTICE	CONTRIBUTION TO THE TEAM
Registered nurse (RN)	A baccalaureate degree from a liberal arts college or university (4 years) OR An associate degree from a junior or community college (2 years) PLUS A license obtained by passing a state board examination	Develops nursing care plans and coordinates all aspects of patient or resident care Provides nursing care to patients or residents Delegates selected aspects of patient or resident care to other team members and supervises these team members as they carry out the delegated tasks
Licensed practical nurse (LPN) OR Licensed vocational nurse (LVN)	A certificate from a 12–18-month training program offered by a vocational school, community college, or hospital PLUS A license obtained by passing a state board examination	Under the supervision of an RN, provides nursing care to patients or residents Delegates selected aspects of patient or resident care to other team members and supervises these team members as they carry out the delegated tasks
Nursing assistant OR Patient care attendant Patient care technician (PCT) Nursing technician Nurse's aide Home health aide	A certificate from a 75–200-hour training program offered by a vocational school, community college, or health care facility, obtained by completing the training and passing a state-administered competency evaluation	Assists the RN or LPN with providing nursing care to patients or residents; responsibilities include basic nursing tasks related to meeting hygiene, safety, comfort, nutrition, exercise, and elimination needs

(Table 2-1). The two types of licensed nurses you will work with most frequently are **licensed practical nurses** or **LPNs** (referred to in some states as **licensed vocational nurses** or **LVNs**) and **registered nurses (RNs)**. The difference between an LPN and an RN is the level of education and training. The RN completes a longer training program that includes a broader scope of knowledge. Because of this training, RNs are able to perform some skills that LPNs may not be allowed to do.

You will work with nurses who have specific job titles and duties to perform within the nursing department.

- **Charge Nurse.** The **charge nurse** is a licensed nurse (an RN or LPN) who supervises the nursing assistants and may supervise another nurse for a particular shift.
- **Unit Manager.** The **unit manager** (sometimes called a *nurse manager* or *head nurse*) is usually an RN who is in charge of a particular floor or section of the facility. The unit manager supervises the charge nurse and has 24-hour-a-day responsibility for the operation of the floor or section.
- **Director of Nursing (DON).** The **DON** is an RN who directs all of the nursing care within the facility. In some facilities, the DON is referred to as the *Chief Nursing Officer,* or *CNO.* The DON hires and manages the nursing staff and is responsible for ensuring that the nursing care provided to patients or residents meets quality and regulatory standards.

- **Coordinator (or Director) of In-Service Education (or Staff Development).** Most health care facilities have a nurse who is in charge of continuing education and staff development. The person in this role is responsible for developing and delivering in-service education sessions and other required training (such as CPR training). This person is also responsible for maintaining records of the educational activities that were offered and the attendance at those activities.
- **Quality Assurance (QA) Nurse** or **Quality Improvement (QI) Nurse.** The nurse in this position is responsible for tracking data that reflect quality-of-care issues and following up on incidents and accidents that occur within the facility. This person also does follow-up and investigation on the numbers of long-term care residents who get infections, have lost weight, or who have fallen and been injured. The QA Nurse then uses this information to identify care practices that may need to be improved.
- **Registered Nurse Assessment Coordinator (RNAC).** Federal law requires an RN to be in charge of the assessment process that is used to complete the Minimum Data Set (MDS). The MDS is a document that is used to determine and record the degree of assistance or skilled care that each resident of a nursing home needs. Other nurses and members of the health care team may contribute to the assessment process, but the RNAC is responsible for ensuring the

accuracy of nursing assessment documentation. The RNAC is also responsible for making sure that the entire MDS is completed, per the requirements of the law. In some facilities, these responsibilities are handled by the charge nurse or a head nurse, instead of by an RNAC.

■ **Certified Registered Nurse Practitioner (CRNP).** A **CRNP** is an RN who has completed additional training for licensure in advanced practice. These highly trained nurses are able to do some tasks that usually only doctors are allowed to do, such as perform advanced health assessments, interpret laboratory results, and manage and treat selected medical conditions. The CRNP may also be allowed to write orders for diagnostic tests or medications and is able to provide more immediate evaluation and treatment when the doctor is not available. The CRNP, although part of the nursing department, does not have any management responsibilities.

The way in which the members of the nursing team work together varies depending on the setting. For example, in the home health care setting, the case manager (an RN) develops a care plan along with the client and their family, and the nursing assistant follows this plan when visiting the client. Often, in this situation, the nursing assistant is the only health care provider who sees the client daily. The nurse may see the client only when visiting the home in a supervisory capacity (for example, every few weeks).

In the hospital or other settings where all of the members of the nursing team are "on-site," care may be given in different ways, depending on the abilities of the team and the types of patients and residents receiving care. Usually, a type of **team nursing** is used. In team nursing, a team leader (an RN) determines all of the nursing needs for the patients or residents under the team's care and assigns tasks according to each team member's skills and level of responsibility. For example, the nurse may assist the nursing assistant with bathing a patient or resident and then the nurse may give that person their medication, or two nursing assistants may work together to complete the tasks typically handled by nursing assistants, such as bathing and bed making.

Regardless of the type of system the nursing team uses to provide care, **patient-centered or patient-focused care** is usually the focus. This method of nursing care is designed around the needs of the patient or resident and works to meet that person's needs more efficiently. Members of the nursing team may be cross-trained to perform tasks that have in the past been done by other departments. For example, a nursing assistant may be trained to draw blood for laboratory tests or do an ECG instead of relying on

technicians from another department to come and perform those tasks.

No matter which nursing care model is used in the health care facility where you work, you will be the team member responsible for providing most of the personal care for your patients or residents. One of your most important duties while providing this care will be to notice changes in a patient's or resident's condition and to report these changes to the nurse.

DELEGATION

To **delegate** a task means to give another person permission to perform that task on your behalf. State nurse practice acts give RNs and LPNs the responsibility of performing nursing tasks and the authority necessary to fulfill this responsibility. In order to ensure that the nursing team functions efficiently, a nurse has the authority to delegate selected tasks to a nursing assistant, but the nurse is still responsible for the quality of the care. For example, if a nurse delegates a task to a nursing assistant that the assistant is not qualified to perform, and the nurse fails to adequately supervise the assistant as they carry out the task, then the nurse is liable for any harm to the patient or resident. However, if the nurse delegates a task to a nursing assistant that is within the assistant's **scope of practice** (the range of tasks the assistant is legally permitted to do), and the assistant fails to perform the task properly, then the nursing assistant is responsible for any injury to the patient or resident that occurs.

Typically, the nurse will delegate nursing tasks related to routine care (hygiene, comfort, exercise) to nursing assistants. An RN can also delegate certain nursing tasks, such as data collection and documentation, to a nursing assistant. However, nursing tasks that require professional judgment, such as assessment, planning, or evaluation, cannot be delegated to a nursing assistant. For example, a nursing assistant can take a person's vital signs and record this information on the person's chart, but the assistant is not qualified to interpret the data.

Understanding how a nurse decides which tasks to delegate will help you to understand why you may be asked to do certain tasks but not others. When delegating a task, the nurse must know the abilities and qualifications of the nursing assistant, and they or another licensed nurse must be available to provide supervision. In addition, they must consider the patient's or resident's individual needs. In order to enable nurses to make good decisions about which tasks to delegate and to whom, the National Council of State Boards of Nursing (NCSBN) has developed guidelines called the **five rights of delegation** (Table 2-2).

TABLE 2-2   Five Rights of Delegation

	QUESTIONS THE NURSE MUST CONSIDER	QUESTIONS THE NURSING ASSISTANT MUST CONSIDER
The right task	Is this a task that can be delegated? Does the nurse practice act allow me to delegate the task? Is the task in the job description for the nursing assistant?	Does the state allow me to perform this task? Have I been trained to do this task? Do I have experience performing this task? Is this task in my job description?
The right circumstance	What is the patient's or resident's condition? Are they stable? What are the needs of the patient or resident at this time?	Can I perform this task safely, given the patient's or resident's condition?
The right person	Does the nursing assistant have the right training and experience to safely complete the task?	Am I confident that I can perform this task safely? Do I have any reservations about performing this task, and if so, what are they?
The right direction	Am I able to give the nursing assistant clear direction regarding how to perform this task? Am I able to explain to the nursing assistant what is expected?	Did the nurse give me clear instructions? Do I understand what the nurse expects?
The right supervision	Will I be available to supervise and answer questions?	Will the nurse be available to supervise and answer questions?

You and the nurse share the responsibility for making sure that delegated tasks are carried out without causing harm to the patient or resident. The nurse is responsible for making good decisions about which tasks to delegate and for providing adequate supervision. You are responsible for recognizing which delegated tasks are within your scope of practice and range of abilities and using this knowledge as the basis for either accepting or refusing the assignment. Just as a nurse uses the five rights of delegation to decide which tasks to delegate and to whom, you can use the five rights of delegation to help you decide whether to accept or decline a delegated task (see Table 2-2). When you agree to perform a task, you accept responsibility for your actions. You must ask for help when you have questions or are unsure about how to proceed, and you must communicate with the nurse by reporting what you have done and what you observed.

You should never refuse an assignment simply because you do not want to do it. You must have a good reason for refusing to carry out an assignment, or you could lose your job. Valid reasons for refusing an assignment include the following:

- The task is not in your job description. Box 2-1 summarizes tasks that are generally outside of the scope of practice of a nursing assistant.
- Carrying out the task could result in harm to the patient or resident.
- The task is illegal or unethical.
- The nurse is not available to supervise your efforts.
- You do not have the proper equipment.
- The directions are not clear.

Box 2-1   Tasks That Are Generally Beyond the Nursing Assistant's Scope of Practice

Administering medications (including oxygen). Some states allow nursing assistants to administer medications to residents in assisted-living facilities, if the nursing assistant has undergone specialized training to do so. In general, only a licensed nurse (RN or LPN) or doctor is allowed to give medications. Nursing assistants may assist patients in taking medication by bringing water or helping to open the medicine bottle.

Receiving verbal orders (in person or over the telephone) from doctors. Licensed nurses (RNs or LPNs) are the only personnel authorized to receive doctors' orders.

Diagnosing illness and prescribing medications. Only doctors can diagnose illness and prescribe medical or surgical treatment.

Supervising other nursing assistants. Licensed nurses (RNs or LPNs) are responsible for supervising nursing assistants.

Performing procedures that require sterile technique. Nursing assistants are permitted to assist a nurse in performing a sterile procedure, but they are not trained to do these procedures themselves.

Inserting or removing tubes from a patient's body (bladder, esophagus, trachea, nose, ears). Nursing assistants generally are not trained in procedures that involve inserting or removing tubes from a patient's or resident's body. Exceptions may be made if the nursing assistant has had the opportunity to practice a procedure under an instructor's supervision.

Guidelines Box 2-1 Guidelines for Accepting or Declining an Assignment

WHAT YOU DO	WHY YOU DO IT
Always ask the nurse for clarification if there is something you do not understand.	It is your responsibility to make sure you know what is to be done and how it is to be done before going to the patient or resident.
Never perform a task that you have not been taught to do or that you feel uncomfortable doing, unless you are supervised by a nurse.	The nurse is ultimately responsible for ensuring the patient's or resident's safety. This means that it is the nurse's responsibility to ensure that whoever is performing the task on their behalf is qualified to do so and capable. It is irresponsible for you to misrepresent your abilities or to proceed unsupervised with a task that you are not fully capable of doing well.
Never ignore an assignment because you do not know how to perform the task or the task is beyond your scope of practice.	The patient's or resident's needs must be attended to, either by you or by someone else. If you feel that you cannot perform the task that you are being asked to do, explain your concerns to the nurse so that they can either help you with the task or reassign it.

- You are not able to perform the task safely.
- You have not received adequate training about the task or the equipment used.

If you do make the decision to decline a task that you have been assigned to do, it is your responsibility to state clearly that you are not going to do the task and your reason why. Failure to communicate your refusal to complete a task to the person requesting your help can jeopardize the care or safety of the patient or resident. The person requesting your help assumes that you are doing the task, unless they hear otherwise. Declining a task is a discussion that you should have privately with the person requesting the task of you. Do not discuss the issue in front of the resident, patient, or visitors.

General guidelines for accepting or declining an assignment are given in Guidelines Box 2-1. A good general rule to keep in mind is that you should not perform any task that is not listed in your job description. Because a nursing assistant's duties can vary from state to state and also from facility to facility, you must be familiar with your formal job description. Ask your supervisor about anything you do not understand. This is important to protect yourself, as well as your patients or residents.

SUMMARY

- No matter what the setting, nursing assistants are an integral part of the nursing team, a subset of the health care team.
  - Like all of the members of the nursing team, nursing assistants undergo training that authorizes them to perform certain tasks.
  - Nursing assistants assist the nurse by performing basic nursing functions, such as those related to hygiene, safety, comfort, nutrition, exercise, and elimination.
- To ensure that the nursing team operates smoothly and efficiently, a "chain of command" exists. This means that licensed nurses (RNs or LPNs) are able to assign (delegate) certain tasks to nursing assistants.
  - The delegation of tasks cannot be taken lightly by either the delegator (the licensed nurse) or the delegatee (the nursing assistant). Both share the responsibility of ensuring that the procedure is carried out without harm to the patient or resident.
  - The nursing assistant must know which tasks are within their scope of practice and which tasks are not.

WHAT DID YOU LEARN?

Multiple Choice

Select the single best answer for each of the following questions.

1. Nursing assistants who work in the long-term care setting must complete a course of training and undergo a competency evaluation. These requirements are set by the:
   a. Centers for Disease Control (CDC)
   b. Food and Drug Administration (FDA)
   c. Omnibus Budget Reconciliation Act of 1987 (OBRA)
   d. Occupational Safety and Health Administration (OSHA)

2. As a nursing assistant, it is your responsibility to:
   a. Plan the patient's or resident's care
   b. Perform the tasks your supervisor assigns to you
   c. Do the best you can without asking for help
   d. Compare assignments with your coworkers

3. If you do not know how to do an assigned task, you should:
   a. Call another nursing assistant for help
   b. Ask the patient or resident how they prefer to have it done

   c. Call the charge nurse and ask for help
   d. Follow the instructions in the procedure manual

4. Nursing assistants work under the supervision of:
   a. A doctor
   b. A registered nurse (RN) or licensed practical nurse (LPN)
   c. Other nursing assistants
   d. The long-term care facility administrator

5. To "delegate" means to:
   a. Do what you are told to do
   b. Give another person permission to perform a task on your behalf
   c. Transfer your duties to another assistant
   d. Have the charge nurse take your assignment

6. What information is included in the registry?
   a. The nursing assistant's full name
   b. The nursing assistant's registry number and date of expiration
   c. Any reported incidents of abuse or theft
   d. All of the above

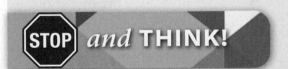

The nurse you are working with has asked you to remove Mrs. Thompson's urinary catheter. Your facility trains nursing assistants to perform this task, and you have just completed that training. Removing Mrs. Thompson's urinary catheter will be the first time you will have a chance to perform this new skill on a "real" person, and you are uncomfortable. What should you do?

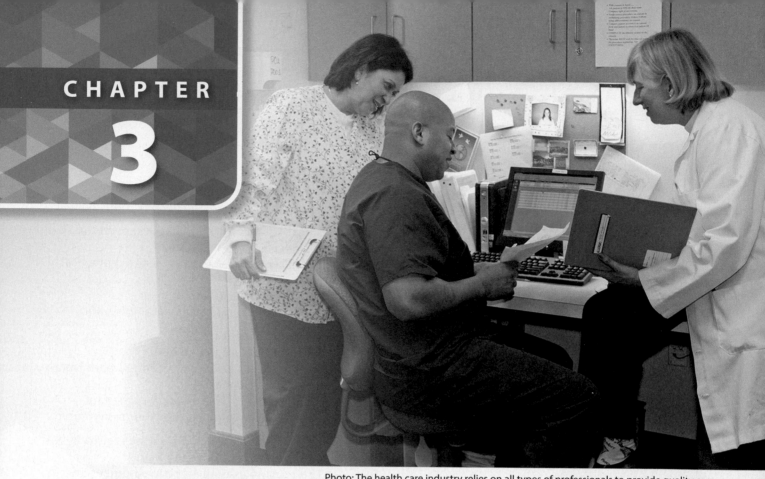

Photo: The health care industry relies on all types of professionals to provide quality care to patients and residents.

Professionalism and Job-Seeking Skills

 WHAT WILL YOU LEARN?

While having the knowledge and ability to perform your duties well is essential, showing professionalism and a strong work ethic are important too. In this chapter, we will explore the qualities of professionalism and a strong work ethic, and how possessing these qualities can help you get a job and excel at it. In addition, we will provide an overview of the process of applying and interviewing for a job. It may seem odd to be talking about how to get a job at the beginning of the book, but knowing what is expected of a good employee helps you make a great impression while you are still a student. When you are finished with this chapter, you will be able to:

1. Define the terms *professional* and *professionalism*.
2. Discuss characteristics that health care workers demonstrate that promote professionalism and explain the importance of each characteristic.
3. Define the term *work ethic* and describe how good work habits promote professionalism.
4. Understand the importance of personal health and hygiene for the health care worker.
5. Describe considerations one must explore when seeking employment.

6. **List several sources of employment information for jobs in the health care industry.**
7. **Discuss the application process necessary for obtaining employment.**
8. **Describe how to make a good impression during a job interview.**
9. **Describe the proper way to resign from a job.**

Vocabulary

Professional
Professionalism
Attitude
Work ethic

Empathy
Hygiene
Résumé

Equal Employment
  Opportunity
  Commission (EEOC)
Reference list

Human resources
  (HR) department
  (personnel)
Interview

WHAT IS A PROFESSIONAL?

What exactly is a professional? And how is professionalism measured? One definition of a professional is "a person with experience and skill in a specified role" who is "engaged in a specific occupation for pay or as a means of livelihood." Another definition relates the word "professional" to "businesslike or conforming to the standards of skill, competence, or character normally expected of a properly qualified and experienced person in a work environment."

The health care industry gives the title of **professional** to those who have credentials, obtained through education and training, that enable them to become licensed or certified to practice a certain profession. This industry certainly relies on all types of professionals, such as physicians, nurses, and nursing assistants, to provide quality care to patients and residents. As a member of the health profession, nursing assistants are considered to be *allied health professionals*. An allied health professional is a person (other than a physician or registered nurse) with special training, certification, or licensing who performs services in the care of patients, residents, or clients in a health care setting. However, many people who are considered professionals do not need a license or a certificate to perform their jobs, and they may not even need a specific educational background. Being a professional also means having a professional attitude, or exhibiting **professionalism**.

An **attitude** is the side of ourselves that we display to the world, communicating outwardly how we feel about things. A person's attitude is apparent from things they say (and the ways they say them), the ways they behave, and the ways they look. You may have heard it said about a person that they "have an attitude," meaning that the person's outward behavior

is unpleasant. Well, an attitude is something we all possess and it can be positive instead of negative.

Possessing a positive attitude in the workplace means that you are caring and compassionate toward your patients or residents and that you demonstrate a commitment to doing your job to the best of your ability at all times. This commitment to doing your best is the attitude that defines professionalism. In other words, professionalism is NOT the job you do, it is HOW you DO the job. While your job as a nursing assistant will allow you to earn a paycheck, a true professional views their work as a reflection of the role they play in society. Income is important but so is the sense of pride you feel as a result of setting high standards for your performance and obtaining satisfaction from the work you do and in knowing that you are helping others. Regardless of the level of education, certification, or experience a health care professional has, professionalism is all about exhibiting the right attitude toward coworkers, patients or residents, and visitors. Professionalism is a choice you make and requires effort. Members of the health care team are often held to higher standards for professional behavior than other professional groups. As a nursing assistant, you become a very visible representative of that team. What attitude will you choose to show?

WHAT IS A WORK ETHIC?

A **work ethic** can be described in many ways and measured by any number of standards, but simply put, it relates specifically to your attitude toward your work. Professionalism and a strong work ethic go hand in hand.

A strong work ethic is what separates an average employee from a great employee (Fig. 3-1). Two

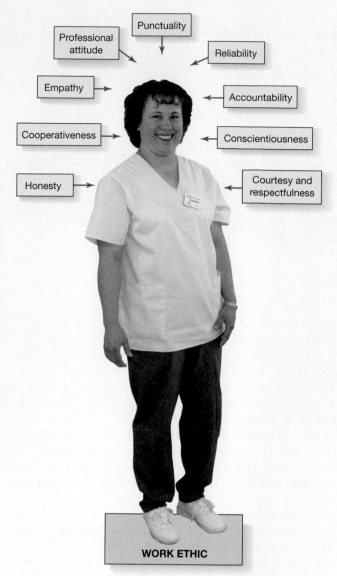

Figure 3-1 Professionalism and a strong work ethic go hand in hand. Many qualities contribute to a strong work ethic.

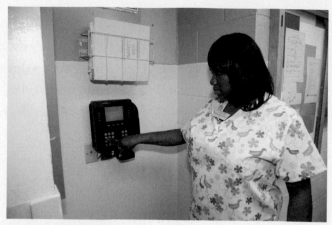

Figure 3-2 Being punctual means that you are on time or a little early. It is important to come to work on time because many people are relying on you!

Punctuality

Being punctual means that you are on time or a little bit early. Arriving to work on time prepared to start your duties is vital in the health care industry (Fig. 3-2). Many people are relying on you! The staff working the shift before yours is anxious for you to relieve them so that they can go home to their families and other responsibilities. If you work a morning shift, patients and residents will need your assistance in getting out of bed and preparing for breakfast, diagnostic tests, or surgery.

Organization is necessary to achieve punctuality. If you work a morning shift, plan ahead the evening before by packing your lunch and making sure your uniform is clean and pressed. If you have children, pack their lunches, lay out their clothes for the next day, and make sure any papers they need for school are completed. Setting the alarm 15 minutes earlier will not significantly affect the amount of sleep you get, but it will allow you that extra time you need to have breakfast before work or tend to any small last-minute crises.

Reliability

Reliability is an essential characteristic for a nursing assistant. Reliability means that others can count on you to come to work every day, as scheduled, and remain there during your entire shift (in other words, that your attendance is consistent). Everyone certainly has to miss a day of work occasionally for sickness or emergencies, but frequent absences are a very poor reflection on your work ethic. Have alternative plans for transportation and childcare in place before the need arises and try to keep yourself healthy to decrease your need to take sick days. Poor attendance

nursing assistants can have solid skills and be very good at getting their work done on time, but the nursing assistant with the strongest work ethic will be the one who enjoys the greatest professional success.

There are many qualities that are associated with a strong work ethic, such as cheerfulness and enthusiasm, a willingness to volunteer for new assignments, and a desire to learn new skills. A nursing assistant with a strong work ethic is someone you can depend on and trust, someone who treats others with kindness, respect, and compassion. People with strong work ethics know how to do their jobs well, like their jobs, and continue to learn and improve. Let's discuss some specific qualities that define a good work ethic.

and chronic lateness are primary reasons employers take corrective action against nursing assistants.

Reliability also means that others can count on you to do your job conscientiously and well, with minimal supervision. Your supervisor should not feel the need to look over your shoulder or "check up" on you to make sure your work has been finished.

Accountability

Accountability is also an essential characteristic for a nursing assistant. An accountable person accepts responsibility for their actions and the results of those actions. Being accountable means that you can accept criticism that is intended to help you improve, admit a mistake, and work to correct the situation. By acknowledging a mistake and taking measures to correct it, you are not only acting in the best interest of your patient or resident, you are letting your supervisors and coworkers know that you can be trusted to do your job to the best of your ability at all times, and that you are interested in learning how to prevent similar mistakes from happening in the future.

Conscientiousness

Conscientious nursing assistants take their assignments seriously and make sure they follow directions carefully. They demonstrate responsibility by asking for additional explanation or clarification when necessary, seeking help with difficult tasks, and admitting that they may not know how to perform a particular task. If you have not been shown how to do a procedure that you have been asked to do, show that you are interested in learning how. A conscientious nursing assistant attends to details and goes the extra mile to complete a task with care. When you act conscientiously, you leave your patients or residents feeling like they are special.

Courtesy and Respectfulness

Always treat other people with respect, both your patients or residents and your coworkers. The phrases *please, thank you,* and *excuse me* can improve the quality of almost any interaction. Avoid using "baby talk" or "talking down" to patients or residents. Address people as they prefer to be addressed. If in doubt, err on the side of formality ("Dr. Flores," "Mrs. Kim," "Mr. Chatterjee," "Miss Thompson"). In some parts of the United States, such as the deep South, older adults prefer to be addressed by their first names, preceded by "Miss" or "Mr." ("Miss Katharine"), and "ma'am" and "sir" are always used. Being polite and having good manners are correct in any situation.

Considering another person's feelings and beliefs shows that you truly care about the person.

Show respect for your coworkers and supervisors by not saying anything negative about them to your patients or residents, or other coworkers. Do not speak poorly about your place of employment to others, even if there are things that you are not happy with. If the person you are speaking to is a patient or resident (or a family member of a patient or resident), they may begin to question the quality of care that is being given.

Honesty

Honesty is a critical quality for health care workers to have. You are expected to accurately record vital signs and other information about the condition of the people you care for. You will have access to people's valuables, especially in the long-term care and home health care settings. You will be trusted with information of a very private nature regarding people's care and medical condition. Patients and residents will come to trust you and confide in you. If you act in a way that gives your patients or residents reason to lose confidence in their ability to trust you, it will be very difficult to reestablish your relationship.

Cooperativeness

Being able to cooperate, or work as part of a team, is essential in the health care industry. Professionals with many different levels of education and areas of training work together to benefit the people they care for. Remember how important your part in the chain of care is and the essential role you play in providing for the care and comfort of your patients or residents, and use this as a driving force. Making an effort to get along with your coworkers will make your work easier and will ease the burden on your coworkers as well. A good nursing assistant does not wait for a coworker to ask for help; they see a need and offer a helping hand. You will undoubtedly have to work with people you may not especially like, but a professional is able to put their personal feelings aside for the benefit of the patient or resident.

Empathy

Empathy means that you are able to try and imagine what it would feel like to be in another person's situation. There are times when coworkers, patients or residents, or the family members of patients or residents will really try your patience, but if you think of how *you* would feel if you were in a similar situation, you may find that you are able to understand the offending behavior better. Empathy gives us another perspective and helps us to be kinder and more tolerant.

A Desire to Learn

Although you may have completed your training as a nursing assistant, you will never stop needing to learn new things. The field of health care is constantly changing, and new techniques and treatments are developed daily. To provide the best possible care to your patients or residents, you must continue to learn new ways of caring for them. It is not the responsibility of your supervisor or your place of employment to keep you up to date on new health care issues. It is your responsibility. There are many professional journals, some specifically for nursing assistants, that cover new information that is important for you to know. Learn about the illnesses or conditions that the people you are caring for have. Ask questions about new techniques or treatments you see being used. This way, you have a better understanding of the care being given and become more involved as a member of the health care team.

PERSONAL HEALTH AND HYGIENE

To care for your patients or residents to the best of your ability, you must first care for yourself. By taking proper care of yourself, you demonstrate that you are a professional who takes their responsibilities seriously.

Maintaining Your Physical Health

The duties of a nursing assistant require much physical effort. You will be constantly lifting, bending, walking, and reaching as you perform your daily tasks at work. As you will learn in later chapters, there are many risks to your health and physical condition in the health care profession. Your employer, your coworkers, your family, and especially your patients or residents rely on you to be able to do your duties. In addition to giving you more energy, staying physically fit keeps your body strong and allows you to avoid many types of job-related injuries (Fig. 3-3). To keep your body in good physical condition:

- **Get enough sleep**. Most people need an average of 7 to 8 hours of sleep to function properly. Not only does rest relax the muscles, it also relaxes the mind and allows you to think clearly. Too little rest can weaken your immune system, making you more likely to get infections, such as cold and flu viruses.
- **Eat well-balanced meals**. A working body needs good nutrition, a subject you will learn more about in Chapter 24. You need fuel for your muscles and for your brain.
- **Exercise regularly**. Regular physical exercise gives you more strength and energy and keeps your heart and lungs healthy. In addition, regular exercise helps reduce the mental stress that sometimes goes along with intensely emotional jobs, such as those in the health care field.
- **Do not smoke**. Smoking causes the blood vessels in the body to narrow, reducing the flow of

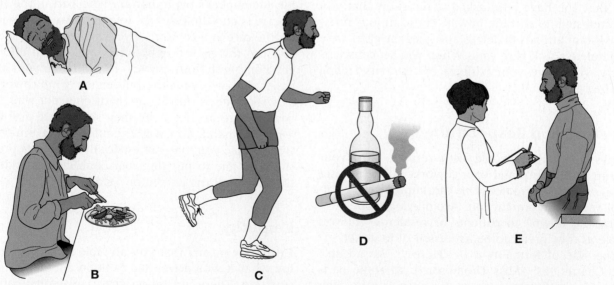

Figure 3-3 There are many things you can do to keep your body in good physical condition. **A.** Get enough sleep. **B.** Eat well-balanced meals. **C.** Exercise regularly. **D.** Avoid smoking, excessive alcohol consumption, and the use of recreational drugs. **E.** Get routine physical examinations to detect health problems early.

oxygen-carrying blood to the body's cells. It is well known that smoking is associated with lung cancer, emphysema, and heart disease. Infertility, impotence, and an increased risk of miscarriage are other negative effects of smoking. In addition to being a health risk, smoking makes your clothes and breath smell bad.

- **Do not take recreational drugs and limit your alcohol intake**. Recreational drugs and the improper use of prescription pain medications are associated with many health problems. Many employers now perform drug screening of potential employees. Although many people feel that there is nothing wrong with occasionally having a drink if this is something you enjoy, drinking too much or too frequently can negatively impact your health and leave you unable to perform your job to the best of your ability. The health care profession needs workers who are clear-headed and able to make good decisions on behalf of others. Do not report to work while under the influence of recreational drugs or alcohol or use these substances while on duty—doing so is dangerous for you, as well as for your patients or residents.
- **Have a routine physical examination**. Many chronic illnesses, such as high blood pressure and diabetes, go undetected until they have caused permanent damage to your body. Many types of cancers can be cured if detected early enough. Uncorrected vision and hearing problems can lead to errors when taking vital signs or reading medication labels. Routine physical examinations can help you to detect problems early, so that actions can be taken to correct them.

Maintaining Your Emotional Health

Caring for others is an emotionally demanding job, as well as a physically demanding one, for many reasons:

- Due to the shortage of health care workers, as well as a need to cut costs, many facilities are understaffed, which means that employees are often overworked.
- Not all patients or residents are happy or grateful for the care they are receiving. Many people in need of care do not feel well and, as a result, may be difficult or hard to manage. Sometimes, a person who is ill or worried will become angry or very critical and will take these feelings out on you, even though you have done nothing wrong.
- As a health care worker, you will have to face the death of some of your patients or residents. This can be difficult, especially in situations where you have had a chance to develop

a relationship with the patient or resident and their family.

Fortunately, there are actions you can take to help keep your emotions in check while on the job and prevent emotional "burnout":

- Maintain your physical health. It is proven that physical activity relieves mental and emotional stress.
- Be sure to schedule time for yourself. Most of us are not just caregivers in the workplace; we are caregivers at home as well. It is important to make time for yourself, to do what you like to do, in order to avoid feeling overwhelmed by your responsibilities at home and at work.
- Take advantage of counseling services offered by your employer or confide in a trusted leader of your faith community. Talking to a professional can help you to manage work-related stress and define your feelings and beliefs about difficult subjects, such as death and dying.
- When a situation becomes particularly "heated" at work, take a physical and emotional break. Have someone relieve you (or make sure your patients are safe) and take a walk outside to calm down.
- Ask to be assigned to different work areas or to different patients or residents, occasionally. Taking a breather from caring for the same patients or residents every day can be emotionally refreshing.

Personal Hygiene and Appearance

Personal **hygiene** or cleanliness addresses several issues. First, it promotes a professional image. If you care enough about yourself to keep yourself clean and neat, the people you care for will feel that you will do the same for them. Second, good personal hygiene helps to prevent the spread of infection, both to your patients or residents and to you and your family. In a health care setting, the potential to come into contact with all types of "germs" is increased, and practicing good personal hygiene is necessary. To practice good personal hygiene:

- Bathe daily and use a deodorant.
- Shampoo your hair regularly and treat dandruff or other scalp conditions.
- Keep your nails short and clean.
- Brush and floss your teeth and use mouthwash. Visit a dentist regularly. Poor dental health can cause breath odors and gum infections.
- Men should shave daily or keep facial hair neatly groomed and trimmed.
- Wear a clean, unwrinkled uniform each day.
- Wash your hands often.

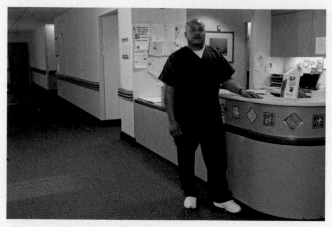

Figure 3-4 In the health care field, many of the traits we have come to associate with a professional image are related to maintaining safety and health.

Practicing good personal hygiene is essential to presenting a professional image. When you picture a health care professional, what do they look like? Are they wearing a wrinkled, stained uniform? Is their hair unkempt? Are their shoes dirty? Of course not! The health care worker you picture in your mind is clean and neat, with an unwrinkled uniform and clean shoes (Fig. 3-4). Hair is neatly styled and held back off the face. Few accessories are worn. A watch with a second hand is an essential part of a nursing assistant's uniform, but bracelets, necklaces, rings, and dangling earrings are not. In the health care field, many of the traits we have come to associate with a professional image are related to maintaining safety and health. Guidelines for a professional appearance are given in Guidelines Box 3-1.

JOB-SEEKING SKILLS

You are currently in the process of training to become a nursing assistant. You may have chosen to take this training for any number of reasons. You may have an interest in the health care profession and are taking this course to explore that interest. You may be entering the workforce after spending years raising a family, or you may find yourself in need of work due to a change in your financial situation. Some students are applying to nursing school and require the nursing assistant training to meet admission criteria. Regardless of your reason or reasons for entering the health care field, you will find many opportunities to put your training to use. The health care field is one of the most rapidly growing areas in industry, and the trend is expected to continue. Long-term care facilities, home health care agencies, hospice organizations, hospitals, doctor's offices, dialysis centers, rehabilitation centers, and many other types of health care organizations employ nursing assistants. Perhaps you already know what type of health care organization you would like to work in, or perhaps you will have to try a few different things before you find your special place.

Defining the Ideal Job

So, you're ready to get a job. Before you begin the process of responding to notices about job opportunities, completing applications, and going on interviews, it is important that you take time to explore what you really want from your employment and what you will be able to offer to your employer (Fig. 3-5). Some questions to consider are:

- **What type of facility do you want to work at?** Do you like working with older adults? If so, you might like working in a long-term care facility. Maybe you have always wanted to work with children who have a disability or you find the idea of caring for people in their homes appealing. Maybe you would thrive as part of the team working in the fast-paced environment of an acute care setting. Focusing on your interests, likes, and dislikes will help you to narrow the search, increasing the chance that you will find a job you will enjoy.
- **Are there limitations on the hours or shifts you are available to work?** If you are a parent with small children, you may be limited to working certain shifts depending on your child-care arrangements. Do not lead an employer to believe that you are available for any shift if you can realistically work only evenings.
- **Do you have reliable transportation to get to work?** Your employer will rely on you to come to work as scheduled and on time. If you rely on public transportation, apply for work at facilities serviced by that particular transportation method.
- **What are some of your personality strengths?** Are you self-motivated and independent, or do you like more supervision and guidance? A nursing assistant who works well independently would be an asset for a home health care agency while one who prefers more supervision would probably be better suited for working in a facility.

Finding Job Openings

Once you have some specific goals in mind, where do you start your search? There are many places to search for job openings. The classified ads in the local newspaper are a place to start, as are telephone books which include the contact information of many organizations. Internet search directories also typically list

Guidelines Box 3-1 Guidelines for a Professional Appearance

WHAT YOU DO	WHY YOU DO IT
Style your hair neatly and away from your face.	Securing your hair away from your face keeps it away from equipment, out of your eyes, and out of your work. If your hair is not secured back, when you move your hair out of your eyes, any germs on your hands will be transferred to your hair and face.
Keep your nails short and clean, with smoothly filed edges.	Germs can hide under the tips of long nails. Long nails can also scratch a person's skin. Frequent handwashing can cause acrylic and false nails to lift, allowing water to become trapped underneath and lead to a fungal infection in the nail bed.
Leave bracelets, necklaces, rings, and dangling earrings at home.	A child or confused person might pull dangling earrings through your earlobes. Necklaces and bracelets get in the way and can get caught in equipment and broken. If you wear rings, germs can become trapped underneath them, which makes hand hygiene less effective. Rings can also scratch a person's skin when you are providing care.
If you wear cologne or perfume, it should be of a light fragrance and lightly applied.	Many people are sensitive to fragrances and may find perfume or cologne that is of a strong scent or heavily applied offensive. In fact, many health care facilities are now requiring that employees be "scent free" and wear no fragrances.
Wear a clean, unwrinkled uniform each day. Make sure that your shoes are clean.	Attention to details, such as making sure that your uniform is wrinkle free and your shoes are clean, says to others that you care about your appearance. A clean uniform is also essential for limiting the spread of infection.
If you have a tattoo or body piercing, try to select a uniform style that will conceal it. If you are thinking about getting a tattoo or body piercing, consider its location carefully.	Many health care facilities that employ nursing assistants have policies that limit the number of earrings a person can wear. The policies may also require that any body piercing jewelry be removed and tattoos be covered while at work.
Practice good personal hygiene and grooming daily.	Good personal hygiene helps to prevent breath and body odors and limits the spread of infection. In addition, if you care enough about yourself to keep yourself clean and neat, the people in your care will feel that you will do the same for them.

facilities and agencies that hire nursing assistants. You could try calling these organizations directly or checking the Internet to see if the organizations you are interested in post job openings on their websites. In addition, you can use the Internet to check sites dedicated to helping people find jobs. The school that you are attending may offer a job placement service where you can check job listings and obtain help with writing a résumé. You could also check for job postings on the bulletin board in the facility where you are receiving clinical training. Last but not least, friends and coworkers may know of openings. Start a list of positions that you hear of that interest you, so that you will have the information readily available.

Preparing Résumés, Cover Letters, and Reference Lists

Résumé

Before actually submitting an application for a particular job, you should prepare a **résumé**, a brief

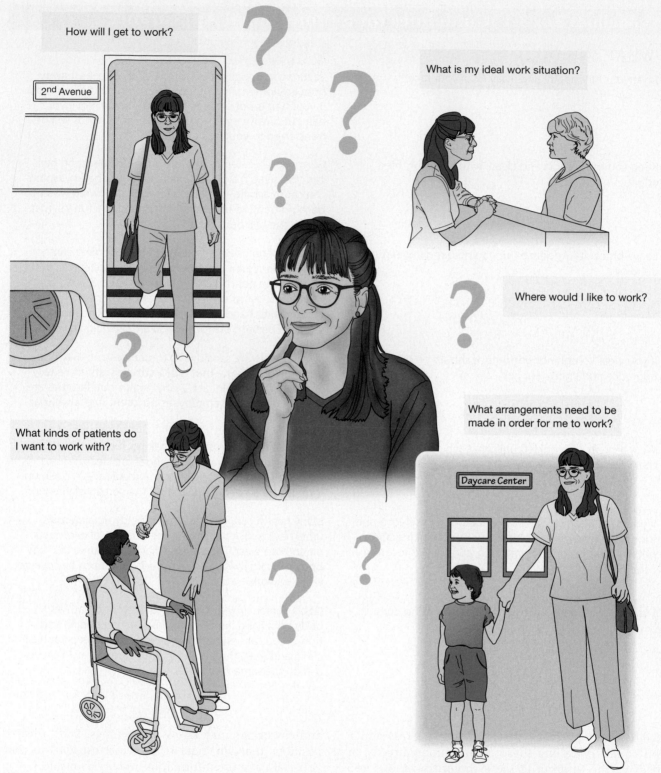

Figure 3-5 The first step to finding a job is thinking about what sort of situation best fits your personality, lifestyle, and interests.

SUZIE SMITH
123 NORTH AVENUE
ANYWHERE, US 12345
(123) 456-7890

Career Objective:

To obtain a position as a Certified Nursing Assistant in a rehabilitation-centered healthcare facility that will allow me to use my skills to assist those in need.

Education:

Anywhere Vocational Center Anywhere, US	May–July 2022 Nursing Assisting Course CNA Certification: August 2022
State Jr. College Anywhere, US	August–December 2021 General Studies
Anywhere High School Anywhere, US	Graduated: June 2020 High School Diploma

Certifications:

Certified Nursing Assistant	August 2022 (Current)
CPR Certification	July 2022 (Current)

Employment History:

Sunshine Assisted Living Anywhere, US	August 2022–Present

CNA, Rehabilitation Unit. Provided assistance with activities of daily living for residents, with an emphasis on rehabilitation. Worked closely with physical therapists to carry out therapy plan with meals and ambulation.

Quality Printing Anywhere, US	July 2020–July 2022

Cashier/Customer Service. Worked part-time while attending college. Responsible for assisting customers with print orders and making end-of-day bank deposits.

Volunteer History:

Hospice Anywhere, US	June 2019–July 2021

Respite Volunteer. Provided respite relief for families receiving hospice care. Sat with patients and read to them.

Figure 3-6 A résumé is a short, precise document with information about you, your work experience, and your education.

document that gives a possible employer general information about you and your education and work experience. Résumés should be typed or printed using a computer on white or off-white paper. With résumés, "plain" is best—no fancy lettering or designs are necessary! A résumé contains only facts and should be kept to one page, if at all possible (Fig. 3-6). Your résumé should include the following:

- Your full name, address, telephone number, and email address.
- A short objective or career goal.
- A history of your education (list the schools you attended most recently first, and for each school,

include the dates you attended the school and the degree you graduated with).
- An employment history (list each of your previous employers, starting with the most recent first, and for each employer, include the dates that you worked there, your job title, and your primary job duties).

Listing volunteer work on your résumé is appropriate, but only if it relates to the job you are applying for. There is some information that should never be included on a résumé, including your age, marital status, weight, religion, sexual preference, and whether or not you have children (or are planning to have

Suzie Smith
123 North Avenue
Anywhere, US 12345
September 1, 2022

Sandra Jones, Director of Human Resources
Sunny Hills Rehabilitation Center
1234 South Avenue
Anywhere, US 12345

Dear Ms. Jones,

 I would like to express my interest in the certified nursing assistant position at Sunny Hills Rehabilitation Center that was listed in the local want ads. In July, 2022, I completed my nursing assistant training at Anywhere Vocational Center. Since that time, I have been employed at Sunshine Assisted Living as a CNA in their rehabilitation unit.

 I am a hard worker and I learn new skills easily. I love working with older adults and have heard that your facility is a very enjoyable place to work.

 Thank you for taking the time to review and consider my application. I am available for an interview at your convenience and look forward to meeting with you soon.

Sincerely,

Suzie Smith

Suzie Smith, CNA

Figure 3-7 A cover letter is a letter that you write to go along with your résumé. Your cover letter allows you to explain more fully why you want to work for a particular organization and what qualities you have that make you the ideal person for the job opening in question.

them). This information should not matter to an employer who is considering you as an employee. In fact, according to the **Equal Employment Opportunity Commission (EEOC)**, it is against the law for an employer to ask a candidate questions related to these subjects at any time during the hiring process.

Cover Letter

You may also want to prepare a cover letter to send out with your résumé. A cover letter is written as a way of introducing yourself to a potential employer. Your résumé contains information about your education, training, and experience, but a cover letter goes beyond the straight facts. A cover letter says, "Hello, this is why I want to work for your organization, and this is why I am the best person for the job" (Fig. 3-7). Your cover letter should be fairly short and printed using a computer on white or off-white paper. Pay special attention to your grammar and spelling.

Reference List

The last document you should prepare before applying for a job is a **reference list**. A reference list is a list of three or four people who would be willing to talk to a potential employer about your abilities. When considering people to include on your reference list, think about people who know you well and have worked with you in a professional capacity, such

as your teachers, coworkers, or previous supervisors. Before listing a person as a reference, make sure you have their permission to do so. Some people may hesitate to act as a reference. For example, they may not want their contact information given out, they may be too busy, or they may not think you did as good a job for them as you thought you did. After a person has agreed to be your reference, make sure you have accurate contact information for that person, including their full name and title (if any), a current and complete mailing address, an email address, and a telephone number. Print your reference list on a sheet of paper that matches your résumé. Some employers will ask for a list of references at the time you turn in an application; others will want you to include your references on the actual application form. Either way, you will be prepared with correct and current information.

Submitting Applications

Now that you have thought about your ideal work situation, prepared a list of job opportunities to pursue, written your résumé and cover letter, and gathered your references, you are ready to place applications. Other required documentation that you may need includes a valid ID (such as a driver's license or government identification card), a copy of your nursing assistant certification, school transcripts or certificate showing completion of your NATCEP training course, and your social security card.

In some facilities, the director of nursing (DON) handles the hiring of nursing assistants. In others, hiring is handled through the **human resources (HR) department** (sometimes referred to as personnel). Most organizations that hire nursing assistants have gone solely to an online application process, although some may still accept written applications in person. You can choose to visit the facility in person to inquire about job opportunities and the application process, or complete the process at home, online. Although it is acceptable and common to just stop by organizations you are interested in and ask to complete an application, you may want to call ahead to ask if there are any positions open for nursing assistants. If you do choose to visit the facility, make sure that you have a professional appearance and have all necessary paperwork with you. Good first impressions are always important.

A job application is a standardized form used to obtain basic pertinent information, such as which position you are applying for, how you can be reached, and what shifts you can work (Fig. 3-8). Whether you are completing your application online or in person at the facility, make sure to have notes available with details that you will need to complete the application. Remember the time you spent earlier thinking about practical factors that needed to be taken into consideration, such as childcare arrangements and transportation? Now you will be able to easily answer the questions on the application about your availability for work. The application form will also require you to provide information about your education, your work history, and the reasons you left your previous job. There are many reasons why a person would leave a place of employment:

- "I left to take a position that is closer to home."
- "I left because I was offered better hours/a pay increase."
- "I left to have children."
- "I left to go to school."
- "I left because we moved to a new city or town."
- "I left because I was laid off."

The reason for leaving a job could be that you were fired. If so, be honest. Your chances of finding new employment are much better if a potential employer hears the truth from you, instead of finding it out by calling your references. When giving a reason for leaving a job, avoid speaking negatively about your previous employer, even if the situation was not ideal. Doing so reflects poorly on you as a potential employee.

If completing a written form, use blue or black ink and write clearly. As with filling out a paper application

form, when completing an online application, make sure that you are careful to fill out each space and use correct spelling and grammar. With online applications, there is usually the ability to also upload copies of your résumé, cover letter, and copies of other required documents that you have saved on your computer.

Know that the application form is a legal document, and your signature at the bottom states that all the information is true and accurate. An employer who finds out that you were not honest about any information on the application form has grounds to fire you without notice.

Ask for an appointment for an interview when you submit your cover letter, résumé, reference list, and completed application. Some facilities will make the appointment at this time. Others may want to review your résumé and application and call, text, or email you for an appointment at a later date. If you have not heard from a potential employer after 1 week, it is appropriate to call or email and ask about the status of your application. A follow-up call shows a potential employer that you have initiative and are interested in the job.

Going on Interviews

You have an appointment for that interview! An **interview** is the chance for a potential employer to meet you personally and learn more about you in an effort to determine if you are the right person for the job. Equally as important, the interview is a chance for *you* to learn more about the employer and the position, in an effort to determine if they are right for you. Being properly prepared for the interview will allow you to gather as much information about the organization and the job as possible during the interview, so that you can make an informed decision about the job if it is offered to you. In addition, being properly prepared can make all the difference in how a potential employer views your potential! Your résumé and application contain all of the "hard" facts about your education and experience, but you are the one responsible for persuading the interviewer of your interest in the job, dedication to your profession, and abilities.

Before going to the interview, make a list of questions you would like answers to, and refer to this list during the interview. This shows that you are interested in the position and are taking the opportunity to interview seriously. Some questions you might want to ask include the following:

- "What are the major responsibilities or duties of the position? May I have a copy of the job description?"

HIGHLAND CARE CENTER
APPLICATION FOR EMPLOYMENT

Highland Care Center is an equal opportunity employer, dedicated to a policy of non-discrimination in employment on any basis, including race, color, age, sex, religion, national origin or disability. Highland supports hiring people who have disabilities and meets all ADA requirements to provide reasonable accommodations for people with disabilities who are qualified to do the job. A mandatory drug test will be performed within 90 days of hire. Criminal background checks will be made on all new employees.

PERSONAL INFORMATION

Name: _____   Date: _____

    Please list any other names you have been known by or employed under: _____

Phone Number: _____   Social Security Number: _____

Position Desired: _____   Salary Desired: _____

Present Address: _____
                Street   City   State   Zip Code

Permanent Address (if different from above): _____
                Street   City   State   Zip Code

Have you ever applied for employment with Highland before? Yes _____ No _____ If yes, when?_____

Have you ever worked for Highland before? Yes _____ No _____ If yes, when?_____

Available for: Full Time _____ Part Time _____ On Call _____ Shifts available for: Morning _____ Afternoon _____ Night _____

If hired, when would you be available to begin work?_____

Are you eligible for employment in the United States? Yes _____ No _____

How did you learn about Highland Care Center?_____

Have you ever been convicted of a felony or misdemeanor? Yes _____ No _____ Do you smoke? Yes _____ No _____

Upon hire a criminal background check will be conducted.

EDUCATION	Name and Location of School	Graduate?
High School		
College		
Business/Trade/Tech.		

List Other Job-Related Skills: _____

_____

Special Skills or Qualifications: _____

_____

Figure 3-8 A job application is a standardized form used to obtain basic information about each person who applies for a job with the organization. It is a legal document, and your signature at the bottom states that all of the information you have provided is true and accurate.

- "Do you have to replace nursing assistants often, here? If so, why?"
- "May I see the unit where I will be working and meet the person who will be supervising me?"
- "What do you think nursing assistants like best about working here? Least?"
- "How many nursing assistants staff each unit?"
- "When would I be eligible for a performance evaluation, and what are the standards I will be evaluated against?"
- "What qualities are you looking for in a nursing assistant?"
- "What opportunities exist for career growth and furthering my education?"

You are interviewing for a job in the health care setting, so help the interviewer see you as a part of their staff. Present yourself as a professional (see Guidelines Box 3-1 and Fig. 3-9). Make sure your clothing is unwrinkled and all repairs, such as missing buttons or loose seams, have been taken care of before the interview. In general, appropriate attire for interviewing includes slacks or dress pants (not jeans), skirts or simple dresses, button-down or polo

shirts and blouses, a belt, and possibly a sport jacket or blazer if the weather is cool. Wear clean dress shoes (not sneakers).

Carrying a small notebook containing the questions you want to ask during the interview and a copy of your résumé, reference list, and your certified nursing assistant certification or registration looks very professional. Do not chew gum during the interview, and make sure your phone is turned off. You only have one chance to make a first impression, so make it a good one!

Give yourself adequate time to get to the interview. Ideally, you will arrive a few minutes early. After being introduced to the interviewer, shake their hand and take a seat when you are invited to do so. Do not address the interviewer by their first name, unless the interviewer specifically asks you to. Thank the person for the opportunity to interview at the beginning of the interview.

During the interview process, sit up straight and try not to fidget. It is certainly understandable to be nervous, but try to appear as confident and comfortable as you can under the circumstances. Maintain good eye contact during the interview and speak clearly. Common questions an interviewer might ask a candidate are listed in Box 3-1. Most interviewers will ask a potential employee about their strengths and weaknesses. Think about this ahead of time and be honest. We all have some terrific strengths and we also have our weaknesses. Remember that a person

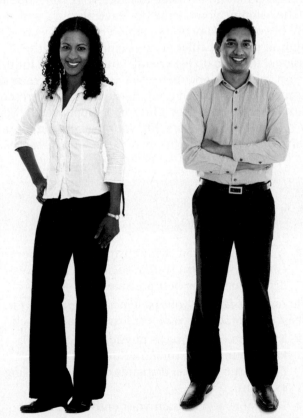

Figure 3-9 Dress like the professional that you are when you go for your interview! Clean, neat hair and nails and clean shoes are appropriate for everyone. Examples of appropriate attire include slacks (or a skirt or simple dress), a button-down or polo shirt, a blouse, and a belt. (**Left:** *ESB Professional\ Shutterstock.com*; **right:** *wong yu liang\Shutterstock.com*)

| **Box 3-1** | **Common Interview Questions** |

"Tell me about yourself. Why did you become a nursing assistant?"

"What part of your last job did you like the most? The least?"

"Why are you leaving your current job?" (or, "Why did you leave your last job?")

"What are you looking for in a manager?"

"How do you describe your work habits?"

"How do you set priorities?"

"How do you handle yourself under stress?"

"How do you handle problems with patients or coworkers?"

"Tell me about a specific situation that interfered with your ability to do your job and how you handled it."

"What is the most satisfying workday you have had this year? Why?"

"Do you have a mentor? What have you learned from this person?"

"Who in your life would you consider to be 'successful'? Why?"

"What do you consider to be your greatest strength? Your greatest weakness?"

"Where do you want to go with your career? What steps have you taken to achieve your goal?"

"What is it about our organization that appeals to you?"

who is aware of a weakness is capable of working to improve it. Try to answer questions concisely yet completely; it is best if you can strike a balance between listening and talking. If you do not know the answer to a question, simply say that you do not know—most interviewers are quick to recognize bluffing.

At the end of the interview, the interviewer will usually give you an opportunity to ask any questions that you may have. Now is the time to refer to your list! Asking questions of your own indicates that you have an active interest in making sure that you are a good fit for the job and the organization. The interviewer may have discussed salary and benefits (medical benefits, dental benefits, retirement plans, holiday and sick time, schedule for pay increases) during the course of the interview, but if they did not, it is best not to ask about these things now. The proper time to discuss pay and benefits is when a job offer is made. When the interview is over, thank the interviewer again for their time and for considering you for the position. If the interviewer did not mention when you can expect to hear from them regarding the position, ask. Then leave! The interview is over, and there is nothing left to do but send a thank-you note.

You should send an email with a short thank-you note within 1 day of interviewing for the position, thanking the interviewer for considering you for the position and briefly explaining why you are excited about the possibility of working for their organization. Everyone wants to be complimented on their organization, and your interest in being a part of that organization is a compliment. As with dropping off the application, if you do not hear from the organization you interviewed with within the amount of time specified at the close of the interview, it is appropriate to follow up with a telephone call or a short email. When a representative of the organization calls to offer you a job, you can take this opportunity to ask any questions that may have occurred to you since the interview or that were not appropriate to ask during the interview. If you need time to think about the offer, it is acceptable to ask the person who has offered you the job if you can call them back with an answer within the next day or so.

Applying and interviewing for jobs can be a time-consuming process that requires a lot of effort. By taking the time to prepare, you increase your chances of finding a situation where you will be happy and satisfied with your work.

Leaving a Job

Chances are, you will accept many different jobs over the course of your career. When leaving a job, give your employer at least 2 weeks' notice so that arrangements can be made to cover your shifts. Write a letter stating your desire to leave the job and the date of your last day on the job. Even if you were not happy at that particular place of employment, the professional thing to do is to thank your employer for the opportunity to work there. Leave on a positive note because you may need a reference from your present place of employment for a future job opportunity. You may even wish to work for your present employer again sometime in the future.

SUMMARY

- The health care industry relies on all types of professionals to provide quality care to patients and residents.
  - Professionals, such as doctors, nurses, and nursing assistants, have certain credentials that are obtained through education and training.
  - Being a professional also means having a professional attitude.
- You must exhibit a strong work ethic in order to be successful and grow professionally.
  - A nursing assistant with a strong work ethic possesses qualities that make them both pleasant to work with and dependable.
  - A nursing assistant with a strong work ethic demonstrates compassion and respect for their patients or residents.

- A nursing assistant with a strong work ethic continues to learn so that their patients or residents receive the best possible care.
- In order to care for your patients or residents to the best of your ability, you must first care for yourself.
  - Take care of the body's physical needs to help keep your body strong, healthy, and able to handle the physical demands of being a nursing assistant.
  - Take steps to maintain your emotional health to prevent emotional "burnout" and help you keep your emotions in check, both at work and at home.
  - Maintain good personal hygiene to prevent the spread of infection and promote a professional appearance.

- Job-seeking skills are useful for finding an employment situation that matches your individual needs.
  - Advance planning about the type of employment you want helps to give your job search direction.
  - Résumés provide potential employers with information about your education and skills.

- Job applications are legal documents that provide pertinent information about your employment history.
  - A job interview is an opportunity for the potential employer to evaluate you and for you to evaluate the potential employer.

WHAT DID YOU LEARN?

Multiple Choice

Select the single best answer for each of the following questions.

1. A person with experience and skill in a specified role who is engaged in a specific occupation for pay or as a means of livelihood is referred to as a(n):
   a. Apprentice
   b. Professional
   c. Graduate
   d. Novice

2. In many states, nursing assistants can be employed at all of the following except:
   a. Hospitals
   b. Long-term care facilities
   c. Research centers
   d. Rehabilitation centers

3. A short, precise document with information about you, your work experience, and your education is called a:
   a. Minimum Data Set (MDS)
   b. Résumé
   c. Reference
   d. Cover letter

4. All of the following information should be included on your résumé, except for your:
   a. Name
   b. Address
   c. Employment history
   d. Religion

5. An organization's human resources (HR) department is also known as:
   a. Personnel
   b. Dietary
   c. Administration
   d. Education

6. Which one of the following is a standardized form that is also a legal document used when applying for a job?
   a. Résumé
   b. Cover letter
   c. Reference list
   d. Application

7. The chance for a potential employer to meet you personally occurs during the:
   a. Application process
   b. Interview process
   c. Job posting process
   d. Reference checking process

8. A nursing assistant can promote their own physical health by doing all of the following except:
   a. Eating well-balanced meals
   b. Getting plenty of rest
   c. Smoking and drinking socially
   d. Working out at a gym

9. A nursing assistant's personal cleanliness is referred to as:
   a. Grooming
   b. Neatness
   c. Hygiene
   d. Fashion

10. Qualities that characterize a good work ethic include all of the following except:
    a. Reliability
    b. Punctuality
    c. Honesty
    d. Tardiness

11. What type of a nursing assistant accepts responsibility for their actions?
   a. An accountable nursing assistant
   b. A respectful nursing assistant
   c. A courteous nursing assistant
   d. A punctual nursing assistant

12. What type of a nursing assistant is able to imagine what it would feel like to be in another person's situation?
   a. A creative nursing assistant
   b. An empathetic nursing assistant
   c. An experienced nursing assistant
   d. An honest nursing assistant

13. What type of a nursing assistant can be counted on to come to work every day?
   a. A punctual nursing assistant
   b. A nursing assistant with access to public transportation
   c. A reliable nursing assistant
   d. An ethical nursing assistant

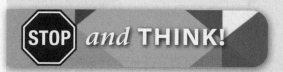
STOP *and* THINK!

Imagine that you have just completed your nursing assistant training and taken the state test. While you are waiting for your test results, you decide to begin searching job postings to see what opportunities are available. At this point, you are considering several options. You are excited about beginning your career in the health care field, and you are anxious to get into the workforce and put your new skills to use. However, you think that you might also want to continue your education and become either a licensed practical nurse (LPN) or a registered nurse (RN) someday. What sorts of organizations may be looking for nursing assistants in your community? How could working as a nursing assistant now help you to further define your career goals?

You are a nursing assistant student completing your training in a local health care facility. Do you think that the nurses and nursing assistants view you as a potential employee? What actions can you take as a student to make a good impression?

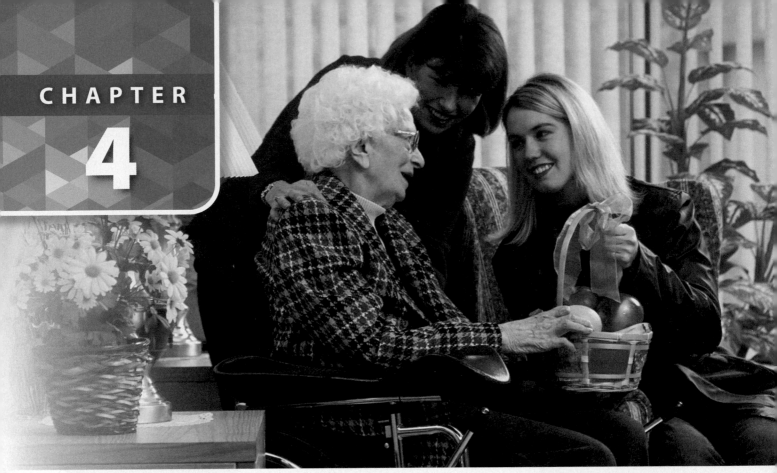

Photo: Residents and their families expect and deserve quality care. Laws exist to protect residents and their families and ensure that they receive quality care.

Legal and Ethical Issues

 WHAT WILL YOU LEARN?

As members of society, we make decisions every day about how to behave. Some of these decisions are dictated by society's laws or rules established by the government. Other decisions are dictated by our own personal ethical code or moral sense of what is right and wrong. Many factors influence an individual's ethical code, including spiritual beliefs and values instilled by the person's family. In general, when we act according to our ethical code, we act a certain way because we believe it is the right way to act. Obeying society's laws and upholding our own personal ethical standards allow us to function as members of society. Just as laws and ethics guide our behavior in society, laws and ethics guide our behavior in the workplace as health care providers. (Recall the discussion in Chapter 3 about the importance of having a "work ethic.") This chapter explores some of the legal issues that can affect you as a nursing assistant, and describes general ethical principles that should guide your behavior in the workplace. When you are finished with this chapter, you will be able to:

1. **List and discuss patients' and residents' rights, as set forth by the American Hospital Association (AHA) and the Federal 1987 Nursing Home Reform Act (OBRA '87), respectively.**

2. **Describe two major types of advance directives and explain why advance directives play an important role in health care.**

3. **Discuss the legal aspects of health care delivery.**

4. List common legal violations that are related to the provision of health care.

5. Define the types of abuse and describe signs that indicate abuse.

6. Discuss the health care worker's obligations in the reporting of suspected abuse.

7. Explain the difference between legal and ethical issues.

8. Describe the ethical standards that govern the nursing profession in particular and the health care profession in general.

9. Discuss awareness that health care workers must have in order to avoid legal and ethical dilemmas.

Vocabulary

Decision-making
  capacity
Advance directive
Durable power of
  attorney for health
  care
Health care agent
Living will
Laws
Civil laws
Criminal laws

Tort
Unintentional tort
Negligent
Malpractice
Intentional tort
Defamation
Slander
Libel
Assault
Battery
Informed consent

Fraud
False imprisonment
Invasion of privacy
Confidentiality
Health Insurance
  Portability and
  Accountability Act
  (HIPAA)
Larceny
Abuse
Vulnerable adult

Physical abuse
Neglect
Abandonment
Psychological
  (emotional) abuse
Sexual abuse
Financial abuse
Elder abuse
Ethics
Value

PATIENTS' AND RESIDENTS' RIGHTS

Patients' Rights

Guidelines have been established to protect patients who receive our care and create an atmosphere of open communication among everyone who is involved in the patient's care: the patient (and their family), the health care workers who are providing the care, and the administrators of the health care organization from which the patient is receiving care. In 1973, the American Hospital Association (AHA) first adopted a series of statements called *A Patient's Bill of Rights*. Since 1973, the health care industry has changed dramatically, and *A Patient's Bill of Rights* has been revised to reflect those changes. For example, *A Patient's Bill of Rights* is now called *The Patient Care Partnership*, to emphasize the partnership that exists between the health care team and the patient and family. Within that partnership, patients have both rights and responsibilities. A brochure, called *"The Patient Care Partnership: Understanding Expectations, Rights and Responsibilities,"* can be found in full on the aha.org website. It is also printed and provided to patients when they receive care in the

hospital. The major points of *The Patient Care Partnership* are as follows:

What to Expect During Your Hospital Stay

- High-quality hospital care
- A clean and safe environment
- Involvement in your care
  - Discussing your medical condition and information about medically appropriate treatment choices
  - Discussing your treatment plan
  - Getting information from you
  - Understanding your health care goals and values
  - Understanding who should make decisions when you cannot
- Protection of your privacy
- Preparing you and your family for when you leave the hospital
- Help with your bill and filing insurance claims

Residents' Rights

Similar guidelines concerning the rights of residents of long-term care facilities are ordered by the federal government and must be followed if a facility receives any federal payments from Medicare. These guidelines are called the *Resident Rights* and are included as part of the Federal 1987 Nursing Home Reform Act (also known as OBRA '87). A simple explanation of these rights can be found on the Centers for Medicare and Medicaid Services website at cms.gov. The major points of the *Resident Rights* portion of OBRA are as follows:

1. The resident has the right to know what rights and responsibilities they have, in a language that they can understand.
2. The resident has the right to exercise their rights as a resident of the facility and as a citizen of the United States. This includes the freedom to make choices about how to live their life (subject to the facility's rules), freedom to vote, and freedom from discrimination.
3. The resident has the right to a dignified existence.
4. The resident has the right to make decisions regarding their care, including choosing their own doctor, participating in planning and implementing their own care, and having their individual needs and preferences accommodated. The resident has the right to refuse treatment and to refuse to participate in experimental research.
5. The resident has the right to privacy, including privacy while receiving treatments and nursing care, making and receiving telephone calls, sending and receiving mail, and receiving visitors. The resident has the right to confidentiality of personal and medical records.
6. The resident has the right to freedom from physical or psychological abuse, including the improper use of restraints.
7. The resident has the right to receive visitors and to share a room with a spouse if both partners are residents in the same facility.
8. The resident has the right to communicate with and have access to people and services both inside and outside of the facility, including advocacy groups. The resident has the right to organize and participate in groups organized by other residents or the families of residents. For example, residents or their families may organize groups dedicated to improving life for residents by suggesting changes that could be made at the facility or by planning group outings and activities. The resident also has the right to participate in social, religious, and community activities of their choosing.
9. The resident has the right to keep and use personal possessions (as space and safety permit).
10. The resident has the right to control their own finances (or, if they wish, have the facility manage personal funds).

11. The resident has the right to information about eligibility for Medicare or Medicaid funds and to be protected from Medicaid discrimination.
12. The resident has the right to information about the facility's compliance with regulations, planned changes in living arrangements, and available services (and the fees for those services).
13. The resident has the right to remain in the facility unless transfer or discharge is required by a change in the resident's health, the resident is unable to pay for the services they are receiving, or the facility is closed. The resident has the right to refuse transfer from a distinct unit (for example, the certified skilled unit) of the facility.
14. The resident has the right to choose to work at the facility, either as a volunteer or a paid employee. Working or helping others gives many people a sense of purpose. However, under no circumstances is a resident obligated to work (for example, in exchange for services).
15. The resident has the right to self-administer medications if the health care team determines that the resident can do so safely.
16. The resident has the right to voice grievances and to have the facility respond to those grievances.

The AHA's *Patient Care Partnership* and the *Resident Rights* portion of OBRA were written to guide the way patients and residents, health care providers, and the administrators of health care organizations interact with one another. In respecting the rights of patients and residents, health care workers behave according to legal standards; they also behave according to ethical standards.

Concerns for Long-Term Care

Advocacy is the process of making a plea or providing support on another's behalf. Because many of the residents of long-term care facilities are vulnerable, federal laws provide advocacy programs for their benefit. An example of a federally funded advocacy program is the Long-Term Care Ombudsman Program. An *ombudsman* (a Swedish word that means "one who speaks on behalf of another") is a person from a state or local Office on Aging who regularly visits residents of long-term care facilities to check on their welfare and overall satisfaction with their care. Ombudsmen gather information from residents and work on their behalf to negotiate solutions to their concerns. These concerns could be related to care issues, misunderstandings between residents and staff, violations of resident rights, or suspected abuse and neglect. While an ombudsman does not have the authority to force a facility to take action, the ombudsman can work with the appropriate people and agencies to ensure that resident issues are addressed.

OBRA requires nursing homes to post information notifying residents of their right to file complaints and listing the contact information for agencies that can assist them (for example, the state agencies that handle licensure of long-term care facilities, Medicare and Medicaid certification, and reports of Medicare or Medicaid fraud). In addition, the contact information for the ombudsman program must also be posted for resident use. As a nursing assistant, you should know where this information is posted in your facility and be able to assist a resident or visitor who asks you how to contact one of these agencies. If a resident or visitor does ask you for this information, you should report the person's request to the nurse. The person's request may indicate that they are unhappy about something that has happened in the facility. By alerting the nurse to the person's request, the nurse may be able to talk with the person about the issue, and perhaps resolve it without involving the state agency.

Advance Directives

Many patients and residents in health care facilities are not able to make their preferences for health care known, or they will become unable to make their preferences known in the future. For example, people with dementia (a medical condition that results in the permanent and progressive loss of the ability to think and remember) lose their decision-making capacity. **Decision-making capacity** is the ability to make a thoughtful decision based on an understanding of the potential risks and benefits of taking a certain course of action. Medical conditions that result in the loss of consciousness also result in a loss of decision-making capacity.

For these situations, state laws make provisions for advance directives. An **advance directive** is a document that allows a person to make their wishes regarding health care known to family members and health care workers in case the time comes when they are no longer able to make those wishes known themselves. One type of advance directive, a **durable power of attorney for health care**, transfers the responsibility for making medical decisions on the person's behalf to a family member, friend, or other trusted individual. The person who is responsible for making decisions on the person's behalf is called the person's **health care agent** (or, sometimes, the

person's *durable power of attorney for health care*). Another type of advance directive, a **living will**, allows the person to give instructions about what medical treatments they would or would not want done in an effort to prolong their life.

Advance directives play a very important role in the health care setting, because many patients and residents have conditions that may result in either the temporary or permanent loss of their decision-making capacity. The Patient Self-Determination Act of 1990 requires health care facilities to educate patients and residents about advance directives and to offer them the opportunity to establish a living will, a durable power of attorney for health care, or both.

LAWS: A WAY OF PRESERVING PATIENTS' AND RESIDENTS' RIGHTS

All people are entitled to certain basic human rights, and the government, which is put in place by the people, plays a role in making sure that these rights are honored.

One way the government works to preserve basic human rights is by making and enforcing **laws**. Laws are rules that are made by a controlling authority, such as the local, state, or federal government, and serve to protect basic human rights for all people, regardless of race, religion, gender, sexual orientation, or income. By formally establishing principles to guide behavior, laws give society a way of settling disputes in a civilized, orderly way. Because many laws are made at the local and state levels, there will be differences from state to state. Some of these laws involve regulation of health care agencies and the professional practice within health care agencies.

There are two types of laws: **civil laws** and **criminal laws**. Civil laws are concerned with relationships between individuals. Criminal laws are concerned with the relationship between the individual and society as a whole. People found guilty of violating civil laws usually must pay a fine or make a financial settlement to the party that was wronged. Those who violate criminal laws may be sentenced to serve time in jail or prison. Each individual is considered responsible and held accountable for their own actions in accordance with the law. This responsibility is known as *liability*.

Violations of Civil Law

When a patient or resident is admitted to a health care facility, they sign a form giving the facility permission to provide medical care. A health care worker employed by that facility likewise agrees to provide that care to the patient or resident. This arrangement

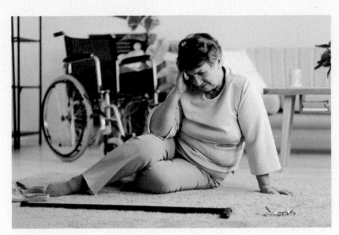

Figure 4-1 The nursing assistant who was responsible for this resident has committed an unintentional tort and would be considered negligent for failing to lock the wheels on the wheelchair, an action that could have prevented the resident from falling. (*Ground Picture\Shutterstock.com*)

is a contractual agreement. Contracts, such as the contract that exists between a nursing assistant and the person they care for, fall under the jurisdiction of civil law. When this civil law is violated, a **tort**, or wrong, is committed. An **unintentional tort** occurs when someone causes harm or injury to another person or that person's property without the intent to cause harm. A person who commits an unintentional tort is considered **negligent** for failing to do what a "careful and reasonable" person would do (Fig. 4-1). For example, in each of the following scenarios, the nursing assistant would be considered negligent:

- A nursing assistant becomes distracted by another resident's needs and forgets to lock the wheels on the wheelchair they have just placed by the resident's bed. As the resident moves from the bed to the wheelchair, the wheelchair rolls, causing the resident to fall.
- While changing a resident's bed, a nursing assistant forgets to check the linens for personal objects. As a result, the resident's dentures are sent to the laundry with the soiled linens, and the dentures are damaged when they go through the washing machine.
- A nursing assistant who is caring for a resident with a reputation for complaining fails to report the resident's complaints of pain to the nurse. It turns out that this time the resident's complaints were valid.

Negligence committed by people who hold a license to practice their profession, such as doctors, nurses, lawyers, dentists, and pharmacists, is considered **malpractice**. Nursing assistants (who receive certification, but not licensure) are not charged with malpractice.

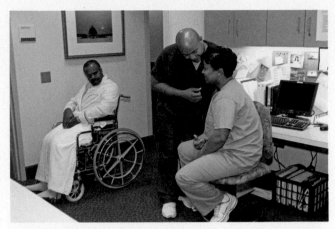

Figure 4-2 Never say negative things or spread rumors about coworkers, patients, or residents. Doing so is unprofessional, and it could get you in trouble with the law!

A violation of civil law committed by a person with the intent to do harm is considered an **intentional tort**. Intentional torts that nursing assistants are particularly at risk for committing in the workplace include defamation, assault, battery, fraud, false imprisonment, invasion of privacy, and larceny.

Defamation

Defamation is making untrue statements that hurt another person's reputation. Statements in oral form are called **slander**, while statements in written form are called **libel**. It is best to avoid saying negative things or spreading rumors about a coworker, supervisor, doctor, patient, or resident (Fig. 4-2). Although it is easy to become hurt, angry, or defensive when you feel that someone has treated you unfairly, making untrue remarks about that person is not the professional way to handle these feelings.

Assault

Assault is threatening or attempting to touch a person without their consent, causing that person to fear bodily harm (Fig. 4-3). A person can be found guilty of committing assault on the basis of an angry statement ("If you get up out of that wheelchair once more without calling for help, I'll tie you down!") or an angry gesture (shaking a fist in someone's face or acting as if you are going to slap them). Even very patient people can become frustrated occasionally. To avoid doing something you will regret later, "take a break" (physically and emotionally) when you feel your emotions get on edge.

Battery

Battery is touching a person without their consent. For example, a health care worker could be accused of battery for physically restraining a person who is

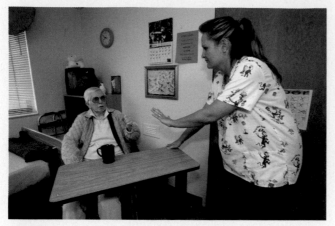

Figure 4-3 Try to avoid letting your emotions get out of check. Making angry gestures toward another is considered assault.

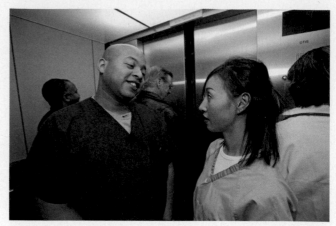

Figure 4-4 It is fine to chat with coworkers in public areas about topics that are not related to work, but never discuss your patients or residents, or their care, in a place where you could be overheard by others.

trying to leave the room, or for performing a procedure that the person or the person's family has not consented to. To avoid being charged with battery, health care providers must obtain **informed consent** from patients and residents before starting a treatment or procedure. Informed consent, which is discussed in detail in Chapter 43, implies that the person has been informed of the need for a procedure or treatment, and has given permission to the health care provider to perform the procedure or administer the treatment. Even if a person initially consents to a treatment or procedure, they are able to withdraw that consent and refuse the treatment or procedure at any time.

Fraud

Fraud is deception that could cause harm to another person. A health care worker who misrepresents their professional qualifications (for example, by telling a patient or resident that they are a nurse when they are not, or lying about previous training or employment on a job application) is committing fraud.

False Imprisonment

False imprisonment is confining another person against their will. In the health care setting, it is sometimes necessary to confine a person to a chair, a bed, or a room to maintain that person's safety (or the safety of others). However, the use of restraints can be considered false imprisonment if the restraints are not justified for the safety of the patient, the resident, or the staff (see Chapter 14).

Invasion of Privacy

Invasion of privacy is violating another person's right to keep certain information and aspects of themselves away from the examination of others. In the

health care setting, discussing a patient's or resident's physical condition, diagnosis, prognosis, or behavior in a public area (such as an elevator, hallway, or cafeteria) violates that person's right to confidentiality, and can be considered an invasion of privacy if someone overhears your discussion (Fig. 4-4).

Confidentiality means keeping personal information that someone shares with you to yourself. Confidentiality applies not only to spoken and observed information, but also to written information. Always make sure that charts, medical records, or computer screens with patient or resident information are not left where others can read them. The only time it is acceptable to discuss a patient or resident is when it is necessary to exchange information about that person's care with someone else who is directly involved in caring for that person. Failure to maintain a person's physical privacy (for example, by leaving a door or curtain open during a procedure, or exposing a person's entire body when it is only necessary to expose a certain part) is also considered an invasion of privacy.

The **Health Insurance Portability and Accountability Act (HIPAA)** originated in 1996. HIPAA is a federal privacy regulation that helps to keep a person's protected health information private and secure. HIPAA:

- Regulates who has the right to view a person's medical records, data, or other private information
- Sets standards on how a person's protected health information is to be stored and transmitted from one place to another
- Requires that health care organizations set policies that allow a patient or resident to have access to their medical records

Larceny

Larceny is stealing. In the health care setting, especially in the long-term care and home health care settings, health care workers have access to patients' or residents' personal belongings. It is never acceptable to take something belonging to another person, even if the item is not of great monetary value or if the person does not seem to "need" it. People who are older or ill are particularly vulnerable to theft, and not just at the hands of health care workers—family members, neighbors, or fellow residents may also commit larceny. As a nursing assistant, it is important for you to be aware of others who may steal from one of your patients or residents and to report any suspicions according to your facility's or agency's policy.

Violations of Criminal Law—Abuse

Abuse, the repetitive and deliberate infliction of injury on another person, is a criminal act and is punishable by a court of law. A person can commit abuse by *actively doing something to* another person or by *failing to do something for* another person, such as providing adequate care or attention. The injury that results from the abuse may be physical or emotional.

Anyone can become the victim of abuse, but those who depend on others for their care (such as infants and children, people with a disability, or older adults) are particularly at risk. The greater the disability, the more at risk the person is for abuse or neglect. Abuse victims can be of any age, sex, race, culture, or religion. Abuse occurs without respect to level of education, employment status, or marital status.

Domestic violence and abuse occur within a relationship by one person's attempts to control the other. Partners may or may not be married and can be heterosexual, gay or lesbian, transgender, living together, separated, or dating. Although people of all genders can be abused, most victims are female. Children who live in homes where there is domestic violence are also more likely to experience abuse or neglect. Child abuse is discussed in detail in Chapter 45.

Another population at high risk for being abused is known as vulnerable adults. A **vulnerable adult** is a person who is 18 years of age or older who may be in need of community care services because they have an intellectual or other disability, an illness, or is at an age (older) that causes them to be unable to care for or protect themselves against significant harm or exploitation.

Forms of Abuse

Abuse takes many forms (Table 4-1).

- **Physical abuse** is the use of force to cause pain or injury to the abused person's body.
- **Neglect** is the failure to provide for a dependent person's basic physical needs. **Abandonment**, which is the act of withdrawing support or help from another person in spite of duty or responsibility, falls under the category of neglect. A health care worker who walks off the job or leaves the unit without telling anyone (even for a short time) has committed abandonment.
- **Psychological (emotional) abuse** is the use of words or actions to cause emotional pain or injury. Psychological abuse can be inflicted in many ways. Making another person fearful by threatening them with physical harm or abandonment is one form of psychological abuse, as is teasing a person in a cruel way or treating a person in an undignified manner. Isolating a person by preventing them from interacting with others (an act called *involuntary seclusion*) is another form of psychological abuse. Keeping a person in a room alone with the door closed can be considered a form of involuntary seclusion.
- **Sexual abuse** involves subjecting a person to unwanted attention of a sexual nature, forcing a person to engage in unwanted sexual activity, or sexually exploiting a person (for example, by taking nude photographs of the person).
- **Financial abuse** involves misusing or stealing another person's money or property. Dishonest people may trick people into giving them money for services that are not provided or charities that do not exist. Older adults are especially vulnerable to this. A common way of doing this is over the phone or through the Internet. A family member may be taking an older person's retirement money and using it for things other than that person's food and medications. There have also been incidents in which health care workers have convinced patients or residents to give them money to help them out of difficult personal situations (for example, to pay for child care, rent, or medication). Discussing personal problems with your patients or residents is not professional behavior and should never be done! Even if a person offers money or property to a health care worker of their own free will, it should never be accepted. Most employers have policies against accepting gifts or money from patients or residents.

Perpetrators of Abuse

There are many reasons why a person may become abusive toward another. Sometimes, abuse is rooted in the desire of one person to overpower and dominate another. Many abusers were victims of abuse themselves and believe that abusive behavior is "normal."

TABLE 4-1 Types of Abuse

TYPE OF ABUSE	EXAMPLES	SIGNS THAT ABUSE MAY BE OCCURRING
Physical abuse: Causing pain or injury to the person's body through the use of force	• Hitting and slapping • Pushing and shoving • Pinching and kicking • Shaking • Burning • Force-feeding • The inappropriate use of medications • The inappropriate use of physical restraints	• Red marks, welts, or bruises, particularly on the face or torso • Broken bones • Broken or bent eyeglasses • Patches of missing hair • Laboratory work that indicates under- or overdosing of medications • Person displays fearful or anxious behavior, especially in the presence of the abuser • Person reports physical abuse
Neglect: Failing or refusing to provide for the person's basic human needs	• Failing to provide food, water, clothing, shelter, or ordered medications • Failing to help the person meet hygiene and toileting needs • Withdrawing support or help from another person, in spite of duty or responsibility (abandonment)	• Unusual weight loss • Dehydration • Pressure ulcers • Poor personal hygiene; unkempt appearance • Incontinence, dried feces on the skin, or skin irritation • Inadequate or inappropriate clothing for environment • Pain • Contractures • Uncontrolled medical conditions (possibly the result of a lack of prescribed medication or treatment) • Person reports improper care
Psychological (emotional) abuse: Causing emotional pain or injury through the use of words or actions	• Insulting or threatening a person • Bullying, humiliating, or harassing a person • Treating a person in an undignified or childlike way • Giving a person the silent treatment • Isolating the person from others (involuntary seclusion)	• Person appears emotionally upset (for example, the person cries frequently) • Person appears withdrawn or apathetic (does not seem to care about anything), or person stops responding • Changes in the person's behavior or unusual behavior (such as rocking or biting) • Person reports psychological abuse
Sexual abuse: Subjecting the person to unwanted attention of a sexual nature, forcing the person to engage in unwanted sexual activity, or sexually exploiting the person (for example, by taking nude photographs of the person)	• Touching personal body parts in an inappropriate way • Making inappropriate, sexually suggestive comments or gestures • Committing sexual assault or battery (for example, forced nudity, inappropriate photography, rape)	• Bruising on breasts or in genital area • Torn or stained underwear • Unexplained bleeding from the vagina or rectum • Person reports sexual abuse or harassment
Financial abuse: Misusing or stealing another person's money or property	• Stealing money or belongings • Withholding a person's Social Security checks or other sources of income • Making withdrawals from a person's bank account or cashing checks without the person's permission • Forging the person's signature on checks or legal documents • Tricking or blackmailing a person into giving away money or property • Tricking or blackmailing a person into signing a legal document or making changes to an existing legal document	• Unexplained disappearance of money or belongings • Sudden change in bank account activity, such as unauthorized withdrawals from the person's account • Unexplained money or property transfers, or changes to the person's will • The inclusion of additional names on the person's bank account • The discovery of forged documents • Person reports mishandling or loss of money or property

Other times, in a situation in which a person requires a great deal of care, the primary caregiver may become overly tired, frustrated, and overwhelmed by the responsibility of providing care (as well as other life demands in addition to caregiving), leading to abuse and neglect. This is often the case with an adult child who finds themselves in the situation of caring for an ill and demanding older parent, without the proper training or support system.

Even people who are trained to administer care may become overwhelmed by their responsibilities or a particular situation. A health care worker is particularly at risk for becoming abusive when a patient or a resident is "difficult" or hard to manage, and the relationship is long term, rather than short term. In long-term care, most relationships with residents last for months, if not years! Any situation can be hard to cope with if you can see no end to the difficulties. As described in Chapter 3, many facilities have counseling services to help employees deal with the emotional stress that caring for others can create. It is a healthy step, not a sign of weakness, to take advantage of these services. Teamwork among coworkers is also essential for helping to reduce work-related stress.

Regardless of the reason abuse occurs, abuse is never an acceptable form of behavior! Be very careful not to place yourself in the position of potentially abusing a patient or a resident. Being found guilty of abuse could destroy your potential for future employment in the health care field.

Elder Abuse

Many older people can be considered vulnerable adults and become victims of abuse. **Elder abuse** is the abuse of an older person. Elder abuse can take any of the forms described in Table 4-1.

Most cases of elder abuse occur in private homes, but elder abuse can and does occur in health care settings as well. Some reports have indicated that episodes of elder abuse have occurred in 30% of our nation's nursing homes. At least 10% of our nation's nursing homes have been charged with abuse as the result of incidents that involved physical harm to a resident. The perpetrators of the abuse may be staff members, other residents, visitors, or family members.

Many factors can place an older person and any other vulnerable adult at risk for abuse:

- **Multiple health conditions**. Older people often have multiple health conditions, which increase their need to depend on others. The older person may require a great deal of care, and the caregiver may become overwhelmed by the demands the person places on their time and energy.

- **An inability to defend oneself**. Physical disabilities, intellectual disabilities, or both can make an older person vulnerable to abuse and unable to defend themselves if abuse occurs.
- **"Difficult" behavior**. An older person in need of care may become "difficult," either as a result of their medical condition (for example, dementia) or because they are having trouble adjusting emotionally to their current situation. For example, the person may fear that their needs will not be met if they are left alone, so they may make constant demands on the caregiver in an effort to keep them close. Or, the person needing care may become resentful or angry about the situation and take these feelings out on the caregiver. This is a common reaction among people who up until this point were very independent.
- **The caregiver's perception of the person needing care**. Sometimes, the caregiver does not fully realize the extent of disability caused by the person's health problem. If the caregiver views the person as being purposefully difficult, this can cause the caregiver to have feelings of anger and resentment toward the person needing care.
- **Social isolation**. Many older people are isolated away from the rest of society, whether they are living in their own homes or living in a long-term care facility. Their daily contact with others is generally limited to a small number of people. This makes it more difficult for the older person to report abuse, and it makes it more difficult for others to detect signs of abuse.
- **A reluctance to report abuse**. Older people are often reluctant to report those who mistreat them. Imagine that you are dependent on someone else to meet your needs, and that person mistreats you. If you report the mistreatment, you will get the caregiver in trouble. Now the caregiver is angry with you. Maybe the other caregivers in the facility (or other members of the family) will turn against you as well, because you got their friend or relative in trouble. But you are still dependent on these people for care. How would you feel in that situation?

Role of the Nursing Assistant in Reporting Abuse

As a nursing assistant, you may find yourself in a situation where you suspect that one of your patients or residents is being abused. (Signs that abuse may be occurring are listed in Table 4-1.) Laws require that any health care worker who suspects the abuse of a child or vulnerable adult must report their suspicions to the proper authorities. Your facility or agency will have specific policies regarding the chain of reporting.

Box 4-1 Reporting Abuse

- Report the incident immediately (for example, do not wait until your next scheduled shift to make your report).
- Set the scene—report what was happening just before the incident.
- Report exactly what you saw or heard.
- Give the names of those involved. If you do not know a person's name, provide a good physical description. If the incident was heard but not seen, describe sounds, including the person's voice, if possible.
- Report the date and time of the incident. If the exact time of the incident is not known, indicate the approximate time by relating it to the routine of the shift (for example, "It occurred after I passed out fresh water, just before dinner.").
- Use exact quotes when reporting what the resident (or someone else) said to you.
- Describe suspicious evidence in detail (for example, if you are describing the appearance of a new injury, such as a bruise, include a description of the location and size of the bruise).
- Keep a written record of what you reported, when you reported it, and to whom.

Examples

- "I am concerned about Mrs. Brewster. I am afraid that something may be occurring between her and her daughter, Ella Franks. I have noticed a change in Mrs. Brewster's behavior, especially when her daughter comes to visit. She doesn't say anything, but she looks at me with pleading eyes whenever her daughter is around, and she often grabs hold of my hand. Mrs. Brewster seems frightened for at least an hour after her daughter leaves. When she hears someone approaching in the hall, she jumps and jerks her head to look at the door with wide eyes and a fearful expression. Sometimes she whimpers. She never used to do that before. Today at about 2:30 pm, just after Mrs. Franks left her mother, I noticed a red mark on Mrs. Brewster's left cheek. I know it wasn't there earlier when I helped her to the bathroom. When I asked Mrs. Brewster what happened, she covered her cheek and just kept shaking her head. She wouldn't say anything."
- "When I did my first rounds after reporting for duty tonight, Mr. Cheng told me that he had observed someone in his room going through his nightstand on the previous shift and now his money is missing. He wasn't sure what time it was, but the room was dark, and he had been asleep for a little while. Mr. Cheng said that he asked the person what he was doing in there, and the person responded, 'None of your business. Shut up and go back to sleep.' The person then quickly shut the drawer. Mr. Cheng said he saw him put something in his pocket. He described the person as tall, with dark hair. His voice was deep. He could not see the person's face, and he did not recognize him as someone he had seen before. He looked like he might have been wearing a blue uniform. Mr. Cheng reports he had about $10.00 in bills that his daughter had given him and probably about $3.00 in quarters from his Bingo winnings. He says that he knows it isn't much, but it was all he had and it gave him a little something to spend at the snack bar. Mr. Cheng is very upset."

Some organizations will require that you report to your supervisor or nurse, while others require reporting to a risk management representative. It is not your responsibility to investigate whether or not abuse has actually occurred, or who has caused it. The state agencies that handle abuse reports will proceed through the proper channels. Your responsibility is to simply report your suspicions (Box 4-1).

Sometimes nursing assistants are hesitant to report suspected, or even witnessed, abuse. They may be fearful of getting a coworker in trouble. However, if you say nothing, you are allowing the abuse, and the harm to the person, to continue. If it becomes known that you were aware of an abusive situation and did not report it, you could find yourself in legal trouble, and your certification may be jeopardized.

ETHICS: GUIDELINES FOR BEHAVIOR

As you have learned, laws serve to preserve basic human rights. As such, laws generally deal with issues that are either "black" or "white": An action is either within the law or outside of it. But what about situations that are not so easily defined? The dramatic changes in health care that have been brought about by advances in technology and research have greatly impacted legal and ethical issues surrounding the medical profession, and have created some unique moral dilemmas. Consider the following questions:

- What should be done with human embryos that have been frozen for future use if the parents decide they do not want to have any more children?
- How does one decide who receives a donor organ, when there are so many people in need but few organs available?
- When does human life begin?
- Should doctors be allowed to end a person's life, at that person's request?

Clearly, these are difficult questions to answer because the answers to these questions depend on the individual's values and beliefs. When definitive

- Treat patients and residents with respect for their individual needs and values.
- Respect the patient's or resident's right to choice in regard to the individual's right to control their own care.
- Hold confidential all information about patients and residents learned in the health care setting.
- Be guided by consideration for the dignity of patients and residents.
- Fulfill the obligation to provide competent care to patients and residents.

answers to questions are not available, we rely on ethical standards to decide what to do. **Ethics** are moral principles or standards that govern conduct. The word "ethics" comes from the Greek word *ethos,* which means "beliefs that guide life." Ethical standards, which are less rigid than laws, help us to determine the difference between right and wrong in areas where the law fears to tread.

Professional Ethics

Each profession has a code of ethics or guidelines pertaining to standards of conduct and practice for that profession. The code of ethics for nursing assistants falls within the American Nurses Association (ANA) code of ethics for nursing (Box 4-2). In addition, there are some general ethical principles that guide all health care workers:

- *Beneficence.* Do good for those in your care by preventing harm and promoting the health and welfare of the person above all else.
- *Nonmaleficence.* Avoid harming those in your care. Use kindness and gentleness when administering care.
- *Justice.* Treat people fairly and equally, regardless of race, religion, culture, disability, or ability to pay.
- *Fidelity.* Act with integrity to earn others' trust.
- *Autonomy.* Respect a person's rights and personal preferences.
- *Confidentiality.* Maintain a person's privacy by allowing the person to discuss sensitive issues with the knowledge that the information will be kept secret.

Personal Ethics

Many factors influence a person's ethics, which are derived from a person's values. A **value** is a cherished

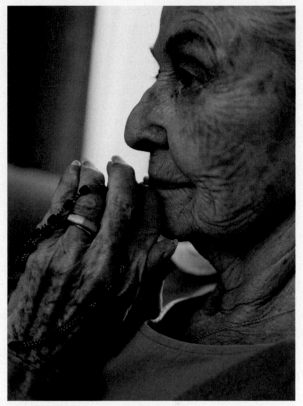

Figure 4-5 Values, which are derived from religious and spiritual beliefs, culture and heritage, and a person's family, are the basis of ethics. Not everyone has the same values. It is important to recognize and respect your patients' or residents' values, even if they are not the same as yours.

belief or principle. Factors that influence a person's values include their religious or spiritual beliefs, level and type of education, culture and heritage, and life experiences. Each person's value system is unique, and as a nursing assistant, you need to think about how you feel about certain moral and ethical issues. Only then will you be able to understand that although another person's values may differ from yours, that person's values are as important to them as yours are to you. Respect for the individual is one of the principles that forms the basis of the code of ethics for nursing (Fig. 4-5).

Ethical Dilemmas

Ethical dilemmas arise when we attempt to judge other people by our own ethical standards. Satisfactory resolutions to ethical dilemmas in the health care field can be difficult to achieve. With so many different types of health care workers involved in patient and resident care, there is always the potential for a clash of viewpoints based on differing values. In the best-case scenario, the patient or resident can speak for themselves with regard to care decisions, either by stating their preferences at the time a decision must be made, or through an advance directive. However, instructions in an advance directive can create an ethical dilemma if they are not clear, or if they do not really apply to the person's clinical situation. Problems can also occur if the patient or resident no longer has the capacity for making decisions and did not prepare an advance directive.

Many states have surrogacy laws, which allow for family members to make health care decisions on behalf of a loved one when the loved one is no longer able to do so. Often, grown children are the ones responsible for making a decision on behalf of their parents. This situation can lead to an ethical dilemma if the children do not agree about what decision should be made. Legally, all of the person's children have an equal say in this situation. These types of disagreements can be very difficult to resolve, and if not handled with care, can lead to family disputes and broken family ties.

Protecting Yourself From Legal and Ethical Difficulties

During your career, you will be exposed to a variety of circumstances and situations. Always bear in mind the legal responsibilities and obligations that you have as a caregiver. There may be many times when you wonder whether a situation poses legal liability issues for you or your employer. Make sure that you are familiar with your employer's policies and with your duties and obligations as listed in your job description. Do not perform duties that are not described in your job description, and always ask your supervisor any

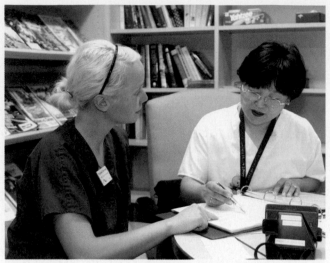

Figure 4-6 In order to stay within the legal limits of your job, know your scope of practice (as defined by the state and your job description), familiarize yourself with your employer's "policies and procedures" manual, and always seek clarification from your supervisor if there is something you do not understand.

questions you may have regarding legal issues. Be aware of the limits of practice for nursing assistants in your state; these limits are set by each state's certification agency and may differ from state to state. Keeping yourself informed is critical to ensure that the care you give is within the legal limits of your job (Fig. 4-6). Finally, if you find yourself in a situation that may pose legal liability issues for you or your employer, or you are facing an ethical dilemma that you are not sure how to resolve, be sure to share your concerns with your supervisor.

SUMMARY

- A professional acts in a way that is legally and ethically appropriate.
- The AHA's *Patient Care Partnership* and the *Resident Rights* portion of the Federal 1987 Nursing Home Reform Act protect the people who receive care and create an atmosphere of open communication among everyone involved in that care.
- Advance directives are legal documents that help to protect patients' and residents' rights by giving the person the opportunity to make their preferences known, in the event that they are unable to state these preferences themselves.

- Laws are rules made by a controlling authority, such as the local, state, or federal government, that serve to protect basic human rights.
  - Civil laws are concerned with relationships between individuals. Criminal laws are concerned with the relationship between an individual and society as a whole.
  - An unintentional tort occurs when someone causes harm or injury to another person or that person's property without the intent to cause harm. A person who commits an

unintentional tort is considered negligent for failing to do what a careful and reasonable person would do.

- A violation of civil law committed by a person with the intent to do harm is called an intentional tort. Examples of intentional torts that may be committed by nursing assistants in the workplace are defamation, assault, battery, fraud, false imprisonment, invasion of privacy, and larceny.

- Abuse, the repetitive and deliberate infliction of injury on another person, is a criminal act and is punishable by a court of law.

  - Child abuse is the abuse of a person under 18 years of age.

  - Domestic abuse occurs when one person in a relationship attempts to control the other.

  - Vulnerable adults often become victims of abuse.

- Abuse can be committed by either actively doing something to another person or by failing to do something for another person.

- Abuse can be physical or psychological (emotional), sexual, or financial. Neglect is a form of physical abuse.

- People who depend on others for their care, such as the very young, the disabled, and the elderly, are particularly at risk for abuse.

- Laws require that any health care worker who suspects the abuse of a child or vulnerable adult must report their suspicions to the proper authorities.

- Ethics are moral principles or standards that govern conduct. Ethical dilemmas in the health care field can be solved only by making sure the patient or resident is an informed, active participant in their care, and by following ethical standards when providing care.

WHAT DID YOU LEARN?

Multiple Choice

Select the single best answer for each of the following questions.

1. All of the following are legal terms that relate to making false statements that injure another person's reputation except:
   a. Defamation
   b. Battery
   c. Slander
   d. Libel

2. If a registered nurse (RN) fails to raise the side rails on the bed of a confused patient, and the patient falls out of bed and is injured, the nurse may be charged with:
   a. Malpractice
   b. Fraud
   c. An intentional tort
   d. Assault

3. *Resident Rights* are a part of which legislation?
   a. American Medical Association (AMA)
   b. Federal 1987 Nursing Home Reform Act (OBRA '87)
   c. Federal Emergency Management Agency (FEMA)
   d. Social Security Act

4. Which ethical principle relates to the concepts of informed consent and a person's right to refuse treatment?
   a. Beneficence
   b. Autonomy

   c. Fidelity
   d. Justice

5. Confidentiality means:
   a. Only sharing information with those directly involved in a patient's or resident's care
   b. Respecting a patient's or resident's right to privacy
   c. Never sharing information with anyone
   d. Both "a" and "b"

6. All residents have basic rights. Which of the following is a basic right of residents?
   a. Right to choice
   b. Right to privacy and confidentiality
   c. Right to be free from verbal abuse or any other abuse
   d. All of the above

7. You are a nursing assistant working in a home health care setting. You suspect that one of your clients is being emotionally and physically abused by their partner. What should you do first?
   a. Call the police
   b. Keep your suspicions to yourself but continue to observe the situation
   c. Immediately report your suspicions to the case manager
   d. Tell another nursing assistant at the agency

8. One of your fellow nursing assistants has been having a very hard time with one of their residents. The resident is confused and, as a result, is being uncooperative. In a moment of complete frustration, your coworker says to the resident, "If you don't shut up and behave yourself right now, I'm going to slap you!" What kind of an intentional tort has this nursing assistant committed?
   a. Assault
   b. Battery
   c. Negligence
   d. Malpractice

9. A nursing assistant answers the phone at the nursing station. The doctor who is calling wants to give a verbal order, and the nursing assistant tells the doctor that they are a nurse and can take the order. What intentional tort has the nursing assistant committed?
   a. Slander
   b. Fraud
   c. Libel
   d. Informed consent

10. What does the Health Insurance Portability and Accountability Act (HIPAA) protect?
   a. The patient's or resident's right to privacy
   b. The patient's or resident's right to sue negligent health care workers
   c. The patient's or resident's right to be free from abuse
   d. The patient's or resident's right to choose who will provide their care

11. A legal document that transfers the responsibility for handling a person's medical decisions to family member, friend, or other trusted individual is known as a:
   a. Living will
   b. HIPAA agreement
   c. Form of consent
   d. Durable power of attorney

12. An ombudsman is a person who:
   a. Advocates to protect residents living in long-term care
   b. Prosecutes long-term care staff guilty of abuse
   c. Lives in a long-term care facility
   d. Is authorized to force a facility to take action to address resident issues when residents have concerns about their care

Matching   *Match each numbered item with its appropriate lettered description.*

_____ **1.** Civil laws

_____ **2.** Liability

_____ **3.** Fraud

_____ **4.** Ethics

_____ **5.** Beneficence

a. The responsibility of an individual to act within the confines of the law

b. A system of moral principles or standards used to govern conduct

c. Protecting a patient or resident from harm

d. Deception that could cause harm to another person

e. Laws that deal with relationships between individuals

STOP *and* THINK!

A licensed practical nurse (LPN) who works with you in a long-term care facility stops in Mrs. Taylor's room to give Mrs. Taylor her daily medications. Mrs. Taylor is in the bathroom, and you are changing the linens on her bed. The nurse hands you the medication cup, which contains three pills and asks you to have Mrs. Taylor take the pills as soon as she comes out of the bathroom. You are aware that in your state, nursing assistants who work in long-term care facilities are not allowed to give medications. When you mention your concern about giving Mrs. Taylor her medication to the nurse, she says, "It's okay; the other nursing assistants do this for me all of the time." What should you do?

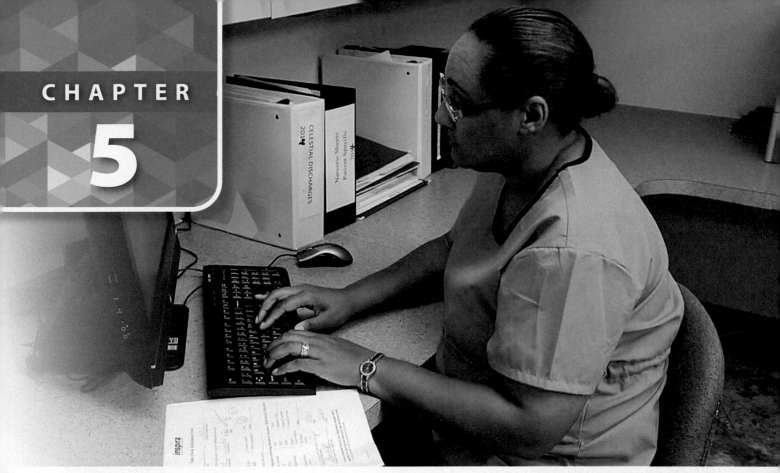

Photo: A nursing assistant checks a resident's medical record. The medical record is one way in which members of the health care team share information with each other.

Communication Skills

 WHAT WILL YOU LEARN?

Being able to effectively communicate, or participate in the exchange of information, is a critical skill for all people in the health care field. Every day, you will need to communicate with your patients or residents, and with other members of the health care team. If just one link in the chain of communication is broken, the quality of care given to the patient or resident can suffer. In this chapter, we will describe techniques for, as well as obstacles to, effective communication. In addition, we will review some of the tools that are commonly used by members of the health care team to ensure that information is readily available to all who are involved with the care of a patient or resident. When you are finished with this chapter, you will be able to:

1. Define communication.
2. Describe the two major forms of communication and give examples of each.
3. Discuss techniques that promote effective communication.
4. Describe obstacles to effective communication and how to avoid them.
5. Identify causes of conflict and ways to resolve it.
6. Demonstrate proper telephone communication skills.
7. Explain how the nursing assistant is a vital link in the communication chain and how they communicate information to other members of the health care team.

8. Discuss the methods of reporting and recording information in a health care setting.

9. Explain how the patient's or resident's medical record facilitates communication among members of the health care team.

10. Describe communication technologies used in the health care field today.

11. List the steps of the nursing process and describe how the nursing team uses them to plan the patient's or resident's care.

Vocabulary

Communication	Objective data	Medical record	Nursing care plan
Verbal communication	Signs	Electronic health record	Nursing process
Nonverbal communication	Subjective data	(EHR)	Nursing diagnosis
	Symptoms	Kardex	Interventions
Conflict	Reporting	Interdisciplinary care	Goals
Observation	Recording	plan	

WHAT IS COMMUNICATION?

Communication is the exchange of information. The key to understanding what communication truly is lies within the word "exchange." If you exchange gifts with another person, you give that person a gift, and in return, you receive one back. In the exchange of information that defines communication, there is a constant back-and-forth flow of information. Communicating is not just about telling someone something (giving information); it is also about listening and observing (receiving information).

For effective communication to occur, all of the people who are involved must actively participate in the exchange of information. Communication involves at least two people, a *sender* and a *receiver*. The sender is the person with information to share, and the receiver is the person for whom the information is intended. The sender delivers the information in the form of a *message*, which the receiver may or may not understand. Through *feedback*, or a return message, the receiver lets the sender know whether the message was received and understood (Fig. 5-1). Note that as information is transmitted back and forth, the sender and the receiver switch roles.

There are two major forms of communication, verbal and nonverbal.

Verbal communication involves the use of language, either spoken or written. Sign language, a system of hand gestures used to make letters of the alphabet and words, is also considered a form of verbal communication. Verbal communication tends to be deliberate—when we use language to express a thought, it is usually with the intent of giving specific information to another person.

Nonverbal communication, on the other hand, tends to be more subtle. In nonverbal communication, a person gives information through the use of facial expressions, gestures, body language, and tone of voice. For example, consider a resident with disabling arthritis. Not wanting to seem a "burden" to the health care staff, the resident may tell you that they feel fine when you ask. However, you note that they make a face when they try to get out of their chair and their voice seems strained. These observations suggest that the resident is not being entirely truthful with you about how they are feeling. Of the two forms of communication, nonverbal communication is perhaps the most reliable method of "reading" another person, especially in the health care field. For various reasons, people may not say what they really mean. Being observant and aware of others' nonverbal cues will give you a greater understanding of what your patients or residents are feeling and thinking.

COMMUNICATING EFFECTIVELY

As a nursing assistant, you must be a successful communicator, both as a sender and a receiver of information, with both those you care for and your coworkers. For example, you will use communication skills to comfort, reassure, and assist your patients or residents. Because nursing assistants typically spend

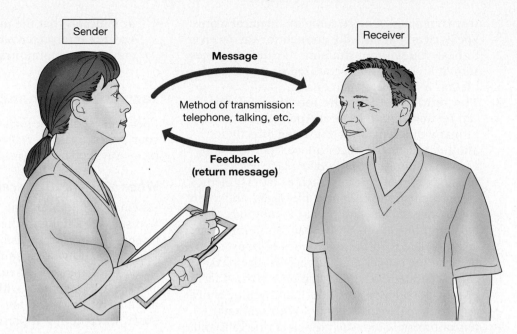

Sender

Receiver

Message

Method of transmission:
telephone, talking, etc.

**Feedback
(return message)**

Figure 5-1 Communication involves the back-and-forth flow of information between a sender and a receiver.

more time with patients and residents and get to know them better than any other member of the health care team, you will become one of the strongest links between the patient or resident and the other health care team members. As you form relationships with your patients or residents, they will talk to you, confide in you, listen to you, and trust you. In addition, by carefully watching your patients or residents for nonverbal communication cues, you may be the first member of the health care team to notice that Mr. Schneider's color is not quite right, or that Mrs. Morales is having abdominal pain after eating, even though she is not complaining verbally.

In addition to communicating well with patients or residents, communicating well with your coworkers is also essential. Supervisors will delegate tasks to you, and you must be sure that you understand what they are asking you to do and how you are to go about doing it. In addition, you will be the "eyes and ears" of the nurses, physical therapists, dietitians, social workers, and other members of the health care team. Relaying vital information about your patient's or resident's condition to the nurse is an essential part of your duties. As a nursing assistant, you are not trained to diagnose and treat medical problems. However, your knowledge of your patient or resident will allow you to gather important information that, when communicated to the nurse, will alert the health care team members to changes in that person's condition and influence the care they receive. Your responsibility as a communication link between the patient or resident and the rest of the health care team is very important (Fig. 5-2)!

Clearly, it is important for a nursing assistant to learn good communication skills. There are many ways that communication can fail. Remember that good

communication is a "two-way street" and involves the *exchange* of information. To see where problems in communication can occur, let's look at each part of the process of exchanging information:

1. **The sender creates a message**. Information needs to be organized and relevant to the person who will be receiving it. Your message, whether it is spoken or written, should convey the relevant facts, organized in an easily accessible manner. Use language that the receiver understands—this could mean getting help from an interpreter, if the receiver does not speak the same language you do, or using simple, common

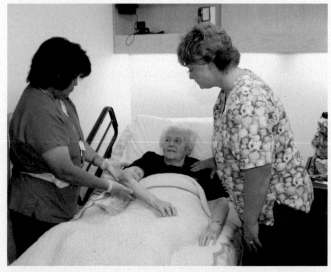

Figure 5-2 As a nursing assistant, you are an important link between the patient or resident and the other members of the health care team.

words in place of more complex, medical words. Speak clearly and loudly enough for the receiver to hear you without straining. Written messages should be legible and organized so that the information is complete and concise.

2. **The sender delivers the message**. Information can be transmitted from one person to another in many different ways. Speaking directly to another person, or "face-to-face," permits nonverbal communication to take place. Other methods of transmission, such as letters, memos, emails, telephone calls, text messages, and intercom conversations, are primarily methods of verbal communication. Nonverbal communication is impossible with these methods of transmission because the sender and the receiver are physically separated. When relying on a written form of transmission, be sure your handwriting is neat and your spelling is accurate. With oral methods of transmission, such as telephone calls and intercom conversations, it is important to ensure that background noise or static does not interfere with the receiver's ability to hear your message.

3. **The receiver receives the message**. For successful communication to occur, the receiver must be physically able to receive the message and mentally engaged in the communication exchange. For example, a person with a hearing loss may have difficulty hearing a spoken message. A person who cannot read would not be able to understand a message sent in written form. A person who has had a stroke may be able to hear your words perfectly but may not be able to understand their meaning. Sign language or communicating through nonverbal means (for example, nodding your head "yes" to a person's question) may not be effective if the person is visually impaired. These are all examples of physical problems that can interfere with a person's ability to receive a message. Communication can also fail when a receiver is mentally distracted, emotionally stressed, or not really paying attention to the sender.

4. **The receiver provides feedback**. Have you ever spoken to someone and had them ignore you? Did you wonder whether or not the person even heard you? You did not receive feedback from that person. Feedback, like other parts of communication, can be verbal (spoken or written) or nonverbal. During an exchange of information, it is important for the receiver to provide feedback to the sender, and it is important for the sender to listen and watch for this feedback. If the receiver does not provide feedback, the sender should make an effort to get a response of some sort. When feedback does not occur

or indicates that the message the sender sent was not interpreted correctly, other methods of enhancing communication may be necessary.

Tactics That Enhance Communication

Good communication skills will serve you well, both in your professional life and your personal life. There are many ways you can enhance communication with others.

When You Are the Receiver, Be a Good Listener

Listening is perhaps the most useful communication skill, especially in the health care setting. Active listening requires focusing your attention on the speaker. Sit down or assume a relaxed posture so that you do not appear rushed or in a hurry to move on, and make eye contact with the person (Fig. 5-3). Do not interrupt or try to finish the person's sentence for them. Interrupting a person may make them forget what they were trying to tell you in the first place. Let the person finish what they were saying before you ask another question or make a comment, and focus on the person and the information they are trying to give you—try not to think about what *you* intend to do or say next. After the person has finished speaking, you should ask questions to help clarify any information that you do not understand. Your comments and questions will let the speaker know whether you understood their message, or whether they need to provide additional information.

When You Are the Sender, Make Sure Your Message Is Clear

Speak clearly and use words that the person you are speaking to understands. A nurse or a fellow nursing

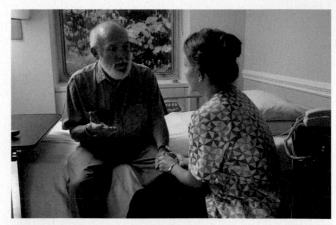

Figure 5-3 Being a good listener is essential to being a good communicator. (Used with permission from Taylor, C., Lillis, C., & Lynn, P. [2014]. *Fundamentals of nursing: The art and science of nursing care* [8th ed., p. 466]. Lippincott Williams & Wilkins.)

assistant will understand medical terminology, and using medical terminology is appropriate when you are communicating with one of your coworkers. However, a patient, resident, or family member may not be familiar with medical terminology. To make sure the patient or family member understands your message, try to use common words instead of technical words whenever it is appropriate to do so. For example, you could say, "Miss Lewis, we're going to go for a walk down the hall now, to get you up and moving" instead of "Miss Lewis, I'm going to ambulate you now."

Sometimes, it is necessary to communicate with someone who does not speak the same language as you do, or who has a physical problem that makes certain forms of communication less effective than others. To meet the regulation that requires patients and residents to give informed consent for treatments and procedures, health care facilities must provide interpreters for patients or residents who speak languages other than English. In fact, approximately one in five residents of the United States speaks a language other than English. And by definition, a person cannot give informed consent unless they understand what they are consenting to! A person who lacks the ability to hear may need a sign-language interpreter to assist with communication, or you could try writing out important questions for the person to read and respond to. Many health care facilities use electronic interpretive services that can be easily accessed through a computer or tablet. A picture board, a tool that allows a person to point to a picture of what they are trying to say, is often useful when trying to communicate on a basic level with someone who speaks a different language or who has difficulty hearing (Fig. 5-4). More information about communicating with patients and residents with specific communication needs can be found in Chapters 33 and 34.

If a patient or resident seems to have difficulty understanding you when you are talking to them, make sure that there is not too much background noise. If the person usually wears glasses or a hearing aid, check to make sure that these aids are in place and the hearing aid is turned on.

Learn Techniques for Encouraging People to Talk

When you need to get information from someone, try asking the person an open-ended question. Questions that can be answered with a simple "yes" or "no" usually get just that response, and the conversation ends. In contrast, open-ended questions encourage the person to talk. Another question that can cause a conversation to end is "Why?" If a patient complains that they do not like their dinner or choice of snack, instead of asking "Why?" (which can be intimidating), you could ask the person to tell you what their favorite food or snack is. For example, consider the following two conversations:

Conversation 1

Nursing assistant: "Good morning, Mr. Hopkins. Did you enjoy your breakfast this morning?"

Mr. Hopkins: "No."

Nursing assistant: "Why not?"

Mr. Hopkins: "I don't know . . . I just wasn't hungry, I guess."

Conversation 2

Nursing assistant: "Good morning, Mr. Hopkins. What did you have for breakfast this morning?"

Mr. Hopkins: "Not much. They sent up scrambled eggs. I don't care for scrambled eggs, so I just had some buttered toast and coffee."

Nursing assistant: "I didn't know you didn't like scrambled eggs! Let me see what I can do

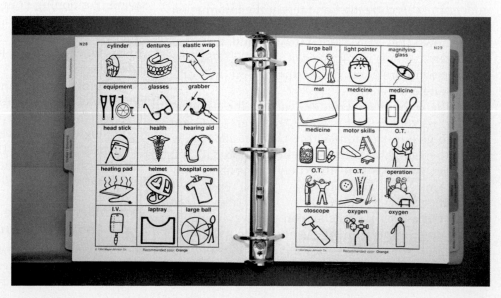

Figure 5-4 A picture board can be used to communicate when illustrations are more effective than words.

about that. Do you dislike eggs in general, or just scrambled eggs? In the meantime, are you still hungry?"

In the second conversation, the nursing assistant achieved two key goals: they engaged Mr. Hopkins in the conversation, and in the process, they made him feel as though they really cared about him as an individual.

Rephrasing what someone says to you is another way to encourage someone to talk. For example, if one of your residents tells you that they feel sad and lonely, instead of asking "Why?" try repeating the person's statement back to them as a question: "You are feeling sad and lonely? Tell me more." By rephrasing and asking an open-ended question, you will invite the person to say more. In addition, encouraging the person to talk more about what they are feeling shows the person that you are actively listening to what they are saying to you.

Usually, asking open-ended questions is better than asking questions that can be answered with a simple "yes" or "no." But in some situations, a "yes or no" question may be better. For example, asking questions that can be answered with a short "yes" or "no" (or a nod or shake of the head) is appropriate when you are caring for a patient or resident who is having trouble breathing or who is having difficulty speaking.

Provide and Seek Feedback

Providing and seeking feedback is a critical communication skill that will come into play with both your coworkers and your patients or residents. Consider two conversations, one between you and the nurse, and the other between you and one of your patients or residents. In the first, you are the "receiver"—the nurse is asking you to do a task. After the nurse has finished speaking, you could say, "Let me make sure I understand this correctly," and repeat the information back to them. What awesome feedback! The nurse now knows that you were listening and that you understand what is being asked of you (Fig. 5-5). The *exchange* of information has occurred. You are communicating effectively.

In the second conversation, you are the "sender" and one of your residents is the "receiver"—you are trying to give instructions to the resident about how to use the call-light control system in the room, and you want to make sure that they understand how the system works. You might say, "Now, repeat that information back to me, so I can make sure you've got it," but asking for feedback in this way could be intimidating to the resident. A more effective way of finding out whether the resident understood your message would be to say, "Now, if you could just repeat these instructions back to me, so I can make

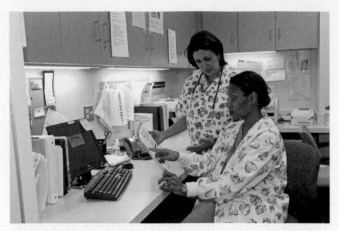

Figure 5-5 By indicating to the nurse that they understand what they are being asked to do, this nursing assistant is providing good feedback.

sure I didn't leave anything out...." This approach makes the resident feel that they are helping you by repeating the information, and in the process, you are able to tell whether or not they understand your instructions clearly.

Be Mindful of Your Body Language and Tone of Voice

Use appropriate body language when listening or talking to other people. Negative body language, such as crossing your arms across your chest, tapping your feet or fingers, rolling your eyes, or constantly looking at your watch or toward the door sends the very clear message that you are bored or uninterested (Fig. 5-6). In contrast, displaying positive body language, such as facing the person, nodding as they speak, smiling or looking serious as appropriate, and making occasional vocal sounds, such as "uh huh" or "hmm" indicates to the person that you are interested in what they are saying. Positioning your body so that you are at eye level with the speaker also shows interest (Fig. 5-7). Children are especially responsive to the adult who comes "down to their level" to listen to what they have to say.

Tone of voice is important too. A sharp or hurried tone of voice suggests to the person that you are impatient or angry. In contrast, speaking slowly in a soothing tone of voice suggests that you are calm, competent, and kind. This relaxes the other person and is a useful technique for calming a person who is frightened or upset.

Remember the Value of Silence and a Comforting Touch

There will be many times throughout your career as a nursing assistant when words will not be enough to communicate your care and concern to a patient

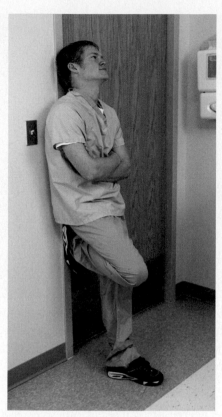

Figure 5-6 If you were a patient or resident, what message would this nursing assistant be sending to you?

or resident or one of their family members. Silence and a comforting touch will say more than words can (Fig. 5-8). In addition to allowing us to communicate when words are not enough, touch is comforting and establishes a bond. So much has been written about the "healing powers of touch"—for example, consider the role of therapeutic massage in the treatment of physical ailments. Research has also shown that

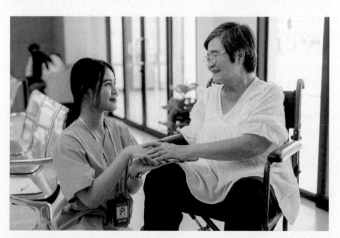

Figure 5-7 Putting yourself at eye level with a patient or resident indicates to the person that you are interested in what they have to say and that you have time to listen. (kelvn\Shutterstock.com)

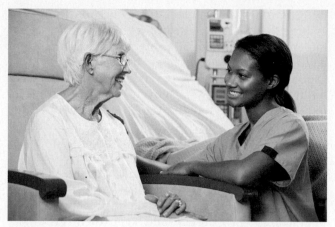

Figure 5-8 Of the many techniques for enhancing communication, nothing says "I care about you and I want to help you" more effectively than a simple touch on a person's hand or shoulder. (Monkey Business Images\ Shutterstock.com)

babies, even when given adequate food and physical care, fail to grow and thrive without human touch and attention.

Touch is perhaps the most universal of all languages, but remember to be sensitive to the individual's comfort level. A person's cultural beliefs also dictate whether touch may be welcomed. Many patients and residents appreciate affection and will enjoy a hug or sitting and holding your hands as you talk. Other people may not be as comfortable with affection and will be satisfied with a light pat on the shoulder or top of the hand as you greet them or say goodbye.

Blocks to Effective Communication

Some behaviors and attitudes can block effective communication. Perhaps the most common obstacle to effective communication is not listening carefully to what another person is saying. You must be especially careful not to "tune out" your patients or residents, despite the fact that you will be busy, and many of the people you will care for could be easily labeled "complainers." Imagine the consequences if you ignore a patient's or resident's complaint and it turns out to be valid.

Being judgmental of others will also block communication. If a person feels that you do not believe or respect what they are trying to tell you, they will most likely stop talking and will probably refuse to answer any questions you may ask later. A judgmental attitude, indicating that you do not really care to hear what the person is trying to tell you, can be revealed through negative body language or comments you may make.

Communication blocks can occur when you assume that someone else knows what you are thinking. Your patient should know that they should not adjust the flow rate on their intravenous (IV) line, shouldn't they? Your coworkers should know without bothering you that Mrs. Nguyen has already been up to the bathroom, shouldn't they? Your romantic partner should know why you are mad at them, shouldn't they? The assumption that other people know what you know, think the way you think, and feel the way you feel presents a major block to effective communication and can lead to conflict and confusion. To avoid this communication pitfall, be proactive in your interactions with others, and keep them informed. For example, give instructions and gentle reminders to patients or residents, tell your coworkers what has already been accomplished and what still needs to be done before you go on break, and ask your partner to take out the trash instead of getting angry because they did not think of it themselves!

Concerns for Long-Term Care

The majority of your residents in the long-term care setting are older adults and may experience difficulty with communication due to hearing loss, aphasia, or dementia. Unfortunately, many people think of older adults as people who are "going through their second childhood" and speak to them accordingly. When speaking with your older adult residents, avoid the use of "baby talk" or calling them all "sweetie" or "honey." These residents, like all people needing health care services, deserve to be spoken to with respect and as the adults they are. If a resident has a specific communication difficulty, learn about why the person has the difficulty and use communication techniques specific for that problem.

Conflict Resolution

Conflict, or discord resulting from differences between people, can occur when one person is unable to understand or accept another's ideas or beliefs. Conflict can also arise when one person's expectations for another differ from that person's expectations for themselves. Other times, conflict arises because one person misunderstands another person's words or intentions. How many times have you been angry with a friend because you thought they said or meant one thing, only to find out after talking with them that what you thought they said or meant is not what they said or meant at all? Conflict can occur when another person's needs or wants conflict with our own needs and wants.

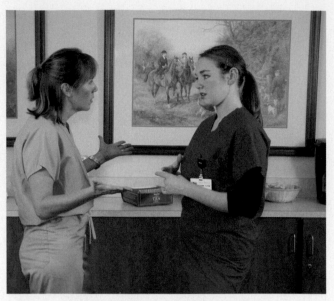

Figure 5-9 Conflict can occur between two members of the health care team or between a member of the health care team and a patient, resident, or visitor. Poor communication is one of the most common reasons conflict occurs!

Some degree of conflict in our lives is inevitable because we are all individuals with unique personalities, feelings, and beliefs. Conflict is a fairly common occurrence in the health care field because health care is a people-oriented business. It is also a very emotional business. Patients and residents are sick, hurting, confused, and frightened. Family members feel helpless and sad. Nursing assistants and other health care workers are often stressed by the emotional and physical demands of their work. As a result, conflicts may arise between a member of the health care team and a patient or resident, between two patients or residents, or between two members of the health care team (Fig. 5-9). Getting along with other people, while a very important part of your job, can sometimes be the hardest part of your job.

Conflict makes the people directly involved, as well as those around them, uncomfortable. This discomfort can affect a patient's or resident's ability to recover or a staff member's quality of work. Good communication is essential to preventing conflict, as well as helping to resolve it. If you find yourself involved in a conflict, remember what it means to be a professional, and take the time to talk calmly with the person you are upset with. It is important to address areas of conflict early, before they have time to get worse and involve more people. Approaches for resolving conflict include the following:

- Ask to speak privately with the person you have a conflict with. Because the two of you may be able to resolve your disagreement on your own,

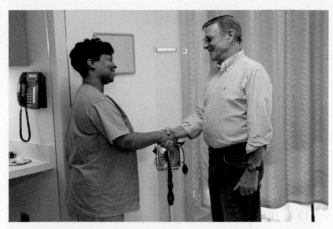

Figure 5-10 Sometimes, the best solution to a conflict is to simply "agree to disagree." Instead of focusing on your differences, focus on your similarities. In the professional setting, for example, even if you and a resident's family member cannot agree about what is "best" for the resident, you can certainly respect the fact that both of you care deeply about the resident and want to do what is best for them.

try this approach before asking a supervisor to mediate, if at all possible. Remain polite and professional and thank the person for their time.

- During your conversation, focus on the specific area of conflict. Do not focus on how you feel about the other person, or how you think they should have acted under the circumstances.
- Be specific about what you understand the problem to be. Express why you are upset in terms of "I," rather than the more accusatory "you." For example, instead of saying, "You really hurt my feelings by what you said the other day," say, "I am bothered by what you said the other day." In this manner, you take responsibility for the emotion and allow the other person to explain their side of the story.
- Be prepared to hear how the other person may feel toward you or the problem, even if it is not pleasant. Perhaps you were the one who was initially misunderstood.
- Be gracious enough to apologize for misunderstanding the other person, or for being the one who was misunderstood.
- Ask the other person for insight into solutions for resolving the conflict. Their suggestions may surprise you!
- Sometimes it is necessary to "agree to disagree." People with differing opinions and beliefs can focus on the things they have in common, such as caring about the patient's or resident's well-being, and still disagree on certain issues (Fig. 5-10). Learning to respect others' beliefs is an important part of being professional.

- If you are unable to resolve a conflict with a coworker, a patient or resident, or a patient's or resident's family member on your own, seek the advice of your supervisor. A conflict that affects the quality of the care you provide must not be allowed to continue!

TELEPHONE COMMUNICATION

The telephone is a primary tool of communication in the health care field. Other departments will call to verify an order or request, doctors will call to ask about a patient or resident or to give orders, and family members will call to get an update on the condition of a loved one. The telephone at the nursing station is in use constantly. As a nursing assistant, you will usually be required to answer the telephone, either at the nursing station or in a patient's or resident's room (Fig. 5-11). Proper telephone etiquette is reviewed in Box 5-1.

When you answer the telephone, make sure your voice is pleasant and unhurried. Believe it or not, a caller can "hear a smile" in your voice. This can be very comforting to an anxious family member who is calling to check on a sick loved one. You must remember to be as professional on the telephone as you are in person. There will be times when a caller may be impatient or angry; resist the urge to respond in a similar manner. You do not know the cause of the caller's impatience or anger, and you certainly do not want to add to it. The way you handle yourself on the telephone reflects directly on your facility. If callers perceive you as kind and professional when they speak to you on the phone, they will feel that the people you are caring for are receiving the same kind, professional care.

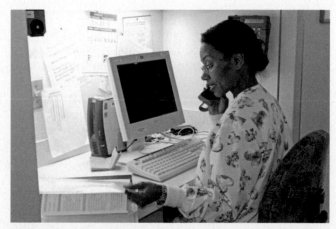

Figure 5-11 Developing a good phone manner is important because you will find yourself using the telephone to communicate frequently!

Box 5-1   Telephone Etiquette

- Answer the phone promptly, within the first three rings.
- Answer with a pleasant greeting, such as "Good morning" or "Good afternoon."
- Identify yourself by name and title and by your unit or floor according to facility policy: "3 West; Mary Smith, CNA, speaking."
- Because the caller obviously needs something (otherwise, they would not be calling), ask "How may I help you?"
- Know how to perform basic functions using your facility's telephone system, such as how to transfer a call or place a caller on hold.
- If you must place a caller on hold, ask for their permission first ("May I put you on hold for a minute?"). Be aware of the length of time a caller has been on hold; if the time becomes excessive (more than 5 minutes), ask the caller if they want to continue to hold, leave a message, or call back later.
- If the person the caller wants to speak to is unavailable, offer to take a message. When taking a message, write down the date and time of the call, the name of the caller, a phone number where the caller can be reached, and your name. Write clearly, and ask the caller to spell their name if you are not sure how to spell it. Deliver the message to the person for whom it was intended.
- A nursing assistant is not to take doctor's orders, receive or give results of diagnostic tests, or release patient or resident information to anyone, even family members. Calls of this nature should be handled by a nurse.
- Do not use the telephone at the nurse's station to make or receive personal calls. Personal calls should be made from your own cell phone, while you are on break or at lunch. Never tie up a telephone used for health care communication by using it for personal business.

Confidentiality is of concern when the telephone is used as a means of communication. When you are discussing a person's care over the telephone, be sure that other patients, residents, or visitors cannot overhear your conversation. Know your facility's policy regarding what information can be provided over the telephone. For example, some facilities, such as those that provide mental health care or substance use rehabilitation, protect their patients' and residents' right to privacy through policies that prohibit staff from confirming or denying that a person is even receiving treatment at the facility. The Health Insurance Portability and Accountability Act (HIPAA), discussed in Chapter 4, specifically regulates who may be given information about a person in a health care facility.

Social Media Concerns

The use of mobile devices has changed the way in which people communicate with each other, both personally and professionally. Almost everyone has a cell phone and takes photos, texts messages, and posts on numerous social media sites. Make sure that you are familiar with your facility's policies related to the use of social media and the confidentiality of the people you care for. While you may think it is a nice idea to take a "selfie" with your favorite resident to post on social media, you may be compromising that person's confidentiality and breaking Federal HIPAA regulations. Be very cautious about posting anything related to where you work, who you work with, and any information about the people you are providing care for. Many facilities and health care agencies are routinely monitoring the social media sites used by their employees and may also examine your social media prior to hiring you.

COMMUNICATION AMONG MEMBERS OF THE HEALTH CARE TEAM

As you have already learned, the nursing assistant plays a very important role in gathering and sharing information about patients and residents with other members of the health care team. As you interact with your patients or residents, you will have the opportunity to make **observations**. An observation is something that you notice about the patient or resident, typically related to a change in the person's physical or mental condition. The amount of time you spend with your patients or residents, combined with the type of duties you are responsible for performing daily (for example, bathing, feeding, ambulating, toileting), will give you a chance to observe things that other health care team members may overlook.

Two types of data, objective data and subjective data, can lead to observations. **Objective data** are information that you obtain directly, through measurements or by using one of your five senses. In the professional setting, the senses you will use most often are sight, hearing, touch, and smell. For example, certain indicators of a person's health, called vital signs, can be objectively measured. (The vital signs are temperature, pulse, respiratory rate, and blood pressure.) You can see the color of a person's skin and feel that it is cool and clammy (Fig. 5-12). You can see the color of a person's urine, smell any foul odor, and measure the amount. You can hear wheezing or gurgling as a person breathes. You can see bruises, swelling, or rashes on the skin when you help a person bathe. You can see how much breakfast the person ate and measure how much juice they

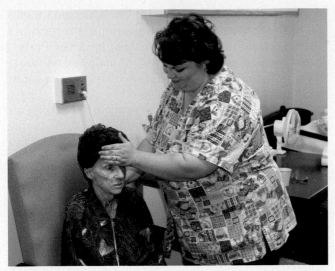

Figure 5-12 When you make an objective observation, you obtain information using one of your five senses. Here, the nursing assistant is feeling the resident's forehead to assess whether or not the skin is hot and dry or cool and clammy.

drank. These are all objective observations. Objective observations, such as an elevated temperature, a rash, or a low urine output, are called **signs. Subjective data**, on the other hand, are information that cannot be objectively measured or assessed. The basis for a subjective observation is usually a person's complaint, or **symptom**. For example, a patient or resident may tell you that they have a headache or stomachache. You cannot see, feel, measure, or hear their pain, but they can describe it to you (Fig. 5-13).

When you are communicating subjective observations to the other health care team members, it is useful to quote the person directly, whether you are

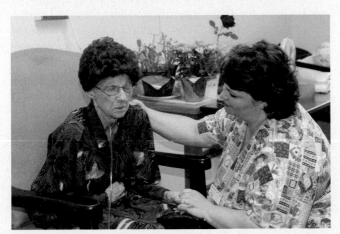

Figure 5-13 A subjective observation is information that is derived "second-hand." This nursing assistant knows that her resident is experiencing stomach pain because the resident is describing it to her, not because she detected the resident's pain using one of her five senses.

relaying the complaint verbally (reporting) or writing the information in the person's medical record (recording). It is also useful to support subjective observations with objective ones. For instance, Mrs. White tells you that she feels dizzy when she stands up (a subjective observation). To gather more information, you ask Mrs. White if she has gotten dizzy before, and whether or not her dizziness is accompanied by a headache or nausea. Her answers to these questions would also be subjective observations. Next, you observe Mrs. White's skin for paleness or redness; touch her skin to see if it is warm, or cool and clammy; measure her blood pressure; and take her pulse. All of these objective observations give you still more information. By gathering objective facts to add to Mrs. White's subjective statements and then organizing this information in a logical way, and relaying it to the nurse, you are truly communicating! Not only have you told the nurse about Mrs. White's symptoms, you have given them objective data that may help them find out what is causing Mrs. White's symptoms.

Once you have made an observation, you must decide on the most effective method of communicating that observation to the nurse. Nursing assistants use two methods of communicating observations about their patients or residents and documenting the care provided so that other health care team members are kept "in the know." These methods are reporting and recording. Some observations need to be reported to the nurse immediately, such as a patient's or resident's complaint of pain or a change in their vital signs. Other observations only need to be recorded in the person's medical record. Throughout this text, observations that need to be reported to the nurse immediately are highlighted as "Tell the Nurse!" notes.

Reporting

Reporting is the spoken exchange of information between health care team members. Reporting is used throughout the shift to communicate changes about a patient's or resident's status to other health care team members (Fig. 5-14). Nursing assistants use reporting to communicate the following information to the nurse:

- Observations that suggest a change in the patient's or resident's condition
- Observations regarding the patient's or resident's response to a new treatment or therapy
- A patient's or resident's complaints of pain or discomfort
- A patient's or resident's refusal of treatment
- A patient's or resident's requests

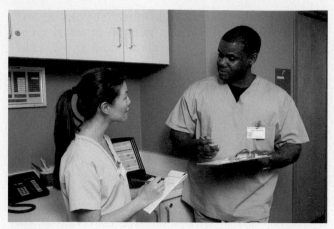

Figure 5-14 This nursing assistant is reporting a change in one of her resident's vital signs to the nurse. (Used with permission from Taylor, C., Lillis, C., & Lynn, P. [2014]. *Fundamentals of nursing: The art and science of nursing care* [8th ed., p. 361]. Lippincott Williams & Wilkins.)

When reporting information, follow the guidelines that help promote effective communication. Make sure the information that you are reporting is accurate—refer to the patient or resident by name and room number, and if you are reporting measurements, such as vital signs, write the numbers down so that you do not forget them or report them incorrectly. Report your observations in an orderly, concise manner. Avoid adding information that is not relevant to what you are trying to communicate. Use correct terminology when reporting, and make sure the person you are reporting to gives you feedback so that you know that they received the information and will act on it.

Reporting is also routinely used when shifts change to keep the staff members who are coming to work aware of all the information that is necessary to ensure a smooth continuation of care for the patient or resident. For example, the end-of-shift report, also known as a "hand-off" report, is when oncoming staff members would be informed of new patients or residents and their care requirements, changes in the care plan for established patients or residents (such as new orders or treatments), and changes in a patient's or resident's status.

Recording

Recording, sometimes referred to as "charting," is communicating information about a patient or resident to other health care team members in written or electronic form. Tools associated with recording include the medical record (chart) and the Kardex.

Medical Record (Chart)

A person's **medical record** (chart) is a legal document that is the formal accounting of the care a person receives from the health care facility. A person's medical record contains information about the person's current condition, the measures that have been taken by the medical and nursing staff to diagnose and treat the condition, and the person's response to the treatment and care.

The medical record is usually organized in sections with specific forms contained in each section. Some of these forms provide general information about the patient or resident. Others are specific to a particular health care department. The forms used may vary depending on the type of facility or health care agency. Typically, however, a medical record contains the following forms:

- **Admission data**. The admission data provides standard information about the person, including the person's name, address, date of birth and age, Social Security number, gender, insurance and employment information, emergency notification information, and advance directive information.
- **Medical history**. Usually, the medical record contains a detailed medical history from the person's doctor. The medical history contains information about the person's previous surgeries and medical conditions, current medications, allergies, and current medical diagnosis.
- **Nursing history**. The nursing history is completed by the nurse at the time of the person's admission to the facility. The nursing history provides information related to the person's care needs, such as information about physical disabilities or limitations, bowel and bladder habits, dietary preferences, and use of assistive devices.
- **Physician's orders**. The physician's orders are used by the doctor to communicate to the other members of the health care team what should be done for the patient or resident. For example, the doctor will use the physician's orders to order treatments (such as medications), specify dietary orders or activity status, or order diagnostic tests.
- **Medication administration record (MAR)**. The medications ordered for the patient or resident are listed here, along with the dosage and the time at which they are to be administered. This form is also used to record when medications are given and by whom. The electronic version of the MAR, sometimes referred to as the eMAR, is used by the person administering the medication at the person's bedside. The recorded information is then immediately saved to the person's electronic health record. Some long-term care and assisted-living facilities provide additional training to allow nursing assistants to give medications. If giving medications is within your scope of practice, then you will record your activities on the MAR.

- **Physician's progress notes**. The doctor uses this form to record their notes and observations about the person's progress and response to treatment.
- **Narrative nurse's notes or nursing progress notes**. The nurse uses this form to document the person's complaints (symptoms) and the actions taken by the nursing staff in response to them. Some facilities allow nursing assistants to make notations in the narrative nurse's notes and some do not.
- **Graphic notes**. This is where information that is gathered routinely—such as vital signs, the frequency of urination and bowel movements, and food and fluid intake—is documented. Some long-term care facilities use a type of graphic notes to record a resident's activities of daily living (ADLs) and exercise therapy. The graphic notes is the form used by nursing assistants most often to document the care that they provide.
- **Miscellaneous documents**. Laboratory reports, radiology reports, and reports related to other diagnostic tests or therapeutic treatments are usually included in specific sections of the person's medical record.

The information recorded on these various forms allows the members of the health care team to communicate with each other efficiently.

Each facility or agency has specific policies about whether or not a nursing assistant is allowed to record information in the medical record. In some agencies or facilities, you may be able to record information on the graphic sheet, but not on the narrative nurse's notes. In others, you will be required to make entries in the narrative nurse's notes as documentation of the care you provide and the observations you make. Whenever you enter information on a person's medical record, date and time your entry correctly. Entries that are made into an electronic record will record the date and time automatically. Most medical facilities and agencies use the 24-hour time clock, also called "military time," for recording the time in a patient's medical record (Fig. 5-15). Guidelines for recording are given in Guidelines Box 5-1.

The way information is organized and entered into a medical record, and the policies dictating who is permitted to enter information into the record, differ from facility to facility. However, two policies regarding the handling of medical records are always the same, no matter where you work:

- The information contained in a person's medical record is considered confidential and is only to be read by members of the health care team who are directly involved in the care of that person and need access to the information in the record to provide that care. For example, you may

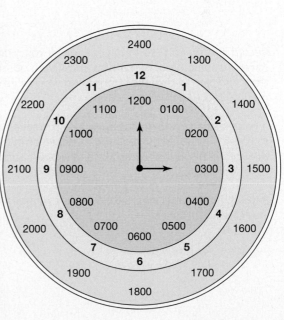

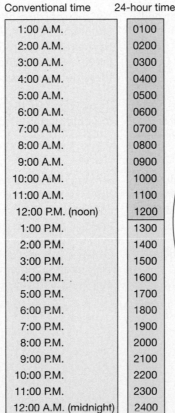

Figure 5-15 Most medical facilities and agencies use the 24-hour time clock, also referred to as "military time," for recording the time in a patient's medical record. The 24-hour time clock eliminates the need to differentiate between morning (AM) and night (PM), thus reducing errors in recording. On the 24-hour time clock, the morning hours are the same as on the conventional clock. To indicate a time in the afternoon, add "12" to the time on the conventional clock. When time is stated according to the 24-hour time clock, the first two numbers indicate the hour and the last two numbers indicate the minute (for example, 8:24 PM conventional time = 20:24 military time). Conventional time = *gray;* morning hours = *orange;* afternoon hours = *blue.*

Conventional time	24-hour time
1:00 A.M.	0100
2:00 A.M.	0200
3:00 A.M.	0300
4:00 A.M.	0400
5:00 A.M.	0500
6:00 A.M.	0600
7:00 A.M.	0700
8:00 A.M.	0800
9:00 A.M.	0900
10:00 A.M.	1000
11:00 A.M.	1100
12:00 P.M. (noon)	1200
1:00 P.M.	1300
2:00 P.M.	1400
3:00 P.M.	1500
4:00 P.M.	1600
5:00 P.M.	1700
6:00 P.M.	1800
7:00 P.M.	1900
8:00 P.M.	2000
9:00 P.M.	2100
10:00 P.M.	2200
11:00 P.M.	2300
12:00 A.M. (midnight)	2400

Guidelines Box 5-1   Guidelines for Recording

WHAT YOU DO	WHY YOU DO IT
Write legibly, using blue or black ink. Your facility may have specific policies regarding the color of ink used.	It is important to write legibly to avoid miscommunication. A pen is used instead of a pencil because pencil can be erased, enabling someone to change the person's medical record. Blue and black ink reproduce best when a document is scanned or photocopied.
Always sign or initial your entry, according to facility policy.	By signing or initialing your entry, you indicate that you are the person who needs to be consulted if further clarification of the information you have entered is necessary. In addition, signing or initialing your entry indicates that you accept legal responsibility for what you have written.
Only record observations that you have made, or care that you have given. Do not make entries for another person.	By making an entry in a medical record, you accept legal responsibility for that entry. Therefore, it is best to record only information that you, personally, can vouch for.
Date and time your entries correctly.	The date and time that actions occurred or observations were made are extremely important elements of the medical record, which is a legal account of care provided.
Check the patient's or resident's name on the medical record and on the form where you are recording.	By verifying the patient's or resident's identification information, you will ensure that you are recording the person's information in the correct medical record.
Use appropriate medical terminology and facility-approved abbreviations when recording.	Using correct terminology and abbreviations will prevent others from having to second-guess your meaning.
Do not record care as given or procedures as performed before you have provided the care or performed the procedure. Only document after the fact.	You may become distracted or involved in another situation that prevents you from carrying out the duties you have already charted. If you record duties as "completed" in the medical record, but then do not actually complete these duties, you will have committed fraud.
Record information in a timely manner. If you must wait to record something, keep notes about your observations and care so that the information you record in the medical record will be accurate.	If you wait until the end of your shift to record, you may forget important information.
If you make an error, do not erase, use correction fluid to cover, or scribble through the mistaken entry. Simply draw a line through the mistake and initial it according to facility policy.	Striking through an error is the only legal way to indicate a change in the medical record. Erasing or using correction fluid to correct an error could be seen as an attempt to hide or change existing information.
Remember that in a legal situation, care not recorded was care not provided.	Proper and conscientious recording of patient or resident information protects the patient or resident, your employer, and you.

notice that a friend or neighbor has been admitted to a different unit at the facility you work at. Unless you are assigned to provide direct care to that person, you may not access their medical record. To do so would violate Federal HIPAA privacy regulations.

- To keep patients and residents safe, each form in the written medical record must be stamped or printed with the patient's or resident's identification information. Accidentally placing a physician's order sheet meant for one person in another person's medical record could cause someone to receive a treatment or medication in error. A miscommunication of this nature could have serious, possibly even fatal, consequences.

Most health care settings manage patient and resident records electronically. An **electronic health record (EHR)** is a computer information system that stores and saves a person's medical information. In contrast to paper recordkeeping, the EHR maintains a person's medical record by having users enter data into a computer in response to the computer's prompts. Medical records created in this way tend to be more accurate and legible because they are typed rather than handwritten. The advantages to using EHR systems are:

- The patient's or resident's health record is easily and quickly accessible to the health care team members involved in the person's care. The doctor can review the person's latest lab results at the nurse's station while the physical therapy team can record notes about the person's progress in that department all at the same time.
- The patient's or resident's admission information, such as address or next of kin, can be updated quickly and the changes are immediately accessible to all of the people involved in that person's care.
- Information such as a person's vital signs and intake and output can be recorded at the person's bedside using portable tablets or bedside computer terminals. Many systems allow the health care team to record progress or nursing notes at the person's bedside insuring that care measures are documented immediately (Fig. 5-16).
- Doctor's orders for dietary changes, medications, lab requests, and treatments are immediately sent to the appropriate departments.

Some facilities may still use a combination of paper recording and computerized recording. For example, you may record all of your patients' or residents' vital signs and other daily care information on a paper flow sheet that is kept at the bedside or at a central location. The information may then be entered into the person's EHR at the end of the day.

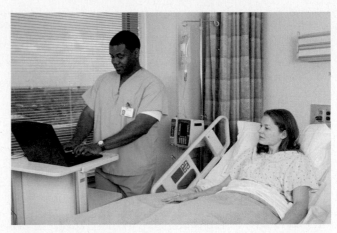

Figure 5-16 Computerized bedside charting is useful for documenting patient or resident information immediately. (Used with permission from Taylor, C., Lillis, C., & Lynn, P. [2014]. *Fundamentals of nursing: The art and science of nursing care* [8th ed., p. 351]. Lippincott Williams & Wilkins.)

Using an EHR information system to maintain and access a patient's or resident's medical record does not require advanced computer training. If your facility or agency uses computerized charting, your employer will provide training as part of your new employee orientation. During this training, you will learn how to enter data about your patients or residents as well as how to quickly retrieve information that you need about a patient or resident in order to provide their care.

Small, handheld computers, known as *tablets, personal digital assistants,* or *PDAs,* are used in many health care facilities. The PDAs can make recording information about a patient or resident more accurate and efficient. For example, the nursing assistant carries the PDA into a person's room and, as soon as the information is obtained, enters information such as vital signs, intake and output, or care assistance. The entered information is then sent electronically to the main computer system and is available for immediate access by other members of the health care team.

Although computerized charting offers many advantages over paper charting, patient and resident confidentiality is still a primary concern when patient data is stored electronically. To promote patient or resident confidentiality, each user is assigned a password, which permits them access to certain patients' or residents' medical records. Never give anyone else your password or leave the computer active after you use it. If you fail to log off after using the computer, the information on the screen may be visible or accessible to people who are not authorized to have it. In addition, if you fail to log off when you are finished with the computer, someone else could enter information under your password, and it will appear that you have entered it. Computer monitors should be positioned

ADVANCED DIRECTIVES

- _X_ Living will
- ___ Do not resuscitate
- ___ Do not hospitalize
- _X_ Organ donation
- ___

- ___ Autopsy request
- ___ Feeding restrictions
- ___ Medication restrictions
- ___ Other treatment restrictions
- ___ NONE OF THE ABOVE

Allergies: **Sulfa** _____

(Write in red or highlight)

Nutritional/Oral

Diet _Regular_ _____

Supplements: _n/a_ _____

Meal Location: Breakfast _Dining room_

Lunch _Dining room_

Dinner _Dining room_

- ___ Swallowing Difficulty   ___ Thicken Liquids
- ___ Tube Feeding   ___ NPO
- ___ I-O   ___ Fluid Restriction
- ___ TPN

Elimination   QOL program(s) ___ _n/a_ ___

Bladder:
- _X_ Continent   ___ Incontinent   ___ Catheter

Bowel:
- _X_ Continent   ___ Incontinent   ___ Ostomy

Cognition
- ___ Short term memory problem
- ___ Decision-making difficulty
- ___ Difficulty expressing self

Oriented to:
- _X_ Person   _X_ Place
- _X_ Time   _X_ Situation

Behavior   QOL program _n/a_
- ___ Verbally Abusive
- ___ Physically Abusive
- ___ Socially Inappropriate
- ___ Resistant to Care
- ___ Wandering/Exit Seeking   QOL program _n/a_

Communication

Primary Language:
- _X_ English   ___ Other: _____
- *Alternative methods used:*
- ___ Communication board   ___ Writing
- ___ Sign language   ___ Gestures
- ___ Other _____

Appliances
- ___ Hearing Aide   ___ R   ___ L
- _X_ Glasses   ___ Contacts
- _X_ Dentures ___ Upper ___ Lower _X_ Partial
- ___ Anti-embolism hose
- _X_ Prosthesis/Splint/Brace (description) _Cast-Rt_ _Forearm_

Respiratory
- ___ Pulse Oximetry
- ___ Tracheostomy   ___ Oxygen
- ___ Ventilator   ___ Suctioning
- Skin Management   QOL program _____
- ___ Turn & Position   ___ Other _____
- ___ Mattress

Additional Quality of Life Program(s) or Medical Specialty Treatment Program(s)

Physical Therapy rt arm

ADL's	Self-Performance	Support (# of Persons)
Bathing	I S (L) E T	(1) 2
Dressing	I S (L) E T	(1) 2
Toileting	(I) S L E T	1 2
Eating	I S (L) E T	(1) 2
Transferring	(I) S L E T	1 2
Walking	I S (L) E T	(1) 2

I - Independent   E - Extensive
S - Supervised   T - Total
L - Limited

Mobility: Weight bearing status _Good_
- ___ Mechanical lift   ___ W/chair
- ___ ROM   ___ Walker
- _X_ AROM   _X_ Cane
- ___ PROM   ___ Other: _____
- ___ Bedfast/chairbound

Weight schedule _X_ mo ___ why ___ other
QOL program _____
Restraint: Type: _____ When: _____
QOL Program _____

Resident Preferences:	Bathing type:	Bathing Day/time:
	___ Shower	M (T) W (Th)
Name: _Miss (Ethel)_	_X_ Tub	F (Sa) Su
Time to arise _7 am_	___ Other:	
Time to rest: _1 pm_		
Time to retire _10 pm_		AM (PM)
Likes/dislikes: ___		

Special Precautions:
Please assist at mealtime by opening milk and cutting food into small pieces

Diagnoses:
Primary: _____
Secondary: _FX Rt radius & ulna_

RESIDENT NAME	ADMISSION DATE	PHYSICIAN	DOB	AGE	Medical Record Number
Ethel Hayes	12/01/22	_Sanders_	03/06/1945	77	1301

Figure 5-17 The Kardex summarizes the most up-to-date information about a patient's or resident's condition and care needs.

so that the screen is not visible to the public when you are working. Your facility or agency will have specific policies (mandated by HIPAA) regarding computer use and confidentiality. Make sure you are familiar with these policies and follow them carefully.

Kardex

The **Kardex** is a card file containing condensed versions of each patient's or resident's medical record. The Kardex may be available to you in paper (hard copy) form or electronically, on the computer or tablet. The Kardex contains a summary of the person's current diagnosis, the diagnostic tests and treatments ordered by the doctor, and information about routine care measures, such as the person's diet, level of assistance, and bathing schedule (Fig. 5-17). The Kardex is updated as the person's condition or doctor's orders change. By providing a one-page summary of the patient's or resident's medical record, the Kardex keeps health care team members from having to search through the entire record every time they need information about the person's status and care plan.

The Nursing Process

There are many members of the health care team who provide care for people in a health care setting. A person's doctor is primarily responsible for diagnosing that person's medical problems, ordering medications and other therapies, and directing that person's medical care, but the actual coordination, planning, and implementation of that care require the efforts of other members of the health care team. Those members involved with the patient's or the resident's care may include nurses, nursing assistants, dietitians, social workers, and physical therapists. The patient or the resident and their family members also play an important role in this process, especially in the long-term care setting. All health care team members meet with the patient or the resident and family members to develop a specific, individualized plan of care called an

interdisciplinary care plan. This plan then directs the efforts of the health care team members who are responsible for carrying out the doctor's orders and providing holistic care to the patient or the resident.

As a part of the interdisciplinary care plan, the nursing team will then develop a specific plan of care for each patient or resident called the **nursing care plan**. The communication method that is used to develop the nursing care plan is called the **nursing process**. The nursing process allows members of the nursing team to communicate with each other regarding the patient's or resident's specific needs (in regard to nursing care), what steps will be taken to meet those needs, and whether or not the steps were effective in meeting the person's needs. The nursing care plan makes sure that all members of the nursing team are "on the same page." The nurse acting as the nursing team leader is responsible for developing the nursing care plan. They accomplish this with the help of other health care team members, including the patient or resident, the nursing assistant, and members of specific departments, such as dietitians, social workers, and physical therapists.

The nursing process is organized into a series of steps:

1. **Assessment**. During this step, information specific to the patient or resident is gathered. Sources of this information are the person's medical history, the nursing history, family members, and most importantly, the person themselves. As part of the assessment process, the nurse examines the patient or resident and asks questions about their abilities, level of discomfort, eating and toileting habits, and specific needs.

2. **Diagnosis**. Using the information gathered during the assessment step, the nurse then develops a **nursing diagnosis**, or a statement that describes a problem the person is having, as well as the cause of the problem. Unlike a medical diagnosis, which states a medical problem that must be identified and managed by a doctor, a nursing diagnosis states a problem that the nursing staff can identify and treat independently. For example, consider a person who has a broken arm. The medical diagnosis for this person might be "fractured radius and ulna." The nursing diagnosis might be "impaired nutritional status due to inability to feed self because of dominant hand being in a cast."

3. **Planning**. The next step in the nursing process involves making a plan for the person's care. Using information obtained from the nursing diagnosis, the nurse develops **interventions** (actions that will be taken to help the person) and **goals** (descriptions of what the interventions are meant to achieve). For example, in order to achieve the goal of improved nutritional status for the person with the cast on their arm, the intervention may be to cut the person's food into bite-sized pieces to make it easier for them to eat. The interventions and goals that have been set for the patient or resident are written down in a formal way. This document (the nursing care plan) becomes part of the patient's or resident's medical record and may be included on the Kardex.

4. **Implementation**. During the implementation step, the interventions detailed in the nursing care plan are carried out. (The nursing care plan specifies the team members who are responsible for doing each intervention.)

5. **Evaluation**. During the evaluation step, the nursing team checks the effectiveness of the nursing care plan and revises it as necessary. Is the care plan working? Are the goals being met? What needs to be improved or changed to meet the goals? Has the patient's or resident's status changed? Is the existing nursing care plan still appropriate for the patient or resident? If certain interventions are not working, or if the goals have been met, the nursing care plan will change.

The nursing process is ongoing. The nursing staff continually assesses the patient or resident and adjusts the nursing care plan as the person's needs change. As a nursing assistant, you will participate in the nursing process by carrying out interventions and communicating observations to the nurse. When you communicate observations to the nurse, you help them with the assessment and evaluation steps of the nursing process. Your observations and communications to the nurse and other health care team members will ensure that the patient or resident remains the focus of quality, compassionate care that is carefully planned, implemented, and evaluated.

SUMMARY

- Communication is the exchange of information.
  - For good communication to occur, a sender must send a clear message directly to a receiver who can understand the message. The receiver must provide feedback that lets the sender know that the message was heard and understood.
  - Effective communication among health care team members is essential to ensure that patients or residents receive top-quality, safe care. Nursing assistants must have good communication skills because the exchange of information with patients, residents, and coworkers is central to their job.
  - Nursing assistants are an important link between the patient or resident and others on the health care team. They are often the first to observe a change in a patient's or resident's condition that could signal something serious.
- There are many ways to improve communication.
  - Listening is one of the most important skills, especially in the health care field.
  - Speaking clearly, asking open-ended questions, and using appropriate body language are other ways to improve communication.

- Reporting and recording are two methods of communication used by the health care team to make sure that everyone involved in the care of a patient or resident has current, reliable information about that person. Observations about a patient's or resident's condition are reported and/or recorded. Observations may be subjective or objective.
  - Reporting is the spoken exchange of information between members of the health care team. Observations about a change in a patient's or resident's condition must be reported to the nurse immediately.
  - Recording is the written exchange of information between members of the health care team. Recording is done in the person's medical record or chart.
- The nursing process is a communication method that allows members of the nursing team to meet a patient's or resident's specific care needs. The nursing assistant plays a role in the nursing process by carrying out interventions and communicating observations to the nurse.

WHAT DID YOU LEARN?

Multiple Choice

Select the single best answer for each of the following questions.

1. Which one of the following is an open-ended question?
   a. "Are you Mrs. Garcia?"
   b. "Mr. Kim, when you were growing up, what was your favorite meal?"
   c. "Are you feeling okay, Mrs. Smith?"
   d. "It's beautiful outside today, Mrs. Devi! Do you want to go for a walk?"

2. Which one of the following is an example of positive body language?
   a. Nodding encouragingly as someone speaks
   b. Crossing your arms across your chest
   c. Tapping your feet or fingers
   d. Rolling your eyes

3. An example of an action that blocks effective communication is:
   a. Interrupting
   b. Not listening carefully
   c. Being judgmental
   d. All of the above

4. Which one of the following is an objective observation?
   a. "Mr. Wohl says that his back hurts when he coughs."
   b. "Ms. O'Connell's urine is cloudy and has a strong odor."
   c. "Mr. McAndrews is complaining of a headache."
   d. "The resident in room 201B is complaining of a stomachache."

5. Which one of the following is an example of nonverbal communication?
   a. Using sign language to communicate
   b. Recording vital sign measurements in a patient's or resident's chart
   c. Gently touching a patient or resident on the shoulder to reassure them
   d. Making a telephone call

6. What usually forms the basis for a subjective observation?
   a. A symptom, or patient complaint
   b. A measurement
   c. A doctor's order
   d. All of the above

7. Which step of the nursing process involves the initial gathering of information about a patient or resident?
   a. Implementation
   b. Assessment
   c. Planning
   d. Evaluation

8. With regard to telephone communication, nursing assistants are responsible for all of the following except:
   a. Writing down the caller's name and telephone number if the person the caller wants to speak to is not available, and delivering this message to the intended recipient
   b. Answering the telephone promptly, with a pleasant greeting
   c. Taking down doctor's orders if the nurse is not available and a doctor calls
   d. Identifying themselves to the caller by name and title, per facility policy

9. When recording information in a person's medical chart, what should you remember to do?
   a. Use a pencil so that errors can be corrected neatly
   b. Sign or initial and date and time your entry, per facility policy
   c. Update all of your patients' or residents' charts at one time at the end of each shift
   d. All of the above

10. What is it called when people have differences and they are unable to come to an agreement?
   a. Communication
   b. Conflict
   c. Culture
   d. Personality difference

Matching *Match each numbered item with its appropriate lettered description.*

_____ **1.** Admission data

_____ **2.** Narrative nurse's notes

_____ **3.** Medical history

_____ **4.** Physician's orders

_____ **5.** Graphic notes

a. Used to record patient complaints and the actions that were taken by the nursing team to provide relief

b. Used to record routine data, such as vital signs, frequency of urination and bowel movements, and food and fluid intake

c. Used to order diagnostic tests and treatments and to specify dietary orders or activity status

d. Document that lists a patient's previous surgeries and medical conditions, current medications, allergies, and current medical diagnosis

e. Document that contains essential information about the patient, including their name and address, birth date, insurance information, advance directives information, and emergency contact information

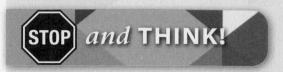

STOP *and* THINK!

- You are caring for Mr. Singh today and notice that he seems distracted and is having difficulty speaking clearly. You know that you should report this to the nurse immediately. What other subjective and objective data should you gather to report to the nurse? How can you make sure that the nurse receives the information from you?

- You work in the rehabilitation unit of a long-term care facility and have become quite comfortable with the electronic health record computer system that they have recently started using. You like that you can use the bedside computer terminals to record your resident's vital signs and other information on the nurse's progress notes. One of your coworkers has struggled with the new computerized charting system and keeps telling you that she would rather keep using the "old-fashioned" method of writing her notes in the person's records.

  Today, your coworker comes to you asking to use your username and password because they cannot remember theirs and they really needs to get their vital signs and care procedures recorded. What should you do?

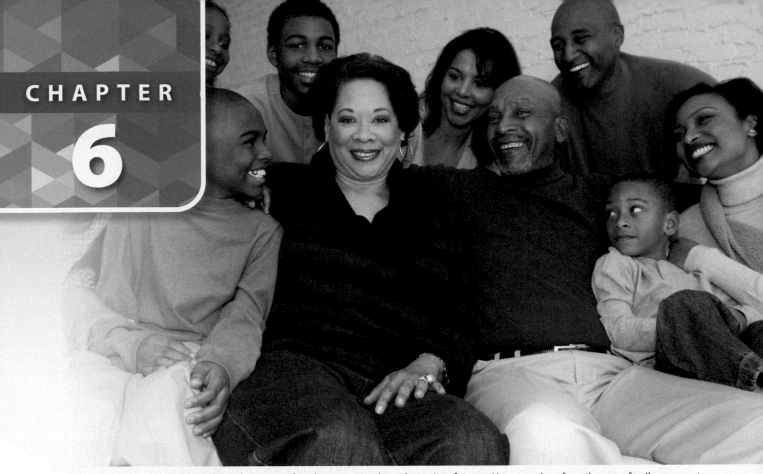

Photo: Throughout the course of our lives, we pass through a series of stages. Here, members from the same family represent the stages of school age, adolescence, young adulthood, and middle adulthood. (Blend Images\Shutterstock.com)

Those We Care For

 WHAT WILL YOU LEARN?

As we start on the final chapter in this introductory unit, you are probably beginning to realize that there is much more to being a nursing assistant than blood pressures and bedpans. A health care worker can go to the most well-known schools, receive the most intense training, and graduate at the top of their class, but if they are not able to connect on a human level with their patients or residents, they will fail. In this chapter, we will explore the qualities that we, as humans, share, as well as the ones that make us unique individuals. When you are finished with this chapter, you will be able to:

1. Discuss why people need health care intervention.
2. Differentiate between acute, chronic, and terminal conditions, and give an example of each.
3. Describe how the health care industry groups people together for the provision of care, and list the types of people you might have the opportunity to work with.
4. List and briefly describe the stages of human growth and development.
5. Illustrate each level of Maslow's hierarchy of basic human needs and ways that a nursing assistant helps patients and residents to meet them.
6. Explain the difference between sex and sexuality and discuss how a person's sexuality can be affected by illness.

7. Explain the concept of diversity, and why it is important for health care workers to recognize their patients' and residents' diversity.

8. Explain the concept of quality of life, and describe ways that nursing assistants help to support a patient's or resident's quality of life.

9. Discuss how family members may be affected by a person's illness or disability.

Vocabulary

Acute illness	Puberty	Sex	Masturbation
Chronic illness	Menarche	Heterosexual	Culture
Terminal illness	Nocturnal emissions	Gay	Race
Growth	Menopause	Lesbian	Religion
Development	Need	Bisexual	
Tasks	Sexuality	Transgender	
Neonate	Intimacy	Coitus	

PATIENTS, RESIDENTS, AND CLIENTS

If someone asked you "As a nursing assistant, who do you care for?", depending on where you work, you might answer "I care for patients," or "I care for residents," or "I care for clients." (As you will recall from Chapter 1, a patient is a person who is receiving health care in a hospital, clinic, or extended-care facility; a resident is a person who is living in a long-term care facility or an assisted-living facility; and a client is a person who is receiving care in their own home, from a home health care agency.) These are all terms for people who need the services that the health care industry offers because they are sick, injured, or unable to care for themselves. At the most basic level, patients, residents, and clients are "those we care for."

There are three general types of illnesses or conditions that can cause a person to need health care services. An **acute illness** is a condition characterized by a rapid onset and a relatively short recovery time. Because the onset is rapid, acute illnesses are usually unexpected. Conditions such as pneumonia, appendicitis, a broken bone, or labor and delivery would be considered acute conditions. In contrast, a **chronic illness** is a condition that is ongoing. A person with a chronic illness generally needs continuous medication or treatment to control the condition. Occasionally, acute flare-ups of the chronic condition lead to hospitalization. Examples of chronic illnesses include diabetes, asthma, arthritis, and high blood pressure (hypertension). Finally, a **terminal illness** is an illness or condition from which recovery is not

expected. People who have a terminal illness will die as a result of their illness, usually within a short period of time. Examples of terminal illnesses include some types of cancer, end-stage emphysema, and some heart conditions.

To make the provision of care more efficient, the health care industry groups people according to their ages, illnesses or medical conditions, or special health care needs (Fig. 6-1). In some cases, specialized training is needed to care for a certain type of patient, so it would make sense to group all of the patients requiring that type of specialized care together. Examples of terms that are often used to describe people, based on the person's age, illness, or special health care needs, include the following:

- **Surgical patients** have illnesses or conditions that are treated by surgery, such as appendicitis or certain types of tumors. Surgical patients are admitted to the hospital for surgery and the recovery period afterward. Many surgical procedures are performed on an outpatient basis, which means that the patient is admitted to the hospital for surgery, but then sent home to recover. The care of surgical patients is discussed in Chapter 43.
- **Medical patients** have an illness or condition that is treated with interventions other than surgery, such as medication, physical therapy, or radiation. Examples of medical conditions include pneumonia, myocardial infarction ("heart attack"), stroke, and some intestinal disorders (such as diverticulitis).

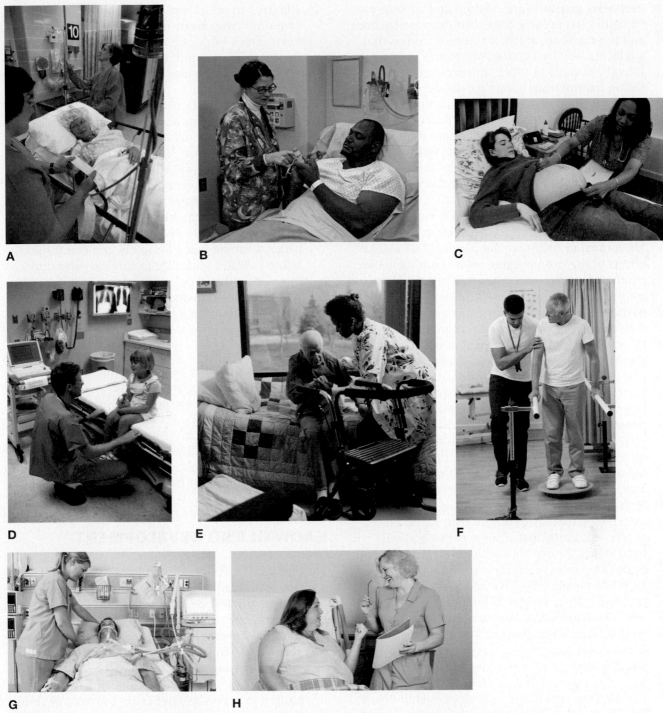

Figure 6-1 Examples of the many ways in which people are grouped by the health care industry. **A.** Surgical patient. **B.** Medical patient. **C.** Obstetrical patient. **D.** Pediatric patient. **E.** Geriatric patient. **F.** Rehabilitation patient. **G.** Intensive care patient. **H.** Bariatric patient. (F, *Monkey Business Images\ Shutterstock.com* G. *Tyler Olson\Shutterstock.com*)

■ **Obstetrical patients** are those who are pregnant or have just given birth. Obstetrical care extends throughout the pregnancy and labor and delivery, and then continues for about 8 weeks after delivery. Although most obstetrical patients are admitted to the hospital for the actual labor

and delivery, and remain hospitalized for a brief time afterward, most of the care before and after the delivery is provided on an outpatient basis (unless the patient or baby experiences complications). The care of obstetrical patients is discussed in Chapter 44.

- **Pediatric patients** are children and adolescents. Pediatrics has become a specialty because children and teenagers are at risk for some disorders that adults are not. In addition, sometimes special considerations must be taken into account when providing treatments and care for younger patients because a child's body does not function in exactly the same way as an adult's does. Sometimes, an entire facility is dedicated to the care of the pediatric patient. Other times, a special unit within the hospital or long-term care facility is designated as the pediatrics unit. The care of pediatric patients is discussed in Chapter 45.
- **Geriatric patients** are older adult patients. Health care workers who specialize in geriatrics are trained to recognize the physical and mental effects of the normal aging process and help older people adjust to these changes. They are also trained to care for people with diseases that are particularly common among this age group. The care of geriatric patients is discussed in Chapter 8.
- **Psychiatric patients** are people with impaired mental health and have been diagnosed with a psychiatric disorder. Psychiatric patients are often treated on an outpatient basis, using a combination of counseling and medication. However, people who have been diagnosed with a psychiatric disorder and are a danger to themselves or others may be admitted to a health care facility for treatment. The care of people with a psychiatric disorder is discussed in Chapter 41.
- **Rehabilitation patients** are those who are undergoing therapy to restore their highest level of physical, emotional or mental, or vocational functioning. People born with physical disabilities or deformities may require physical rehabilitation. So might people who have had a stroke or are recovering from surgery or an injury. Emotional or mental rehabilitation may be necessary for people with substance use disorder. Vocational rehabilitation focuses on providing the person with special training after an injury or surgery so that they can return to a particular type of work. Rehabilitation facilities or units provide services both on an inpatient and outpatient basis. Rehabilitation and restorative care is discussed in Chapter 39.
- **Subacute or extended-care patients** are usually recovering from an acute illness or condition. They do not need the total care provided by a hospital, but are not quite ready to return home. They may continue to have a need for intravenously administered medications, physical therapy, or other treatments that cannot be provided by untrained caretakers.
- **Intensive care patients**. Patients needing very specialized, or intensive, care are usually admitted to an intensive care unit or a special care unit. After heart or brain surgery, or after a heart attack or stroke, a patient will stay in the special care unit until their condition improves. They will then be moved to a regular hospital unit.
- **Bariatric patients**. *Bariatrics* is a branch of medicine that treats and manages obesity. Class I obesity is defined as having a Body Mass Index (BMI) ranging from 30 to 35; Class II obesity is defined as having a BMI ranging from 35 to 40; and Class III obesity is defined as having a BMI of 40 or higher. Many health care facilities have specialized units containing larger-sized beds, chairs, toilets, and stretchers so that bariatric patients can be cared for safely and comfortably. Many facilities specialize in surgical procedures that are used to treat patients and help them lose weight. A person with a BMI of 30 or higher may also be a patient in a facility for other medical or surgical reasons, either related or not related to obesity.

As you can see, the people we care for can be classified in many different ways. However, those in need of health care services are not merely defined by their illnesses and disabilities. First and foremost, patients, residents, and clients are human beings. In the rest of this chapter, we will take a closer look at some of the things that all people have in common, as well as some of the things that make us different.

GROWTH AND DEVELOPMENT

Throughout the course of our lives, we pass through a series of stages. We are constantly changing, from conception until the time of death. Changes that occur physically are known as **growth**. Changes that occur psychologically or socially are known as **development**. Growth is demonstrated by changes in height and weight and by physical maturation of the body's organ systems. Development is evidenced by changes in a person's behavior and way of thinking. Both growth and development generally occur in an orderly fashion and progress from the simple to the complex. Physically, a baby must develop the muscle strength and coordination that will enable them to sit, then stand, and finally to walk. Developmentally, that baby will smile at their parents, then coo, say their first word, and soon speak in complete sentences.

The process of growth and development is divided into stages of normal progression (Fig. 6-2). Although all people progress through the stages of growth and development in a series of expected steps, they do not progress through the stages at the same rate. For

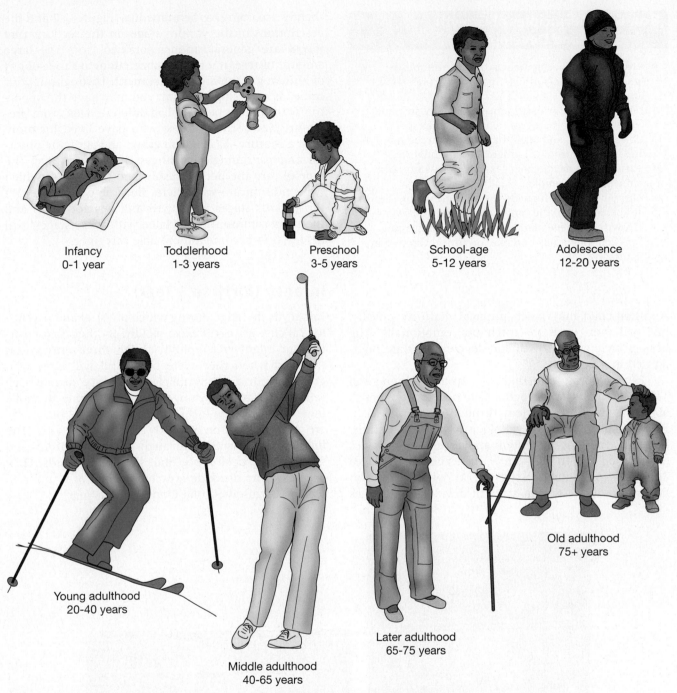

Infancy
0-1 year

Toddlerhood
1-3 years

Preschool
3-5 years

School-age
5-12 years

Adolescence
12-20 years

Young adulthood
20-40 years

Middle adulthood
40-65 years

Later adulthood
65-75 years

Old adulthood
75+ years

Figure 6-2 Everyone passes through the same stages of growth and development.

example, one child may walk at 8 months and speak their first word at 10 months. That child's sibling, on the other hand, may talk relatively early at 7 months, but not walk until the age of 14 months. Although the stages of growth and development can be generalized by age, it is important to note that each person, like the siblings described here, progresses through the stages at their own pace. A person cannot progress to the next stage without successfully completing the **tasks**, or growth and development milestones,

associated with the stage they are currently in. With young children and teenagers, it is quite common to see some overlap in the stages. This is because growth and development occur unevenly, or in spurts, with one part occurring faster than the other. A 5-year-old may have matured quickly emotionally and prefer the company of older children, but lack certain motor skills that would allow them to ride a bike or play baseball. This can be quite frustrating for the child until they have physically grown enough to keep up.

Box 6-1	Principles of Growth and Development

- Growth and development occurs continuously throughout a person's life span, from conception until death.
- Growth and development occurs step by step and in an orderly progression. Each stage has specific characteristics and tasks that must be accomplished before the person can progress to the next stage.
- Growth and development tasks progress from the simple to the complex.
- Growth and development tasks progress from head to toe, and from the center of the body outward.
- Growth and development occurs at variable rates for each individual, and may occur unevenly or in spurts.

Another child may reach physical maturity quickly, but will then need to "catch up" emotionally. The basic principles of growth and development are highlighted in Box 6-1.

Psychologists are people who study the mind and behavior. Many psychologists have developed theories about human development throughout the lifespan. Depending on which psychologist's work you study, you may find that the growth and development stages are defined slightly differently, in terms of age ranges and tasks. In addition, the age at which a person begins or ends a certain stage of development varies slightly according to the individual. Figure 6-2 and the descriptions of the various stages in the sections that follow are generalizations, obtained from the large amount of research that has been done on the subject of human growth and development. Throughout your career as a nursing assistant, you may have the opportunity to care for people of all different ages, from premature newborns to those who have lived for more than a century. As a person grows and ages, the physical and psychological changes that occur affect the type of care the person needs, and the way in which we communicate with them. Becoming familiar with the various stages of growth and development, and the tasks commonly associated with these stages, will help you to become a more able caregiver.

Infancy (Birth to 1 Year)

Infancy is the stage during which physical and psychological changes occur most rapidly. By their first birthday, an infant will typically weigh three times what they did when they were born, and will have progressed from a totally helpless **neonate** (a newborn infant, 28 days or younger) to a child able to move independently (Fig. 6-3). During this stage, new tasks are accomplished on a weekly and monthly basis. The infant begins to smile and laugh, recognize parents and siblings, play peek-a-boo, and say simple words. They progress from drinking only breast milk or formula to feeding themselves solid foods. What a year!

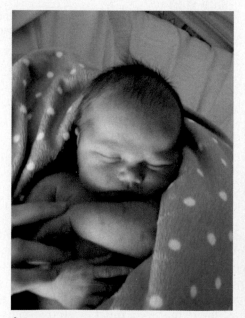
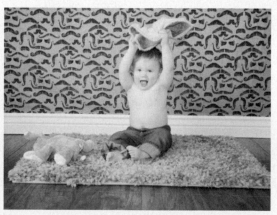

A　　　　　　　　　　　**B**

Figure 6-3 During the infancy stage, growth and development tasks are accomplished in leaps and bounds. Within the space of a year, an infant goes from being totally helpless (**A**) to being able to move around independently (**B**).

Toddlerhood (1 to 3 Years)

Physical growth slows down during toddlerhood, but development of the muscular and nervous systems allows the toddler to become quite active. The toddler can walk, run, climb, jump, and peddle a tricycle easily (Fig. 6-4). Suddenly, parents and caretakers must work hard to remove unsafe objects and curb the natural curiosity of the toddler! In addition to permitting increased mobility, development of the muscular and nervous systems permits greater control of the bladder and bowels, so this is when toilet training begins.

Developmentally, the toddler learns the words to express emotions, such as "sad" or "scared," and is able to express themselves in short, complete sentences. Toddlers become quite independent and sometimes have trouble following rules of behavior. The toddler's world revolves around the toddler! Toddlers will engage actively in play, but usually play alone or alongside another child without many interactions. Toddlers do not separate from a parent or familiar caregiver easily. Therefore, medical procedures that require separation of the child and the caregiver can be very frightening for a toddler.

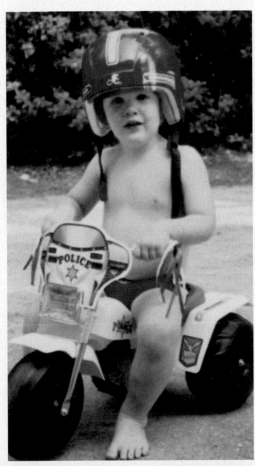

Figure 6-4 During the toddler stage, development of the nervous and muscular systems leads to increased mobility.

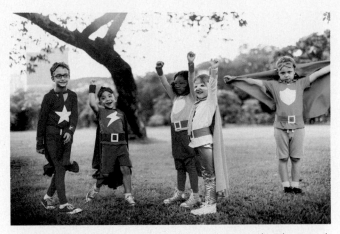

Figure 6-5 Preschoolers enjoy interacting with others and playing "make-believe." (*Rawpixel.com\Shutterstock.com*)

Preschool (3 to 5 Years)

The preschooler is an adventure waiting to happen! The preschooler's physical coordination improves a great deal, and they learn to dress themselves and tie their own shoes. Toileting becomes more independent. Preschoolers become involved in playing with other children and will use their active imaginations to create detailed play stories and scenes (Fig. 6-5). During this stage, children become aware of gender differences and roles and are very curious about the differences between boys and girls. They ask questions all the time and love to have stories told or read to them. As the preschooler begins to know the difference between right and wrong behavior, they begin to develop a conscience and are able to follow rules more easily.

School-Age (5 to 12 Years)

The school-aged child experiences several major physical growth spurts, which lead to increases in both height and weight. As their fine motor skills develop, the child's ability to write and draw improves. Play usually involves groups of same-sex friends, and a sense of gender identity begins to develop. Participation in team sports, scouting groups, and other physical activities are common at this age (Fig. 6-6). With school attendance comes an increased ability to follow society's rules. Children in this age group actively seek approval from authority figures and peers. They develop logical thinking patterns and learn to incorporate other people's perspectives into their own thinking. Morals develop, and school-aged children may feel very strongly about issues being either right or wrong, with no gray area. Spirituality and religious beliefs, as well as a concern for other living things, also take root during this developmental stage.

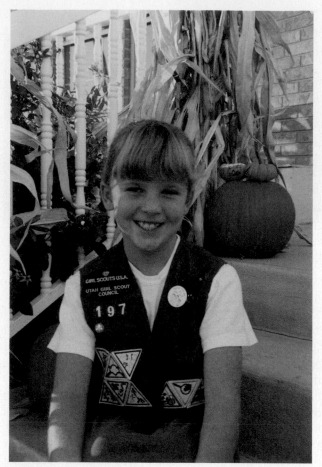

Figure 6-6 School-aged children like activities that allow them to interact with members of the same gender.

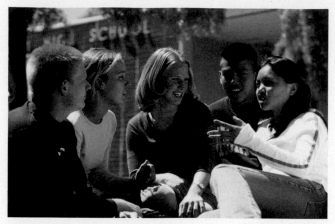

Figure 6-7 Adolescence can be a difficult yet exciting time.

Adolescence (12 to 20 Years)

The ages of children in this developmental stage vary considerably. Adolescence begins at the onset of **puberty**, when the secondary sex characteristics (such as enlarged breasts and facial hair) appear and the reproductive organs begin to function. In females, the onset of puberty usually occurs between the ages of 10 and 14 years, and in males, it usually occurs between the ages of 12 and 16 years.

Physical growth and development during adolescence is considerable. In females, the development of breasts and the growth of hair in the pubic and armpit (axillary) regions occur before the onset of menstruation, or **menarche**. Throughout adolescence, a female's breasts continue to develop and the hips broaden. In males, the genitals increase in size. Pubic, axillary, and facial hair develops, and the voice deepens. Ejaculation, or the release of semen, signals the onset of puberty; adolescent males often experience **nocturnal emissions** (commonly known as "wet dreams") while sleeping. A growth spurt occurs, and the adolescent male may gain more than a foot in height over the course of a few months. The

shoulders broaden and the muscles become more developed.

Psychologically, the period of adolescence is stormy. Adolescents may be self-conscious about their changing bodies and increased awareness of their own sexuality. They are torn between wanting to be treated as grown-ups and being afraid to make their own decisions. Adolescents experiment with new styles of dress and hair, and follow very closely with their friends (Fig. 6-7). They generally begin to date and to question the moral teachings of authority figures and parents. As a result, experimentation with alcohol, drugs, and sex may occur during this stage. As a reflection of their increasing emotional maturity, adolescents may take jobs, learn to drive, or begin to make plans for their future education or the beginning of a career.

Young Adulthood (20 to 40 Years)

After the turmoil of adolescence, young adulthood comes as a relief. Young adults typically enjoy stable, supportive friendships and good health. The primary developmental tasks of this stage include completing one's education, starting a career, and, possibly, finding a partner or spouse. The young adult learns to be successful on their own and possibly cohabitates with a partner or spouse. Many young adults choose to start families (Fig. 6-8). For many females, the most significant physical change that will occur during young adulthood is pregnancy. Otherwise, the physical changes that occur in young adults are generally minor.

Middle Adulthood (40 to 65 Years)

Middle adulthood frequently finds people at the height of their careers and productivity. Many middle adults find themselves in the role of caregiver for their children as well as to their aging parents. This is sometimes

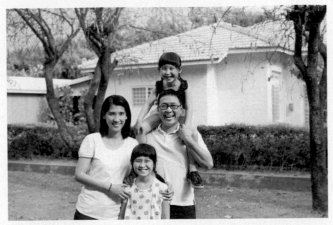

Figure 6-8 Many young adults choose to get married and begin families of their own. (*Tom Wang\Shutterstock.com*)

referred to as the "sandwich generation." As the children grow up and become less reliant, many middle adults find that they have more time to travel or participate in leisure activities (Fig. 6-9). During middle adulthood, many people become grandparents. Physically, the middle adult begins to show signs of aging, such as wrinkles or a few gray hairs. Females typically experience **menopause** (cessation of menstruation and fertility) in their early 50s. Although good health is usually still enjoyed, some chronic illnesses, such as hypertension and diabetes, become apparent during this stage.

Later Adulthood (65 to 75 Years)

During this stage, the physical signs of aging and the development of chronic illnesses become more prevalent. Strength diminishes, as do many senses, such as hearing and sight. Retirement may place the older

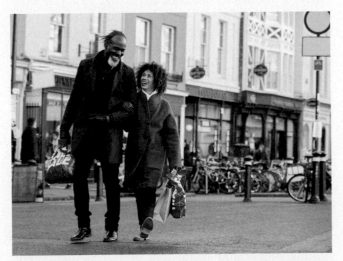

Figure 6-9 Many middle adults have raised their families and now have more time to reconnect as a couple and pursue their own interests and hobbies. (*Monkey Business Images\Shutterstock.com*)

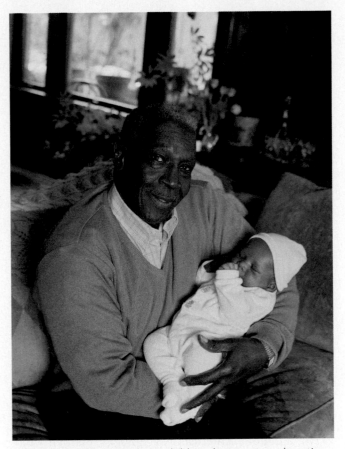

Figure 6-10 During late adulthood, many people retire from their careers and begin to enjoy the results of a lifetime of hard work, such as grandchildren and travel.

adult on a fixed income, but some are able to travel and pursue hobbies that they did not have time for when they were employed (Fig. 6-10). During this stage, many people must cope with the loss of friends or a partner or spouse due to death.

Older Adulthood (75 Years and Beyond)

During this stage, a primary task is preparing for one's own death. Although some older adults continue to be relatively healthy and independent, many must adjust to failing health and a growing dependency on others. Even if their health or physical abilities prevent them from being totally independent, many older adults continue to feel fulfilled and needed until death, and enjoy sharing the wisdom of their years with younger people (Fig. 6-11).

BASIC HUMAN NEEDS

Clearly, all patients and residents are not alike. The people you will care for will be in different growth

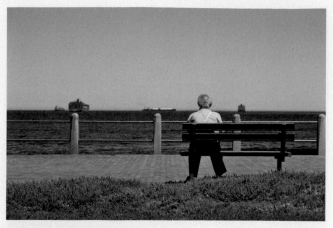

Figure 6-11 Many older adults feel that they have lived a good life. (*Alzbeta\Shutterstock.com*)

and development stages, and as such, they will have different needs. The primary mission of health care is to tend to the physical and emotional needs of those we care for. But what exactly are needs?

Maslow's Hierarchy of Human Needs

A **need** is something that is essential for a person's physical and mental health. Abraham Maslow (1908–1970), a famous American psychologist, defined what he thought to be the basic human needs, and then arranged them in a pyramid to show that certain needs are more basic than other needs (Fig. 6-12). Maslow's pyramid, called *Maslow's hierarchy of human needs,* reflects Maslow's belief that the more basic, lower-level needs must be met, at least to some degree, before the higher-level needs can be met. Many

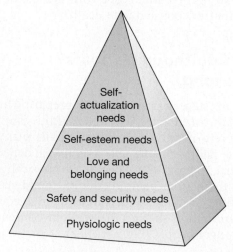

Figure 6-12 Maslow's hierarchy of human needs. A "hierarchy" shows the relationship of one idea to another. By arranging the basic human needs in a pyramid shape, Maslow created a visual representation of the idea that basic needs must be fulfilled before more complex ones.

people can meet their needs with little or no outside help. But people who have an illness, injury, or disability must rely on the help of the health care team to make sure that their needs are met.

Physiologic Needs

The most basic level in Maslow's hierarchy of needs is the physiologic (physical) needs, such as oxygen, water, food, shelter, elimination, rest and sleep, physical activity, and sexuality. Meeting the physiologic needs is essential for survival. Therefore, meeting these needs is of the highest priority. A person must have enough oxygen or they will die within minutes. Water and food are essential for life, as is the ability of the body to eliminate waste products, such as carbon dioxide, urine, and feces. Shelter protects a person from the elements and extremes in temperature. Rest and sleep are essential for preventing physical exhaustion, which can lead to disability and illness. Physical activity keeps the nervous, skeletal, and muscular systems functioning and prevents wasting. Sexuality involves both the individual's need to have a sexual identity, as well as the need to engage in sexual activity, which allows for a species to reproduce and avoid extinction. Nursing assistants perform many duties that assist patients in meeting their physiologic needs: Assisting with meals, toileting, ambulating, and providing a relaxing environment in which to sleep are just some of the many ways you will help people to meet their most basic needs (Fig. 6-13).

Safety and Security Needs

Safety and security needs are both physical and emotional. Not only must we *be* safe, we must also *feel* safe. For example, parents of young children take measures, such as covering electrical outlets, padding sharp surfaces, and keeping household cleaners and medications out of reach, to make sure that their children remain physically safe from harm. Nursing assistants follow policies and procedures that are designed to ensure their own safety, as well as that of their patients or residents. For example, to prevent the spread of infection, a nursing assistant follows the procedure for hand hygiene. To protect a resident who is at risk for falling, the nursing assistant always makes sure that the resident has their walker close at hand. In Units 3 and 4, you will learn about the many ways in which nursing assistants work to ensure their own safety, as well as that of the people they care for.

The emotional part of safety and security involves trusting others and being free of fear of harm. For example, parents and guardians help children feel safe and secure by tucking them into bed at night, establishing routines, and letting them know that they will always "be there." A nursing assistant can help a patient

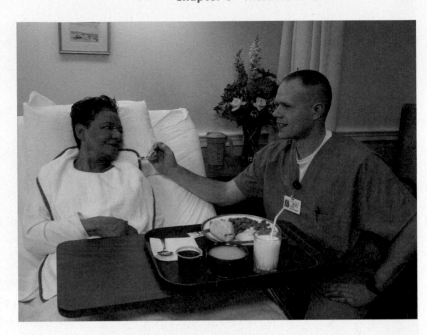

Figure 6-13 The nursing assistant shown here is helping his resident to meet her need for nutrition, one of the most basic human needs.

or resident feel safe by remembering that the entire experience of being in an unfamiliar place and having unfamiliar tests and treatments done is very frightening for many people. By explaining procedures and having questions answered promptly, the nursing assistant can help relieve much of this anxiety (Fig. 6-14).

Love and Belonging Needs

All people need to feel loved, accepted, and appreciated by others. People meet this need for one another by showing affection and forming close (intimate) relationships. Family life helps us to meet our love and belonging needs. We need to feel that we are part of an accepting group. When this need is unmet, feelings of loneliness and isolation develop. Babies and children fail to grow, and older people can actually "die of loneliness." Being a patient or a resident in a

health care facility can cause a person to feel isolated, unlovable, and unappreciated. Patients and residents often feel that they have become a medical condition, instead of a person. By taking an interest in the person and showing respect for the person's specific likes and dislikes, nursing assistants can help to meet that person's need to feel loved, accepted, and appreciated by others. A smile, a kind word, or a gentle touch can go a long way toward making someone feel loved, appreciated, and like they "belong" (Fig. 6-15).

For more information relating to the different ways you can help show respect to your patients and residents and their unique needs, see the new "Respect" feature you will find at the end of each unit.

Self-Esteem Needs

Self-esteem is influenced by how a person perceives themselves and how they think others perceive them.

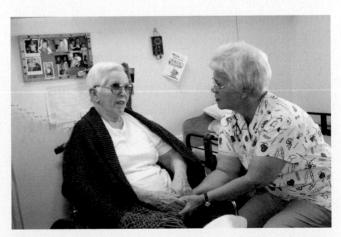

Figure 6-14 Understanding how the bed-positioning controls work can make a nervous patient or resident feel more secure in her unfamiliar environment.

Figure 6-15 All human beings need to feel that they are loved and needed by others.

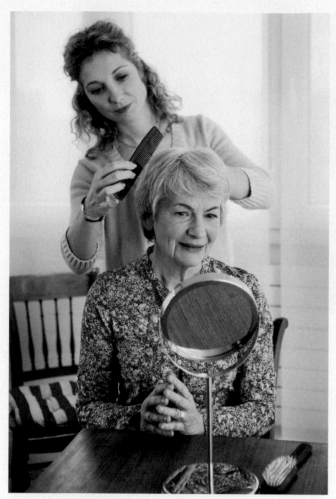

Figure 6-16 By helping this resident to look her best, this nursing assistant is helping to foster the resident's self-esteem. (*Image Point Fr\Shutterstock.com*)

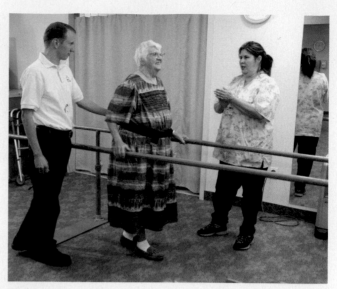

Figure 6-17 Helping patients and residents to set small, realistic goals lets them to meet their need for self-actualization.

Everyone wants to be respected and thought well of by others. Many realities of being hospitalized or moving to a long-term care facility can affect a person's self-esteem, such as:

- Having to wear a hospital gown
- Having surgery that might cause the person's physical appearance to change
- Having to depend on others for something one used to be able to do for oneself

Nursing assistants help to preserve their patients' and residents' self-esteem by providing for privacy when it is necessary to expose someone's body, by allowing people to wear their own clothing (as opposed to a hospital gown) whenever possible, and by assisting people with basic grooming (Fig. 6-16).

Self-Actualization Needs

The highest level on the hierarchy of needs is self-actualization. To achieve self-actualization, a person must reach their fullest potential. Most of us try throughout life to meet this need, constantly setting new goals for ourselves. As a health care worker, you will have the unique opportunity to help the people you care for achieve self-actualization by helping them set small, realistic goals for a positive outcome (Fig. 6-17). Examples of goals that patients or residents may have include taking one step (for a person who has had a stroke), delivering a healthy baby (for a pregnant patient), or returning home (for a person who has broken a hip).

The needs of the people you care for will change as their conditions improve or decline. By helping people to meet their most essential needs first, you will enable them to meet their higher-level needs. For example, it is difficult to work on a person's self-esteem if they are struggling to breathe! Recognizing and helping people meet needs that they have difficulty meeting on their own is one of the most valuable contributions you will make as a nursing assistant.

Human Sexuality and Intimacy

All human beings are sexual beings. Sexuality differs from **intimacy**, which is a feeling of emotional closeness to another, and **sex**, which is the physical activity one engages in to obtain sexual pleasure and reproduce. **Sexuality** is a broad concept that includes our sexual feelings and behaviors, including how a person perceives of their gender and sexual identity. A person's sexuality can be influenced by many social and psychological factors, including societal norms and values and a person's attitudes and beliefs.

An individual's attraction to another individual is called *sexual orientation*. For example, **heterosexual** or straight individuals include women with an attraction to men and men with an attraction to women. **Gay** and **lesbian** individuals include men with an attraction to men and women with an attraction to women. **Bisexual** individuals have the capacity to form attractions to men and women alike.

Sexual orientation is independent of gender identity. *Gender identity* is an individual's psychological sense of themselves with respect to being male/masculine or female/feminine, a combination of both, or neither, and relates directly to how a person chooses to express themselves. People express their gender identity in the way they dress, the cosmetics they choose to wear, how they style their hair, and how they present themselves to other people. Gender identity does not always correspond with assigned sex or biology, nor is it necessarily visible to others.

Sometimes, a person's feelings about their gender do not correspond with the person's sex assigned at birth. These individuals are known as **transgender** (often abbreviated as *trans*) individuals. A transgender woman is an individual who was assigned male at birth who now lives as a woman, and a transgender man is an individual who was assigned female at birth who now lives as a man. A transgender person may prefer to be called by a different name or pronoun (for example, he/him, she/her, or they/them) with which they identify. It is always respectful to ask a person how they prefer to be addressed. Some transgender individuals choose to undergo gender-affirming surgery to have the physical appearance and functional abilities of the gender they identify with, while other trans individuals may only receive hormone therapy or dress according to the gender they identify with.

As a nursing assistant, you will meet people whose feelings about their gender and sexuality, and the ways in which they express these feelings, might differ from your own feelings and the way you express them. You must avoid being judgmental or critical of how another person chooses to express their gender and sexuality. Acceptance of another person involves respecting that person's right to make their own decisions.

Although sexual activity is a part of some intimate relationships, it is not necessarily a part of all. Many people share intimacy by just cuddling or caressing. Sometimes, illness or physical disabilities make **coitus** (sexual intercourse) difficult or impossible, but there are other ways in which two people can express love for each other.

There are many ways that, as a nursing assistant, you can help patients and residents to fulfill their need to be thought of as sexual beings, and to engage in intimate relationships with others:

- Avoid being judgmental.
- Help your patients and residents with rituals that allow them to express their gender identity, such as dressing and applying make-up, perfume, or aftershave lotion.
- Allow for privacy. If the person is in a private room, close the door and use a "do not disturb" sign as the person requests. If the person has a roommate, suggest to the roommate that the two of you take a walk or participate in another activity, outside of the room. Privacy is necessary for people in intimate relationships, whether or not they involve coitus (sexual intercourse). It is also necessary for people who want to engage in **masturbation** (stimulation of the genitals for sexual pleasure or release, by a means other than sexual intercourse).
- If a person is masturbating in a public room (some confused patients or residents will do this), take the person to their room and provide for safety and privacy.
- Always knock before entering a person's room. If you do interrupt a sexual encounter, excuse yourself quietly and say you will return later.

Some people become sexually aggressive and will behave in an unpleasant or unwelcome way toward you or another patient or resident. It is important for you to be able to recognize situations that could be considered sexual abuse or assault. However, before you get upset and report the person's inappropriate behavior to a supervisor, stop and think about a few things. Although an older patient or resident may not seem attractive to you, think about what that person sees when they look at you. You may be young and very attractive to them. You may remind the patient or resident of their spouse or significant other, when that person was young. The patient or resident may have poor eyesight and mistake you for someone else, or they may be confused or disoriented as a result of a disease process. Although it is totally inappropriate for you to attend to the sexual needs of your patients or residents, it is important to avoid being unkind or hateful in your response. Depending on the situation, tell the patient or resident kindly, yet firmly, that you are not going to do what they are asking you to do, or that they must not touch you in that manner. Avoid giggling or teasing the patient or resident in a flirtatious manner. This will only serve to reinforce the inappropriate behavior. If the behavior does not stop, or if the behavior is directed at another patient or resident, you should discuss the matter with your supervisor.

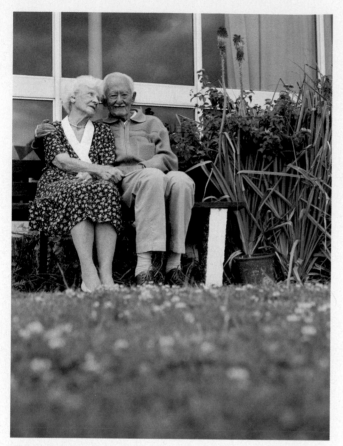

Figure 6-18 Sexuality and intimacy are basic human needs for everyone, young and old.

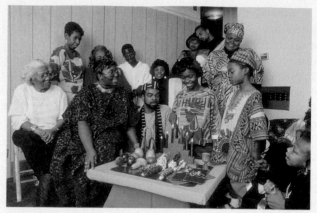

Figure 6-19 This African-American family is celebrating Kwanzaa, a holiday celebrated by Africans and people of African descent throughout the world. Kwanzaa, a celebration of African history and culture, with a special emphasis on family life, occurs from December 26 through January 1. Kwanzaa is a cultural holiday, not a religious one. Celebrants are united by their African heritage, not their religion. (© *Lawrence Migdale*.)

Concerns for Long-Term Care

Because society so often associates youth and beauty with sexuality, we often do not consider the sexual needs of aging people. Sexuality and intimacy are basic human needs, common to all people, young and old (Fig. 6-18). Many older adults in long-term care facilities have lost their sexual partners, either as a result of death, divorce, or separation. Quite often, they have the chance to find happiness again in their golden years with someone they meet in a nursing facility.

CULTURE AND RELIGION

You can see that there are many things that, as human beings, we all have in common. For example, everyone has the same basic needs, although some needs may be more pressing than others at any given time for any one individual. Similarly, we all pass through the same stages of growth and development, although not at the same time or at the same rate. Culture, the subject of this section, is another thing that makes human beings human. All people have a culture, although everyone's culture is not the same. **Culture** is made up of the beliefs (including religious or spiritual beliefs), values, and traditions that are customary to a group of people. It is a view of the world that is handed down from generation to generation. A culture can be shared by people of the same race or ethnicity, by people who live within the same geographic area or speak the same language, or by a combination of these two (Fig. 6-19).

One of the most unique things about the United States is the diversity of cultures that are represented here. **Race** refers to physical differences that groups and cultures consider socially significant. It is important to be aware that race has a social, not biologic, basis. Racial identity is an important aspect of a person's culture, and each individual may identify as a member of multiple racial, ethnic, or cultural groups. In all cases, always view each person as an individual, not as a "representative" of any specific cultural group, which leads to stereotypes. Diversity has enriched this country, yet problems can arise when people are not sensitive to, or respectful of, the unique identity of each individual. As a health care worker, it is important for you to learn as much as possible about the characteristics of other cultural or ethnic groups because your patients or residents may have cultural differences that affect their preferences regarding health care. In addition, a primary goal of the nursing team is to provide for the comfort of those we care for. A person who feels that their culture is not understood or respected by the people who care for them will feel uncomfortable.

There are many ways in which a health care worker can accidentally be disrespectful of a patient's or resident's culture, which can lead to conflict. Sometimes, misunderstandings occur simply because a health care worker is not aware of how a certain person's culture influences their behavior. Although it is difficult to make generalizations about culture—not everyone from the same geographic region, or with the same skin tone, necessarily has the same beliefs or value system—being aware of what a patient or resident is telling you can help you to know when cultural differences need to be taken into account. Areas where culture and health care often intersect include beliefs and practices associated with food and meals; religious beliefs and practices; and attitudes toward health, sickness, and death.

Liking certain types of food, or food prepared a specific way, is very cultural. For example, a person from the southern United States may prefer "grits" (cornmeal) to oatmeal. Sometimes, a patient or resident may request or refuse a certain food or combination of foods in order to follow religious beliefs or practices. For example, a person of the Catholic faith may not want to eat meat on Fridays during Lent, and a person of the Jewish faith may follow the practice of not drinking milk with a meal that contains meat. In some cultures, it is believed that certain combinations of foods can aid or inhibit healing. For example, according to Taoism (a philosophy that originated in Asia), illness occurs when the body is out of balance. To restore balance, certain foods may be chosen over others. If one of your patients or residents requests or denies a certain food or combination of foods for religious or other reasons, be sure to tell the nurse. The nurse will work with the dietary department to help meet the person's request.

A person's spiritual beliefs, or **religion**, are often very closely linked with their culture. Members of some cultural groups have certain rituals that they feel will bring them good luck or aid in healing. For example, you may encounter a person who believes hanging an "evil-eye" talisman will ward off bad spirits. A person might want to light candles while praying to a specific saint or deity. Many people are very spiritual and find comfort and solace in prayer, reading scriptures or spiritual books, singing, and meditation. If a patient or resident asks to see a spiritual leader or clergy member, communicate the request promptly and according to your facility's policy, and allow for privacy during the visit. Another person's religious beliefs may be very different from yours, but you can be certain that their beliefs are as important to them as yours are to you. You do not have to believe in a person's religion to offer the kind of care shown by reading their scriptures or spiritual books to them when they cannot (Fig. 6-20).

There are other examples of cultural practices that we must be respectful of, even if we do not agree

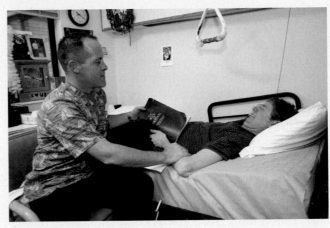

Figure 6-20 A nursing assistant can help people to obtain comfort from their religious beliefs, even if they do not share those same beliefs.

with them. Remember, your culture influenced your value system, and your patient's or resident's culture influenced theirs. Respecting another person's values does not mean that you have to agree with that person or their values. For example, greater emphasis is placed on modesty during medical examinations in some cultures than others, and you might encounter a reluctance among some patients or residents to expose their bodies. Sometimes, they will also have a preference for the examination to be conducted instead by a member of the gender with which they identify. Although it would be tempting to try to go ahead with the procedure, you know that your patient or resident would not be comfortable if you were to put them in a difficult situation. You would be devaluing their belief system by trying to overrule it. Instead, do everything you can to respect the person's cultural beliefs and meet their needs and preferences. Ask for permission before proceeding, slowly, with the examination. If necessary, arrange to get a staff member of the gender they prefer to conduct the examination.

Throughout your career, you may be lucky enough to care for people from many different cultural and religious backgrounds. You will most likely encounter situations, practices, and beliefs that no book could have prepared you for! Take time to listen to your patients or residents, and to learn from them. Exposure to cultures other than your own is enriching, both professionally and personally.

QUALITY OF LIFE

Treating illness and promoting good physical health are two primary goals of all health care providers. However, sometimes we are so focused on treating a patient's or resident's problems, we forget to consider the desires of the individual. As you have learned, a humanistic approach to health care takes into account a person's emotional, social, and spiritual needs in addition to their physical ones. Making an effort to accommodate a person's cultural beliefs and practices is one way that health care workers provide humanistic care. Another way is by allowing patients and residents to make decisions related to their own quality of life.

As a nursing assistant, you will encounter patients who have diabetes and must control their diet carefully. You will encounter patients with heart disease who should eat fewer foods high in cholesterol and stop smoking. But what if your patient or resident does not comply with the recommendations of the health care team? Is the woman with diabetes a bad person if she truly loves sweets and does not want to give them up? Is the man with heart disease a bad person if he cannot bear to give up his daily breakfast of eggs and bacon? What if a person refuses a treatment or surgery that may prolong their life? Should the health care worker simply write that person off and focus only on those willing to follow medical advice?

If a health care worker gives a person the proper information about their illness or condition and educates them about the steps to take to treat or resolve it, then the health care worker has provided the person with the information they need to make a conscientious decision concerning their own health. The person must make these decisions according to their own personal values and sense of what is best for themselves as an individual. This is where the idea of *quality of life* comes into play. Quality of life has to do with getting satisfaction and comfort from the way we are living. The idea of what quality of life means differs for each person and may vary as a person's situation changes. For example, during your career as a health care worker, you will care for people with terminal illness who want every treatment available to help them fight for life, even if the procedures are dangerous or painful. You will also care for people with terminal illness who decline painful or risky treatments because they feel that their ability to enjoy life and derive pleasure from living will be too compromised by the treatments. Each of your patients and residents must be allowed to make decisions concerning their quality of life. In order to provide holistic care for your patients or residents, you must respect their decisions related to maintaining their quality of life.

Helping Hands and a Caring Heart

Focus on Humanistic Health Care

Think for a moment, What is it like to be a patient? Patients feel scared and lonely. They feel sick. They are unsure about their health, now and in the future. Some worry about whether they will be able to return to work and are concerned about their illness affecting their family's financial future. Some medical treatments cause a change in a person's physical appearance and some patients worry about how they will look afterward. Patients worry about spouses, children, and pets at home, and whether they are being cared for properly. They worry about the emotional effects of their illness on their family members. The hospital environment itself can be frightening and uncomfortable, full of strange noises and smells. If you were in this situation, how would you feel and how might this affect your behavior?

Similarly, what is it like to be a resident? Imagine what it would be like to have to move from a home you loved to a long-term care facility. You have lived a long, full, independent life. Now, you are not managing as well as you once did—you have fallen twice, and left the teakettle on numerous times and forgotten about it. Even though, logically, you know it makes sense to move to a place where there is always someone around to "take care of you," when you gave up your home, you gave up a certain amount of your independence along with it. You cannot take all of your furniture, and you must find a new home for your pets. You have a roommate (at your age!) and you have to eat the meals that are prepared for you, when they are served to you. Gone are all your favorite things and your favorite pastimes at home. How would you feel about this loss of independence, and how might this affect your behavior?

People who find themselves as patients and residents often feel that they are at the mercy of the health care industry. While some patients and residents are cheerful, compliant, and grateful, others may be depressed, angry, anxious, or just downright mean. When you must care for a patient or resident who makes you wish you had never chosen to be a nursing assistant (and you can be certain you will encounter patients or residents like this), stop and think for a moment about the reasons that person may be acting out of sorts. When you look beyond the illness or condition, past the technical duties and procedures, and into that person's eyes, you will find your reason for choosing to be a nursing assistant…a person who needs you very much.

A PERSON'S FAMILY

Families, like your patients and residents, may also be very diverse. We often think of a family in terms of being related by blood or marriage, or that a family unit consists of parents, their children, and other relatives. However, modern families can be made up of many different members. Single parents frequently raise their children without the support of a spouse or the other parent. Grandparents or other relatives may raise children when their parents are unable to. A person's significant other may be a same-sex partner. In many circumstances, a very close friend may become the family member that a person relies upon for both physical and emotional support. Many families are very close to each other, visiting regularly and displaying outward affection. Other families are not as close and may have histories of abuse or other turmoil that has caused the members to distance themselves from each other. Regardless of who a patient or a resident considers to be "family," we must always remember the importance of respecting that relationship.

Illness, injury, or disability, especially if it involves an admission to a health care facility, not only affects the patient or the resident but can have a significant impact on that person's family members. If family members have previously been actively involved in caring for the patient or the resident at home, they may have a lot of difficulty giving up the role of caregiver and may feel that you and the other health care workers will not care for their family member as well as they did. Many family members feel guilty, especially if the person is being admitted to a long-term care facility. They may feel that they have failed their loved one by not being able to continue caring for them at home. The family members may experience feelings of helplessness that the situation has become out of their control. Some family members will question you and second-guess the care you are providing. It is important that you consider how stressful it is for them to have a loved one who is now a patient or a resident and not take their behavior personally.

If the patient or the resident consents, it is very important for family members to be included in their care decisions. If the person is a resident of a long-term care facility, family members are encouraged to participate in the interdisciplinary care planning meetings and to be involved in helping to develop the resident's care plan. Frequent visits and calls from family members can help keep a patient or a resident from becoming depressed. Allowing family members to participate in the patient's or the resident's care as much as possible helps them to regain some sense of usefulness and control. It is also helpful to make sure that you listen to a family member's suggestions and input about the person's preferences. In reality, you do not just provide care for the patient or the resident, you also must consider the needs of that person's family.

SUMMARY

- Patients, residents, and clients are people who need the services of the health care industry because they are sick, injured, or unable to care for themselves.
  - Acute, chronic, or terminal illnesses can cause a person to need health care services.
  - People in health care settings are grouped according to their ages, illnesses or medical conditions, or special health care needs.
- The process of growth and development is divided into stages of progression: infancy, toddlerhood, preschool, school-age, adolescence, young adulthood, middle adulthood, later adulthood, and older adulthood. Everyone passes through these, but not necessarily at the same rate.
  - The growth and development changes that occur affect the type of care the person needs

and the way we communicate with them. Become familiar with the various stages of growth and development.
- People in health care settings have many different physical and emotional needs.
  - Basic needs must be met before higher-level needs can be met.
  - Maslow's hierarchy of human needs includes physiologic, safety and security, love and belonging, self-esteem, and self-actualization needs.
  - Sexuality is a broad concept that includes our sexual feelings and behaviors, including how a person perceives of their gender and sexual identity. Sexuality differs from intimacy and from sex. Sexuality and intimacy are basic human needs.

- Patients and residents who are not able to meet their needs on their own rely on the health care team to recognize and help meet these needs for them.
- The people you will care for are individuals, with unique feelings, memories, goals, and personalities.
    - You will care for people in varying stages of growth and development.
    - You will care for people from different cultural and religious backgrounds.

- Recognizing and respecting the differences in the people you care for will allow you to provide humanistic care, which makes a difference in the lives of your patients or residents and their family members.
- It is important for you to recognize the impact that illness or disability has on a patient's or a resident's family members.

WHAT DID YOU LEARN?

Multiple Choice

Select the single best answer for each of the following questions.

1. Sandra is caring for Mrs. Norville, who lives in a long-term care facility. Sandra encourages Mrs. Norville to make her own decisions about what to do each day. She helps her with dressing and grooming, but lets her do as much as she can for herself. These activities help fulfill Mrs. Norville's need for:
   a. Security
   b. Shelter
   c. Spirituality
   d. Self-esteem

2. When caring for people from different cultures, you should try to:
   a. Understand and respect their special needs
   b. Encourage them to change their beliefs while in your facility
   c. Pretend that the cultural differences do not exist
   d. Avoid asking them about their culture

3. Which one of the following is an example of an acute condition?
   a. Appendicitis
   b. Emphysema
   c. Diabetes
   d. High blood pressure (hypertension)

4. A resident's religion forbids them from eating pork. Pork chops are being served for dinner. What should you do?
   a. Tell the resident that religious restrictions on diet do not count in times of illness
   b. Inform the nurse so the dietary department can be called

   c. Insist that the resident eat the pork, because it contains protein, an essential nutrient
   d. Reassure the resident by telling them that the doctor ordered this diet

5. A resident in a long-term care facility may show her sexuality by doing all of the following except:
   a. Desiring sexual intercourse
   b. Engaging in public fondling
   c. Giving her granddaughter a doll for her birthday
   d. Applying make-up and scented powder before receiving a male visitor

6. Which one of the following is not a basic human need?
   a. Fear
   b. Self-actualization
   c. Self-esteem
   d. Water

7. Which one of the following is a basic social need?
   a. Food
   b. Water
   c. Air
   d. Love

8. What term describes a person who identifies with a gender that does not correspond with their sex assigned at birth?
   a. Heterosexual
   b. Transgender
   c. Bisexual
   d. Gay

Matching *Match each numbered item with its appropriate lettered description.*

_____ **1.** Infancy

_____ **2.** Toddlerhood

_____ **3.** Preschool

_____ **4.** School-age

_____ **5.** Adolescence

_____ **6.** Middle adulthood

_____ **7.** Older adulthood

a. A 16-year-old boy going to the junior prom

b. A 42-year-old executive running her own company

c. A 2-year-old boy starting toilet training

d. A 6-month-old girl learning to sit up

e. A 92-year-old great-grandmother moving to a long-term care facility

f. A 4-year-old boy learning to tie his shoes

g. An 11-year-old Girl Scout participating in her troop's annual volunteer day

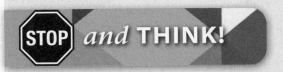

You are caring for Mr. Adichie, who was admitted to your long-term care facility yesterday. Yesterday, he was quiet and polite. Today, however, he is hostile and mean. He refused to go to the dining room for lunch and knocked the tray you brought him to the floor. He keeps yelling at you, saying, "This feels like a prison!" Why do you think Mr. Adichie is acting this way? What could you do to help him?

Respect

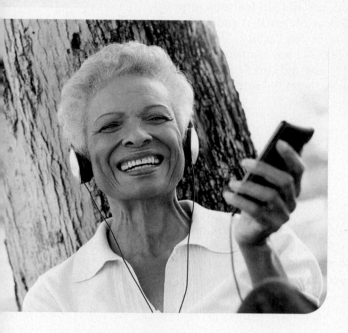

I work at a large long-term care facility, where I have been a CNA for about a year now. I love our residents and try very hard to get to know each one individually so I can provide the best care for them. Although I am still very young myself, I find myself learning so much from their life experiences and the stories they tell.

I have been trying hard to get to know one of our newer residents, Mrs. Jackson. She is a lovely older lady who has been pretty quiet and seems a little sad since moving here. Yesterday, I knocked on the door to her room to bring her some clean linens for her bed and I found her listening to music and singing softly to herself. The song was "Respect," sung by Aretha Franklin, and I shared with Mrs. Jackson how much I loved that song.

Mrs. Jackson's face lit up and she turned the music down and started talking about how much she admired the "Queen of Soul" and the work she did throughout her career to promote the Civil Rights Movement and the rights of women. She went on to tell me that this particular song helped send a message to Americans about peace, equality, and justice, and became an anthem for personal freedom, sexual revolution, and freedom from racial oppression.

Mrs. Jackson then told me that she had grown up in Memphis, Tennessee around the same time that Aretha Franklin and the Reverend Martin Luther King, Jr. did, and that she herself had marched for the equal rights that are so essential to us all. I was inspired hearing the story of Mrs. Jackson's social justice activism and important role in our nation's history!

After hearing Mrs. Jackson's stories about her life, Aretha Franklin's anthem "Respect" has a whole new meaning for me. It has helped me develop a better awareness of who our residents are and what they have been through in their lives. It makes me want to learn more about them so I can not only come to know them better, but also come to know myself. I know this experience has helped me become a better CNA, and developed a better awareness of the unique needs of my residents.

At the end of each unit in this textbook, we will pause for a moment to reflect on the people you will care for. Learning to respect each person as the unique individual they are is one of the most important things a health care worker can do.

As Aretha sang...*R-E-S-P-E-C-T, find out what it means to me*!

(Monkey Business Images\Shutterstock.com)

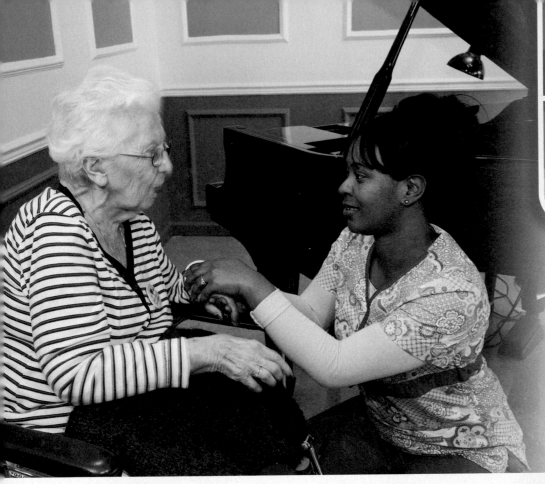

Long-Term Care

THE MAJORITY OF NURSING ASSISTANTS ARE EMPLOYED BY LONG-TERM CARE FACILITIES. In fact, in some states, the long-term care setting is the only place where nursing assistants may work. The population of older adults continues to increase dramatically due to advances and improvements in health care. It is estimated that on any given day, about 5% of this population resides in a long-term care facility. And, almost half of people who are 65 years old or older are likely to spend some time in a long-term care facility.

The focus of this unit is on long-term care; the types of long-term care facilities, the people who reside in long-term care facilities, and people who have dementia.

Photo: Here, a nursing assistant pauses to visit with a resident.

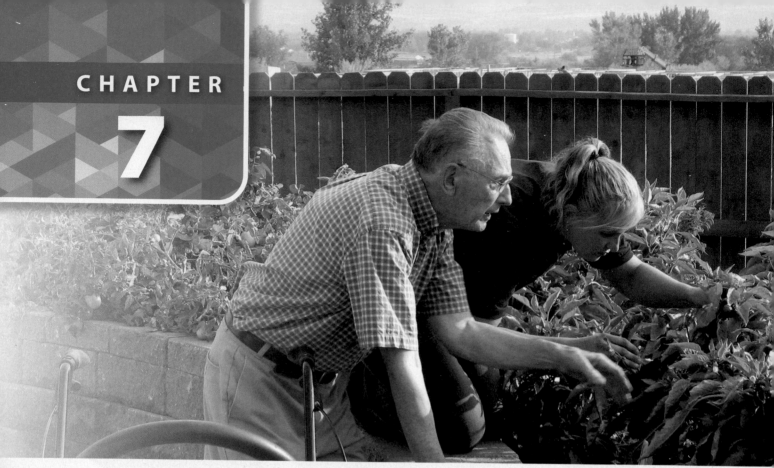

Photo: A resident of a Green House® home enjoys gardening. The Green House® project is an example of how long-term care is changing. (Photo courtesy of THE GREEN HOUSE® Project.)

Overview of Long-Term Care

 WHAT WILL YOU LEARN?

In this chapter, we will take a closer look at the long-term care setting. We will review the different types of long-term care settings that exist in the United States today. In addition, we will discuss the history of long-term care in the United States, as well as its future. You will learn more about the regulatory and accreditation organizations that help to ensure the quality of long-term care provided in the United States today. Finally, we will discuss how long-term care is paid for. When you are finished with this chapter, you will be able to:

1. Explain the different types of long-term care settings.
2. Describe some of the government and private agencies that provide oversight of long-term care.
3. Discuss how long-term care is paid for.
4. Discuss the past, present, and future of long-term care.

Vocabulary

Continuing care retirement community (CCRC)

Continuum of care

For-profit facility

Nonprofit (not-for-profit) facility

Free-standing facility

Chain facility

Centers for Medicare and Medicaid Services (CMS)

Continuing Care Accreditation Commission (CCAC)

Benefit period

Private pay

Long-term care insurance

TYPES OF LONG-TERM CARE SETTINGS

As you remember from Chapter 1, a long-term care setting is a place where health care is provided for people who require ongoing nursing care, personal assistance, or both as a result of illness or disability. The three major types of long-term care settings are nursing homes, assisted-living facilities, and continuing care retirement communities (CCRCs). Some people also consider adult day care and home health services part of long-term care.

Nursing Homes

Nursing homes, also called *nursing facilities*, provide residents with around-the-clock nursing care and supervision. Typically, residents live in private rooms grouped along a common hallway (Fig. 7-1). Some older nursing homes may still offer semiprivate rooms. All rooms have access to a toilet (either private or shared between two rooms). Often, a communal bathing area (with bathtubs, showers, or both) is located down the hall. Some rooms may have private

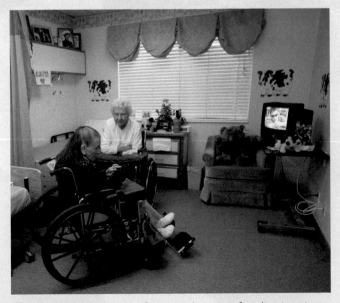

Figure 7-1 Residents of nursing homes often live in private or semiprivate rooms.

bath and toilet facilities that are used only by the resident occupying the room. Usually, there are also common areas where residents gather to socialize (such as dining rooms and activity rooms), a special area set aside for religious services, and patios and gardens that allow the residents access to outdoor activities.

Nursing homes require that a registered nurse (RN) or licensed practical nurse (LPN) be on-site at all times. In addition to providing basic medical care and nursing services, nursing homes must also provide rehabilitation therapies, podiatry, dental, and medical specialty consultation services (for example, a cardiologist consult for a resident with a heart condition).

Care in a nursing home is usually categorized as *intermediate care* (usually long term) or *skilled* (usually short term). Intermediate care is provided for people who are chronically ill and need assistance with the activities of daily living (ADLs). In addition, an increased focus on rehabilitation or restorative care (discussed in more detail in Chapter 39) helps residents to maintain or even improve their level of function and independence so that their abilities do not decline.

Many nursing homes contain nursing units that provide skilled care. Skilled care (sometimes referred to as skilled rehabilitation care) is provided for people who have recently required some type of acute care for an illness or injury. Typical reasons that a resident may be admitted for skilled care include stroke, fractured hip, and rehabilitation after an acute illness such as pneumonia or a heart attack. If a person who is a resident in the intermediate care part of the facility falls and breaks their hip, they can be cared for in the skilled care unit after they are released from the hospital. When they no longer require the skilled care, they will then return to their intermediate care room. Many nursing homes also provide skilled nursing care for people who will be returning to their own private homes after they have rehabilitated.

Another growing trend for long-term care facilities is the establishment of special care units (SCUs). These units are separate areas in the facility designed to meet the needs of residents with specific types of disorders. Rehabilitation, and dementia care units, or Alzheimer's units, are examples of SCUs (Fig. 7-2). Other disorders that may have designated SCUs include oncology, ventilator-dependent, pressure ulcers, and traumatic brain injury.

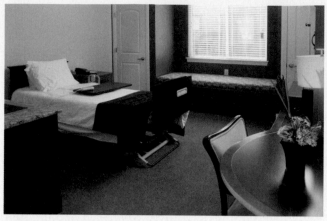

Figure 7-2 A private rehabilitation room. (Photo courtesy of Legacy Village, Layton, UT—A Continuing Care Senior Living Community.)

Assisted-Living Facilities

Assisted-living facilities provide residents with limited assistance with tasks such as personal care, medication administration, transportation, meals, and housekeeping. Residents of assisted-living facilities often live in small apartments that have a kitchen or kitchenette, a bathroom, a living area, and a bedroom (Fig. 7-3). Most assisted-living facilities also have common areas where residents can go to socialize and eat.

Continuing Care Retirement Communities

Continuing care retirement communities (CCRCs) provide many different levels of care and multiple services on the same campus. The CCRC campus provides a **continuum of care** by including facilities for independent living, assisted living, skilled care, and nursing

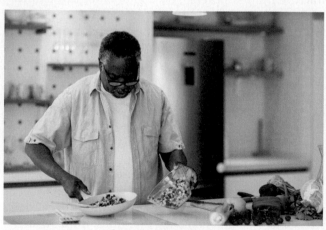

Figure 7-3 Residents of assisted-living facilities often have a small apartment with areas for eating, living, and sleeping. (*astarot\Shutterstock.com*)

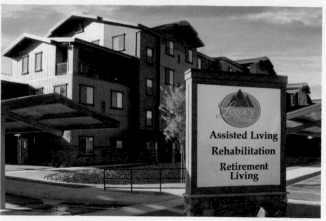

Figure 7-4 A continuing care retirement community (CCRC) has facilities for independent living, assisted living, and nursing home care, all on the same campus. As residents' needs change, they can obtain the care they need without moving away from the campus. Other buildings on campus might include restaurants, recreational facilities, worship facilities, stores, and a health center where residents can go for medical care. (Photo courtesy of Legacy Village, Layton, UT—A Continuing Care Senior Living Community.)

home care (Fig. 7-4). As age, health problems, or both cause a resident of a CCRC to become less independent, they are able to stay within the CCRC to obtain the care they need. In addition, the CCRC campus may include restaurants or dining facilities, recreational and social facilities, facilities for worship, a small market where food and other items can be purchased, and a health center where residents can go for medical care.

OWNERSHIP AND OPERATION OF LONG-TERM CARE FACILITIES

Long-term care facilities differ from one another in terms of the types of services they provide. They also differ from one another in terms of how they are owned and operated.

For-Profit Facilities Versus Nonprofit (Not-For-Profit) Facilities

A facility may be "for-profit" or "nonprofit" (not-for-profit). A **for-profit facility** is one owned by a company or organization that operates the facility as a business, with the intention of making money (a profit). In contrast, a **nonprofit (not-for-profit) facility** is owned and operated by a service organization, like a church or charitable group. Its primary goal is to provide a service to fulfill a need in the community. Although a nonprofit facility still has to make money to stay in business, money-making for the purpose of financial gain is not the primary intent. The profits are often put back into the services provided by the organization.

Free-Standing Facilities Versus Chain Facilities

Long-term care facilities may be free-standing or part of a chain. A **free-standing facility** is independently owned and operated. A **chain facility**, on the other hand, is owned and operated by a corporation that owns multiple facilities. Facilities that are part of a chain tend to be very similar to each other because they are run by the same corporation. If you have ever visited a McDonald's or a Wal-Mart in another city, you are already familiar with this concept. By the name, you basically know what to expect when you go inside the restaurant or store. The same is true of long-term care facilities that are part of a chain. Each facility in the chain follows the same corporate policies and procedures, so the services offered and the care provided are similar from facility to facility within the chain. Chain facilities are often for-profit facilities, although some nonprofit organizations may also run multiple facilities.

OVERSIGHT OF LONG-TERM CARE

Many different agencies—including the federal, state, and local government, as well as independent nonprofit organizations—are responsible for making sure that the care provided in long-term care facilities in the United States is safe and of high quality.

Oversight by the Federal Government

All types of long-term care facilities must follow the requirements of agencies such as the Occupational Safety and Health Administration (OSHA), the Food and Drug Administration (FDA), and the Centers for Disease Control and Prevention (CDC). The functions of these agencies were reviewed in Chapter 1. In addition, federal OBRA laws apply to every nursing home in the United States. (These laws apply only to nursing homes, not to assisted-living facilities.) Each nursing home is subject to routine inspection by the government. These inspections are called *surveys*. The purpose of the survey is to make sure the facility is following OBRA regulations and meeting the government's standards. The **Centers for Medicare and Medicaid Services (CMS)** is the government agency responsible for monitoring nursing homes to make sure that they are following OBRA regulations and meeting the government's standards. Government payment for services depends on whether or not the facility is meeting the required standards. If a facility is found through the survey process not to meet the required standards, government payment for services becomes jeopardized.

Under the federal OBRA laws, nursing homes must make their most recent survey results readily available to residents, families, and anyone else who wants to review them. In addition, CMS posts survey results on the Internet. Because survey results are easily available to anyone who is interested, the facility has an additional incentive to provide quality services, beyond just avoiding regulatory problems. Survey results that indicate a high quality of care can make the facility more attractive to potential residents and their families. As a nursing assistant, you will play a very important role in ensuring that your facility meets or exceeds survey requirements by doing your job well and always following facility policy.

Oversight by State Governments

All long-term care facilities must have a state-issued license to operate. To maintain *licensure*, long-term care facilities must undergo an inspection. The state officials who perform this inspection are responsible for checking to make sure the facility is meeting the state's requirements. In addition, they may be responsible for making sure that the facility is following any federal regulations that may apply.

Assisted-living facilities are regulated by the state. Because no federal laws apply to assisted-living facilities, assisted-living services can vary greatly from state to state. However, nursing homes must comply with state laws in addition to federal laws. Many state laws that apply to nursing homes follow OBRA, but some states have additional requirements that OBRA does not include.

Nursing homes that wish to participate in the Medicare and Medicaid programs must be certified. In order to achieve and maintain *certification*, the facility must undergo inspections. These inspections are usually carried out by state officials who are contracted by the federal government (for example, CMS). These officials check to make sure that the facility is meeting federal regulations, as well as state regulations.

Oversight by Local Governments

Local agencies (such as city or county health departments) are responsible for ensuring that long-term care facilities are in compliance with any regulations that the local government has established for them. Local officials may also have a role in checking to make sure that the facility is providing care according to state or federal standards.

Independent Nonprofit Organizations

In Chapter 1, you learned about accrediting organizations that set national standards for all types of health care organizations and officially recognize (accredit) organizations that meet these standards. Many long-term care facilities seek accreditation from these organizations.

Another organization, the **Continuing Care Accreditation Commission (CCAC)**, grants accreditation to CCRCs, as well as to some other types of organizations that provide long-term care services (such as adult day care centers). The CCAC is the only accrediting organization specifically for CCRCs. A CCRC (or other health care organization) seeking accreditation by the CCAC requests and pays for routine inspections. Organizations that have been accredited by the CCAC are permitted to display the CCAC's accreditation seal, which is recognized nationwide as a symbol of quality.

PAYING FOR LONG-TERM CARE

Long-term care is very expensive and not easily paid for by individuals or by the government (Fig. 7-5).

Paying for Nursing Home Care

In the United States, the average cost for nursing home care is more than $6,000 per month. By *average,*

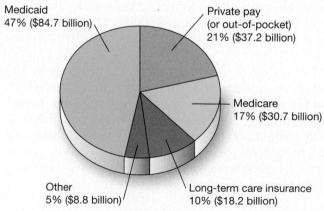

Medicaid 47% ($84.7 billion)

Private pay (or out-of-pocket) 21% ($37.2 billion)

Medicare 17% ($30.7 billion)

Long-term care insurance 10% ($18.2 billion)

Other 5% ($8.8 billion)

Figure 7-5 Long-term care is expensive! This graph shows the billions of dollars that are spent each year on long-term care in the United States, as well as where that money is coming from.

we mean that in some areas it may cost less, but in other areas it may cost more. Many Americans underestimate the cost of nursing home care. As a result, many do not have the savings to pay for nursing home care if it is needed.

Medicare

Many people assume that Medicare will pay for nursing home care. In reality, what Medicare pays for is extremely limited. For Medicare to pay, several requirements must be met:

- The person must meet strict criteria for skilled health care services. Skilled health care services are those provided by nurses or other licensed health care professionals.
- Care must follow a hospital stay.
- Care must be provided in a nursing facility licensed to provide skilled care.

A **benefit period** begins when the person is hospitalized and ends when the person has not received any skilled health care services, either in the hospital or nursing home, for 60 days. The Medicare program uses benefit periods as a way of tracking how many days of skilled health care services a person uses, and how many are still available. A person can have up to 100 days of skilled care in one benefit period. Once the person uses those 100 days, the current benefit period ends. A new benefit period cannot begin until the 60 days without skilled services is completed. During a benefit period, only the first 20 days are fully covered by Medicare. The remaining days (days 21 to 100) require a co-pay of approximately $100 per day. Medicare can end a person's coverage when the person no longer meets the strict criteria for coverage, even if the 100-day period is not over.

Medicaid

So, what happens to those who need nursing home care but do not have Medicare coverage? Many are admitted to a nursing facility as "**private pay**," meaning that they pay for care using their own money (Fig. 7-6). With care in a nursing home costing an average of more than $6,000 per month, you can see that it may not take very long to go through a lifetime of savings. Many people do exhaust all of their savings, and then must rely on Medicaid to pay for their care. Approximately 70% of those currently living in nursing homes are relying on Medicaid to pay for their care.

Although Medicaid eases the financial burden for the person receiving care, the financial burden is transferred to the nursing facility, and to the state that is distributing the Medicaid payments. For facilities, Medicaid causes a financial strain because Medicaid

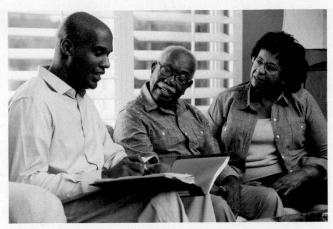

Figure 7-6 Most people are not prepared to pay for nursing home care for an extended period of time. Here, a member of the nursing home admissions staff reviews options for paying for care with the family of a resident. (*Monkey Business Images\Shutterstock.com*)

payments have not been able to keep up with the rising costs of care. As a result, it often costs the facility more to provide the services than the facility receives as payment in return. For states, Medicaid causes a financial strain as well. The state must accommodate Medicaid costs within its budget. This is becoming hard to do because Medicaid costs are consuming a greater percentage of state budgets every year.

Long-Term Care Insurance

Long-term care insurance is a private insurance policy that can be purchased by an individual to help pay for long-term care in the future, should it be needed. The benefit of long-term care insurance is that it can help to pay for long-term care services, which help to protect the person's savings and assets. The disadvantages are that long-term care insurance is very expensive and somewhat risky.

Long-term care insurance, like Medicare, does not pay for all costs associated with nursing home care. Even if the insurance pays for the nursing home stay, it may not cover additional expenses related to medications, supplies, or other special services and therapies. These additional expenses can add up very quickly. Many policies also require the person to pay a *deductible* (that is, a sum of money paid "out-of-pocket" before actual insurance benefits are paid).

Paying for Assisted-Living Care

The average cost for assisted-living care is approximately half the cost of nursing home care. Even though assisted-living care is less expensive, it is primarily a private pay expense. Medicare does not cover any portion of assisted-living care, and in most

cases, Medicaid does not either. Payment by long-term care insurance depends on the type of policy that was purchased. In general, long-term care insurance only covers certain expenses related to assisted living.

LONG-TERM CARE: PAST, PRESENT, AND FUTURE

In past years, public opinion of long-term care, specifically nursing homes, was very low. Throughout history, there have been many problems with long-term care in the United States, so it is understandable how such an opinion developed. However, it is important to recognize that today's long-term care facilities provide a significantly improved quality of care and quality of life for residents. Only by understanding our past can we truly understand the present and appreciate the future of long-term care, so let's start by reviewing some key historical developments.

The Journey From the Past to the Present

For as long as there have been older, chronically ill, and disabled people, society has sought different ways to care for them. Throughout history, family members or friends of those in need often took on the responsibility of caring for them. Taking care of those without family or friends (or the money to hire help) became the responsibility of the community. The community responded to this need by establishing *poorhouses* (community-supported facilities that provided shelter for those without the means of supporting themselves, also known as *almshouses* or *poor farms*). From the mid-1800s, up until the Social Security Act was passed in 1935, many people with chronic illness or disability lived in poorhouses. Conditions in the poorhouses varied quite a bit, and unfortunately, overcrowding, filth, and disease were common. Nevertheless, poorhouses can be thought of as an early version of the types of long-term care facilities covered in this chapter.

Modern nursing home care is a great improvement upon these older institutions, and the course of its development has been influenced by many factors, including many acts of federal legislation. See Box 7-1 for a brief timeline of this history. Not only has this history improved access to nursing home care for the people who need it, but the quality of care in the nursing home environment has also improved.

An especially important development in modern nursing home care occurred in the 1980s, when the Institute of Medicine (IOM) was given the task of

Box 7-1   The Past, Present, and Future of Long-Term Care in the United States

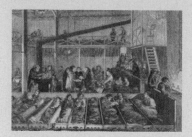

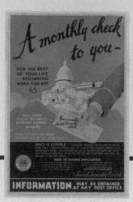

More private dwellings begin to open up to provide board and care for older people, decreasing the number of poorhouses from 135,000 to 72,000.

1935–1950

Mid-1800s

Poorhouses provide shelter for older people who are no longer able to work to pay for housing and who have no families to take care of them. The poorhouses are often crowded and dirty.

Photo by Mansell/Time & Life Pictures/Getty Images

1900–1930s

Shelters dedicated solely to housing the elderly begin to appear and are called "homes for the aged," "convalescent homes," or "rest homes."

1935

President Franklin D. Roosevelt signs the Social Security Act into law, providing monthly pensions for older people.

1965

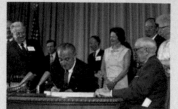

President Lyndon B. Johnson signs the Medicare/Medicaid programs into law, making it possible for more people to afford long-term care.

LBJ Library, photo by Unknown. Source: http://www.lbjlibrary .net/collections/photo-archive/ photolab-detail.html?id=96.

studying it to look for improvements. The result of their report was the Omnibus Budget Reconciliation Act (OBRA) of 1987 (also now called the Federal 1987 Nursing Home Reform Act), which was put into effect in 1990. The strict OBRA legislation improved the quality of life for nursing home residents by making sure that they received a certain standard of care that took into account residents' physical, emotional, spiritual, and social needs. In addition, OBRA set standards for the physical environment in the nursing home, as well as for the training and evaluation of the nursing assistants who worked there (Box 7-2). These important standards remain in effect today.

Costs have also been a challenge in nursing home care throughout history. However, in the late 1990s, less costly alternatives to the traditional nursing home began to emerge. One of these alternatives was the assisted-living facility. Because assisted-living facilities provide care for people who need support but do not need skilled nursing care, their services are not as costly. Currently, we are also seeing a trend toward more caregiving occurring within a person's home, reducing costs even further, which helps to decrease the financial burden on residents and families.

The Future

In 1997, a small group of professionals working in long-term care met to share ideas and create a new vision for the future of long-term care. This group of long-term care professionals, which in 2000 officially became known as the *Pioneer Network*, developed several models for long-term care known as *Pioneer Models for Culture Change* (Box 7-3). In terms of long-term

Box 7-2   The Omnibus Budget Reconciliation Act (OBRA)

An understanding of OBRA standards is an absolute must for nursing assistants who work in nursing homes. As you read this book, look for the OBRA icon 🗹, which highlights key information related to this law. OBRA legislation is reviewed and passed by Congress each year. If you work in a nursing home, your employer may provide informational sessions to update the staff on new requirements. It is important for you to attend these sessions so that you can stay current on the most up-to-date information regarding your role in resident care.

Nursing homes are recognized as a new kind of business. There is an increase in the number of for-profit and chain facilities. Many facilities are poorly managed and provide poor care, and public concern grows.

1965–1970s

The Omnibus Budget Reconciliation Act (OBRA) of 1987 establishes standards that improve the quality of care and quality of life for residents of nursing homes. The culture change movement begins.

1987–1990

President Bill Clinton signs the Balanced Budget Act (BBA) of 1997, resulting in the most significant cut to the Medicare budget in the program's history and establishing the prospective payment system (PPS). Alternatives to nursing homes, such as assisted-living facilities, start to emerge. A small group of long-term care professionals meet to share ideas about the future of long-term care.

1997

1980s

The Institute of Medicine (IOM) studies nursing home care and reports unsatisfactory care and poor quality of life.

1990s

Health care costs are increasing at a rapid rate. To control costs, hospitals begin to discharge patients "sooner and sicker." Sub-acute care facilities that specialize in immediate post-acute care start to emerge.

2003

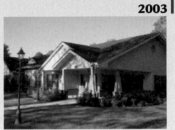

The first nursing homes are built following The Green House® Project model in Tupelo, Mississippi.

Photo courtesy of THE GREEN HOUSE® Project.

Box 7-3   Pioneer Models for Culture Change

Individualized Care. In this model, each resident's personal history is used as the basis for an individualized plan of care. The plan of care is based on an understanding of what has been important to the person throughout their life, and how the person wants to live life. Staff members are permanently assigned to residents to foster this individualized knowledge and understanding.

Regenerative Community. This model fosters a sense of community within a facility among residents, staff, families, and volunteers. It moves away from the traditional medical model, which focuses on tasks. Instead, the regenerative community model focuses on understanding and meeting needs. Focusing on each resident's strengths and abilities, regardless of their physical or mental status, is emphasized.

Resident-Directed Care. This model focuses on the idea of creating a "neighborhood." Neighborhoods are made up of small groups of residents who live in a home-like environment that has a kitchen, laundry facility, and family gathering room. Residents are

encouraged to contribute to daily routines related to daily life and the care of the facility (for example, gardening, helping to prepare meals, light housekeeping). This helps to provide a sense of meaning and purpose in their lives. Resident care is based on individual choice, rather than facility routine and schedules. This allows the resident more independence (for example, in bedtime, mealtime, and leisure activities).

The Eden Alternative®. This model also focuses on creating a sense of community. The surroundings are designed in a way to support life and eliminate loneliness, helplessness, and boredom. Plants and companion animals (such as birds, dogs, cats, and fish) are part of the facility environment. Daycare centers for children may be located on the same site. These features provide the residents with opportunities to participate in the care of the facility pets and environment and to enjoy the companionship of children. Staff members work together to ensure that the services provided meet each individual resident's needs and desires.

care, *culture change* is an ongoing process that focuses on changing attitudes, goals, and practices in order to improve the long-term care environment and the way care is delivered.

The Green House® project is representative of culture change in long-term care. It was founded in 2003 by Dr. Bill Thomas, the creator of The Eden Alternative®, to be a place of warmth and growth for residents and staff. The design of a Green House home is much like that of a private home. Only 7 to 12 residents live in each Green House home. Each resident has a private bedroom and bathroom. Because only 7 to 12 residents live in each Green House®, there are no long hallways, so many residents are able to get around without using wheelchairs. Other features of the house include a large common living area called "The Hearth" (which contains a fireplace, an open kitchen, and a dining area), a laundry area, and an open patio and outdoor garden (Fig. 7-7). Residents are encouraged to help in the preparation of meals, which are served at a large common table where residents and staff can eat together in a family-style arrangement. Daily routines are based on individual choice, just as if the person was in their own home. This helps to foster a greater sense of independence and individuality for residents.

The first Green House® project, built in Tupelo, Mississippi, has been very successful. Some of the problems that residents frequently experience in more traditional long-term care settings, such as urinary incontinence (an inability to control urination), unexplained weight loss, depression, and a decline in abilities, are seen less frequently among residents of

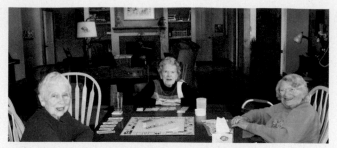

Figure 7-7 Residents of a Green House® home enjoy a board game together in the large common living area called "The Hearth." (*Photo courtesy of THE GREEN HOUSE® Project.*)

The Green House® homes. The Green House® model has other benefits as well. For example, nursing assistants receive additional education that enables them to make decisions and plan care. Nursing assistants are called *Shahbazim*, (a universal worker who performs housekeeping, laundry, cooking, and elder care) and their role is to protect and nurture the residents and each other. Staff turnover rates remain well below the national average, and there have been fewer work-related injuries.

These successes have gained attention. The Robert Wood Johnson Foundation, a major funding organization that is devoted to supporting education and research projects to improve health care, has provided a $10 million grant to help develop other Green House® homes. Today, there are hundreds of Green House homes open or under development across the United States, adding to a visionary future of long-term care.

SUMMARY

- The three major types of long-term care settings are nursing homes, assisted-living facilities, and CCRCs. Some consider adult day care and home health care services part of long-term care.
  - Nursing homes provide residents with around-the-clock nursing care and supervision.
  - Assisted-living facilities provide residents with limited assistance with certain tasks, such as meals and housekeeping.
  - CCRCs provide residents with multiple levels of services, ranging from independent living to nursing home care, all on the same campus.
- A long-term care facility can be "for profit" (operated with the intent of making money) or

"nonprofit" (operated with the intent of meeting a need in the community). A long-term care facility can be free-standing (independently owned and operated) or part of a chain (owned and operated by a corporation that owns and operates other similar facilities as well).

- Government agencies, as well as independent nonprofit organizations, provide oversight of the long-term care industry.
  - Nursing homes in the United States must follow federal, state, and local regulations. Currently, no federal laws govern assisted-living facilities; each state has its own regulations.
  - Independent nonprofit organizations set standards for health care organizations and grant

accreditation to organizations that meet them. Participation is voluntary.

- Long-term care is very costly and is not easily paid for by either the individual or the government.
  - Most people do not have adequate funds for long-term care. At an average cost of more than $6,000 per month for nursing home care, a lifetime of savings may not last very long.
  - Medicare coverage for nursing home care is minimal. Those qualifying must meet very strict criteria for skilled health care, and the coverage is limited. Medicare provides no payment for assisted-living care.
  - Medicaid pays for most nursing home care. This causes financial strain for both the facilities and the government, as the cost of care continues to rise. Medicaid usually does not pay for assisted-living care.

- Long-term care insurance is private insurance that can help pay for long-term care. Premiums are expensive, benefits may be limited, and the policyholder may never actually benefit from the policy.
- Only by understanding the past can we understand the present, and future, of long-term care.
  - In the past, long-term care in the United States had many problems. As a result, many people today still hold poor opinions of long-term care facilities (especially nursing homes).
  - Legislation, such as OBRA has greatly improved the quality of care provided in nursing homes.
  - Today, leaders in long-term care continue seeking ways to improve the long-term care environment and the way care is delivered.

WHAT DID YOU LEARN?

Multiple Choice

Select the single best answer for each of the following questions.

1. What is the name of the law that called for the biggest cut in the Medicare budget in history?
   a. Balanced Budget Act of 1997
   b. Deficit Reduction Act of 2005
   c. Omnibus Budget Reconciliation Act (OBRA) of 1987
   d. Social Security Act of 1935

2. Which one of the following is an insurance policy for long-term care that can be purchased by an individual?
   a. Long-term care insurance
   b. Medicaid
   c. Medicare
   d. Pension

3. How is most assisted-living care paid for?
   a. Medicaid
   b. Medicare
   c. Private pay
   d. Long-term care insurance

4. What did the members of the Pioneer Network do?
   a. They started a movement to get older people out of poorhouses in the late 1800s
   b. They met to share ideas and create a new vision for the future of long-term care
   c. They investigated nursing home care and wrote the report that led to the Omnibus Budget Reconciliation Act (OBRA) in 1987
   d. They developed the Social Security program in the 1930s

5. What is a benefit period?
   a. The period of time when a person receives nursing home care after using up all private funds
   b. The period of time when long-term care insurance benefits are paid out to a person who has purchased a policy
   c. The period of time when a person is eligible for Medicare benefits
   d. The period of time that Medicaid pays for a person's nursing home care

Matching   *Match each numbered item with its appropriate lettered description.*

_____ **1.** Pension

_____ **2.** For-profit facility

_____ **3.** Continuing care retirement community (CCRC)

_____ **4.** Poorhouse

_____ **5.** Centers for Medicare and Medicaid Services (CMS)

_____ **6.** Omnibus Budget Reconciliation Act (OBRA)

_____ **7.** Continuing Care Accreditation Commission (CCAC)

_____ **8.** Culture change

_____ **9.** Chain facility

_____ **10.** Continuum of care

a. A long-term care facility that provides multiple levels of care and multiple services on one campus

b. A facility that is operated with the intent of making money for the business owners

c. Community-supported facilities that provided shelter for those without the means of supporting themselves from the mid-1800s until the 1930s in the United States

d. The delivery of health care over time as a person moves from being independent to needing assistance with personal care, medical care, or both

e. A facility owned by a corporation that owns other similar facilities

f. An ongoing process that focuses on changing attitudes, goals, and practices in order to improve the long-term care environment and the way care is delivered

g. Tough regulations put into action to improve the quality of care and quality of life for residents of nursing homes

h. The government agency that provides oversight to ensure nursing home compliance with Omnibus Budget Reconciliation Act (OBRA) regulations

i. Monthly income provided to older Americans as a result of the Social Security Act of 1935

j. An organization that provides voluntary oversight of continuing care retirement communities (CCRCs) and offers accreditation to those meeting their quality standards

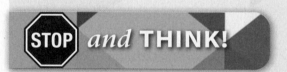

How would your life change if you had to take in an older, dependent family member because there were no other options available to provide care?

What difficulties would you encounter? What would be the benefits?

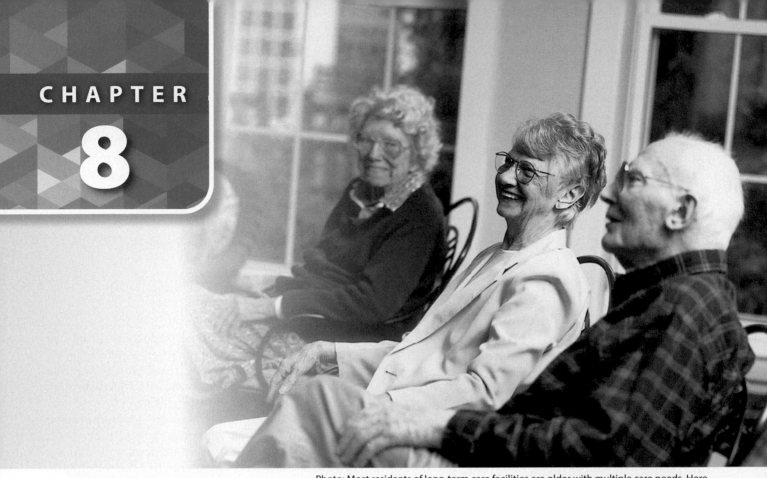

Photo: Most residents of long-term care facilities are older with multiple care needs. Here, a group of residents enjoy an activity together. (Photo courtesy of Copper Ridge.)

The Long-Term Care Resident

 WHAT WILL YOU LEARN?

In Chapter 6, you learned about human growth and development and meeting human needs. In this chapter, you will build on this knowledge by learning more specifically about the residents and the families that you will care for in the long-term care setting. As you begin your nursing assistant career in long-term care, it is important that you have knowledge about the people in this setting as well as their circumstances. Who are they? Why are they here? What do they need? When you can answer these questions, you will be better able to meet their needs. When you are finished with this chapter, you will be able to:

1. Discuss why the number of people 65 years and older living in the United States is increasing and the effect this could have on the long-term care industry.
2. Explain why a person might need long-term care.
3. Identify the expected length of stay for someone in long-term care.
4. Describe the challenges a person may face when admitted to a long-term care facility.
5. Describe the challenges a family may face when one of its members comes to live in a long-term care facility.
6. Explain how chronic illness can affect a person.

7. List reasons why a younger person might become a resident of a long-term care facility and some of the special considerations to take into account for their care.

8. Explain the importance of quality of life for long-term care residents and how assisting with activities helps to promote it.

Vocabulary

Chronic condition
Degenerative condition
Activities of daily living (ADLs)

Instrumental activities of daily living (IADLs)
Coexistent medical conditions

Cognitive impairment

OUR AGING POPULATION

According to a 2019 study conducted by the National Center for Health Statistics, there are over 65,600 regulated long-term care (LTC) facilities in the United States. These facilities currently care for approximately 8.3 million residents. People of all ages are cared for in LTC facilities, but most of the residents of LTC facilities are 65 years and older, with the highest number of people being 85 years and older. Although only about 4.1% of the older adult population resides in an LTC facility at any given time, a higher percentage will need some form of long-term care at some point in their lives; each year, the number of people living in the United States who are 65 years and older increases, and those 85 years and older are most likely to require care in an LTC facility. As a society, we need to be prepared to care for this growing segment of the population.

So, why is the number of older people in the United States steadily increasing each year? One major reason is advances in health care, which have made it possible for people to recover from (or continue to live with) conditions that at one time would have caused them to die because there were no treatments. For example, many people with acute heart conditions who have open heart surgery today would not have survived in the past because that treatment was not available. Similarly, in the early 1900s, the major cause of death in the United States was infectious disease, such as tuberculosis, influenza, and pneumonia. Because of advances in public health and medical care, we have significantly reduced the risk of death from these diseases. Public sanitation and hygiene are better now, reducing the spread of infection. Antibiotics, which were not generally available before the 1940s, made treatment of infection possible, thus reducing the risk of death. Once the risk of death from infection was reduced, more people had a chance to live longer.

Conditions that are now considered chronic or degenerative might have also caused a person to die sooner in the past. A **chronic condition** is one that is ongoing and often needs to be controlled through continuous medication or treatment (for example, diabetes, heart failure, or hypertension). A **degenerative condition** is one that gets progressively worse over time (for example, arthritis or dementia). Today, we have medications and treatments that help people to live with chronic or degenerative conditions, while in the past we did not.

These changes are reflected in our current population. We have large numbers of people who are living longer lives, but with chronic conditions. According to government figures, 80% of all people 65 years and older have at least one chronic condition, and 50% have at least two. Keep in mind that these figures describe the general population, not just the segment of the population living in long-term care. As more and more people live longer lives, many with one or more chronic conditions, the need for LTC services will increase.

FACTORS LEADING TO LONG-TERM CARE ADMISSIONS

There are several reasons why a person might be admitted to an LTC facility. Specifically, a person may be admitted to an LTC facility because:

- They need to recover on a temporary basis from the lingering effects of an acute illness (such as a stroke) or injury (such as a broken hip).
- They need continuous monitoring and treatment as a result of one or more chronic conditions.
- They need help meeting their physical needs as a result of a degenerative condition.
- It is no longer safe for the person to live on their own, due to physical or mental impairment (or both).

Short-Stay Admissions

The use of LTC facilities for short-stay admissions (3 months or less) has been steadily increasing. As discussed in Chapter 1, this increase in short stays is primarily due to changes in how health care is paid for, which lead hospitals to discharge patients "quicker and sicker." Many of these patients are admitted to LTC facilities to receive the care they need until they are well enough to return home. Providing this care in an LTC facility instead of in a hospital saves government insurance programs significant money and thus helps to control overall health care spending.

Extended-Stay Admissions

Although the use of LTC facilities for short-stay admissions has been increasing, most people cared for in LTC facilities are there for longer periods of time (1 year or more). However, it is important to recognize that of all the people 65 years and older living in the United States, only 4.1% require some type of long-term care. If most older people are able to live in the community, what are the factors that make LTC admission necessary?

People come to live in LTC facilities because they have physical or mental impairments that make it impossible for them to care for themselves properly. Many times, the level of care they require is beyond what family members are able to provide, or there simply are no family members to provide care.

Most residents of LTC facilities need help with routine tasks of daily life, called **activities of daily living (ADLs)**. These tasks include bathing, dressing, eating, moving, and toileting (Fig. 8-1). At least 75% of LTC residents need help with three or more of their ADLs. **Instrumental activities of daily living (IADLs)** are more complex tasks that a person must be able to do in order to continue living independently, such as using the telephone, handling money, and obtaining groceries and preparing meals. About

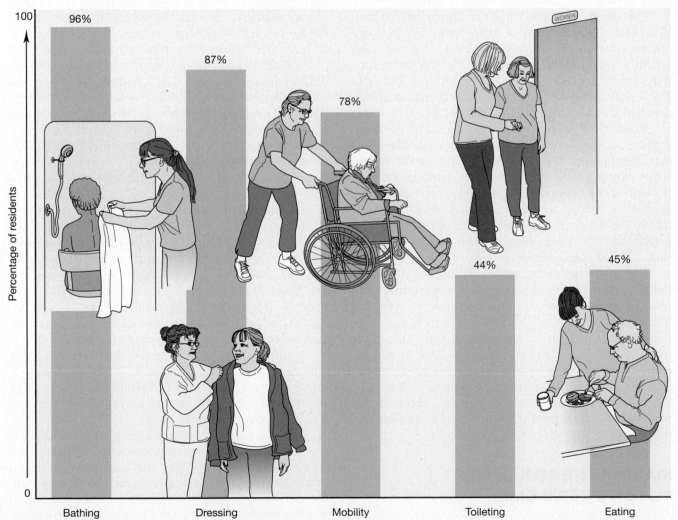

Figure 8-1 Most residents need help with their activities of daily living (ADLs) such as bathing, dressing, moving, toileting, and eating.

75% of LTC residents need help with at least some IADLs, and more than 50% need help with all of them. Several factors can cause a person to need help with their ADLs and IADLs:

- Medical conditions or the effects of aging can affect the person's strength, endurance, or coordination.
- Medical conditions that affect a person's ability to think and remember (such as dementia) can cause the person to forget how to do these routine tasks.
- Sensory deficits, such as impaired vision or hearing, can make it harder for the person to function independently.

It is very common for a resident to have **coexistent medical conditions** (more than one medical condition at the same time). For example, the person might have both an acute and a chronic condition. Or, the person could have more than one chronic condition. Nearly all residents of LTC facilities have more than one medical condition at the time of admission. More than half of them have three or more.

The most common medical conditions among LTC residents are cardiovascular disease, respiratory disease, stroke, dementia, depression, diabetes, and arthritis. These are all examples of chronic conditions that require continuous medical monitoring and care. These conditions may also significantly impact a resident's ability to perform ADLs and IADLs.

Cognitive impairment (problems processing, learning, or remembering information), especially when it is accompanied by physical problems, is the reason why many people come to live in LTC facilities. Seventy percent of the residents in long-term care have either short-term or long-term memory loss, or both. Almost half of the residents have some form of dementia (the permanent and progressive loss of mental functions caused by damage to the brain tissue).

Nursing assistants are responsible for providing most hands-on care in the LTC setting. In many instances, the resident requires special consideration when receiving that care, often due to advanced age. You will see sections titled "Concerns for Long-Term Care" throughout this textbook that will point out areas of special consideration related to the topic being discussed. Pay special attention to these concerns. Your role as a caregiver in this type of health care setting is very important and you have the opportunity to improve the comfort and quality of life for each person you care for.

MAKING THE ADJUSTMENT TO LONG-TERM CARE

The move to an LTC facility is often preceded by some crisis, such as an unexpected accident or illness. For example, an older widow living alone may have a stroke. Suddenly, she is taken from her home to the hospital for intensive medical care. She needs extensive rehabilitation that the hospital cannot provide, so she is transferred to a skilled nursing facility for that care. Despite months of therapy, she is unable to regain enough self-care skills to live independently anymore. Living with her son or daughter is not an option because their homes are not set up for someone with a disability and besides, no one is at home during the day. Without much time for emotional preparation, this woman must adjust to the loss of her independence and the loss of her home. Her son and daughter must also adjust to the changes brought on by their mother's stroke.

Consider a different situation. Perhaps an older man is living with family members because he has dementia and diabetes. He is no longer able to take care of any of his own needs. As the dementia progresses, he becomes more and more difficult to care for. The family struggles to get him to take his medication. He is no longer able to find the bathroom and has begun to urinate in inappropriate places throughout the house. His odd behaviors are scaring the grandchildren. He requires supervision 24 hours a day. He has wandered away from home several times, once in the middle of the night. The last time the police had to be called to help find him. The family is exhausted and family relationships are suffering. The family can no longer continue to provide the care that the man needs so they decide to admit him to an LTC facility. Even though this situation is not as sudden as the situation described in the first example, there is still a crisis (in this case, calling the police for assistance in locating him) that spurs action toward LTC placement.

Can you imagine what it would be like if you suffered an unexpected injury or medical crisis that made it impossible for you to return home? Perhaps someone else made the decision about where you would live, and you did not even get a say in the matter. This happens frequently—most residents are "placed" in the LTC facility; they do not choose to come live there. How would you feel? How would you react?

Similarly, how would you feel if you were the one who had to make the decision to admit your parent, sibling, spouse, partner, or child to an LTC facility? Would it be a hard decision to make? Would you feel a sense of loss or possibly guilt?

When a person comes to live in an LTC facility, it is often a difficult adjustment for both them and their family members (Fig. 8-2). As a nursing assistant, there are many things that you can do to help ease the transition to long-term care for both the resident and the family (Box 8-1). Let's take a closer look at the impact admission to an LTC facility can have on both the resident and the family.

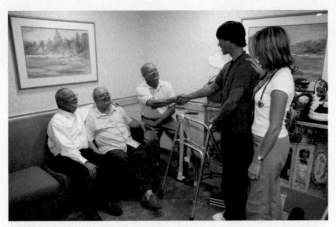

Figure 8-2 Being admitted to a long-term care facility is often stressful for the resident, as well as their family members. As a nursing assistant, it is important for you to take steps to make the transition easier for everyone. The first step is understanding what the resident and family may be feeling.

The Resident

Most people do not *plan* to come live in an LTC facility, and to be honest, it is not something most people *want* to do. People do not choose illness or infirmity. All of us, given the choice, would prefer to remain healthy and in our own homes.

Many of your residents are coping with multiple losses and life changes. For example, in the case of the widow who suffered a stroke, she must not only cope with the loss of her home, but with the fact that her body no longer functions as it used to. She has to relearn many tasks that she took for granted before. The man with dementia from the second example is thoroughly confused in his new environment. He is unable to understand the reason for the change, and he does not recognize anything or anybody. How upsetting and frightening this must be!

Box 8-1 Helping Residents and Family Members Adjust

- Be knowledgeable about the resident's condition.
- Be knowledgeable about the circumstances that necessitated the move to the long-term care facility.
- Know your resident. Learn about their likes, dislikes, relationships, and interests.
- Allow the resident to make choices about their care.
- Be sensitive to both resident and family needs.
- Be flexible!
- Welcome family members and include them in the resident's care when appropriate.
- Be sensitive to the resident's environment. Accommodate needs for privacy.

Residents of LTC facilities often have many fears and anxieties. They may worry about how their medical problems will affect their health and independence in the future. Because long-term care is expensive, they may have concerns about finances. They worry about how the move to the LTC facility will affect their family members, and they may be sad to be separated from them.

The LTC environment itself can be frightening and uncomfortable, full of strange noises and smells and unfamiliar people. The resident must learn to develop trusting relationships with many new people under very difficult circumstances. Imagine what it would be like to have staff members you do not know well asking personal questions about your life, poking and prodding your body with strange equipment, or seeing and touching private parts of your body during care. Staff, and sometimes even other residents, come into your room and handle your personal belongings. People may be coming in and out of your room at all hours of the day and night. You might find it disheartening to be surrounded by so many other people in various stages of sickness and disability.

Moving to an LTC facility means having to give up your home. Think about your own home. What does it mean to you? What makes it home? What are your favorite belongings? What is your favorite thing to do at home? Now, imagine having to give that up. Your new home will be a room that you may have to share with someone you do not know. Since space is limited, you will have to leave most of your belongings behind. What would you bring with you? Do you think that will make your new room feel like home? What would you miss the most?

Moving to an LTC facility also means having to adjust to the loss of a certain amount of independence. It means not being able to do whatever you want to do, whenever you want to do it. You may have to adapt your usual routines to your new situation. How difficult will it be for you to do the things that you are used to doing in a different place, with different people, and perhaps on a different schedule?

People who become residents of LTC facilities often feel that they are at the mercy of the health care industry. While some are cheerful, compliant, and grateful, others may be depressed, angry, anxious, or unpleasant. You must understand that residents will not always see you as an "angel of mercy" who is there to provide help. To some residents, you may be an unwelcome reminder of all the things they can no longer do! When you must care for a resident who makes you wish you had never chosen to be a nursing assistant (and you can be certain you *will* encounter residents like this), stop and think for a moment about the reasons that person may be acting out of sorts. When you look beyond the illness or condition, past the technical duties and procedures, and into that person's eyes, you will find your reason for choosing to be a nursing assistant … a *person* who needs you very much.

The Family

Admitting a family member to an LTC facility is often a traumatic event for the family as well as for the person who is actually being admitted. Like the resident, the family may have a hard time adjusting to the fact that admission to an LTC facility is necessary. They may be struggling to accept the change in the resident's condition that made admission to long-term care necessary in the first place. It may be difficult for them to accept that their loved one is in declining health or is no longer able to be independent. Finally, family members do not always get along with each other. When this is the case, it may be hard for the family members to agree on a course of action, especially when they are under stress, and this can lead to conflict within the family. Also, keep in mind that some family members may take out their stress on the person being admitted to the facility, leading to abuse. Family members struggle with many things when a loved one is admitted to an LTC facility, including changing roles within the family, giving up the responsibility of "primary caregiver," and losing a life partner.

Adjusting to Changing Roles Within the Family

Within a family, each family member has familiar and expected roles. For example, imagine that your mother has had a stroke. As a result, she can no longer talk. Your mother has always been the person that you could tell your troubles to. She has always had words of wisdom for you and sound advice about what to do. Now that she is unable to talk, who do you turn to for needed advice in difficult times? How will what has happened change your relationship with your mother?

A decline in health or function for any one member of the family often disrupts expected roles and relationships for all of the family. Many adult children experience "role reversal" as their parents become more dependent, meaning in a way, the child becomes the parent and the parent becomes the child. We are used to our parents caring for *us*. It is physically and emotionally difficult to assume basic care for a parent. Sometimes the change in roles causes problems among other members of the family. If there are several children in a family with older parents, it often happens that one child assumes primary responsibility for the parent's care. This can lead to resentment and jealousy among siblings. If you are the child who takes on the primary responsibility for caring for a parent, perhaps you are angry that your siblings are not doing their fair share and that you have such a heavy burden. If you are not the child who takes on primary caregiving responsibility, perhaps you feel jealous of the close relationship that the caregiving sibling seems to have with your parent. Caregiving responsibilities take a lot of time, and sometimes even financial resources, away from other family members. This can also create tension, conflict, and stress within the family.

As you can see, admission of a family member to an LTC facility affects the whole family. Family members may look to you for direction and support. (Unfortunately, some will also look to you as a target for their stress and frustration.) As a nursing assistant, it is your responsibility to care for the resident as well as the family.

Giving Up the Role of "Primary Caregiver"

You might think that admitting a loved one to an LTC facility is a relief to family members because it relieves them of their caregiving responsibilities. In reality, it is not a relief, just a change. Family members must learn to trust other people—usually people they do not know—with providing care for their loved one. This is not always easy, no matter how competent and caring the staff may be! To further complicate matters, because many admissions to long-term care are brought on by a crisis like a medical emergency, often the choice of facility is made rapidly. In this situation, the family may not feel like they had time to make the best decision.

Family members often feel guilty about not being able to provide care themselves. They may feel like they have let their loved one down. Because they are no longer in control of the care being provided, some family members may assume the role of "watchdog" to monitor the quality of care being given. Family members who provided care to their loved one before the person was admitted to the LTC facility usually have a great deal of knowledge about how to care for the person. Adjusting to a new role (that of "visitor" instead of "primary caregiver") may be particularly difficult for these family members. When the family member tries to share knowledge about the resident's care with a staff member, the staff member may feel that the family member is interfering or lacks confidence in their abilities. This may create tension and conflict between the family and the staff.

Families want to see that staff members are interested in their loved one as a human being. They expect staff members to ask questions about their loved one's preferences and dislikes. They want to feel as if their input provides the staff with welcome and valuable knowledge. As a nursing assistant, you can help family members adjust by making them feel included and involved in their loved one's ongoing care (Fig. 8-3).

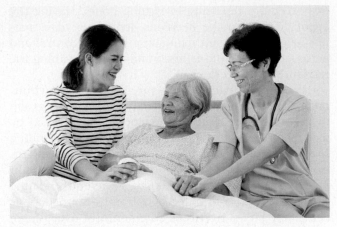

Figure 8-3 As a nursing assistant, you can help family members adjust by helping them to feel included and involved in the ongoing care of their loved one. (*StudioByTheSea\Shutterstock.com*)

Losing a Life Partner

For couples, admission of one partner to an LTC facility can be particularly difficult, for both the partner who is left behind and for the partner who is moving to the facility. No longer being able to live together can trigger a tremendous sense of loss for both partners. The need to share intimate moments with a life partner, whether sexual or not, is important throughout one's entire life. As a nursing assistant, you can help to make the transition easier by ensuring that couples have privacy during their visit.

LIVING WITH A CHRONIC CONDITION

As you have learned, most residents have one or more chronic conditions. A chronic condition affects our self-image (how we see or feel about ourselves). Many people with chronic conditions find it difficult to accept that their bodies no longer function as they did. Some people have a "Why me?" attitude. Others are thankful for what they can still do or experience.

A chronic condition often affects how others act toward the person with the condition. Some people become overprotective. This may cause problems with roles and relationships, particularly if the person does not want to be treated any differently. The opposite can also happen; the person with the chronic condition may let others do everything for them, when in reality they are capable of doing many things independently. This can also cause problems with relationships, as those around the person with the chronic condition become frustrated and impatient.

Medications for a chronic condition are usually taken over a very long period of time. The person may have to learn to live with unpleasant side effects. In many instances, numerous medications may interact with each other, causing serious complications. Some people have a hard time accepting the fact that they must take medication every day, sometimes multiple times a day, in order to prevent acute symptoms. In addition, many medications are very expensive, particularly for people who are living on a fixed income. Worrying about how to pay for medication can be a source of stress.

Living with a chronic condition often necessitates making lifestyle changes that are not always welcome. For example, a person with diabetes must change the way they eat. The person may have to begin to exercise, an activity they might not enjoy. A person with a cardiovascular or respiratory disease should stop smoking, but they may not want to or be able to. Making changes to the way we live can be difficult even when we *want* to make these changes. Imagine how it must feel to be told that you *must* make these changes, or risk further health problems.

It is common for people with chronic conditions to experience problems with mental health. Some see the disease as taking over their lives and become angry, frustrated, or depressed. Some will just continue to deny that they have the disease. Some chronic conditions, such as arthritis, are painful. Living with pain can disrupt a person's life. Constant pain or discomfort reduces a person's physical abilities and limits the person's ability to interact socially with others and is, therefore, often associated with depression. The battle for pain relief may become the primary focus of every single day!

For a person with a chronic condition, there will be good days when the person feels well and there will be bad days when symptoms make it hard to function. This can become very tiresome for the person. The person may have to be hospitalized repeatedly for acute flare-ups. The person may worry about the outcome of these flare-ups. For example, the person may wonder if they will be able to regain the same level of function that they had before, or whether they will have to adjust to a reduced level of health or function.

As a nursing assistant, it is important to understand the roller-coaster ride of living with a chronic condition. You cannot expect your residents to perform at the same level every day. You must adapt to their good and bad days by being flexible with your approach and the amount of assistance that you provide. Knowledge of each resident's *conditions* will help you understand that resident's struggles and limitations. Knowledge of each *resident* will help you understand the resident's strengths and triumphs. Your encouragement and support can help your residents maintain their sense of self and their dignity, despite any limitations caused by disease.

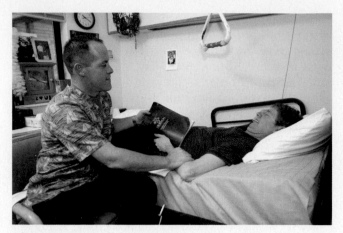

Figure 8-4 Not all residents are older adults.

THE YOUNG RESIDENT

Although most people living in LTC facilities are 65 years of age or older, younger people receive long-term care as well. You may care for residents who are in their 20s, 30s, or 40s (Fig. 8-4). (Children and adolescents with severe disabilities may also require long-term care, but usually they are cared for in LTC facilities that specialize in the care of children and adolescents.) Traumatic injuries (such as severe brain and spinal cord injuries), degenerative neurologic conditions (such as multiple sclerosis), and developmental disabilities (such as cerebral palsy or Down syndrome) are reasons why a younger person may require long-term care.

For many younger residents, the disease or injury that results in the need for long-term care is an unexpected life event. As you learned in Chapter 6, people in their 20s to 40s are often busy completing their educations, starting or advancing in their careers, and possibly finding life partners and starting families. Can you imagine what it would be like to have your life upended by disease or injury and to find yourself living in a facility where most of the other residents are significantly older than you are?

Understandably, many younger residents experience anger, frustration, and depression. It may take a younger person a lot longer to adjust to placement in an LTC facility. Younger residents may feel like they have lost all control over their lives. As a result, younger residents may "act out" (for example, by breaking rules, using foul language, or making unrealistic demands) in an effort to gain some kind of control over their situation. When caring for a younger resident, you will need to have empathy and patience. Be flexible, and give the person opportunities to exercise personal choice whenever possible. Ask the younger resident how they would like to plan the day, and try to accommodate these wishes. For example, a younger resident may want to stay up later at night and sleep later in the morning,

or have more flexibility in visiting hours. Having the opportunity to make decisions about everyday matters helps the resident maintain a sense of control and personal identity and is important for maintaining the resident's self-esteem.

Because younger residents are living in an environment that is generally not reflective of their age group or interests, special accommodations will need to be made. For example, food choices often differ according to age. A younger person living in an LTC setting might want pizza, subs, or spicy foods, while an older person might prefer more traditional fare. Preferences relating to activities will also differ significantly. Younger residents may prefer electronic entertainment over Bingo, and popular music over Frank Sinatra. They may enjoy action and thriller movies more than classic movies. Scheduling a movie and pizza night for a younger resident or providing head phones so they can listen to their own choice of music are examples of ways to meet the unique needs of a younger resident.

Younger residents still need to connect with life outside of the facility. Looking stylish and dressing in an age-appropriate manner is just as important for many younger residents as it is for you. If complete flexibility with clothing choices is not possible because of the resident's physical or medical needs, jazzing up sweat suits, pajamas, or hospital gowns with modern accessories or jewelry may help younger residents feel a connection with their peers. Phone and computer access can help younger residents keep up with the outside world, and a pleasant area where younger residents can "hang out" with friends should be available (Fig. 8-5). If the resident is able, it may even be possible for the resident to participate in some activities outside of the facility, such as attending club meetings, sporting events, or taking a class. Helping a younger resident find ways to enjoy and participate in life and interests outside of the facility greatly enhances the

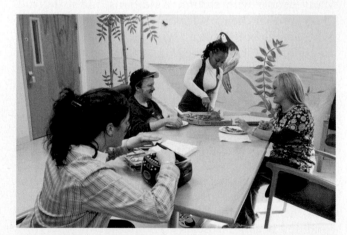

Figure 8-5 Providing opportunities for younger residents to enjoy the same things that others their age enjoy can greatly improve the younger resident's quality of life.

resident's quality of life and provides a sense of hope for the future.

Being involved in life outside of the LTC facility also includes being involved in family life. Being separated is hard on all members of the family. Family members' roles usually have to change when one member of the family is absent from the home. For example, when one parent is admitted to an LTC facility, the children may need to assume more responsibility in the home to help the other parent keep things running smoothly. Family relationships can be strained by these changes. Family members at home may even feel "abandoned" by the family member who was admitted to the LTC facility. Finding ways to help the resident continue to participate in family life is very important. Providing for phone and e-mail access, ensuring that a private space is available for family visits, and encouraging the family to participate in events held at the facility are all measures you can take to help maintain connections among family members.

As you learned in Chapter 6, sexuality and intimacy are basic human needs for everyone, young and old. Younger residents face many of the same challenges older residents face in meeting these needs. For young residents who are married or in a committed relationship, admission to an LTC facility disrupts the normal intimate relationship between the two partners. Other young residents will not be married or in committed relationships, but will still have the need to establish and maintain intimate relationships with others. In an LTC environment, it can be especially difficult for a younger resident to find someone to develop an intimate relationship with, and privacy can be an issue. As a nursing assistant, you will need to recognize the importance of sexual expression as part of the human experience and take measures to help your younger residents meet their needs related to sexuality and intimacy.

Caring for a younger resident can pose some unique challenges for a nursing assistant. Sometimes a younger resident may take out their anger on you because you are the same age, but you still have a so-called "normal" life. You may find it emotionally difficult to take care of someone who is close to your own age. The feeling that "this could be me" can be very frightening. You may also find it difficult to maintain professional boundaries. Younger residents often interact more with staff members than with the other older residents or even with their friends outside of the facility. As a result, a younger resident may interpret your professional interest and caring as a sign of personal friendship, and become interested in developing a personal, or even a sexual, relationship with you. Although it is important for you to have a friendly and warm attitude toward all of your residents, you must make sure that you keep your relationships with your residents professional at all times.

QUALITY OF LIFE IN THE LONG-TERM CARE SETTING

Quality of life has to do with getting satisfaction and comfort from the way we are living. As you recall, the Omnibus Budget Reconciliation Act (OBRA) was put into place to protect residents' quality of life. As you have learned, the changes a person experiences when faced with being admitted to an LTC facility take away many of the things that they felt gave life quality. Many factors contribute to quality of life, including:

- The ability to be free from physical and emotional discomfort.
- The ability to make decisions for oneself, based on one's own personal values and sense of what is best for oneself.
- The ability to engage in activities that one finds enjoyable.

When you take a humanistic approach to health care, you help to ensure that your residents enjoy a good quality of life. Respecting residents' rights, as outlined in the Residents' Rights portion of OBRA, also helps to protect your residents' quality of life.

Activities

In order to enjoy a good quality of life, we must get pleasure from life. One of the ways that we get pleasure from life is by engaging in hobbies or activities that interest us. An *activity* is a hobby or pursuit (pastime) that engages the mind, body, or both. Participating in activities that we enjoy benefits us physically as well as mentally; it provides an outlet for our creativity, prevents boredom, reduces stress, improves sleep, and allows us to feel a sense of purpose and accomplishment. Many activities also give us the opportunity to interact with people who share similar interests, so they help us to meet our need to socialize with others.

Because participation in activities has so many benefits, and is so important for maintaining quality of life, OBRA specifies that LTC facilities must provide for meaningful activity for residents (Fig. 8-6). The activity program must include a variety of activities that allow residents to socialize with others and pursue personal interests.

The activity program of an LTC facility is developed and managed by the Activities (or Therapeutic Recreation) Department. However, all staff members

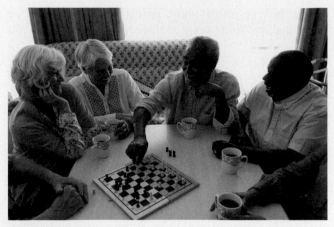

Figure 8-6 Activities provide entertainment and an opportunity to socialize with others. (*wavebreakmedia\ Shutterstock.com*)

play an important role in making sure that each resident has the opportunity to participate in activities that provide pleasure and increase the resident's satisfaction with their quality of life. As a nursing assistant, you will support the facility's activity staff by ensuring that residents are ready on time for scheduled activities (for example, by helping residents select and put on appropriate clothing and assisting residents with toileting before the activity begins), and by helping to transport residents to the area where the activity is taking place.

Not all activities must be coordinated through the Activities Department. As a nursing assistant, you can also help residents enjoy activities throughout the day. Some activities, such as reading to the resident from a favorite book or playing a game of cards together, will require you to set aside some special time. Other activities can just be worked into your normal routine. For example, it is easy to ask a resident what the score is and cheer along for their favorite team when they are watching a ballgame on TV or sing along with a resident who is listening to their favorite tunes.

Many residents will express the need to feel useful, rather than just sitting around watching other people work. While it is not acceptable to require a resident to perform work in a facility, it is acceptable to allow a resident to help wipe tables, water plants, and perform other simple chores on the unit, if that is what the resident wants to do. Productive activities like this often do a great deal to help boost a resident's self-esteem and sense of worth. The resident's desire to assist with chores on the unit should be documented appropriately in the resident's care plan, so that it is clear that the resident's participation in these sorts of activities is voluntary.

SUMMARY

- The population of the United States is aging.
  - People are living longer because of improvements in public health and advances in medical care and technology. The number of people 65 years and older is increasing each year.
  - One third to one half of all people aged 65 years and older will need long-term care. People 85 years and older are the most likely to require long-term care.
- Medical need, triggered by acute, chronic, or degenerative illness, often necessitates long-term care. Most residents have three or more coexistent medical conditions.
- Most people who live in LTC facilities need help with ADLs and IADLs because of physical or mental impairment, or both.
  - At least 75% of residents need help with three or more ADLs such as bathing, dressing, moving, eating, and toileting.

- At least 75% of residents need help with at least some IADLs, such as using the telephone or paying bills.
- Adjusting to admission to an LTC facility is difficult for both the person being admitted and their family.
  - Adjustment is complicated by the fact that admission to an LTC facility is often necessitated by a crisis, such as an unexpected illness or injury.
  - The resident must adjust to changes in their health at the same time that they are learning to adjust to a new home.
  - The loss of privacy and independence is very difficult.
  - The resident must learn to trust new people in new surroundings.
  - Not everyone learns to adapt to these changes in a positive way.

- Admission is often just as traumatic for the family as it is for the resident.
    - Family members must adjust to their loved one's health status and new surroundings.
    - Family roles and relationships change when a loved one moves to a long-term care facility.
    - Family members may have a hard time learning how to be "visitors." Their tendency to monitor the quality of care and attempts to share information may lead to conflict and tension with staff.
    - Families need to be welcomed and included to the best extent possible.
    - Families expect facility staff to show interest in their family member as a person.
    - Provision of privacy for family visits is essential, particularly for couples.
- Most residents of LTC facilities are living with one or more chronic health conditions.
    - Chronic conditions affect how we feel about ourselves and how other people feel about us.
    - The strain of living with a chronic condition can affect mental health.
    - Physical health and functioning can be variable and unpredictable. Nursing assistants must adapt care approaches to accommodate the person's "good days" and "bad days."
    - Knowledge of both the disease as well as the person is necessary to help the person with a chronic condition maintain their sense of self and dignity.
- Although people 65 years and older make up most of the population, younger people may also live in LTC facilities. Give the younger resident the opportunity to socialize with peers, engage in age-appropriate activities, and connect with the world outside of the facility.
- We are responsible for helping our residents maintain a good quality of life.
    - Participating in enjoyable activities benefits residents physically, emotionally, and socially, and contributes to their overall quality of life.

WHAT DID YOU LEARN?

Multiple Choice

Select the single best answer for each of the following questions.

1. Which of the following is a reason why people are living longer than they ever have before?
   a. Advances in public health and medical care
   b. Antibiotics
   c. Improvements in public sanitation and hygiene
   d. All of the above

2. As more people live into old age, you would expect:
   a. All of them to need long-term care
   b. An increase in long-term care use
   c. A decrease in long-term care use
   d. No change in long-term care use

3. Most residents of LTC facilities fall into what age group?
   a. Younger than 65 years
   b. 65 to 74 years
   c. 75 to 84 years
   d. 85 years and older

4. Mrs. Papadopoulos was admitted to the Golden Harvest Nursing Center following a fall that resulted in a broken hip. She had been living alone in her own home, where she had lived for more than 50 years. She could not return home because she experienced complications from her broken hip and was unable to regain her ability to walk. She cried a lot when she was first admitted to the facility and often was impatient with the staff. What could be the cause of these behaviors?
   a. Mrs. Papadopoulos' LTC admission occurred with little warning or preparation
   b. Mrs. Papadopoulos had to cope with multiple changes and losses at one time
   c. Mrs. Papadopoulos had to get used to being cared for by people she did not know
   d. All of the above

5. Mrs. Papadopoulos has been a resident at the Golden Harvest Nursing Center for almost 2 years. You know that this length of stay is:
   a. Typical for most LTC facility residents
   b. Unusual (most people stay for 3 months or less)
   c. Longer than most stays (the average stay is 6 months to 1 year)
   d. Shorter than most stays (the average stay is 2.5 years or more)

6. Which of the following are reasons that someone might need long-term care?
   a. The family can no longer provide for care at home
   b. The person needs to recover from the lingering effects of an acute accident or illness
   c. The person is no longer able to care for themselves
   d. All of the above

7. Which of the following statements about family members' reactions to a loved one's LTC admission is NOT true?
   a. Family members are relieved, knowing that they no longer have to worry about the person
   b. Family members must adjust to changes in roles and relationships
   c. Family members often feel guilty about admitting a loved one to an LTC facility
   d. Family members may not trust staff members to provide adequate or proper care

8. Which of the following is true about the challenges a person must face when living with a chronic condition?
   a. The chronic condition changes how the person feels about themselves and how others feel about them
   b. The person must adapt to repeated episodes of illness
   c. The person may have to make lifestyle changes to control the chronic condition
   d. All of the above

9. A younger resident may live in an LTC facility because of:
   a. A spinal cord injury from a diving accident
   b. A developmental disability
   c. Progressive multiple sclerosis
   d. All of the above

10. Most of the residents at Seaside Village Nursing Home are "typical," in that they are older people. However, today Mr. Leroy, a 35-year-old married father of two with progressive multiple sclerosis, was admitted to Seaside Village. To meet Mr. Leroy's needs, staff members at Seaside Village should:
   a. Help Mr. Leroy to stay connected with his family and friends outside of the facility
   b. Make a special effort to plan activities of interest to someone Mr. Leroy's age
   c. Recognize that Mr. Leroy may have difficulty coping emotionally as a result of his admission to Seaside Village
   d. All of the above

Matching *Match each numbered item with its appropriate lettered description.*

_____ **1.** Acute illness

_____ **2.** Chronic condition

_____ **3.** Degenerative condition

_____ **4.** Activities of daily living (ADLs)

_____ **5.** Instrumental activities of daily living (IADLs)

_____ **6.** Coexistent medical conditions

_____ **7.** Cognitive impairment

a. Problems processing, learning, or remembering information

b. A condition that gets progressively worse over time

c. Examples include dressing, eating, bathing, toileting, and moving

d. More than one illness at the same time in the same person

e. A condition that is ongoing

f. Examples include using the telephone and balancing a checkbook

g. An unexpected illness with a rapid onset and a relatively short recovery time

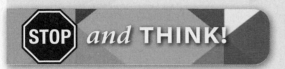

- You are working the day shift on a very busy day. One of your coworkers went home sick so everyone had to pick up the care for additional residents. You are behind in your work, and the charge nurse has just told you that Ms. Wilkins, a new resident, is arriving any minute and you have been assigned to her care. You wish the charge nurse would have told you this earlier. There is only an hour left on your shift, and you have to leave on time because you have a doctor's appointment after work. You still need to answer Mr. Diaz's call light, and now you see Ms. Wilkins arriving in a wheelchair. How are you feeling about this new admission? What mood will you be in when you enter Ms. Wilkins' room to greet her? If you are not careful, what impression could you give Ms. Wilkins and her family members? What impression do you want to give Ms. Wilkins and her family members?

- After helping Mr. Diaz, you enter Ms. Wilkins' room and greet her. She is very quiet. You ask Ms. Wilkins a few questions to get to know her, and she replies, "What do you want to know for?" As you begin to put Ms. Wilkins' belongings away, she questions you about what you are doing and then says, "Leave those alone! Those are mine!" You explain how the call light control works and ask Ms. Wilkins to use it when she needs help to go to the bathroom. You notice that Mr. Diaz's call light is on again, so you go across the hall to help him. When you return to Ms. Wilkins' room, you find her alone in the bathroom, barefoot, and without her walker. There is urine on the floor. You ask Ms. Wilkins why she didn't put her call light on, and she tells you that she did not know about the call light. How are you feeling about Ms. Wilkins? What might be some reasons that she is acting this way? What could you do to make Ms. Wilkins' adjustment to her new environment easier?

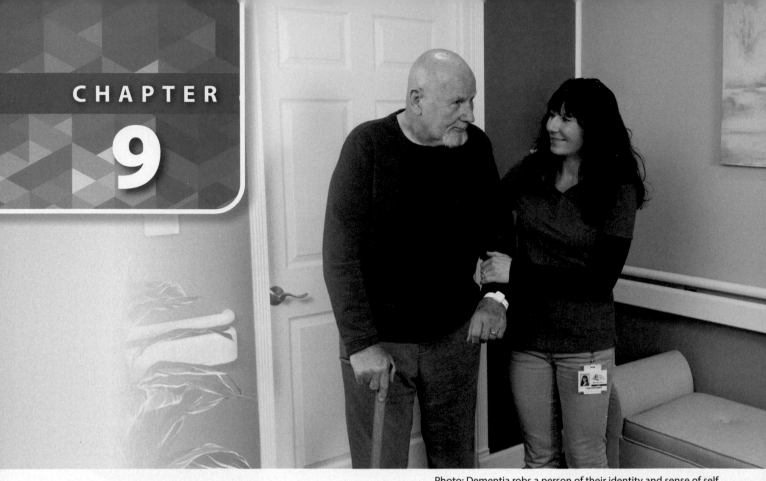

Photo: Dementia robs a person of their identity and sense of self.
(Courtesy of STANLEY Healthcare, Waltham, MA.)

Caring for People With Dementia

 WHAT WILL YOU LEARN?

Can you imagine what it would be like to know that there is something terribly wrong with your ability to remember or to think? For example, you are out to lunch with friends and when the check comes, you can't remember how to figure out the tip. Or you leave your house to go to the grocery store, a place you have been many times before, and you can't remember how to get home. Or you can't remember the middle name of the person you have been married to for the last 40 years. For a person with dementia, a frightening experience like this is often the first sign that something is wrong. Dementia, which is caused by changes in the brain tissue, affects a person's ability to remember and think. As the disorder progresses, the person loses the ability to perform even the most basic tasks related to self-care. Dementia is devastating, both for the person who has it and for their family members.

More than 50% of the residents in long-term care facilities are there because they have dementia and are no longer able to care for themselves. In this chapter, you will learn about some of the causes of dementia and the special care needs of people with dementia. When you are finished with this chapter, you will be able to:

1. **Explain the difference between dementia and delirium.**
2. **Describe the three major stages of dementia.**
3. **Describe four major causes of dementia.**

4. List and define the "four As" of dementia: amnesia, aphasia, agnosia, and apraxia.
5. Describe behaviors that are common in people with dementia.
6. Discuss strategies for managing difficult behaviors in people with dementia.
7. List special considerations to keep in mind while helping a person with dementia with activities of daily living (ADLs), such as bathing, eating, and toileting.
8. Describe special care measures to take to help maintain quality of life for a person with dementia.
9. Discuss the effects of caring for a person with dementia on the caregiver, and strategies for coping.

Vocabulary

Dementia	Lewy body dementia	Aphasia	Catastrophic reaction
Delirium	Frontotemporal	Agnosia	Sundowning
Alzheimer disease	dementia	Apraxia	Validation therapy
Vascular dementia	Amnesia	Perseveration	Reminiscence therapy

WHAT IS DEMENTIA?

Dementia is the permanent and progressive loss of mental functions (such as thinking, reasoning, and remembering), caused by damage to the brain tissue. A person with dementia experiences the following:

- Problems with memory, especially short-term memory
- Difficulty communicating
- Problems with judgment (the person is not able to make good decisions)
- Disorientation (the person is not oriented to person, place, or time)
- An inability to manage activities of daily living (ADLs)

Dementia typically has a gradual onset, with symptoms appearing over a period of several months or a few years. On average, a person with dementia will live 8 to 10 years after the first symptoms appear. During this time, the person will pass through three major stages (Box 9-1). Although medications are available that may help to slow the progression of the dementia, there is currently no cure for dementia. Studies have shown that an estimated 5% of older adults suffer from some form of dementia.

Dementia must not be confused with **delirium**, which is a temporary state of confusion. Delirium is a symptom of an underlying disorder, such as an infection. It may also be caused by nutritional deficiencies or a side effect of medication. Once the underlying

---

Box 9-1 Stages of Dementia

Early Stage
- The person begins to experience memory loss. Because the person is aware of these memory changes, they may become fearful, anxious, or depressed. The person may become angry at other people.

Middle Stage
- The person begins to have difficulty communicating. They may have difficulty using words, understanding words, or both.
- The person begins to have difficulty recognizing familiar people and things.
- The person begins to have difficulty remembering the steps that are necessary to complete familiar tasks, such as getting dressed.
- The person's personality may change, and they may begin to behave differently, often in challenging ways.
- The person begins to experience incontinence.

Late Stage
- The person loses the ability to walk and sit independently and eventually becomes bedridden.
- The person is no longer able to speak, swallow, or smile.
- The person becomes totally incontinent of urine and feces.
- The person dies.

disorder is treated or the medication is stopped, the delirium goes away. In some cases, the person may die if the underlying cause of the delirium is not identified and treated.

CAUSES OF DEMENTIA

Many different disorders can cause dementia. Some neurologic disorders, such as Parkinson disease and Huntington's disease, are associated with the development of dementia. Dementia may also be a part of some infectious disorders, such as HIV/AIDS, syphilis, and "mad cow disease." However, four of the most common causes of dementia are Alzheimer disease, vascular dementia, Lewy body dementia, and frontotemporal dementia.

Alzheimer Disease

Alzheimer disease is the most common cause of dementia, accounting for more than 60% of all cases. In the United States today, Alzheimer disease is a leading cause of death. More than 5 million people in the United States have Alzheimer disease. If no cure is found, it is estimated that 11 to 16 million people will have the disease by the year 2050.

Alzheimer disease usually occurs in people older than 65 years; however, people as young as 40 years may also get the disease. Because the risk for developing Alzheimer disease increases with age, people 85 years and older are at the highest risk for developing Alzheimer disease.

Alzheimer disease is named after Alois Alzheimer (1864–1915), a German doctor who discovered the disease in 1906. One of Dr. Alzheimer patients, a 51-year-old woman, died after showing unusual mental changes and behaviors. To learn why these changes occurred, Dr. Alzheimer performed an autopsy on her brain. He found that certain areas of her brain seemed soft and shrunken. In addition, he saw abnormal deposits of protein, especially in the parts of the brain that function in memory. He called these abnormal deposits *plaques* and *tangles* (Fig. 9-1). We now know that these plaques and tangles affect the ability of the nerve cells in the brain to communicate with each other. The nerve cells start to die. As a result, the brain shrinks in size, and brain activity decreases (Fig. 9-2).

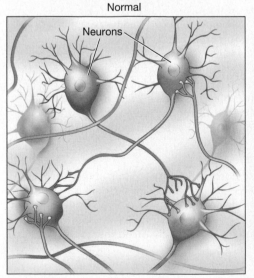
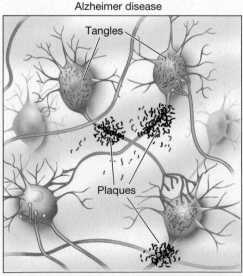

Figure 9-1 Protein deposits, called plaques and tangles, are found in the brains of people with Alzheimer disease.

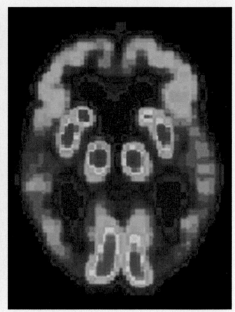

Figure 9-2 Dementia is the permanent and progressive loss of the ability to think and remember. **A.** Brain scan of a healthy person. **B.** Brain scan of a person with Alzheimer disease, the most common type of dementia. The *blue areas* indicate areas where brain activity is lost. (Alzheimer's Disease Education Referral Center, a service of the National Institute on Aging.) **A** **B**

Although we do not know exactly what causes Alzheimer disease, researchers have identified a number of risk factors. The most significant risk factor for developing Alzheimer disease is age. Another known risk factor is family history; those who have a parent, child, or sibling with Alzheimer disease are more likely to get the disease themselves. If more than one family member has the disease, the risk increases. Researchers have also found that those who have had serious head trauma are at increased risk for developing Alzheimer disease. Finally, risk factors for heart disease (such as high blood pressure, high blood cholesterol levels, and diabetes) have also been linked to the development of Alzheimer disease.

Most people with Alzheimer disease are cared for by family members during the early stages of the disease. However, as it progresses, many people with Alzheimer disease must move to a long-term care facility because they become very difficult to care for. The person needs more and more assistance with basic activities, such as bathing and toileting. In addition, the disease can cause the person to behave in disruptive or frustrating ways, which can place a great deal of emotional stress on the caregiver. The emotional pain suffered by a person with Alzheimer disease, as well as their family members, is immeasurable (Fig. 9-3).

Vascular Dementia

Damage to the blood vessels that supply the brain can affect the delivery of oxygen and nutrients to the brain tissue and may contribute to the onset of **vascular dementia**, also known as multi-infarct dementia. (An *infarction* is death of tissue due to lack of oxygen and nutrients.) Vascular dementia is thought to be the cause of dementia in approximately 20% to 25% of people with dementia. Vascular dementia often coexists with other types of dementia.

Vascular dementia most often affects people between the ages of 55 and 75 years, most commonly occurring in people who are about 70 years old. It is more common in males than in females. Conditions that put a person at risk for developing vascular dementia include:

- A history of myocardial infarction (heart attack)
- Hypertension (high blood pressure)
- Diabetes mellitus
- Peripheral vascular disease
- Transient ischemic attacks (TIAs)
- Obesity
- Smoking
- High blood cholesterol levels

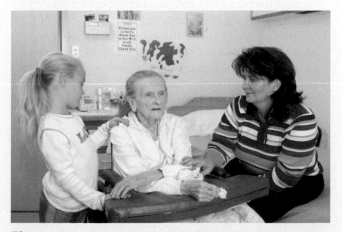

Figure 9-3 The emotional pain suffered by a person with dementia, as well as their family members, is immeasurable.

Symptoms may appear suddenly and they may vary from person to person, depending on which areas of the brain are affected. Like Alzheimer disease, vascular dementia is irreversible and incurable. Keeping the person's blood pressure, blood glucose, and blood cholesterol levels within normal limits can help to slow the progression of the dementia.

Lewy Body Dementia

Lewy body dementia is caused by the build-up of abnormal protein deposits (called *Lewy bodies*) in areas of the brain that are responsible for thinking and movement. In addition to a decline in mental abilities, people with Lewy body dementia develop problems controlling body movement (for example, muscle rigidity, a shuffling gait, slow movements, and tremors), similar to those seen in people with Parkinson disease. People with Lewy body dementia also tend to experience visual hallucinations (that is, they see things that do not really exist) and distinct changes in mental alertness. For example, one day a person

with Lewy body dementia will be alert and capable of participating in their own care but the next day they will be very confused and need more assistance to complete their ADLs. Lewy body dementia accounts for approximately 20% of all cases of dementia.

Frontotemporal Dementia

Frontotemporal dementia is caused by damage to the frontal and temporal lobes of the brain. The frontal lobe is the area of the brain that is responsible for personality and behavior. The temporal lobe is the area of the brain that is responsible for language. As a result, a person with frontotemporal dementia may show extreme changes in personality and behavior, have difficulties with language, or both. Caring for a person with frontotemporal dementia can be particularly challenging because the disease may cause the person to say or do things that are socially inappropriate. For example, the person may undress in a public area or make comments that are insulting or rude. Other people with frontotemporal dementia become bored and listless. They no longer seem to care about anything, and they lack motivation and energy. These behavioral difficulties are a common reason why a person with frontotemporal dementia may require long-term care.

Frontotemporal dementia accounts for about 5% of all cases of dementia. Symptoms of frontotemporal dementia generally appear at a younger age than in other types of dementia, often between the ages of 40 and 65 years. Also, unlike other forms of dementia, the effects on memory may not be experienced until later in the disease process.

THE "4 As" OF DEMENTIA

No matter what the underlying cause of dementia is, all people with dementia experience changes in the brain that lead to the "4 As" of dementia: **amnesia** (difficulty remembering), **aphasia** (difficulty using language), **agnosia** (difficulty recognizing information obtained using the five senses), and **apraxia** (difficulty coordinating the steps needed to complete a task). Understanding these "4 As" will allow you to provide better care for your patients and residents with dementia because you will better understand what they are experiencing, thinking, and feeling.

Amnesia

Amnesia is memory loss. During the early stage of dementia, memory loss generally only affects short-term (recent) memory, and long-term memory remains intact. So, although the person may not

Helping Hands and a Caring Heart

Focus on Humanistic Health Care

For family members, having a loved one with dementia can be particularly hard. Because dementia may last for many years, dementia is sometimes referred to as "the long goodbye." Throughout the course of the person's illness, family members will constantly have to deal with loss, as the person they knew and loved slowly slips away. Imagine how hard it would be if someone you loved no longer remembered or recognized you.

As a nursing assistant, you can support the family members of a patient or a resident with dementia by helping them make the most of their time with their loved one. Encouraging family members to bring in photographs or other mementos to share with the person benefits the person and also benefits the family members by allowing them to remember and talk about experiences they shared together. Sometimes, simple things, such as just sitting together as a family in the sunshine and listening to the birds, can form the basis for special memories in the future. Helping family members create special memories during this difficult time can help them deal with the feelings of loss they will experience as the person's disease progresses and after the person dies.

remember who they had lunch with last Thursday, they will still be able to tell you the name of their high school sweetheart. As time passes and more and more of the brain becomes diseased, long-term memory is also lost, eventually robbing the person of all memory.

Short-Term Memory Loss

The loss of short-term memory can cause a person with dementia to behave in puzzling ways. For example, the person may:

- Accuse others of stealing a personal belonging (because they cannot remember where they put it)
- Ask for a meal after they have already eaten (because they cannot remember eating)
- Stop in the middle of a task (because they cannot remember what they were doing)
- Ask the same question over and over again (because they cannot remember asking the question and cannot remember the answer you gave them)

Because of the short-term memory loss that a person with dementia experiences, as a nursing assistant, you will need to provide lots of reminders and redirections. Be sure to introduce yourself each time you see the person, and explain what you will be doing. Do not expect the person to remember you, even if they just saw you 5 minutes ago! It is also important to maintain a structured routine. Because of amnesia, people with dementia have a limited ability to think through the changes in their routine and to remember what they are supposed to be doing. As a result, a change in the normal routine causes a person with dementia a great deal of stress. Find out about the person's usual routine and try to adapt your care approaches to that routine as much as possible. This helps the person feel more comfortable by minimizing stress caused by change.

Long-Term Memory Loss

As dementia progresses, the person's long-term memory will begin to be affected as well. The person can lose years of memory, causing them to forget about entire periods of their life. Sometimes time periods blend together. For example, a married person with several children may believe that she is 16 years old and still living at home with her parents. She may not recognize her married name, and she may tell you she has no children (yet another time, she may tell you that she is waiting for her husband). Because this person is literally living in the past, they will not be able to understand references to their current situation. Trying to orient the person to their current reality can embarrass or upset them. If you insist that what the person believes to be true is not real, they may lose their trust in you. Instead, it is better to use a technique called validation therapy.

Validation therapy stresses the importance of acknowledging the person's reality. Rather than correcting the person, you respond to the person within their own reality. For example, let's say you are trying to get one of your residents, Mrs. Pyne, to go to the dining room for lunch, but she tells you that she does not want to go because her father is coming to the facility to pick her up. You know that Mrs. Pyne's father died many years ago, but in Mrs. Pyne's mind, he is still very much alive. Instead of telling Mrs. Pyne the truth, which is likely to cause her significant emotional distress, you could respond by suggesting that she have a little snack in the dining room while she waits because her father is going to be late. You can also acknowledge Mrs. Pyne's reality by asking her questions about her father, such as "What does your father look like?" or "What kind of work does your father do?" This supports Mrs. Pyne's current reality and gives her the opportunity to connect with fond thoughts about her father. Validation therapy protects the feelings and beliefs of the person with dementia and helps the person retain a sense of self-worth and dignity. Validation therapy also helps the caregiver understand what the person with dementia is experiencing.

Aphasia

Aphasia is difficulty in communicating. During the middle stage of dementia, the person begins to experience aphasia. The person may have *expressive* aphasia (difficulty using words), *receptive* aphasia (difficulty understanding words), or both. The inability to make oneself understood, or to understand others, can be a great source of stress and frustration for the person with dementia. For example, Mr. Ochoa, a resident with dementia, really needs to use the bathroom, but because of his aphasia, he cannot explain his need to anyone. In addition, no one is recognizing his need. You are asking Mr. Ochoa to join the others in the activity room, but his need to use the bathroom has not been taken care of. As this becomes more urgent, Mr. Ochoa becomes increasingly uncomfortable and stressed, suggesting he may lash out. Behaviors are often the person's way of telling us that there is an unmet need. It is up to us to be observant of our patient's or resident's behavior and body language and use this information to figure out what they are trying to tell us.

Allow extra time when communicating with your patients and residents who have dementia. Because of aphasia, it will take a person with dementia longer to process what you are telling them and to find the words they want to say. When possible, eliminate distractions to help the person focus on the conversation. It is also important to maintain eye contact during communication. If the person is not looking at you, they may forget that you are there! Remember what you learned about good communication in Chapter 5. Even if a person with dementia does not understand your words, they do understand your tone of voice and body language. If the person detects that you are impatient, irritated, or angry, they are going to respond in a similar manner. A calm, soothing tone of voice and a helpful attitude will help you be more successful when working with patients and residents with dementia.

Expressive Aphasia

A person with expressive aphasia may have difficulty finding the right word. Sometimes a word will come out that is related to what the person is trying to say, but it is not the right word. For example, a person with expressive aphasia may refer to their husband as their brother. "Brother" is a word for a male family member, but it is not the right word for the relationship the person is describing. The person may group words together that do not make sense (for example, "My twig had a cap and the nose was had indeed!"), or utter nonsense sounds in a tone and pattern that mimics normal conversation. Do not laugh at the person or tell them that they are talking nonsense. Instead, when you cannot understand the words or sounds, respond to the mood or feeling that the person is conveying through their body language and tone of voice. For example, if they are smiling and pleasant, respond in a lighthearted, pleasant manner. If they seem worried or distressed, respond with concern and care.

Receptive Aphasia

A person with receptive aphasia may not respond appropriately to your questions or directions. For example, you are asking the person to go with you to the dining room, but instead the person opens their closet to show you something. You may think that the person is being difficult, but it is more likely that the person just does not understand what you are asking them to do. Using gestures may help the person understand your message. For example, you could point toward the door, and mimic picking up a fork and eating so that the person gets the idea. If you need the person to sit, you could point to the chair and bend at the knees to demonstrate the sitting position.

Agnosia

Agnosia is difficulty in recognizing sensory input (that is, information received through the eyes, ears, nose, taste buds, or sense of touch). For example, when a person with agnosia looks at a pencil, their eyes see the pencil, but the part of the brain that tells the person that they are seeing a pencil is not working. By the size and shape of the pencil, the person may think that the pencil is a straw, put it in a cup, and try to drink through it.

Difficulty Recognizing Objects

We rely on our senses to protect us from harm. People with dementia who have agnosia will not be able to recognize potential danger and could easily harm themselves. For example, because of agnosia, a person with dementia may not be able to tell the difference between shampoo and lemonade, and as a result, may try to drink the shampoo. When caring for people with dementia, you must be very careful to keep cleaning solutions, personal care items, medications, equipment, and other potentially dangerous items in a secure place.

Difficulty Recognizing People

Because of agnosia, a person with dementia may not recognize people they know (such as family members, friends, and caregivers), which can be very frightening and frustrating. Imagine how not being able to recognize people can affect a person with dementia who lives in a long-term care facility. Each shift change brings many new "strangers" onto the unit! You can help minimize some of the stress your resident may feel by taking the time to introduce yourself and others at each interaction.

In addition to not recognizing others, a person who has agnosia may not even recognize themselves in a mirror. They may think their reflection is a stranger spying on them through the window. Putting a towel over the mirror to "close the curtain" can help to reassure and calm the person.

Apraxia

Apraxia is difficulty coordinating the steps needed to complete a task. Simple, everyday activities become very difficult for a person with dementia. For example, the person may have difficulty getting dressed because they might put clothes on in the wrong order. Or, they cannot remember how to use the knife and fork. The frustration the person experiences because of the inability to perform these tasks can contribute to a behavioral outburst. It is important to observe the person to determine what they are capable of doing and what they need help to accomplish. Although it may be easier and faster to just do the task for the person, it is important to allow the person to do as much as they can for themselves for as long as possible.

When you are coaching a resident through daily care, break the task down into individual steps. For example, if you are helping the resident brush their teeth, you could break that task down into the

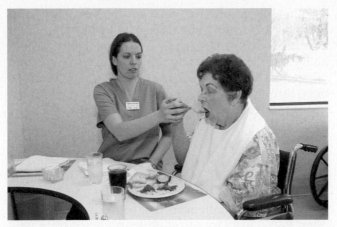

Figure 9-4 Hand-over-hand cueing may be useful when assisting a person with dementia at mealtime.

following individual steps: Take the cap off the toothpaste…Pick up your toothbrush…Put toothpaste on the toothbrush…Turn on the water…and so on. You will need to remind the person at each step what they need to do next. If you give the person too many instructions at once, they will not remember what you said (because of amnesia) and they will not be able to complete the task.

Hand-over-hand cueing is another technique that may help a patient or resident complete their care routines (Fig. 9-4). For example, you could use hand-over-hand cueing to help a person remember how to eat. First, you would put the fork in the person's hand. Then you would place your hand over the person's hand, and together you would move the fork to the plate to pick up a bite of food. Finally, you would guide the fork to the person's mouth. Sometimes, the familiar feel of the movement will come back to the person and they will be able to continue with the task by themselves, with occasional reminders.

Never rush a person who has dementia. Plan your care to allow the extra time the person needs to think about how to coordinate and complete their care routines. Rushing a person with dementia increases the person's confusion and frustration, and it will most likely result in a behavioral outburst.

BEHAVIORS ASSOCIATED WITH DEMENTIA

People with dementia often show a wide range of behaviors, especially as the dementia progresses. Some of these behaviors can be dangerous for the person, such as the tendency to wander. Others are not dangerous, but they can be very frustrating to caregivers or other residents. When you are caring for a person with dementia, you will come to know the behaviors

that are "normal" for that person. Be aware that a change in a person's "normal" behavior is a cause for concern. As the dementia progresses, the person loses the ability to communicate effectively, and a change in their behavior may be a sign that they are trying to tell you something. For example, they may be experiencing an acute physical problem, such as a bladder infection, pain, dehydration, or constipation.

Types of Behaviors

Common behaviors in people with dementia include the following.

Wandering

A person with dementia may stray away from home. This can be very dangerous because the person is often confused and disoriented. They might get lost, walk into the path of an oncoming car, or drown in a body of water, such as a lake or river. Depending on the weather and climate, the person may not be dressed appropriately to be outside. For example, if it is raining or cold, the person may not have a coat.

Because this tendency to wander cannot be stopped, many long-term care facilities have developed ways to allow residents to wander safely. Many facilities have outside courtyards with high fencing, which allow the resident to wander outside while still keeping them within the safe environment of the facility (Fig. 9-5). A resident who tends to wander may also wear a bracelet or an anklet that will set off an alarm if the resident tries to leave the facility through a doorway that leads to an unsafe area. When the alarm sounds, staff members are alerted and can guide the person back to safety.

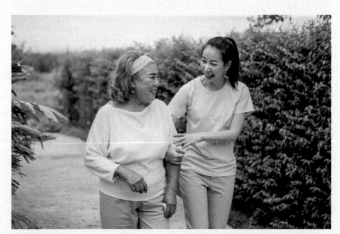

Figure 9-5 Wandering and pacing are two very common behaviors in people with dementia. Many long-term care facilities that specialize in the care of people with dementia have enclosed areas outdoors where people can wander and pace safely. (*Iammotos\Shutterstock.com*)

Pacing

A person with dementia may pace back and forth. Often, the person is pacing because they have a physical need that is not being met. For example, they may be hungry or need to use the bathroom. A person might also pace in response to a noisy, over-stimulating environment, or because they are feeling scared or lost. If one of your residents is pacing, try to figure out what is causing the behavior, and take steps to relieve the cause of the behavior. Sometimes there is nothing to do but to let the person pace. In this case, you might take the person to a safe place (for example, a fenced-in garden) and walk alongside them until the behavior has run its course.

Repetition

A person with dementia may do the same thing over and over again. This is called **perseveration**. For example, the person might repeat the same phrase or question constantly. Or they might constantly move a piece of cloth around on a table, as if dusting. Although these behaviors are usually not physically harmful to the person, they can be a sign that the person is bored. These behaviors can also be frustrating to caregivers and other residents. Distracting the person by offering to take them for a walk, or by getting them involved in an activity such as looking through a magazine, may help to break the cycle.

Rummaging

A person with dementia may go through drawers or closets, searching for an item that they are never able to find. If you notice that a resident is rummaging, ask the person what they are trying to find, and offer help in finding it. If the person tends to rummage through other residents' belongings or every single drawer in their own dresser, it may be necessary to make certain areas "off-limits" by locking them. You can then show the person a special drawer or a box filled with small personal items that they can rummage through.

Delusions and Hallucinations

A person with dementia may think that they are someone they are not, such as the Queen of England. Thoughts like these are called *delusions*. If one of your residents is delusional, do not try to correct the person. This will only upset them because they honestly believe that they are the Queen of England. It would be like someone telling you that you are not who you think you are! Instead, just try to redirect the conversation. For example, you might say, "Tell me about your day" or "Would you like to take a walk now?"

Hallucinations are also common in people with dementia. A *hallucination* is seeing, hearing, tasting, or smelling something that is not really there. For example, a person with dementia may tell you that there is a cat in the hallway or insects on the bed. If a person is hallucinating, reassure the person. For example, you might tell the person that you will ask the cat to leave, or go through the motion of sweeping the bugs off the bed. Then, gently redirect the person's attention.

Agitation

People with dementia often become very upset and excited. When a person with dementia is agitated, they may pace, shout, or lash out at caregivers or other residents. Remember that people with dementia often lose the ability to communicate effectively with others, so they express themselves through behavior (Fig. 9-6). Many things can cause agitation, including pain or an infection, an unmet physical need (for example, hunger, a full bladder, or lack of sleep), or a noisy environment.

Catastrophic Reactions

A person with dementia may over-react to something that would cause a healthy person minimal or no stress. This is called a **catastrophic reaction**. For example, a person with dementia may become very agitated or begin to scream or sob loudly when you try to give them a bath. Catastrophic reactions often occur when the person feels threatened. For example, the person may feel that their privacy is

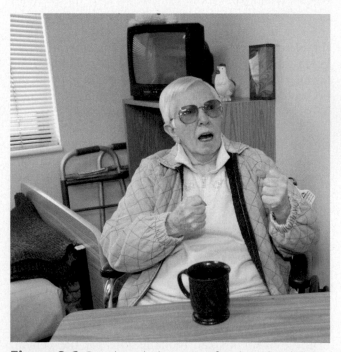

Figure 9-6 People with dementia often lose the ability to communicate effectively with others, so they express themselves through behavior. Agitation is often a sign that a physical or emotional need is not being met.

being threatened when you attempt to give them a bath. Feeling overwhelmed can also cause a person to have a catastrophic reaction. For example, a ringing telephone in a room where the television is on and people are talking might be too much commotion for a person with dementia to handle.

Sundowning

Sundowning is the worsening of a person's behavioral symptoms in the late afternoon and evening, as the sun goes down. For example, the person may become more agitated, restless, and confused in the evening hours, and may have trouble getting to sleep.

No one knows for sure exactly why sundowning behavior occurs. Some people think that it might be brought on by fatigue, especially if the person frequently wanders, paces, or engages in other repetitious behavior of a physical nature. Ensuring periods of quiet and rest during the day might help reduce fatigue, in turn reducing sundowning. Another theory is that sundowning occurs because the person cannot see as well in the evening hours when the sun starts to go down, which can increase their confusion and agitation. Turning on lights earlier in the evening may help prevent or reduce sundowning behavior.

Inappropriate Sexual Behaviors

A person with dementia may attempt to have sexual intercourse with another resident. Sometimes the person will begin to masturbate or undress in a public area, such as the dining room. These behaviors occur because the person is disoriented to person, place, and time.

You must take measures to stop inappropriate sexual behaviors, especially if the person is making unwelcome sexual advances toward another person. Gently, but firmly, lead the person back to their room and redirect the person's attention by introducing another activity. Although OBRA specifically says that a resident of a long-term care facility must be allowed to fulfill their sexual needs with another consenting resident, another resident with dementia is not able to give that consent. Therefore, you have a responsibility to protect all of the residents of the facility from unwelcome sexual advances.

Managing Difficult Behaviors

Many of the behaviors demonstrated by people with dementia can be difficult to deal with on an ongoing basis. Try to remember that the person with dementia does not want to act this way and cannot help it. Often, there is some physical or emotional reason for the behavior (Box 9-2).

In many cases, finding the underlying cause of the behavior and addressing it causes the behavior to stop,

---

> **Box 9-2   Situations That Can Cause Dementia-Related Behaviors**
>
> - The person is in a room that is too large or too small.
> - The person is in a room that is over-stimulating (cluttered, noisy, or decorated with fabrics and wallpapers with "busy" patterns).
> - The person is in a place that is new or unfamiliar (for example, the person is hospitalized for treatment of an acute problem).
> - The person is being asked to do something that is too complicated, has too many steps, or is unfamiliar.
> - The person is trying to express a physical or emotional need.

---

providing relief to you and the person. Also remember that for a person with dementia, a change in behavior might be the first and only sign of a medical problem. For example, a urinary tract infection or constipation can cause a person with dementia who is normally pleasant and calm to become agitated and lash out at a caregiver. Therefore, it is important to try and determine the cause of the behavior, rather than just accepting it as a normal part of the person's disease process.

When caring for a person with dementia who is demonstrating a particular behavior, you must use your observation skills to try and answer the following questions:

- **What** is the behavior? Describe the behavior in as much detail as possible.
- **Who** is the behavior associated with? For example, does the person act this way only in the presence of certain people?
- **When** does the behavior occur?
- **Where** does the behavior occur?

Having answers to these questions can help you answer the biggest question of all: "Why is the behavior happening?" Once you have a few ideas about what is causing the behavior, you can try different things to see if the person's behavior improves. For example, if you suspect that the person is acting a certain way because they are hungry or need to use the bathroom, you can try offering a snack or taking the person to the restroom. If you observe that the room is noisy and there is a lot of activity, you might try taking the person to a quieter place. If you suspect that the person is behaving in a certain way because they have a medical problem or is in pain, report your suspicions to the nurse so that the nurse can investigate further. Knowing your resident is the key to stopping (and sometimes preventing) difficult behaviors.

The way that you interact with a person with dementia can also affect the person's behavior. Many years ago, caregivers used a technique called *reality orientation* with people with dementia. Reality orientation

TABLE 9-1 Reality Orientation Versus Validation Therapy

EXAMPLE	REALITY ORIENTATION APPROACH	VALIDATION THERAPY APPROACH
Mrs. Rivera is trying to leave the facility. She is very agitated. She keeps repeating that she needs to go home to take care of her mother.	Nursing assistant: "Don't you remember? Your mother died 20 years ago. You are staying here with us." Mrs. Rivera's agitation increases. She may continue to insist on going home, or begin to grieve her mother's death.	Nursing assistant: "You want to go home to see your mother. Aren't mothers wonderful? Here, sit down and tell me about your mother." Mrs. Rivera is diverted from wanting to go home. She happily sits down with the nursing assistant to discuss mothers.
Dr. Carroll, a retired family doctor, believes that he needs to leave the facility and go to the hospital to deliver babies and make rounds on his patients.	Nursing assistant: "I'm sorry. Don't you remember that you are retired? You live here in the nursing home with us now. We can't let you leave because you might get lost or hurt." Dr. Carroll becomes agitated because what the nursing assistant is saying does not match his current reality.	Nursing assistant (leading Dr. Carroll to the nurse's station): "I bet we can find you a nurse who would love to have you make rounds with her and see the patients here." Dr. Carroll is diverted while still thinking that he has some value as a doctor.

was based on the idea that it is important to bring the person back to the "here and now" by constantly orienting the person to time, place, people, and things. If the person was given enough information to stay on track, then they could be brought back to the present. We now know that although reality orientation is useful for people who are experiencing temporary confusion that is reversible and treatable (that is, delirium), it is not an effective technique to use with a person who has dementia. People with dementia often cannot remember what they have been told just a few minutes earlier. Because of this, attempting to orient the person to reality can embarrass the person and increase their irritation and agitation.

Using validation therapy when working with people who have dementia is much more effective (Table 9-1). As you recall, validation therapy stresses the importance of acknowledging the person's reality. Rather than correcting them, you attempt to distract them and redirect the conversation whenever possible, such as by encouraging them to talk about things from their past. Pay special attention to the words, phrases, and body language that they use so you can better understand what they are trying to communicate. What they are saying may seem like nonsense to you, but there may be an important meaning behind the words.

CARING FOR A PERSON WITH DEMENTIA

As a person's dementia progresses, they will need more and more help with all ADLs. In addition to physical needs, the person will have emotional needs that must be met as well. General guidelines for caring for a person with dementia are given in Guidelines Box 9-1.

Meeting the Physical Needs of a Person With Dementia

For a person with dementia, everyday activities such as bathing, dressing, eating, and using the bathroom can be challenging. The person cannot remember how to do these things, and as a result, may become frustrated. Sometimes the person will resist doing what you need them to do.

When you are helping a person with dementia with their ADLs, there are several general things you can do to make the task go more smoothly:

- **Speak clearly, in a calm tone of voice**. Also, consider gently resting one of your hands on the person's arm or hand. Many people with dementia respond positively to touch (Fig. 9-7).
- **Remind the person at each step what they need to do next**. The person may be able to

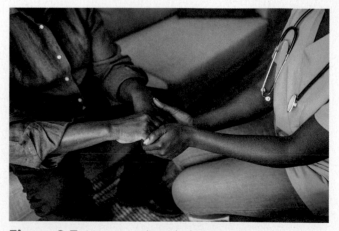

Figure 9-7 Many people with dementia respond well to touch. (*Dragana Gordic\Shutterstock.com*)

Guidelines Box 9-1   Guidelines for Caring for a Person With Dementia

WHAT YOU DO	WHY YOU DO IT
Maintain a calm, structured environment.	A person with dementia can become overwhelmed very easily. When the person becomes overwhelmed, difficult or dangerous behaviors such as wandering, agitation, or a catastrophic reaction are likely to increase.
Approach the person with dementia slowly, announcing yourself before touching them.	Many people with dementia also have hearing problems, vision problems, or both. If you approach quickly without warning, you may startle the person, triggering a catastrophic reaction.
Avoid arguing or disagreeing with the person.	A person with dementia exists in a different reality from the rest of the world. Trying to force the person with dementia to understand or acknowledge anything other than their own reality will increase the person's agitation.
When asking a person with dementia to do something, use short words and short sentences. Avoid negatively worded instructions (such as, "Don't put that there!"). Avoid instructions that require the person to remember more than one action at a time.	Because a person with dementia has problems with short-term memory, they will not be able to remember or process long words and sentences. A positively worded command ("Please put that here") is easier to understand than a negative one. Failing at a task increases the person's frustration. When you give the person instructions in a way that they can understand, you increase the person's chances of successfully completing the task.
Give a person with dementia enough time to respond to questions and directions.	It may take the person a while to think of the word or words they need to answer your question, or the action they must take to follow your directions. Feeling rushed can cause the person to become agitated or upset.
"Listen" to the person by paying attention to body language. Make good use of your observation skills.	As a person's dementia gets worse, they lose the ability to communicate effectively. Often, body language and behaviors become the person's main way of expressing themselves
When managing difficult behaviors, be aware that solutions that work today may not work tomorrow. Be creative, and do not give up.	Dementia is a progressive disease. Therefore, the person's abilities, disabilities, and needs change over time, and your approaches to managing difficult behaviors may also need to change.
Help the person with dementia to feel secure and loved by showing affection (kind words, a gentle touch) and smiling.	Like all people, people with dementia have emotional needs that must be met.
Allow the person with dementia to do as much as they can for themselves, for as long as possible.	This is important for maintaining the person's dignity and self-esteem. No one likes to feel helpless or useless.
Help the person to maintain independence for as long as possible by using visual cues to orient the person to place and time. For example, place a large-faced clock in the person's room, decorate for the holidays, and post names and other reminder signs in prominent, meaningful places (for example, if a person keeps trying to walk out the front door, apply a big, red and white "stop" sign to the inside of the door).	Using visual cues can help the person to maintain their independence longer, which is important for the person's self-esteem.

(continued)

Guidelines Box 9-1 Guidelines for Caring for a Person With Dementia (*continued*)

WHAT YOU DO	WHY YOU DO IT
Help the person to exercise their mind by getting the person involved in activities that relate to the person's former interests and experiences.	Participating in activities helps to prevent boredom and increases the person's sense of purpose and accomplishment.
Protect the person from physical injury.	People with dementia often become clumsy as a result of their disease, which increases their risk of falling. In addition, they lose the ability to make good decisions related to their well-being. For example, a person with dementia might walk in front of an oncoming car, leave the house without a coat in the middle of a snowstorm, or drink the contents of a bottle found under the sink.
Maintain the person's hygiene and good grooming habits.	This is important for the person's health as well as for their self-esteem.
Be as tolerant as possible of the person.	The person's behaviors are a result of their dementia and are beyond the person's control. The person is not purposely trying to frustrate or annoy you.
When you become tired and frustrated, take time out, be good to yourself, and share your feelings with the nurse. Know that these emotions and thoughts are normal.	Caring for a person with dementia is emotionally draining and physically difficult. If you do not take measures to protect your own mental health, you run the risk of "burnout." In addition, you place the resident at risk for abuse, should you lose your temper.

complete tasks such as dressing, shaving, or brushing their teeth with your guidance. Allowing a person to complete tasks independently for as long as possible is important for their self-esteem.

- **Use hand gestures in addition to spoken instructions**. For example, if you are trying to get the person to sit down at the table and eat, pat the seat of the chair as you ask the person to come sit down.
- **Plan for the procedure in advance**. "Getting ready" steps are always important, but especially when you are caring for a person with dementia. Many routine procedures, such as bathing, are very stressful for a person with dementia. Being prepared and having everything you need before you begin a procedure will allow you to accomplish the task as quickly as possible, which can help reduce the amount of stress the person feels.
- **Keep to a regular schedule**. A person with dementia responds best to a very structured environment. To a person with dementia, the world is very confusing. Structuring the person's world as much as possible, by following an established routine, can reduce their confusion and fear.

Assisting With Bathing

Bath time can be a frightening time for a person with dementia. The person may not remember what a bath or shower is, or why they need to take one. The sound of running water, the bright lights, and the shiny surfaces in the tub room can be upsetting. Being naked makes the person feel exposed and vulnerable. The person may be very afraid of falling.

As a result, the person may become agitated when you tell them that it is "time to take a bath." If this is the case, try to avoid the word "bath." Instead, say "Let's go freshen up" or "It's time for an activity you will enjoy." If the person seems very agitated, you might try singing to the person. Singing can have a very calming effect on people with dementia.

It may also be very useful to find out from the family what the person's daily bathing routine was like prior to coming to the long-term care facility. The person's resistance to a morning shower may only be due to the fact that they have always taken a tub bath in the evening before going to bed.

Bath time will generally go more smoothly if you prepare the tub room in advance. Make sure that the room is warm, and fill the tub ahead of time so that the person does not become frightened by the sound

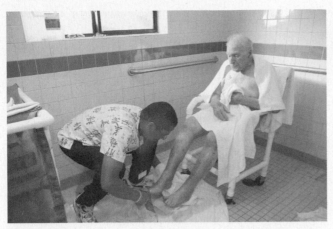

Figure 9-8 Bath time can be very frightening for a person with dementia. Making every effort to maintain the person's modesty is important.

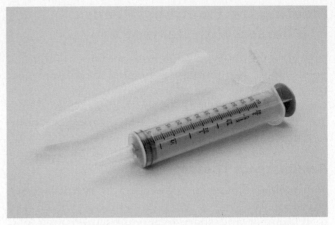

Figure 9-9 A feeding syringe is sometimes used instead of a spoon to feed people in the advanced stages of dementia.

of the running water. Put a folded towel on the shower chair for comfort. Allow the person to wear their robe as long as possible, and consider draping a bath blanket or towel over the person's shoulders while they are bathing (Fig. 9-8). The bath blanket or towel will make the person feel less exposed and it will also provide some warmth. Hand the person a washcloth and let the person assist as much as possible.

Assisting With Dressing

Many people with dementia have trouble selecting an outfit to wear. They often want to wear the same clothes every day. Limiting the number of outfits the person has to choose from and asking family members to purchase several identical outfits for the person can help to solve these problems.

For a person with dementia, putting on and fastening clothing can also be difficult. To help make dressing less frustrating for the person, select articles of clothing that are simple, rather than complex. For example, a shirt that pulls over the head is easier to manage than a shirt that buttons up the front. Pants with elastic waistbands are easier to manage than pants with zippers and buttons.

Assisting With Eating

You might find that it is difficult to get a person with dementia to focus on eating at mealtimes. The person may forget why they are at the table or become distracted by others at the table. A quiet setting and limited food choices can help. Many times, the person will not recognize eating utensils, or they will forget how to use them. Using hand-over-hand assistance during mealtime may be useful. Make sure that the person swallows the food after chewing it. People with dementia often have a tendency to chew and then pack the food in the cheeks, increasing the risk of choking. If the person cannot focus long enough to eat a proper meal, try offering the person "finger foods" such as sandwiches, cut-up vegetables or fruit, or a nutrition bar. A plastic cup with a lid and a straw or a spout can help to ensure that the person drinks enough fluids.

People in the advanced stages of dementia eventually lose the ability to eat independently. When we eat, the tongue pushes the food to the back of the throat so that we can swallow it. People with advanced dementia often "forget" how to do this. Most of the food placed in the mouth of a person with advanced dementia just comes right back out again. Because a person with advanced dementia loses the ability to use their tongue to move food to the back of the throat, sometimes a special syringe with a nozzle-shaped tip is used for feeding instead of a spoon (Fig. 9-9). The food is semi-liquid and the syringe is used to place the food further back in the mouth so that the person can swallow it more easily. The food is given slowly in small amounts to prevent choking. Using a feeding syringe may allow the person with advanced dementia to continue taking food by mouth for a longer period of time, instead of through a feeding tube, which can be very uncomfortable. Some facilities consider using a feeding syringe to be outside the nursing assistant's scope of practice, so before using a syringe to feed a person, check with the nurse.

Assisting With Elimination

Elimination can present many problems for the person with dementia. The person may forget where the bathroom is, or fail to recognize the toilet. Sometimes, the person will have an accident because they are unable to move the necessary clothing out of the way fast enough. Taking the person to the bathroom on a regular schedule (for example, every 2 hours) can help, as can helping the person to select clothing with fasteners that are easy to manage. If a person suddenly seems to be having a lot of accidents, report this to the nurse. The person may have a medical problem, such as a urinary tract infection, that needs to be addressed.

Meeting the Emotional Needs of a Person With Dementia

Helping a person with dementia meet their emotional needs is just as important as helping the person meet their physical needs. Just like everyone else, a person with dementia needs to feel loved and needed. There are several helpful approaches to meeting the emotional needs of a person with dementia.

Reminiscence Therapy

To *reminisce* means to remember. In **reminiscence therapy**, the person with dementia is encouraged to remember and share experiences from their past with others (Fig. 9-10). For example, if a person with dementia insists that they need to go see their mother (who has been dead for years), you might say, "What does your mother look like?" or "Tell me about a favorite food that your mother used to make when you were growing up." Talking about the past diverts the person's attention and increases their self-esteem. Reminiscence therapy can be used in a "one-on-one" or group setting. When done in a group setting, reminiscence therapy gives the person a chance to socialize with other residents.

Activity Therapy

Like all people, people with dementia need to exercise their minds. Even though a person with dementia is confused, they still can become bored. In fact, boredom may be an underlying cause of some difficult behaviors, such as wandering or rummaging. Activities are so important to a resident's well-being that many facilities display a large calendar with daily planned activities on the wall. Engaging in activities helps the person feel useful and gives them a sense of purpose and accomplishment.

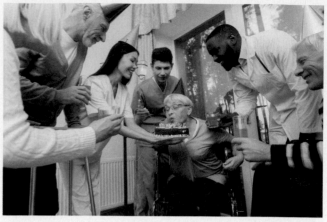

Figure 9-11 Activity therapy is an important part of caring for people with dementia. Activities can be planned for an individual or for a group of residents. (*VGstockstudio\Shutterstock.com*)

Activities may be planned for a single resident or group of residents (Fig. 9-11). There are many different types of activities that a person with dementia can enjoy:

- Creative activities (flower arranging, painting, baking)
- Intellectual activities (looking at a book of photographs, reading the news aloud together, attending a play)
- Social activities (singing with other residents, going on a picnic)
- Physical activities (taking a walk, participating in a group exercise class or dancing)

When planning an activity, take care to choose one that relates to the former interests and abilities of the person or people who will be participating in it. For a group activity, assign tasks according to each resident's abilities and interests.

Music Therapy

Music can be very beneficial for people with dementia. Research has shown that when we listen to music we enjoy, our heart and respiratory rates slow, and our blood pressure becomes lower. In this way, music can calm an agitated person. Holiday music, religious music, or music from a certain time period that holds special meaning to them may be particularly appealing to residents with dementia.

Pet Therapy

Spending time with companion animals, such as dogs and cats, can have many benefits for people with dementia (Fig. 9-12). The facility may participate in a visiting pet program, in which volunteers bring specially selected animals to the facility for a few hours each week to share with the residents. Or the facility

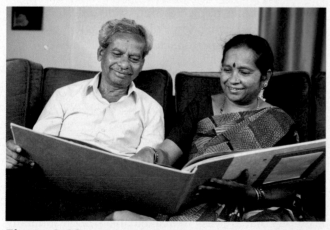

Figure 9-10 Reminiscence therapy increases a person's self-esteem and happiness by encouraging them to remember the past. (*WESTOCK PRODUCTIONS\Shutterstock.com*)

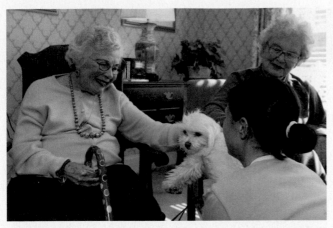

Figure 9-12 Pet therapy can improve the quality of life for many residents with dementia.

may have a pet cat or dog that lives on the unit. A person with dementia may benefit from pet therapy in many different ways. The person may get pleasure simply by watching the animal. Some people may like to stroke the animal's fur, or sit with the animal in their lap. This can be very calming. Other people will benefit from pet therapy by remembering and talking about pets they had in the past.

Caring for the Person With Late-Stage Dementia

In the final stage of dementia, the person loses the ability to walk and sit independently. Immobility puts the person at risk for problems such as pressure ulcers, contractures, and pneumonia.

The person also loses the ability to swallow, affecting their ability to eat. When the person can no longer eat on their own, it usually signals the final phase of the disease process before death occurs. The person may have an advance directive that specifies whether or not a feeding tube should be inserted to provide nourishment. If no advance directive is in place, the person's health care agent will need to decide whether or not nutrition will be artificially supported with a feeding tube. This is not an easy decision to make. There is no research that suggests that tube feeding really benefits a person at this stage in the disease process, and it often leads to complications, such as aspiration pneumonia. Although family members may understand the reasons for not placing a feeding tube, it is still emotionally difficult to watch a loved one go without nourishment. Families need a tremendous amount of support at this time.

Because a person with dementia will eventually die from the disease, care efforts during the final phase of the disease process are directed toward ensuring that the person is as comfortable as possible until death occurs. For example, oxygen therapy might be provided to make breathing easier. The doctor will often

discontinue orders for medications and laboratory work that are no longer beneficial. Routine measuring of the person's weight is also usually discontinued at this time because weight loss is expected. Your responsibilities during this time will be the same as they are when caring for any person who is dying (see Chapter 27).

EFFECTS ON THE CAREGIVER OF CARING FOR THE PERSON WITH DEMENTIA

Caring for people with dementia is very important work. The difference you make in the life of the person with dementia, as well as those of their family members, is significant. However, caring for a person with dementia can take its toll on you, physically and emotionally.

- A person with dementia is prone to outbursts of anger and can become agitated very easily. Therefore, it is likely that on any given day, you may be cursed at, spit on, slapped, hit, scratched, or pinched. Because you will most likely develop a fondness for the residents in your care, it can be very difficult when a resident has a "bad day" and that affection is not returned!
- Many of the behaviors of people with dementia can be very frustrating because they are repetitious. It is not always easy to figure out what you can do to make the behavior stop, and until a solution is found, the behavior can really try your patience.
- Caring for a person is hard physical work. As the dementia progresses, the person becomes completely dependent. Exhaustion and fatigue can put you on edge, making it difficult for you to keep your emotions in check.

If you feel yourself becoming overwhelmed by your responsibilities or a particular situation, take a deep breath and remind yourself that a person with dementia cannot be held responsible for their actions. If you still feel angry, make sure that the person is safe and walk away. Ask a coworker or the nurse for help with the person. Sometimes you may need to ask to be assigned to another resident for a while. If your frustration or anger moves you to the point of actually causing a resident physical harm, you will lose your job (as well as all chances of future employment in the health care field). You could even be charged with abuse, depending on the situation. Remember, a member of the health care team is particularly at risk for becoming abusive when the resident is "difficult" or hard to manage, and the relationship is a long-term relationship. When you become tired and frustrated, take time out, be good to yourself, and share your feelings with the nurse. To provide the best care to your residents, you need to care for yourself.

SUMMARY

- Dementia is caused by changes in the brain tissue and affects a person's ability to think, remember, and communicate.
    - Dementia must not be confused with delirium, which is confusion in a person who is normally alert and oriented. Delirium goes away when the underlying cause is treated.
    - The most common causes of dementia are Alzheimer disease, vascular dementia, Lewy body dementia, and frontotemporal dementia.
    - Most types of dementia follow a similar course and ultimately lead to death. Currently, there is no cure for dementia.
- All people with dementia experience changes in the brain that lead to the "4 As" of dementia: amnesia, aphasia, agnosia, and apraxia.
- A person with dementia often shows a wide range of behaviors, especially as the dementia progresses.
    - A change in a person's behavior is often a sign of an unmet physical or emotional need.

- Nursing assistants use observation to try and figure out the underlying cause of behavior. If it can be determined, then actions can be taken to stop the behavior.
    - The way you interact with a person with dementia can affect their behavior. Try to understand what is "real" for the person with dementia, and do not try to correct them. This communication technique is called *validation therapy*.
- A person with dementia has physical and emotional needs that must be met.
    - As the person's dementia gets worse, they need more and more help with ADLs such as eating, bathing, dressing, and toileting.
    - Reminiscence therapy, activity therapy, music therapy, and pet therapy are used to help meet their emotional needs.
- Caring for a person with dementia is a very demanding yet very important work. Dementia is a terrible disease that is devastating both to the person who has it, as well as their family members.

WHAT DID YOU LEARN?

Multiple Choice

Select the single best answer for each of the following questions.

1. Which one of the following is experienced by a person with dementia?
   a. Problems with memory, especially short-term memory
   b. Confusion and disorientation
   c. An inability to manage activities of daily living (ADLs)
   d. All of the above

2. When caring for a person with dementia, it is helpful to:
   a. Be understanding and see the person's behaviors as part of the disease
   b. Take the same approach with every resident
   c. Correct the person to bring them back to the "here and now"
   d. Avoid acknowledging your own feelings

3. When communicating with a person with dementia, what is the best approach to take?

   a. Speak loudly and quickly to get the person's attention
   b. Speak clearly, in a calm tone of voice
   c. Avoid touching the person or using hand gestures
   d. Avoid talking about the past

4. Which statement about validation therapy is true?
   a. Validation therapy stresses the importance of bringing the person with dementia back to the "here and now."
   b. Validation therapy is based on the belief that people with dementia are able to return to the present, if given enough information to do so.
   c. Validation therapy stresses the importance of acknowledging the person's reality.
   d. Validation therapy encourages the caregiver to correct the person, to help the person to stay on track.

5. A person with dementia may show which one of the following behaviors?
   a. Pacing and wandering
   b. Hallucinations
   c. Agitation
   d. All of the above

6. When you come on duty at 3:00 pm, Mr. Antonio asks you what time dinner will be served. You tell him that dinner is served at 5:30 pm and show him where "5:30" is on the clock. When you return to his room at 3:30 pm, he asks you again what time dinner will be served. You give him the same response as you did before. He leaves the room and heads toward the dining room. You hear him ask another staff member what time dinner will be served. You understand this behavior is most likely a symptom of:
   a. Aphasia
   b. Apraxia
   c. Agnosia
   d. Amnesia

7. What is sundowning?
   a. Increased confusion, restlessness, and insecurity that occur late in the day, as it becomes darker outside
   b. Aimless wandering after dark
   c. Repeating the same action over and over
   d. Crying inconsolably for a long time

8. Mr. Greene, one of the residents in your care, has Alzheimer disease. For the last hour, Mr. Greene has been folding and unfolding a piece of paper, and he is showing no signs of stopping. What should you do?
   a. Let him keep doing it; perseveration is a normal behavior in a person with dementia.
   b. Try to distract Mr. Greene by starting a new activity with him, such as reading the newspaper together or going for a walk.
   c. Tell the nurse, who will be able to give Mr. Greene a sedative to make the behavior stop.
   d. Tell Mr. Greene firmly that the behavior is unacceptable and it must stop, immediately.

9. What is a catastrophic reaction?
   a. A response to a situation that is more extreme than would normally be expected
   b. An abnormal protein deposit that is found in the brains of people with Alzheimer disease
   c. The belief that you are someone you are not (for example, the President of the United States)
   d. The reaction family members have on learning that a loved one has Alzheimer disease

10. When helping a person with dementia with their activities of daily living (ADLs), such as bathing, eating, and dressing, what should you remember?
   a. Keep to an established routine as much as possible
   b. Prepare for the procedure ahead of time
   c. Many ADLs are very frightening or frustrating for the person with dementia
   d. All of the above

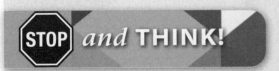

STOP *and* THINK!

- You work in the dementia unit of a long-term care facility. Ms. Darden, one of the residents you are responsible for, needs a great deal of help with all of her activities of daily living (ADLs). Lately, Ms. Darden has started having a catastrophic reaction every time you help her to bathe. What are some things you could do to make bathing easier and less frightening for Ms. Darden?

- You work in a long-term care facility. One day, you go to the room of one of your residents, Mrs. Craven, to answer her call light. When you enter the room, Mrs. Craven cries out to you in a frightened voice, "Get them out of here! Get them out of here now!" You don't know what she is talking about—you don't see anybody or anything in the room. You ask Mrs. Craven to explain what she means, and she tells you that there are spiders crawling all over the walls. Normally, Mrs. Craven is alert and oriented, but today, she definitely seems "out of it." What do you think is wrong with Mrs. Craven? What should you do?

- Mr. Nagy has Alzheimer disease. You have cared for Mr. Nagy for a long time and know pretty much what to expect from him in terms of behavior. Although he does tend to pace and rummage quite frequently, he is usually calm and pleasant. Today in the dining room, however, when you are trying to help Mr. Nagy eat lunch, he becomes angry and lashes out at you. What might be the explanation for this behavior?

Respect

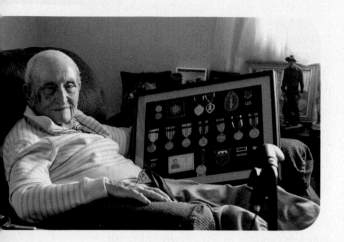

I work as a Nursing Assistant in a Veteran's nursing home. I chose to work with Veterans because I also served in the military and it gives me a sense of pride to work with people who served our country in this way. Most of our residents are older and served in the Vietnam War. But there are some my age who are here because of medical and emotional injuries they recently received while in service. Some of these young vets have suffered severe injuries from explosive devices and have lost limbs or suffered serious brain injuries. Others suffer from debilitating PTSD as a result of combat. The people I care for are my family.... my comrades.

One of our older residents, Mr. Solis, is one of my favorites. He doesn't talk much about his tour of service. One day, I walked past his room and saw him sitting in his favorite chair, holding something and crying softly. I went and sat down in a chair beside him and just waited for him to speak. When he did, he told me that his father was also a military man. He had served in World War II and fought in Germany. Mr. Solis said his father came home to a hero's welcome, but he was never the same. He lost a leg in combat and suffered the effects of exposure to mustard gas, and ended up dying about 10 years later. Mr. Solis was holding one of his father's medals in his hands as he spoke.

Then he looked at me and continued to tell me about his own service in Vietnam. He said he still felt guilt that he had come home with only minor injuries when almost all the others in his platoon had been killed in an ambush. Once home, he said that there was no hero's welcome for his service. Political tensions and anti-war protests made life pretty hard for a while. He said he was really depressed for a long time, but with the help of his wife and other veteran support groups, he managed get better emotionally and build a happy life. He then took my hand and told me that he appreciated my service, both for my service in the military and especially for my continued service as a Nursing Assistant showing care to fellow veterans like him.

Mr. Solis passed away in his sleep about a month after our conversation, but he will always be remembered for the quiet respect he showed for his fellow veterans. He certainly made an impression on me and my plans to continue serving fellow veterans.

(Layne V. Naylor\Shutterstock.com)

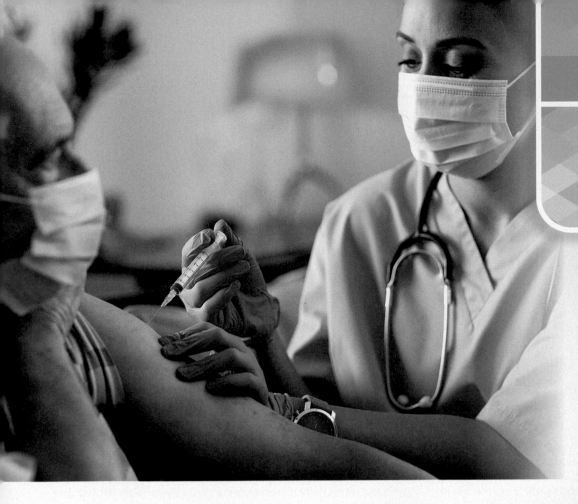

Infection Control

AS YOU HAVE LEARNED, being a Nursing Assistant places you in very close contact with those you care for. Communicable illnesses are present, both in the health care facility and in the outside world. Many of the people you will care for will have health concerns that put them more at risk for catching communicable illnesses. Not only must you know how to protect those entrusted to your care, you must also know how to protect yourself. Controlling the spread of infection is the focus of Unit 3.

Photo: Immunizations help to control the spread of infection, both within the health care setting and in the outside world.

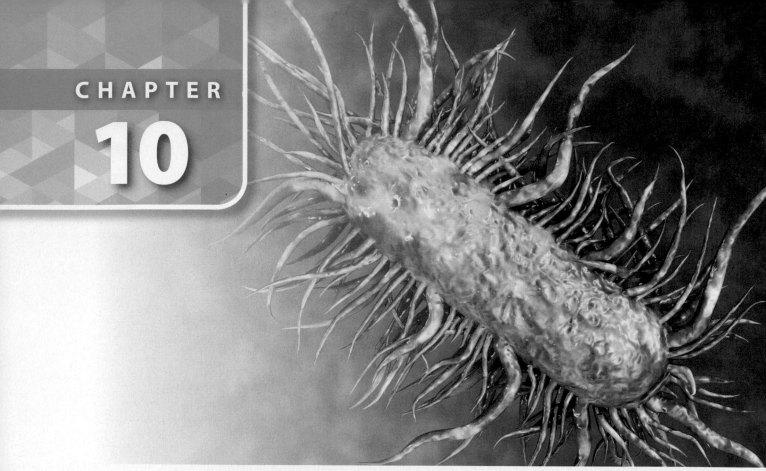

CHAPTER

10

Photo: *Escherichia coli,* a microbe that can cause disease. Color was added to this photograph, which was taken with a special microscope (a tool that is used to see things that are not visible to the naked eye). (MichaelTaylor3d\Shutterstock.com)

Communicable Disease

WHAT WILL YOU LEARN?

Communicable diseases are diseases that can be spread from one person to another. There are many factors that come together in the health care setting to make it easy for communicable diseases to spread. In this chapter, you will learn about the causes of communicable disease and the ways our bodies protect us from catching these diseases. You will also learn why some people are more likely than others to catch a communicable disease. When you are finished with this chapter, you will be able to:

1. **List the different types of microbes that cause disease and discuss the conditions that are essential for their survival and growth.**
2. **Define the terms *normal flora* and *pathogen*.**
3. **Explain the defense mechanisms the body uses to help keep us from getting sick.**
4. **Define the term *infection* and describe the chain of events required for infection to occur.**
5. **List factors that can make a person more likely to get an infection.**

Vocabulary

Communicable disease	Aerobic	Methicillin-resistant	Chain of infection
Microbe (microorganism)	Anaerobic	*Staphylococcus aureus*	Contaminated
Normal (resident) flora	Antibodies	(MRSA)	Fomites
Pathogens	Multidrug-resistant	Vancomycin-resistant	Vector
Opportunistic microbes	organisms (MDROs)	enterococcus (VRE)	Virulence
Colonies		Infection	

WHAT IS A MICROBE?

A **microbe**, also called a **microorganism**, is a living thing that cannot be seen with the naked eye. Many (but not all) microbes consist of just one cell. (To give you an idea of how small a cell is, consider that it is estimated that the adult human body is composed of approximately 50 *million* cells!) Microbes are found in air, soil, water, food, and in and on the bodies of plants and animals, including humans.

Most microbes cause no harm and are actually essential for healthy living. For example, some of the microbes that live in the human digestive tract help us to get certain vitamins from the foods that we eat. Others help maintain an environment that is unfriendly to harmful microbes. The harmless microbes that help the human body function properly are called **normal (resident) flora**.

Some microbes, however, can cause illness and are known as **pathogens**. Sometimes microbes can be considered normal flora in one part of the body and pathogens in another. For example, *Escherichia coli* (*E. coli*) is a microbe that normally lives in our large intestines, where it is harmless. However, when *E. coli* finds its way out of the intestine and into another part of the body where it is not normal flora, such as the bladder, it can cause an infection. These types of microbes are called **opportunistic microbes**. Given the chance, opportunistic microbes can change from harmless to pathogenic.

There are many different types of microbes that live and prosper among us. Microbes can generally be classified as bacteria, viruses, fungi, or parasites (Table 10-1).

Bacteria

Many scientists believe that bacteria lived on Earth long before any other life forms. Bacteria have been found in polar ice caps and in deep cracks in the ocean floor. The ability of bacteria to adapt to all sorts of environments is proof of this life form's ability to survive.

Most bacteria consist of only one cell and reproduce by dividing in half. Although bacteria usually consist of only one cell, they often group together to form **colonies**. Scientists classify and name bacteria by:

- Their shape
- The way they arrange themselves in a colony
- The way they stain (how they react to the dye scientists use to make microbes visible under a microscope)

For example, round bacteria are called *cocci*, rod-shaped bacteria are called *bacilli*, and spiral-shaped or curved bacteria are called *spirilla* (Fig. 10-1). Bacterial colonies may consist of pairs of bacteria (indicated by the prefix *diplo-*), chains of bacteria (indicated by the prefix *strepto-*), or grape-like clusters of bacteria (indicated by the prefix *staphylo-*). So, what would you know if you saw the word *Staphylococcus aureus* on a person's medical record? You would know that this person had an infection caused by a round bacterium (*-coccus*) that arranges itself in clusters (*Staphylo-*)! There are thousands of types of bacteria and not all of them are named using this method. However, this example illustrates how you can learn the meaning of a word that might be unfamiliar to you by taking it apart. In Appendix B, "Introduction to the Language of Health Care," you can learn about many more prefixes, suffixes, and roots that are used to form words commonly used in the health care setting.

Like all living things, bacteria have certain basic requirements for survival. These requirements vary according to the type of bacteria. For example, **aerobic** bacteria need oxygen to live. On the other hand, **anaerobic** bacteria die if oxygen is present. Most bacteria that cause illness need a warm, moist, dark environment, and a source of nutrition to grow—requirements that the inside of the human body meets perfectly! Some types of bacteria can surround themselves with a protective shell, called an *endospore*, and enter a state of inactivity. If the inactive bacterium's best growing conditions become available, the bacterium will become active again. Because of

TABLE 10-1 Types of Microbes

	TYPE	EXAMPLES OF COMMONLY CAUSED INFECTIONS
 (Kateryna Kon\Shutterstock.com)	Bacteria	"Strep throat," urinary tract infections, abscesses, tuberculosis (TB), bacterial meningitis, Lyme disease, Rocky Mountain spotted fever, syphilis
 (nobeastsofierce\Shutterstock.com)	Viruses	HIV/AIDS, hepatitis, fever blisters, common cold, flu, COVID-19
 (David Litman\Shutterstock.com)	Fungi	Ringworm, "athlete's foot," vaginal yeast infections (candidiasis), oral yeast infections (thrush)
 (Devil79sd\Shutterstock.com)	Parasites insects	Scabies, pediculosis (lice)
 (Jeephotoghapher\Shutterstock.com)	Helminths (worms)	Pinworm infestation
 (Rattiya Thongdumhyu\Shutterstock.com)	Protozoa	Malaria, amebic dysentery

Cell Shapes

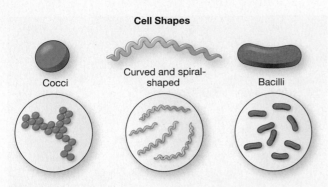

Cocci

Curved and spiral-shaped

Bacilli

Figure 10-1 Categories of bacteria based on the shape of their cells. (Redrawn from Cohen BJ. *Memmler's The human body in health and disease.* 11th ed. Lippincott Williams & Wilkins; 2009.)

their protective endospores, these types of bacteria are very difficult to kill using the standard techniques described in Chapter 12. Examples of illnesses caused by bacteria that form endospores include tetanus (lockjaw) and botulism (food poisoning).

Bacteria are the most common cause of infection in the health care setting. Some common illnesses caused by bacteria include "strep throat" (caused by *Streptococcus pyogenes*), some bladder infections (such as those caused by *E. coli*), and some skin infections (such as those caused by *Staphylococcus aureus*). Several types of small, rod-shaped bacteria are transmitted by ticks and fleas and cause diseases such as Rocky Mountain spotted fever and typhus. Bacteria are also responsible for some types of pneumonia and some infections of the reproductive and urinary systems.

Viruses

Viruses, the smallest of all microbes, can only be seen using a special kind of microscope called an electron microscope. Viruses are not even complete cells—they are just small bundles of protein. Because viruses are not complete cells, they cannot carry out normal cellular activities, such as reproduction, by themselves. Instead, they must take over a host cell, usually a plant or animal cell. Once inside the host cell, the virus uses the host cell's "machinery" to make copies of itself. Eventually, the virus and all of its copies (called *progeny*) break through the host cell's wall, killing the host cell and freeing the viruses to infect other, neighboring host cells. Many illnesses are caused by viruses, including the common cold, flu, COVID-19, fever blisters (caused by herpes simplex virus), chickenpox (caused by varicella zoster virus), hepatitis, and acquired immunodeficiency syndrome (AIDS, caused by human immunodeficiency virus, or HIV). Even smaller protein particles, called prions, can cause illnesses. Creutzfeldt–Jakob disease, sometimes known

as "mad cow disease," is caused by a prion. Many of the illnesses caused by viruses are easily spread from person-to-person.

Fungi

Fungi are a group of plant-like organisms that scientists have classified together because of certain characteristics, including the makeup of their cell walls. Not all fungi are microscopic—for example, mushrooms are a type of fungus! Other types of fungi you may be familiar with include yeasts (such as the yeast that is used to make bread rise and beer foamy) and molds (such as the mildew that grows inside a shower stall or the growths that appear on bread and cheese if left too long). Many fungi help us (or, at least, do not harm us). However, some fungi are capable of causing illness. If you have ever had ringworm (caused by *Tinea corporis*), athlete's foot (caused by *Tinea pedis*), thrush (a yeast infection in the mouth), or candidiasis (a vaginal yeast infection), then you have been the victim of a fungus!

Parasites

Parasites live in or on a host, such as a plant or animal, and use that host for food and protection. Some parasites can be transmitted from one person to another through physical contact. For example, scabies, an itchy skin condition, is caused by a mite that burrows under the skin. Pediculosis (lice) is caused by wingless insects that live on the scalp or body and feed on the host's blood. Both scabies and lice are often seen in the health care setting. Other parasites are transferred from one person to another through feces or blood.

Helminths, a type of parasite, are worm-like organisms that live in the human body (as well as the bodies of other animals). Examples of helminths include pinworms, tapeworms, and roundworms. Although the way these organisms are transmitted from one host to another varies, transmission usually involves eating or inhaling the worm eggs, which then grow in the host's digestive tract. The mature worms produce eggs or larvae of their own, which are then passed out of the host's body with the feces. Once the eggs reach the outside world again, they are free to be eaten or inhaled by another host, and the life cycle of the helminth continues.

Protozoa, another type of parasite, are said to be "animal-like" because they can take in food. Protozoa causes illnesses such as malaria (transmitted by a mosquito bite) and amebic dysentery (a type of diarrhea caused by drinking water contaminated with protozoa).

DEFENSES AGAINST COMMUNICABLE DISEASE

Many, many microbes share the Earth with us. Fortunately, our bodies have protective mechanisms to help shield against harmful microbes, and modern medicine has brought us many powerful medications to help combat infections.

The Immune System

If microbes (commonly referred to as "germs") are everywhere, and some of them can make us sick, then why aren't we all always sick? The answer to this question lies in the body's immune system, the wonderful defense system that protects us from infection. Some of the body's defenses are nonspecific, which means that they help to protect us from all pathogens. Other defenses are specific, which means that they help to protect us only from certain pathogens.

Nonspecific Defense Mechanisms

Our main nonspecific defense mechanism is healthy, intact skin and mucous membranes. Skin that is without cuts, scrapes, or wounds physically prevents pathogens from entering the body. In addition, the natural lubricants on our skin contain substances that help prevent the growth of pathogens. Mucous membranes line all of the organ systems that come in contact with the outside world (the respiratory, digestive, urinary, and reproductive systems). The special cells of the mucous membranes secrete mucus, a sticky substance that creates a physical barrier by trapping and destroying pathogens. Keeping the skin clean helps reduce the number of pathogens on the skin. Good oral hygiene and drinking plenty of fluids help to keep mucous membranes functioning properly. These are important measures to take for yourself as well as your patients or residents. Stomach acid (which kills many of the microbes contained in the food that we eat), tears (which contain a substance that kills microbes), and the acts of coughing and sneezing (which remove inhaled microbes) are also nonspecific defense mechanisms that prevent microbes from "setting up shop" in our bodies.

If a pathogen manages to get past these first lines of defense and an infection results, the body activates a general immune response that helps fight off the infection. Blood vessels around the site of the infection dilate (widen), allowing more blood flow to the area. The increased blood flow brings more oxygen and nutrients to the tissues, along with large numbers of white blood cells (leukocytes). White blood cells destroy pathogens that invade the body, either by eating them (Fig. 10-2) or by secreting substances that

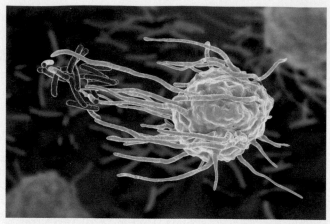

Figure 10-2 In this photograph, a white blood cell has trapped and is preparing to engulf and kill a pathogen by eating it. This is a process called phagocytosis (*phago-* means "eat" and *cyt-* means "cell"). (*Kateryna Kon\Shutterstock.com*)

cause them to die. The increased blood flow causes the infected area to become red, warm, swollen, and painful (Fig. 10-3). A person who is fighting off an infection may have a high body temperature (fever). If you remember, most pathogens prefer a nice, normal body temperature. The fever helps to destroy the pathogens and is a normal response for many infections.

As a nursing assistant, it is important for you to watch for signs of infection in your patients or residents. Many patients or residents may not be able to communicate that they do not feel well or that they have pain. If not treated at an early stage, some infections can be very dangerous. If one of your patients or residents has signs or symptoms of an infection, the doctor may order a diagnostic test, called a *culture and sensitivity*, to find out which microbe is causing the infection and which medication is best suited to

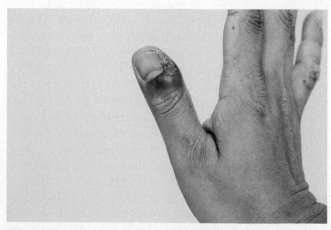

Figure 10-3 The site of infection is typically hot, red, swollen, and painful. This means the body's general immune response is at work! (*Shidlovski\Shutterstock.com*)

fight it. The culture and sensitivity may be performed on urine, wound drainage, or other body fluids or substances.

Specific Defense Mechanisms

The body's nonspecific defense mechanisms, including physical barriers and the general immune response, are one way our immune system helps prevent and fight off infections. The immune system also has the ability to develop specialized proteins called **antibodies**, which help our bodies fight off specific microbes. A person develops antibodies following exposure to the microbe, which come from a previous infection with the microbe, or through a vaccination. For example, the antibodies that build up in the body following a case of measles or chickenpox are the reason most of us only get these "childhood diseases" once. Now, routine vaccinations have almost eliminated many of these infections. Similarly, when you get your annual "flu shot," you are getting a dose of the virus strains that cause the flu. The viruses have been weakened or killed, so that you do not actually get sick, but the exposure is enough to cause your immune system to begin producing antibodies against those particular strains of the virus. That way, if you are exposed later, you will be less likely to become sick.

Antibiotics

Many times, our immune systems can fight off invading pathogens on their own. Other times, however, some outside help is required. An *antibiotic* is a medication that is able to kill bacteria or make it difficult for them to reproduce and grow. The first antibiotic, penicillin, came into widespread use during World War II and completely changed how we treat infectious disease. Today, there are many types of antibiotics used to treat many different types of bacterial infections. Antimicrobial agents (used to treat fungal and parasitic infections) and antiviral agents (used to treat some viral infections) are other drugs that we use to treat infection.

However, not all antibiotics and other medications used to treat infection are effective. As you will recall, bacteria are very adaptable organisms that have been around since the beginning of time. As such, some bacteria have evolved to develop resistance to the antibiotics used to fight them. In particular, **multidrug-resistant organisms (MDROs)** are resistant to one or more classes of antibiotics that may have previously been effective against them. Be aware that two particular MDROs, **methicillin-resistant *Staphylococcus aureus* (MRSA)** and **vancomycin-resistant enterococcus (VRE)**, are easily spread from person to person in a health care setting, usually via the hands of health care workers.

Staphylococcus aureus and enterococci are common microbes. *Staphylococcus aureus* is often found on a person's skin and upper respiratory tract and is transmitted easily through person-to-person contact. *Enterococci* are commonly found in a person's digestive tract and are transmitted through contact with feces. In a health care setting, these pathogens can be very dangerous because many patients and residents do not have healthy immune systems and are therefore less able to fight off infection. If infection occurs, it is difficult to treat because these microbes have become resistant to the drugs used to treat them in the past. In addition to MRSA and VRE, it is reasonable to expect that in the future other bacteria will become resistant to antibiotics as well.

On occasion, powerful antibiotics that are used to treat infections destroy other bacteria that help keep us healthy. When this happens, other bacteria that are not destroyed by the antibiotic will grow rapidly. One such bacterium, *Clostridium difficile (C. diff)*, is a major cause of health care–associated diarrhea. *C. diff* is easily spread from person to person in a health care setting and has been responsible for large outbreaks that can be fatal for patients or residents already weakened by illness or advanced age.

Although antibiotics have given us more options for treating infectious disease, they do not work against all pathogens all of the time, and the best policy is to avoid infection in the first place. You can keep your immune system strong and healthy through proper nutrition, adequate rest, and regular exercise. You can also take steps to limit your exposure to pathogens. In the next few sections, we will look at how pathogens are spread from one person to another and what you can do to help control their spread.

COMMUNICABLE DISEASE AND THE CHAIN OF INFECTION

An **infection** is an illness caused by a pathogen. Infections can be local (affecting a small, defined area of the body), generalized (affecting a general area or an organ), or systemic (affecting the entire body). Many (but not all) infections are communicable, which means that they can be transmitted either directly or indirectly from one person to another. Sometimes the terms *communicable* and *contagious* are used to refer to the same thing, but the two terms do not truly have the same meaning. *Contagious* is more accurately used to describe an infection that can be easily transmitted from one person to another through casual contact, such as a common cold or the flu. For example, you can get a cold just by touching a button in an elevator after someone who has a cold has touched it, or by sitting next to someone with a cold on a crowded bus. Therefore, a common cold is not only communicable, it is contagious. On the other hand, infections such as AIDS and hepatitis, while still communicable, are not referred to as *contagious* because they are not transmitted through casual contact.

For a person to get a communicable infection, six key conditions must be met, known as the **chain of infection** (Fig. 10-4).

1. A *pathogen* must be present. A microorganism capable of causing an infection must be present that is strong enough and in large enough numbers to cause an infection.
2. A *reservoir* must be present. A reservoir is a place where something is stored. In this case, a reservoir is a place that is suitable for the pathogen's survival. Pathogens collect in the reservoir and sometimes multiply there as well. Possible reservoirs of pathogens include humans and other animals, food, water, milk, and objects that come in contact with an infected person's secretions or body fluids.
3. A *portal of exit* must be available. The portal of exit is the way the pathogen leaves the reservoir. (The word *portal* means "door.") The way a pathogen leaves its reservoir varies, depending on the type of pathogen and the reservoir. For

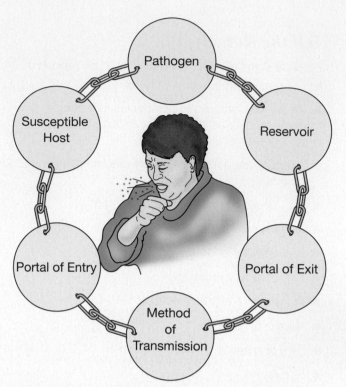

Figure 10-4 The chain of infection. For a person to get an infection, all six links in the chain must be present.

example, when the reservoir is a human being, common portals of exit for pathogens include the digestive tract (through feces, saliva, or vomitus), the respiratory tract (through mucus), the urinary and reproductive tracts (through urine, semen, or vaginal secretions), and the skin (through blood, pus, or other drainage from wounds).

4. A *method of transmission* must be available. After the pathogen leaves its reservoir via the portal of exit, it must have a way of physically getting from one person to another. This is called the pathogen's method of transmission, and it may be direct or indirect. Direct transmission requires close contact between an infected and a noninfected person. Pathogens can be directly transmitted when a noninfected person makes physical contact with an infected person, or inhales or ingests droplets exhaled by the infected person (for example, when that person coughs, talks, or sneezes). Indirect transmission occurs when a noninfected person comes into contact with a nonliving object that has been **contaminated** (soiled) by pathogens. These objects are called **fomites**. For example, a water glass or a bed sheet can become a fomite if it becomes contaminated by pathogens from a person with an infection, because if a noninfected person

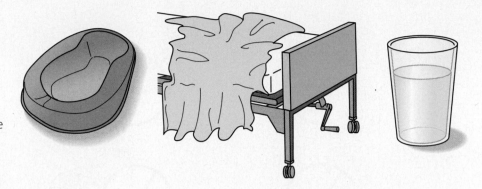

Figure 10-5 Pathogens can live on objects such as linens, bedpans, and drinking glasses. When an uninfected person touches or uses these items, they might pick up some of the pathogens on them and become sick. Nonliving objects that are capable of transmitting disease are called fomites.

uses the contaminated water glass or sleeps on the contaminated bed linens, they could become infected (Fig. 10-5). Also, surfaces that an infected person touches can become contaminated, causing a noninfected person who touches it afterward to pick up the pathogen. Other pathogens, such as the protozoan that causes malaria, are transmitted by way of a **vector** or a living creature (in the case of malaria, a mosquito). Some pathogens can be transmitted by more than just one method.

5. A *portal of entry* must be available. Now that the pathogen has left its reservoir and been successfully transmitted to another person, it must have a way of entering the new person's body. The respiratory, urinary, digestive, and reproductive systems are common portals of entry. So are breaks in the skin. A pathogen can leave one person's body and be transmitted to another person, but if the pathogen is not able to enter the new person's body, infection will not occur.

6. A *susceptible host* must be available. Microbes that can cause infection enter the human body continuously. The defense systems of the body we are born with and those we acquire (such as vaccines) can fight off most of these pathogens. However, many factors can place us at risk for infection. This is when the pathogen "makes its move." Risk factors that make a person more likely to get an infection include:

- **Very young or very old age**. People who are very young or very old are more likely to get an infection. Very young children have not had time to develop an effective defense mechanism for fighting infections, and older adults lose their defenses as they age, especially if they also have other chronic health conditions.
- **Poor general health**. A person who is sick or debilitated ("worn down") is more at risk for infection because the body's defenses are

already weakened by illness. Therefore, the person is not able to fight off the pathogen as easily. In addition, certain medical treatments, such as chemotherapy or radiation therapy, can affect the functioning of the body's immune system and put a person more at risk for infection.

- **Stress and fatigue**. Lack of rest and emotional stress can affect the body's ability to defend itself from pathogens.
- **Indwelling medical devices**. Medical devices, such as catheters, feeding tubes, and intravenous (IV) lines increase a person's risk of infection by providing a portal of entry for pathogens.

Many of the people you will care for as a nursing assistant have risk factors for infection. Your patients or residents will be sick, recovering from surgery, older, or have chronic illness or conditions that increase their risk of getting an infectious disease. A major part of your responsibility in caring for other people involves protecting them from infection.

The chain of infection can be broken by taking away just one of the six required elements (Fig. 10-6). For example, taking the right antibiotic for a bacterial infection quickly turns a person's body into an unfriendly reservoir for bacteria. Covering an infected wound with a dressing eliminates a pathogen's portal of exit by containing the pathogen within the dressing. Good hand hygiene and making sure that linens, utensils, glassware, surfaces that are touched frequently, and other possible fomites are properly cleansed eliminate a method of transmission. Wearing gloves and keeping your skin healthy and intact remove one potential portal of entry available to pathogens. Receiving required immunizations and maintaining general good health make you a less susceptible host. All of these actions break a link in the chain of infection, stopping the infection from being transmitted. Other factors that determine whether

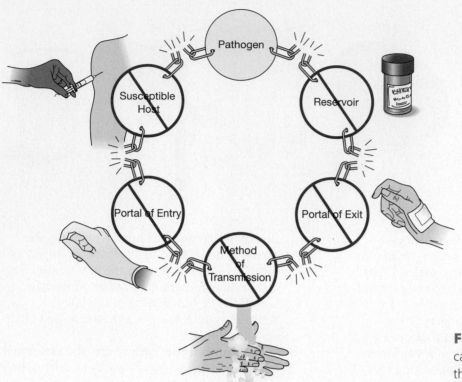

Figure 10-6 The chain of infection can be broken by removing just one of the six elements that must be present for infection to occur.

or not an infection will be transmitted are the **virulence** (strength or disease-producing potential) of the pathogen and the actual number of pathogens that enter the body.

In Chapter 12, you will learn more about important measures to take in the health care setting that control infections and help keep you and your patients and residents safe.

SUMMARY

- A huge variety of microbes share our planet.
  - Major types of microbes include bacteria, viruses, fungi, and parasites.
  - Some microbes cause disease while others are harmless.
- Our immune systems help us fight off infections.
  - Nonspecific defense mechanisms include physical barriers (skin and mucous membranes) and the general immune response.
  - Specific defense mechanisms include antibodies.

- Health care facilities provide the perfect environment for the spread of infection.
  - The chain of infection describes the elements that must be present in order for infection to occur. The six elements of the chain of infection are pathogen, reservoir, portal of exit, method of transmission, portal of entry, and susceptible host.
  - Breaking just one link in the chain of infection stops the spread of infection from one person to another.

WHAT DID YOU LEARN?

Multiple Choice

Select the single best answer for each of the following questions.

1. Bacteria may enter the body through:
   a. The mouth
   b. The nose
   c. Cuts in the skin
   d. All of the above

2. Microbes can be spread by:
   a. Looking at a person with a communicable disease
   b. Coughing or sneezing
   c. Touching a person with a communicable disease
   d. Both "b" and "c"

3. Which one of the following could be a fomite?
   a. A water glass that has been used
   b. A mosquito
   c. Linens that have just come back from the laundry
   d. A cut in the skin

4. Which one of the following must be present in order for infection to spread?
   a. A nursing assistant
   b. An indwelling medical device
   c. A susceptible host
   d. A patient or resident who looks ill

5. Infections such as the common cold and the flu are usually caused by:
   a. Bacteria
   b. Viruses
   c. Fungi
   d. Parasites

6. The most common cause of infection in the health care setting are due to:
   a. Bacteria
   b. Viruses
   c. Fungi
   d. Parasites

Matching   *Match each numbered item with its appropriate lettered description.*

_____ **1.** Communicable disease

_____ **2.** Pathogen

_____ **3.** Leukocyte

_____ **4.** Opportunistic microbe

_____ **5.** Fomite

_____ **6.** Aerobic

_____ **7.** Contagious

_____ **8.** Vector

_____ **9.** Anaerobic

_____ **10.** Antibody

a. Describes bacteria that need oxygen to survive
b. Special proteins that help fight specific pathogens
c. Can be transferred from one person to another
d. Microbe that can cause illness
e. Nonliving object that is contaminated
f. White blood cell
g. Can change from harmless to pathogenic, given a chance
h. Infection that is very easily spread from person to person
i. A living creature that transmits disease
j. Describes bacteria that die if oxygen is present

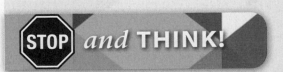

Several residents in your care have come down with a nasty intestinal virus that causes diarrhea. One resident, Mrs. Grande, is so weak that she was unable to get out of bed in time and soiled her clothing and bedding.

Where is the most likely portal of exit for this pathogen? What steps should you take when cleaning up Mrs. Grande that will help to keep this virus from being spread to other residents, your coworkers, and you?

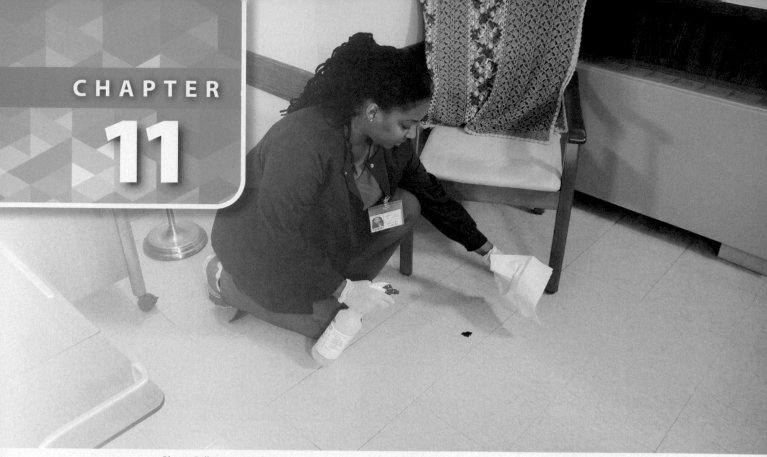

Photo: Following standard precautions, such as wearing personal protective equipment (PPE) whenever contact with blood or other body fluids is likely, helps to protect you from bloodborne pathogens.

Common Communicable Diseases and Transmission in the Health Care Setting

 ## WHAT WILL YOU LEARN?

As a nursing assistant, you will have close contact with patients and residents, some of whom will have communicable diseases. Many of these diseases can be spread easily to other patients and residents, and even to yourself. In this chapter, you will learn about some of the communicable diseases that pose the most risk of being transmitted in the health care setting, and how these diseases are transmitted. You will learn what you can do to minimize your risk of getting one of these infections. And you will also learn about the standards that have been developed by the Occupational Safety and Health Administration (OSHA) with the goal of protecting you at work while you provide quality care for your patients or residents. When you are finished with this chapter, you will be able to:

1. **List reasons why communicable diseases may be more easily transmitted in a health care setting.**
2. **Discuss how pathogens are transmitted by contact methods.**
3. **Identify infectious diseases that are commonly transmitted by contact in the health care setting.**

4. **Explain how bloodborne pathogens are transmitted.**

5. **Describe two major bloodborne diseases that pose a threat to the health care worker.**

6. **Describe how HIV/AIDS affects a person physically.**

7. **Discuss the risks of infection for HIV and AIDS.**

8. **Describe measures health care workers and employers take to protect against exposure to bloodborne pathogens.**

9. **Describe how airborne pathogens are transmitted.**

10. **Describe major airborne diseases that pose a threat to the health care worker.**

Vocabulary

Bloodborne pathogen
Body fluids
Hepatitis
Hepatitis A virus (HAV)
Oral–fecal route
Hepatitis B virus (HBV)
Carrier

Centers for Disease
   Control and Prevention
   (CDC)
Hepatitis C virus (HCV)
Hepatitis D virus (HDV)
Hepatitis E virus (HEV)

Human
   immunodeficiency
   virus (HIV)
Acquired
   immunodeficiency
   syndrome (AIDS)
T cell

HIV positive
OSHA Bloodborne
   Pathogens Standard
Exposure control plan
Airborne pathogen
Tuberculosis (TB)

COMMUNICABLE DISEASES IN THE HEALTH CARE SETTING

You learned in Chapter 10 that in order for a communicable disease to occur, there must be a method of transmission from an infected person to another person. Understanding how certain diseases are transmitted from person to person is vital so that you can take measures to both protect yourself and your patients and residents from infection.

In the health care setting, it is common to have a large number of patients and residents living in a small area. There are also numerous people providing care for those people, both directly and indirectly. Add to this mix the visitors who come into a facility on a daily basis. Just this sheer number of people under one roof dramatically increases the types of communicable diseases and the methods in which they can be transmitted. Because many of your patients and residents will have risk factors that make them more susceptible to infection, protecting them from transmission is very important.

COMMUNICABLE DISEASES SPREAD BY CONTACT

As you learned in Chapter 10, communicable diseases are often spread by contact, such as through person-to-person contact or contact with contaminated materials or substances. It is important to be aware of how contact transmission occurs in health care settings and what diseases are commonly transmitted in these settings.

Contact Transmission

Bacteria are the cause of most common diseases spread by contact in the health care setting. As you recall, contact transmission can occur by both direct and indirect methods. Interestingly, the most common direct contact transmission occurs from the hands of the health care workers themselves! As a nursing assistant, you will care for many people during your shift, going from person to person and touching most of them with your hands. Failure to perform good hand hygiene (discussed in detail in Chapter 12) can result in picking up bacteria from one patient or resident and then passing it to many others as you provide care. Patients and residents themselves can also transmit communicable diseases through direct contact by touching other people.

Indirect transmission occurs when a person who has the infectious organism on their hands touches areas, such as door handles, elevator buttons, handrails, or other high-touch areas, that may later be touched by another person. Contaminated items, such as soiled dressings, clothing, or medical equipment can also contaminate surfaces they come in contact with or the hands of people touching them.

Diseases Commonly Transmitted by Contact in the Health Care Setting

Wound infections, especially those caused by MRSA, are easily spread by contact in the health care setting. Any items that have come in contact with drainage from an infected wound must be disposed of carefully and surfaces that may have come into contact with those items must be cleaned carefully. In many instances, your patient or resident with a wound infection may also be confused and pull their dressing loose, which allows the spread of infection to other people and surfaces they touch. Since many healthy people may still carry MRSA on their skin and upper respiratory tract, those bacteria can be transmitted into another person's wound through touch and cause an infection.

Other communicable diseases, such as VRE and *C. diff*, are easily spread through contact transmission in a health care setting from contact with contaminated feces. Most people suffering from these infections will have diarrhea and may soil their clothing, bedding, chairs, and other surfaces. Hands that come in contact with these items or the diarrhea can then spread the organisms easily to other people. Other types of intestinal viruses can be spread in this manner also.

BLOODBORNE DISEASES

As a nursing assistant, you will be exposed to your patients' and residents' blood (and other body fluids), and will need to be aware of the risks of bloodborne transmission and the serious diseases that can result.

Bloodborne Transmission

A **bloodborne pathogen** is a disease-producing microbe that is transmitted to another person through blood or other body fluids. **Body fluids** are liquid or semiliquid substances produced by the body, such as blood, urine, feces, vomitus, saliva, drainage from wounds, sweat, semen, vaginal secretions, tears, cerebrospinal fluid, amniotic fluid, and breast milk. For a bloodborne pathogen to be transmitted from one person to another, blood or body fluids from an infected person must enter the bloodstream of a person who is not infected. There are several ways this could occur in the workplace:

- Needlesticks (puncture wounds caused by used hypodermic needles)

- Cuts from contaminated, broken glass (such as that from a broken blood tube)
- Direct contact between infected blood and broken skin, mucous membranes, or the eyes

In addition, bloodborne pathogens can be transmitted via sexual intercourse or through blood transfusions.

Several diseases are caused by bloodborne pathogens. The most common are:

- Hepatitis B and C
- Human immunodeficiency virus (HIV), which causes acquired immunodeficiency syndrome (AIDS)
- Malaria
- Syphilis
- Ebola

Of these, hepatitis and HIV pose the greatest occupational risk to the health care worker in most countries. However, previous outbreaks of the Ebola virus in Africa have shown that Ebola is also a substantial occupational risk to health care and aid workers.

Hepatitis

Hepatitis is inflammation of the liver, the organ that removes toxic substances from the bloodstream (Fig. 11-1). Hepatitis is most commonly caused by a viral infection, but it may also be caused by chemicals, drugs, or drinking alcohol. Some infections with a hepatitis virus are mild, producing no lasting effects on the liver. Others are chronic and affect the liver's ability to function over time. If the liver failure is severe, the person will die unless they receive a liver

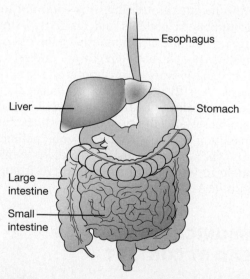

Figure 11-1 Hepatitis is inflammation of the liver, the organ that removes toxic substances from the blood.

transplant. Currently, five types of hepatitis virus have been identified: the hepatitis A, B, C, D, and E viruses.

Hepatitis A Virus

Hepatitis A virus (HAV) is not a bloodborne pathogen. This virus is transmitted through the **oral–fecal route**, which means that the virus lives in the digestive tract of an infected person and leaves the person's body through the feces. The feces can contaminate food or water, then is transmitted orally (by mouth) when a person eats or drinks the contaminated food or water and becomes infected. For example, HAV can be passed on when a food service worker who has the virus uses the restroom but fails to wash their hands properly before returning to work and handling a customer's food. Hepatitis A outbreaks are also found in areas where raw sewage comes into contact with bodies of water where shellfish, such as oysters, live. The virus infects the shellfish and is then passed on to unsuspecting people who eat the contaminated shellfish raw. Fortunately, the illness caused by HAV (commonly referred to as *infectious hepatitis*) is usually acute and the person usually recovers fully. An effective vaccine against this virus is available and recommended for the general public.

Hepatitis B Virus

Hepatitis B virus (HBV), a bloodborne pathogen, is a serious threat for the health care worker. The virus is found in blood, as well as in other body fluids, such as semen and vaginal secretions. This means that HBV can be transmitted through transfusion of infected blood or blood products, across the placenta from birthing parent to infant, and through unprotected sexual intercourse. In addition, body fluids known to carry high amounts of HBV include wound drainage and cultures, cerebrospinal fluid, amniotic fluid, and breast milk. Other body secretions do not typically have high viral counts unless there is visible blood present.

Infection with HBV causes an acute illness in most people, but some people can be infected by the virus and never develop symptoms. These people are considered **carriers**. Because they do not have symptoms of the disease, carriers may be unaware that they have it. However, the virus lives in their bodies and can be transmitted to another person. Between 5% and 10% of HBV infections become chronic. People with chronic infections may never have symptoms and become carriers. Or, they may have flare-ups of symptoms every so often, resulting in months of disability.

Health care workers who have any direct contact with patients or residents can be exposed to body fluids that contain HBV. Health care workers are at risk for getting HBV through:

- Needlestick injuries
- Cuts from contaminated objects
- Exposure of broken skin or mucous membranes to contaminated blood or other body fluids (Fig. 11-2)

Although the virus is not known to be transmitted in saliva, the gums of people with periodontal (gum) disease may bleed during oral care and tooth brushing, exposing the health care worker to potentially contaminated blood. There is always the risk of nicking a patient or resident with the razor during shaving, and patients or residents may fall and injure themselves, resulting in wounds that bleed. A used hypodermic needle could be lost in the bed linens or accidentally tossed in the trash, placing an unsuspecting health care worker at risk for a puncture injury.

Because of these occupational risks, the **Centers for Disease Control and Prevention (CDC)** recommends that all health care workers who have even the slightest potential for being exposed to blood or contaminated body fluids should receive the hepatitis

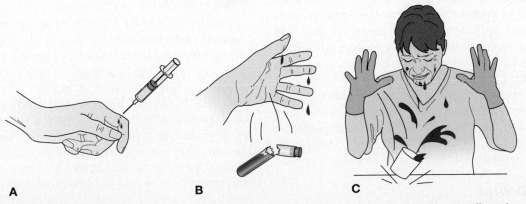

A   **B**   **C**

Figure 11-2 In the workplace, hepatitis B virus (HBV) can be transmitted by (**A**) a needlestick injury, (**B**) cuts from contaminated glass, or (**C**) direct contact with blood, for example, through a blood splash to the face.

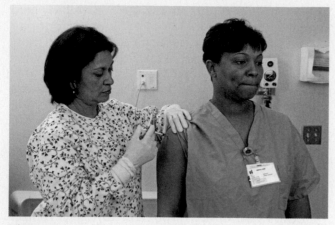

Figure 11-3 A vaccine against hepatitis B virus (HBV) is available. The Occupational Safety and Health Administration (OSHA) requires employers to make the vaccine available to nursing assistants free of charge.

B vaccination, which provides immunity to the virus. OSHA requires employers to offer this vaccine to employees free of charge (Fig. 11-3) and recommends the vaccine for the general public as well.

Hepatitis C Virus

Hepatitis C virus (HCV) is also a bloodborne pathogen and is the most common cause of chronic viral hepatitis in the United States. Prior to 1992, when screening donated blood for HCV became routine practice, blood transfusions were a major source of transmission. Now, IV drug use is the most common mode of transmission. Although transmission of HCV can occur for a health care worker through a needle-stick injury, the risk is much lower than for HBV. Other possible, but unlikely, methods of transmission can occur from an HCV-infected birthing parent to baby during birth and through unprotected sexual intercourse. Although the mode of HCV transmission is mainly bloodborne, in more than 40% of people who are diagnosed with HCV, no obvious route of transmission is found. The illness that results from infection with HCV tends to be more chronic and serious than that resulting from infection with HBV. As many as 85% of people with hepatitis C develop chronic disease, and of these, 20% go on to develop end-stage cirrhosis (a fatal liver disease), liver failure, or liver cancer. Hepatitis C is the leading cause for liver transplantation in the United States. Currently, no vaccine against HCV is available, but new treatments have been successful in curing HCV in many people.

Hepatitis D Virus

Hepatitis D virus (HDV), also known as "delta hepatitis," is found only in people who are already infected with HBV. Hepatitis D is uncommon in the United States. There is no vaccine for HDV, but HDV can be prevented by vaccination against HBV.

Hepatitis E Virus

Hepatitis E virus (HEV) is not a bloodborne type of hepatitis. Like HAV, HEV is spread through the oral–fecal route of transmission. HEV infection is most common in countries with limited resources for sanitation control. There is no vaccination for this virus.

HIV/AIDS

Human immunodeficiency virus (HIV) is the virus that causes **acquired immunodeficiency syndrome (AIDS)**. HIV is a bloodborne pathogen and is transmitted in the same way as HBV. Its effect on the body, however, is very different.

As described in Chapter 10, the human immune system recognizes and destroys pathogens (microbes that can enter the body and cause illness). One way the immune system does its job is through **T cells**, special white blood cells (leukocytes) that play a role in the immune response to invading pathogens. There are two main types of T cells. One type of T cell recognizes cells that are foreign to the body, such as those infected by viruses, and kills them by producing substances that cause the foreign cells to burst. The other type of T cell produces substances that help other cells in the immune system to defend the body against pathogens.

T cells are the main target of HIV (Fig. 11-4). The virus invades the T cell, but instead of killing it immediately, it uses the T cell to make copies of itself and increase its numbers. Eventually, the virus kills the T cell and then the virus (and all of its copies) moves on to repeat the process in other T cells. Over time, this process results in an increase in the virus count and a decrease in the T cell count.

What Is AIDS?

Currently, more than 1.2 million people in the United States are infected with HIV, and of those who are currently infected, nearly one in five people do not know that they are. Approximately 30,000 people become newly infected each year. A person who is infected with HIV is said to be **HIV positive** because they have tested positive on the blood test for HIV antibodies. In invading a person's T cells, the virus destroys the cells that are responsible for protecting the body. As HIV takes over the body's immune system, the infected person begins to have more and more health problems, such as severe infections and aggressive cancers. Many HIV-positive people eventually develop AIDS, an advanced stage of HIV infection. AIDS is said to occur when the person's weakened immune system

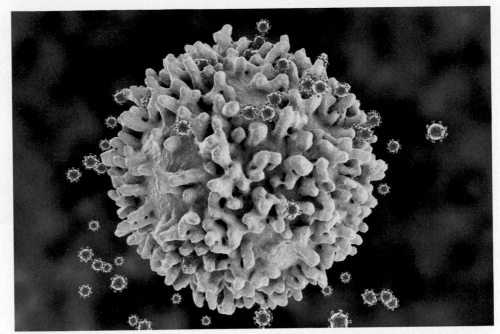

Figure 11-4 This photograph was taken by a special microscope, and color was added to enhance it. It shows a T cell (*green*) that is infected with the human immunodeficiency virus (HIV), shown in *red*. Infection with HIV can lead to the development of acquired immunodeficiency syndrome (AIDS), a fatal disease. (*Kateryna Kon\ Shutterstock.com*)

is no longer able to fight off infections and malignancies. People with AIDS do not die from the virus that has infected their bodies. Rather, they die from infections and malignancies that the body is no longer able to fight.

Most people who become infected with HIV experience a brief, flu-like illness about 2 to 4 weeks after they are first exposed to the virus. During this brief illness, the person may have a fever, swollen lymph nodes, a sore throat, a rash, or any combination of these signs and symptoms. These signs and symptoms eventually go away and may be forgotten. In many cases, if the person is tested for the virus within the next 3 to 6 months, the test will not be positive, even though the person is infected with the virus. A person can be infected with HIV for many years before developing AIDS, or they may never develop AIDS. The amount of time that it takes before AIDS develops and death occurs varies greatly from person to person. For example, in children and people in poor health, HIV infection is likely to progress to AIDS more quickly. As HIV infection progresses, the person is likely to experience:

- Loss of appetite, nausea, vomiting, or diarrhea
- Weight loss
- Fever (with or without night sweats)
- Pain or difficulty swallowing (dysphagia)
- Fatigue
- Swollen lymph nodes in the neck, armpits, and groin
- A cough or recurrent episodes of pneumonia
- Sores or white patches in the mouth
- Bruises or dark bumps on the skin that do not heal, called Kaposi's sarcoma (Fig. 11-5)

- Forgetfulness and confusion
- Dementia
- Vision loss

To date, there is no cure for HIV/AIDS; however, early diagnosis of HIV infection and early treatment with antiretroviral therapy (ART) is becoming very successful in helping delay the onset of HIV and reduce the risk of transmission of the virus to other people. In many individuals who have tested positive for HIV, ART can reduce the viral load to undetectable

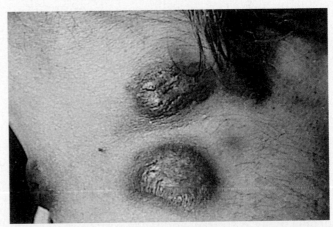

Figure 11-5 As a result of their weakened immune systems, people with AIDS often develop malignancies, such as Kaposi's sarcoma. The lesions of Kaposi's sarcoma are often seen on the skin and mucous membranes of people with advanced HIV infection (AIDS). (Photograph courtesy of Goodheart HP. *Goodheart's Photoguide of Common Skin Disorders: Diagnosis and Management.* Lippincott Williams & Wilkins; 2003: p. 374.)

levels, allowing HIV infection to become a manageable chronic health condition. Currently, no medication can kill HIV and offer a complete cure for AIDS. And, for many people who are unaware that they are infected with HIV, ART is not effective because the infection is too far advanced.

What Are the Risks of Infection for HIV/AIDS?

Anyone who comes into direct contact with HIV is at risk of getting infected. Earlier in this chapter, you learned that HIV is transmitted from one person to another through body fluids, such as blood, semen, and vaginal secretions. Exposure to HIV can also occur either before or during birth, or through breast milk. Behaviors and situations that increase a person's risk for becoming infected with HIV include the following:

- **Having unprotected sex.** Unprotected sexual intercourse (such as without barrier methods) is the most common method of HIV transmission.
- **Sharing of needles.** Sharing of needles among people who use intravenous drugs is the second most common method of transmission.
- **Receiving tissue transplants or transfusions of blood or blood products.** Before 1985, people who received blood transfusions may have been exposed to HIV. This method of transmission is less common now in nations with more health care resources and systems because donated blood is screened for the virus. However, blood supplies are still not screened in some countries.

In the United States, the highest rate of HIV infection is found among males who have sex with males who are between the ages of 25 and 34 years. However, this is not the only age group at risk. Younger people, aged 13 to 25 years, are seeing an increasing occurrence of HIV infection.

A Global Health Issue

Today, HIV/AIDS continues to be considered a global public health issue. The rate of infection continues to increase in some parts of the world, and there is no cure for this devastating disease. The World Health Organization (WHO) reports that the number of people living with HIV worldwide continues to grow, reaching an estimated 37.7 million people at the end of 2020, with over two thirds of those living in the WHO African Region. It is estimated that 1.5 million new HIV infections occurred and an estimated 680,000 people died as the result of AIDS-related illnesses in 2020. AIDS awareness programs, which teach people about AIDS and how to lower their risk of becoming infected with HIV, have helped to lower

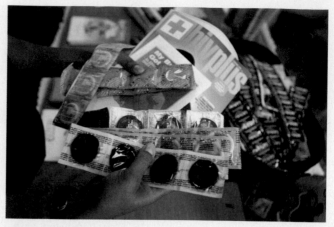

Figure 11-6 AIDS awareness programs provide information about HIV infection and AIDS to the general public. These programs provide free advice about the disease, how it can be prevented, and where a person can go to get tested for HIV. (*Joe Raedle\Getty Images.*)

the rate of infection in resource-abundant countries, such as the United States and many European nations (Fig. 11-6). In addition, people who live in resource-abundant countries often have better access to health care if they do become infected with HIV.

Protecting Yourself from Bloodborne Diseases

To protect yourself and others in the workplace from the risk of bloodborne diseases, it is crucial to follow the specific precautions and standards designed for your and your patients' and residents' health and safety.

Standard Precautions

As a health care worker, you will come in contact with substances that carry the HIV, HBV, and HCV viruses and therefore pose a risk to you. In addition, in many cases, you will not be able to easily identify patients or residents who have these diseases. For example, HIV can be present in the blood of an infected person for a long time without causing symptoms or being detected using the diagnostic tests that are currently available. Similarly, the viruses that cause hepatitis B and hepatitis C can live in a person's body without causing signs or symptoms. For these reasons, we in the health care field *must* treat each patient or resident we have contact with as if they *may* be infected with a bloodborne pathogen. This is why standard precautions, discussed in detail in Chapter 12, are taken with each patient or resident. *For standard precautions to be effective, they must be used consistently with every patient or resident.*

It is important to remember that although those who choose to work in the health care field place themselves at risk for exposure to substances that can cause disease, the risk of encountering these substances outside of the workplace also exists. In fact, your behavior outside of the workplace could put you at much higher risk for getting one of these diseases. For example, having unprotected sexual intercourse is the most common way of getting HBV and HIV, and the rate of new HBV and AIDS cases is growing fastest among young people. Your job exposes you to risks, such as needlesticks, that people in other professions do not need to worry about. But, if you follow the standard precautions, your risk of getting a bloodborne disease in the workplace will probably be lower than your risk of getting a bloodborne disease outside of it!

OSHA Bloodborne Pathogens Standard

Your safety in the workplace is a shared responsibility. You are responsible for following the standard precautions. Your employer is responsible for making sure that you have the equipment and training you need to maintain your safety in the workplace. To help employers to meet their responsibilities toward their employees, OSHA has created certain standards that all employers must follow, called the **OSHA Bloodborne Pathogens Standard** (Box 11-1).

Any health care facility that does not follow the OSHA standards for bloodborne pathogens may risk heavy fines and serious penalties, such as closure of the facility. For health care workers who do not follow standard precautions, the penalty can be even greater—a deadly illness. In addition, if you have an exposure accident and were not following the recommended precautions, you may not be covered by worker's compensation if you become sick as a result of the exposure. The consequences of not following proper procedures in the workplace are not worth the risk.

Box 11-1	OSHA Bloodborne Pathogens Standard

- People working in an area where exposure to bloodborne pathogens is possible must receive training on the risks associated with bloodborne pathogens and on the methods they can use to safeguard themselves. Proof of initial training (at orientation) is to be on file in the employee's records, and training must be updated annually.
- Employers must make the hepatitis B vaccine available to workers who are at risk, free of charge. If an employee refuses the vaccination, a disclaimer signed by the employee must be kept on file. If the employee decides to accept the vaccine at a later date, the employer must provide it.
- The employer must provide adequate personal protective equipment (PPE), as required by the employee's duties. This includes gloves (nonlatex, if the employee has allergies), face and eye protection, gowns and aprons, and scrub attire. It is the employee's responsibility to use the PPE consistently and conscientiously.
- Environmental control methods must be used to protect both the employees and the patients or residents. Environmental control methods include special ventilation systems to keep the air clean, procedures for the disposal of liquid waste, the availability of sharps disposal containers, and procedures for handling contaminated linen and trash. Housekeeping and cleaning methods must also meet OSHA's standards.
- Each health care facility must have an **exposure control plan** in place in case an employee is exposed to blood or other body fluids from a patient or resident. The exposure control plan states what actions must be taken if an employee is exposed to blood or other body fluids while on the job. This plan must be up to date, available in written form, and available to all employees. It is the employee's responsibility to report any exposure incidents so that the employer can arrange for appropriate medical tests and treatment.

AIRBORNE DISEASES

In addition to transmission of disease through contact or body fluids, there is also risk of transmission of diseases by air. These diseases are called airborne diseases.

Airborne Transmittal

Airborne pathogens are disease-producing microbes that are transmitted through the air. When an infected person coughs or sneezes, the pathogens leave the body through particles of saliva or sputum (Fig. 11-7).

As these particles spray through the air, they dry out and remain in the air for a long time (much like particles of dust caught in a shaft of sunlight). Like dust, the dried-out droplets containing pathogens are in the air we breathe and on the surfaces we touch. Infection spreads when a person breathes the air containing the suspended pathogens. Infections that are transmitted in this way include measles, chickenpox, SARS, smallpox, and TB.

Other airborne pathogens are transmitted in a similar fashion, called droplets. These microbes are suspended in larger droplets of saliva or sputum, but the pathogen usually does not remain alive or active after drying out. Like other airborne pathogens, they

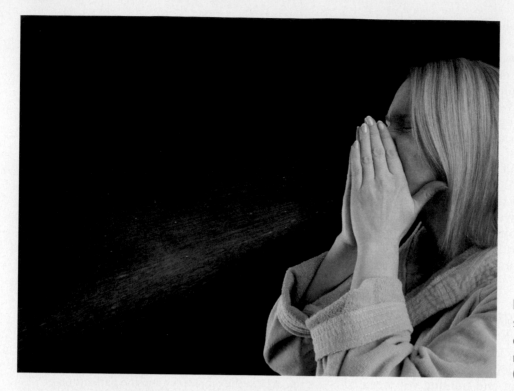

Figure 11-7 A typical sneeze sends several thousand droplets of microbe-containing mucus and saliva into the air. (*Riopatuca\Shutterstock.com*)

are released from the infected person during coughing, sneezing, or talking, but because they are heavier particles, most only remain suspended in the air for about 3 to 6 feet from the person. Infections that are transmitted in this way include mumps, influenza, whooping cough, strep throat, scarlet fever, rubella, meningitis, some types of pneumonia, diphtheria, epiglottitis, and COVID-19. However, because the virus that causes COVID-19 is found in very fine droplets that an infected person exhales, it can remain suspended in the air longer than other types of microorganisms.

Close and/or extended contact with a person who has an airborne infection increases your chances of catching that infection from them. Crowded conditions, such as those on public transportation or in elevators or busy indoor spaces, increase exposure to airborne infections.

It is important to understand that although these infections are primarily transmitted from one person to another through the air, they can also be transmitted through contact. When an infected person sneezes or coughs into their hands and then touches another person's hand or surface that is then soon touched by another person, that person can transmit the microorganism to themselves by then touching their face.

Tuberculosis

Tuberculosis (TB) is an infection caused by a bacterium that usually infects the lungs but may also infect the kidneys or bones. The bacteria are present in the sputum of an infected person and are spread by airborne droplets when the person coughs, sneezes, speaks, or sings. People who have close, frequent contact with a person who has TB are most likely to get the disease. A person infected with TB may have the disease for years before they show any symptoms.

In the early 1900s, TB caused many deaths. It was often called "consumption" because the disease progressed slowly and caused a wasting effect on the person. (In other words, the person grew very thin, and appeared to be eaten, or "consumed," by the disease.) During this time, people with TB were usually sent to special hospitals called *sanatoriums*, which offered treatment and served as a way of limiting the spread of the disease by keeping people with TB away from others. In the early 1950s, the development of antibiotics that worked against the bacterium that causes TB resulted in a decrease in the number of people with the disease. However, since the mid-1980s, there has been an increase in the number of new cases of TB.

Many factors seem responsible for these new cases:

- Strains of the bacterium that cause TB have become resistant to the antibiotics used to treat the infection, making the antibiotics less effective.
- People with immunodeficiency syndromes, such as AIDS, are more at risk for infections such as TB, and the number of people with immunodeficiency syndromes has increased.
- More people are traveling to developing nations, where TB is still common.

■ People who live in crowded conditions or who lack easy access to medical care, such as people experiencing homelessness who are living in a shelter, are at increased risk for TB.

People who get TB need to be treated for a long time, with many different antibiotics. Unfortunately, the people who are most likely to get the disease are least likely to complete the course of treatment for it because they lack money, a stable home, or both.

Because the number of new TB cases is increasing, and because the disease may go undiagnosed, a very real potential for exposure to TB in the workplace exists. Because health care workers are at risk for getting TB from patients or residents, health care facilities regularly screen employees for TB using a simple skin test. Testing positive on a skin test does not mean that you have TB, just that you have been exposed to it. People who have lived in other countries may have received a type of TB immunization and will test positive on a skin test. Additional tests, such as blood tests and a chest x-ray, may be necessary to determine if a person actually has TB.

Protecting Yourself from Airborne Diseases

If a patient or resident is known or suspected to have an airborne disease such as TB, take airborne precautions, discussed in detail in Chapter 12.

SUMMARY

■ HBV, HCV, and HIV are bloodborne pathogens that a health care worker may be exposed to. These viruses cause serious, possibly life-threatening diseases.

  ■ For a bloodborne pathogen to be transmitted from one person to another, blood or body fluids from an infected person must enter the bloodstream of a noninfected person.

    ■ Needlesticks, cuts from contaminated glass, and splashes and sprays of contaminated blood can put a health care worker at risk for a bloodborne disease.

    ■ Bloodborne diseases can also be transmitted through sexual intercourse and blood transfusions.

    ■ A person who is infected with a bloodborne pathogen may not appear to be ill.

■ Acquired immunodeficiency syndrome (AIDS) is caused by infection with the human immunodeficiency virus (HIV). HIV invades the body's immune system, leaving it unable to do its job. As a result, the person eventually dies from infections or cancers that take over the body.

  ■ A person who has tested positive for having antibodies to HIV in their blood is said to be *HIV positive.*

  ■ Many HIV-positive people eventually develop AIDS, an advanced stage of HIV infection. A person who is infected with HIV may live for many years before AIDS develops.

■ HIV/AIDS is a global public health issue. Since it was first identified in the early 1980s, HIV/AIDS has spread rapidly, killing a large number of people throughout the world in a short period of time.

  ■ In the United States, Canada, and England, rates of HIV infection and death from AIDS are decreasing due to the efforts of AIDS awareness programs and the availability of funding for research and health care.

■ Anyone can get HIV/AIDS, regardless of race, sex, gender, sexual orientation, or age.

  ■ Behaviors that increase a person's risk of becoming infected with HIV include having unprotected sexual intercourse and sharing needles used to inject drugs with other people.

  ■ The virus can also be transmitted through tissue transplants or transfusions of blood or blood products, and from a birthing parent to a child during birth or through breast milk.

  ■ You and your employer share the responsibility for maintaining your safety in the workplace.

    ■ Employers must follow OSHA standards to ensure that the work environment is safe (the OSHA Bloodborne Pathogens Standard).

    ■ Employees must follow the recommended precautions for preventing the spread of disease (standard precautions). Following the standard precautions is the single most important thing you can do to ensure your own safety.

  ■ An HBV vaccine is available and offers protection against HDV as well. Currently, there is no vaccine available for HCV or HIV.

- TB is caused by an airborne pathogen, which is spread when an infected person coughs, sneezes, speaks, or sings.
    - The number of TB cases is on the rise. A person with TB may not appear to be ill.
    - Although antibiotics are available to treat TB, treatment is difficult, time consuming, and expensive. There is currently no vaccine available for TB.

- You will face exposure to many infections, some life threatening, while caring for others. Learning about these infections and how they are transmitted, as well as staying well informed about new developments and treatments for these diseases, will allow you to provide quality care to those you are responsible for.

WHAT DID YOU LEARN?

Multiple Choice

Select the single best answer for each of the following questions.

1. Hepatitis B virus (HBV), a bloodborne pathogen, can be found in all of the following body fluids except:
   a. Blood
   b. Semen
   c. Wound drainage
   d. Sweat

2. Human immunodeficiency virus (HIV) can be transmitted through all of the following means except:
   a. Blood splash to mucous membrane
   b. Sexual intercourse
   c. Sharing needles
   d. A mosquito bite

3. A vaccination against which one of the following bloodborne diseases is available?
   a. Lyme disease
   b. AIDS
   c. Hepatitis C
   d. Hepatitis B

4. Hepatitis B is a viral disease of the:
   a. Spleen
   b. Liver
   c. Blood
   d. Heart

5. When are standard precautions used?
   a. When a person who is HIV positive develops AIDS
   b. When a person is HIV positive or has AIDS
   c. When caring for a patient or resident who has just returned from international travel
   d. When caring for any patient or resident and contact with blood or body fluids is possible

6. Which one of the following statements about HIV infection is true?
   a. Anyone who comes into direct contact with HIV is at risk of becoming infected.
   b. Infection can occur during the birth of a baby to a parent who has HIV.
   c. Blood transfusions of unscreened blood can risk exposing people to HIV and infecting them.
   d. All of the above.

7. TB, influenza, and COVID-19 are infections that are primarily transmitted through:
   a. Blood
   b. Skin-to-skin contact
   c. Airborne droplets
   d. Needlestick injuries

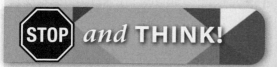

STOP *and* THINK!

You are walking past the TV room of the nursing facility where you work. You hear a call for help. As you enter the room, you see that Mr. Torres has a pretty bad nosebleed. There is blood on his hands and clothes, and some has puddled on the floor. What should you do as you rush to help Mr. Torres? How will you clean up the blood afterward?

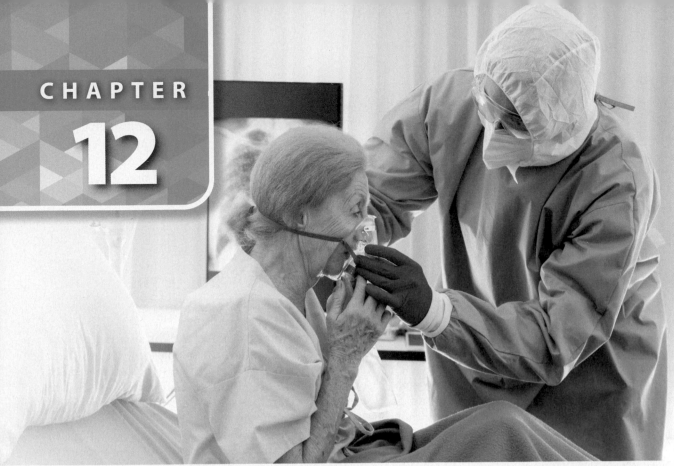

Photo: The COVID-19 pandemic caused an increased focus on measures that are taken to help prevent the spread of infection, both in the health care setting and for the general public. (Narint Asawaphisith\Shutterstock.com)

Infection Control Measures

 WHAT WILL YOU LEARN?

You have learned in the previous chapters in this unit that many communicable diseases can be easily spread from person to person, especially in the health care setting. In this chapter, you will learn methods that are used to protect yourself, your family members, and your patients and residents from catching a communicable disease. When you are finished with this chapter, you will be able to:

1. Explain the differences between communicable diseases that are considered *endemic, epidemic,* and *pandemic.*
2. Define the term *health care–associated infection (HAI)* and discuss ways a person could get an infection within the health care system.
3. List the four major methods of infection control.
4. List the four techniques of medical asepsis.
5. State how personal protective equipment (PPE) is used in infection control.
6. Explain the standard precautions that are taken with every patient or resident.
7. Describe the three types of transmission-based precautions and explain when they are used.
8. Demonstrate proper hand hygiene, gloving, masking, gowning, and double-bagging techniques.

Vocabulary

Endemic
Epidemic
Pandemic
Health care–associated
  infections (HAIs)
Nosocomial infections
Infection control

Medical asepsis
Sanitization
Antisepsis
Disinfection
Sterilization
Transient flora

Personal protective
  equipment (PPE)
Isolation precautions
Standard precautions
Transmission-based
  precautions

Airborne precautions
Airborne infection
  isolation room (AIIR)
Droplet precautions
Contact precautions

COMMUNICABLE DISEASES AND HOW THEY AFFECT US

Communicable diseases are always present in our general population, and for most of us, they are just an occasional disruption in our daily lives. We catch the common cold, intestinal bugs, and the flu on what seems like a regular basis. Then, we recover and go about business as usual. Most of the communicable diseases we catch are considered **endemic**, which means that they are always present to some extent in our general population. That's why there are always a few cases of the flu at any time of the year.

However, there are some conditions that can make any particular communicable disease more prevalent. For instance, the flu (influenza) usually increases in the number of cases, sometimes greatly, between November and February each year. This is a time of year that is colder, people spend more time indoors (often in crowded environments), and they go to holiday parties and family gatherings. Since the flu is highly contagious, it is easily transmitted and can infect a large group of people in a specific population all at once, therefore becoming an **epidemic**. Many healthy people get sick and recover; however, as you have learned, individuals who receive care in a health care setting may be affected more severely by a common illness.

Many epidemics in the past, and illnesses such as the bubonic plague, smallpox, polio, and the influenza outbreak of 1918, infected and killed many people. Many of these epidemics were so widespread that they affected populations worldwide and therefore were known as **pandemics**. Unfortunately, we are still experiencing communicable diseases on the pandemic level. HIV/AIDS infected people globally and is still uncontrolled in some parts of the world. Our most recent pandemic illness has been from the COVID-19 virus (SARS-CoV-2 virus), and because it is so contagious and easily transmitted, it has greatly influenced how we view the measures we take to control the spread of infection within the general public and in the health care setting especially.

INFECTION CONTROL IN THE HEALTH CARE SETTING

What do you think when you think of a health care facility? Health care professionals in clean, fresh uniforms, a smell of antiseptic in the air, and miles of shiny tile floors? Most of us think of health care facilities as clean, possibly even sterile, environments. Maintaining cleanliness in health care facilities is essential because exposure to pathogens is high in these settings. In addition, most of the people in health care facilities are there because they are not in good overall health. Therefore, their potential to become infected is increased.

Health care–associated infections (HAIs) are infections that people get while they are in the hospital or other health care settings. A patient or resident can get an HAI while they are receiving care, or a health care worker can get an HAI while providing care. Infections acquired by patients or residents while they are in a health care facility are also called **nosocomial infections**. The most common method of transmission for HAIs, including the very dangerous VRE, is through the hands of health care workers. Other infections, such as COVID-19, are easily spread through the air when an infected person coughs or speaks. According to statistics from the Centers for Disease Control and Prevention (CDC), approximately 2 million people (1 in 20 people) get an HIA each year!

All health care facilities follow basic practices that are designed to decrease the chance of an infection spreading from one person to another. These practices are called **infection control**. There are four major methods of infection control—medical asepsis, surgical asepsis, barrier methods, and isolation precautions.

Medical Asepsis

Medical asepsis involves physically removing or killing pathogens, primarily achieved through processes involving soap, water, antiseptics, disinfectants, or heat.

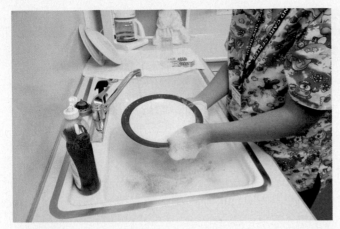

A Sanitization

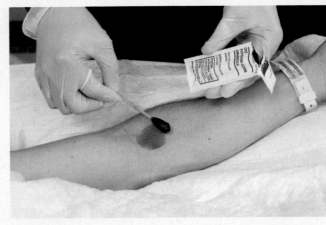

B Antisepsis

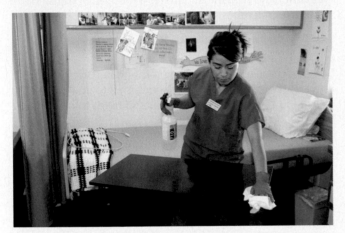

C Disinfection

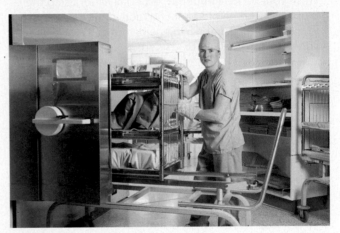

D Sterilization

Figure 12-1 There are many approaches to medical asepsis, a general term used to describe techniques used to remove or kill microbes. **A.** Sanitization is physically removing microbes from surfaces. Here, a home health aide washes dishes. **B.** Antisepsis involves the use of agents that kill microbes or slow down their growth, such as iodine (Betadine) or rubbing alcohol. Here, a nurse cleans a patient's skin with a Betadine swab. **C.** Disinfection also involves the use of agents that kill microbes. Because disinfectants are strong chemicals, disinfection is used only to clean nonliving objects. This nursing assistant is using a disinfectant to clean an overbed table. **D.** Sterilization involves the use of pressurized steam heat or very strong chemicals to kill microbes. This technician is removing sterile supplies from a steam autoclave, a device used to sterilize instruments and equipment. (*Lopolo\Shutterstock.com*)

The goal of medical asepsis is to remove pathogenic microbes from surfaces, equipment, and the hands of health care workers. There are four techniques that make up the practice of medical asepsis: sanitization, antisepsis, disinfection, and sterilization (Fig. 12-1):

- **Sanitization** describes practices associated with basic cleanliness, such as handwashing, cleansing of eating utensils and other surfaces with soap and water, and providing clean linens and clothing. Sanitization practices physically remove pathogens, thereby preventing their spread. General guidelines for maintaining a sanitary environment in a health care setting or home are given in Guidelines Box 12-1.

- **Antisepsis** takes sanitization one step further by actually killing microbes or stopping them from growing. Antisepsis involves the use of antiseptics, or chemicals capable of killing a pathogen or preventing it from growing, which can be used on the skin or other surfaces. Rubbing alcohol and iodine are common antiseptics used on the skin to prevent infection. Many soaps used in health care settings now also contain an antiseptic agent. The use of an alcohol-based hand rub is a type of antisepsis.
- **Disinfection** involves the use of stronger chemicals to kill pathogens. The chemicals used for disinfection are too strong to be used on the skin. Instead, disinfectants are used to clean nonliving

Guidelines Box 12-1 Guidelines for Maintaining a Sanitary Environment

WHAT YOU DO	WHY YOU DO IT
Wash your hands instead of using an alcohol-based hand rub, after contact with any body fluid or substance, whether it is your own or another person's. Examples of body fluids and substances include blood, saliva, vomitus, urine, feces, vaginal discharge, semen, wound drainage, pus, mucus, and respiratory secretions.	Pathogens often leave the body through the gastrointestinal tract, genitourinary tract, respiratory tract, or breaks in the skin. In addition, some pathogens are transmitted through blood and other body secretions, such as breast milk.
Handwashing, instead of hand hygiene with an alcohol-based rub, should be used when caring for a person who may have certain infections, such as *C. diff*.	Alcohol-based hand rubs may not be effective against certain microorganisms.
Wash your hands frequently, especially after using the bathroom and before handling food, drink, or eating utensils. Perform hand hygiene before and after any contact with a patient or resident.	Frequent hand hygiene eliminates a method of transmission for microbes.
Cough or sneeze into a tissue or into your sleeve at the elbow, and teach your patients and residents to do the same. Dispose of tissues properly by placing them in a waste container.	Some microbes are transmitted through particles of saliva or sputum. Coughing or sneezing into your sleeve or a tissue contains these particles and helps to prevent the spread of infection.
Provide each patient or resident with individual personal care items, such as toothbrushes, drinking glasses, towels, washcloths, and soap. Disposable items are preferred when possible.	If not properly cleaned after use, these items can act as fomites. Therefore, it is better to limit their use to one person.
Keep contaminated or dirty items, such as soiled linens, away from your uniform.	Microbes can be transferred from the dirty item to your uniform, which can then act as a fomite.
When cleaning, take care not to stir up dust. For example, wiping dusty surfaces with a damp cloth or mop helps prevent the movement of dust and lint into the air. Do not shake linens when making beds.	Dust can act as a fomite and carry microbes from one area to another.
Dispose of trash properly.	If not disposed of properly, trash can provide an ideal environment for microbial growth, especially if the trash contains food or other materials susceptible to rotting.
Follow established procedures for preparing dirty linens and clothing for the laundry.	Soiled linens and clothing act as fomites and must be handled in a way that will lessen the chance of someone else coming in contact with the contaminated item.
Maintain good personal hygiene and help your patients or residents to do the same. Bathing, washing hair, brushing teeth, and wearing clean clothing are all grooming practices that help prevent the spread of infection.	Personal grooming practices help to reduce the number of microbes present on the skin.

objects that come in contact with body fluids or substances, such as bedpans, urinals, and over-bed tables.

- **Sterilization** is the most thorough method of killing microbes. Sterilization is used on objects that must be completely free of any microbes,

such as surgical instruments, hypodermic needles, or IV catheters. These objects must be sterilized because they are placed in the patient's or resident's body. Therefore, they can act as portals of entry for microbes. Many disposable items used in health care settings, such as hypodermic needles, IV catheters, and urinary catheters, are sterilized and packaged by the manufacturer. Reusable items, such as surgical instruments, are usually cleaned and sterilized in the health care facility. Items are sterilized either by placing them in an autoclave (a machine that uses pressurized steam heat to kill microbes) or by soaking them in chemicals that destroy all microbes. Although covering items in boiling water will kill most microbes, boiling is not an effective method of sterilization.

Before disinfecting or sterilizing an object, the object must be cleaned first using basic sanitization methods. The chemicals used to disinfect or sterilize an object cannot work properly unless the surface to be disinfected or sterilized is clean and free of any organic material (material from a living organism, such as blood, urine, or feces). Organic materials contain fats and proteins that coat the surface of the object, much like how an egg yolk coats the surface of a plate; if the plate is not washed with detergent and warm water before the egg yolk dries, the hardened yolk becomes very difficult to remove. The same principle applies to dirty bedpans, urinals, and other pieces of equipment—if the piece of equipment is not washed first using soap and water, any organic material that is present can harden, making it difficult for the disinfectant or sterilization agent to kill the microbes underneath the dried material. Therefore, equipment must be properly cleaned using basic sanitization methods before moving on to disinfection or sterilization.

Hand Hygiene

As a nursing assistant, the medical asepsis technique that you will use most frequently is hand hygiene. Hand hygiene consists of both thoroughly washing your hands using soap and water and the use of alcohol-based hand rubs. According to the CDC in 2002, *handwashing is still the best method of decontaminating the hands and the consistent use of both methods of hand hygiene is the most important method of preventing the spread of infection.* This is true in everyday life as well as in the health care setting. However, in the health care setting, hand hygiene takes on a special importance because the chance of picking up a pathogen and passing it on to someone else is greater than in normal, everyday life. In addition, many of the people who are in health care facilities are less able to fight off an infection, should they get one. The easiest way to protect yourself and your patients or residents is to be conscientious about performing hand hygiene!

In the process of taking care of your patients or residents, you will collect microbes on your hands. These microbes could then be easily transferred to the next patient or resident you care for, yourself, or one of your family members. Before you move from one person's room to another in a health care facility, you must always perform hand hygiene. Failing to perform good hand hygiene before giving care to a patient or resident could even be considered negligence.

There are two main types of microbes found on a person's hands. Earlier in Chapter 10, you learned about the first type, normal (resident) flora. These are the microbes that normally live on a person's skin and usually do not cause infections. Normal flora lives deep in the pores of the skin and cannot be totally removed. The other type of microbe typically found on a person's hands is called **transient flora**. Transient flora is picked up from touching contaminated objects or people who have an infectious disease. Most HAIs are caused by transient flora—the hands of the health care worker serve as the method of transmission from one person to another. Transient flora lives on the surface of the skin and is easily removed by proper hand hygiene.

There are differences in opinion about handwashing techniques, such as the time required, the type of cleaning agents that should be used, and the frequency with which handwashing should occur. Certain situations may require specific handwashing techniques. For example, health care workers who work in the operating room, intensive care unit, neonatal unit, or labor and delivery units may be required to use an antiseptic cleaning agent, a scrub brush, or both, because patients in these settings have higher infection risks (Fig. 12-2). Antiseptic cleaning agents remove the transient flora from the surface of the skin. They also slow down the growth of the normal flora, which can be helpful in certain areas of health care. Procedure 12-1 describes the basic handwashing procedure. Although the specifics of how handwashing is performed vary from setting to setting, one aspect of handwashing always remains the same—it

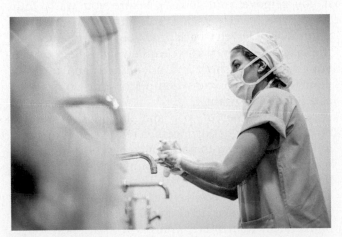

Figure 12-2 This person is performing a surgical scrub in preparation for entering an operating room. (*Carrastock\ Shutterstock.com*)

must be performed thoroughly, properly, and consistently. Handwashing, instead of using an alcohol-based rub, is required:

- When you first arrive at your facility
- When hands are visibly dirty
- When hands are visibly soiled with or in contact with blood or other body fluids
- When caring for patients or residents who may have certain infections, such as *C. diff*
- Before you go on break and before you leave your shift
- Before and after drinking, eating, or smoking
- Before and after inserting contact lenses
- After using the bathroom
- After coughing, sneezing, or blowing your nose
- After touching anything that may be contaminated with blood or other body fluids or substances
- After handling your hair or applying makeup or lip gloss

When washing your hands, make sure you clean those areas where microbes love to hide, under and around the fingernails and between the fingers. As you learned in Chapter 3, long fingernails can be a health issue in the nursing assistant profession. Long fingernails trap microbes underneath them and therefore are harder to clean. Nail polish cracks and peels, providing many places for transient microbes to hide. False nails, acrylics, and wraps often lift, creating an excellent breeding ground for microbes. Many health care facilities ban the use of these types of nail treatments by anyone involved in providing hands-on care for patients or residents.

It is also not a good idea to wear rings and bracelets while on the job. Many health care workers think that by removing their jewelry before performing hand hygiene, they can remove any microbes trapped underneath the jewelry. But, think about this: even if you remove your jewelry before you wash your hands, the jewelry itself is still dirty, so you will be putting dirty jewelry back onto your clean hands. For the sake of efficiency and cleanliness, it is best to keep your fingernails short and unpolished, and to leave your jewelry at home when performing your duties as a nursing assistant.

A good lather of soap and the physical motion of rubbing your hands together remove skin oils and lotions which can harbor microbes. Rinsing thoroughly removes microbes, along with the dirt and lather. Because frequent handwashing can cause the skin to become excessively dry, leading to cracking, applying a lotion or hand cream after washing is recommended. Remember, your own intact skin too is important to help protect you from infection.

While nothing can replace the effectiveness of good handwashing to remove visible dirt, blood, or other body fluids or substances, the CDC issued guidelines in October, 2002, recommending the use of alcohol-based hand rubs for routine hand decontamination. (These CDC guidelines are continuously reviewed and remain current.) Alcohol-based hand rubs have several advantages:

- Using an alcohol-based hand rub is quicker than washing your hands at the sink, which means that during duties that require frequent handwashing, using an alcohol-based hand rub can save time.
- Alcohol-based hand rubs are gentler on the skin than soap and water.
- Alcohol-based hand rubs are used without water, so they can be used anywhere. In many facilities, alcohol-based hand rubs can be dispensed at the patient's or resident's bedside, saving many trips back and forth to the sink. Many even come in containers small enough to be carried in your uniform pocket.

It is very simple to use an alcohol-based hand rub. The label on the product will tell you how much product to use. Apply this amount to one of your palms and rub your hands together, covering your hands and fingers (front and back) with the product. Continue rubbing your hands together until your skin is dry. That's all there is to it! Procedure 12-2 describes how to use an alcohol-based hand rub.

Remember, if your hands are visibly soiled with dirt, blood, or other body fluids or substances, you must wash them at the sink, using soap and water. However, if your hands are not visibly soiled, then it is acceptable to use an alcohol-based hand rub to decontaminate your hands, instead of handwashing.

Alcohol-based hand rubs are appropriate to use:

- When hands are not visibly soiled
- Before entering a patient's or resident's room
- Before and after patient or resident contact or contact with surfaces in the patient's or resident's room
- Before entering a "clean" supply room
- Before obtaining clean linen from a linen cart
- Before handling a person's meal tray
- After picking up an object from the floor
- After removing or changing disposable gloves, including those times when you are replacing a torn glove
- When moving from a dirty body site to a clean body site when providing care

Surgical Asepsis

Surgical asepsis is used for procedures that involve entering a person's body. Examples of procedures that require surgical asepsis include surgical procedures, injections, sterile dressing changes, the insertion of IV catheters, and the insertion of urinary catheters. Because these procedures disrupt the body's natural protective barriers, all instruments and equipment used must be sterile, or totally free from microbes. In most states, performing procedures that require surgical asepsis is not within a nursing assistant's scope of practice. However, some facilities will provide extra training in this area if performing procedures that require surgical asepsis is part of your job description.

Taking It to the Next Level:

Advanced Skills

More in-depth information related to advanced skills used when performing procedures requiring sterile technique can be found in *Lippincott Acute Care Skills for Advanced Nursing Assistants*.

Visit thePoint® at thepoint.lww.com for access to the ebook.

Barrier Methods

In addition to medical asepsis and surgical asepsis, barrier methods are used to control infection in the health care setting. A *barrier* is an object that physically prevents microbes from reaching a health care provider's skin or mucous membranes. Examples of barriers used in infection control, called **personal protective equipment (PPE)**, include disposable gloves, gowns, masks, respirators, and protective eyewear. While in use, the barrier becomes contaminated with microbes and must be removed in a way that prevents transmission of the microbes onto the skin of the health care worker.

Gloves

Gloves are the most commonly used barrier method. Gloves are worn when:

- There is a possibility of coming in contact with body fluids or substances
- Providing care for a patient or resident who has a communicable disease that could be transmitted by contact
- Performing or assisting with perineal care (cleaning of the area between the legs)
- Performing or assisting with mouth care
- Shaving a patient or resident
- Performing care on a patient or resident who has an open wound or other break in the skin
- Handling soiled linen or clothing
- Cleaning equipment that may have come in contact with body fluids or substances
- You have a cut or abrasion on your hands

To effectively prevent contamination of your hands, gloves must be intact (without holes or tears), and they must fit properly. Gloves that are too tight are uncomfortable. Gloves that are too loose will not stay on your hands. Many people are allergic or sensitive to latex, the material that is most commonly used to make disposable gloves. If you or someone you are caring for is sensitive to latex, then you should use gloves made from another synthetic material, such as vinyl. Health care facilities must provide nonlatex barrier methods for people who are sensitive to latex.

The most common error made by people who wear gloves for barrier protection is becoming too comfortable with the fact that they are protecting themselves and forgetting to protect others! If you are wearing gloves and you touch a surface that is contaminated, then your gloves become contaminated. If you then touch another surface, such as the side rail, light switch, or doorknob, with your contaminated gloves, the pathogens will be transferred from your gloves to that surface. The next person who touches the surface could then pick up the microbes you deposited there with your dirty gloves (Fig. 12-3). Gloves that become contaminated with material that may contain pathogens should be removed before touching any other surface. You may need to change gloves several times during one procedure to prevent the transfer of microbes from dirty areas to clean areas (such as, when cleaning feces from a person who has soiled themselves or when changing soiled sheets). You should remember to perform hand hygiene by using an alcohol-based hand rub in between glove changes during a procedure. And always wash your hands after removing your gloves. Procedure 12-3 describes the proper way to remove gloves.

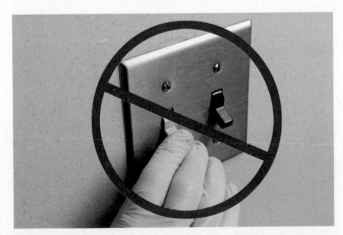

Figure 12-3 Do not make this mistake! By touching the light switch with their gloved hands, this nursing assistant has transferred whatever microbes were on their gloves onto the light switch, where they could be easily transferred onto the hands of the next person who turns on the light.

Gowns

A gown (fabric or paper) should be used when it is possible that your uniform could be soiled with body fluids or substances. Many gowns that are used for PPE are fluid resistant. The use of the gown prevents contamination of your uniform. Each gown is worn only once. Any gown, fabric or paper, is considered contaminated if it becomes wet. Procedures 12-4 and 12-5 describe how to put on and take off a gown, respectively.

Masks

Masks prevent you from breathing in microbes through your nose or mouth and are worn when there is a chance that you will be exposed to pathogens that are transmitted through the air or droplets of saliva. For example, the pathogens that cause measles, COVID-19, and tuberculosis (TB) are airborne pathogens, and the pathogens that cause pneumonia, strep throat, and meningitis are transmitted through droplets of saliva. You could be exposed to these pathogens when a person with one of these diseases talks, coughs, or sneezes.

Masks are also worn to protect patients and residents from microbes that you exhale. You may need to wear a mask when assisting the nurse during a sterile procedure.

Surgical masks are most commonly used, but if you are caring for a person with COVID-19 or TB, you will be required to wear a special high-filtration mask (Fig. 12-4). Surgical masks are "one size fits all," but high-filtration masks are available in various sizes, and you must be fitted for them in advance. Surgical masks are used only once and should never be lowered around the neck and then brought back up on your face for reuse. You must discard and replace your mask if it becomes wet or soiled. Because the

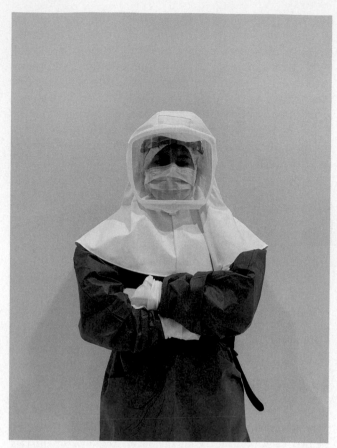

Figure 12-5 A PAPR mask may be necessary when providing care for some patients with certain respiratory infections such as COVID-19. (*nymphoenix\Shutterstock.com*)

mask will be considered contaminated in the front, you will need to be careful to only handle the mask by the ties or straps when you remove it. Procedure 12-6 explains how to put on and take off a mask.

When providing care to some patients who are infected with viruses such as COVID-19, you may be required to wear a special ventilation hood or ventilator. These are called powered air-purifying respirator (PAPR) masks and have special units that provide filtered air to the wearer (Fig. 12-5). A PAPR mask provides protection from organisms that can be inhaled as well as splashed, since it provides full face coverage. If you are required to wear a PAPR mask, you will receive training in the use and care of these devices.

Protective Eyewear

Goggles, face shields, and other types of protective eyewear are used to protect your eyes from substances that may splash (Fig. 12-6). Blood and other body fluids, as well as the fluid used to clean wounds, may contain pathogens which can enter your body through your eyes. Goggles fit close to your face and can be worn over prescription eyeglasses. Face shields

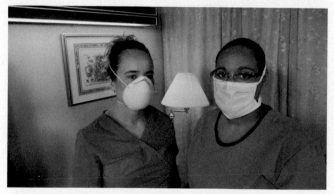

Figure 12-4 Masks cover your nose and mouth and protect you from inhaling pathogens that are transmitted through the air or saliva. (**Left**) A high-filtration respirator mask, worn when caring for people with tuberculosis (TB). (**Right**) A surgical mask.

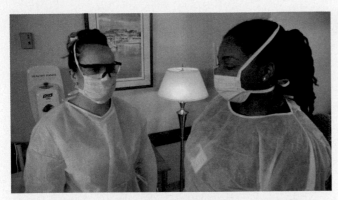

Figure 12-6 Face shields (**right**) and goggles (**left**) are used to protect your eyes from substances that may splash.

may be attached to a mask or to an elastic band that fits around the head. Your employer is required to provide you with appropriate protective eyewear.

In many situations, you may need to wear more than one article of PPE. The best sequence for putting these items on is as follows: gown, mask, protective eyewear, gloves. The order for removal of PPE is gloves, protective eyewear, gown, mask. Procedure 12-7 describes how to remove PPE when more than one article is being used. After use, PPE is considered contaminated. Removal of PPE in the correct sequence helps to protect you from infection. For instance, you would not want to remove your mask first because this would mean that you would have to touch your face with your contaminated gloves.

Isolation Precautions

The last major method of controlling the spread of infection throughout a health care facility is by using **isolation precautions**. Isolation precautions are guidelines, based on a pathogen's method of transmission, that we follow to contain the pathogen and limit others' exposure to it as much as possible.

Standard Precautions

As you will recall from Chapter 11, **standard precautions** are precautions that health care workers take with every patient or resident to protect themselves and others from pathogens that are transmitted through blood and other body substances. Standard precautions involve the use of barrier methods, as well as certain environmental control methods, to protect the health care worker (Box 12-1). *For these methods to be effective, they must be used consistently.*

Three new elements have been added to existing standard precaution guidelines. Although standard precautions were initially developed to protect health care workers, these new elements are focused on protecting patients and residents. These new standard precautions are as follows:

- *Respiratory hygiene/cough etiquette* is used to help prevent the spread of any undiagnosed respiratory infection from patients, residents, and also any visitors in a health care facility to others. The person with a cough or other symptoms should cover their mouth and nose with a tissue when coughing or sneezing, dispose of used tissues in a waste receptacle, wear a mask when within 3 feet of other people, and wash their hands or use an alcohol-based hand cleaner frequently. Masks and gloves should also be worn by health care workers when providing care for patients or residents with signs of a respiratory infection.
- *Safe injection practices* are used to prevent the spread of infection by using a new, sterile syringe and needle each time medication is drawn from a multiuse vial for IV injection.
- *Infection control practices for special lumbar puncture procedures* require that health care workers wear a surgical mask when assisting with any type of lumbar puncture procedure.

Transmission-Based Precautions

Transmission-based precautions are used in addition to standard precautions when a person is known to have a disease that is transmitted a certain way, for example, via the air, through droplets, or by direct contact. Any of the three types of transmission-based precautions can be used in combination with the others. Equipment that you use during routine patient and resident care should be disposable (when possible), kept in that person's room, and not used for other patients or residents. Required PPE for the precautions should be put on before entering the patient's or resident's room for all interactions. PPE should be removed when leaving the room and remember to also wash your hands.

- **Airborne precautions** are used when caring for people infected with pathogens that remain infectious when suspended in air. Airborne pathogens enter the respiratory tract of people breathing the same air as the infected person. Therefore, airborne precautions include placing the person in a private room, called an **airborne infection isolation room (AIIR)**, that is equipped with special ventilation and filtration systems. Health care workers caring for a person on airborne precautions should put on a mask or high-filtration respirator before entering the room. Gloves should also be worn if you will be touching any surfaces within the room. Anyone who visits an infected person should also wear a mask.

Box 12-1   Standard Precautions

1. Gloves must be worn if the *possibility* exists that the hands could come in contact with blood or other body fluids. Gloves must also be worn when touching any surface or linen that could be contaminated with infected materials. Remember that you cannot see a virus with the naked eye.

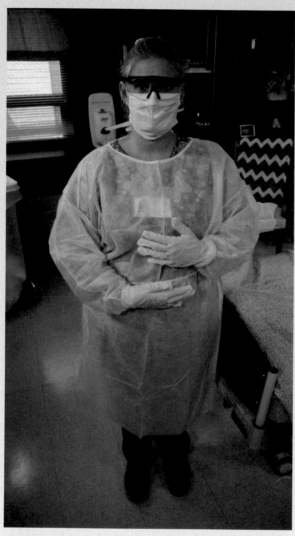

2. A waterproof (impervious) gown must be worn if the *possibility* exists that your clothes could become soiled with blood or other body fluids.

3. A mask, face shield, and eye goggles must be worn if the *possibility* exists that blood or other body fluids could splash or spray.

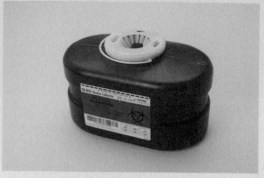

4. Sharps, such as used needles, razors, or broken glass, must be disposed of properly in labeled, OSHA-approved containers. Contaminated, broken glass items should not be handled, even with gloved hands. They should be swept or vacuumed up for disposal.

5. Spills of blood or other body fluids must be cleaned up promptly with an approved viricidal cleaning agent or a solution of 1 part household bleach to 10 parts water. Personal protective equipment (PPE), such as gloves and a gown (if necessary, for large spills), should be worn while cleaning up spills.

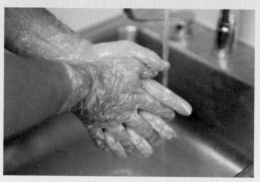

6. Hands must be washed when you remove your gloves. If accidental exposure to blood or other body substances occurs, hands must be washed thoroughly and immediately. Alcohol-based hand rubs should not be used if your gloves or hands have been in contact with blood or other body substances.

When it is necessary for the infected person to leave their room, they must wear a mask. Diseases caused by pathogens that can be transmitted through the air include TB, COVID-19, chickenpox, measles, and possibly severe acute respiratory syndrome (SARS). Airborne precautions are listed in Box 12-2.

■ **Droplet precautions** are used when caring for people with diseases caused by pathogens that are transmitted by direct exposure to droplets released

from the mouth or nose (for example, when the person coughs, sneezes, or talks). Droplet precautions must also be taken when performing procedures that involve contact with an infected person's mouth or nose. Diseases caused by pathogens that can be transmitted through droplets include mumps, influenza, whooping cough, strep throat, scarlet fever, rubella, meningitis, pneumonia, diphtheria, and epiglottitis. Droplet precautions are the same as airborne precautions,

Box 12-2	Airborne Precautions

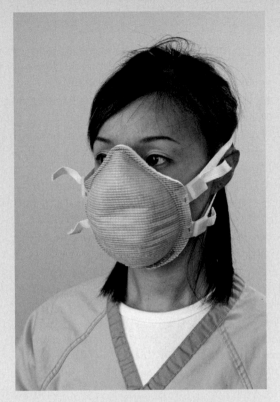

1. Patients or residents known or suspected to be infected with an airborne pathogen are to be placed in an airborne infection isolation room (AIIR).

2. Health care workers should wear gloves and high-filtration respirators when caring for patients or residents with known or suspected COVID-19 virus or tuberculosis (TB). If the health care worker has not been exposed to measles or chickenpox (and is, therefore, not immune), then they are at risk for these diseases and should wear a mask when caring for patients or residents with measles or chickenpox.

3. Health care workers should wear a gown when changing linens or providing care which would cause their uniforms to be against bed linens or the person's body.

4. A surgical mask should be placed over the patient's or resident's face if they must be transported from one location to another. Transport of the patient or resident should be kept to a minimum.

5. All precautions for preventing transmission of COVID-19 or TB should be implemented if the patient or resident is known or suspected to have a respiratory infection.

Helping Hands and a Caring Heart

Focus on Humanistic Health Care

When caring for a person with a communicable disease, it is very important to remember the person. We work hard to follow all of the procedures that help prevent the spread of infection, and this is a very important part of providing care. However, sometimes it is easy to forget about how the person with the infection might feel. A person with a communicable disease often feels dirty or unwanted. Think about it—how would you feel if a health care worker had to wear gloves or a mask every time they came near you? Very young children or people who are confused or disoriented may become frightened by a health care worker decked out in a mask and eye protection. When airborne or droplet precautions are in effect, the person with the communicable disease may feel isolated and lonely, and desperately miss the company of other people. Friends and family members may not be allowed to visit the person. When you are caring for a patient or resident with a communicable disease, checking on the person frequently and taking the time to talk with the person when you are providing care can help to make the person feel better.

except that a regular mask, instead of a high-filtration mask is worn.

■ **Contact precautions** are used when caring for people with diseases caused by pathogens that are transmitted directly (by touching the person) or indirectly (by touching fomites). Diseases that can be transmitted by contact include skin and wound infections, digestive tract infections, and some respiratory tract infections. Contact precautions involve wearing a gown and gloves when providing care for the infected person or touching items contaminated with wound drainage or body substances. Contaminated linen and waste materials must be contained and disposed of properly. Procedure 12-8 describes how to transfer contaminated items out of a person's room when contact precautions are being followed.

SUMMARY

- Communicable diseases are always present in the population but can become more widespread under certain conditions.
  - Many communicable diseases throughout history have reached epidemic and pandemic proportions, causing illness and death for large numbers of people.
- Some of the people you will care for will be receiving care because they have a serious communicable disease. Others may have a serious communicable disease and not even know it. In addition, many of the people you will care for will be more at risk for catching a communicable disease because they are already not in good health. Therefore, infection control is very important.
  - Health care workers take many approaches to infection control. As a nursing assistant, it is your ethical and legal responsibility to protect your patients or residents from infectious disease. You must also protect yourself and your family members. The techniques to help control the spread of infection are effective only if performed properly and consistently.
- Medical asepsis involves physically removing or killing pathogens.
  - Methods of medical asepsis include sanitization, antisepsis, disinfection, and sterilization.
  - Proper hand hygiene, a form of medical asepsis, is the single most important method of controlling the spread of infection.
- Surgical asepsis is required for procedures that involve entering a person's body.
- Barrier methods prevent a pathogen from gaining access to a health care worker's body. Commonly used barrier methods include gloves, gowns, masks, and protective eyewear.
- Isolation precautions are based on a pathogen's mode of transmission (blood, air, droplet, direct contact).

> **Procedure 12-1**

Handwashing

WHY YOU DO IT   According to the CDC, handwashing continues to be the best method of decontaminating the hands.

---

1. Gather needed supplies if not present at the handwashing area: *soap or the cleansing agent specified by your facility, hand lotion* (optional), *paper towels, an orangewood stick or disposable nail cleaner* (optional).

2. Stand away from the sink, so that your uniform does not touch the sink. Push your sleeves up your arms 4 to 5 inches; if you are wearing a watch, push it up too.

3. Turn on the water and adjust the force so that it does not splash on your uniform. Use warm, not hot water.

4. Wet your hands, keeping your fingers pointed down. This will cause the water to run off your fingertips and into the sink. Do not allow water to run up your forearms.

5. Press the hand pump or step on the foot pedal to dispense the cleaning agent into one cupped hand.

6. Lather well, keeping your fingers pointed down at all times. Make sure the lather extends at least 1 inch past your wrists.

7. Rub your hands together in a circular motion, washing the palms and backs of your hands. Interlace your fingers to clean the spaces between your fingers. Continue for at least 20 seconds.

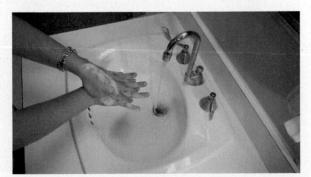

STEP 7   Interlace your fingers.

8. Rub the fingernails of one hand against the palm of the opposite hand to force soap underneath

the tips of the fingernails, *or* clean underneath the tips of the fingernails with the blunt edge of an orangewood stick or a disposable nail cleaner.

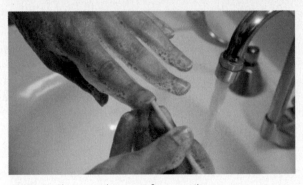

STEP 8   Clean under your fingernails.

9. Rinse your hands, keeping your fingers pointed down at all times.

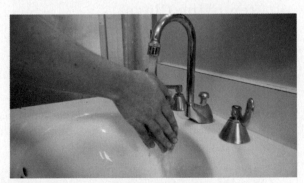

STEP 9   Always point your fingertips down.

10. Dry your hands thoroughly with a clean paper towel, beginning with the fingers and moving upward to the wrists. Dispose of the paper towel in a facility-approved waste container, being careful not to touch the container.

11. With a new paper towel, turn off the faucet. Carefully dispose of the paper towel without touching it to the other clean hand.

12. As you leave the handwashing area, if there is a doorknob, open the door by covering the

(*continued*)

175

doorknob with a clean paper towel. If there is no doorknob, push the door open with your hip and shoulder to avoid contaminating your clean hands.

13. After leaving the handwashing area, apply a small amount of hand lotion to keep your skin supple and moist.

 Procedure 12-2

Using an Alcohol-Based Hand Rub

WHY YOU DO IT   Proper hand hygiene is the most important method of preventing the spread of infection.

1. Gather needed supplies: *facility-approved alcohol-based hand rub, hand lotion* (optional).

2. Check the product label for the correct amount of product you should use.

3. Apply the correct amount of the hand rub to the palm of one hand.

4. Rub your hands together, covering your hands and fingers (front and back) and in between the fingers with the product. Make sure to clean the fingertips and rub the fingernails against your palms to force the product under the nails.

5. Continue rubbing your hands together until they are dry.

6. Apply hand lotion if desired.

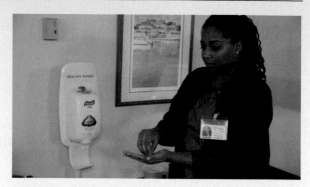

STEP 4 Rub your fingernails against your palms to force the product under the nails.

Procedure 12-3

Removing Gloves

WHY YOU DO IT   Removing your gloves properly prevents you from contaminating your skin or uniform.

1. With one gloved hand, grasp the other glove at the palm and pull the glove off your hand. Keep the glove you have removed in your gloved hand. (Think, "glove to glove.")

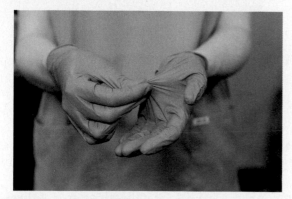

STEP 1 "Glove to glove."

2. Slip two fingers from the ungloved hand underneath the cuff of the remaining glove, at the

wrist. Remove that glove from your hand, turning it inside out as you pull it off. (Think, "skin to skin.")

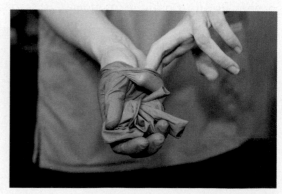

STEP 2 "Skin to skin."

3. Dispose of the soiled gloves in a facility-approved waste container.

4. Perform hand hygiene.

Procedure 12-4

Putting on a Gown

WHY YOU DO IT Putting on a gown properly prevents your uniform from becoming soiled with body fluids.

1. Gather needed supplies: *a gown, gloves.*
2. Remove your watch and place it on a clean paper towel or in your pocket. (If you are wearing jewelry, remove that as well.) Roll up the sleeves of your uniform so that they are about 4 to 5 inches above your wrists.
3. Perform hand hygiene.
4. Put on the gown by slipping your arms into the sleeves.

5. Secure the gown around your neck by tying the ties in a simple bow or by fastening the Velcro strips.
6. Reach behind yourself and overlap the edges of the gown so that your uniform is completely covered. Secure the gown at your waist by tying the ties in a simple bow or by fastening the Velcro strips.

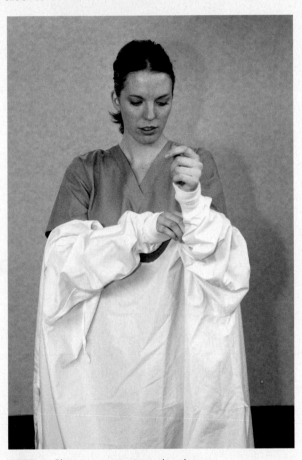

STEP 4 Slip your arms into the sleeves.

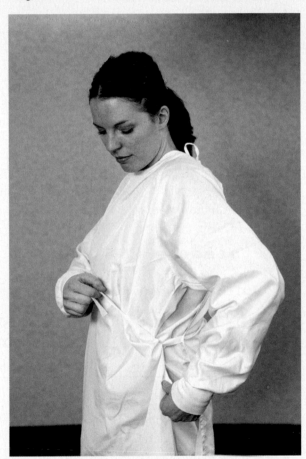

STEP 6 Overlap and tie.

7. Put on the gloves. The cuffs of the gloves should extend over the cuffs of the gown.

Procedure 12-5

Removing a Gown

WHY YOU DO IT   Removing a gown properly prevents you from contaminating your skin or uniform.

1. Remove and dispose of your gloves as described in Procedure 12-3. (If your gown ties in the front, untie the waist strings before removing your gloves.)
2. Untie the waist ties (or undo the Velcro strips at the waist).
3. Untie the neck ties (or undo the Velcro strips at the neck). Be careful not to touch your neck or the outside of the gown.
4. Grasping the gown at the neck ties, loosen it at the neck and allow the gown to fall away from the shoulders.
5. Be careful to touch only the inside of the gown and pull it away from your body and off your arms.
6. Holding the gown away from your body, roll it downward, turning it inside out as you go. Take care to touch only the inside or uncontaminated side of the gown.
7. After the gown is rolled up, contaminated side inward, dispose of it in a facility-approved container.
8. Perform hand hygiene.

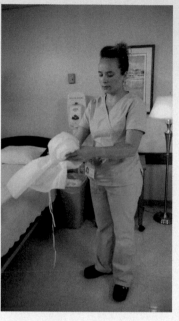

STEP 6 Hold the gown away from your body and roll it downward, turning it inside out.

Procedure 12-6

Putting on and Removing a Mask

WHY YOU DO IT   Putting on a mask properly prevents pathogens that are transmitted through the air or droplets from entering your nose and mouth. Removing a mask properly prevents you from contaminating your skin or uniform.

Putting on a Mask

1. Gather needed supplies: *a mask*.
2. Perform hand hygiene.
3. Place the mask over your nose and mouth, being careful not to touch your face with your hands.

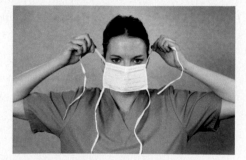

STEP 3 Be careful not to touch your face with your hands.

4. Tie the top strings of the mask securely behind your head.

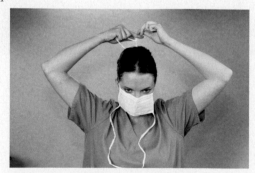

STEP 4 Tie the top strings securely.

5. Tie the bottom strings of the mask securely behind your neck. Make sure that the mask fits snugly around your face. You want to breathe through the mask, not around it.

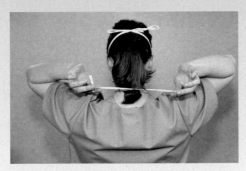

STEP 5 Tie the bottom strings securely.

Removing a Mask

1. Perform hand hygiene. (You do not want to touch your face with dirty hands.)

2. Untie the bottom strings first, and then untie the top strings. The front of the mask is considered to be contaminated, so touch only the strings.

3. Remove the mask by holding the top strings. Dispose of the mask, holding it by its ties only, in the facility-approved container located inside the patient's or resident's room.

4. Perform hand hygiene.

▶ Procedure 12-7

Removing More Than One Article of Personal Protective Equipment

WHY YOU DO IT Remove personal protective equipment (PPE) at the doorway before leaving the patient room.

---

1. Remove and dispose of your gloves as described in Procedure 12-3.

2. Remove your protective eyewear. Handle only by the "clean" headband or earpieces.

3. Untie the gown's waist ties (or undo the Velcro strips at the waist). *If the gown ties in the front, untie the waist tie before removing your gloves.*

4. Untie the gown's neck ties (or undo the Velcro strips at the neck), and loosen the gown at the neck. Remove and dispose of the gown as described in Procedure 12-5.

5. Remove and dispose of the mask as described in Procedure 12-6.

6. Perform appropriate hand hygiene immediately after removing PPE.

▶ Procedure 12-8

Double-Bagging (Two Assistants)

WHY YOU DO IT Double-bagging helps to keep any pathogens that may be on the outside of the bag from spreading to other places.

---

1. The nursing assistant inside the person's room places the contaminated items into an isolation bag (usually a color-coded plastic bag) and secures the bag with a tie.

2. Another nursing assistant, referred to as the "clean" nursing assistant, stands outside of the person's room, holding a plastic bag cuffed over their hands. The cuff at the top of the bag protects the "clean" nursing assistant's hands.

3. The nursing assistant inside the isolation unit deposits the bag of contaminated items into the bag held by the "clean" nursing assistant.

4. The "clean" nursing assistant secures the top of the plastic bag tightly and disposes of the double-bagged items according to facility policy.

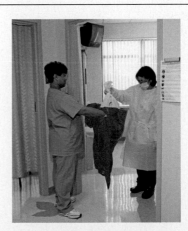

STEP 3 The assistant inside the room places the bag of contaminated items in the bag held by the nursing assistant outside of the room.

WHAT DID YOU LEARN?

Multiple Choice

Select the single best answer for each of the following questions.

1. When you wash your hands, you should:
a. Use the hottest water possible
b. Scrub with a brush for 3 minutes
c. Rinse with your fingers pointed up
d. Rinse with your fingers pointed down

2. When should you wash your hands instead of using an alcohol-based hand rub when performing hand hygiene?
a. When hands are not visibly soiled.
b. When hands have come in contact with blood or other body substances.
c. After performing routine care such as taking a person's blood pressure.
d. When changing gloves during a care procedure.

3. You have been told to follow contact precautions with one of your residents. Therefore, this resident's soiled linen should be:
a. Thrown away
b. Bagged prior to removing it from the room
c. Taken directly to the laundry
d. Placed in the linen hamper

4. Which of the following procedures best destroys all bacteria?
a. Sterilizing
b. Washing with bleach
c. Soaking in alcohol
d. All of the above

5. A communicable disease that is always present to some extent in the general population is said to be a/an:
a. Pandemic
b. Plague
c. Epidemic
d. Endemic

6. Which statement about the handwashing procedure is correct?
a. As long as soap is used, the temperature of the water does not matter
b. The faucet and sink are clean and may be touched during handwashing
c. Wash at least 1 inch above the wrist
d. All of the above

7. Which one of the following statements about protective gowns is true?
a. The outside is considered the "clean" side
b. The gown opens in the front
c. A gown may be used more than once
d. A gown is considered contaminated when wet

8. When are goggles a necessary part of personal protective equipment (PPE)?
a. Whenever blood is present
b. Whenever blood may splash or spray
c. Whenever you are taking care of a person with tuberculosis (TB)
d. Goggles are not really a necessary part of PPE

9. For health care workers, which of the following is the most important method of preventing the spread of infection?
a. Standard precautions
b. Proper hand hygiene
c. Wearing gloves
d. Wearing gowns and goggles

10. Personal protective equipment (PPE) refers to:
a. Sterilization and disinfection
b. Security personnel
c. Disposable gloves, face masks, and gowns
d. Isolation precautions

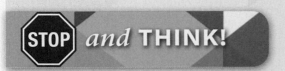

You work in a rehabilitation unit of a large CCRC facility that recently spent time in lockdown due to the spread of COVID-19. It seems things are starting to return to a more "normal" state of affairs. Your residents can once again have family and friends visit, the big dining room where everyone can enjoy each other's company at mealtimes is open again, and group movie night has returned…popcorn and all.

Last week, however, a couple of your new residents were admitted showing signs of a respiratory infection and have since been diagnosed with COVID-19. This has placed your facility under lockdown again. How can you help your residents feel less lonely and isolated during this 2-week isolation period until they can visit with family members and socialize with other residents again?

Respect

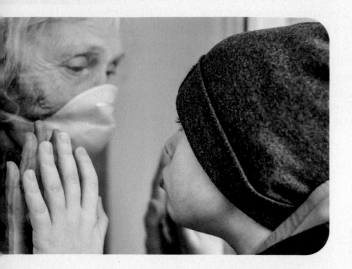

I am a caregiver aide in a retirement and rehabilitation facility. Most of our residents still enjoy fairly good health and our facility offers many activities to help keep them active and healthy. We have a big open dining room that has a huge fireplace and overlooks the mountain valley. Not only do our residents enjoy dining there together, but they gather for movie night, game night, and lots of birthday parties thrown by their families.

Things changed dramatically a couple of years ago when the COVID-19 pandemic hit. About half of our residents got sick, and a number of them died from their infection. Staff went into strict isolation mode to help protect our residents and ourselves from further infection. Everyone was made to stay in their rooms, all meals were served to the residents in their rooms, and we allowed absolutely no visitors. And of course, there were no group activities.

In our attempts to further protect those we cared for, we minimized our own contact with them. We would check on them and attend to their needs briefly, then sanitize our hands and move on quickly.

Later in the pandemic, after the residents and staff had been fully vaccinated and we had no new cases of COVID-19, we slowly relaxed some of our restrictions. One thing we did was open our small hair salon and schedule our residents one-at-a-time. Mrs. Zolenski was one of our first salon clients. I seated her at the hair wash station and proceeded to lather her hair and massage her scalp gently. As I did, she started to cry. When I asked if she was okay, she said, "Yes, but this is the first time I have felt a touch by an ungloved hand in over 10 months." She went on to tell me that she knew how hard we had worked to keep her and the rest of the residents safe, and she certainly appreciated it. She said she had really missed seeing her family and being able to enjoy the company of her fellow residents. But, she had not realized how much she had missed just a simple touch from another person.

I cried as I listened to her talk, because I realized how important a simple touch can mean to a lonely resident. That we have to learn to respect those simple, basic needs and find ways to meet those for the people we care for, even in the midst of isolation. I know Mrs. Zolenski will always have a special place in my heart for teaching me that.

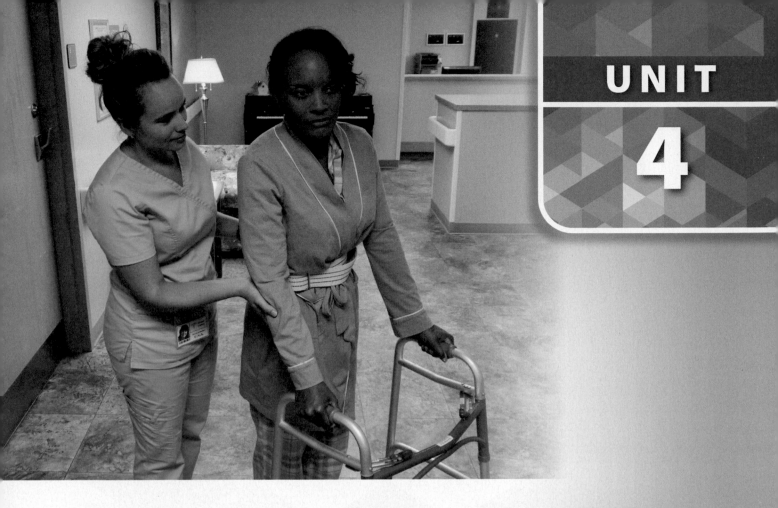

Safety

13 **Workplace Safety**

14 **Patient Safety and Restraint Alternatives**

15 **Positioning, Lifting, and Transferring Patients and Residents**

16 **Basic First Aid and Emergency Care**

As You Have Learned, Being a Nursing Assistant Is physically demanding work that places you in close contact with people. Many of the people you will care for will be ill, injured, frail, or a combination of the three. Not only must you know how to protect yourself in the workplace from physical injury, you must also know how to protect those entrusted to your care. Maintaining safety is the focus of Unit 4.

Photo: A nursing assistant helps a resident to walk safely.

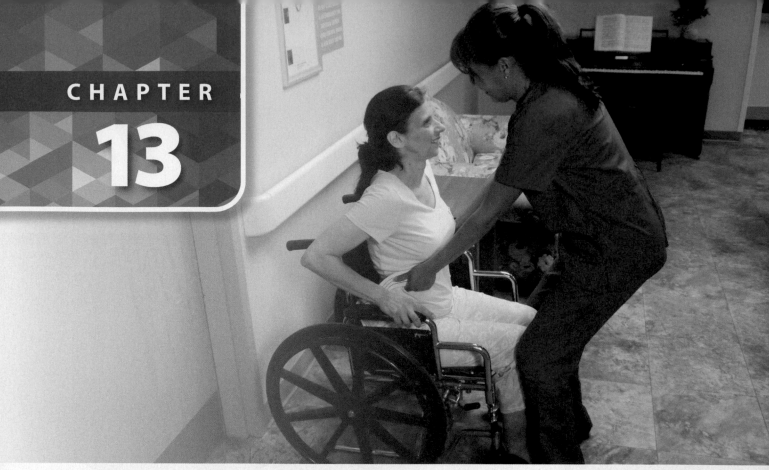

Photo: A nursing assistant uses good body mechanics to protect herself from injury while assisting a resident to stand.

Workplace Safety

 WHAT WILL YOU LEARN?

As you have learned in Unit 3, the risk of infectious disease is a work-related hazard faced by all people in the health care system—patients and residents, family members and visitors, and health care workers. Although minimizing the spread of infectious disease is a major safety concern for health care workers, it is not the only one. In this chapter, we will explore other threats to the safety of people who work or live in a health care setting, and the measures you can take to minimize these threats. When you are finished with this chapter, you will be able to:

1. Define the term *ergonomics* and discuss why people who work in a health care setting are at an increased risk for developing musculoskeletal disorders.
2. Define the term *body mechanics* and the "ABCs" that make the body more effective when working.
3. Demonstrate proper lifting technique and ways to prevent back injury.
4. Explain the importance of following procedures when providing patient or resident care.
5. List and explain the steps to take before and after every patient or resident care procedure.
6. Describe hazards that increase the risk of falls in the health care setting and how to assist a person who is falling.
7. Describe chemical hazards found in the health care setting and ways to avoid them.

8. **Discuss electrical hazards found in the health care setting and ways to avoid them.**

9. **List the elements necessary for a fire to start and continue to burn.**

10. **Demonstrate the RACE fire response plan and how to use a fire extinguisher.**

11. **Identify disaster situations that may affect a health care facility, and describe the focus of a disaster preparedness plan in a hospital versus in a long-term care facility.**

12. **Discuss factors that may lead to workplace violence in the health care setting.**

Vocabulary

Ergonomics

Body mechanics

Alignment

Balance

Coordinated body
   movement

Procedures

Pre-procedure actions

Post-procedure actions

Grounded

Safety Data Sheets
   (SDS)

RACE fire response
   plan

Disaster

Workplace violence

PROTECTING YOUR BODY

Performing the same action over and over again places stress on the body—for example, think of the stress on a baseball catcher's knees as they squat, then stand, then squat again hundreds of times throughout a single game. In addition, moving a large, awkward, or heavy object also places strain on the body and can lead to injury. As a nursing assistant, you will place stress on your body as you lift, push, pull, stoop, and bend repeatedly on a daily basis. In addition, in many cases, you will need to move a person or a piece of equipment that is larger and heavier than you are. There is no doubt about it—being a nursing assistant is extremely physically demanding! Fortunately, by practicing good body mechanics and learning proper lifting techniques, you can minimize your risk for physical injury.

Ergonomics

The Occupational Safety and Health Administration (OSHA) recognizes that health care workers encounter many physical hazards when performing routine duties in the health care setting. These hazards include being exposed to bloodborne pathogens and other infectious diseases, hazardous chemicals, unsafe walking surfaces, and the threat of violence from combative patients, residents, and visitors. The physically demanding nature of duties performed by nurses and nursing assistants, such as manual lifting and transferring and repositioning patients or residents, places these health care workers at an increased risk of injury, particularly back injury. Workers in long-term care facilities, especially nursing assistants, have

been identified as being more than twice as likely to be injured on the job. The most common types of injuries are muscle strains and tears, ligament sprains, joint and tendon inflammation, pinched nerves, and herniated discs in the spinal column. These conditions are referred to as *musculoskeletal disorders (MSDs)*. For this reason, OSHA has developed a set of guidelines specifically focused on prevention of these types of injuries.

OSHA defines **ergonomics** as the practice of designing equipment and work tasks to conform to the capability of the worker. This involves adjusting the work environment and how workers perform work-related practices so that injuries are prevented. Work-related practices that nursing assistants face on a daily basis in the health care setting include:

- *Force*, which is the amount of physical effort that is required to perform a task, such as during heavy lifting or repositioning a patient or a resident.
- *Repetition*, where the same motion or series of motions are performed continually or frequently.
- *Awkward postures*, where a person assumes positions that place stress on the body, such as reaching above shoulder height, kneeling, squatting, leaning over a bed, or twisting the torso while lifting.

To better protect workers in health care settings, OSHA guidelines recommend that workers should be provided with ergonomics training. The material you will read in the following sections of this chapter contains important guidelines on how to safely use your body to perform daily work tasks. OSHA also recommends that manual lifting of residents in long-term care facilities be minimized in all cases and eliminated whenever possible by using mechanical lifts. You will receive ergonomics training specific to the type of health care setting you work in. However, it is your responsibility to follow the recommended practices of this training to avoid injury. Injuries sustained by workers in the health care setting are usually avoidable and should never be thought of as just a routine occurrence.

The "ABCs" of Good Body Mechanics

The efficient movement and use of the body is accomplished through good **body mechanics**. The basic components (the "ABCs") of good body mechanics are **A**lignment, **B**alance, and **C**oordinated body movement.

Alignment is simply good posture. For the body to work most efficiently, proper alignment is necessary to ensure that no excess strain is placed on the joints and muscles. The back is held in a "neutral" position, with the natural curvature of the lower back intact. Imagine that you are looking at a person who is holding their body in proper alignment (Fig. 13-1). On the side view, you would be able to draw a straight line connecting the person's ear, shoulder, hip, knee, and ankle. From the front view, you would be able to draw a straight line that connected the nose, the sternum (breastbone), and the navel, and then continued between the legs, dividing that space equally in half.

Balance is stability produced by the even distribution of weight. Balance involves holding your center of gravity or area of largest mass, close to your base of support. For example, when you are standing, your base of support is your feet (which are placed squarely on the floor), and your center of gravity is your torso, the heaviest part of your body. The larger your base of support, and the closer the heaviest part of your body is to that base of support, the more balanced you will be. How, then, can you stabilize your body and maximize your ability to remain balanced? There are two ways:

- Increase your base of support by spreading your feet further apart.
- Bring your center of gravity closer to your base of support by bending at the knees and hips, so that your torso is closer to your feet.

Imagine that you are standing with your legs together and your ankles touching. If someone pushed you, you might lose your balance and fall. Now imagine that you are standing with your feet about shoulder-width apart. The same shove might not cause you to lose your balance. And if you were then to lower your body into a squat, it would be even harder to push you over! Increasing your base of support by standing with your feet apart and positioning yourself so that your center of gravity (your torso) is close to your base of support (your feet) improves your balance and is a very important part of practicing good body mechanics (Fig. 13-2).

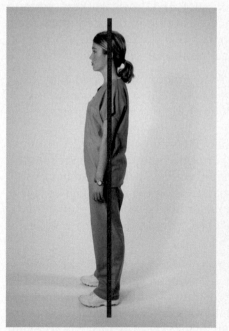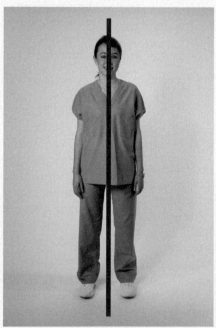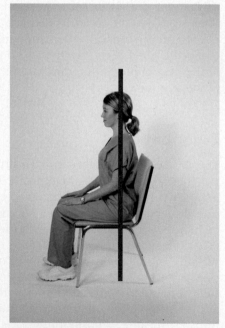

Figure 13-1 When the body is held in proper alignment, the back is in a "neutral" position, with the curve of the lower spine intact. Holding the body in proper alignment prevents strain on the joints and muscles.

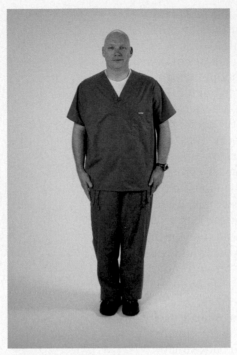 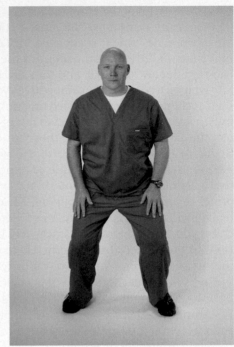

Figure 13-2 Maintaining balance. Spreading your feet apart and bending at the hips and knees improve your ability to stay balanced.

Coordinated body movement involves using the weight of your body to help with movement. For example, when moving a person up in bed, you stand facing the bed, with your feet apart. As you step sideways to move the person's head and shoulders up, you transfer your weight from one foot to the other and the momentum helps you to move the person (Fig. 13-3).

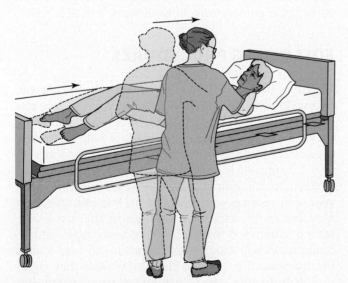

Figure 13-3 Coordinated body movement involves using the weight of your body to help with movement. When the nursing assistant steps sideways, shifting their weight from their left foot to their right, the momentum of their body helps to move the person up in bed.

Lifting and Back Safety

Practicing good body mechanics is important, especially when you must lift heavy equipment or move people who have trouble moving on their own. Lifting is a required task for nursing assistants who provide direct care to patients or residents. Therefore, it is important to learn the proper technique. Failure to use good body mechanics when lifting something or someone can result in back injuries. Back injuries are the most common work-related injury in the nursing field. Injuries of the back range from muscle strains and soreness to ruptured vertebral discs (a condition that may require surgery and a long recovery period). Back injuries are painful and costly (in terms of medical care and missed work), and they can be serious enough to end your career and prevent you from participating in other activities that you enjoy. If you do not take precautions to prevent back injuries, you could find yourself in the position of being the patient instead of the care provider!

If you have ever watched the weightlifting event in the Olympics, you know that competitive weightlifters can lift more than 500 pounds. The weightlifter's lifting technique is an excellent example of good body mechanics being used. The athlete squats low to the ground, using their arms and shoulders to pull the weight close to their body at chest level. They then use their hips and legs to stand up with the weight. After becoming upright, they widen their base of support by moving one foot ahead of the other. These maneuvers allow the large, strong muscles of the body to do the work of lifting and also protect the back from injury.

The muscles of the arms and legs are attached to the long bones in our limbs. The muscle contracts by pulling against the bone it is attached to. This allows us to move and to lift weight. In contrast, the muscles of the back are flat and fan-like, and they are not designed to lift weight. When the competitive weightlifter lifts their weights, they use their leg muscles, not their back muscles. As they raise themselves out of the squat, they use the powerful muscles in their buttocks, hips, and thighs to move themselves, and the weight, upward. Although you will not be required to practice competitive weightlifting at work, you should try to imitate the professionals with your technique! For example, if you had to move a patient or resident from the bed to a chair, you would bend your knees and hold the person close to the center of your body. Then, you would use the muscles in your thighs and hips to lift and move the person from the bed to the chair. Proper lifting technique is summarized in Figure 13-4.

Some health care workers prefer to wear a back support when lifting. Be sure that you use the support correctly. Improper or prolonged use of a back support can actually weaken the back muscles. But, when used correctly, the back support will remind you to hold your body in proper alignment when lifting,

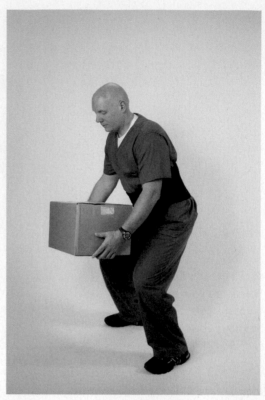

Figure 13-5 A back support can help to hold your body in proper alignment when lifting.

because bending at the waist with a tight back support around you is very uncomfortable (Fig. 13-5).

Guidelines for protecting yourself from injury as a result of the physical nature of your job are summarized in Guidelines Box 13-1. To protect your health, remember the principles of good body mechanics and apply them consistently, both at work and at home.

FOLLOWING PROCEDURES

To ensure that the care you provide is safe and correct, you will follow specific **procedures**. A procedure is a series of steps followed in a particular order. Following the recommended steps of a procedure helps to protect the person you are caring for, and it protects you.

The steps of the procedures you learn may differ somewhat depending on where you work and what state you receive your training in. For example, you may use more disposable supplies in the acute care setting compared with the long-term care setting. Some states will require you to be able to read a glass thermometer for your skills test, while other states may only require you to use an electronic thermometer. The steps of the procedures in this book reflect general practice and may be a little different than what your instructor teaches. Always be sure to follow the policies of the facility or the state where you work so that the care you provide is safe and consistent.

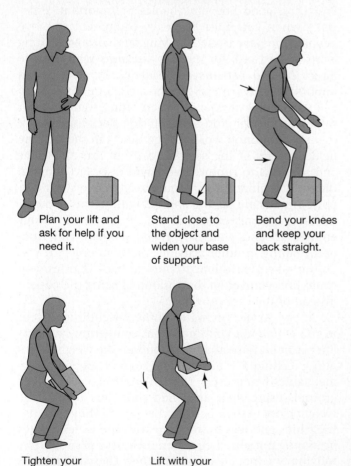

Plan your lift and ask for help if you need it.

Stand close to the object and widen your base of support.

Bend your knees and keep your back straight.

Tighten your abdominal muscles.

Lift with your leg muscles.

Figure 13-4 Proper lifting technique.

Guidelines Box 13-1 Guidelines for Protecting Yourself From Physical Injury

WHAT YOU DO	WHY YOU DO IT
Make a habit of practicing good posture.	Keeping the body in proper alignment, regardless of the activity, reduces stress and fatigue to the muscles and joints.
Create a solid base of support by moving your feet apart, either by widening your stance or by placing one foot in front of the other.	A solid base of support improves your balance, reducing the chance that you will injure yourself during the maneuver.
Allow the weight of your own body to assist in pulling or pushing heavy objects.	Using coordinated body movement to move something minimizes the stress on your body while making the task you are trying to accomplish easier.
When moving or lifting people or objects, place your body as close as possible to the object being moved.	Bringing your body's center of gravity closer to the object improves your balance and allows the strong muscles of the shoulders and upper arms to assist in the move.
Squat, do not lean over, to lower your center of gravity when lifting.	Lowering your center of gravity improves your balance. However, this lowering should be accomplished by squatting, rather than leaning over. Squatting allows you to use the strong muscles of your lower body to move yourself, and the weight, upward. Leaning over while lifting weight strains the back joints and muscles.
Use the large, strong muscles of the hips, buttocks, and thighs to do the lifting.	Using the strong muscles of the hips and legs to move yourself upward is preferable to placing strain on the muscles of the back, which are not meant to be used to lift substantial amounts of weight.
Do not lift heavy objects from a position higher than your head. Use a step stool or a short safety ladder to raise your entire body closer to the desired level.	Attempting to lift a heavy object from an awkward position (for example, with your arms raised above your head) interferes with your ability to balance and places you at risk for injury.
If an object is very heavy, do not attempt to lift it. Instead, pull, push, or roll the object.	Pushing, pulling, or rolling a heavy object places less strain on your body because you can use your body weight to help you accomplish the task. In other words, you can use the principle of coordinated body movement.
Use assistive devices whenever possible to make the job easier.	Handcarts and dollies permit the easy movement of objects by placing them on wheels. Gait belts, draw sheets, and mechanical lifts (discussed in detail in Chapter 15) help make moving people easier.
Ask for help when lifting or moving heavy people or objects. You should also get help when you need to move a person who cannot offer any assistance or is combative.	Heavy or awkward loads increase your risk of injury (and, if you are attempting to lift a person, increase that person's risk of injury as well). A person who is "dead weight" or uncooperative is both heavy and awkward.
Keep your body in good physical condition by exercising regularly, eating nutritious foods, and getting enough rest.	Your body can be compared to an automobile. It must be properly maintained in order to provide you with years of solid performance.

Certain steps, called **pre-procedure actions**, are followed before performing any procedure on a patient or resident. In this book, we call these actions "Getting Ready" steps (Guidelines Box 13-2). The "Getting Ready" steps promote efficiency, safety, courtesy, and respect of the patient's or resident's rights.

"Getting Ready" always begins with checking the patient's or resident's care plan. The care plan will tell you the specifics about providing care for each individual person. Care plans change, sometimes frequently, so that they correlate with changes in the patient's or resident's condition and abilities. That is why you will

Guidelines Box 13-2 Guidelines for Getting Ready (Pre-procedure Actions) WEAVERS

WHAT YOU DO	WHY YOU DO IT
To prepare for any type of care you provide, always check the person's care plan.	The person's care plan gives you specific information about the type of care you need to provide and will change as the person's condition and abilities change.
WASH Perform proper hand hygiene. Apply gloves and follow standard precautions if contact with blood or body fluids is possible.	Proper hand hygiene and taking standard precautions prevent the spread of infection.
EQUIPMENT Gather all needed supplies.	Having everything you need before you start promotes efficiency.
ANNOUNCE Knock on the door and identify yourself by name and title to the person.	Knocking before you enter protects the person's right to privacy. Identifying yourself respects the person's right to know who is providing care.
VERIFY Identify the person, and greet them by name. Methods of identifying patients and residents will vary depending on where you work. Common methods of identifying people in health care facilities include wrist bands and photographs.	Identifying the person ensures that the procedure is being done on the correct patient or resident. Greeting the person by name is courteous.
EXPLAIN the procedure and encourage the person to participate as appropriate.	Explaining the procedure lets the person know what to expect and helps them to understand how they can help.
RESPECT the person's privacy by showing any visitors where they may wait, if necessary, until you have completed the procedure. Close the door and the curtain. Drape the person for modesty as appropriate.	Asking visitors to leave the room, closing the door and curtain, and draping the person for modesty protect the person's right to privacy.
SAFETY Take safety precautions by following standards of body mechanics, equipment use, and infection control. In procedures that involve getting a person out of bed, lower the bed to its lowest position. This decreases the distance between the bed and the floor, should the person fall. In procedures that involve providing care while the person remains in bed, raise the bed to a comfortable working height, usually around elbow level of the caregiver. This protects your back. When using a bedside table to hold items used to provide personal care, keep the table close to the bed so you do not have to turn or move away from the patient or resident.	Following standards of body mechanics, equipment use, and infection control keeps you and your patients or residents safe.

Guidelines Box 13-3   Guidelines for Finishing Up (Post-procedure Actions) ALSO Wash & Document

WHAT YOU DO	WHY YOU DO IT
ALIGNMENT Confirm that the person is comfortable and in good body alignment.	Proper body alignment is most comfortable for the person. It relieves strain on the muscles and joints, promotes good heart and lung function, and helps prevent contractures and pressure ulcers.
LIGHT Leave the call light control, telephone, and fresh water within easy reach of the person.	Having necessary items nearby promotes independence and helps to prevent falls.
SAFETY Return the bed to the lowest position, lock the wheels, and raise the side rails (if side rails are in use).	Lowering the bed, locking the wheels, and raising the side rails (if side rails are in use) help to prevent falls.
OPEN the curtain and door if desired by the patient or resident, and inform visitors that they may return to the room.	Opening the curtain and door and letting visitors know that they can return help to prevent feelings of isolation.
WASH Perform hand hygiene. If gloves were worn during the procedure, remove them, discard according to facility policy, and perform hand hygiene before touching clean items. Perform hand hygiene again before leaving the patient's or resident's room.	Performing proper hand hygiene helps to prevent the spread of infection.
DOCUMENT Report and record actions as required by your facility.	Reporting lets the nurse know that you have completed the task and allows you to update the nurse about any changes in the patient's or resident's status. Recording formally documents the care that was provided and ensures that all members of the health care team have the same information about the patient's or resident's status and care.

need to check the care plan frequently, especially if you work in an acute care type of setting.

A simple mnemonic has been created to help you remember the "Getting Ready" steps: "WEAVERS." Guidelines Box 13-2 lists and explains each of these actions.

Similarly, there is a group of actions that are routinely performed at the end of each procedure, called **post-procedure actions**. In this book, we call these actions "Finishing Up" steps (Guidelines Box 13-3). The "Finishing Up" steps promote comfort, safety, and communication among members of the health care team. The mnemonic to help you remember the "Finishing Up" steps is "ALSO Wash & Document." As you review the procedure boxes throughout this book, you will see references to these "Getting Ready" and "Finishing Up" steps in each of them. You must learn these steps and perform them before and after every procedure.

PREVENTING FALLS

In Chapter 14, you will learn about situations that increase a patient's or resident's risk for falling, such as poor vision, a limited ability to move, or confusion. But what about factors that increase a nursing assistant's chances of falling?

Nursing assistants work hard and have many duties that must be completed during a shift. Being in too much of a hurry can increase your risk of falling. Even in an emergency situation, when you need to move quickly, be aware of your surroundings and move only as fast as you are safely able. You cannot help during an emergency if you fall and hurt yourself!

Wet floors also increase your risk of falling. Helping patients and residents with showers and baths often results in water on the floor. A resident who is incontinent (unable to control their bladder) can leave a puddle of urine in the hallway that you could slip

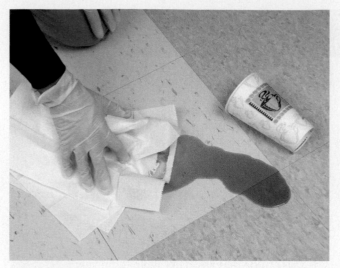

Figure 13-6 Mopping up spills is an important safety measure. Failing to do so can lead to falls.

in, especially if you are in a hurry. If you see water or other fluids or substances on the floor, you should immediately stop what you are doing and dry the area (Fig. 13-6). Failure to do so puts you, your patients or residents, visitors, and coworkers at risk for falling.

Be aware of objects in your path that could cause you to trip. Electrical cords can also pose a tripping hazard. Try to position furniture so that the electrical cords for lamps and other appliances are close to the outlet.

Make sure that you can see clearly. Night lights positioned near the floor are useful in a health care setting. They allow you to see where you are going without disturbing the patient or resident by turning on the overhead light.

Helping a very weak, unsteady, or uncooperative person to walk or transfer from one place to another without help can cause both of you to fall. You may not want to ask a busy coworker for help, but resist the temptation to "go it alone." If the patient or resident you are attempting to help falls, they will take you with them, potentially resulting in serious injury to you both. Attempting to prevent a patient or resident from falling can also result in a back injury for you. Please ask for help whenever you feel you need it in order to safely continue. If you are assisting a person who begins to fall, follow the steps in Box 13-1 to minimize the risk of injury for everyone involved.

PREVENTING CHEMICAL INJURIES

Health care facilities use many chemicals on a daily basis—for example, cleaning solutions and disinfectants, sterilizing agents, and chemotherapeutic drugs. Many of these chemicals can be harmful if they are inhaled, swallowed, absorbed through the skin, or splashed in the eyes. Some chemicals are relatively harmless alone but can become dangerous if accidentally mixed with another product.

OSHA requires all employers to maintain a list of the chemicals that are used in the facility, from household cleaners to highly toxic solutions, and to inform and educate all workers about the chemicals that are in use in their workplace. One way of communicating information about chemicals to employees is through **Safety Data Sheets (SDS)**, which the manufacturer of the chemical is required to supply (Fig. 13-7). These SDSs were previously called Materials Safety Data Sheets (MSDS), but OSHA revised their Hazard Communication Standard in 2013 to simplify and standardize labels and information about materials that may be hazardous to people. This will help to improve a worker's understanding of the chemicals they may be exposed to in the workplace and allow them to better protect themselves and those they care for from these hazards. The SDS for each chemical in use must be kept on file and be readily available in each unit of the health care facility. The manufacturer must renew the SDS every 3 years (or sooner, if there is a change in the product). The SDS summarizes key information about the chemical, such as what it is made from, which exposures may be dangerous, what to do if an exposure occurs, and how to clean up spills. Container labels also provide information about the chemicals in the container, and all containers must be clearly labeled. Most container labels now contain symbols, known as *pictograms*, that are used to help communicate specific information and hazards about the contents. As a nursing assistant, it is your responsibility to be familiar with the chemicals that you may come in contact with in your facility and to know the proper, safe way to handle each chemical in use.

PREVENTING ELECTRICAL SHOCKS

There are many types of electrical equipment used in the health care setting, from complex monitoring devices to the common hair dryer. Knowing how to safely operate and maintain electrical equipment in the workplace will help create a safe working environment for you and a safe living environment for your patients or residents.

Precautions, such as using grounded appliances and power strips, help to minimize the risk of electrical shock. Most electrical equipment used in the health care setting are **grounded**. This means that it has a way of returning stray electrical current to the outlet so that the risk of electrical shock is reduced. Grounding may be achieved through a three-prong plug (Fig. 13-8A) or a safety outlet with a ground-fault breaker (Fig. 13-8B). The use of extension cords is not recommended, and outlets should not be overloaded. If more than two items must be plugged into an outlet, a facility-approved power strip should be used (Fig. 13-8C). Some types of

Box 13-1 Minimizing the Risk of Injury as a Result of a Fall

1. If the person complains of dizziness or seems unsteady, help them to sit in a chair. If a chair is not close by, help the person to sit on the floor. Stay with the person and call for assistance. This action can prevent a fall completely.

2. If a fall cannot be avoided, place your body behind the person and place your arms around their torso, pulling them close to your body. Do not grab the person's arm in an attempt to prevent the fall because doing so may actually cause more extensive injuries in some people (such as elderly people, who may have brittle bones, and people with weaknesses on one side of the body).

3. With the person's body pulled close to yours, widen your base of support by placing one foot behind the other, and allow the person to slide down your body toward the floor.

4. As the person slides down, squat while still supporting their body and gently lower them to the floor. Lower yourself to the floor and assume a sitting position with the person's head in your lap.

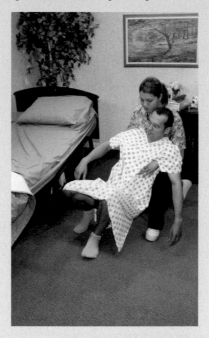

5. Stay with the person and call for assistance.

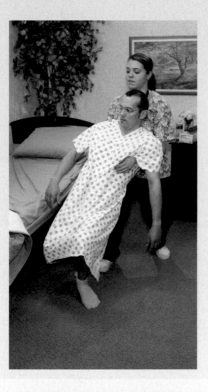

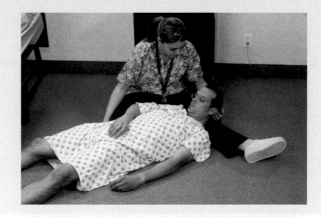

electrical equipment used in a health care setting may be intended to be plugged directly into the wall outlet. For example, some types of specialty beds used in acute care settings may not be plugged into a power strip. Be sure that you follow the manufacturer's instructions.

As a nursing assistant, you must be alert for electrical items that pose potential shock or fire hazards. Residents of long-term care facilities often bring small electrical items with them to furnish their rooms, such as radios, televisions, and table lamps. Most facilities require items like these to be inspected by the maintenance or biomedical engineering department before the resident can use them. However, if you notice anything unsafe about an electrical appliance that is being used, such as frayed

wires or loose plugs, you should remove the appliance from use immediately. This is true of facility-owned equipment as well, such as electrically controlled hospital beds and call light controls. Most health care facilities have a system for tagging a defective item and sending it for repair (Fig. 13-9). Follow your facility's policy. Failure to properly tag a defective electrical device could result in injury or even death to the next person who uses it.

When using electrical equipment, be aware of the safety hazard posed by operating an electrical appliance around water. Do not operate hair dryers, electric razors, curling irons, radios, or other electrical appliances around showers and bathtubs. The risk of electrical shock or electrocution must be taken seriously.

MATERIAL SAFETY DATA SHEET 3M (TM) Avagard (TM) Antiseptic hand Rub with Chlorhexidine Gluconate 0.5%w/v in 70% v/v Ethanol 9250H & 9250P 06/12/13

3.2 POTENTIAL HEALTH EFFECTS

Eye Contact:
Moderate Eye Irritation: Signs/symptoms may include redness, swelling, pain, tearing, and blurred or hazy vision.

Skin Contact:
Allergic Skin Reaction (non-photo induced): Signs/symptoms may include redness, swelling, blistering, and itching.

Avagard Antiseptic Hand Preparation should not be used by persons who are known to be hypersensitive to chlorhexidine gluconate or any of its components.

Inhalation:
Respiratory Tract Irritation: Signs/symptoms may include cough, sneezing, nasal discharge, headache, hoarseness, and nose and throat pain.

May be absorbed following inhalation and cause target organ effects.

Ingestion:
Gastrointestinal Irritation: Signs/symptoms may include abdominal pain, stomach upset, nausea, vomiting, and diarrhea.

May be absorbed following ingestion and cause target organ effects.

Target Organ Effects:
Central Nervous System (CNS) Depression: Signs/symptoms may include headache, dizziness, drowsiness, incoordination, nausea, slowed reaction time, slurred speech, giddiness, and unconsciousness.

Prolonged or repeated exposure may cause:
Liver Effects: Signs/symptoms may include loss of appetite, weight loss, fatigue, weakness, abdominal tenderness, and jaundice.

NOTE: This product contains ethanol. There are data associating human consumption of alcoholic beverages with developmental toxicity, and the California Environmental Protection Agency has classified ethanol in alcoholic beverages as a developmental toxicant (for purposes of Proposition 65). Exposure to ethanol during the foreseeable use of this product is not expected to cause developmental toxicity.

NOTE: This product contains ethanol. Alcoholic beverages and ethanol in alcoholic beverages have been classified as human carcinogens by the International Agency for Research on Cancer, the U.S. National Toxicology Program, and the California Environmental Protection Agency (for purposes of Proposition 65). Exposure to ethanol during the foreseeable use of this product is not expected to cause cancer.

SECTION 4: FIRST AID MEASURES

4.1 FIRST AID PROCEDURES

The following first aid recommendations are based on an assumption that appropriate personal and industrial hygiene practices are followed.

Eye Contact: Flush eyes with large amounts of water. If signs/symptoms persist, get medical attention.
Skin Contact: No need for first aid is anticipated. If signs/symptoms develop, get medical attention.

Inhalation: Remove person to fresh air. If signs/symptoms develop, get medical attention.
If Swallowed: Rinse mouth. Do not induce vomiting. Get immediate medical attention.

SECTION 5: FIRE FIGHTING MEASURES

Figure 13-7 Part of a Safety Data Sheet (SDS). The SDS provides important information about each chemical in use in the workplace.

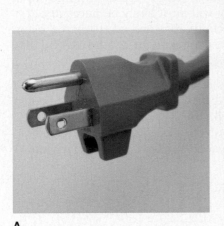
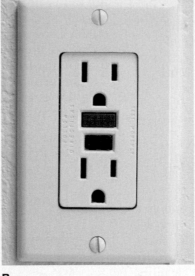
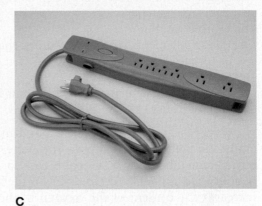

A   **B**   **C**

Figure 13-8 **A.** Three-prong plugs, (**B**) outlets with ground-fault breakers, and (**C**) power strips help to reduce the risk of electrical shock and fire.

FIRE SAFETY

In a health care facility, a fire that gets out of control can have tragic consequences. Not only does the facility house a large number of people, many of these people are relatively unable to help themselves in the event of an emergency. As a health care worker, you must know how to prevent fires in the workplace, and what to do in the event that a fire does occur.

Preventing Fires

For a fire to occur, three elements must be present: fuel (something that burns), heat (something to ignite the fuel), and oxygen (Fig. 13-10).

Common sources of fuel in the health care setting include:

- Cloth, such as bed linens, mattresses, and clothing
- Paper
- Substances that easily catch fire and burn quickly, such as cooking oil, gasoline, chemicals, and nail polish remover
- The building itself

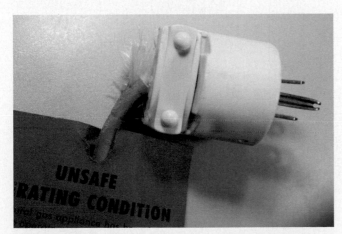

Figure 13-9 If you notice that a piece of electrical equipment is malfunctioning or presents a safety hazard, follow your facility's policy for removing it from use and getting it repaired.

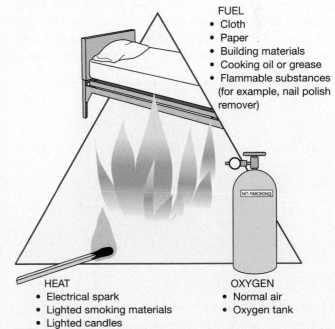

FUEL
- Cloth
- Paper
- Building materials
- Cooking oil or grease
- Flammable substances (for example, nail polish remover)

HEAT
- Electrical spark
- Lighted smoking materials
- Lighted candles

OXYGEN
- Normal air
- Oxygen tank

Figure 13-10 Three things must be present for a fire to occur: fuel, heat, and oxygen.

Heat can be provided by:

- An electrical spark (such as may occur with a frayed electrical cord, a "short" in a piece of electrical equipment, or even a lightning strike)
- Lighted smoking materials (such as cigarettes, cigars, or matches)
- Lighted candles
- Heating elements (such as radiators, space heaters, or furnaces)
- Stoves
- Personal care appliances (such as hair dryers and curling irons)

Oxygen is found in the air around us, and generally the better the air supply, the better a fire will burn. Remember that in a health care facility, many patients and residents receive oxygen therapy, which increases the content of the oxygen in the air in the immediate area. Safety precautions that are used to prevent fires (Guidelines Box 13-4) are extremely important when oxygen therapy is in use. The patient or resident and any visitors should be made aware of the added risks (Fig. 13-11).

Reacting to a Fire Emergency

Sometimes, despite taking precautions, a fire will occur. In some cases, the fire will be small and can be dealt with rather easily if the situation is addressed promptly and correctly. For example, imagine a fire that begins in a resident's room because a visitor drops a half-lit cigarette in a wastebasket full of paper, or a stovetop fire that begins in the hospital kitchen. In both of these situations, an alert person who knew what to do could control the fire, and it is possible that others outside of the immediate area would not even be aware of the disturbance. However, sometimes a

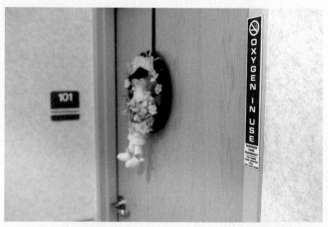

Figure 13-11 Oxygen therapy is common in health care facilities. "Oxygen In Use" signs are posted to warn patients or residents and their visitors that extra precautions are needed when oxygen therapy is in use.

fire can begin on a much larger scale, for example, as a result of faulty electrical wiring in the walls of the building, a gas leak, or even a natural disaster. In situations like these, a large-scale evacuation (removal) of those in the facility will most likely be necessary.

The general actions that are taken in the event of a fire emergency are known as the **RACE fire response plan** (Fig. 13-12):

Rescue or remove any patients or residents who are in immediate danger to safety. Escort people who can walk. Use wheelchairs for unsteady people. To prevent a confused or disoriented person from accidentally wandering back into

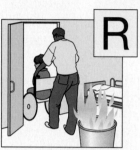

Rescue/remove

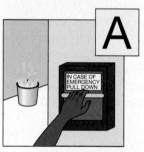

Alarm

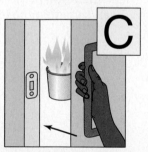

Contain

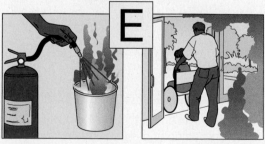

Extinguish   or   Evacuate

Figure 13-12 The RACE fire response plan.

Guidelines Box 13-4 Guidelines for Preventing Fires

WHAT YOU DO	WHY YOU DO IT
Supervise patients or residents who are disoriented or who may fall asleep while smoking, any time that they smoke.	A sleepy or disoriented person is not paying close attention to the lighted smoking material, which increases the chance that a fire will start.
Do not allow any patient or resident to smoke in bed, especially if the person is receiving oxygen therapy.[a]	A person who smokes in bed is bringing all three elements necessary for a fire together (fuel = bed linens; heat = lighted smoking material; oxygen = surrounding air). Smoking in bed is especially dangerous because the person is more likely to fall asleep and forget about the lighted smoking material. In addition, the use of oxygen therapy increases the oxygen content of linens and bedding in the immediate area. If burning ashes from a cigarette should happen to drop on the bed, a fire would be more likely to start and would burn much faster as a result of the added oxygen.
Do not provide patients or residents who are receiving oxygen therapy with wool or mohair blankets.	These materials can produce sparks of static electricity, which could lead to a fire.
If smoking is permitted in the facility, make sure that all smoking occurs only in designated smoking areas.	Designated smoking areas have ashtrays for properly extinguishing lit smoking materials. They are also located in a part of the building where oxygen therapy is not in use.
Keep smoking materials, lighters, and matches in a place where children and confused patients or residents cannot reach them.	Children do not understand that playing with these materials can be dangerous. A confused person is not able to use these materials responsibly on their own and should be supervised.
Keep all electrical equipment in good working order.	A spark from a frayed wire, an improperly grounded plug, or an electrical "short" can start an electrical fire.
Handle flammable substances safely and clean up any spills immediately. Do not use flammable substances near a heat source such as a hair dryer, curling iron, or heater, or while smoking.	Flammable substances ignite easily and burn quickly. Therefore, if they come in contact with a heat source, a fire is likely to start.
Report any malfunctioning smoke detectors immediately.	A smoke detector is the best early fire detection device available, but only if it is functioning properly.
Investigate smoke or smells of anything burning promptly. Be aware of the location of fire alarms and fire extinguishers and know how to activate and use them.	Early investigation and quick action can help to contain a fire before it gets out of control.
Be familiar with your facility's fire safety policies and know the location of all exits.	If a fire does occur, you may need to evacuate patients or residents. You will be much more effective in your duties if you are able to remain calm, and your calmness will also help to calm others.

[a]Although health care facilities prohibit smoking in patient or resident rooms, some people may forget or disregard the rules.

the fire area, assign another, alert patient or resident or a visitor to attend to the person. People who cannot get out of bed should be moved in their beds, if possible. If the bed cannot be moved out of the room, or if stairs must be used, the patient or resident can be pulled to safety using a carry device or the linens from the bed (Box 13-2). Some facilities will train you in special techniques that are used to carry a person to safety.

Activate the **A**larm if the alarm has not been sounded. Follow your facility's policy for

Box 13-2	Using Bed Linens to Evacuate a Bedridden Person

1. Loosen the bottom sheet from the foot of the person's bed.
2. Make sure that the bed is lowered to its lowest position and that the wheels are locked.
3. Grasp the top of the bottom sheet near the person's head and shoulders. Have a coworker grasp the bottom sheet at the foot of the bed. Using the sheet, gently lower the person to the floor, feet first.
4. Pull the sheet, with the person cradled in it, toward the nearest exit.
5. If it is necessary to move the person downstairs, support the person's upper body by pulling up on the sheet and proceed down the steps backward. Do not allow the person's body to bump against the steps.

reporting a fire. For example, you may be required to pull the fire alarm or use the intercom or telephone system.

Contain the fire by closing doors and windows. This action helps to slow the spread of the fire.

Extinguish the fire if possible, or, if the fire is large or spreading quickly,

Evacuate the building.

Extinguishing Fires

As you know, there are three elements that must be present for a fire to continue burning—fuel, heat, and oxygen. If you remove just one of these elements, you can put out (extinguish) the fire. Not all fires are alike. Fires are classified as either "A" type, "B" type, or "C" type fires (Table 13-1). This classification determines the best way to put them out.

TABLE 13-1   Types of Fires

TYPE	DESCRIPTION	METHOD OF EXTINGUISHING
A	Fueled by ordinary material such as wood, paper, cloth, leaves, and grass	Water effectively extinguishes a Type A fire by removing the heat.

B	Fueled by a petroleum product (for example, gasoline, automotive oil), cooking oil, or grease	Do not try to put these fires out with water! Instead, smother the fire by sprinkling powder (such as baking soda) on it or by using a fire extinguisher made for a Type B fire. A stovetop fire that starts in a pan can be extinguished by covering the pan and removing it from the heat source.
	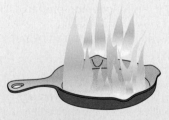	
C	An electrical fire	Attempting to put an electrical fire out with water can result in shock or electrocution. Use a fire extinguisher that is specific to an electrical fire instead.
	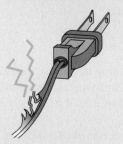	

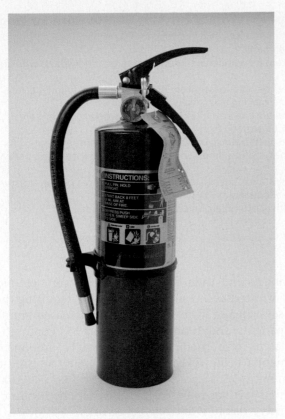

Figure 13-13 An ABC fire extinguisher is effective against all types of fires.

A commonly used tool for putting out fires is a fire extinguisher (Fig. 13-13). There are fire extinguishers that are specific for each type of fire, but the most common type of fire extinguisher, an ABC extinguisher, can be used for all types of fires. ABC fire extinguishers use carbon dioxide to remove the oxygen from the fire. This smothers the fire, putting it out. All health care facilities must have easily accessible fire extinguishers in case a fire should occur. You are responsible for knowing where fire extinguishers are kept in your facility. During your orientation, you will be trained in the use of your facility's fire extinguishers, and these instructions will be reviewed with you each year. In the event of a small fire, you should be able to use a fire extinguisher to put the fire out safely and effectively. When using a fire extinguisher, remember the word **PASS**:

Pull the safety pin out.
Aim the hose toward the base of the fire.
Squeeze the handle.
Spray the contents of the fire extinguisher at the base of the fire, sweeping from side to side.

Evacuating the Building

If a large, uncontrollable fire breaks out, you will need to know how to get your patients or residents and yourself to safety. Health care facilities must regularly practice and evaluate fire safety plans. You should take these fire drill exercises seriously so that if a fire emergency should occur, your actions will be almost second nature. By knowing what to do and acting calmly, you will increase the efficiency of the evacuation and help to calm those around you.

DISASTER PREPAREDNESS

A **disaster** is a sudden, unexpected event that causes injury to many people, major damage to property, or both. Disasters can be caused by acts of nature (such as tornadoes, earthquakes, hurricanes, floods, wildfires, blizzards, or ice storms), or they may be the result of explosions, accidents, or acts of war or terrorism. Acts of terrorism can easily be targeted at vulnerable areas such as health care facilities and schools. These acts could include the use of explosives, the use of rapid-fire automatic guns, the release of chemicals (for example, nerve gas agents), radiation exposure (dirty bombs), or the release of biologic agents (such as anthrax).

Your facility or agency will have a disaster preparedness plan that will direct the actions of the health care team in the event of such an occurrence. If you work for a hospital, your facility's disaster plan may focus on preparing staff to handle the simultaneous admission and treatment of multiple people with injuries. If you work in a long-term care facility, the focus of your facility's disaster plan may be more on how to provide safe care for your residents in the event of a power failure. In the event of a disaster, you may have to help evacuate residents and patients to safer quarters. Know the particular duties that will be required of you in the event of a disaster and remain calm.

WORKPLACE VIOLENCE

Violent acts are increasing in areas where the victims are the most vulnerable, such as schools, churches, and health care facilities. Not only are seemingly random attacks against large numbers of people at one time taking place, but personal, one-on-one violence also occurs. As a result of this increased threat to people who work in health care settings and to those they care for, OSHA and the National Institute for Occupational Safety and Health (NIOSH) have issued recommendations and guidelines aimed at preventing workplace violence for health care workers.

Workplace violence is defined by the NIOSH as "violent acts (including physical assaults and threats of assaults) directed toward persons at work or on duty." This definition also includes acts of terrorism, as a

TABLE 13-2 Factors That Increase the Risk of Workplace Violence in the Health Care Setting

- The prevalence of handguns and other weapons among patients, their families, or friends
- The increasing use of hospitals by police and the criminal justice system for criminal holds and the care of individuals who are acutely disturbed or pose a threat of violence
- The increasing number of patients with acute or chronic mental illness being released from hospitals without follow-up care
- The availability of drugs or money at hospitals, clinics, and pharmacies, making them likely robbery targets
- Factors such as the unrestricted movement of the public in clinics and hospitals and long waits in emergency or clinic areas that lead to client frustration over an inability to obtain needed services promptly
- The increasing presence of gang activity, drug or alcohol use, patients with trauma, or distraught family members
- Low staffing levels during times of increased activity such as mealtimes, visiting times, and when staff are transporting patients
- Isolated work with clients during examinations or treatments
- Solo work, often in remote locations with no backup or way to get assistance, such as communication devices or alarm systems
- Lack of staff training in recognizing and managing escalating hostile and assaultive behavior
- Increasing incidence of domestic abuse violence involving both health care workers and patients or residents
- Poorly lit parking areas

result of the terroristic acts that took place on September 11, 2001 that took the lives of 2,886 people in the workplace in New York, Virginia, and Pennsylvania. These guidelines are intended to advise employers on the risks of violent acts that may occur in their specific types of work environment and how to train their employees to recognize and respond to these risks.

Health care workers may be victims of violent acts from many sources. External parties such as robbers or muggers can attack a worker as they walk from the parking lot to the building going to and from work. Domestic violence incidents, either aimed at a health care worker or a patient or resident, have increased. In many of these situations, the perpetrator not only targets their intended victim, but any others who may be nearby.

Internal parties that may inflict violence include coworkers, patients and residents, and their family members or other visitors. While acts of violence that result in death attract more attention, the vast majority of workplace violence is made up of nonfatal assaults. Interestingly, data have shown that up to 48% of all nonfatal injuries on the workplace occur in health care and social service settings. Of these injuries, nurses, nursing assistants, orderlies, and attendants were the most likely victims.

Why then is the risk of workplace violence so high for health care settings? As you have learned in previous chapters, people who are sick, injured, or disabled, and their families, may be very emotionally stressed as a result of whatever is requiring them to seek health care services. An increased number of patients and residents who may be confused or agitated from medications, medical conditions, or dementia being cared for by an already stressed-out staff may play a significant role. Table 13-2 lists factors that NIOSH has released that increase the health care worker's risk of work-related assaults.

Employers in health care settings take the NIOSH guidelines very seriously and provide training specific to the setting so that you and other health care workers will be more aware of potential risks of workplace violence. Locked facilities and units are becoming more common, and visitors must request entrance, and in some instances, show proper identification before being allowed to enter.

Be aware of your surroundings and the people around you. Most facilities are promoting the "See Something, Say Something," method of awareness that asks workers to notice and immediately report anything or anyone that seems out of place or suspicious. You will learn how to recognize situations that may escalate to violence and how to react in ways that can help prevent violence from happening. You will also learn ways to protect yourself personally from an attack of violence. Pay attention and take this training very seriously because what you learn could help protect both you and those you care for.

SUMMARY

- Many factors contribute to workplace safety and workplace safety affects many people.
  - It is your responsibility to help make your workplace safe for you and others by following guidelines and reporting unsafe conditions.
  - The Occupational Safety and Health Administration (OSHA) oversees safety regulations in all types of workplaces and addresses everything from safe lifting techniques to the control of hazardous materials.
    - OSHA mandates that employers inform workers of all workplace safety risks.
    - OSHA requires employers to provide regular training about workplace safety risks and how to avoid injury. Your employer must keep records of any training you have received that meets OSHA regulations.
  - Ergonomics involve making adjustments in the work environment and how workers perform work-related duties to help prevent injuries.
  - Work-related practices that nursing assistants face daily that increase the risk of musculoskeletal disorders include force, repetition, and awkward postures.
- Practicing good body mechanics allows for effective lifting and moving patients and equipment and helps protect you from injury in your daily duties.
  - The "ABCs" of good body mechanics are alignment, balance, and coordinated body movement.
  - Proper lifting technique is especially critical to preventing back injuries.
- Following procedures when providing patient or resident care helps to ensure that the care is safe and correct.
  - Pre-procedure actions ("Getting Ready" steps) are taken before every patient or resident care

procedure. They promote efficiency, safety, and respect of the patient's or resident's rights.
  - Post-procedure actions ("Finishing Up" steps) are taken after every patient or resident care procedure. They promote comfort, safety, and communication among members of the health care team.
- Falling poses a risk to both the health care worker and the patient or resident. Asking for assistance and knowing how to properly assist a person who is falling can help to prevent injuries to everyone involved.
- Most health care facilities use chemicals in daily operation. Information about how to respond to a chemical exposure is found in the SDS, which each chemical manufacturer must supply, and on the labeled container.
- Malfunctioning or improperly used electrical appliances can lead to electric shock, electrocution, and electrical fires.
- A fire in a health care facility can have tragic consequences because many people who are housed in health care facilities are unable to move independently or quickly.
  - Three elements are necessary to start a fire and keep it burning: fuel, heat, and oxygen.
  - The RACE fire response plan describes the general actions that are to be taken in the event of a fire emergency: **R**escue or remove people in the immediate area, Activate the **A**larm, **C**ontain the fire, and **E**xtinguish or **E**vacuate as indicated by the situation.
- In the event of a disaster, follow your facility's disaster preparedness plan.
- Workplace violence is increasing as a risk to the health care worker.
  - Nurses, nursing assistants, orderlies, and attendants are most likely to be injured as the result of workplace violence.

WHAT DID YOU LEARN?

Multiple Choice

Select the single best answer for each of the following questions.

1. In the event of a fire in a resident's room, your first action should be to:
   a. Remove the resident to a safe place
   b. Get the fire extinguisher
   c. Sound the fire alarm
   d. Notify the head nurse

2. When lifting, remember to use the large muscles of your:
   a. Chest
   b. Hips, buttocks, and thighs
   c. Back
   d. Shoulders

3. You accidentally knock over a water pitcher, spilling water on the floor of a patient's room. What should you do?
   a. Call housekeeping
   b. Continue with your assignment and make a mental note to wipe up the spill later
   c. Throw a towel over the spill to absorb the liquid and alert others to be careful
   d. Wipe the spill up immediately

4. While you are walking with Ms. Nakamura in the hallway, she complains of dizziness. Your first response should be to:
   a. Assist her into a nearby chair and call for help
   b. Assist her to the floor and go get help
   c. Ask Ms. Nakamura to breathe deeply and reassure her that everything will be fine
   d. Encourage Ms. Nakamura to continue walking because she needs the exercise

5. As you come around the corner on your unit, you hear Mrs. Petersen shouting in alarm, and you see smoke and flames coming from the wastebasket in her room. You should:
   a. Run to the telephone and call the fire department
   b. Take Mrs. Petersen's cigarettes away
   c. Assist Mrs. Petersen out of the room and close the door
   d. Throw water on the flames

6. Using good body mechanics to lift an object off the floor means that you would:
   a. Use a mechanical lift
   b. Kneel down to get the broadest base of support and lift up
   c. Squat and lift with your legs
   d. Lean over at the waist, keeping your back flat

7. Unsafe conditions in a health care facility can be caused by:
   a. Health care workers who allow patients or residents to get out of bed
   b. Health care workers who stop doing an assigned task to clean up a spill
   c. Overloaded outlets and extension cords
   d. Patients and residents who smoke in "smoking only" areas

8. All of the following actions could cause a fire except:
   a. Using a three-prong plug
   b. Emptying an ashtray into a wastebasket
   c. Smoking in a room where a person is receiving oxygen therapy
   d. Placing a stack of linens on a heating unit to warm them

9. Where should you direct the foam when using a fire extinguisher to put out a fire?
   a. At the base of the fire
   b. In a circle around the fire, to prevent the fire from spreading
   c. At the top of the fire
   d. Anywhere in the general area of the fire

10. What are the "ABCs" of good body mechanics?
   a. Assess, Balance, Complete
   b. Assign, Begin, Complete
   c. Alignment, Balance, Coordinated body movement
   d. Attempt, Brace, Change

11. You are a new nursing assistant and have been assigned to clean the room of a resident who has just been discharged. The nurse shows you the cleaning closet, which contains towels, rags, and containers holding liquids and powders of various colors and odors. How can you find out what cleaning products are appropriate for your assigned task?
    a. Read the nursing care plan
    b. Read the product label
    c. Use your senses—smell the contents of each container and use whichever has the most pleasant smell
    d. There is no need to find out which product is most appropriate—the cleaning closet contains only products used for cleaning

12. Following pre- and post-procedure actions before and after each procedure is important to:
    a. Prevent the patient or resident from becoming confused
    b. Ensure that the care you give is safe and correct
    c. Make the nurse happy
    d. Pass the certification exam

13. Which one of the following is a pre-procedure ("Getting Ready") step?
    a. Report and record
    b. Identify the person
    c. Confirm that the person is comfortable and in good body alignment
    d. Open the curtain or door

14. How do you "see to safety" before and after performing a procedure?
    a. Use good body mechanics
    b. Use equipment properly
    c. Practice infection control
    d. All of the above

15. Workplace violence can result from either internal or external parties. Which of the following is an example of an external party?
    a. Confused resident
    b. Mugger in the parking garage
    c. Angry coworker
    d. Mentally ill patient

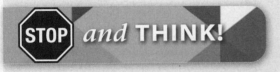

You work on the second floor of a long-term care facility. As you are walking down the hall toward the nursing station, you hear one of your residents, Miss Verna, call for help. When you look into her room, you see that her wastebasket is on fire. What should you do? Is it possible to accomplish more than one step of the RACE plan at once?

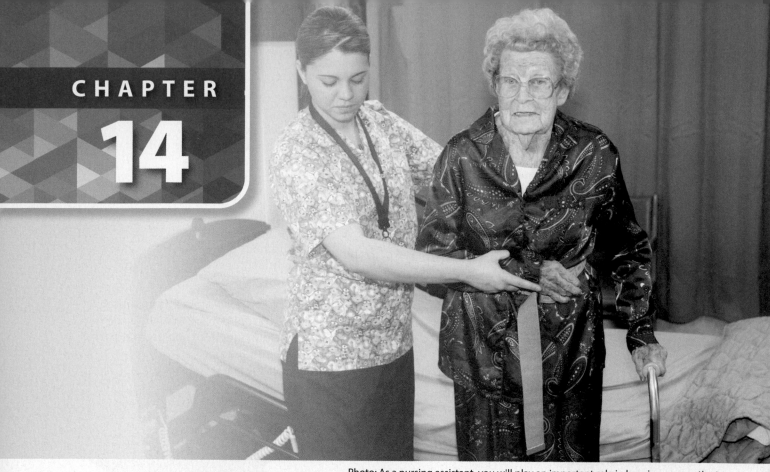

Photo: As a nursing assistant, you will play an important role in keeping your patients or residents safe. Here, a nursing assistant helps a resident to get out of bed safely.

Patient Safety and Restraint Alternatives

 WHAT WILL YOU LEARN?

Life has taught us many lessons in safety. When you were a child, your parents reminded you to look both ways before crossing the street. As a teen learning to drive, you were cautioned to wear your seat belt and to observe the rules of the road. As an adult, you remember to lock the door at night and turn off the coffeepot before you leave home. As you remember from Chapter 6, safety is a basic human need. If we feel safe, we can relax and rest and we feel secure and comfortable. The previous chapters have explained principles and procedures designed to help keep you safe while you perform your duties as a nursing assistant. In this chapter, we will focus on principles and procedures that help to keep those you care for safe. When you are finished with this chapter, you will be able to:

1. Define the terms "accident" and "incident," and discuss how each can threaten the safety of a person in a health care setting.

2. Identify risk factors that may put people in a health care facility at higher risk for accidents and injury.

3. List and describe special needs that residents in a long-term care setting may have related to safety.

4. **Describe basic safety methods designed to prevent accidents and incidents in a health care facility.**

5. **Explain the importance of reporting and recording accidents and incidents.**

6. **List the different types of restraints.**

7. **Identify safety concerns of restraint use.**

8. **Describe methods used to reduce the need for restraints.**

9. **Demonstrate the proper application of a vest restraint, a wrist or ankle restraint, and a lap or waist (belt) restraint.**

Vocabulary

Accident	Tetraplegia (quadriplegia)	Entrapment	Physical restraint
Incident	Hemiplegia	Incident (occurrence)	Chemical restraint
Paraplegia	Comatose	report	Restraint alternatives

ACCIDENTS AND INCIDENTS

The Omnibus Budget Reconciliation Act (OBRA) defines an **accident** as an unexpected, unintended event that has the potential to cause bodily injury. An **incident** is an occurrence that is considered unusual, undesired, or out of the ordinary, and that disrupts the normal routine for the patient or resident, the health care facility, or both (for example, a resident wanders away from a long-term health care facility, or a person's personal property is lost). Accidents and incidents can involve patients or residents, staff, or visitors to the facility.

All accidents are considered incidents. For example, if a patient or a resident trips and falls, an accident has occurred because the fall was unintended and could cause injury to the person. An incident has also occurred because the fall is an undesired event that disrupts the normal routine. On the other hand, not all incidents are accidents. For example, if a resident in a nursing facility becomes angry with another resident and hits them, an accident has not occurred because the angry resident intended to hit the other resident. However, an incident has occurred because the action is undesired, out of the ordinary, and disrupts the normal routine.

Risk Factors

For many reasons, certain groups of people are at more risk than others to have an accident (Fig. 14-1). Recognizing the factors that can increase a person's chances of having an accident will help you to minimize the chance that an accident will occur.

Age

Infants and young children are at high risk for accidents. Infants are helpless. As a result, they are prone to accidental suffocation and falls. Young children are not helpless, but they lack knowledge and judgment about things that are dangerous. As a result, young children are at risk for injuries such as falls, burns, poisoning, and drowning. You can find out more about safety issues related to children in Chapter 45.

Older adults are at high risk for accidents also. Although an older person can recognize a dangerous situation, some of the physical and mental effects of the aging process can affect their ability to remain safe.

Medication

The effects of medications, especially pain medications or sedatives, can affect a person's ability to be safe, regardless of age or other factors. For example, under the influence of a pain medication (which has a sedative effect), a person who normally smokes a cigarette while watching the evening news could fall asleep in front of the television while smoking, causing a fire. Driving and operating machinery are dangerous under the influence of some medications. Medications can also cause a person to become dizzy when standing or walking, causing a fall.

Paralysis

Paralysis (an inability to move or to feel) can be caused by a spinal cord injury or a stroke ("brain attack"). Depending on where a spinal cord injury occurs, a

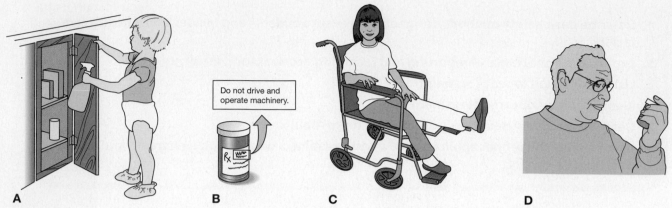

Figure 14-1 Some factors that place people at risk for accidents: (**A**) very young or very old age; (**B**) medication effects; (**C**) impaired mobility (an inability to move easily); and (**D**) sensory impairment (an inability to see, hear, smell, taste, or detect pain or changes in temperature).

person can be paralyzed from the waist down, or from the neck down. Paralysis from the waist down is known as **paraplegia**. Paralysis from the neck down is known as **tetraplegia (quadriplegia)**. A tetraplegic or paraplegic person's abilities vary, according to the exact level of the spinal injury. A stroke can cause **hemiplegia**, or paralysis on one side of the body. Not only is a person with paraplegia, tetraplegia, or hemiplegia unable to move the affected areas of their body, they may also be unable to sense pain, heat, or cold in these areas. The inability to move properly increases the person's risk for falling. The lack of sensation increases the person's risk for other injuries, such as burns.

Poor Mobility

An inability to move easily can put a person at risk for falling. Pain and stiffness from arthritis can make it difficult for a person to get around easily. Although older people tend to have more trouble with mobility than younger people, this is a risk factor that can affect all age groups. For example, a person recovering from knee surgery or a broken leg will be more likely to fall because of difficulty with mobility.

Sensory Impairment

We rely on our five senses (vision, hearing, touch, smell, and taste) to give us information about our environment and to keep us safe. Perhaps the sense we rely on the most is sight—not being able to see clearly can put anyone at risk for accidents. Poor vision increases the risk of falls, especially on stairs or over objects left on the floor. A person who wears bifocals may misjudge distance when stepping on or off curbs and steps, leading to falls. In addition, poor vision can increase the chances of accidental poisoning from

medications if the person is not able to clearly read the directions on the medication label.

Our sense of hearing also plays a large role in keeping us safe. A person with hearing difficulties may not be able to hear signs of danger approaching, such as the sound of an oncoming car. They may also miss warning alarms, such as the sound made by a smoke or carbon monoxide detector. When receiving instructions or directions (for example, regarding how to take a medication), a hearing-impaired person may be able to hear part of what is being said, but not enough to understand completely.

Touch and smell play a role in informing us about our environment as well. Certain conditions, such as diabetes, can decrease a person's sense of touch. People with an impaired sense of touch may not be able to tell that their bath water is too hot, leading to increased risk for burns. Because their ability to feel pain is lessened, they may be unaware that a favorite pair of shoes is causing blisters, leading to infection. Similarly, a decreased ability to smell (which often occurs as part of the normal aging process) can leave a person unable to detect spoiled food, a natural gas leak in the home, or smoke.

Limited Awareness of Surroundings

There are many reasons a person may not be aware of their surroundings. Confusion and disorientation can be caused by reactions to medication, head injuries, dementia, and other medical conditions. It can also be caused by something as simple as a change in environment or forgetting to put one's glasses on. Confusion can cause a person in a health care facility to forget to call for help when they need to get up. A person who is unconscious or **comatose** is totally unable to respond to their environment and will also need your assistance to remain safe.

Concerns for Long-Term Care

Residents in long-term care settings often have special needs regarding safety. ☑

In fact, OBRA requires the facility to maintain an environment that lowers the risk of accidents and incidents to the greatest extent possible. In addition, OBRA requires that all residents receive the supervision and assistance needed to prevent accidents and incidents from occurring. To fulfill those requirements, all facility staff must be alert for any potentially unsafe conditions that exist in the environment and for each resident.

Physical Changes of Aging

The majority of people who reside in a long-term care facility are older. The normal physical changes that occur with aging can affect a resident's ability to be safe. For example:

- **Neurologic changes.** It takes an older person longer to regain balance if they start to fall, or to change course to avoid running into another person or tripping over an object in their path.
- **Sensory changes.** Vision, hearing, taste, and smell decrease with age. These changes can make it more difficult for an older person to detect and respond to dangerous situations.
- **Musculoskeletal changes.** Loss of muscle tissue causes an older person to become weaker, which means the person becomes fatigued during physical activity more easily. When a person is fatigued, they are at increased risk for accidents, such as falling.

- **Urinary changes.** The amount of urine the bladder is able to hold before the person feels the urge to urinate decreases with age, leading to urinary frequency (the need to urinate more often). Rushing to the bathroom or failing to take necessary safety measures (such as waiting for help, using a walker, or turning on a light) can put the person at higher risk for falls.
- **Respiratory changes.** With age, lung capacity decreases. This can cause an older person to feel short of breath and weak during physical activity, putting the person at risk for falls.
- **Skin changes.** Older people are at very high risk for experiencing bruises and skin tears, often during routine care. In older people, the blood vessels become more fragile, which increases the tendency to bruise. In addition, an older person's skin is very thin, dry, and fragile. These changes can cause the skin to tear very easily (Fig. 14-2). Residents who are very dependent on the staff for care are at the highest risk for bruises and skin tears because they require the most "hands-on" care.

Effects of Medical Conditions or Treatments

Most of the residents in the long-term care setting will have chronic health conditions. The health condition, its treatment, or both can increase the resident's risk for accidents or incidents. For example, diabetes can decrease a person's sense of touch, putting the person at risk for burns and other injuries. Pain and stiffness from arthritis can affect a person's mobility, putting the person

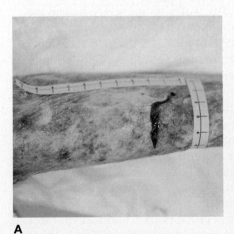
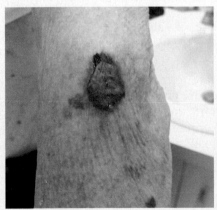
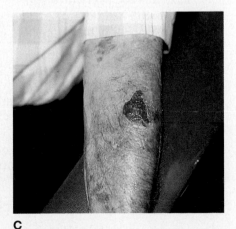

A   B   C

Figure 14-2 Because skin becomes thin and fragile with age, older residents are at high risk for experiencing skin tears during routine care. (Used with permission from Baranoski, S., & Ayello, E. A. [Eds.]. [2008]. *Wound care essentials: Practice and principles* [2nd ed., p. C2]. Lippincott Williams & Wilkins.)

at increased risk for falling. Neurologic disorders, such as stroke or Parkinson disease, can cause a person to shuffle their feet when they walk, increasing the person's risk for tripping and falling. An irregular heartbeat can cause a person to suddenly lose consciousness and fall. An accident involving incontinence (an inability to control one's bowel, bladder, or both) can cause the person to slip and fall in urine or feces on the floor.

Many of your residents will take one or more medications to treat their chronic health conditions. These medications can affect a person's ability to be safe. For example, a medication that affects blood pressure can cause a person to become dizzy if they stand up quickly, leading to a fall. Some medications cause confusion in older adults, especially if they are not taken properly.

Environmental Conditions

The risk for accidents and incidents is also increased simply by the nature of the long-term care environment itself. Consider the following points:

- Something as simple as a change in living environment (such as a move to a long-term care facility) can cause a new resident to become confused or disoriented, increasing the resident's risk for an accident or incident.
- In a long-term care facility, there are many residents living under the same roof, each with varying degrees of mental disability, physical disability, or both. Each resident needs a different level of supervision and assistance to remain safe.
- Long-term care facilities are very busy places. The hustle and bustle of people and equipment creates an environment where accidents and incidents are likely to occur.
- Environmental hazards (such as clutter, slippery surfaces, poor lighting, and sun glare) can also affect resident safety.

As you can see, there are many factors that can affect a person's safety in the health care setting. When several of these risk factors are combined, complex safety issues can result. As a nursing assistant, you must evaluate each patient or resident and situation individually so that you can provide a safe environment for those you care for.

Avoiding Accidents and Incidents

Many accidents and incidents that occur in health care facilities could have been prevented. Most safety measures do require an extra step or two, meaning more work for already overworked staff members.

However, remember your obligation to provide the same quality of care for your patients or residents that you would want for a member of your own family. Take that extra step to help ensure the safety of those you care for.

Preventing Falls

Falls are the leading cause of nonfatal and fatal injuries in the United States and of accidental death among older adults. One third of older adults living in the community and more than one half of those who reside in a long-term care facility fall every year. Falls are the most common cause of functional decline, hospital admission, emotional trauma, and eventual placement in some type of nursing facility for older people. Falls are also the most common type of accident that occurs in the health care setting. In Chapter 13, you learned how to assist a person who is falling. However, preventing a fall is always the best policy.

The Joint Commission requires hospitals to evaluate each new patient or resident for risk factors that increase the person's risk for falls (Fig. 14-3). Because most falls, especially those in a long-term care facility, are preventable, the Centers for Medicare and Medicaid Services (CMS) identifies falls as "never events" as they should never occur. Measures that can be taken to prevent falls are then included in the person's nursing care plan. Guidelines for preventing falls are given in Guidelines Box 14-1.

Preventing Burns

As you learned earlier, people who have a reduced sense of touch (reduced sensation) may be at risk for burns. A burn can be life threatening to a patient or resident. Measures for preventing burns include the following:

- If a person will be taking a tub bath or shower, always check the water temperature first using a bath thermometer. The water temperature should be 105°F (40.5°C). If the person is older, the water temperature should be slightly lower. Many long-term care facilities have whirlpool tubs that allow you to set the water temperature before filling the tub.
- If you will be giving a person a bed bath, you should measure the temperature of the water in the basin. The water in the basin can be warmer than the water in a bathtub or shower because it cools off quickly and the person will not be immersed in it. The temperature range for a bed bath is between 110°F (43.3°C) and 115°F (46°C).
- Teach patients or residents who will be bathing themselves to check the water temperature with a thermometer or a hand or wrist before getting into the bathtub or shower.

FALL RISK ASSESSMENT FORM

Resident Name:			Rm:
Check off reason for assessment			
Initial Assessment		Re-Assessment after fall	
Re-Assessment (periodic)		Change in Status	

Categories	Circle reference number(s) in each category	Description	Total reference numbers by category
Recent Fall History	0	NO FALLS in past 3 months	
	2	1–2 FALLS in past 3 months	
	4	3 OR MORE FALLS in past 3 months	
Ambulation/Continence	0	AMBULATORY/CONTINENT	
	2	CHAIR BOUND - Requires assist with elimination)	
	4	AMBULATORY/INCONTINENT	
Mental Status	0	ALERT (oriented X 3) OR COMATOSE (no voluntary or involuntary movement)	
	2	DISORIENTED X 3 at all times	
	4	INTERMITTENT CONFUSION/forgets limitations	
Vision	0	ADEQUATE (with or without glasses)	
	2	POOR (with or without glasses)	
	4	LEGALLY BLIND	
Balance	To assess, have resident stand on both feet without holding onto anything; walk straight forward; walk through a doorway; and make a turn.		
	0	Gait/Balance normal	
	1	Balance problem while standing	
	1	Balance problem while walking	
	1	Decreased muscular coordination	
	1	Change in gait pattern when walking through doorway	
	1	Unstable when making turns	
	1	Requires use of assistive devices (that is, cane, w/c, walker, furniture)	
	1	Inappropriate use of assistive device/footwear	
Blood Pressure (Systolic)	0	NO NOTED DROP between lying and standing	
	2	Drop LESS THAN 20 mm Hg between lying and standing in 3 minutes	
	4	Drop MORE THAN 20 mm Hg between lying and standing in 3 minutes	
Medications	Diuretics (somnolence, volume depletion, electrolyte disturbance, urgency to rush to bathroom), Psychoactives: Benzodiazepines (that is, Ativan, Halcion), Narcotics, Anticonvulsant stabilizers, Cardiovascular medications, Corticosteroids (can adversely effect muscle function), or any medication that adversely affects muscle function, coordination, and physical stability.		
	0	NONE of these medications taken currently for within last 7 days	
	2	TAKES 1–2 of these medications currently and/or within last 7 days	
	4	TAKES 3–4 of these medications currently and/or within last 7 days	
	1	If resident has had a change in medication and/or change in dosage in the past 5 days = score 1 additional point	
Predisposing Conditions or Diseases	Gastrointestinal: Bleeding, Diarrhea, Defecation Syncope, Postprandial Syncope, Genitourinary: Micturition syncope, Incontinence, Nocturia (80% of the elderly experience nocturia and going to the bathroom at night is a major risk factor), Cardiovascular: Myocardial Infarction, Arrhythmia, Orthostatic Hypotension, Musculoskeletal disorders: Arthritis, Inflammatory Joint Disease, Osteoarthritis Proximal Myopathy, Deconditioning, Neurologic: Parkinsonian, Dementia, Stroke, Transient Ischemic Attack, Delirium, Myelopathy, Vertebrobasilar Insufficiency, Carotid Sinus Supersensitivity, Cerebellar Disorder, Peripheral Neuropathy, Diabetes, B12 Deficiency, Multiple Myeloma, Vasculitis, Chronic dehydration		
	0	NONE PRESENT	
	2	1–2 PRESENT	
	4	3 OR MORE PRESENT	
A TOTAL SCORE OF 10 OR MORE INDICATES A RESIDENT "AT RISK" FOR FALLS.		TOTAL SCORE --->	

Figure 14-3 Many health care facilities use a form like this one to assess a new patient's or resident's risk of falling. Once the risk factors are known, precautions can be taken to decrease the person's risk of falling.

Guidelines Box 14-1 Guidelines for Preventing Falls

WHAT YOU DO	WHY YOU DO IT
Check the person's clothing and shoes. Clothing should fit properly. Shoes should provide good foot support and have nonskid soles.	Long or loose clothing (such as a robe) or shoes that provide inadequate foot support or have slippery soles could lead to tripping.
Encourage the person to use rails along hallways and stairways while walking.	The additional support offered by rails may be all that is needed to allow a person to move about safely and independently.
Observe the person for signs of unsteadiness and offer physical assistance as needed.	Offering assistance as needed allows the person to remain as independent as possible while minimizing the risk of falls.
Encourage and assist the person to ambulate and exercise according to their care plan and abilities.	Gait and balance training, along with exercise and restorative care can help reduce falls in the older person by improving strength and mobility.
Observe the person's ability to use walking aids, such as canes and walkers, and correct incorrect use.	Using a piece of equipment improperly can be just as hazardous as not using it at all.
Check equipment, such as walkers and wheelchairs, to ensure that it is in good condition. Nonskid tips should be intact on walkers. Wheelchair wheel locks should function properly.	Malfunctioning or broken equipment increases a person's risk for accidents.
Make sure a patient or resident who needs glasses is wearing them when they are out of bed.	A person who cannot see clearly is more at risk for falls.
Remove any clutter or obstacles from walkways and provide adequate lighting.	Proper lighting enhances the ability to see. Removal of obstructions is an easy way to minimize falls.
Create clear pathways in the person's room leading to the door and the bathroom. Keep heavy or large pieces of furniture away from the bed side and walkways.	Keeping walkways clear of obstacles reduces the risk of falling. It also prevents a person from hitting their head against a piece of large furniture in the event of a fall.
Keep beds in the lowest position. Keep bed wheels locked. Use beds that lower closer to the floor for older people who are at an increased risk of falling out of bed.	Keeping the bed in the lowest position minimizes the distance from the bed to the floor, should the person fall out of bed. Keeping the wheels on the bed locked prevents the bed from rolling. A rolling bed could result in injury to the nursing assistant, the patient or resident, or both.
Keep side rails up or down, according to the care plan for that particular person.	Side rails can prevent a person from falling out of bed. Because side rails are considered a form of restraint, they should always be lowered, unless the person's medical condition is such that they need the protection that is offered by having the side rails raised. Some patients or residents will benefit from having the side rails raised on one side of the bed so that they can be used to assist with repositioning or getting out of bed.
Use cushioned floor mats beside the bed for people who are likely to fall out of bed.	Floor mats can help prevent or lessen an injury caused by falling out of a low bed. However, they should be used with caution because they can actually cause a person to fall when they stand up.
Always make sure the call light control is within easy reach of the person. Answer call lights promptly, and offer to help the person with toileting frequently.	Many falls are the result of a person trying to make it to the bathroom without assistance.

Guidelines Box 14-1 Guidelines for Preventing Falls (*continued*)

WHAT YOU DO	WHY YOU DO IT
Wipe up any spills immediately.	Wet surfaces may not be obvious (especially to people with some degree of visual impairment) and greatly increase the risk of slipping.
Keep people who are at risk for falling and disoriented close to the nursing station. Offer frequent assistance with walking.	Keeping a person who is disoriented and at risk for falling close to the nursing station allows staff to "keep an eye" on the person and also minimizes the chance that a person who feels lonely will try to get up to look for company. A person who is offered help with walking on a regular basis is less likely to try to get up on their own, thereby minimizing the chance of a fall.
Orient a newly admitted patient or resident to the unit and their room.	Falls and other accidents often occur when a person is unfamiliar with their surroundings.

- Use extreme care with heat applications (discussed in detail in Chapter 21).
- Warn people that a food or beverage is hot before giving it to them. Many burns occur when hot liquids (such as soup, coffee, or tea) spill. Some people may need a cup with a lid for their coffee or tea if weakness or unsteadiness puts them at risk for spilling.
- Follow the guidelines for using electrical appliances that are given in Chapter 13. Electrical burns can occur if an appliance malfunctions or is used near water.

Entrapment

Beds in health care settings usually have side rails, which can be raised to help prevent the person from falling out of bed. Some patients or residents may also use a raised side rail as an assistive device for repositioning themselves in bed or for getting up. Although the use of side rails is often ordered to help protect a patient or a resident or to promote independence, the use of side rails can also put the person at risk for **entrapment**. Entrapment occurs when a person becomes trapped in the side rail or between the side rail and the mattress (Fig. 14-4). Severe injury, or even death, can occur, especially if the person's head, neck, or chest becomes trapped.

Any time the side rails are in use, there is a risk for entrapment. Patients and residents who are confused (for example, as a result of medications or dementia) and those with physical disabilities (such as a lack of muscle control) are at the highest risk for entrapment. A person who is small or who has uncontrolled body movement also has an increased risk of entrapment. Mattresses that do not fit the bed frame properly increase the risk of entrapment because it results in extra space left in between the mattress and the side rail.

To help lower a person's risk for entrapment, always use the side rails as ordered in the person's care plan. If the use of side rails has been ordered, check on the person frequently, especially if they have risk factors for entrapment. Devices that are designed to reduce the risk for entrapment by covering open spaces between the side rails or between the side rail and the mattress are available. If the patient's or resident's care plan specifies that these devices should be used, make sure the devices are properly in place.

Preventing Accidental Poisonings

Many people think of accidental poisonings as a problem that affects only children, but older people are at risk for accidental poisonings too. Poor eyesight, confusion, or a decreased sense of taste or smell can cause an older person to eat or drink something that causes harm. Accidental poisonings can also occur if a person takes too much, or the wrong, medication. An older person might not be able to read the medication label, or they might forget that they have already taken their medication that day and take it again. To minimize the risk of accidental poisonings:

- Never store household cleaners or other chemicals in containers meant for food or beverages.
- Keep household cleaners and chemicals in a locked cabinet.
- Make sure the contents of all containers are clearly marked on the outside.
- Provide help with reading labels as necessary.

Reporting Accidents and Incidents

Accidents and incidents will happen despite the precautions taken by even the most conscientious of health

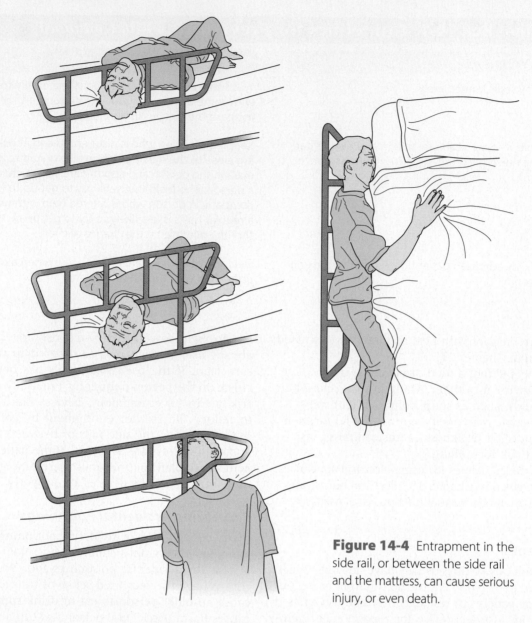

Figure 14-4 Entrapment in the side rail, or between the side rail and the mattress, can cause serious injury, or even death.

care workers. Some accidents and incidents occur as a result of faulty equipment or from unfamiliarity with new equipment. Other accidents and incidents are the result of carelessness on the part of a health care worker or family member of the patient or resident involved. When accidents or incidents do occur, you must know exactly how to report the accident or incident at your particular facility or organization.

All accidents and incidents are to be verbally reported immediately to the nurse. In addition, most facilities require the accident or incident to be reported in written or electronic form as well. This report is called an **incident (occurrence) report**. Some facilities are now calling these a *safety event report*. It generally takes the form of a preprinted or electronic document that must be completed. Information about the accident or incident should be provided in a straightforward and factual manner, without opinion or blame.

The completed incident (occurrence) report is used by the quality assurance department and is very important for follow-up. For example, consider a situation where an accident has occurred because a wheelchair's brakes did not hold properly. Following the completion of the proper forms by the nursing assistant, the quality assurance department might find that several similar accidents have occurred with wheelchairs of the same type, or after repairs from the same shop, or on the same shift of work scheduling. This would show a trend that could help prevent accidents like this from happening in the future.

Some health care workers hesitate to report an accident or incident because they feel responsible for the accident or are afraid they will be blamed for the accident. Other times, they know that a coworker will be blamed for carelessness and do not want to report the coworker's error to a supervisor. As described in

Chapter 3, the nursing assistant must be honest and dependable in carrying out their duties. Reporting accidents and incidents promptly helps to protect your patients, your facility, and yourself.

RESTRAINTS

Restraints, referred to as "reminder devices" in some facilities, are sometimes necessary to help keep a person safe. For example, a restraint might be used for an agitated, disoriented patient who continually tries to remove an intravenous (IV) line from their arm. A device is not considered a restraint if a person has the physical and mental ability to release the fastener. For example, a safety strap that is fastened across a person's lap in a wheelchair that they can unfasten if they wish is not considered a restraint.

Restraints can be either physical or chemical. A **physical restraint** is a device that is attached to or near a person's body to limit a person's freedom of movement or access to their body (Fig. 14-5). Physical

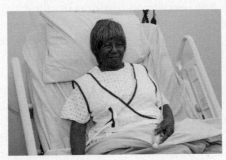

A. Vest restraint

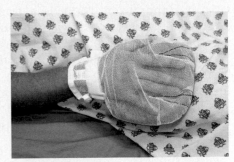

D. Mitt restraint

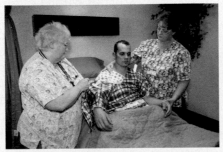

B. Jacket restraint

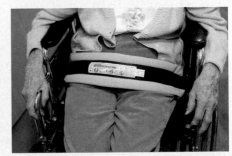

E. Lap restraint

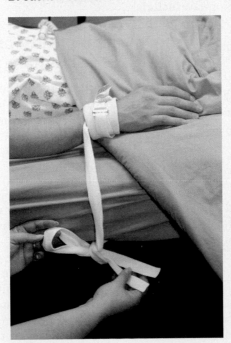

C. Wrist restraint

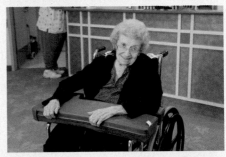

F. Lap buddy

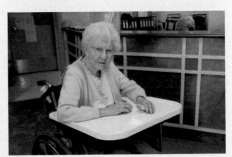

G. Chair with a tray table

Figure 14-5 Physical restraints are attached on or near a person's body. They limit freedom of movement. Some examples of physical restraints are shown here. **A.** A vest restraint. **B.** A jacket restraint. **C.** A wrist restraint. **D.** A mitt restraint. **E.** A lap restraint. **F.** A lap buddy and (**G**) a chair with a tray table are considered restraints if the person cannot remove the lap buddy or tray table independently.

restraints confine a person to a bed or a chair or prevent movement of a specific body part and cannot be easily removed by the restrained person. Physical restraints can be applied to parts of the body, such as the wrists, ankles, chest, waist, or elbows. In addition, some types of chairs or attachments to chairs can act as restraints. So can the side rails of beds or tightly tucked sheets. Not permitting a person free access to other rooms or parts of the facility is also considered a form of physical restraint.

A **chemical restraint** is any medication that alters a person's mood or behavior, such as a sedative or tranquilizer. There is a fine line between using medications to help calm an anxious, combative (physically aggressive), or agitated (very upset) person and using medications for staff convenience. These medications should assist in the control of anxiety, combative behavior, or agitation. They should not be used in so high a dose as to make the person sleepy or unable to function in a normal fashion.

Use of Restraints

Restraints are never used as punishment or for the staff's convenience. They are used to provide postural support, to protect the patient or resident from harm, and/or to protect the staff from harm (in the case of a combative or violent patient). Restraints are to be used only if all other methods have failed (see "Restraint Alternatives" on p. 216) and the person is considered to be a danger to themselves or others if restraints are not applied. Examples of situations where the use of restraints may be appropriate include but are not limited to:

- A person who does not have the ability to walk but repeatedly tries to get out of the bed or chair without calling for assistance
- A person who cannot control body movements or maintain proper posture due to a medical condition (for example, a nervous system disorder)
- A person who attempts to remove or pull out tubing necessary for medical treatment (this is particularly common among small children, confused patients or residents, and patients or residents who are intubated and uncomfortable)
- A person who is demonstrating combative behavior that poses a serious threat to the welfare and safety of themselves, other patients or residents, or staff
- A person who has overdosed on alcohol or medications and is demonstrating combative behavior (due to withdrawal symptoms) or is on suicide precautions

The use of restraints is clearly defined in guidelines issued by the Omnibus Budget Reconciliation Act (OBRA), the Joint Commission on Accreditation of Healthcare Organizations (JCAHO), and the Food and Drug Administration (FDA). The *Resident Rights* portion of OBRA addresses a person's right to be free from physical and chemical restraints. According to OBRA, the improper use of restraints can be considered holding a person against their will, or false imprisonment. Current standards of care set forth by JCAHO and the Centers for Medicare and Medicaid Services (CMS) require that health care facilities minimize their use of restraints. Today, many health care facilities, especially long-term care facilities, are almost restraint-free.

Before deciding that restraint use is appropriate, especially in the long-term care setting, the health care team must perform a thorough assessment. As part of this assessment, there must be evidence that less restrictive measures have been tried and proven unsuccessful in meeting the person's needs. In addition, the health care team must carefully consider the risks and benefits of restraint use, and agree that in this particular situation, the benefits of restraint use outweigh the risks.

Each health care facility has policies and procedures detailing the use of restraints for patients and residents. As a nursing assistant, you must understand these for your facility. Failure to follow these policies can result in a situation that is dangerous for your patient or resident. In addition, failure to follow these policies can leave you and your facility open for litigation. Guidelines for the use of restraints are given in Guidelines Box 14-2.

Complications Associated With Restraint Use

Many complications can result from the use of restraints. Restraints are dangerous even when used properly but doubly so if they are not. A person who is restrained is eight times more likely to die than a person who is not restrained. Consider the following:

- Strangulation (cutting off the person's air supply) can occur if a vest restraint is improperly applied or if the restraint gets tangled in a piece of furniture.
- Bruises, nerve damage, and skin abrasions can result if a restrained person pulls at the restraint or if the restraint is applied too tightly.
- Permanent tissue damage as a result of impaired blood flow can occur if a restraint is placed incorrectly or too tightly. All of the tissues of the body require oxygen to live, and oxygen is

Guidelines Box 14-2 Guidelines for Using Restraints

WHAT YOU DO	WHY YOU DO IT
Do not use a restraint without a written doctor's order that states the reason for the restraint.	OBRA and state laws protect patients and residents from being unnecessarily restrained.
Never use a restraint to "punish" a patient or resident, or for your own convenience.	Physically and emotionally, the use of restraints has a very negative impact on the person's quality of life. Therefore, restraints are only used when absolutely necessary, after all other methods of ensuring the person's safety have failed.
Use the least restrictive restraint for the least amount of time.	Minimizing the use of restraints is important to preserve the person's quality of life.
Follow the manufacturer's instructions, nurse's direction, and facility policy for applying restraints.	Improper application of restraints can lead to serious medical complications, injury, or even death.
Use a restraint that is the correct size and In good condition.	If the restraint is too large, the person may be able to remove it, either completely or partially. This puts the person at risk for falling and strangulation. If the restraint is too small, complications such as restriction of blood supply to areas beyond the restraint can result. If the restraint is in poor condition, it may not properly restrain the person, or the person may be injured when the restraint is applied.
Use commercial restraints. Do not use makeshift restraints, such as bed sheets or locks.	Using anything other than a commercial restraint to restrain a person is unprofessional and dangerous.
Restraints are always applied over clothing, pajamas, or a gown.	Clothing offers a layer of protection between the restraint and the person's skin.
Restraints are tied in simple, quick-release knots placed out of reach of the patient's or resident's hands. Some restraints are manufactured with quick-release buckles or airline-type buckles instead of ties.	Quick-release knots or buckles must be used in case a person needs to be released from the restraint quickly due to an emergency (for example, choking).
Ensure that you have enough help when applying a restraint.	Attempting to apply a restraint to an uncooperative, combative person can lead to injury of the person, you, or both.
Check on the restrained person every 15 minutes to make sure that feeling and blood flow are normal in any restrained extremity (arm or leg).	A restraint that is applied too tightly can lead to poor blood flow, which "in turn" can lead to permanent tissue or nerve damage. In addition, checking on the person regularly helps to prevent them from feeling abandoned.
Make sure wheelchair wheels are locked and the front swivel wheels are facing forward when a person is restrained in a wheelchair.	Locked wheels and forward-facing front wheels help make the wheelchair more stable and less likely to tip over.
Side rails should always be raised when a person is restrained in bed.	Raising the side rails decreases the chances that a restrained person could slide out of bed and become tangled in the restraint.

(continued)

Guidelines Box 14-2   Guidelines for Using Restraints (*continued*)

WHAT YOU DO	WHY YOU DO IT
Completely remove the restraint every 2 hours, for a total of 10 minutes. Provide range-of-motion exercises and reposition the person.	Releasing the restraint allows you to reposition the person and perform exercises to prevent loss of mobility and skin breakdown. All patients and residents should be repositioned at least every 2 hours, whether they are restrained or not.
Attend to the person's needs for nutrition, hydration, toileting, and general comfort.	A restrained patient or resident is unable to get a drink of water or go to the bathroom if they need to.
Record any care given to a restrained person promptly and according to your facility's policy.	In a litigation situation, any action not recorded is considered not done. You can provide the best care possible, but if you do not record it, your effort will not protect you or your facility if legal action is taken.
Make sure that the call light control is within the restrained person's reach and respond to the call light promptly.	The ability to call for help if needed and knowing that someone will respond quickly help to make the restrained person feel safe.
Use restraints only if you have been properly trained in their use.	**Incorrect use of restraints can result in death!**

carried to the tissues in the blood. If something stops blood from flowing to a certain part of the body, the affected tissues can be permanently damaged from lack of oxygen. In some cases, amputation (removal of a limb) may even be necessary.

- Broken bones and other serious injuries can occur if a restrained person tries to get out of the restraints. For example, a person restrained in a chair may still try to get up, which could result in injury if the chair overturns. Similarly, a person who is improperly restrained in a bed could slide between the bed and the side rails, or attempt to climb over the side rails, actions that could lead to injury or death if the restraint gets caught in the side rails.
- Physical restraints do not prevent falls. They do increase the possibility of serious injury if a person who is restrained does fall.
- Pneumonia, pressure ulcers, and blood clots (complications of immobility) can occur if a person is left in a restraint for too long.
- Incontinence can occur if a person is not taken to the bathroom regularly.
- Loss of independence can occur when decreased mobility from restraint use leads to a decrease in bone and muscle strength, affecting the person's ability to stand, transfer, and walk.
- The mental effects associated with the use of restraints can be serious and include agitation,

increased confusion, humiliation, embarrassment, and depression.

Helping Hands and a Caring Heart

Focus on Humanistic Health Care

Physically and emotionally, restraints have a very negative impact on a person's quality of life. Imagine how you would feel if you had to be "tied down." You might feel embarrassed, frightened, or humiliated. As a nursing assistant, there are many things you can do that may eliminate or reduce the need for restraints. These things require planning and effort, but the effort is considered part of the quality, individualized care that should be given to each person.

Restraint Alternatives

Although the use of physical or chemical restraints is not forbidden by any regulating agency, measures must be taken to avoid their use. In other words, **restraint alternatives** must be sought and used. The measures taken to avoid the use of restraints on a person must be documented before resorting to the use of restraints to protect that person's safety.

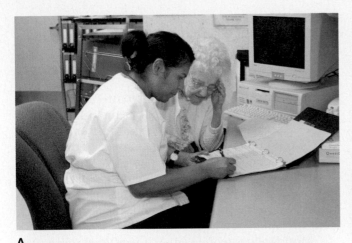

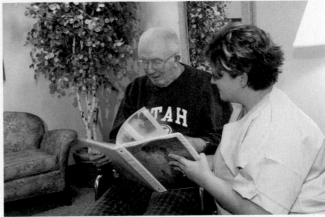

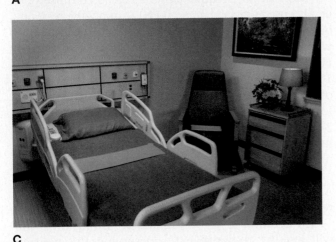

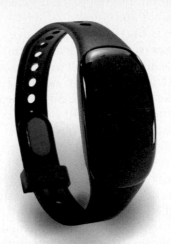

Figure 14-6 Alternatives to physical and chemical restraints should always be tried first. **A.** Moving the person to a place, such as the nurses' station, can help ease feelings of loneliness. Sometimes all people want is company or to be where the action is. **B.** Volunteers, other residents, or family members can be called on to provide company to a person too. **C.** A pressure-sensitive bed monitoring system is shown here. The pressure-sensing mat is secured across the mattress (under the sheet), located where the person's buttocks will be. The monitor, shown here next to the mat, is then usually hung from the headboard, out of the person's reach and sight. If the person tries to get out of bed, an alarm may sound, alerting the staff that the person needs help. Systems like this are helpful for patients or residents who are likely to fall if they try to get up unassisted. Similar systems are available for chair or wheelchair seats as well. **D.** A wanderer monitoring system is a sensor that is attached to the person's wheelchair or worn around the wrist. If the person tries to leave the facility through a doorway or hallway that leads to an unsafe area, it is designed to sound an alarm, alerting the staff so that someone can guide the person back to safety. Systems like this are useful for patients or residents who are likely to stray away from the facility, such as those with dementia. (*C and D, Courtesy of Securitas Healthcare, Lincoln, NE.*)

Some alternatives to using chemical or physical restraints are shown in Figure 14-6. For example, a nursing assistant can:

■ Provide an environment in which the person feels safe and secure. Placing a confused person close to the nurses' station, where they can be observed and the person can, in turn, watch others and not feel left alone, is often helpful. Taking time to speak to the person often or sitting beside them while you complete paperwork offers the person company and companionship. Soft music, television, or other methods of entertainment can be calming.

■ Provide frequent attention to the person's physical needs. Take the person to the bathroom and offer a drink or snack regularly, per facility policy or more frequently if necessary. Assist the person with walking or change their position frequently, to help maintain comfort. Answer call lights promptly and make sure that the call light control is within easy reach of the person.

■ Explain procedures and reassure the person. Being in a situation or having a condition that requires the use of restraints can be confusing and embarrassing.

■ Get help from family members, volunteers, or other residents of the facility. Providing companionship can be an effective alternative to the use of restraints. In addition, this approach improves the quality of a person's life.

■ Use restraint methods that are less restrictive. For example, pressure-sensitive alarm systems are placed on a person's wheelchair seat or bed. If the person tries to get up without help, the alarm will sound, alerting the staff. Sometimes the alarm will remind the person to call for help when they need to get up. Another type of alarm system, called a wanderer monitoring system, involves a small sensor that is worn around the wrist or ankle, or placed on the person's wheelchair. If the person tries to leave the facility, an alarm will sound, alerting the staff so that the person can be gently and safely led back inside. These sensors work the same way as anti-shoplifting devices in shopping malls work. *However, remember that motion and pressure detection devices are effective as restraint alternatives only if caregivers respond to the alarms in a timely manner.*

■ Using postural supports, such as lateral supports, nonskid material on seat cushions, and wedge cushions in wheelchairs can eliminate the need for a restraint device.

■ Use bed control bolsters instead of side rails to help prevent falls out of the bed.

Applying Restraints

In some situations, restraint alternatives will not be enough to keep the patient or resident safe, and it will be necessary to apply a physical restraint. Only a doctor can order a restraint for a patient or resident. If a doctor orders a restraint for one of your patients or residents, always follow your facility's policies regarding the application and use of restraints in order to protect yourself, your facility, and, most importantly, your patient or resident.

Most facilities require either a registered nurse (RN) or a licensed practical nurse (LPN) to apply the restraint, but as a nursing assistant, you will be responsible for providing care for the person while they are restrained. For example, you must check on the person every 15 minutes and help them with repositioning, range-of-motion exercises, and meeting nutritional and toileting needs. The restraint must be removed every 2 hours. Be sure to consider how frightening and humiliating it can be for a person to be restrained. Do not forget to provide the care necessary to meet the person's emotional, as well as their physical, needs. All care that you give to a restrained person must be recorded promptly.

In addition to providing and recording care, you will also be responsible for observing the person's response to the restraint and reporting any signs of trouble to the nurse immediately.

Any restraint that is tied should be tied with a "quick-release" knot (Fig. 14-7). A quick-release knot, or slip knot, will hold tightly if the restrained person pulls against it but can be undone quickly by pulling on its "tails." The use of a quick-release knot will allow you to free a person from a restraint quickly in the event of an emergency.

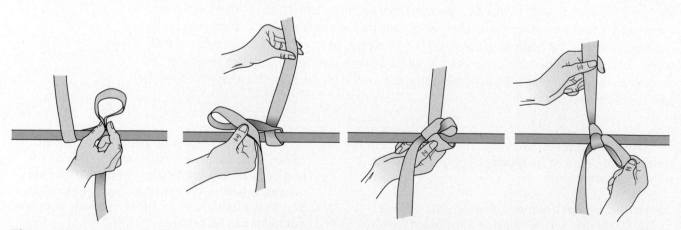

Figure 14-7 To make a quick-release knot, make a regular overhand knot, but slip a loop (instead of the end of the strap) through the first loop.

Tell the Nurse!

Each time you attend to a person who is wearing a restraint, you should be alert to signs and symptoms related to the use of the restraint. Tell the nurse immediately if:

● The restrained person complains of, or shows any signs of, shortness of breath or difficulty breathing

● The hand or foot beyond the restraint is pale, blue, or cold

● The restrained person complains of pain, numbness, or tingling at or below a restrained body part

● The skin beneath a restraint device is red, blistered, broken, or bruised

● The restrained person has become more confused, disoriented, or agitated

Applying a Vest Restraint

A vest restraint is applied to a person's chest to protect the person from falling out of bed or a chair. The person's arms are placed through the armholes of the vest, and the flaps of the vest are crossed over each other, across the person's chest. A vest restraint should never be put on backward (that is, with the back of the vest on the person's chest and the flaps crossed across their back). Putting the vest on backward can cause the person to strangle if they slide down against the improperly placed restraint because the back of the restraint is higher than the front. The procedure for applying a vest restraint is given in Procedure 14-1.

A jacket restraint is similar to a vest restraint, in that it is applied to the chest, but a jacket restraint has sleeves and closes in the back.

Applying Wrist or Ankle Restraints

In some cases, wrist or ankle restraints are applied to keep a person from moving their arms, legs, or both. When keeping a person in bed is the goal, the doctor may specify the number of extremities that are to be restrained. For example, a two-point restraint would involve two extremities (for example, both wrists), a three-point restraint would involve three extremities, and a four-point restraint would involve all four extremities.

Although wrist restraints are sometimes used to confine a person to bed, a more common use is to prevent a person from removing tubes and catheters. When preventing a person from removing a tube or catheter is the purpose of the wrist restraint, a mitt restraint may be used instead. This mitten-like variation of a wrist restraint restricts finger movement. A mitt restraint prevents the person from grasping tubes or catheters but allows for more freedom of arm movement.

The procedure for applying wrist or ankle restraints is given in Procedure 14-2.

Applying Lap or Waist (Belt) Restraints

Lap restraints are used to prevent a person from sliding out of a chair. Waist (belt) restraints can be used to secure a person in a chair or in a bed. The procedure for applying a lap or waist (belt) restraint is given in Procedure 14-3.

Be sure to study Procedures 14-1 through 14-3 closely. It is your duty as a nursing assistant to ensure the safety of your patients and residents, and proper restraint use is of the utmost importance.

SUMMARY

- Safety is a basic human need.
  - If we feel safe, we can relax and rest because we feel secure and comfortable.
  - Nursing assistants are responsible for helping to ensure the safety of those they care for.
- Many factors put a person at increased risk for an accident, including age, impaired mobility, use of certain medications, and sensory impairment.
  - Residents in long-term care settings are at increased risk for accidents and incidents as a result of age-related changes, medical conditions, and their treatments. When combined with environmental conditions, these factors increase the likelihood of accidents.
- Most accidents that occur in a health care facility are avoidable.
  - Providing for the safety of those we care for is never-ending.
  - A nursing assistant must be continuously aware, observing patients and residents and their environment for safety risks. Nursing assistants must also perform their duties in accordance with specified safety policies and procedures.
- If an accident or incident does occur, it should be reported immediately and an incident (occurrence) report should be completed promptly. Proper reporting and recording of accidents and incidents help to protect your patients and residents, your facility, and yourself.
- Restraints are sometimes necessary to ensure a person's safety. Because their use can be associated with complications (and possibly even death), restraints are used only when all other measures have failed.
  - Restraints are never used to punish a person, or for the convenience of the staff.
  - Physically and emotionally, restraints have a very negative impact on a person's quality of life. The use of restraints requires extra care from the nursing assistant to protect the patient's or resident's safety and dignity.

> **Procedure 14-1**

Applying a Vest Restraint

WHY YOU DO IT A vest restraint is applied to a person's chest to prevent the person from falling out of bed or a chair.

Getting Ready

1. Complete the "Getting Ready" steps.

Supplies

■ vest restraint in proper size

Procedure

2. Get help from a nurse or another nursing assistant, if necessary.

3. Assist the person to a sitting position by locking arms with them.

4. Support the person's back and shoulders with one arm while slipping the person's arms through the armholes of the vest using your other hand. Apply the restraint according to the manufacturer's instructions. The vest should cross in the front, across the person's chest.

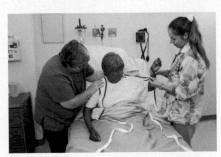

STEP 4 Support the person's back and shoulders while slipping their arms through the armholes of the vest.

5. Make sure there are no wrinkles across the front or back of the restraint.

6. Bring the ties through the slots.

7. Help the person to lie or sit down.

8. Make sure the person is comfortable and in good body alignment.

9. If the person is in a chair, thread the straps under the armrests and tie behind the chair (to keep the person seated) according to the manufacturer's directions. If the person is in bed, attach the straps to the bed frame out of the person's reach, never the side rails. Always use the quick-release knot approved by your facility.

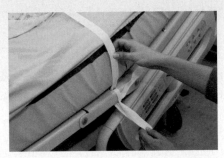

STEP 9 Attach the straps to the bed frame, never the side rails.

10. Make sure the restraint is not too tight. You should be able to slide a flat hand between the restraint and the person. Adjust the straps if necessary.

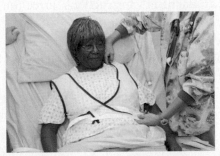

STEP 10 Check to make sure the restraint is not too tight.

11. a. Raise the side rails if the person is in bed.

b. Lock the wheels and make sure front wheels are facing forward if the person is in a wheelchair.

Finishing Up

12. Complete the "Finishing Up" steps.

(continued)

13. Check on the restrained person every 15 minutes.

14. Release the restraint every 2 hours and:

    a. Reposition the person.

    b. Meet the person's needs for food, fluids, and elimination.

    c. Give skin care and perform range-of-motion exercises.

15. Reapply the restraint.

What You Document

- Type of restraint used
- Time restraint was applied
- Person's response to restraint
- Position of patient or resident (when repositioned)
- Food or fluids taken by the person
- Elimination results
- Skin care given
- Range-of-motion exercises completed

 Procedure 14-2

Applying Wrist or Ankle Restraints

WHY YOU DO IT Wrist or ankle restraints are applied to limit movement of a person's arms, legs, or both.

Getting Ready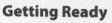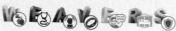

1. Complete the "Getting Ready" steps.

Supplies

- appropriate number of wrist restraints, ankle restraints, or both

Procedure

2. Get help from a nurse or another nursing assistant, if necessary.

3. Apply the wrist or ankle restraint following the manufacturer's instructions. Place the soft part of the restraint against the skin.

4. Secure the restraint so that it is snug, but not tight. You should be able to slide two fingers under the restraint.

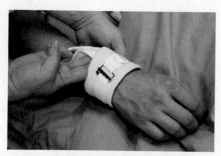

STEP 4 You should be able to slip two fingers between the person's wrist and the restraint.

5. Attach the straps to the bed frame. Always use the quick-release knot approved by your facility.

6. If applying more than one restraint, repeat steps 3 through 5.

7. Raise side rails if person is in bed.

Finishing Up

8. Complete the "Finishing Up" steps.

9. Check on the restrained person every 15 minutes.

10. Release the restraint every 2 hours and:

    a. Reposition the person.

    b. Meet the person's needs for food, fluids, and elimination.

    c. Give skin care and perform range-of-motion exercises.

11. Reapply the restraint.

What You Document

- Type of restraint used
- Time restraint was applied
- Person's response to restraint
- Condition of the person's skin underneath the restraint
- Position of patient or resident (when repositioned)
- Food or fluids taken by person
- Elimination results
- Skin care given
- Range-of-motion exercises completed

▶ Procedure 14-3

Applying Lap or Waist (Belt) Restraints   ▶

WHY YOU DO IT   Lap restraints are used to prevent a person from sliding out of a chair. Waist (belt) restraints can be used to secure a person in a chair or in a bed or to remind the person to not get up without assistance.

Getting Ready

1. Complete the "Getting Ready" steps.

Supplies

■ lap or waist restraint in proper size

Procedure

2. Get help from a nurse or another nursing assistant, if necessary.

3. If the person is in a chair, assist them to a proper sitting position, making sure that the person's hips are as far back against the back of the chair as possible. (If the person is in a wheelchair, make sure the brakes are locked first, the front wheels are facing straight forward, and position the footrests to support the person's feet.)

4. Wrap the restraint around the person's abdomen, crossing the straps behind the person's back.

5. Bring the ties through the loops at the sides of the restraint, according to the manufacturer's directions.

6. Make sure the person is comfortable and in good body alignment.

7. Thread the straps under the armrests and secure the straps out of the person's reach, at the back of the chair. If the person is in the bed, secure the straps to the bed frame, not the side rails, out of reach of the person. Always use the quick-release knot approved by your facility.

8. Secure the restraint, making sure it is not too tight. You should be able to slide a fist between the restraint and the person.

9. Raise side rails if person is in bed.

Finishing Up

10. Complete the "Finishing Up" steps.

11. Check on the restrained person every 15 minutes.

12. Release the restraint every 2 hours and:
    a. Reposition the person.
    b. Meet the person's needs for food, fluids, and elimination.
    c. Give skin care and perform range-of-motion exercises.

13. Reapply the restraint.

What You Document

■ Type of restraint used
■ Time restraint was applied
■ Person's response to restraint
■ Position of patient or resident (when repositioned)
■ Food or fluids taken by person
■ Elimination results
■ Skin care given
■ Range-of-motion exercises completed

WHAT DID YOU LEARN?

Multiple Choice

Select the single best answer for each of the following questions.

1. After applying a restraint to a patient or resident:
   a. Try to ignore the person's complaints; they just want attention
   b. Check the restraint every 6 hours
   c. Change the restraint once a day
   d. Remove the restraint at least every 2 hours

2. Vest restraints are applied so that the flaps:
   a. Cross in the back
   b. Cross in the front
   c. Are left open
   d. Are wrapped tightly around the person's chest

3. Which one of the following should not be done when applying a restraint to a patient or resident?
   a. Explain the procedure to the patient or resident
   b. Introduce yourself by name and title
   c. Make sure the patient or resident is asleep
   d. Make sure you have a written doctor's order for the restraint

4. A person with tetraplegia is paralyzed:
   a. From the waist down
   b. From the neck down
   c. On the left side
   d. On the right side

5. What is the leading cause of accidental death among older adults?
   a. Burns
   b. Falls
   c. Poisonings
   d. Drowning

6. Maria is helping a patient get out of bed when the patient becomes dizzy, loses their balance, and falls. How should Maria report this accident?
   a. Maria should tell the nurse about it
   b. Maria should fill out an incident (occurrence) report
   c. Maria should tell the nurse about it and fill out an incident (occurrence) report
   d. Maria should tell the doctor about it

7. Why is a restraint used?
   a. To make caregiving easier for the staff
   b. To punish residents or patients who refuse to follow the rules
   c. To protect a person from harming themselves or others, when all other methods of keeping the person safe have failed
   d. All of the above

8. You work in the pediatrics unit of a hospital. One of your small patients has a nasogastric feeding tube that is causing them discomfort, and they keep trying to pull it out. What should you do to prevent the child from removing the feeding tube?
   a. Apply a mitt restraint
   b. Report your observations to the nurse
   c. Explain to the child that they have to leave the tube alone
   d. Use a sensor alarm

9. What is entrapment?
   a. The patient or resident cannot leave the facility without the knowledge of the staff
   b. A type of restraint alternative
   c. The person becomes trapped in the side rail or between the side rail and the mattress
   d. A type of physical restraint

10. In which situation would a seat belt on a wheelchair not be considered a restraint?
   a. The seat belt can easily be removed by the staff
   b. The seat belt is fitted to the patient or resident snugly, but it is not too tight
   c. The patient or resident is not able to unfasten the seat belt
   d. The patient or resident is able to unfasten the seat belt when they want to

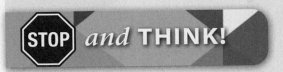

Mr. Lovell, one of the residents with dementia at the long-term care facility where you work, has become very agitated. He is prone to falling and should not get up without help. However, today he is refusing to stay in his bed or his wheelchair. You get him situated, and then as soon as you leave the room, he tries to get up again. This has happened twice, and you are only in the first hour of your shift. You are very concerned that Mr. Lovell will fall and hurt himself, but you cannot stay with him all day because you have other residents to attend to. Describe some things that you could do to help protect Mr. Lovell.

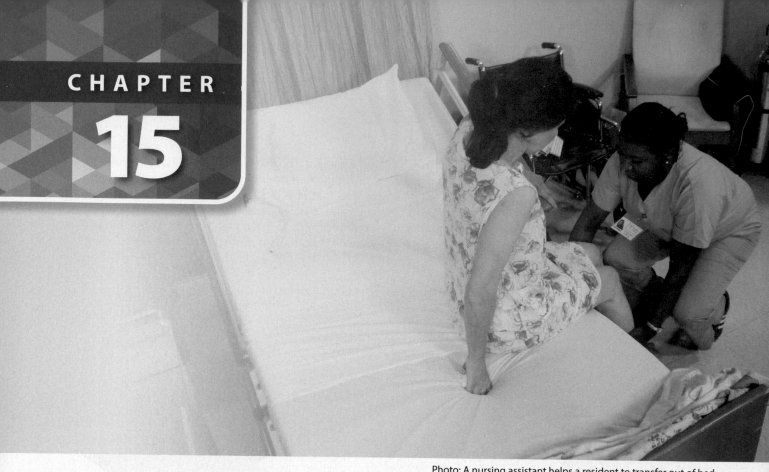

Photo: A nursing assistant helps a resident to transfer out of bed.

Positioning, Lifting, and Transferring Patients and Residents

 WHAT WILL YOU LEARN?

Have you ever been awakened from sleep because the position you were in was uncomfortable? If so, you probably rolled over, found a more comfortable position, and went back to sleep. Can you imagine what it would be like to be unable to change positions, especially if the position you were in was uncomfortable? Most of the people you will care for as a nursing assistant will be able to move with little or no help. But others will need help to reposition themselves or get out of their bed or chair.

Repositioning, lifting, and transferring people are a major part of the nursing assistant's daily routine. You will do this many times a day. By following the guidelines for body mechanics and back safety that you learned in Chapter 13, you can protect yourself from fatigue and injury. In this chapter, you will learn how to keep your patients or residents safe while assisting them with movement. When you are finished with this chapter, you will be able to:

1. List the complications of immobility.
2. Describe proper body alignment and explain its importance.
3. Identify the different body positions and explain the purpose of regular, frequent repositioning.

4. **Discuss safety measures related to lifting and transferring people.**

5. **Demonstrate safe lifting and transferring techniques.**

Vocabulary

Pressure ulcers
Contractures
Body alignment
Supportive devices
Supine (dorsal recumbent) position

Fowler's position
Semi-Fowler's (low-Fowler's) position
High-Fowler's position

Lateral position
Prone position
Sims' position
Shearing
Friction
Logrolling

Transfer
Weight bearing
Transfer belt (gait belt)
Ambulate

POSITIONING PATIENTS AND RESIDENTS

Changing position frequently helps us to stay comfortable while we are sitting or lying down. It also prevents complications that can result from spending long periods of time in the same position. Additionally, in a health care setting, a person may need to get into a certain position to have a procedure done, or to recover from one. Although many of your patients or residents will be able to reposition themselves, some will need your help. For these reasons, helping people who must stay in bed or a wheelchair to reposition themselves is an important responsibility of the nursing assistant.

There are many reasons why a person may not be able to shift positions without help. For example, the person could be recovering from surgery, wearing a body cast, or in traction. They may be totally or partially paralyzed, unconscious or in a coma, or very weak from a disease or illness. For these people, the inability to change positions regularly can lead to discomfort and, potentially, serious complications. For example, consider a person with limited mobility who has been positioned in a sitting position in bed. With time, this person will begin to slide down in the bed, leading to discomfort and an inability to breathe easily (Fig. 15-1).

In addition to discomfort, a person who cannot reposition themselves is at risk for developing complications (Fig. 15-2). Some of the most serious complications affect the skin, bones and muscles, lungs, and heart:

■ **Integumentary system (skin).** The most common complication of immobility is pressure ulcers. **Pressure ulcers**, also known as *decubitus ulcers* or *bed sores*, form when bony areas press against the mattress. The pressure slows down blood flow to the tissues that are pressed between the bone and the mattress. This results

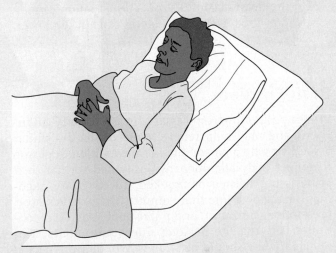 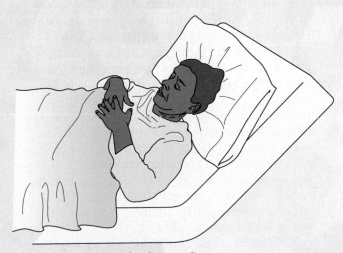

Figure 15-1 Gravity causes a person who is sitting in bed to slide down over time, leading to discomfort and interfering with the person's ability to breathe.

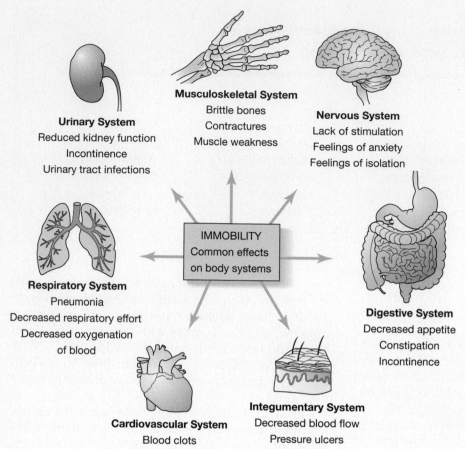

Urinary System
Reduced kidney function
Incontinence
Urinary tract infections

Musculoskeletal System
Brittle bones
Contractures
Muscle weakness

Nervous System
Lack of stimulation
Feelings of anxiety
Feelings of isolation

IMMOBILITY
Common effects
on body systems

Respiratory System
Pneumonia
Decreased respiratory effort
Decreased oxygenation
of blood

Digestive System
Decreased appetite
Constipation
Incontinence

Cardiovascular System
Blood clots
Reduced blood flow

Integumentary System
Decreased blood flow
Pressure ulcers

Figure 15-2 Immobility can cause complications in almost every body system.

in a wound , which can be very difficult to heal and might even be fatal. Pressure ulcers are discussed in detail in Chapter 29.

- **Musculoskeletal system (bones and muscles).** **Contractures**, discussed in detail in Chapter 30, occur when a joint is held in the same position for too long a time. Contractures cause stiffness and shortening of the tendons, leading to loss of motion of the joint that may be permanent. Long-term immobility can also cause loss of muscle mass and strength. Finally, immobility can cause the loss of calcium from the bones, making the bones brittle and more likely to break.
- **Respiratory system (lungs).** Lying in one position for a long period of time can prevent the lungs from completely filling with air when the person breathes. This causes the small air sacs in the lungs, called *alveoli*, to close. As a result, the person's ability to get oxygen into their bloodstream is decreased. In addition, decreased filling of the lungs with air allows fluids and mucus to collect in the lungs. This fluid and mucus creates an environment that is favorable for the types of bacteria that cause pneumonia.

- **Cardiovascular system (heart and blood vessels).** When we walk, the large muscles in our legs contract. Contraction of the leg muscles squeezes the veins, helping to move blood from the legs back up to the heart. People who must stay in bed are not using their leg muscles. Therefore, the blood flow from the legs back up to the heart becomes slow. This situation can lead to the formation of blood clots in the lower legs.

Basic Positions

Proper positioning is necessary for good **body alignment** and may help relieve some of the discomfort associated with a person's medical condition. A person in proper body alignment is positioned so that their spine is not twisted or crooked. To check for alignment, imagine a line that connects the person's nose, breastbone (sternum), and pubic bone, and then continues between the person's knees and ankles. This imaginary line should be straight whether the person is lying on their back, side, or abdomen (Fig. 15-3). If the person's legs are spread apart, each leg should

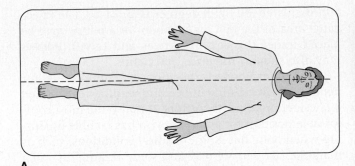

A

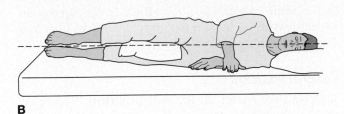

B

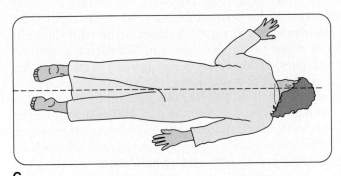

C

Figure 15-3 When a person is in proper body alignment, an imaginary straight line can be drawn connecting the person's nose, breastbone (sternum), and pubic bone. **A.** Proper body alignment for a person who is lying on their back in bed (supine). **B.** Proper body alignment for a person who is lying on their side in bed (lateral). **C.** Proper body alignment for a person who is lying on their abdomen in bed (prone).

be the same distance from the imaginary line. When helping to position one of your patients or residents, imagine yourself in that particular position and think of how your body is most comfortable.

Proper body alignment is most comfortable for the patient or resident. It relieves strain on muscles and joints, promotes good heart and lung function, and helps prevent contractures and pressure ulcers. Sometimes **supportive devices**, such as pillows; rolled sheets, towels, or blankets; and devices designed specifically for the purpose of offering support (Fig. 15-4), are needed to keep the person in proper body alignment. Learning to position these supports correctly is essential. Proper use of supportive devices helps to keep your patients or residents both safe and comfortable. Make sure you ask the nurse or physical therapist

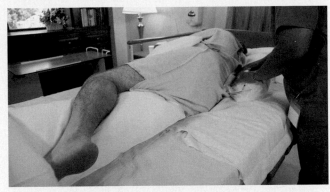

Figure 15-4 Some people require extra support to maintain proper body alignment. This support can be achieved by using pillows; a rolled-up towel, sheet, or blanket; or a supportive device made especially for this purpose.

about the proper use of any supportive devices for your patients or residents.

There are several basic positions that are used when a person must stay in bed or seated for long periods of time (Fig. 15-5). As you work as a nursing assistant, you may see variations on these positions for reasons specific for your patient or resident. A doctor may order restrictions on positions for a person after some surgeries or diagnostic procedures. Refer to the person's care plan or ask the nurse if there are any limitations or special positioning needs that the person may have.

Supine (Dorsal Recumbent) Position

When a person is in the **supine (dorsal recumbent) position**, they are lying on their back. The bed is flat and the person's head is supported by a pillow. Sometimes, pillows are placed to support the arms and hands as well. Some people may be more comfortable with a pillow under their knees and lower legs to take strain off the lower back. Others may ask for a small pillow under their lower back. In an older person, the supine position can lead to skin breakdown on the heels, which puts the person at risk for developing pressure ulcers. To prevent this complication, "float" the person's heels above the surface of the bed by placing a pillow underneath the person's calves (from the knees to the ankle). You should be able to slide your hand in the space between the mattress and the person's heels.

Fowler's Position

A variation of the supine position is **Fowler's position**, in which the head of the bed is elevated to between 45 and 60 degrees. In **semi-Fowler's (low-Fowler's) position**, the head of the bed is elevated approximately 30 to 45 degrees. In **high-Fowler's position**, the head of the bed is elevated

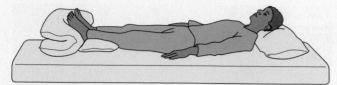

A Supine (dorsal recumbent) position

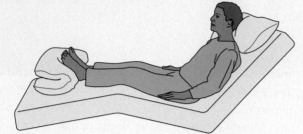

B Fowler's position

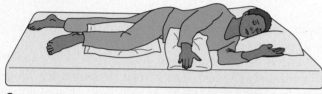

C Lateral position

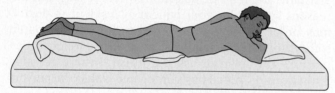

D Prone position

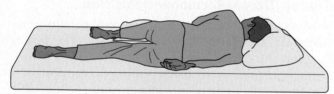

E Sims' position

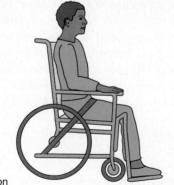

F Sitting position

Figure 15-5 There are several basic positions that are used when a person must remain in bed or seated for a long period of time. **A.** Supine position. **B.** Fowler's position. **C.** Lateral position. **D.** Prone position. **E.** Sims' position. **F.** Sitting position.

approximately 60 to 90 degrees (Fig. 15-6). The knee-gatch area of the bed may be bent or a pillow may be placed under the person's knees and calves. Pillows may also support the arms and hands.

The semi-Fowler's position is comfortable for people who are resting in bed and want to read, watch television, or talk with visitors. It is also the most comfortable position for a person who has trouble breathing when lying flat. Some medical conditions, such as hiatal hernia with reflux, and some treatments, such as tube feedings, require the person to be positioned in the semi-Fowler's position. High-Fowler's position is useful when a person is eating a meal in bed, and during grooming procedures.

Lateral Position

A person who is in the **lateral position** is lying on their side. When documenting the lateral position, the side of the person that is on the bed is used as the descriptor. For example, a person lying with their left side down on the mattress is in "left lateral position." The person's lower leg is straight and their upper leg is slightly bent at the knee, so that the knees are not pressed together. Pillows are placed under the person's head and neck, between the legs, and under the upper arm to keep the spine in alignment. A small pillow or rolled sheet may be placed close against the back to keep the person from rolling backward.

A variation of the lateral position may be used to keep pressure off the side of the hip. In the *semi–side-lying position*, pillows are placed either against the person's back and hip or along the front of their body. The pillows cause the person to lie either a little more forward or a little more toward the back. When the pillows are placed along the person's back and hip, they will lie a little more on their back, leaning toward the pillows. When the pillows are placed along the person's front, they will lie a little more on their abdomen.

The lateral position is often used for people with back pain, to relieve pressure on the spine, and for those in a body cast. Also, the lateral position is part of the cycle of positions for people who are unable to reposition themselves—the person is moved from the supine position to the lateral position, then back to the supine position, and then to the lateral position on the other side every 2 hours, routinely.

Prone Position

A person who is in the **prone position** is lying on their abdomen with their head turned to one side. A small pillow is placed under the person's head. Another small pillow is placed under the lower abdomen and pelvis to allow room for the chest to expand when the person breathes. (Alternatively, a rolled towel can be

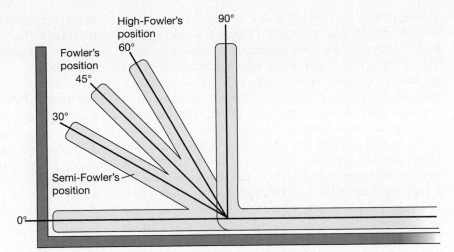

Figure 15-6 In Fowler's position, the head of the bed is elevated. Variations of Fowler's position include semi-Fowler's (low-Fowler's) position and high-Fowler's position.

placed under each of the person's shoulders to reduce pressure on the chest.) A pillow is also placed under the person's shins to keep the feet in proper position. The person's arms are bent at the elbows and their hands are placed on either side of the head, palms facing down. Many people, especially older people, are not comfortable in the prone position. Make sure you check with the nurse before placing a person in this position.

Sims' Position

Sims' position is an extreme side-lying position that is almost prone. The person's head is turned to one side and their knee on that side is bent sharply and supported by a pillow. The corresponding arm is bent at the elbow with the hand in front of the face, palm down, resting on a pillow. The lower leg is straight and the lower arm extends out from the side with the hand down near the hips and the palm turned upward. Sims' position is used for people who are receiving enemas, and to relieve pressure on areas that may be prone to developing pressure ulcers, such as the coccyx (the "tailbone") and the greater trochanter of the femur (the "hip bone").

Sitting Position

Positioning and body alignment are important for everyone, not just people who must stay in bed. Proper sitting position holds a person's body in correct alignment while they are sitting in a chair. The person's feet should rest flat on the floor or on the footrests of the wheelchair. Their knees are bent at approximately 90 degrees and the calves of their legs do not touch the chair. The person's buttocks and back rest against the back of the chair. Paralyzed or weak arms should be supported on pillows or in appropriate support devices. A person who cannot hold their body upright for long periods of time may need postural supports to assist in good body alignment.

Repositioning a Person

Some people will have conditions that require repositioning as frequently as every hour, but most people will require repositioning every 2 hours. Each time you reposition a person, you should be alert to signs and symptoms of complications related to immobility.

Tell the Nurse!

Possible signs and symptoms of complications related to immobility that should be reported to the nurse immediately include:

- Reddened skin, especially over bony areas, that does not return to its normal color after gentle massage of the surrounding tissue

- Pale, white, or shiny skin over a bony area

- Tears, scrapes, or skin that looks burned

- Hot, reddened, painful areas in the lower legs (do not rub these areas because doing this could dislodge a blood clot, which could then move to a vital organ such as the heart, lungs, or brain)

- New occurrence of urinary or bowel incontinence

- New complaints of pain on movement

- Any disconnected or heavily draining tubes or drains

To assist a person who is in bed into a new position, you will need to know how to lift and turn the person without causing injury to yourself or the person you are trying to move. People who are being moved in bed are particularly at risk for shearing and friction injuries if they are not moved properly. Perhaps you remember sliding across a vinyl car seat or down a metal sliding board while wearing shorts and feeling pain as you moved and your skin "stuck to" the vinyl or metal. That pain is similar to the pain caused by shearing and friction. **Shearing** is caused by pulling a person across a sheet or other surface that offers resistance. When a person is pulled against a surface that offers resistance, the skin is dragged in a direction opposite that of the underlying tissues and muscles, injuring the blood vessels and connective tissue under the skin and starting the process of skin breakdown. Shear actually separates the skin from the underlying tissues. **Friction** occurs when two surfaces, such as a sheet and the person's skin, rub against each other. The rubbing action can injure the skin and contribute to skin breakdown. The risk of shearing and friction can be minimized by rolling or lifting, instead of pulling or dragging, a person who needs to be moved. Guidelines for repositioning a person are given in Guidelines Box 15-1.

Moving a Person to the Side of the Bed

There are many reasons why you may need to reposition a person so that they are lying closer to one side of the bed or the other. For example, if you want to turn a person, you first want to move the person to the side of the bed so that when the turn is completed, they are in the middle of the bed (not on one side). You might also need to move a person to the side of the bed before performing a personal care procedure, so that the person is closer to you during the procedure. Depending on the situation, you may be able to move the person to the side of the bed by yourself (Procedure 15-1), or you may need help (Procedure 15-2). Generally speaking, you should get help from a coworker if the patient or resident is large, seriously ill or injured, or uncooperative.

Helping a Person to Move Up in Bed

As mentioned earlier, people who are sitting up in bed tend to slide down, toward the foot of the bed, over time. To keep a person who is sitting in bed comfortable and in proper body alignment, you must help them with moving up in the bed periodically. Many people will be able to move up in bed by themselves with the use of a trapeze bar or by grasping the side rails of the bed after the head of the bed has been lowered. However, if the person is unable to move up in the bed, you will need to assist them. In order to move a dependent person up in bed safely, you will need to have another person assist you. This is not a one-person task. Procedure 15-3 explains how to move a person up in bed.

Raising a Person's Head and Shoulders

Often, you will need to lift a person's head and shoulders away from the bed. For example, you may need to do this to help a person with drinking or to rearrange the pillow. Procedure 15-4 explains how to lift a person's head and shoulders away from the bed safely.

Turning a Person Onto Their Side

Helping a person to roll over in bed helps to keep the person comfortable. It also helps to prevent many of the complications associated with remaining in a single position for a long period of time. The person may be turned away from you (Procedure 15-5) or toward you, depending on the situation. Make sure that the side rail on the opposite side of the bed is raised whenever you are turning a person away from you.

Logrolling a Person

Logrolling is performed whenever it is necessary to move a person who has had back surgery or an injury to the neck or spine. In logrolling, the person is rolled in one fluid motion so that the head, torso, and legs move as one unit and the body (the "log") is kept in alignment, without twisting or bending. At least three assistants, plus a lift sheet, are necessary to logroll a person. Procedure 15-6 explains how to logroll a person safely.

Concerns for Long-Term Care

Many people who reside in a long-term care setting will only need minimal assistance with moving and repositioning in bed or a chair. Some residents only need to be reminded to change position at regular intervals. Even though it may be faster to reposition the resident yourself, make sure that you encourage the person to do as much as they are able to. For example, if the person is able to reach across and grasp the side rail of the bed with their hand while you help them roll onto their side, it helps to promote independence and prevent loss of function.

It is also important to remember that an older person's skin is fragile and can be easily torn or bruised during routine care. Always use a lift sheet when moving a resident up in bed or during repositioning to help prevent injuries from shearing and friction. Use a gentle touch and move the person slowly and smoothly. After repositioning, always check underneath the person to make sure that there are no wrinkles in their bedding or clothing. Lying for a while on wrinkled sheets or clothes can cause the skin to begin to break down, especially for an older person.

Guidelines Box 15-1 Guidelines for Repositioning a Person

WHAT YOU DO	WHY YOU DO IT
Plan how you will reposition the person and get help from others if necessary.	Depending on the person's medical condition or size, extra equipment or people may be necessary. Planning ahead helps to ensure that the procedure will be carried out efficiently, and with the most consideration for the person's safety and comfort.
Know the specific positioning guidelines for each person in your care. Refer to the person's care plan or ask the nurse as necessary.	Depending on the person's medical condition, some positions may be required and others may not be allowed. Failure to follow your patient's or resident's specific positioning guidelines can cause the person injury or discomfort.
Reposition the person at least every 2 hours, or according to the person's care plan.	Regular repositioning is necessary to prevent complications of immobility, such as pressure ulcers.
Explain the procedure to the person, even if they are unconscious.	Understanding how the procedure is done builds trust and helps the person feel like an active participant. Although an unconscious person will not be able to assist in the procedure, the person may still be aware that they are being moved. Telling the person what you are doing as you are doing it helps to reassure the person.
Make sure that you allow the person to assist in the repositioning to the full extent of their ability.	Being able to assist with one's own repositioning promotes feelings of independence and lessens the embarrassment some people may feel over having to rely on someone else for assistance.
Provide for the person's modesty by keeping their body covered.	Keeping the person's body covered preserves their dignity.
Take care to protect any tubes or drains from being pulled out while the person is being moved.	Dislodging tubes or drains is painful for the person. In addition, if tubes or drains become dislodged, it is necessary to reinsert them, which can cause additional discomfort.
Use good body mechanics when helping to reposition a person.	Using good body mechanics will protect you, as well as the patient or resident, from injury.
Use a gentle touch to avoid injury to delicate skin and fragile bones. Use a lift sheet to reposition the person whenever possible. (A lift sheet, also called a draw sheet or a "friction-reducing sheet," is a small sheet that is placed over the bottom sheet so that it extends from the person's shoulders to below their buttocks. Lift sheets are discussed in detail in Chapter 19.)	A lift sheet allows you to lift the person (instead of dragging them across the sheets). This helps to prevent shearing and friction injuries.
Avoid moving or lifting someone by holding onto their arm or leg.	You could dislocate the arm or leg, or stretch the joint beyond its range of motion.
After repositioning a person, make sure that the bed linens are free of wrinkles, and that the person's clothing is not twisted or wrinkled up underneath the person.	Lying on wrinkled bed linens or clothing can lead to skin breakdown. Skin breakdown increases the person's risk of getting a pressure ulcer.
Gently move the person's clothing aside to check the person's skin, especially on the part of the body the person was just lying on.	Reddened or pale skin can be a sign that a pressure ulcer is starting.

TRANSFERRING PATIENTS AND RESIDENTS

To **transfer** means to move from one place to another. As a nursing assistant, you will help people with transfers many times each day. For example, people transfer from the bed to a chair and back again, or from a wheelchair to a dining chair or toilet and back again. Many people are able to transfer from one place to another with little or no help, while others require a lot of help. The assistance you offer will vary from just providing a steadying hand to totally lifting a person from one place to another.

A person's ability to assist with their own transfers may be affected by the person's ability to bear weight. **Weight bearing** refers to a person's ability to stand on one or both legs. A limited ability to bear weight could be caused by surgery that affects the legs; injury to the hip, leg, or foot; pain; weakness; or paralysis. Some people with paraplegia have learned to transfer themselves by using their arms to support the weight of their body as they move from one surface to another.

A **transfer belt** is a webbed or woven belt with a buckle that is used to assist a weak or unsteady person with standing, walking, or transferring. (When used to help a person walk, a transfer belt is called a **gait belt**.) The belt is approximately 1.5 to 2 inches wide, and it is 54 to 60 inches long and may have hand grips attached to the outer surface. Most health care facilities require nursing assistants to use a transfer belt when helping people to stand, walk, or transfer. The transfer belt is applied around the person's waist (Procedure 15-7), giving the nursing assistant a place to grasp and support the person (other than by the person's arms or ribcage). When using a transfer belt, remember:

- Some patients or residents may have medical conditions that make it dangerous to use a transfer belt on them. For example, a transfer belt should not be applied to a person who is recovering from abdominal surgery. Transfer belts are also not used with people with certain heart disorders. If you are in doubt about using a transfer belt on a patient or resident, check the nursing care plan or ask the nurse for specific directions.
- A transfer belt is only an assist device and should never be used to "lift" a person who is unable to bear weight. A person who is unable to bear weight should be moved with a mechanical lift device.

Before beginning a transfer, advance planning is always necessary. Ask the nurse or physical therapist about any specific limitations the patient or resident has and what the recommended transfer method is. Many nursing care plans will also have this information. Gather any needed equipment (for example, a mechanical lift or wheelchair) and make sure the equipment is in good working condition. If necessary, move the furniture in the room to make space for a safe transfer. Finally, ask others for help as necessary.

Transfer-Assist Devices

The use of assist devices when transferring, lifting, and repositioning patients and residents is an effective way to help prevent work-related injuries for the health care worker. When used correctly, these devices not only help protect you from injury, they are safer for those you care for also. Many of these devices help patients and residents to move and reposition themselves with minimal assistance. This helps to promote their independence and, because they are more likely to continue to use their muscles and joints during the process, helps to prevent complications of immobility.

There are many different types of devices that will be used to assist with moving and transferring people in a health care setting. Some are as simple as a lift sheet placed on a person's bed. Although side rails on a person's bed can be considered a restraint if they keep a person from being able to get out of bed, leaving one side rail or the upper half of a side rail up can allow a person to grasp it to help themselves roll over or even steady themselves as they stand up from the bed or a bedside chair. It is important to carefully follow the person's care plan or ask the nurse what type of assist devices the patient or resident should use.

Other types of stand-assist devices attach to the side of the bed. The person can grasp it to steady themselves while they stand, either alone or with your assistance. Powered stand-assist devices can be used for a patient or resident who can bear weight on at least one leg and is cooperative. The device mechanically lifts the person to a standing position and then can be wheeled to a chair or the toilet where they are then lowered into a sitting position (Fig. 15-7).

Lateral transfer-assist devices, such as a sliding board (Fig. 15-8), allow a person who has good upper-body strength to slide across from a bed to a chair, or from a wheelchair to the toilet, often with minimal assistance. Other types of lateral transfer-assist devices can be used to move a dependent patient or resident from a bed to a stretcher. These devices, such as transfer boards or roller boards, are placed underneath a person's draw sheet and allow the health care worker to use the draw sheet to gently slide the person across onto the stretcher. Lateral-assist devices significantly reduce the friction between a person and the sheet during lateral transfers.

Mechanical lift devices are used to lift a person from one place to another when they are unable to bear weight, are weak or unsteady, or large in size. Different

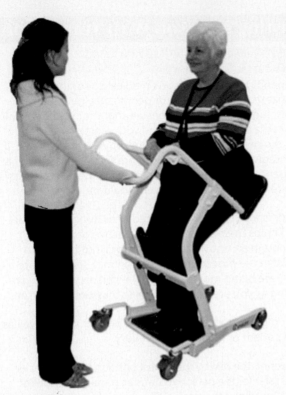

Figure 15-7 Stand-assist devices are used to assist people into a standing position.

Helping Hands and a Caring Heart

Focus on Humanistic Health Care

Remember that a person who needs your assistance during a transfer may feel weak and shaky. The person may be frightened, or embarrassed about having to rely on others to help them do something that always seemed so easy before. Always explain the transfer procedure to the person and make certain they understand how they are expected to help. Allow the person to assist as much as possible. Encouragement and reassurance from you, along with firm, steady assistance, will help your patient or resident gain confidence in their own abilities and learn to trust that you will be there to offer help as necessary. Promoting a person's independence is an important part of providing humanistic care.

types of mesh slings are available that can be used with a tub or shower chair to bathe a patient or resident. Toileting slings allow a person to be moved onto a bedside commode or toilet. Many health care settings provide each patient or resident with their own individual sling that is used only for that person. This helps to prevent the spread of infection. If slings are used for multiple people, covers are placed on them during use, and they must be cleaned properly between uses.

It is important that you learn safe transfer techniques to protect yourself and your patients or residents. Many long-term care and rehabilitation facilities are utilizing "lift teams" that function to lift and transfer residents whenever necessary. Accidents are common during the act of transferring, for both the nursing assistant and the person being transferred. Regardless of the particular type of transfer, the safety measures summarized in Guidelines Box 15-2 should always be followed. Specific procedures for various types of transfers are described in the sections that follow.

Transferring a Person to and From a Wheelchair or Chair

Wheelchair use, although a common practice, presents some specific safety issues. Wheelchairs, like any other piece of equipment, need to be checked before use to ensure safety. Check to make sure that there are no broken or missing parts, that the wheels turn smoothly, that any safety straps are secure, and that the brakes hold well. Trying to transfer a person into or out of a wheelchair with unlocked or poorly locked wheels is a common cause of accidents. You should always remember to position the front swivel wheels of a wheelchair facing to the front. This makes the wheelchair more stable and less likely to tip over during a transfer. Also,

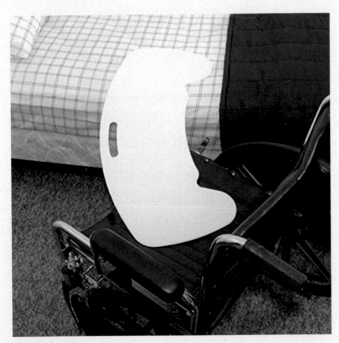

Figure 15-8 Sliding boards allow a person with good upper body strength to move from one surface to another with minimal assistance.

Guidelines Box 15-2   Guidelines for Assisting a Person With Transferring

WHAT YOU DO	WHY YOU DO IT
Plan how you will transfer the person and get help from others if necessary.	Depending on the person's medical condition, ability, or size, extra equipment or people may be necessary. Planning ahead helps to ensure that the procedure will be carried out efficiently, and with most consideration for the person's safety and comfort. As a general rule, if a caregiver is required to lift more than 35 pounds of a patient's or resident's weight, assistive devices and assistance from another caregiver should be used.
Explain the procedure to the person, even if they are unconscious.	Understanding how the procedure is done builds trust and helps the person feel like an active participant. Although an unconscious person will not be able to assist in the procedure, the person may still be aware that they are being moved. Telling the person what you are doing as you are doing it helps to reassure the person.
Use correct body mechanics. Keep your body close to the person and bend at the knees. Use a transfer belt.	Using good body mechanics will protect you, as well as the patient or resident, from injury.
Make sure that beds are lowered to their lowest position and wheels are locked on beds, stretchers, and wheelchairs.	Lowering the bed to the lowest position makes it easier and safer for the person to transfer, because the lowest position allows the person to put their feet on the floor. Locking the wheels on equipment prevents the equipment from moving out from under the person as they transfer.
Make sure front swivel wheels on wheelchairs face forward in line with the back wheels.	Having front wheels facing forward makes the wheelchair more stable and less likely to tip over.
Make sure that footrests on a wheelchair are removed or folded back to the side of the chair.	Keeping the footrests out of the way can help prevent the person from tripping over them during a transfer or bumping into them and receiving an injury.
Check the person's clothing and shoes. Clothing should fit. Shoes should provide good foot support and have nonskid soles.	Long or loose clothing and shoes that do not provide enough support or have slippery soles could lead to tripping.
Plan the transfer so that the person is leading with their strongest side, if possible.	Doing so allows the person to bear weight in the direction they are going.
Do not allow a person to hold onto you during a transfer. Instead, have an unsteady person grasp the arm of the chair or a transfer bar for support.	If the person stumbles or falls while holding on to you, you could be injured.
Do not place your hands under a person's arms to help support them.	If the person stumbles or falls, they may be injured when you lift up as they are falling down.

make sure that the footrests are either removed or folded up and swiveled to the side of the chair so that the person does not trip over them or bump into them during the transfer. Procedure 15-8 describes how to transfer a person into a wheelchair or chair by yourself. Procedure 15-9 explains how to transfer a person from a wheelchair or chair to a bed.

Transferring a Person to and From a Stretcher

Stretchers are used to transport people to other parts of the facility for surgery or diagnostic testing. Critically ill and comatose people are also transported on stretchers. Procedure 15-10 describes how to transfer

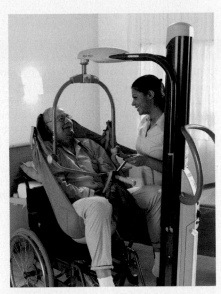

Figure 15-9 A mechanical lift is used to move a person who is very heavy, completely unable to assist with the move, or both. There are many different types of mechanical lifts in use. You should be trained how to operate the lift at the facility where you work before using it. (*Courtesy of Arjo AB, Malmö Sweden.*)

a person from a bed to a stretcher. Procedure 15-11 describes how to transfer a person from a stretcher to bed.

Transferring a Person Using a Mechanical Lift

A mechanical lift is used to move people who are very heavy or who are unable to assist in the transfer (Fig. 15-9). Because using a mechanical lift is safer for both the patient or resident and the staff, many facilities encourage the use of these devices for all transfers. Before using a mechanical lift, always make sure the person you need to transfer weighs less than the weight limit specified on the lift. Some facilities require two staff members to operate the mechanical lift. Make sure you know your facility's policy. Procedure 15-12 describes one method of transferring a person using a mechanical lift. Because lifts from different manufacturers may vary greatly in their procedures for use, do not use a mechanical lift until you have been taught specifically how to use that lift.

Assisting a Person With Walking (Ambulating)

Some patients and residents may be able to transfer without using a wheelchair or stretcher, if they are offered assistance with ambulating. To **ambulate** means to walk. It is important to encourage people who are able to walk (either with or without assistance) to do it on a regular basis. Although using a wheelchair to transfer a person to the dining room or activity room may be quicker or easier for you, it can result in unnecessary dependence and a decline in a person's overall abilities. Walking helps to preserve mobility, improves heart and lung function, and promotes digestion. In addition, walking helps the person to remain as independent as possible for as long as possible. A person who feels weak or unsteady benefits, both physically and emotionally, from being encouraged to walk with assistance.

Sitting on the edge of the bed, also called "dangling," is the first step for someone who is going to get out of bed and walk. Procedure 15-13 explains how to help a person to sit on the edge of the bed. When a person has been resting in bed, especially for a long time, sitting up and then standing cause blood to flow to the legs and away from the head. This can lead to dizziness and fainting. Dangling allows time for the heart and blood vessels to make up for the change in position. Blood flow is sent to the head. This reduces the person's risk of falling due to dizziness or loss of consciousness.

There are many different devices people use to help them walk (Table 15-1). These devices are specially fitted to the individual and, therefore, should not be shared.

Procedure 15-14 describes how to assist a person with walking. Be alert to potential problems and be sure to report these to the nurse. Safety guidelines for assisting a person with walking are summarized in Guidelines Box 15-3.

Tell the Nurse!

Each time you assist a person with a transfer, tell the nurse immediately if:

- The person complains of dizziness, shortness of breath, chest pain, a rapid heartbeat (palpitations), or sudden head pain

- The person complains of pain when they try to bear weight, and this is new

- You observe any changes in the person's usual grip, strength, or ability

- A usually cooperative person refuses to participate ("I just don't feel like it today")

- The equipment is not working properly or is broken

TABLE 15-1 Assistive Devices for Walking (Ambulating)

DEVICE	WHO USES IT	HOW IT IS USED
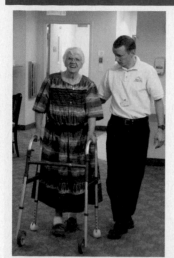 Walker	People who can bear weight but may be weak or unsteady	**Proper fit:** Handgrips level with the person's hips **Proper technique:** The person grasps the top of the frame, lifts the walker up, and places it squarely on the ground 10–18 inches in front of their body. The tips of the walker are placed flat on the floor. Using the top of the frame for support, the person moves one leg forward and then the other, stepping into the frame of the walker. The process is then repeated. The person can use the top of the frame for support between steps if necessary. A walker should never be used on stairs.
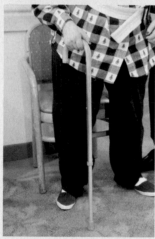 Cane (may have one tip, three tips, or four tips)	People who can bear weight but are weak on one side	**Proper fit:** Handle level with the person's hip **Proper technique:** The person holds the cane on their strong side, placing it in front of the body and using it to support their weight while moving. The tip of the cane is placed flat on the floor. If the person is using a three- or four-tipped cane, all of the tips are placed flat on the floor at the same time. The weaker leg is moved forward first, followed by the stronger leg. The nursing assistant stands slightly behind and to the side of the person, on the person's weak side.
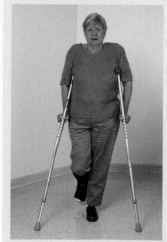 Crutches	People who cannot bear full weight on one leg	**Proper fit:** Top of the crutches rests against the person's sides, not underneath the arms **Proper technique:** The person supports their weight with hands on the handgrips (not under the arms). The tips of the crutches are placed flat on the floor. The nurse or physical therapist will teach the person how to move using the crutches.

Guidelines Box 15-3 Guidelines for Assisting a Person With Walking (Ambulation)

WHAT YOU DO	WHY YOU DO IT
Use correct body mechanics.	Using good body mechanics will protect you, as well as the patient or resident, from injury.
Use a transfer belt on the person according to your facility policy and the person's care plan.	The transfer belt gives you a safe place to grasp and support the person.
Watch the person for fatigue or discomfort.	A person who is tired or uncomfortable is at greater risk for tripping or fainting.
Check the person's clothing and shoes. Clothing should fit. Shoes should provide good foot support and have nonskid soles.	Long or loose clothing and shoes that do not provide enough support or have slippery soles could lead to tripping.
Check ambulation devices to ensure that they are in good condition. Tips on canes and walkers should not be cracked, worn, or missing.	The tips on canes and walkers provide traction. If they are cracked or worn, they can slip, causing the person to fall.
Request help from a coworker as necessary when you must assist a weak, unsteady, or uncooperative person with walking.	A person who is weak, unsteady, or uncooperative is likely to fall, injuring both of you. Having help from a coworker makes a fall less likely.
Allow the person to "dangle" for the specified amount of time before assisting the person to stand up.	Allowing a person time to "dangle" before getting out of bed reduces the person's risk of falling due to dizziness or loss of consciousness.
Ensure that the person is using ambulation devices correctly.	Using an ambulation device correctly reduces the person's risk of slipping and falling.

SUMMARY

- People in a health care setting may be unable to reposition themselves without assistance.
  - The resulting immobility can cause pressure ulcers, contractures, pneumonia, and blood clots in the legs.
  - Preventing the complications of immobility, through frequent repositioning and transferring, is a major responsibility of the nursing assistant.
    - Some people will have conditions that require regular repositioning as often as every hour, but at least every 2 hours.
    - Several basic positions are used when a person must remain in bed for extended periods: the supine (dorsal recumbent), Fowler's, lateral, prone, and Sims' positions. Proper positioning is essential for comfort and helps ensure proper body alignment, which relieves muscle and joint strain, promotes good heart and lung function, and helps prevent contractures and pressure ulcers.
    - When repositioning a person, it is important to prevent shearing and friction injuries to the skin.
- Nursing assistants also help people transfer from one place to another throughout the day.
  - Advance planning and proper technique help to ensure a safe transfer.
  - Using transfer-assist devices is safer for both the health care worker and the patient or resident.
  - Some patients and residents may be able to walk on their own, with help. Encouraging and assisting patients and residents to walk enhances their quality of life by providing both physical and emotional benefits.

Procedure 15-1

Moving a Person to the Side of the Bed (One Assistant)

WHY YOU DO IT Moving a person to the side of the bed is a necessary first step in many procedures, such as the procedures for turning a person onto their side, assisting a person to sit on the edge of the bed, or assisting a person to get out of bed.

Getting Ready

1. Complete the "Getting Ready" steps.

Procedure

2. Make sure that the bed is positioned at a comfortable working height, usually elbow height of caregiver (to promote good body mechanics), and that the wheels are locked.

3. Place the pillow at the head of the bed, on its edge against the headboard. This gets the pillow out of the way.

4. If the side rails are in use, lower the side rail on the working side of the bed. The side rail on the opposite side of the bed should remain up. Lower the head of the bed so that the bed is flat (as tolerated). Fanfold the top linens to the foot of the bed.

5. Stand at the side of the bed with your feet spread about 12 inches apart and with your knees slightly bent to protect your back.

6. Gently slide your hands under the person's head and shoulders and move the person's upper body toward you.

7. Gently slide your hands under the person's torso and move the person's torso toward you.

8. Gently slide your hands under the person's hips and legs and move the person's lower body toward you.

9. Now, position the person as planned (for example, in the prone or lateral position).

10. Reposition the pillow under the person's head and straighten the bottom linens. Draw the top linens over the person. Raise the head of the bed as the person requests.

11. Make sure that the bed is lowered to its lowest position and that the wheels are locked. If the side rails are in use, return them to the raised position.

Finishing Up

12. Complete the "Finishing Up" steps.

What You Document

- Position the person was placed in
- Any special support devices used
- Personal care given
- Appearance of skin, especially over bony prominences

> **Procedure 15-2**

Moving a Person to the Side of the Bed (Two Assistants)

WHY YOU DO IT This method of moving a person to the side of the bed is safer for both you and the person if the person is large, very ill or injured, or uncooperative. Using a lift sheet also helps to prevent shearing and friction injuries.

Getting Ready

1. Complete the "Getting Ready" steps.

Supplies

- lift sheet (if one is not already on the bed)

Procedure

2. Make sure that the bed is positioned at a comfortable working height, usually elbow height of caregiver (to promote good body mechanics), and that the wheels are locked.

3. Place the pillow at the head of the bed, on its edge against the headboard. This gets the pillow out of the way.

4. If the side rails are in use, lower the side rails. Lower the head of the bed so that the bed is flat (as tolerated). Fanfold the top linens to the foot of the bed.

5. If the lift sheet is already on the bed, make sure that it is positioned so that it is under the person's shoulders and hips. (If a lift sheet is not already on the bed, position one under the person's shoulders and hips.)

6. Stand at the side of the bed, opposite your coworker, with your feet spread about 12 inches apart and with your knees slightly bent to protect your back.

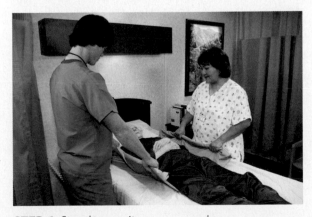

STEP 6 Stand opposite your coworker.

7. Grasp the edge of the lift sheet and roll it over as close to the person's body as possible. This will provide for a better grip. (Your coworker does the same.)

8. Grasp the rolled edge of the lift sheet with both hands, palms and fingers facing down. One hand should be level with the person's shoulders and the other should be level with their hips.

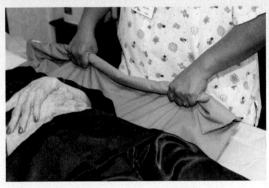

STEP 8 Grasp the rolled lift sheet with both hands, palms and fingers facing down.

9. On the count of "three," slowly and carefully lift up on the lift sheet in unison and move the person to the side of the bed.

10. Now, position the person as planned (for example, in the prone or lateral position).

11. Reposition the pillow under the person's head and straighten the bottom linens. Draw the top linens over the person.

12. Make sure that the bed is lowered to its lowest position and that the wheels are locked. If the side rails are in use, return them to the raised position.

Finishing Up

13. Complete the "Finishing Up" steps.

What You Document

- Position the person was placed in
- Any special support devices used
- Personal care given
- Appearance of skin, especially over bony prominences

Procedure 15-3

Moving a Person Up in Bed (Two Assistants)

WHY YOU DO IT Gravity causes a person who is sitting in bed to slide down over time, leading to discomfort and interfering with the person's ability to breathe. Helping the person to move up in bed promotes comfort and makes it easier for the person to breathe. This method of moving a person up in bed is safer for both you and the person. Using a lift sheet also helps to prevent shearing and friction injuries.

Getting Ready

1. Complete the "Getting Ready" steps.

Supplies

- lift sheet (if one is not already on the bed)

Procedure

2. Make sure that the bed is positioned at a comfortable working height, usually elbow height of caregiver (to promote good body mechanics), and that the wheels are locked.

3. Place the pillow at the head of the bed, on its edge against the headboard. This gets the pillow out of the way. It also pads the headboard in case you move the person up a little too much or too fast!

4. If the side rails are in use, lower the side rails. Lower the head of the bed so that the bed is flat (as tolerated). Fanfold the top linens to the foot of the bed.

5. If the lift sheet is already on the bed, make sure that it is positioned so that it is under the person's shoulders and hips. (If a lift sheet is not already on the bed, position one under the person's shoulders and hips.)

6. Stand at the side of the bed, opposite your coworker, with your feet spread about 12 inches apart and with your knees slightly bent to protect your back.

7. Grasp the edge of the lift sheet and roll it over as close to the person's body as possible. This will provide for a better grip. (Your coworker does the same.)

8. Grasp the rolled edge of the lift sheet with both hands, palms and fingers facing down. One hand should be level with the person's shoulders and the other should be level with their hips. If the person is able to assist, have them bend their knees and push during the move upward.

9. On the count of "three," slowly and carefully lift up on the lift sheet in unison and move the person toward the head of the bed. Avoid dragging the person across the bottom linens.

10. Reposition the pillow under the person's head and straighten the bottom linens. Draw the top linens over the person. Raise the head of the bed as the person requests.

11. Make sure that the bed is lowered to its lowest position and that the wheels are locked. If the side rails are in use, return them to the raised position.

Finishing Up

12. Complete the "Finishing Up" steps.

What You Document

- Amount of assistance needed
- Personal care given

▶ Procedure 15-4

Raising a Person's Head and Shoulders

WHY YOU DO IT　Raising the person's head and shoulders away from the bed is necessary when you need to adjust the pillow and during some care procedures, such as dressing. Knowing how to perform this procedure safely prevents injury to you and your patient or resident.

Getting Ready

1. Complete the "Getting Ready" steps.

Procedure

2. Make sure that the bed is positioned at a comfortable working height, usually elbow height of caregiver (to promote good body mechanics), and that the wheels are locked.

3. Place the pillow at the head of the bed, on its edge against the headboard. This gets the pillow out of the way.

4. If the side rails are in use, lower the side rail on the working side of the bed. The side rail on the opposite side of the bed should remain up. Fanfold the top linens to the person's waist if necessary.

5. Face the head of the bed. Position your outside foot (that is, the foot that is farthest away from the edge of the bed) 12 inches in front of the other foot, and bend your knees slightly to protect your back.

6. Slide one hand under the person's shoulder that is nearest to you.

7. Slide the other hand under the person's upper back.

8. On the count of "three," slowly and carefully lift the person's head and shoulders.

9. Reposition the pillow under the person's head and straighten the bottom linens. Draw the top linens over the person. Raise the head of the bed as the person requests.

10. Make sure that the bed is lowered to its lowest position and that the wheels are locked. If the side rails are in use, return them to the raised position.

Finishing Up

11. Complete the "Finishing Up" steps.

▶ Procedure 15-5

Turning a Person Onto Their Side

WHY YOU DO IT　The lateral position is part of the cycle of positions for people who are unable to reposition themselves. The person is moved from the supine position to the lateral position, then back to the supine position, and then to the lateral position on the other side.

Getting Ready

1. Complete the "Getting Ready" steps.

Supplies

- additional pillows or other supportive devices (if not already in the room)

Procedure

2. Make sure that the bed is positioned at a comfortable working height, usually elbow height of caregiver (to promote good body mechanics), and that the wheels are locked.

3. Place the pillow at the head of the bed, on its edge against the headboard. This gets the pillow out of the way.

4. If the side rails are in use, lower the side rail on the working side of the bed. The side rail on the opposite side of the bed should remain up. Lower the head of the bed so that the bed is flat (as tolerated). Fanfold the top linens to the foot of the bed.

(continued)

5. If the lift sheet is already on the bed, make sure that it is positioned so that it is under the person's shoulders and hips. (If a lift sheet is not already on the bed, position one under the person's shoulders and hips.)

6. Stand at the side of the bed with your feet spread about 12 inches apart and with your knees slightly bent to protect your back.

7. Move the person to the side of the bed opposite the side to which they will be turned.

8. Cross the person's arm that is nearest to you over the person's chest. If the person is able to assist, have them reach over and grasp the side rail on the side of the bed toward which they are turning.

9. Roll the person onto their side:

   a. **To roll the person away from you:** Making sure that the side rail is raised on the side in which the person is being rolled toward, roll the lift sheet close to the person's body and grasp with one hand near the person's shoulder and the other hand near the person's hips. Gently roll the person away from you, toward the opposite side of the bed.

   b. **To roll the person toward you:** Raise the side rail and move to the other side of the bed. Lower that side rail. Reaching across the person, roll the lift sheet close to the person's body and grasp with one hand near the person's shoulder and the other hand near the person's hips. Gently roll the person toward you.

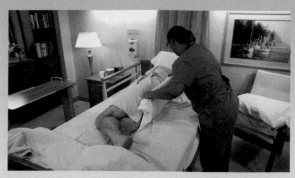

STEP 9 Gently roll the person away from you, toward the opposite side of the bed.

10. Reposition the pillow under the person's head and straighten the bottom linens. Support the person by placing a pillow lengthwise between the person's legs. The person's lower leg should be straight, and the upper leg should be slightly bent at the knee. Place additional pillows under the person's upper arm, and behind their back. Draw the top linens over the person.

11. Make sure that the bed is lowered to its lowest position and that the wheels are locked. If the side rails are in use, return them to the raised position.

Finishing Up

12. Complete the "Finishing Up" steps.

What You Document

■ Position the person was placed in
■ Any special support devices used
■ Personal care given
■ Appearance of skin, especially over bony prominences

▶ Procedure 15-6

Logrolling a Person (Three Assistants)

WHY YOU DO IT Logrolling is done whenever it is necessary to move a person who has had back surgery or an injury to the neck or spine. The person is rolled in one fluid motion so that the head, torso, and legs move as one unit and the body is kept in alignment.

Getting Ready

1. Complete the "Getting Ready" steps.

Supplies

■ lift sheet (if one is not already on the bed)

Procedure

2. Make sure that the bed is positioned at a comfortable working height, usually elbow height of caregiver (to promote good body mechanics), and that the wheels are locked.

3. Keep the pillow in place underneath the person's head to keep the neck aligned.

4. If the side rails are in use, lower the side rails. Lower the head of the bed so that the bed is flat (as tolerated). Fanfold the top linens to the foot of the bed.

5. Stand with another assistant on the side of the bed toward which the person will be moved. The third assistant stands on the opposite side of the bed. Stand facing the bed with your feet spread about 12 inches apart and with your knees slightly bent to protect your back. One assistant is aligned with the person's head and shoulders; the other is aligned with the person's hips and legs. The third assistant is on the opposite side of the bed.

6. Roll the lift sheet close to the person's sides and grasp it. Lifting in unison, gently move the person toward the side of the bed opposite to that which the person will be turned.

7. Place a pillow lengthwise between the person's legs and fold the person's arms across their chest.

8. The two assistants on the side of the bed toward which the person is being moved should roll the lift sheet in close to the person's body. The third assistant should gently support the person's head during the move to prevent twisting of the person's neck and should grasp the lift sheet with their lower hand near the person's shoulders. The assistants on the other side of the bed should grasp the lift sheet close to the person's shoulders and hips and near the person's hips and place the lower hand behind the person's knees. The third assistant will assist from behind the person.

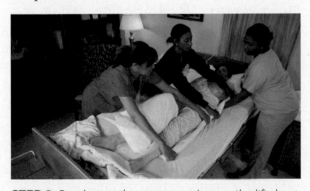

STEP 8 Reach over the person and grasp the lift sheet.

9. On the count of "three," roll the person as a unit toward the side of the bed with the two assistants in a single movement, being sure to keep the person's head, spine, and legs aligned.

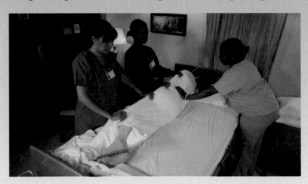

STEP 9 On the count of "three," roll the person in one fluid movement.

10. Reposition the pillow under the person's head and straighten the bottom linens. Make sure the person is in straight alignment. Support the person by bolstering their back with pillows. The pillow between the person's legs should remain in place, and additional pillows or folded towels should be used to support the person's arms. Draw the top linens over the person.

11. Make sure that the bed is lowered to its lowest position and that the wheels are locked. If the side rails are in use, return them to the raised position.

Finishing Up

12. Complete the "Finishing Up" steps.

What You Document

- Position the person was placed in
- Number of people assisting
- Any special positioning or support devices used
- Personal care given
- Appearance of skin, especially over bony prominences

Procedure 15-7

Applying a Transfer (Gait) Belt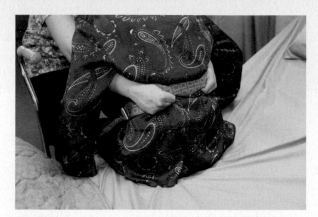

WHY YOU DO IT   The transfer belt gives you a safe place to grasp and support the person when assisting the person with standing, transferring, or walking.

Getting Ready

1. Complete the "Getting Ready" steps.

Supplies

■ transfer belt

Procedure

2. If the person is in bed, make sure that the bed is lowered to its lowest position and that the wheels are locked. If the side rails are in use, lower the side rail on the working side of the bed. The side rail on the opposite side of the bed should remain up. Fanfold the top linens to the foot of the bed. Assist the person to sit on the edge of the bed.

3. Apply the belt around the person's waist, over their clothing. Buckle the belt in the front by threading the tongue of the belt through the side of the buckle that has "teeth" first, and then placing the tongue of the belt through the other side of the buckle.

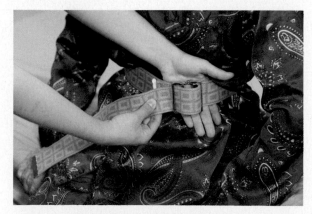

STEP 3 Thread the tongue of the belt through the side of the buckle that has "teeth" first.

4. Before tightening the belt, turn it so that the buckle is off-center in the front or to the side.

5. Tighten the belt and check for fit. The belt should be snug, but you should be able to slip your fingers between the belt and the person's waist. If the patient has breasts, make sure that they are not trapped underneath the belt.

6. Use an underhand grasp when holding the belt to provide greater safety.

STEP 6 Use an underhand grasp to hold the belt.

Finishing Up

7. When the person has finished transferring and is ready to return to bed, reverse the procedure.

8. Complete the "Finishing Up" steps.

What You Document

■ That a transfer belt was used
■ Nature of transfer (for example, from bed to wheelchair, wheelchair to toilet, to ambulate)
■ How the person tolerated the transfer (any complaints of dizziness, pain, or other discomfort)

Procedure 15-8

Transferring a Person From a Bed to a Wheelchair (One Assistant)

WHY YOU DO IT   Wheelchairs are used to transport people who are unable to walk. Using proper technique helps to keep both you and the person safe during the transfer from bed to wheelchair.

Getting Ready

1. Complete the "Getting Ready" steps.

Supplies

- wheelchair
- lap blanket (optional)
- person's robe
- person's slippers or shoes
- transfer belt

Procedure

*Note: This technique can be used with two assistants, having one on either side of the patient or resident during the transfer.

2. Determine the person's strongest side, and then place the wheelchair alongside the bed. (You may need to move other items of furniture or equipment out of the way so that you can maneuver safely.) Position the wheelchair so that the person will move toward the chair "strong side first." Whenever possible, position the wheelchair so that it is against a wall or a solid piece of furniture so that it will not slide backward during the transfer.

3. Lock the wheelchair wheels, and either remove the footrests or swing them to the side.

4. Fanfold the top linens to the foot of the bed.

5. Make sure that the bed is lowered to its lowest position and that the wheels are locked. Raise the head of the bed as tolerated. If the person uses the side rail to assist themselves to sit up or stand, leave the top half of the rail in the up position.

6. Help the person to move toward the side of the bed where the wheelchair is located.

7. Assist the person to dangle.

8. Allow the person to rest on the edge of the bed. The person should be sitting squarely on both buttocks, with their knees apart and both feet flat on the floor (to offer a broad base of support). The person's arms should rest alongside their thighs. Watch for signs of dizziness or fainting. Position yourself in front of the person so that you can offer assistance in case they lose balance.

9. Help the person to put their shoes or slippers on and help them to get into a robe. Apply a transfer belt.

10. Help the person to stand. (If the person uses a stand-assist device, have them grasp this to come to a standing position.)

    a. Stand facing the person.

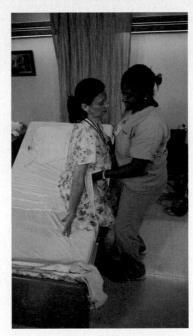

STEP 10 Help the person to stand. Brace the person's knees with your knees, and the person's feet with your feet.

    b. Have the person put their hands on the edge of the bed, alongside each thigh.

    c. Make sure the person's feet are flat on the floor.

    d. Have the person lean forward.

    e. Grasp the transfer belt at each side, using an underhand grasp. (If you are not using a transfer belt, pass your arms under the person's arms and rest your hands on their upper back.)

(continued)

f. Position your feet alongside the person's feet, flexing your knees. Place your shins against the person's shins to block the person's feet and keep their knees from buckling as they stand up.

g. Have the person push down on the bed with their hands or grasp the stand-assist device and stand on the count of "three." Assist the person into a standing position by pulling on the transfer belt as you straighten your knees. (If you are not using a transfer belt, assist the person into a standing position by gently pulling them up and forward as you straighten your knees.) Remember to keep your back straight.

11. Support the person in the standing position by holding the transfer belt or by keeping your hands on their upper back. Continue to block the person's feet and knees with your feet and knees.

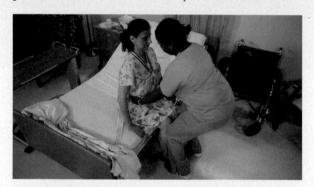

STEP 11 Support the person in the standing position.

12. Help the person to turn by pivoting on the stronger leg toward the chair. This will allow the person to grasp the far arm of the wheelchair.

13. Continue to assist the person with turning until they are able to grasp the other armrest. The backs of the person's legs should touch the edge of the chair.

14. Lower the person into the wheelchair by bending your hips and knees.

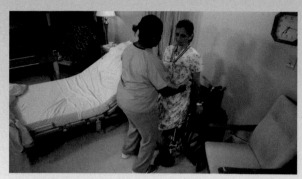

STEP 14 Lower the person into the wheelchair by bending your hips and knees.

15. Make sure the person's buttocks are at the back of the chair. Make sure the person is comfortable and in good body alignment.

16. Remove the transfer belt.

17. Position the person's feet on the footrests of the wheelchair. Buckle the wheelchair safety belt (if ordered) and cover the person's lap and legs with a lap blanket, if desired. Make sure that the lap blanket does not drag on the floor.

Finishing Up

18. Position the wheelchair according to the person's preference.

19. Complete the "Finishing Up" steps.

What You Document

■ Whether or not a transfer belt was used
■ How the person tolerated the transfer

 Procedure 15-9

Transferring a Person From a Wheelchair to a Bed

WHY YOU DO IT Wheelchairs are used to transport people who are unable to walk. Using proper technique helps to keep both you and the person safe during the transfer from wheelchair to bed.

Getting Ready

1. Complete the "Getting Ready" steps.

Supplies

■ transfer belt

Procedure

2. Make sure that the bed is lowered to its lowest position and that the wheels are locked. Raise the head of the bed, fanfold the top linens to the foot of the bed, and raise the opposite side rail. (You may need to move other items of furniture or equipment out of the way so that you can maneuver safely.)

3. Position the wheelchair close to the side of the bed so that the person's strong side is next to the bed. Lock the wheelchair wheels and either remove the footrests or swing them to the side.

4. Remove the person's lap blanket (if one was used) and release the wheelchair safety belt, if in use. Apply a transfer belt.

5. Stand facing the person with your feet spread about 12 inches apart and with your knees slightly bent to protect your back. With your back straight, slide the person to the front of the wheelchair seat.

6. Grasp the transfer belt (or pass your arms under the person's arms, placing your hands on their upper back). Position your feet alongside the person's feet, flexing your knees. Place your shins against the person's shins to block the person's feet and keep their knees from buckling as they stand up.

7. Have the person place their hands on the armrests of the wheelchair and press down as you assist them to stand by pulling on the transfer belt as you straighten your knees. (If you are not using a transfer belt, assist the person into a standing position by gently pulling them up and forward as you straighten your knees.) Remember to keep your back straight. Alternatively, a person who requires less assistance can make use of a stand-assist device to stand while you offer support.

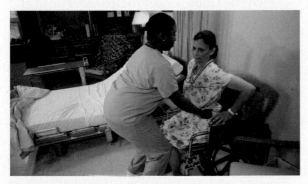

STEP 7 Help the person to stand.

8. Slowly help the person to turn toward the bed by pivoting on their strong leg. Help the person to sit on the edge of the bed.

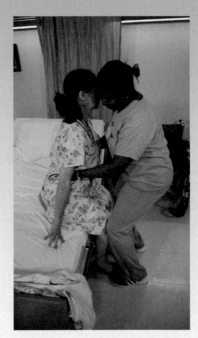

STEP 8 Help the person to sit on the edge of the bed.

9. Remove the transfer belt and the person's robe and slippers, if appropriate.

10. Move the wheelchair out of the way.

11. Place one of your arms around the person's shoulders and one arm under their legs. Swing the person's legs onto the bed.

12. Help the person to move to the center of the bed and position them comfortably.

13. Straighten the bottom linens and make sure the person is comfortable and in good body alignment. Draw the top linens over the person.

14. If the side rails are in use, return them to the raised position.

Finishing Up

15. Complete the "Finishing Up" steps.

What You Document

- How long the person has been in the chair
- Whether or not a transfer belt is used
- Position the person was placed in once in bed
- Any personal care given
- Appearance of skin, especially on buttocks
- How the person tolerated the transfer

Procedure 15-10

Transferring a Person From a Bed to a Stretcher (Three Assistants)

WHY YOU DO IT Stretchers are used to transport people to other parts of the facility for surgery or diagnostic testing. Critically ill and comatose people are also transported on stretchers. Using proper technique helps to keep both you and the person safe during the transfer from bed to stretcher.

Getting Ready

1. Complete the "Getting Ready" steps.

Supplies

- stretcher
- lift sheet (if one is not already on the bed)
- lateral-transfer device (transfer board or roller board)
- blanket

Procedure

2. Raise the bed so that it is level with the height of the stretcher. Lower the head of the bed so that the bed is flat. Make sure that the bed wheels are locked. Lower the side rails. Fanfold the top linens to the side of the bed opposite the stretcher and cover the person with the blanket.

3. If the lift sheet is already on the bed, make sure that it is positioned so that it is under the person's shoulders and hips. (If a lift sheet is not already on the bed, position one under the person's shoulders and hips.)

4. Two assistants should stand on the stretcher side of the bed. A third assistant should stand on the side of the bed without the stretcher. Have the person fold their arms across their chest. Rolling and grasping the lift sheet close to the person's body, the assistants should move the person toward the side of the bed where the stretcher will be.

5. Position the stretcher alongside the bed. Place the lateral-transfer device on the stretcher. Lock the stretcher wheels and move the stretcher safety belts out of the way.

6. The assistant on the side opposite the stretcher reaches across the person and, using the lift sheet, slightly rolls the person over toward them so that the other two assistants can place the lateral-transfer device across the space between the stretcher and the bed, slightly underneath the person. The person is then gently rolled back onto their back.

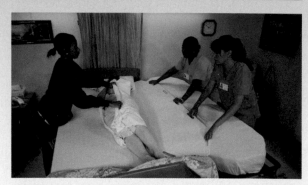

STEP 6 Place the lateral-transfer device across the space between the stretcher and the bed.

7. Each assistant now grasps the lift sheet, and on the count of 3, gently slides the person across the lateral-transfer device onto the stretcher.

8. Once the person is centered on the stretcher, remove the transfer device. Unlock the stretcher wheels and move it away from the side of the bed.

9. Position the person on the stretcher and make sure they are in good body alignment. Reposition the pillow under the person's head and cover the person with a blanket for modesty and warmth. Buckle the stretcher safety belts across the person and raise the side rails on the stretcher. Raise the head of the stretcher as the person requests.

Finishing Up

10. Transport the person to the appropriate site. A person on a stretcher should always be transported "feet first." Remain with the person; never leave someone alone on a stretcher.

11. Complete the "Finishing Up" steps.

What You Document

- The time of the transfer
- Number of people assisting
- Transfer aids used (lift sheet, roller board, mechanical lift)
- Use of side rails/safety strap on stretcher
- Where the person is being transported

Procedure 15-11

Transferring a Person From a Stretcher to a Bed (Three Assistants)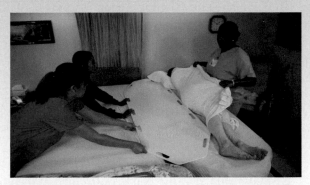

WHY YOU DO IT Stretchers are used to transport people to other parts of the facility for surgery or diagnostic testing. Critically ill and comatose people are also transported on stretchers. Using proper technique helps to keep both you and the person safe during the transfer from stretcher to bed.

Getting Ready
1. Complete the "Getting Ready" steps.

Supplies
- lift sheet (if one is not already on the stretcher)
- lateral-transfer device (transfer board or roller board)

Procedure

2. Raise or lower the bed so that it is level with the height of the stretcher. Lower the head of the bed so that the bed is flat. Place the lateral-transfer device on the bed. Make sure that the bed wheels are locked. Lower the side rails. Fanfold the top linens to the side of the bed opposite the stretcher.

3. If the lift sheet is already on the stretcher, make sure that it is positioned so that it is under the person's shoulders and hips. (If a lift sheet is not already on the stretcher, position one under the person's shoulders and hips.)

4. Unbuckle the stretcher safety belts and lower the side rails on the stretcher.

5. Position the stretcher against the bed and lock the stretcher wheels.

6. Two assistants stand at the far side of the bed facing the third assistant, who is positioned along the outside edge of the stretcher. (Some facilities allow the assistants on the far side of the bed to kneel on the bed to complete the transfer; follow your facility's policy.)

7. Grasp the edge of the lift sheet and roll it over as close to the person's body as possible. This will provide for a better grip.

8. The assistant on the stretcher side will reach across the person and, using the lift sheet, roll the person up slightly while the other two assistants place the lateral-transfer device across the space between the stretcher and the bed, partially underneath the person. Roll the person back onto their back.

STEP 8 Roll the person up slightly while the two other assistants place the lateral-transfer device across the space between the stretcher and the bed.

9. Grasping the lift sheet close to the person's body, on the count of "three," all three assistants slowly and carefully pull the lift sheet in unison and move the person to the bed. Move the stretcher away from the bed and remove the lateral-transfer device from the bed.

10. Help the person to move to the center of the bed and, if desired, remove the lift sheet by turning the person first to one side, then the other. Position the person comfortably.

11. Straighten the bottom linens and make sure the person is comfortable and in good body alignment. Draw the top linens over the person.

12. Make sure the bed is lowered to its lowest position and that the wheels are locked. If the side rails are in use, return them to the raised position.

Finishing Up
13. Complete the "Finishing Up" steps.

What You Document
- The time of the transfer
- Number of people assisting
- Transfer-assist devices used
- Position the person placed in once in bed
- Personal care given

▶ **Procedure 15-12**

Transferring a Person Using a Mechanical Lift (Two Assistants)

WHY YOU DO IT   Using a mechanical lift to move a person who is helpless or very heavy is safer for both you and the person.

Getting Ready

1. Complete the "Getting Ready" steps.

Supplies

- wheelchair or chair
- mechanical lift
- sling in proper size
- lap blanket (optional)
- lap restraint (if ordered)

Procedure

2. Make sure that the bed is positioned at a comfortable working height, usually elbow height of caregiver (to promote good body mechanics), and that the wheels are locked. Move other equipment or furniture out of the way to clear room for the lift and the wheelchair or chair.

3. If the side rails are in use, lower the side rails.

4. Fanfold the top linens to the foot of the bed.

5. Center the sling under the person. If the sling is for use with more than one patient or resident, place a cover or pad on the sling. (To get the sling under the person, move the person as if you were making an occupied bed.) The sling should be positioned evenly underneath the person, from shoulders to mid-thigh.

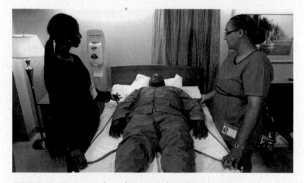

STEP 5 Center the sling under the person.

6. Move the chair or wheelchair to the side of the bed. Lock the wheels.

7. Roll the base of the lift underneath the side of the bed nearest the chair. Center the frame over the person and lock the wheels of the lift.

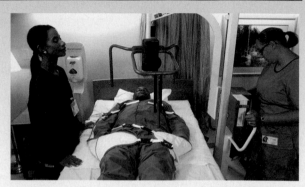

STEP 7 Move the lift into position over the person.

8. Widen the legs of the lift to provide a solid base of support. The legs must be locked in this position.

9. Lower the arms of the lift down toward the person, close enough to attach the sling to the frame.

10. Fasten the sling to the straps or chains of the lift. Make sure the hooks face away from the person.

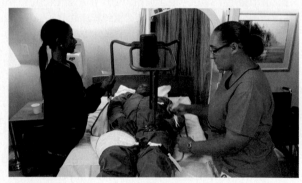

STEP 10 Fasten the sling to the lift according to the manufacturer's instructions.

11. Attach the sling to the swivel bar with the short straps attached to the top of the sling and the long straps attached to the bottom of the sling.

12. Have the person cross their arms across their chest. Check to make sure all tubes and drains are free and will not be pulled out during the transfer.

13. With an assistant standing on each side of the lift, raise the lift until the person and the sling are about 6 inches above the bed.

14. Unlock the wheels of the lift and carefully wheel the person straight back and away from the bed.

15. Have your coworker support the person's legs as you move the lift into position over the wheelchair.

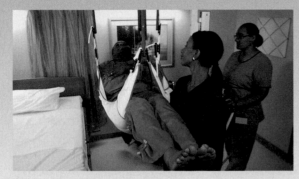

STEP 15 A coworker supports the person's legs as you move them into position over the wheelchair.

16. Position the person over the chair with the base of the lift straddling the chair.

17. Gently lower the person into the wheelchair. Make sure the person's buttocks are at the back of the chair.

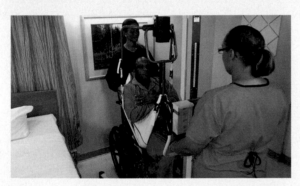

STEP 17 Gently lower the person into the wheelchair.

18. Lower the swivel bar so that you can unhook the sling. Leave the sling under the person unless it is needed for use with another patient or resident prior to moving this person back into bed.

19. Make sure the person's buttocks are at the back of the chair. Make sure the person is comfortable and in good body alignment.

20. Position the person's feet on the footrests of the wheelchair. Buckle the wheelchair safety belt (or place a lap restraint, if ordered). Cover the person's lap and legs with a lap blanket, if desired. Make sure that the lap blanket does not drag on the floor.

Finishing Up

21. Position the wheelchair according to the person's preference.

22. Follow the "Finishing Up" steps.

23. When the person is ready to return to bed, reverse the procedure.

What You Document

- Type of mechanical lift used
- Number of people assisting
- Where the person was transferred to (wheelchair, geri chair, bathtub, stretcher)
- Any special positioning aids used
- How the person tolerated transfer

> ## Procedure 15-13

Assisting a Person With Sitting on the Edge of the Bed ("Dangling")

WHY YOU DO IT Allowing a person time to "dangle" before getting out of bed reduces the person's risk of falling due to dizziness or loss of consciousness.

Getting Ready

1. Complete the "Getting Ready" steps.

Procedure

2. Make sure that the bed is lowered to its lowest position and that the wheels are locked.

3. If the side rails are in use, lower the side rail on the working side of the bed. The side rail on the opposite side of the bed should remain up. If the person uses the side rail as an assistive device to sit, leave the top half of the side rail in the up position. Fanfold the top linens to the foot of the bed.

4. Help the person into a side-lying position, facing you.

5. Raise the head of the bed into a sitting position.

(continued)

6. Gently slide one arm behind the person's upper back. Slide the other arm under their knees and rest your hand on the side of their thigh.

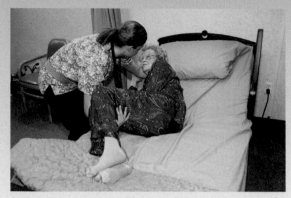

STEP 6 Slide one arm behind the person's upper back. Slide the other arm under their knees.

7. With a single smooth movement, slide the person's legs over the side of the bed while moving their head and shoulders upward so that they are sitting on the edge of the bed.

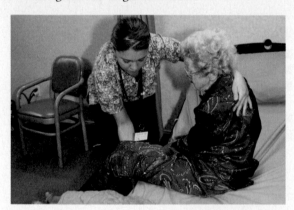

STEP 7 Help the person to sit on the edge of the bed.

8. Have the person put their hands on the edge of the bed, alongside each thigh, for support or raise the upper section of the side rails for them to hold on to. Watch for signs of dizziness or fainting. If the person feels faint, help them to lie down and call for the nurse.

9. Allow the person to "dangle" their legs over the side of the bed for the specified period of time, and then either take their vital signs (if indicated), help them to lie back down, or assist them to a standing position. Stay with the person during the entire time.

Finishing Up

10. Complete the "Finishing Up" steps.

What You Document

- How long the person dangled
- How much assistance was needed
- How the person tolerated dangling

▶ Procedure 15-14

Assisting a Person With Walking (Ambulating) ▶

WHY YOU DO IT Assisting a person to ambulate regularly helps to meet the person's need for exercise and helps prevent complications of immobility. It also helps to keep a person as independent as possible for as long as possible.

Getting Ready

1. Complete the "Getting Ready" steps.

Supplies

- transfer belt
- cane or walker (if indicated)
- person's robe
- person's slippers or shoes (nonskid soles)

Procedure

2. If the person is in bed, make sure that the bed is lowered to its lowest position and that the wheels are locked. Make sure that furniture and

equipment are moved aside so the person will have a clear path.

3. Assist the person to "dangle." Check the person's pulse; a weak pulse could lead to lightheadedness. If the person's pulse is weak, stay with them and alert the nurse before attempting ambulation.

4. Help the person put on their shoes or slippers, and help them into a robe. Apply a transfer belt.

5. Help the person to stand.

   a. Stand facing the person.

   b. Have the person put their hands on the edge of the bed, alongside each thigh.

   c. Make sure the person's feet are flat on the floor.

   d. Have the person lean forward.

   e. Grasp the transfer belt at each side, using an underhand grasp. (If you are not using a transfer belt, pass your arms under the person's arms and rest your hands on their upper back.)

   f. Position your feet alongside the person's feet, flexing your knees. Place your shins against the person's shins to block the person's feet and keep their knees from buckling as they stand up.

   g. Have the person push down on the bed with their hands or grasp the stand-assist device and stand on the count of "three." Assist the person into a standing position by pulling on the transfer belt as you straighten your knees. (If you are not using a transfer belt, assist the person into a standing position by gently pulling them up and forward as you straighten your knees.) Remember to keep your back straight.

6. Have the person grasp the cane or walker, if they are using one, in order to maintain balance. The person should hold the cane on their strong side.

7. Help the person to walk, reminding them to keep their head up, looking forward. Stand slightly behind the person on their weaker side. Grasp the transfer belt with an underhand grip from the back. If the person is using an ambulation device, make sure they are using it correctly.

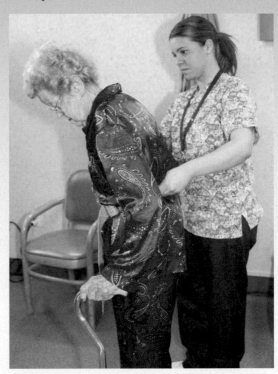

STEP 7 Grasp the transfer belt with an underhand grip from the back.

8. After returning to the person's room, help them back into bed or a chair.

Finishing Up

9. Complete the "Finishing Up" steps.

What You Document

- Whether or not gait belt was used
- What ambulation devices (if any) were used
- How far or where the person ambulated
- How the person tolerated ambulating

WHAT DID YOU LEARN?

Multiple Choice

Select the single best answer for each of the following questions.

1. Which of the following describes good standing posture when helping to reposition or transfer a person?
a. Feet 12 inches apart
b. Abdominal muscles relaxed
c. Arms out straight
d. Feet close together

2. When assisting a person to move to the head of the bed, you should:
a. Face the head of the bed
b. Unlock the bed wheels
c. Place a pillow under the person's head
d. Place the foot that is farthest away from the bed edge behind the other foot

3. Which person is likely to need help moving and turning in bed?
a. A person who is ambulatory
b. A person who has Alzheimer disease
c. A sleeping person
d. An unconscious person

4. To transfer a person correctly from a bed to a stretcher, you must:
a. Use a mechanical lift
b. Get help from at least five coworkers
c. Use good body mechanics
d. Raise the far side rail of the stretcher first

5. When moving and positioning people, you should:
a. Avoid friction and shearing
b. Use good body mechanics
c. Use pillows and rolled towels to maintain the position
d. All of the above

6. Sitting a person on the side of the bed is called:
a. Semi-sitting
b. Proning
c. Supining
d. Dangling

7. When transferring a person from one place to another, you should:
a. Use a transfer belt (unless the person has a condition that prevents the use of a transfer belt)
b. Adjust the bed to the lowest possible height
c. Lock the brakes of the bed, wheelchair, or stretcher
d. All of the above

8. A person in the prone position is lying on their:
a. Right side
b. Left side
c. Abdomen
d. Back

9. When moving a person by yourself and the person is wearing a transfer belt:
a. Lift from the side
b. Use an underhand grasp
c. Use an overhand grasp
d. Stand behind the person

10. A nurse asks you to place a patient in the semi-Fowler's position while their tube feeding is running. You know the head of the bed should be elevated:
a. 90 degrees
b. 60 degrees
c. 30 degrees
d. 15 degrees

11. A mechanical lift can be used to:
a. Move a patient or resident who is very heavy
b. Move a patient or resident who is very weak
c. Help a nursing assistant carry out their duties without injuring themselves
d. All of the above

12. When transferring a person from a bed to a stretcher, you should position the bed:
a. At its lowest level
b. Level with the stretcher
c. In the high-Fowler's position
d. In the supine position

13. A person who cannot reposition themselves independently is at risk for developing:
   a. Pressure ulcers
   b. Blood clots
   c. Pneumonia
   d. All of the above

14. What is it called when a joint is held in one position for too long, and the tendons shorten?
   a. A pressure ulcer
   b. A bed sore
   c. A contracture
   d. A shearing injury

15. Why is it important to ensure that your patients or residents are in good body alignment every time you reposition them?
   a. Good body alignment is most comfortable for the patient or resident
   b. Good body alignment helps prevent complications, such as pressure ulcers and contractures
   c. Good body alignment helps the person to breathe easier and improves blood flow to tissues
   d. All of the above

16. What technique would you use to reposition a patient who has just had spinal surgery?
   a. Logrolling
   b. A mechanical lift
   c. Dangling
   d. Turning

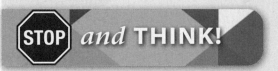

- Sofia, a new nursing assistant, has been assigned to take care of Mrs. Adkins. Mrs. Adkins weighs more than 250 lb and has had a stroke, so she is paralyzed completely on her left side. Sofia has to transfer Mrs. Adkins from her bed to a wheelchair so she can go to the shower room. What steps should Sofia take to help ensure a safe transfer for Mrs. Adkins?

- You have been assigned to the north hall and have five residents you must assist to the dining room for breakfast. Mr. Ali is recovering nicely from a fractured hip and is eager to walk to the dining room with the aid of his new walker. What words of advice can you give Mr. Ali to help him use his walker more efficiently?

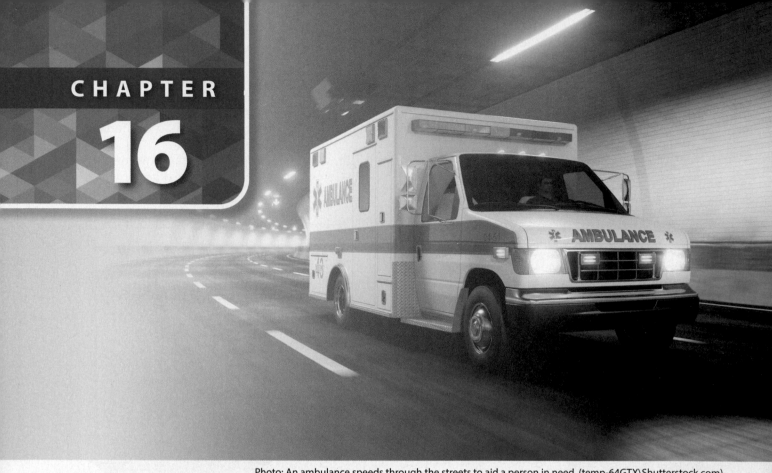

Photo: An ambulance speeds through the streets to aid a person in need. (temp-64GTX\Shutterstock.com)

Basic First Aid and Emergency Care

 WHAT WILL YOU LEARN?

Any condition that requires immediate medical attention to prevent a person from dying or having a permanent disability is an **emergency**. An emergency can occur as a result of an accident (such as a fall) or as a result of a medical condition (such as a heart attack or stroke). Emergency situations can occur anywhere, even in a health care setting. As a nursing assistant, you must be prepared to provide safe, compassionate care for a person in an emergency situation. When you are finished with this chapter, you will be able to:

1. Explain your role in an emergency situation.
2. List and discuss basic life support (BLS) measures.
3. List the signs and symptoms of a "heart attack" and describe the actions that a nursing assistant would take to assist a person with these signs and symptoms.
4. List the signs and symptoms of a stroke.
5. Describe how you would assist a person who complains of feeling faint, or who has fainted.
6. Describe how you would assist a person who is having a seizure.
7. Describe how you would assist a person who is bleeding uncontrollably (hemorrhaging).
8. Describe some of the types and causes of shock and how you would assist a person who is in shock.

9. **Demonstrate how to clear the airway of a choking adult or child older than 1 year by using abdominal or chest thrusts.**

10. **Demonstrate the method used to clear the airway of a choking infant.**

11. **Describe the steps of the chain of survival.**

Vocabulary

Emergency
Oriented to person, place, and time
Disoriented
Unresponsive
Emergency response system
First aid

Respiratory arrest
Cardiac arrest
Basic life support (BLS)
Rescue breathing
Cardiopulmonary resuscitation (CPR)
Automated external defibrillator (AED)

Syncope
Grand mal (tonic–clonic) seizures
Petit mal (absence) seizure
Hemorrhage
Pulse points
Shock

Cardiogenic shock
Hemorrhagic shock
Septic shock
Anaphylactic shock
Aspiration
Chain of survival

RESPONDING TO AN EMERGENCY

As you learned in Chapter 5, the nature of your daily duties will bring you in close and frequent contact with your patients or residents. This unique relationship gives you insight that others might not have. Through your interactions with your patients or residents, you become aware of their individual qualities, personalities, and habits. For example, you know that Ms. Smith typically has an above-average blood pressure reading, even though she is taking medication. You know that Mr. Martinez complains about his arthritis, especially in the morning. You know that Mr. Kim always says that he is starving after eating a full meal. You know which of your patients or residents are "morning people," and which are grumpy and slow until after they have had their first cup of coffee. Your familiarity with your patients or residents makes you more likely to notice when something is not quite right.

For example, the first sign of a stroke is often just a slight slurring of speech or a small change in a person's personality. Heart attacks may be signaled by complaints of fatigue or indigestion. Other emergency situations are recognized by changes in vital signs (such as respiratory rate, heart rate, and blood pressure) or behavior. The people you care for will have varying levels of ability and awareness, and you will come to learn what is normal for each person. A change in a person's usual abilities or level of awareness can be a sign that something is wrong. A person who is usually alert and **oriented to person** (able to tell you who they are and who you are), **place** (able to tell you where they are), and **time** (able to tell you the year,

the day of the week, and the time of day) can suddenly become **disoriented**, or unable to answer those basic questions. A person is said to be **unresponsive** if they are unconscious and cannot be aroused, or conscious but not responsive when spoken to or touched. Either of these conditions should be reported to the nurse immediately. By conscientiously reporting signs or symptoms that seem unusual or give you cause for alarm to the nurse, you may prevent an emergency situation from worsening (Fig. 16-1).

In an emergency situation, your responsibilities as a nursing assistant are clear. You should:

1. **Recognize that an emergency exists.** Use your observation skills and familiarity with the patient or resident to detect changes in behavior or physical condition.

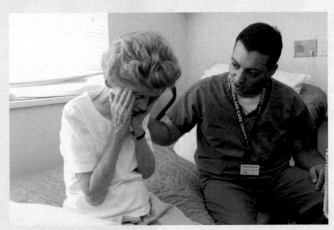

Figure 16-1 Being able to recognize an impending emergency is a life-saving skill.

2. **Decide to act.** Stay calm and organize your thoughts. Check the scene to make sure that you are not entering a situation that is potentially dangerous for you, or for other members of the health care team. For example, a person who has been electrocuted may still be tangled in live electrical wires, which could shock you. Or, you could be entering an area that is contaminated with hazardous materials or gases. Acting hastily can make the problem worse in some situations. For example, someone who has fallen from a ladder may have injuries to the spinal column that would be made worse if the person was moved.

3. **Check for consciousness.** If it is safe to do so, gently shake the person and call to them. The person may have just fainted ("passed out"), in which case you will need to call the nurse for help. Keep the person lying down, and stay with the person until the nurse arrives. The nurse will make sure that no other injuries are present and work to find out why the person fainted. If the person does not respond when you gently shake their arm and call to them, then you will need to . . .

4. **Activate the emergency response system.** An **emergency response system** is a network of resources (including people, equipment, and facilities) that is organized to respond to an emergency. Hospitals typically have a code or procedure for calling for emergency assistance from within the facility. Home health care agencies, assisted-living facilities, and long-term care facilities may require you to dial "911" or some other emergency telephone number. Know your facility's or agency's policy so that you can get help quickly. Early activation of the emergency response system allows a person in an emergency situation to get advanced medical care as soon as possible. This greatly increases the person's chances of survival. When you call, be prepared to give accurate information about your location and the condition of your patient or resident. If you work in a long-term care facility, an assisted-living facility, or for a home health care agency, the people who respond to your call may be emergency medical technicians (EMTs) or paramedics. In an acute care facility, such as a hospital, the people who respond will be a specially trained group of nurses, doctors, and other health care workers, known as the *rapid response team (RRT)*.

5. **Provide appropriate care until the emergency response personnel arrive.** Provide **first aid** (the care given to an injured or sick person while waiting for more advanced help to arrive) according to the situation and your level of training. (As in any situation, you should perform only those procedures that you have been trained to do and that are within your scope of practice.) Speak gently and calmly to the person, and reassure them that more help is on the way.

6. **Record the care you provided.** As always when you provide care, you must accurately record your observations and the care that you provided.

Helping Hands and a Caring Heart

Focus on Humanistic Health Care

An emergency can be very frightening for the person experiencing it. Although you will be focused on the person's physical needs, try not to forget about the other needs that the person and their family members have. Remain calm. Reassure the person and family members that more help is on the way. While the situation may be too serious to say something like, "Everything will be OK," you can certainly tell the person that you will "do everything you can to help."

BASIC LIFE SUPPORT MEASURES

Emergency situations often result when something occurs that affects breathing or circulation. The body's cells need oxygen to live. When we inhale, we take air, which contains oxygen, into our lungs. Once in the lungs, the oxygen in the air passes from the tiny air sacs of the lungs (called the *alveoli*) into the blood in the blood vessels that surround the alveoli. Each time the heart beats, the oxygen-containing blood is sent to all of the cells in the body.

Any process that affects our ability to take air into our lungs or to send oxygen-containing blood to the cells of the body is an emergency. Without oxygen, the cells of the body begin to die. Humans can live for days without food and water but only for a few minutes without oxygen.

Respiratory arrest means that breathing has stopped (*arrest* means "stop"). There are many reasons that a person could stop breathing. Some of these reasons include:

- *Obstructed airway.* The airway could become obstructed by food, loose dentures, a foreign object, or the person's tongue.
- *Stroke or head trauma.* A person who has had a stroke or has fallen and injured their head could stop breathing.

- *Medications.* Some medications, especially narcotic pain medications, can cause a person to stop breathing.
- *Drowning.* Drowning or near-drowning can cause a person to stop breathing.
- *Cardiac arrest.* A person who has had a heart attack or experienced sudden cardiac arrest may not be breathing.
- *Other trauma.* Trauma from an accident, fall, electrocution, seizure, or other condition can cause a person to stop breathing.

When breathing stops, the oxygen content of the blood decreases, and there is not enough oxygen for the cells of the body to function properly. Soon, key organs such as the brain and the heart stop functioning.

A person who is in respiratory arrest may have a heartbeat initially, but if breathing is not started again soon, their heart will stop beating. This condition is called **cardiac arrest**. Cardiac arrest can be the result of prolonged respiratory arrest, or it can occur from other causes. Some of these reasons include:

- *Heart attack.* A person who has a heart attack can go into cardiac arrest.
- *Medication overdoses.* Some medications can cause a person's heart to stop beating.
- *Severe bleeding.* A person who is bleeding profusely (either internally or externally) can go into cardiac arrest if the bleeding is not stopped.
- *Electrocution.* Accidents involving electrical current and severe shock can cause sudden cardiac arrest.
- *Irregular heartbeat (arrhythmia).* The normal electrical signals within the heart can become abnormal resulting in an irregular heartbeat that can cause sudden cardiac arrest. This can also result from changes in the heart muscle itself.

Regardless of the cause of cardiac arrest, it can only be reversed if action is taken quickly to both get the heart started beating again and to correct the underlying cause of cardiac arrest.

Basic life support (BLS) measures are taken to prevent respiratory arrest, cardiac arrest, or both. If the person is already in respiratory or cardiac arrest, BLS is used to keep the person alive until advanced medical assistance arrives. BLS measures include rescue breathing, cardiopulmonary resuscitation (CPR), and the use of an automated external defibrillator (AED).

- In **rescue breathing**, the rescuer blows air into the person's mouth to perform the function of breathing for the person until the person begins breathing again on their own.
- In **cardiopulmonary resuscitation (CPR)**, the rescuer uses a combination of rescue breathing and chest compressions to sustain breathing and circulation for a person who has gone into respiratory or cardiac arrest.
- An **automated external defibrillator (AED)** is a small, portable device that automatically detects a person's heart rhythm and delivers an electrical shock to the heart to stop fast, abnormal heartbeats and restore the heart's normal rhythm. If the facility where you work has an AED, you should know exactly where it is located. Often, the AED is stored in a closet or on a cart with other emergency equipment. In the event of a cardiac emergency, it is important to get the AED to the person as quickly as possible. The person's chances of survival decrease with every minute that passes without its use.

Recent revisions made by the American Heart Association (AHA) have changed the sequence of BLS. You will find the updated 2020 AHA guidelines for BLS in Box 16-1.

Your facility may require first aid and BLS training as a requirement for employment. In some states, first aid and BLS training are provided as part of nursing assistant training. However, because improvements are periodically made in the way some of these techniques, such as CPR, are taught, we have not provided specific instructions for all first aid and BLS techniques in this text. If training in first aid and BLS is not included as part of your nursing assistant training course, you can learn these techniques in courses offered by organizations such as the American Red Cross (ARC), the National Safety Council (NSC), and the AHA. The courses these organizations offer are taught by certified instructors, using approved teaching methods (Fig. 16-2). This additional training will better prepare you for emergency situations that may arise in your workplace, home, or community.

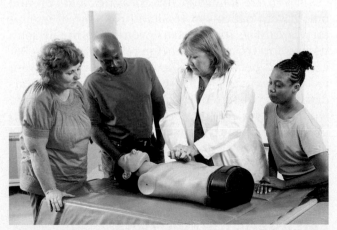

Figure 16-2 Students practice rescue breathing and cardiopulmonary resuscitation (CPR) on a mannequin during a basic life support (BLS) training course. (*Lisa F. Young/ Shutterstock.com*)

Box 16-1 | 2020 American Heart Association Guidelines for BLS[a]

"C" is for "compressions." Initially check for unresponsiveness. If the person is unresponsive, shout for nearby help and active the emergency response services. Check the person's pulse. You can feel an adult's or child's pulse by placing your fingers on either side of the Adam's apple, over the carotid artery in the neck. An infant's pulse is felt over the brachial artery, in the upper arm. A person in an emergency situation may have a rapid, weak, erratic (irregular), or very slow pulse. As you are checking the pulse, also check by looking at the person's chest to see if they are breathing normally. If the person does have a definite pulse but is not breathing normally, you should proceed to open the airway and give one breath every 3 seconds. Recheck the pulse every 2 minutes.

A person with no pulse needs immediate chest compressions and defibrillation. Chest compressions should be started within 10 seconds.

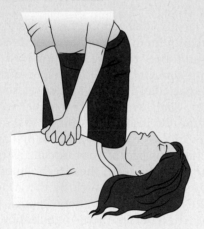

"A" is for "airway." After completing one cycle of 30 chest compressions (100–120 compressions in a minute), open the person's airway by tilting the head back and lifting the chin. This prevents the person's tongue from falling backward against the back of the throat, blocking the flow of air into the lungs.

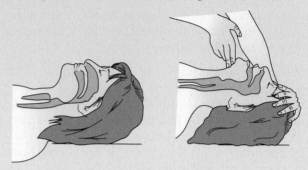

"B" is for "breathing." Give the person two breaths and continue on with chest compressions. You should perform cycles of 30 compressions and 2 breaths. As soon as an AED arrives, it should be used.

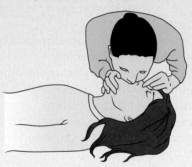

[a]These recommendations by the AHA have changed the sequence of BLS from "ABC" to "CAB," have eliminated the "Look, Listen, and Feel" step, and should be used for all adult and pediatric patients with the exclusion of newborns.

If you are trained in BLS measures and you find one of your patients or residents in a state of respiratory or cardiac arrest, be sure you know the person's wishes for resuscitation before beginning BLS. For example, a person who is terminally ill may not want to be resuscitated if they go into respiratory or cardiac arrest. In this case, the person's medical record would carry a no-code or do not resuscitate (DNR) order. (See Chapter 26, where the subject of advance directives is covered more fully.) If a person is on DNR status, follow your facility's or agency's policy accordingly.

EMERGENCY SITUATIONS

Many different emergency situations can occur, both in the home and community and in the health care setting. In this section, we will review some of the most common emergency situations, as well as what you should do to help a person in one of these situations.

"Heart Attacks" and Strokes

Both heart attacks and strokes can occur suddenly. These are life-threatening situations that require emergency care. Perhaps the classic emergency situation is that of a "heart attack," or myocardial infarction (MI). The myocardium is the muscular wall of the heart. An infarction occurs when blood flow to a part of the body is blocked, depriving the cells of oxygen and causing them to die. So when a person has an MI, blood flow to the muscular wall of the heart is blocked, and part of the heart muscle dies. As a result, the heart is unable to pump blood effectively throughout the body, creating an emergency situation. If the damaged area of the heart is large enough, cardiac arrest can occur. (More information about myocardial infarction can be found in Chapter 32.)

The signs and symptoms of a heart attack can vary greatly from one person to the next. Symptoms can occur suddenly and be intense, or they can start slowly and persist for days or weeks. Signs and symptoms of a heart attack may include:

- Pain, pressure, or tightness in the chest, which may extend to the neck, back, or arm
- Pale or grayish skin
- Excessive sweating
- Trouble breathing
- Nausea or heartburn-like pain
- Fatigue

If you observe that a person is having signs or symptoms of a heart attack, have the person lie down. Raise the person's head to help make breathing easier, and call the nurse or activate the emergency response system immediately. Prompt medical intervention can help minimize damage to the heart muscle. If the person goes into respiratory or cardiac arrest, you will need to begin BLS.

Strokes are also known as "brain attacks" or cerebrovascular accidents (CVAs). A stroke can be caused by a blocked blood vessel in the brain or by a blood vessel that suddenly ruptures. In either circumstance, blood supply to a part of the brain is cut off, causing that part of the brain to die from lack of oxygen. (More information about strokes can be found in Chapter 33.) Like a heart attack, a stroke can cause different signs and symptoms in different people. For example, a stroke might cause only mild physical changes in some people. In others, it might cause loss of consciousness or a coma. Signs and symptoms of a stroke can easily be remembered with "*Spot A Stroke FAST*," published by the American Heart Association, wherein FAST stands for the following:

Face drooping: Does one side of the face droop or is it numb? Ask the person to smile.
Arm weakness: Is one arm weak or numb? Ask the person to raise both arms. Does one arm drift downward?
Speech difficulty: Is speech slurred, are they unable to speak, or are they hard to understand?
Time to call 911: If the person shows any of these symptoms, even if the symptoms go away, call 911 and get them to the hospital immediately.

If you think that a person is having or has had a stroke, report your observations to the nurse and activate the emergency response system. Keep the person lying down and watch for signs of respiratory arrest until advanced care arrives. New advances in the treatment of stroke have resulted in improved outcomes for some patients, especially when treatment is started early.

Fainting (Syncope)

Fainting (**syncope**) occurs when the blood supply to the brain suddenly decreases, resulting in a temporary loss of consciousness. Although fainting may be an early sign of a serious medical condition, such as a heart problem, it can also be the result of hunger ("low blood sugar"), pain, extreme emotion, fatigue, medication side effects, a "stuffy" room (poor ventilation), excessive heat, or standing for a long time. Fainting is not life threatening in and of itself, but because a person who faints is at risk for injury from falling, it is important to act quickly if you believe a person is about to faint. A person who is about to faint may complain of dizziness or a temporary loss of vision. Their skin may be pale and clammy and they may sweat excessively. The person may breathe shallowly, and their pulse may be weak.

If you think that a person is about to faint, have the person lie down in the supine position and elevate their legs 12 inches, or ask them to sit down and bend forward, placing their head between their knees (Fig. 16-3). These actions will increase blood flow to the brain, which may prevent the person from losing consciousness. Loosen any restraints or tight clothing (such as a belt or necktie), and have the person remain in the supine or sitting position

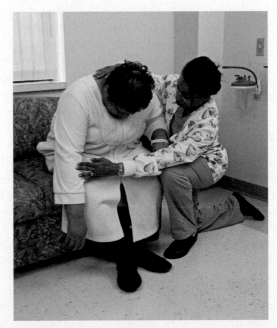

Figure 16-3 Having a person sit with their head between their knees increases blood flow to the brain and may prevent a fainting episode.

Tell the Nurse!

Because fainting may be a sign of a serious medical condition, it is important to report and record the following for the nurse:

- What time the person fainted
- Whether there was a change in the person's level of consciousness, and if so, how long this change lasted
- Whether the person vomited
- The person's appearance at the time of the incident (for example, overheated, pale, sweaty)
- Whether the person complained of anything before the incident (for example, loss of vision, dizziness, nausea)
- The actions you took to assist the person

(with their head between their knees) for at least 5 minutes. Do not leave the person unattended during this time. If necessary, use the call light control to call the nurse.

If a person you are assisting does faint, lower them to the floor or other flat surface, remembering to use good body mechanics (see Chapter 13, Box 13-1). Position the person on their back with their head turned to the side, in case they vomit. If you are sure that the person does not have any injuries to the head, neck, or spinal cord, raise their legs 12 inches, and loosen any tight clothing or restraints. Make sure the person is breathing, and call for help. Then check the person's vital signs. Even if the person recovers from the episode quickly, have them continue to lie down until the nurse arrives.

Seizures

Seizures, also known as *convulsions,* occur when brain activity is interrupted. Seizures can result from head injuries (either recent or past), strokes, infections, high fevers, low blood sugar, poisonings, brain tumors, and epilepsy.

The severity of a seizure can vary. **Grand mal seizures**, also called *tonic–clonic* seizures, are characterized by violent jerking of the muscles all over the body. A person who is having a **petit mal (absence seizure**, however, may simply stop speaking in mid-sentence and stare into space.

Although absence seizures are not an emergency situation, tonic–clonic seizures usually are. Tonic–clonic seizures cause a loss of consciousness and,

because of the violent jerking of the muscles, place the person who is having the seizure at risk for injuring themselves. If a person is standing or sitting when a seizure begins, they could be injured when they fall as the result of losing consciousness. A person who is having a seizure is also at risk for injuring themselves by striking nearby objects or by severely biting their own tongue and lips. A tonic–clonic seizure may last for just a few seconds, or it may go on for as long as 5 to 10 minutes.

First aid for a person having a tonic–clonic seizure involves protecting the person until the seizure is over, and keeping the airway open during the period of unconsciousness afterward. If a person is standing or sitting when a seizure begins, gently help the person to the floor and move furniture or other objects that might cause injury out of the way. Protect the person's head by placing a pillow or folded towel underneath it and call for help while allowing the seizure to run its course. Although in the past, it was common practice to insert a tongue blade into the person's mouth to prevent the person from biting their own tongue, you should not do this. Never attempt to place anything in the person's mouth or between the teeth. You may hurt the person or get bitten. It is common for a person who is having a tonic–clonic seizure to lose control of their bladder or bowels. Because the gag reflex may also be temporarily lost, saliva may pool in the mouth. After the seizure is over, turn the person to their side (place them in the recovery position) and allow any secretions to drain from the mouth to prevent choking. Provide warmth and a quiet environment (Fig. 16-4). A person who has just had a seizure may be very disoriented, tired, or both, and may have no memory of the episode at all.

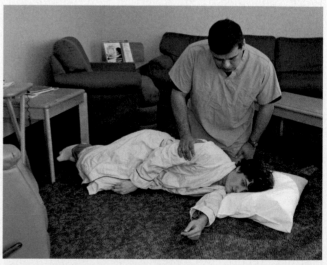

Figure 16-4 After the seizure has passed, place the person in the recovery position and allow secretions to drain from the mouth.

Hemorrhage

Hemorrhage (severe, uncontrolled bleeding) can be caused by trauma to a blood vessel or by certain illnesses, such as gastric ulcers. Ordinarily, when a blood vessel wall is injured, a blood clot forms to prevent the loss of blood. However, if the trauma to the blood vessel wall is major, or if the person lacks the clotting factors needed to form blood clots, the bleeding will not stop. It should be noted that people who are taking medications to prevent blood clotting are at high risk for hemorrhage as well, because the medication decreases the body's normal clotting response.

Hemorrhage can be either external (plainly visible) or internal (occurring within the body). Internal hemorrhage may be hidden unless the person vomits blood or passes blood through the rectum. Hemorrhage can be either venous or arterial, depending on the type of blood vessel that is injured. Venous hemorrhage flows steadily. Arterial hemorrhage spurts or pulses with the heartbeat. If hemorrhage is not controlled quickly, death will result.

If a person is hemorrhaging, call for help and make sure the person is lying down. Take standard precautions to protect yourself from exposure to bloodborne pathogens. Apply firm, steady pressure directly to the wound using a sterile dressing, a clean towel, or whatever else is clean and available for use as a compress. Continue to apply pressure to the wound until more advanced medical help comes. If the direct pressure does not stop or slow the flow of blood, raise the affected body part (if it is an arm or leg) and apply pressure to a pulse point between the wound and the heart. **Pulse points** are the points where large arteries run close enough to the surface of the skin to be felt as a pulse (see Chapter 20, Fig. 20-8). At these points, the artery can be compressed against a bone by applying direct pressure, helping to slow blood loss from a wound. A tourniquet is a device that is placed tightly around an arm or leg to cut off nearly all blood supply. A tourniquet is only used as a last resort to control bleeding, and should always be applied by a specially trained emergency responder.

Shock

Shock results when the organs and tissues of the body do not receive enough oxygen-containing blood. There are many different causes and types of shock. For example:

- **Cardiogenic shock** can occur when the heart is unable to pump enough blood throughout the body to meet the tissues' need for oxygen.
- **Hemorrhagic shock** results from massive blood loss, which means that there is not enough blood in the vessels to supply the tissues of the body.

- **Septic shock** is caused by severe bacterial infections that involve the entire body. The toxins produced by the bacteria cause the blood vessels to dilate (widen), leading to pooling of blood away from the heart and poor circulation.
- **Anaphylactic shock** is caused by a severe allergic reaction (for example, to medications, bee stings, or certain foods, such as nuts). As in septic shock, widening of the blood vessels occurs, causing the blood to pool away from the heart. In addition, the tiniest tubes in the lungs (called bronchioles) close off, preventing the oxygen in the air from passing into the lungs and reaching the blood.

To treat shock, the underlying cause of the shock must be addressed. For example, if a person is in shock because of hemorrhage, the bleeding must be stopped and the fluid replaced intravenously to prevent death. If the pumping action of the heart is too weak or erratic to circulate blood to the organs and tissues, the heart's ability to pump must be restored through medications or other measures, such as the implantation of a pacemaker.

A person entering a state of shock will have low blood pressure that continues to decrease. Their pulse will be rapid and weak. The skin will be cool, clammy, and pale. The person will be confused or disoriented. They will breathe rapidly, and if conscious, may complain of thirst. Make sure that advanced emergency medical care has been called and keep the person warm and calm. The treatment for anaphylactic shock is the immediate administration of a medication called epinephrine (adrenaline). People who know that they are allergic to something that could cause them to go into anaphylactic shock (for example, bee stings) often carry this medication with them (Fig. 16-5). If a person who is in anaphylactic shock is unable to give themselves this medication, someone else will need to.

Foreign-Body Airway Obstruction (FBAO)

Foreign material, such as food, a foreign object, or vomitus, can become lodged in the airway ("windpipe"), blocking the flow of air to the lungs. The accidental inhalation of foreign material into the airway is called **aspiration**. Aspiration is very common during meal times. People with poorly fitting dentures or who are missing teeth cannot chew their food properly, which puts them at risk for aspiration. In addition, talking or laughing with food in the mouth can lead to aspiration.

Children are at high risk for aspiration. Children often do not chew their food well, and they can

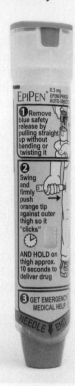

Figure 16-5 The EpiPen Auto-Injector, a self-injectable cartridge of epinephrine, is used to treat anaphylactic shock. (*Amy Kerkemeyer/Shutterstock.com*)

choke on very small pieces of food. Foods that do not usually cause problems for adults, such as hard candies, hot dogs, popcorn, apples, grapes, carrots, and nuts, can be choking hazards for children. Children may put small toys or other objects in their mouths. They often try to eat while running, playing, laughing, or crying. All of these actions increase the risk for aspiration.

People who are not conscious or who have weak coughing or swallowing reflexes as a result of paralysis or the effects of a medication (for example, some pain medications) are also at an increased risk for aspiration. Most people who are vomiting can keep their airway clear and will choke and gag easily, but people with an impaired gag reflex may aspirate vomitus. This is why, when you are assisting a person who is vomiting or at risk for vomiting, you turn the person's head to the side to help keep the airway clear.

An airway obstruction can be either partial or complete. In a partial airway obstruction, the object is not totally blocking the airway and some air can pass through. A person who is coughing strongly and has good skin color most likely has a partial airway obstruction with good air exchange (that is, an adequate ability to breathe). Stay with the person and allow them to continue to cough. If the person is not already sitting up, help them sit up to make breathing

easier. If the person does not quickly cough up the object, call for help because advanced emergency medical assistance may be necessary to remove the item. Also, there is the risk that the item will move and totally obstruct the airway, in which case the person will need immediate assistance. A partial airway obstruction with poor air exchange (that is, an inadequate ability to breathe) is demonstrated by a weak, ineffective coughing effort; high-pitched, "crowing" sounds as the person tries to breathe; and a bluish skin color (cyanosis). A person with this type of airway obstruction needs immediate help.

A complete airway obstruction is one that totally blocks all airflow to the lungs. The person cannot cough, speak, or breathe and will lose consciousness quickly if the object that is blocking airflow is not removed. The person will be frightened, and may run to the bathroom if the obstruction occurs in a public place, such as in a restaurant or dining room. (If you suspect that someone who has left the table is choking, please follow them.) The person may grab their throat in what is considered the universal choking sign (Fig. 16-6).

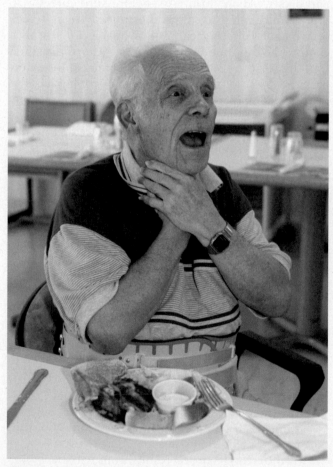

Figure 16-6 Grasping the throat is the universal sign for "I'm choking!"

Clearing the Airway in Adults and Children Older Than 1 Year

Abdominal thrusts, known in the past as the *Heimlich maneuver*, are used to clear an obstructed airway in an adult or a child older than 1 year who is choking. The thoracic (chest) cavity, which contains the heart and lungs, is separated from the abdominal cavity, which contains the stomach and other organs, by the diaphragm, a flat muscle. When performing abdominal thrusts, the area beneath the diaphragm (the abdominal cavity) is compressed, forcing the air out of the lungs. This dislodges the object that is blocking the airway (Fig. 16-7). The procedure for performing abdominal thrusts on a person who is conscious is given in Procedure 16-1. In 2020, the AHA made revisions on how to relieve FBAOs in an unconscious person. The changes have been included in Procedure 16-2.

Abdominal thrusts are done the same way in children older than 1 year and in adults, except that in children, less force is applied to the abdomen. This is to avoid injuring the child's ribs, sternum (breastbone), and internal organs. In people who are pregnant or very heavy, the procedure is modified so that chest thrusts and back blows, rather than abdominal thrusts, are used. This is because in these situations, giving abdominal thrusts would be either impossible or dangerous. In the case of a very heavy person, it is too hard to get your arms around the person. In the case of a pregnant person, applying pressure to the abdomen could harm the baby. Procedure 16-3 explains how to give chest thrusts to both conscious and unconscious people.

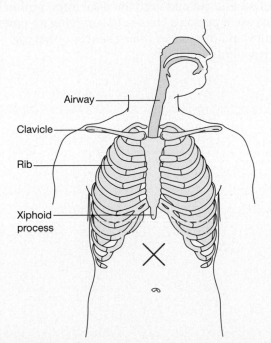

Figure 16-7 Applying pressure to the abdominal cavity (*red X*) forces the air out of the lungs, which in turn forces the object out of the person's airway.

Airway

Clavicle

Rib

Xiphoid process

When a person is choking, the emergency response system should be activated as soon as possible. While you wait for help, perform abdominal thrusts repeatedly, until the airway is open again and the person starts breathing on their own. If the person becomes unresponsive, lower the person to the ground and begin CPR, starting with compressions (do not check for a pulse).

Clearing the Airway in Infants

In children younger than 1 year, abdominal thrusts are not used because of the risk for damaging the baby's internal organs. Instead, a combination of backslaps and chest thrusts is used. Clearing the airway in a conscious infant is described in Procedure 16-4. Clearing the airway in an unconscious infant is described in Procedure 16-5. You can give back blows and chest thrusts while kneeling or sitting.

THE CHAIN OF SURVIVAL

A person's ability to survive an emergency, without any permanent damage, relies on a series of events called the **chain of survival:**

1. Someone must recognize that an emergency situation exists and activate the emergency response system.
2. First responder care (basic first aid, including BLS with rapid defibrillation if applicable) must be given by able people at the scene of the emergency.
3. Advanced medical intervention, such as that provided by an EMT, a paramedic, a nurse, or a doctor, must be provided as soon as possible.
4. After the immediate crisis passes, hospital care may be needed to help the person survive. As the person's condition improves, they may be transferred to a subacute care unit or return to a long-term care facility or private home for further recovery.
5. Rehabilitation, the final step in the chain of survival, focuses on improving the general health status of the person. One goal of rehabilitation may be to help the person to recover abilities that may have been lost as a result of the emergency. For example, a person who has suffered a stroke may need to relearn skills such as walking or speaking. Another goal of rehabilitation may be to help the person learn how to prevent further progression of a disease. For example, a person who has had a heart attack may be taught new diet management skills and started on an exercise program.

As a nursing assistant, you can play a vital role in helping to see a person through the immediate crisis (steps 1 and 2). You may also care for someone who is in the recovery phase (steps 4 and 5).

SUMMARY

- An emergency is any situation in which a person needs immediate medical attention to prevent death or permanent disability. Emergencies can result from medical conditions (such as a heart attack or stroke) or from an accident (such as a fall).

  - Knowing your patient's or resident's usual condition may help you recognize a potential emergency. By communicating your observations to the nurse, you could prevent the emergency from getting worse.

  - In an emergency situation, you will be responsible for (1) recognizing that an emergency exists, (2) deciding to act, (3) checking for consciousness, (4) activating the facility's emergency response system, (5) providing appropriate care per your training and scope of practice until the emergency personnel arrive, and (6) recording your observations and the care you provided.

- The AHA guidelines for BLS involve checking the person's pulse to make sure the heart is beating and blood is circulating throughout the body, and making sure that the person is breathing.

  - BLS measures include rescue breathing, CPR, and the early use of an AED.

  - Training in first aid and BLS measures, whether required by your employer or not, will prepare you for emergency situations in your workplace, home, or community.

- Common emergency situations include heart attacks and strokes, fainting, seizures, hemorrhage, shock, and FBAO.

  - Early recognition of the signs of a heart attack or stroke is very important so that prompt treatment can be used to help minimize damage to the heart or brain.

  - Although fainting is not life threatening, it could put the person at risk for injury from falling. If a person complains of feeling faint, have them lie down or place their head between their knees to increase blood flow to the brain.

  - First aid for a person having a seizure involves protecting them from injury during the seizure and keeping the airway open after the seizure.

  - Hemorrhage is controlled by applying direct pressure to the wound or a pulse point between the wound and the heart.

  - Shock results when the organs and tissues of the body do not receive enough oxygen-rich blood. Keep a person who is in shock warm and calm until emergency personnel arrive.

  - Airway obstructions block the flow of oxygen into the lungs and if not cleared can quickly result in death.

- Skilled first aid and early medical intervention increase a person's chance of surviving an emergency and minimizes their chances of having permanent disabilities.

Procedure 16-1

Relieving Foreign-Body Airway Obstruction in Conscious Adults and Children Older Than 1 Year

WHY YOU DO IT   If the object is not removed from the airway, allowing air to get to the lungs, the person will die.

1. Check the person's ability to breathe and speak by tapping them on the shoulder and saying, "Are you okay? Can you talk? I can help you." A person who cannot breathe or speak needs immediate help.

2. If the person starts to cough, wait and see whether the coughing will dislodge the object. If the person's cough is weak and ineffective, or if the person is in obvious distress, continue with step 3.

3. Stay with the person and call for help. Have the person who is helping you activate the facility's emergency response system.

4. Stand behind the person with the obstructed airway and wrap your arms around their waist. The person may be sitting or standing.

5. Make a fist with one hand and place the thumb of the fist against the person's abdomen, just above the navel and below the sternum (breastbone). Grasp your fist with the other hand. (Do not tuck your thumb inside your fist.)

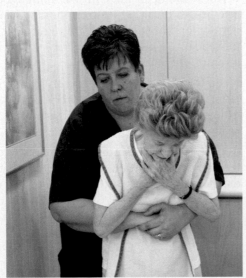

STEP 5 Place your fist just above the person's navel and below the sternum.

6. Being careful not to put pressure on the person's ribs or sternum with your forearms, press your fist inward and pull upward, using quick thrusting motions, until the object is expelled, the person begins to cough forcefully, or the person loses consciousness. (Give each thrust with the intent of relieving the obstruction.) If you have difficulty administering abdominal thrusts, or if the object is not expelled quickly, alternate giving 5 abdominal thrusts with 5 back blows between the shoulder blades with the heel of your hand.

   a. If the object is expelled, stay with the person, and follow the nurse's directions.

   b. If the person begins to cough, wait and see whether the coughing results in expulsion of the object. If it does not, continue giving abdominal thrusts.

   c. If the person loses consciousness, lower the person to the floor and begin Procedure 16-2, beginning with step 6.

7. The person should be evaluated by a doctor following the choking incident.

8. Record your observations and actions according to your facility's policy.

Procedure 16-2

Relieving a Foreign-Body Airway Obstruction in Unconscious Adults and Children Older Than 1 Year

WHY YOU DO IT   If the object is not removed from the airway, allowing air to get to the lungs, the person will die.

1. **Responsiveness:** Check the person's state of consciousness by gently shaking or tapping them. Quickly check to see if the person is breathing (at least 5 seconds, but no more than 10 seconds).

2. Stay with the person and call for help. Have the person who is helping you activate the facility's emergency response system.

3. Check for a pulse (no more than 10 seconds). If there is no pulse, go on to step 6.

4. **Rescue breathing:** If you feel a definite pulse, open the airway, using a head tilt–chin lift maneuver, and deliver one breath into the person's mouth through a ventilation barrier device. Deliver enough air into the person to make the person's chest rise.

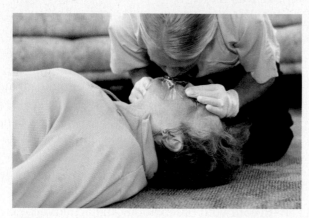

STEP 4 Rescue breathing.

5. If the chest does not rise, repeat the head tilt–chin lift maneuver and give a second breath. If you are unable to ventilate the person after two attempts, promptly begin chest compressions.

6. Chest compressions: If the person does not have a pulse, or if you are unable to ventilate the person after two attempts, begin chest compressions. To give chest compressions:

   a. Kneel beside the person.

   b. Place the heel of your hand closest to the person's head on their sternum (breastbone) and place your other hand on top and interlock your fingers.

   c. Position your body forward so that your shoulders are over the center of the person's chest and your arms are straight. You will want to compress straight down and up. Do not rock back and forth.

   d. **Push hard, push fast:** Compress the chest at a rate of at least 100–120 compressions per minute with a depth of at least 2 inches for adults and approximately 2 inches for children. Allow the chest to recoil completely after each compression.

7. After you have given 30 chest compressions, quickly open the person's mouth wide and look for the object. If you see an object that can easily be removed, remove it with your fingers.

8. Perform the head tilt–chin lift maneuver. Blow one breath into the person's mouth through a ventilation barrier device. If the air does not go in, repeat the head tilt–chin lift maneuver and attempt one breath again.

9. If the breath does not go in, continue with the chest compressions, object check, and ventilation attempt cycle until the obstruction has been relieved or advanced help arrives.

10. Repeat the chest compression–object check–rescue breathing sequence until the object is expelled, rescue breathing is successful, or other trained personnel arrive and take over.

Procedure 16-3

Performing Chest Thrusts in Conscious Adults and Children Older Than 1 Year

WHY YOU DO IT   If the object is not removed from the airway, allowing air to get to the lungs, the person will die.

If the Person Is Conscious

1. Stand behind the person and place your arms under the person's armpits and around their chest.

2. Make a fist with one hand and place the thumb of the fist against the center of the person's sternum. Be sure that your thumb is centered on the sternum, not on the lower tip of the sternum (the xiphoid process) and not on the ribs.

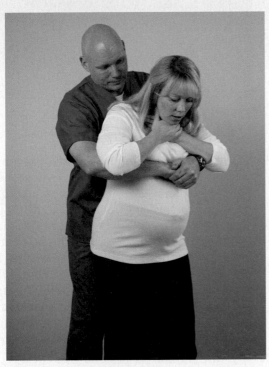

STEP 2 Place your fist over the person's sternum.

3. Give up to five quick chest thrusts by grasping your fist with your other hand and pressing inward five times. Each thrust should compress the chest at least 2 inches. Then deliver 5 back blows with the heel of your hand between the person's shoulder blades.

4. Continue to alternate giving chest thrusts and back blows until the object is expelled, the person begins to cough forcefully, or the person loses consciousness.

   a. If the object is expelled, stay with the person, and follow the nurse's directions.

   b. If the person begins to cough, wait and see whether the coughing results in expulsion of the object. If it does not, continue giving chest thrusts in groups of five.

   c. If the person loses consciousness, lower the person to the floor and begin Procedure 16-2, beginning with step 6.

5. The person should be evaluated by a doctor following the choking incident.

6. Record your observations and actions according to facility policy.

Procedure 16-4

Relieving a Foreign-Body Airway Obstruction in a Conscious Infant

WHY YOU DO IT   If the object is not removed from the airway, allowing air to get to the lungs, the infant will die.

1. Check the infant's ability to breathe and cry. An infant who cannot breathe or cry needs immediate help.

2. Stay with the infant. Call for help and have the person who is helping you activate the emergency response system.

3. Kneel or sit with the infant in your lap.

4. Hold the infant facedown with the head lower than the chest, resting on your forearm. Rest your forearm on your lap or thigh and support the infant's head and jaw with your hand. Be careful to not put pressure on the soft tissues of the infant's throat.

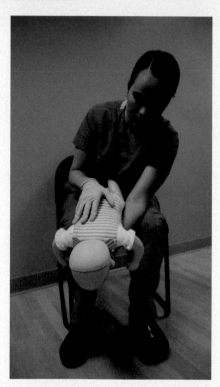

STEP 4 Hold the infant facedown with the head lower than the chest.

5. Give up to five backslaps forcefully (between the infant's shoulder blades), using the heel of your hand. Be sure that you continue to support the infant's head and neck by firmly holding the baby's jaw between your thumb and forefinger.

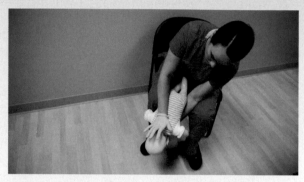

STEP 5 Use the heel of your hand to deliver backslaps while supporting the infant's head and neck.

6. If the backslaps do not dislodge the foreign object, you must turn the infant over in preparation for administering chest thrusts. Turn the infant over by placing your free hand and forearm along the infant's head and back so that the infant is sandwiched between your hands and forearms. Continue to support the infant's head between your thumb and forefinger from the front, while you cradle the back of the head in the palm of your other hand. Turn the infant onto their back. Lower your arm onto your thigh so that the infant's head is lower than the chest.

7. To locate the correct place to give chest thrusts, imagine a line running across the infant's chest between the nipples. Place the pads of your first two fingers on the infant's sternum (breastbone), right below this imaginary line. If you feel the notch at the end of the infant's sternum, move your fingers toward the infant's head so that your fingers are over the center of the sternum.

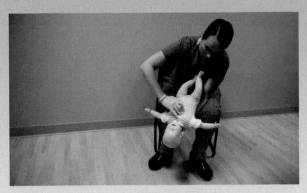

STEP 7 Place the pads of your first two fingers on the infant's sternum to give chest thrusts.

8. Perform up to five quick chest thrusts at the rate of about 1 per second, compressing the sternum approximately 1½ inches.

9. Repeat the backslap–chest thrust sequence until the foreign body is expelled, the infant begins to cough forcefully, or the infant loses consciousness.

   a. If the foreign body is expelled, stay with the infant, and follow the nurse's directions.

   b. If the infant begins to cough, wait and see if the coughing results in expulsion of the object. If it does not, continue giving five backslaps followed by five chest thrusts.

   c. If the infant loses consciousness, initiate Procedure 16-5, beginning with step 4.

10. The infant should be evaluated by a doctor following the choking incident.

11. Record your observations and actions according to facility policy.

 Procedure 16-5

Relieving a Foreign-Body Airway Obstruction in an Unconscious Infant

WHY YOU DO IT   If the object is not removed from the airway, allowing air to get to the lungs, the infant will die.

1. Check the infant's responsiveness by gently shaking the infant and speaking to them. An unresponsive infant needs immediate help. If there is no response and no breathing or only gasping, shout for help.

2. Stay with the infant and have anyone who responds to your shout activate the emergency response system.

3. Place the infant on a flat surface and check the infant's pulse by finding the brachial artery located on the inside of their upper arm. Check for a pulse for at least 5 seconds but no more than 10 seconds.

4. If there is no pulse, or if the pulse rate is less than 60 beats per minute, place your first two fingers in the middle of the infant's sternum, just below the nipple line and begin chest compressions. Push hard and fast, compressing the infant's sternum down at least one third the depth of the chest (approximately 1½ inches), at a rate of at least 100–120 compressions per minute.

5. After delivering 30 chest compressions, open the infant's airway by tilting the head back slightly and lifting the chin until the infant's nose points toward the ceiling. Look for the object in the back of the throat. If you see an object you can easily remove, remove it.

6. Maintaining the head tilt–chin lift maneuver to keep the airway open, cover the infant's nose and mouth with your mouth or an airway device and blow two slow breaths into the infant's mouth, removing your mouth and inhaling between each breath. You should see the infant's chest rise with each breath.

7. If the chest does not rise, repeat the head tilt–chin lift maneuver and attempt to deliver breaths again.

8. If the chest still does not rise, repeat steps 4 through 7 until the foreign object is expelled, rescue breathing is successful, or other trained personnel arrive and take over.

9. The infant should be evaluated by a doctor following the choking incident.

10. Record your observations and actions according to facility policy.

WHAT DID YOU LEARN?

Multiple Choice

Select the single best answer for each of the following questions.

1. A person with an airway obstruction will usually:
   a. Have a seizure
   b. Vomit
   c. Be able to speak and breathe normally
   d. Clutch at their throat

2. The first step in the chain of survival is:
   a. Rehabilitation
   b. Recognizing that an emergency exists and calling for help
   c. Giving first aid
   d. Initiating basic life support (BLS) measures

3. In the guidelines for BLS, the "C" stands for:
   a. Cardiac
   b. Consciousness
   c. Compressions
   d. Check for bleeding

4. You are helping to prepare a holiday dinner at your mother's house, when suddenly your sister misses the vegetable she is trying to slice and cuts deeply into her finger instead. Blood is spurting from the cut, which indicates to you that your sister:
   a. Is hemorrhaging internally
   b. Has cut a vein
   c. Has cut an artery
   d. Requires the application of a tourniquet

5. Where do you place your fist while clearing an obstructed airway in a conscious adult?
   a. On the person's back
   b. Above the person's navel
   c. On the person's chest
   d. Below the person's navel

6. If a person with a partial FBAO is coughing but able to breathe, you should:
   a. Administer oxygen
   b. Use a finger sweep to remove the object that is obstructing the person's airway
   c. Perform abdominal thrusts
   d. Stay with the person and allow them to continue coughing

7. Which is a sign or symptom of shock?
   a. Low blood pressure
   b. A weak, rapid pulse
   c. Cool, clammy, pale skin
   d. All of the above

8. Which of the following actions should you take to assist a person who is having a grand mal seizure?
   a. Protect the person's head by placing a pillow underneath it
   b. Clear the area by moving furniture out of the way
   c. Avoid placing anything in the person's mouth
   d. All of the above

Matching *Match each numbered item with its appropriate lettered description.*

_____ **1.** Emergency response system

_____ **2.** First aid

_____ **3.** Basic life support (BLS)

_____ **4.** Hemorrhage

_____ **5.** Respiratory arrest

_____ **6.** Cardiac arrest

_____ **7.** Grand mal (tonic-clonic) seizure

_____ **8.** Petit mal (absence) seizure

_____ **9.** Anaphylactic shock

_____ **10.** Fainting (syncope)

a. Occurs when the blood supply to the brain suddenly decreases, resulting in a loss of consciousness

b. Severe bleeding

c. Breathing has stopped

d. A potentially deadly allergic reaction (for example, to a bee sting or certain foods, such as nuts)

e. Heart has stopped

f. Care given to an injured person before more advanced medical assistance arrives

g. A network of resources, including people, equipment, and facilities, that is organized to respond to an emergency

h. The person stares off into space or stops speaking for a moment

i. Measures taken to prevent respiratory arrest, cardiac arrest, or both

j. Generalized and violent contraction and relaxation of the body's muscles

STOP *and* THINK!

- You work as a nursing assistant in a nursing home. One of your responsibilities is to check on the residents while the nurses are attending the change-of-shift report. You enter Mrs. Oblonsky's room and find her on the floor. She has no roommate, so no one witnessed what happened. It does not appear that Mrs. Oblonsky fell out of bed. Her color is pale, and her lips are turning blue. What should you do first?

- One of your responsibilities is to oversee the residents of the long-term care facility where you work while they are in the recreation room. Today, the residents are gathered and getting ready for an activity. Everyone is busy talking, selecting teams, and generally having fun. Everyone, that is, except for Mr. Grant. Normally outgoing and friendly, today Mr. Grant is just sitting in his wheelchair, staring into space without moving. You speak to Mr. Grant and notice that he seems confused and is having difficulty forming his words. The left side of his mouth looks droopy and he's drooling a bit. These observations may be signs of what emergency situation? What should you do?

Respect

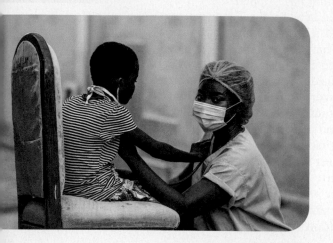

My name is Lacindra and I have been working as a CNA for about 10 years. I have worked in both long-term and acute care settings and I love what I do! When my church decided to go on a medical and dental mission, I was one of the first to volunteer. I could hardly wait for the experience to go to another country and help others in need.

As we planned for our trip, we learned some basic Spanish, the language spoken in the small Caribbean village we were planning to visit. None of us mastered it very well, but fortunately we had medical interpreters going with us to help. The day finally arrived, and we set up a little clinic in a small mobile home next to an elementary school. Most of the homes the residents lived in nearby lacked plumbing and electricity. The people, however, were so welcoming. Many stood in line for hours to be seen in our clinic. I loved the children most, who laughed at our attempts to speak their language and helped us learn to communicate with them better.

One day, as we were working, I looked out the window and saw a woman carrying a limp child running toward us across the school yard. I met her at the door, took the little boy, and tried to find the words to ask what was wrong. Fortunately, the children had taught us the word for lollipop (since we had brought them to give as treats), and I heard the mother keep saying that word and pointing to her throat. It was then that I realized that her child had aspirated a piece of candy. I acted automatically by giving a couple of chest compressions, and the candy flew out of his mouth. His eyes opened and he started crying! I think I was crying too as we checked him over and made sure that he was okay. As we handed him back to his mother, she kept saying gracias, gracias, over and over again. Even if I hadn't learned the meaning of that word, my heart certainly understood what she was saying.

Working and providing care for the people in this small village impacted my life in a way that no other experience has. It helped me realize that happiness has nothing to do with what we have, it has everything to do with sharing yourself with others. It helped me learn to respect and communicate with others of different backgrounds more deeply. In this case, it even helped save a life!

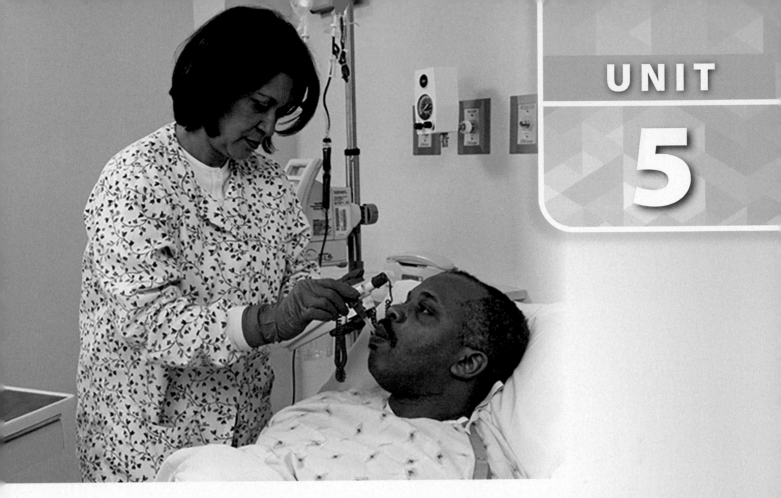

Basic Patient and Resident Care

YOU MAY HAVE CHOSEN TO PURSUE A CAREER as a nursing assistant for many reasons, but chances are good that at least one of those reasons had to do with a desire to help and care for others. As a nursing assistant, you will have the chance to fulfill this desire many times over! In Unit 5, we will explore the skills and responsibilities that form the basis for the daily care you will provide for your patients and residents.

Photo: Measuring vital signs is a skill you will use every day.

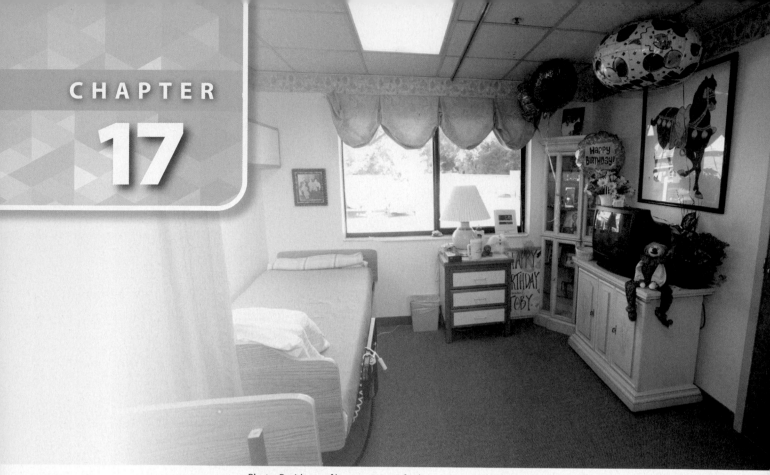

Photo: Residents of long-term care facilities are encouraged to make their rooms as "home-like" as possible.

The Patient or Resident Environment

 WHAT WILL YOU LEARN?

Have you ever moved into a new house or apartment? If so, you probably remember how strange the place felt, until you managed to get some boxes unpacked and make it your own. After you had added your own personal touch, even if it was just to hang a picture, then the place probably felt more like "home." For a person who is entering a health care facility, whether just for a few nights' stay or for the rest of their life, the idea of "home" takes on a whole new meaning. Suddenly, "home" may only be one room, or even half of one room, and everything that the person has always associated with "home" is gone, except for perhaps a few select items. Items that were never part of the person's home environment before, such as special beds and medical equipment, may now be present. In this chapter, we will take a closer look at the physical environment in a health care facility, and how that environment can affect a person's well-being. We will also provide an overview of the standard equipment and furniture that are typically found in a patient's or resident's room. When you are finished with this chapter, you will be able to:

1. Describe the types of rooms and areas that are commonly found in different health care settings.
2. List the Omnibus Budget Reconciliation Act (OBRA) regulations related to the physical environment in long-term care facilities.

3. Discuss the importance of allowing a person to have and display personal items.

4. Explain your role in helping to keep the patient's or resident's environment clean and comfortable.

5. Describe the standard equipment and furniture found in a person's room in a health care facility.

6. Explain the importance of adapting the environment to meet the individual needs of a patient or resident and how to make modifications.

Vocabulary

Unit

Hopper

Ventilation system

General lighting

Task lighting

Gatches

Trendelenburg position

Reverse Trendelenburg position

Over-bed table

Call light system

THE PATIENT OR RESIDENT UNIT

In Chapter 1, you learned about the many different types of health care facilities, such as hospitals, long-term care facilities, and assisted-living facilities. You also learned that some people receive health care in their homes, from home health care agencies or hospice organizations. A patient's or resident's room, also referred to as a patient's or resident's **unit**, will vary in the way it is set up according to the type of facility and the needs of the person. However, no matter what form the person's room takes—whether it is a single room, a room shared with a roommate, or an apartment-like suite of rooms—the room is considered the person's home.

Hospitals

Several different types of rooms are usually found within a hospital (Fig. 17-1). Patients who are recovering from an illness or surgery will most likely stay in private, single-occupancy rooms. Patients who are very ill usually have private rooms in the intensive care unit (ICU) or critical care unit (CCU). These rooms contain special equipment that helps the health care team monitor and care for very ill patients. On the maternity ward, new mothers and babies may receive care before, during, and after the birthing process in a room called a birthing suite. A birthing suite is typically very home-like, with curtains, attractive furniture, and attractive cabinets that contain monitoring equipment and an entertainment center. Other special accommodations include an attached room for waiting family members, a special bed designed to

make the process of labor and delivery easier, and possibly even a whirlpool bath! Some hospitals, rehabilitation, and long-term care facilities have subacute care (skilled nursing) units for patients who are not quite well enough to go home but not quite sick enough to be in a typical hospital room. The subacute care unit is usually designed to be more home-like and may include a common (communal) dining room and activity rooms for the patients.

All patient rooms have some form of bathroom. However, the setup varies according to the type of room. Usually, the bathroom is attached to the patient's room and will include a shower or bathtub, a toilet, and a sink. Some attached bathrooms may contain only a sink and a toilet, with communal bathing facilities located down the hall. The bathrooms in health care facilities usually have special features, such as handrails and a toilet that is higher than a regular toilet, to help people who may be unsteady or have limited mobility. There may also be more "open space," to accommodate a wheelchair. Finally, there will be a call light or an intercom system to ensure that a person can obtain help if necessary (Fig. 17-2).

Long-Term Care Facilities

As you will recall, long-term care facilities provide care for people who are not able to care for themselves independently. In most cases, a person moving into a long-term care facility is making a permanent move into what is truly a new home. For most people, moving into a long-term care facility represents a major change. For example, a person who once enjoyed an apartment or home with several rooms would now have to adjust

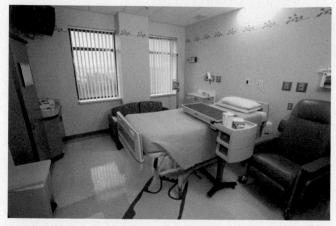

A. Typical hospital room

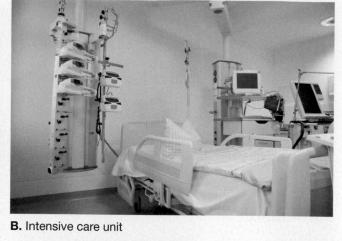

B. Intensive care unit

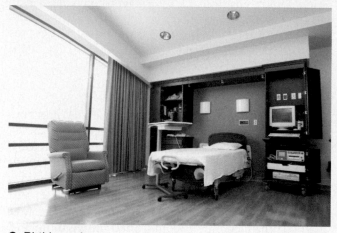

C. Birthing suite

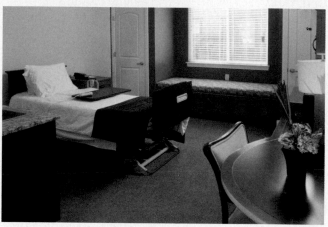

D. Sub-acute care unit

Figure 17-1 Patient rooms in the hospital vary, depending on the needs of the patient. **A.** A typical hospital room. **B.** A room in the intensive care unit (ICU). **C.** A birthing suite in the maternity ward. **D.** A room in the subacute care unit. (*B, Daniel Donciu\Shutterstock.com*)

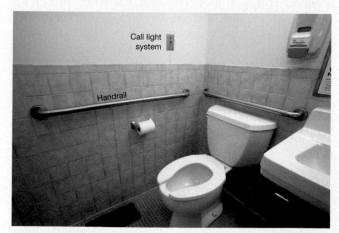

Call light system

Handrail

Figure 17-2 Most bathrooms in health care facilities have modifications for people who have trouble with mobility. For example, the bathroom usually has handrails, an elevated toilet, or both to make it easier for a person to get up and sit down. The bathroom also has a call light or intercom system, so that a person can call for help if necessary.

to living in a single room, possibly with a roommate. To help ease the transition, people who are moving into a long-term care facility are usually allowed to furnish their rooms with one or two favorite pieces of furniture and various personal items (Fig. 17-3).

Many residents bring their own bedspreads or comforters to make up the standard facility bed. They may have their own clothing, jewelry, books, and favorite wall hangings. Some residents bring a television, a stereo, or even a personal computer to their new home, and many have a private telephone line installed in their rooms so that they can keep in touch with loved ones and friends. You may see plants, drawings from grandchildren, and maybe even a small pet, such as a bird or fish, in your residents' rooms!

Each room in a long-term care facility may have a full private bath, consisting of a shower or tub, a toilet, and a sink. Or it may have a partial bath, consisting of a toilet and a sink that is shared between two

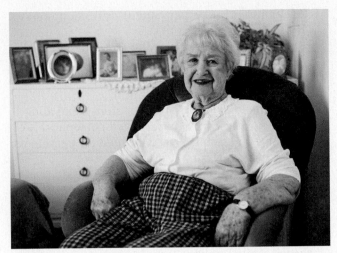

Figure 17-3 People moving into a long-term care facility are often encouraged to bring one or two favorite pieces of furniture, as well as small decorative items, to furnish their new home.

rooms. In this case, a communal bath area, designed to accommodate the bathing of several residents at the same time, is located down the hall. Like a bathroom in a patient room, a bathroom in a resident room will have special modifications, such as handrails and a means of calling for help.

In addition to resident rooms, long-term care facilities usually have common rooms where residents gather to socialize, such as the dining room, day (or activity) rooms, and a small chapel where religious services are held. Long-term care facilities may also be designed with patios and gardens to allow the residents access to outdoor activities (Fig. 17-4).

Assisted-Living Facilities

Assisted-living facilities are a type of long-term care facility. However, the residents of assisted-living facilities are usually still somewhat independent. In assisted-living facilities, the word "unit" usually refers to the individual resident's living quarters. Residents of assisted-living facilities often live in small apartments that have a kitchen or kitchenette, a bathroom, a living area, and a bedroom (Fig. 17-5). In other assisted-living facilities, residents live in suites consisting of a private bedroom and bath, with communal dining and activity rooms. Some units may also provide private access to a balcony or patio. As in a nursing home, bathing facilities (a tub, shower, or both) might be included in the resident's private bathroom, or they may be located down the hall and shared by many residents. Communal bathing rooms are equipped with privacy stalls or curtains to allow several residents to bathe at the same time.

Many of the same areas for staff use that are found in the nursing home setting are present in the assisted-living setting as well. However, these areas are usually not as prominent because residents of assisted-living facilities do not require the same level of nursing and medical care. For example, while nursing homes must have a prominent nurses' station on each unit, an assisted-living facility may have only one health center or nursing office in the building.

Concerns for Long-Term Care

Although the long-term care facility is a health care facility, it is also the resident's home. OBRA requires that the facility provide a

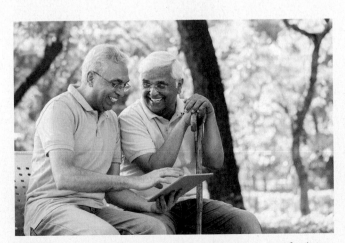

Figure 17-4 The living spaces in long-term care facilities are designed to enrich the daily lives of residents. These residents are enjoying nature and the opportunity to socialize in this pleasant outdoor space. (*IndianFaces\Shutterstock.com*)

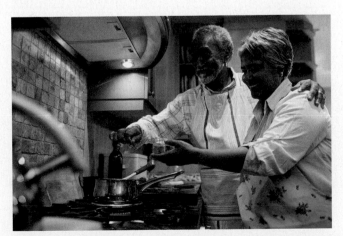

Figure 17-5 Residents of assisted-living facilities may have an apartment with a kitchen. (*wavebreakmedia\Shutterstock.com*)

home-like environment that reflects the individuality of each resident and minimizes the institutional nature of the setting to the best extent possible. OBRA regulations protect each resident's right to personalize their own living space and to have and to use personal items. Personal items help to create a living space that is as home-like as possible for the resident and foster the resident's sense of independence and individuality. You should help your residents to decorate their rooms according to their own individual taste and preference while making sure that they stay within the safety standards established by OBRA and your facility.

Home Health Care

Some people receive health care services in their homes. Usually in this situation, the person's bedroom, living room, or dining room becomes the patient care unit (Fig. 17-6). The home health care setting is discussed in more detail in Unit 10.

Staff Work Areas

In addition to patient and resident rooms, both acute care and long-term care facilities have similar work areas for staff use:

- The *nurses' station* serves as the central base of operations for the nursing staff. Staff members use the nurses' station to complete documentation and charting, receive and make telephone calls, and monitor activity in that particular care area. The nurses' station is usually centrally located because staff members must be able to

see hallways and other patient or resident areas from the station.
- The *medication room* is used to store medications and the supplies for administering medications. The medication room is often part of, or located very close to, the nurses' station.
- The *clean utility room* is used to store clean and sterile supplies, such as packaged personal care products and supplies used for medical treatments and procedures.
- The *soiled utility room* is where dirty items are handled or stored. Bins for trash and soiled linens are usually found here. This is also the room where used equipment (such as a bedside commode) is placed until it can be cleaned and disinfected. Soiled utility rooms often have a **hopper**, a sink-like fixture that flushes like a toilet and is connected to a sewer line. The hopper is used for tasks such as cleaning bedpans and rinsing clothing or linens that have been soiled with feces. In many facilities, liquids that contain body fluids (such as drainage emptied from a wound drainage device) are disposed of in the hopper.
- The *nourishment room* is where snacks and beverages are stored and prepared for patients and residents. The nourishment room is equipped with a refrigerator and freezer for items like milk, juice, and ice cream. Other basic equipment usually include a microwave, toaster, coffee maker, and ice machine. Many facilities keep a selection of fruits, cookies, crackers, cereal, and beverage supplies (such as tea bags, hot chocolate mix, and creamer) there for patient and resident use as well. Supplies for serving snacks (such as cups, spoons, and straws) are also kept in the nourishment room.

ENSURING COMFORT

Environmental conditions, such as a room's cleanliness, temperature, noise level, and quality of light, affect how we feel. Imagine what it would be like if you were confined to bed in a dirty room, or one that smelled bad or was too hot or too noisy or too dark. To enhance the comfort and well-being of patients and residents, hospitals and long-term care facilities have policies designed to regulate the environment within the health care facility. In long-term care facilities, these policies are set by OBRA regulations and enforced by CMS (see Chapter 7). Facilities that receive federal funding from Medicare must follow these regulations. ☑ The following aspects of the resident's environment are regulated by OBRA:

- The size of the room
- The lighting that must be available

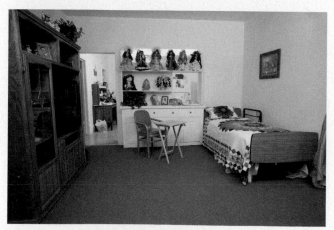

Figure 17-6 When a person is receiving health care at home from a home health care agency, the bedroom, living room, or dining room becomes the person's "unit."

- The temperature at which the facility must be maintained
- The measures that must be taken to maintain air quality
- The measures that must be taken to control noise
- The types of furnishings and equipment that must be present
- The types of modifications to the room that must be present to ensure safety (such as handrails and a call light or intercom system in the bathroom)
- The minimal amount of personal space for storage of belongings that each resident is allowed to have
- The ability to provide privacy for each resident

Cleanliness

Cleanliness is essential for controlling the spread of infection and odors. In addition, a facility's cleanliness and overall appearance is something that people who are receiving health care at the facility, as well as their family members and other visitors, notice. The appearance of the facility is a reflection on the quality of service provided. To make a good impression, a facility does not need to be new or filled with state-of-the-art equipment, but it does need to be kept clean and neat.

Each member of the health care team is responsible for keeping the facility clean (Fig. 17-7). The housekeeping or custodial staff does major, routine cleaning of the facility (such as mopping floors,

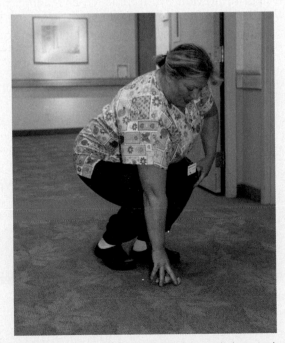

Figure 17-7 Keeping the facility neat and clean is the responsibility of each member of the health care team.

emptying waste containers, and cleaning bathrooms). However, each member of the health care team also has specific duties related to maintaining cleanliness. For example, nursing assistants are responsible for changing the bed linens according to facility policy. In addition, if you notice something out of place, then it is your responsibility to correct the problem. For example, if you notice something spilled on the floor or a countertop, you should wipe it up. If you see a piece of trash on the floor, you should pick it up and dispose of it properly. If you notice that there is an ongoing problem, such as wastebaskets not being emptied or bathrooms not being cleaned properly, you should report this observation to the nurse, so that they can follow up with the appropriate people.

In the long-term care setting, nursing assistants are responsible for helping residents keep their personal belongings neat and clean. We all have the tendency to accumulate things over time. Periodically, you may have to help your residents go through their belongings and either put them away neatly or dispose of them. Excessive clutter makes it difficult to keep the room clean and can be a safety hazard. Residents, visitors, or staff members can trip over objects left in pathways. An excessively crowded room can also make it difficult to exit the room safely and quickly in the event of an emergency, such as a fire.

Odor Control

There are many potential sources of bad odors in a health care setting. The smell of vomit (emesis), wound drainage, urine, or feces can make any environment unpleasant! However, there are things you can do to help minimize odors and maintain a pleasant environment:

- Follow your facility's policy regarding the handling of waste and soiled linens.
- Keep the lids on laundry and waste receptacles closed.
- Empty and clean emesis basins, urinals, bedside commodes, and bedpans promptly.
- Use a facility-approved air freshener when appropriate.
- Assist your patients and residents with routine personal care. Clean skin and good oral hygiene are essential for controlling odors.
- Pay attention to your personal hygiene (see Chapter 3). Scented products, such as cologne, aftershave, or perfume, can be nice, but they must be used sparingly. If you apply too much, the scent may be overpowering, and many people are sensitive to strong scents. If you are a smoker, be aware that the odors from smoking can cling to your clothes and hair and are

considered unpleasant by many people. Make sure you wash your hands after smoking and use a mint or breath freshener before continuing your patient or resident care duties.

Ventilation

A **ventilation system** provides fresh air and keeps air circulating. A well-functioning ventilation system is essential for carrying away unpleasant odors, for keeping the air from seeming stale, and for preventing rooms from feeling stuffy. However, good ventilation systems can also create drafts (chilly currents of air), especially near the circulation vents. Infants, older adults, and people who are ill may become easily chilled and may require an extra blanket, a sweater, or a lap robe to stay warm (Fig. 17-8). Also, be sure to position chairs and beds so that your patient or resident is not in a drafty area. For example, avoid placing furniture and wheelchairs right underneath a circulation vent.

Room Temperature

Most people prefer a room temperature that is somewhere between 68°F and 74°F. However, people who are ill, older, or relatively inactive may prefer a warmer room temperature. OBRA regulations require the temperature in a long-term care facility to be kept between 71°F and 81°F. Although this temperature may seem quite warm to you, especially when you are moving around and busy with your daily duties, remember that the temperature regulations are intended to ensure the comfort of the people you care for.

Lighting

There are two major types of lighting used in the health care setting: general lighting and task lighting. Usually, both lighting types are used in a single room. **General lighting** provides overall illumination (light), allowing a person to see and move about safely. Sunlight is one common source of general lighting. Usually the general light provided by an uncovered window is supplemented by light from a ceiling fixture or floor and table lamps. Many people prefer to have the drapes or blinds covering the windows in a room opened during the day, to allow natural light in. Others may prefer a darkened room, or to illuminate the room with light from a lamp or ceiling fixture instead of sunlight. You should ask each of your patients or residents what they prefer, and act accordingly (Fig. 17-9).

Task lighting directs bright light toward a specific area. In a patient or resident room, task lighting is usually provided by a fixture mounted over the head of the bed. Some of these fixtures provide both general and task lighting with dual switches. The patient or resident may use task lighting for activities that require good light to prevent eyestrain, such as reading, needlework, or doing a crossword puzzle. You would use task lighting when providing patient or resident care,

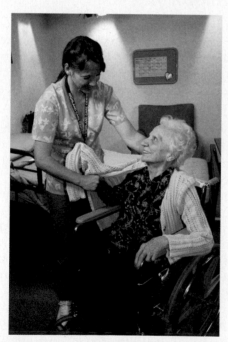

Figure 17-8 Although good ventilation is essential for health and comfort, older adults, infants, and people who are ill often "catch a chill." Provide additional layers as needed, and be sure to position people away from drafts created by the ventilation system.

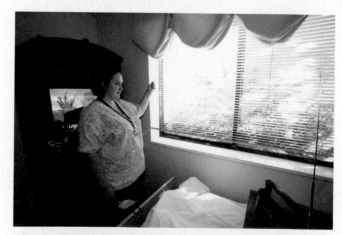

Figure 17-9 Some people prefer to have the blinds or drapes opened during the day to let in the sunlight. Others prefer a darkened room and will want to have the blinds or drapes drawn. Always ask the patient or resident about their preference.

so that you could see clearly while carrying out the procedure. The focused illumination provided by task lighting also helps you to notice changes that should be reported to the nurse. For example, you may notice a change in a person's skin tone or a strange new rash that might otherwise go unnoticed.

Lighting helps us to orient ourselves to the time of day. If a patient or resident prefers to have their blinds or drapes closed during the day and the overhead light fixture or a lamp is in constant use, they may find it difficult to tell the difference between day and night. During the evening and night hours, overhead lights should be dimmed, and the use of bright task lighting should be kept to a minimum. These measures help patients and residents maintain orientation to the time of day.

Noise Control

Health care facilities can be such busy, noisy places! Imagine that you are a patient on a typical floor in a hospital. It is about 11:30 in the morning, and there is a lot of activity. The telephone is ringing at the nurse's station. Here comes the person with the cart carrying the food trays up from the kitchen. You know they are coming because their cart has a squeaky wheel. A nurse and a nursing assistant are having a conversation in the hallway about what needs to be done that afternoon. A patient down the hall, who is a little bit hard of hearing, has the volume turned all the way up on their television set. Several visitors are going down the hallway to visit a friend who is recovering from surgery, and they are laughing and talking as they go. You are not feeling very well, and you wonder if things will ever quiet down enough for you to get some rest!

Although a certain level of noise in a busy place is to be expected, too much noise can affect the comfort of patients and residents. OBRA OBRA regulations require long-term care facilities to take measures to control noise. Because a quiet environment is known to promote rest and sleep and aid healing, many health care facilities have programs designed to remind people of the importance of keeping noise levels down inside the facility (Fig. 17-10). As a nursing assistant, there are many things you can do to help minimize noise and maintain a pleasant environment:

- Encourage patients or residents to use headsets or earphones when watching television or listening to the radio
- Answer telephones promptly
- Report noisy equipment that needs to be adjusted or oiled
- Be aware of the volume of your voice

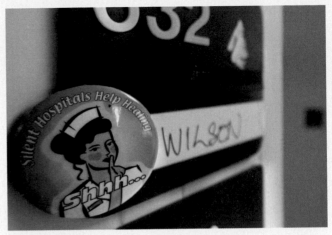

Figure 17-10 A quiet environment is so important for the well-being of patients or residents that some health care facilities, like this one in New York, have posted signs designed to remind staff and visitors to keep quiet. "Shhh" is an acronym for Silent Hospitals Help Healing. (*Frank Franklin II/AP*)

During the evening and night hours when patients and residents are sleeping, it is especially important to take precautions to minimize noise.

FURNITURE AND EQUIPMENT

The furniture and equipment that are considered "standard" for a patient's or resident's room will differ according to the facility and to the specific needs of the patient or resident. To ensure your own safety, as well as that of your patients' or residents', you must make sure that you know how to operate and adjust any furniture and equipment that are considered standard in the facility where you work. The furniture and equipment described in this section would be considered standard for a typical room in a hospital or a long-term care facility. In a facility that offers specialized care (for example, a burn unit or rehabilitation center), items considered standard might vary from this list.

Beds

An adjustable bed, commonly referred to as a *hospital bed*, is used in most health care settings (Fig. 17-11). The frame of an adjustable bed can be raised or lowered, moving the entire bed either further away from, or closer to, the floor. This helps health care workers maintain good body mechanics when performing care procedures. It also helps the patient or resident get into or out of the bed. The mattress platform on an adjustable bed can also be positioned in a variety of ways to keep the patient or resident comfortable.

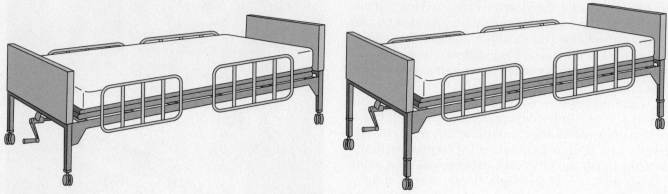

A. The bed can be moved up or down in terms of distance from the floor.

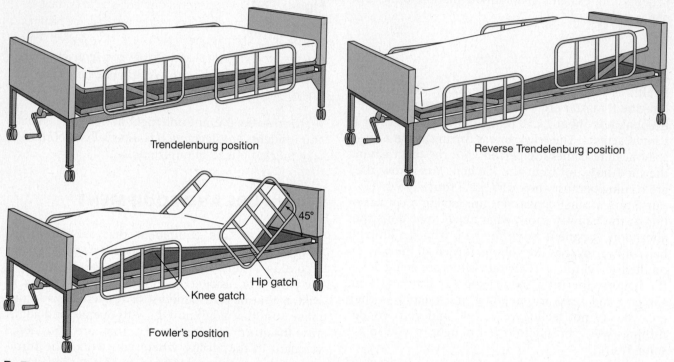

Trendelenburg position

Reverse Trendelenburg position

45°

Hip gatch

Knee gatch

Fowler's position

B. The mattress can be adjusted to assist with positioning of the patient or resident.

Figure 17-11 Most beds used in health care settings are adjustable, both in terms of (**A**) their height from the floor and (**B**) the position of the mattress.

Sometimes, the doctor will order a specific mattress position for a patient or resident.

The mattress platforms of most adjustable beds have joints at the hips and knees, which allow the mattress to "break" or bend. These joints are called **gatches**, after Willis Gatch, the surgeon who developed the first bed that was adjustable at the hips and knees. The hip gatch raises the person's upper body to a semi-sitting position (Fowler's position; see also Chapter 15). The knee gatch raises the person's knees to help prevent the person from sliding toward the end of the bed while in the Fowler's position. In addition to having hip and knee gatches, most adjustable beds permit the mattress to be "tilted" without

bending the person at the waist. In **Trendelenburg position**, the foot of the mattress is raised so that the person's head is lower than their feet. Trendelenburg position is sometimes used for a person who has gone into shock or has a very low blood pressure, to encourage blood flow to the heart. In the **reverse Trendelenburg position**, the head of the mattress is raised so the person's head is higher than their feet. The reverse Trendelenburg position is useful for people who are recovering from spinal cord injury or back surgery, or who are in traction.

Most health care facilities use adjustable beds that are adjusted electrically, using control buttons located on or near the side rails (Fig. 17-12). However, some

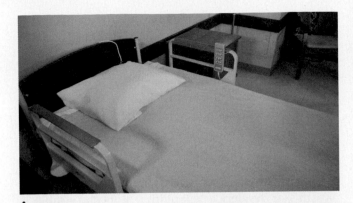

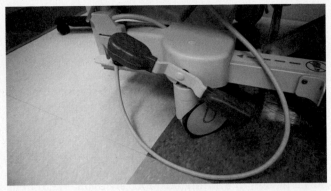

Figure 17-13 Wheel locks help to prevent unintentional movement of the bed. There are different types of wheel locks. In the type shown here, the red pedal locks the wheel, and the green pedal unlocks it.

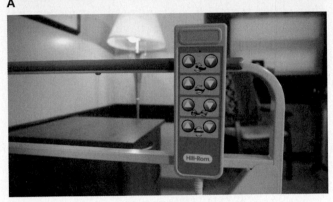

A

B

Figure 17-12 Adjustable beds may be adjusted using electrical controls.

long-term care facilities may still use beds that are adjusted manually, using a system of cranks located at the foot of the bed. One advantage of electrically operated beds is that the control buttons are located in a place that is accessible to the patient or resident, as well as to members of the health care team. When using an electrically operated bed, remember that it is a piece of electrical equipment. Appropriate safety precautions should be taken when operating it to avoid electrical shock (see Chapter 13). When using a manually operated bed, remember to fold the cranks down and away under the bed after you are finished using them so that people who are walking near the foot of the bed do not bump into them.

In addition to being adjustable, adjustable beds usually have two other features that regular beds do not—side rails and wheels (casters). The side rails on a bed are raised to help prevent a person from falling out of the bed. Always remember, however, that side rails can be considered a form of restraint and should only be used according to your facility's policies and the person's individual care plan. Some of your patients or residents may want to have one of the side rails raised, so that they can use it as an assistive device for repositioning. The patient or resident can grab the side rail and use it to reposition themselves in bed or to get up.

Wheels make the bed easier to move from place to place, which is sometimes necessary when a person needs to be moved from one part of the facility to another without leaving their bed. Wheels are also useful when it is necessary to move the bed to clean underneath it. The wheels have locking devices that are used to keep the bed steady and prevent it from rolling. Always make sure the bed's wheels are locked, unless you are moving it (Fig. 17-13)! A person could be injured while getting into or out of the bed if the bed shifts out from underneath them. In addition, you may be injured if the bed suddenly shifts away from you while you are providing care to a patient or resident.

A "low bed" (that is, a bed specially designed to lower to a height very close to the floor) is often found in the long-term care environment (Fig. 17-14). A low bed is very useful for residents who may roll out of bed or get out of bed without calling for assistance when needed. Because the bed is so low to the floor,

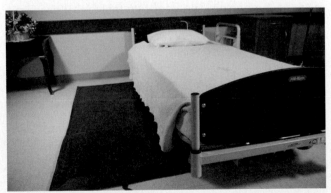

Figure 17-14 A low bed can minimize the risk for serious injury as a result of a fall and can be useful for residents who may roll out of bed or get out of bed without calling for assistance when needed.

the risk for serious injury as a result of a fall from the bed can be minimized.

In some cases, you may care for a person who is in a regular bed, instead of an adjustable bed. For example, some assisted-living and long-term care facilities allow people to bring their own beds from home, if they prefer. Also, a person who is being cared for in their home may not have an adjustable bed. When you are caring for a person in a regular bed, you can use blocks to elevate the head of the bed. Positioning devices, such as pillows and wedges shaped to support a person in a sitting position, are available to help achieve the other positions.

Chairs

A person's room should be furnished with one or two chairs that are comfortable for the person and will accommodate any visitors. Some people with disabilities require special chairs, such as Geri chairs, wheelchairs, or chairs with special lifting devices that help the person to get in and out of the chair easily. A person who is recovering from hip or spinal surgery may need a chair that has firm upholstery, a straight back, and no armrests. Many residents of long-term care facilities will bring a favorite chair or two from home. These chairs may recline or have a rocking action that the person finds very comfortable.

Over-Bed Tables

Most health care facilities furnish patient and resident rooms with **over-bed tables**, which fit over the bed or a chair and can be raised or lowered as needed (Fig. 17-15). You will use the over-bed table to hold basins and other articles when carrying out personal care for a patient or resident. The patient or resident may use the over-bed table as a surface for writing a letter, or for eating a meal or snack. When kept in easy reach of the person, the over-bed table is an excellent

place to keep a water pitcher or any other items the person may want close by. Because the over-bed table is considered a "clean" area, items placed there should be either sterile or clean. One way to help remember this is to consider the over-bed table the person's dining room table—you would never place dirty items, such as bedpans or soiled linens, there.

Storage Units

Various types of storage units are used to house a patient's or resident's belongings. A bedside table is often placed next to the bed and used to store personal care items. Most bedside tables have drawers or a combination of drawers and closed shelves. The person's toothpaste and toothbrush, lotion, soap, deodorant, and other personal hygiene items are usually stored in the top drawer while basins, clean bedpans, and other care equipment are stored neatly underneath in the lower drawers or shelves. The telephone, a flower arrangement, and other personal items may be placed on top of the bedside table (Fig. 17-16).

Additional storage for a person's personal items may be provided in the form of a closet, a wardrobe, or a chest of drawers. OBRA regulations require long-term care facilities to provide each resident with enough storage space for their clothing and other personal items. The resident must have free access to this storage space and the items it contains. Because the resident's closet, wardrobe, or chest of drawers is considered private, personal property, you must

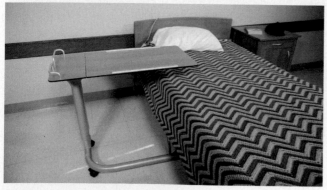

Figure 17-15 The over-bed table fits over the bed or a chair.

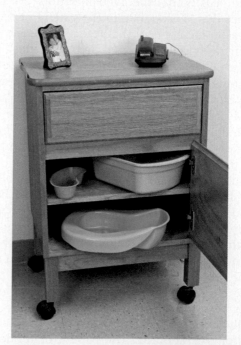

Figure 17-16 Personal care items are usually stored in the bedside table.

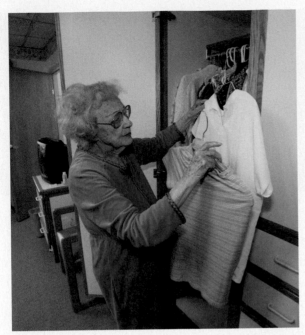

Figure 17-17 The resident's closet is considered private, personal property.

have the person's permission to remove items from it (Fig. 17-17).

Occasionally, you will need to inspect a resident's personal storage area. For example, you may suspect that a resident is keeping something in the storage area that is not permitted, such as food. Food can spoil and may attract insects and rodents. In this situation, you would be permitted to inspect the personal storage space, but first you must inform the resident of your intent to do so, and the search must be conducted in the resident's presence. If you must carry out an inspection of a resident's personal storage space, it may be a good idea to have another staff member present during the inspection to verify that you acted appropriately and within the regulations.

Call Light and Intercom Systems

Patients and residents must have a way of communicating with the health care staff at all times. Most health care facilities have a **call light system**, which patients or residents can use to alert a staff member that they need help. Many also have an intercom system, which allows staff members to speak to a patient or resident in their room from the nurses' station.

A call light system consists of a call light control (usually either a cord that is pulled or a hand-held button device), a light in the hall (over the doorway of the patient's or resident's room), and a panel of lights at the nurses' station or some other central location. When the person pulls the cord or pushes the button

on the call light control, the light over the doorway blinks and the light on the panel at the nurses' station lights, alerting the staff that the person needs help. A staff member who is at the nurses' station could then use the intercom system to communicate with the patient or resident before going to the person's room (Fig. 17-18). Newer systems connect the call light and intercom systems into individual headsets worn by staff members, leading to better communication between patients or residents and staff members as well as reduced noise levels on the unit.

The call light control must always be within a person's reach, whether the person is in the bed or in a chair. An unconscious or comatose person will be unable to call for help and should be checked on very frequently. It is also important to note that a person who is hearing impaired will have difficulty communicating with an intercom system. The person will not be able to understand what you are saying, so remember to respond in person to a hearing-impaired person's calls. Answer all requests for assistance promptly, even though it can be frustrating to respond to numerous, seemingly silly requests from any particular person, especially when you are very busy. Sometimes people who use the call light system excessively are feeling scared and lonely. What they are really seeking is reassurance that if a problem actually does occur, someone will come quickly to their aid. Part of helping to meet a person's safety and security needs is your quick response to a request for help.

Privacy Curtains and Room Dividers

Each patient or resident unit will have privacy curtains (which are usually hung from the ceiling) or room dividers. The privacy curtain should be closed, or a room divider used, when you are providing care for your patients or residents. The door to the room should also be closed, as the privacy curtains do little to keep voices and other sounds private. OBRA regulations require long-term care facilities to use privacy curtains or room dividers to protect the privacy of each resident.

Pay attention to the cleanliness of privacy curtains or room dividers. Although privacy curtains or room dividers are cleaned routinely, they are not cleaned every day. Report any stains to the proper person so that the privacy curtain or room divider can be cleaned or replaced, as needed.

Other Equipment

Depending on the type of facility and the purpose of the room, other equipment may be present. For example, many rooms have hanging intravenous (IV)

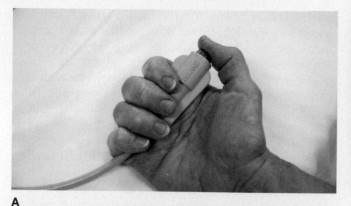

A

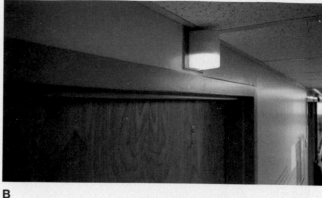

B

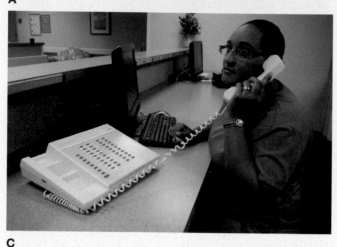

C

Figure 17-18 Call light and intercom systems allow patients and residents to communicate with members of the health care team. (**A**) The resident pushes a call light control button or pulls a cord, (**B**) the light above the person's door and the corresponding light on the panel at the nurses' station light up, and (**C**) a nurse or nursing assistant can use the intercom system to communicate with the person before going to the person's room.

poles and outlets for oxygen and suction devices. The Occupational Safety and Health Administration (OSHA) requires personal protective equipment (PPE), such as alcohol-based handrub, gloves, and disposal equipment, such as sharps containers, to be kept in every patient or resident care area for your use. Therefore, the room may be equipped with a wall-mounted sharps disposal box and a wall-mounted box of disposable gloves.

ADAPTING THE ENVIRONMENT TO THE INDIVIDUAL

Overall, the basic furniture and equipment in each patient's or resident's room will be the same depending on the particular type of unit within the health care facility. However, patients and residents have many different needs. For example, an orthopedic unit in a hospital or rehabilitation unit may equip all beds with an overhead trapeze device to assist patients with repositioning. Per OBRA regulations, long-term care facilities are expected to provide care in a manner that promotes residents' independence. Being able to do as much as possible independently

helps any person in a health care setting reach the important goal of attaining (or maintaining) their highest level of function and well-being. Environmental factors can get in the way of the patient or resident functioning at their best. The health care environment can and should be adapted as necessary to suit the patient's or resident's individual needs and to promote independence, safety, and comfort. For example:

- The hanging rod in a closet may need to be lowered so that a patient or resident in a wheelchair can independently remove articles of clothing from the closet.
- An elevated seat can be installed on a toilet to make it easier for a patient or a resident who has difficulty sitting down and standing up to use the toilet independently. This is especially important for someone who may have recently had surgery on the hip, knee, or lower back.
- For a person with visual problems, a white toilet in a bathroom with light walls and a light floor may tend to "disappear." A toilet seat in a color that contrasts with the bathroom floor and walls can help a patient or resident with visual problems identify the toilet more easily.

Helping Hands and a Caring Heart

Focus on Humanistic Health Care

Our homes are decorated with things that have special meaning to us. In the same way, many of the items a resident chooses to bring to a long-term care facility will hold special meaning. You may notice items in a person's room that represent the person's cultural background, spiritual beliefs, or mementos from a career or a hobby. Take an interest in these things. Ask the resident to tell you about them. This lets the resident know that you care about them as an individual.

Always respect a person's personal items as if they belonged to you. Remember that even a small scrap of paper can be very precious to a resident, especially if it is a note from someone the person loves. While you may consider a resident's personal things quite a bit of clutter, especially if you have to help keep these things neat, remember that each one of those items represents a piece of that person's life. When you show respect for, and take an interest in, a patient's or resident's personal belongings, you are letting the person know that you truly care for them. The "Respect" feature at the end of this unit gives an example of how residents may wish to add their own personal touches to their rooms to reflect their personal heritage.

■ Placing signs on dresser drawers to identify the contents of each drawer can help a person with dementia find what they are looking for without opening all of the drawers. Similarly, a picture of a toilet on the bathroom door may help the person remain independent in toileting for a period of time.

■ A patient or resident who is very petite (small) may benefit from a low bed and a chair that is lower than a standard chair so that they can get in and out of them safely. Similarly, a pediatric (child-sized) wheelchair may be safer and more comfortable for the person.

■ A patient or resident who is very large may also need special furniture and equipment to promote comfort and safety. For example, bariatric beds, chairs, and wheelchairs are designed and constructed to meet the comfort and safety needs of people with obesity. (*Bariatrics* is the branch of medicine that specializes in the treatment of obesity.)

As you are helping your patients and residents with their care, it is important for you to report any environmental barriers to their comfort and independence that you see. Share your observations with the nurse and other team members. Together, you may be able to find a creative solution to the person's challenges!

Tell the Nurse!

You are responsible for making sure that the patient's or resident's room is home-like, clean, and safe. Report the following situations to a nurse immediately:

● You notice that a piece of equipment or furniture in the room is not working properly

● A patient or resident has been injured by a piece of equipment or furniture in the room

● You have been injured by a piece of equipment or furniture in the room

● You suspect that a patient or resident is storing unwrapped food in a drawer or closet area

● A patient or resident, or one of their family members, complains that personal items are missing from the room

● You accidentally break a personal item belonging to a patient or resident

● Bathroom fixtures and floors do not appear to be properly cleaned or wastebaskets are not emptied

● There is an odor in the room that cannot be eliminated

● Environmental factors are affecting the patient's or resident's ability to function independently

SUMMARY

- Patient or resident rooms will vary according to the purpose of the facility and the needs of the person receiving care.
  - A patient room in a hospital is a person's temporary home.
  - A resident room in a long-term care or assisted-living facility usually becomes a person's permanent home.
- The physical environment of a health care facility contributes to overall comfort, health, and well-being. Long-term care facilities that receive federal funding must follow OBRA regulations concerning the physical environment of the resident's room.
  - A clean environment is essential for odor and infection control. In addition, many people judge a facility according to its level of cleanliness.
    - All members of the health care team are responsible for providing a clean and comfortable environment.
    - Nursing assistants are responsible for helping patients and residents keep their rooms neat and clean.
  - Odor is controlled by promptly removing and cleaning dirty emesis basins, urinals, bedpans, and linens. Assisting patients and residents with bathing and brushing their teeth also helps prevent odors.
  - Good ventilation helps carry away unpleasant odors and prevents stale air. However, it is important to protect your patients and residents from becoming chilled by drafts.
  - The temperature of a patient's or resident's room should remain between 71°F and 81°F.
  - Adequate light must be provided for all activities that take place in a person's room.
    - General lighting, such as from sunlight or an overhead ceiling fixture, provides overall illumination.

- Task lighting focuses bright light on one particular area.
  - Too much noise interferes with a person's ability to rest.
- Most patient and resident rooms contain the same basic furniture and equipment.
  - All patient or resident rooms contain a bed, which in most cases will be electrically or manually adjustable.
  - All patient or resident rooms contain at least one chair, to accommodate a visitor and to provide a "change of scenery" for the patient or resident. Many residents in long-term care facilities bring a favorite chair from home.
  - Over-bed tables fit over a person's bed to provide a work surface for both the patient or resident and the health care worker. The over-bed table is considered a "clean" area.
  - Personal care items, such as toiletries, are usually stored in the bedside table.
  - In long-term care facilities, a closet, wardrobe, or chest of drawers is used to provide private storage space for the resident's personal belongings.
  - Call light and intercom systems are used for communication.
    - The call light system allows patients or residents to signal that they need help.
    - The intercom system allows members of the health care team to communicate with patients or residents without leaving the nurses' station.
  - Privacy curtains or room dividers are used to help maintain a resident's or patient's privacy when care is being given.
- The environment should be adapted to help each patient or resident remain as independent as possible and to ensure comfort and safety.

WHAT DID YOU LEARN?

Multiple Choice

Select the single best answer for each of the following questions.

1. In the long-term care setting, how should a resident's room look?
   a. Functional and sparsely decorated
   b. Like a hospital room
   c. As home-like as possible
   d. Like a hotel room

2. You show respect to a patient or resident when you:
   a. Knock before entering their room
   b. Close the door and pull the privacy curtain when you are providing care
   c. Handle the person's personal belongings with care
   d. All of the above

3. The nurse tells you that Mr. Haskill's bedside table is looking a little bit disorderly and asks you to clean it up a bit. You should:
   a. Search the shelves for hidden food and throw anything that you find away
   b. Remove the bedpan and washbasin because these items do not belong there
   c. Straighten the items on the top of the table and on the shelves, removing any dirty items so that they can be cleaned and returned
   d. Wait for housekeeping staff to make their rounds

4. Which regulations state that a resident's unit must be clean, safe, orderly, and free of obstacles in the pathway?
   a. Occupational Safety and Health Administration (OSHA) regulations
   b. Omnibus Budget Reconciliation Act (OBRA) regulations
   c. State regulations
   d. Medicaid regulations

5. One of your patients has had back surgery, and the nurse asks you to position their bed so that the head of the bed is elevated. The patient's body needs to remain flat against the mattress. What position would the nurse tell you to put the patient in?
   a. Reverse Trendelenburg position
   b. Fowler's position
   c. Prone position
   d. Trendelenburg position

6. You are working in a nursing home. As you are preparing Mrs. Everly for bed, she tells you that she is feeling a bit hungry because she did not really eat much at dinner. She asks you if she can have some graham crackers and a glass of milk. Knowing that Mrs. Everly does not have any dietary restrictions, how you should respond to Mrs. Everly?
   a. You should tell Mrs. Everly that you are sorry, but the kitchen has closed for the evening.
   b. You should tell Mrs. Everly that you will have to run to see if you can get into the kitchen and look for a snack for her.
   c. You should tell Mrs. Everly that you will go to the nourishment room and get a snack for her.
   d. You should tell Mrs. Everly that snacking in the room is not allowed. You will be glad to assist her back to the dining room for a snack.

7. How can you help to control unpleasant odors in the workplace?
   a. Empty emesis basins promptly
   b. Assist your patients or residents with skin care and oral hygiene
   c. Use facility-approved air fresheners as necessary
   d. All of the above

Matching *Match each numbered item with its appropriate lettered description.*

_____ **1.** Side rails

_____ **2.** Patient or resident unit

_____ **3.** Over-bed table

_____ **4.** Task lighting

_____ **5.** Bariatric bed

a. The patient's or resident's pitcher and meal trays may be placed here

b. Light source that can be directed to a specific area and used during care tasks

c. Special bed for a patient or resident with obesity

d. The space where a patient or resident lives in a health care facility

e. Used to prevent a person from falling out of bed, and as an assistive device; may also be considered a form of restraint

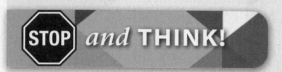

- One of your residents, Mrs. Kishore, is complaining that she is cold even though you are feeling a bit too warm. What are some measures that you can take to help make Mrs. Kishore more comfortable?
- Mrs. Tinetti is a new resident at the long-term care facility where you work. She is 86 years old and still able to walk on her own with the help of her walker. Mrs. Tinetti is only 4 feet 9 inches tall and weighs 96 pounds. You notice that she seems to have a great deal of difficulty getting out of her bed and her chair. When she is seated on either one, her feet do not touch the floor. You see her struggling to get out of bed and go over to offer her assistance. She accepts the assistance, but snaps that this just should not be. She has always prided herself at being able to do for herself, despite her age. She does not want to lose that just because she has moved into this facility! What can be done to help Mrs. Tinetti maintain the independence that she is so proud of?

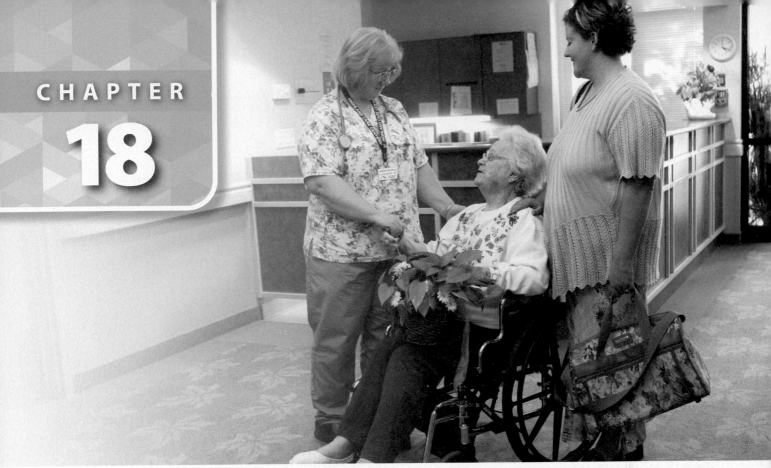

Photo: A new resident arrives at a long-term care facility.

Admissions, Transfers, and Discharges

 WHAT WILL YOU LEARN?

Checking people into and out of a health care facility is a routine event in many health care settings. Routine, that is, unless you are the person being admitted ("checked in"), discharged ("checked out"), or transferred (moved from one room in the facility to another, or moved to another facility altogether). All of these events cause a major change to the patient's or resident's daily routine and normal lifestyle. For many people, this is very upsetting. In this chapter, you will learn how admissions, transfers, and discharges are carried out. You will also learn about things you can do to help make these times of change easier for your patients or residents. When you are finished with this chapter, you will be able to:

1. Explain why admission to a health care facility may be emotionally difficult for a person and their family members.
2. Discuss how the nursing assistant can help make a person's admission into a health care facility more pleasant.
3. List the nursing assistant's responsibilities during the admission process.
4. Explain why a person in a health care facility might need to be moved to another room or to another facility.

5. List the nursing assistant's responsibilities when assisting with the transfer of a patient or resident.

6. Discuss the purpose of discharge planning.

7. List the nursing assistant's responsibilities during the discharge process.

Vocabulary

Admission
Nursing history
Resident inventory sheet

Transfer
Discharge

Against medical advice (AMA)
Discharge planning

ADMISSIONS

An **admission** is the official entry of a person into a health care setting. A person who needs health care must be formally admitted to the health care facility that will be providing the care, whether the length of the stay is:

- A few hours (for example, a person entering an outpatient surgical unit for same-day surgery)
- A few days or weeks (for example, a person entering a hospital to receive treatment for a complication of diabetes)
- A few months, or
- The rest of the person's life (for example, a person entering a long-term care facility because of advanced Alzheimer disease)

In the case of a home health care agency, the health care setting is the client's home, but there will still be an admissions process. This is because admission is a time of orientation, for both the new patient, resident, or client and the health care team. During the admissions process, the patient, resident, or client is informed of their rights and the policies of the facility or agency and is introduced to the people who will be caring for them. At the same time, the members of the health care team are introduced to the person and their family, and the process of gathering the information that the health care team needs to care properly for the person begins.

The members of the health care team may regard the admission process as routine. To the person being admitted, however, this "routine" event can be very stressful. It means they must take on a new role—that of a patient, resident, or client—which can be stressful, because most people are used to thinking of themselves as independent, unique individuals, not as dependent people in need of the services of the health care industry. The person may feel a loss of identity as the illness or condition takes "center stage," causing all of their other unique qualities to fade into the background. This is why the members of the health care team must always make an effort to treat each new patient or resident as if they are a guest in the facility. Make the person feel welcome, not like they are just another body to wash. Ask the person how they prefer to be addressed. This helps maintain the person's sense of identity and individuality. Never refer to a patient or resident by their condition, such as "the hemiplegic in room 212." If you cannot remember the person's name, at least say "the person in room 212 who has had a stroke."

In addition to feeling stressed by the need to adjust to a new role, a person who is being admitted to a health care facility may also be feeling fear and anxiety about the future. For example, a person who is entering a long-term care facility may worry that they will not like their new home and may be sad about giving up their old one. A person who is being admitted to the hospital may worry that diagnostic tests will reveal bad news or that a surgery will not be successful. Even if the reason for the admission to a health care facility is joyous (for example, to deliver a baby), there may still be some lingering fear and anxiety (for example, about what labor and delivery will actually be like, or whether the baby will be healthy). The health care setting itself may be frightening. Imagine how you would feel if you were entering an environment filled with strangers asking personal questions about your life and poking and prodding your body with strange equipment! One way to help ease the fear and anxiety felt by patients or residents is to include their family members in the admissions process. Make sure that family members know that

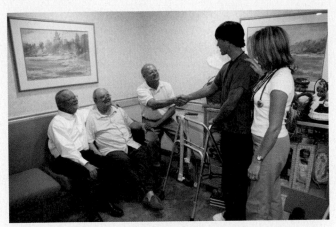

Figure 18-1 Being admitted to a health care facility is often stressful for the patient or resident, as well as their family members. Involving family members in the admissions process can help to put everyone at ease.

they are welcome and that their support benefits the patient or resident (Fig. 18-1).

Family members will have many of the same fears and worries about the future as the person being admitted. They may feel helpless. If the person is being admitted to a health care facility because family members are no longer able to provide the proper care at home, the family members may feel guilty. Stress can make people behave differently than they would under normal circumstances. Some family members may become demanding, bossy, or critical when they are under stress. Understanding the feelings that might cause a person to act this way can help you make allowances for the person's behavior. Showing empathy and kindness and involving family members in the admissions process can help family members feel better about the situation.

Concerns for Long-Term Care

As you learned in Chapter 8, most people do not choose to be admitted to a long-term care facility. Many admissions, especially those to nursing homes, are preceded by some sort of a crisis, such as an unexpected accident or illness. In many cases, the accident or illness results in the person being hospitalized. It is common for the person and the family to learn during this time that because of the person's condition, the person will need ongoing care following discharge from the hospital. The person and family must now decide, in a very short period of time, how and where that ongoing care will be provided.

In many situations, such as when a person whose health or mental abilities have been slowly declining over time, that person's family members may have been providing the care. A point in time comes when the family realizes that caregiving needs are becoming more than they can handle. By the time the decision is made to place the loved one into a long-term care setting, the family is physically, emotionally, and financially drained. These feelings add to the guilt and frustration they are already feeling because they can no longer care for their loved one.

The Admissions Process

Because the admissions process is an emotional time for the patient or resident and their family members, you must focus on the person and their needs, as well as on the process and the paperwork. Most admissions follow a process established by the health care facility:

1. The admissions process usually begins in a doctor's office, unless the admission is caused by an emergency. In the case of an emergency, the person may arrive at the health care facility without seeing the doctor first. Normally, however, the admissions process begins when a doctor writes orders regarding the specific needs of the person. These orders usually include the doctor's diagnosis of the person's condition and specify dietary orders, activity status, medications, diagnostic tests, and the type of room required by the person.

2. On arrival at the health care facility, the person first goes to the admissions office, where they meet with an admissions coordinator or a nurse who is responsible for admissions. The health care team member who is handling the admission will help the person complete the facility's standard admission information process, which gathers information electronically about the person, such as name, address, date of birth and age, social security number, gender, insurance and employment information, emergency notification information, and advance directive information. The admissions coordinator or nurse will also have the person sign a consent form giving the facility permission to treat the person's medical condition. When the admissions information is completed, the admissions coordinator or nurse will provide the patient or resident with a way of being identified. In a hospital, an identification bracelet will be issued

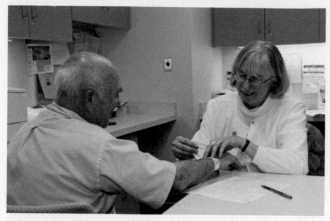

Figure 18-2 Each patient receives an identification bracelet in the admissions office.

(Fig. 18-2). In a long-term care facility, a photograph of the person will be taken for identification purposes (Fig. 18-3).

3. After completing the admissions information, the person will be escorted to their room by the admissions coordinator or nurse, a volunteer, or a nursing assistant. Depending on the situation, the person may be able to walk to their room, or they may be taken in a wheelchair or on a stretcher.

4. A nursing assistant is usually responsible for helping the person unpack and for taking and recording the person's vital signs, height, and weight. If you work in a hospital, you may need to help the person change into a hospital gown or pajamas. Make sure that the person is comfortable by helping them into the bed or a chair. Next, a nurse will come to the patient's or resident's room to complete the **nursing history**. As you will remember from Chapter 5,

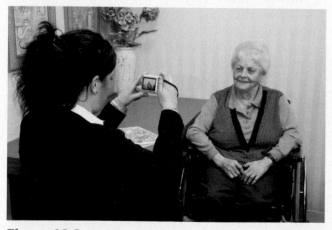

Figure 18-3 A photograph of the resident is usually taken for identification purposes.

the nursing history is used to gather information about the person's preferences, abilities, disabilities, and habits. The nurse completes this document by interviewing the patient or resident (or, in some cases, a family member of the patient or resident).

Helping a New Patient or Resident Feel Welcome

When a new patient is being admitted to a hospital, the admissions staff will usually notify the nursing staff as soon as the person arrives in the admissions office. This gives the nursing team time to prepare for the person's arrival. When a person is being admitted to a long-term care facility, the nursing staff typically has a few days' advance notice of the new arrival. As a member of the nursing team, you will play a very important role in making sure that the person feels expected and welcomed when they arrive at the facility. A good first impression can go a long way toward easing a person's anxiety, especially if one of the things the person is anxious about is the quality of care that they will be receiving while staying at your facility. As a nursing assistant, there are several things you can do to make sure that the admission goes as smoothly as possible.

Prepare the Person's Room in Advance of Their Arrival

Ask the nurse about any special requirements that your new patient or resident may have. Does the person use a walker or some other ambulation device, or will they be arriving in a wheelchair or on a stretcher? If so, you will want to check the placement of the furniture in the room and move it as necessary to ensure easy entry into the room. If necessary, adjust the lighting and temperature of the room. Open the blinds or drapes and prepare the bed by turning the sheets back, lowering the bed to the lowest position, and making sure the wheels are locked (see Chapter 19). If the person is arriving by stretcher, you would prepare the bed in a slightly different manner (also described in Chapter 19).

Gather the equipment you will need for taking and recording the person's vital signs (see Chapter 20). Make sure any other equipment needed by the incoming patient or resident, such as oxygen tubing, a suctioning device, or an intravenous (IV) pole, is in the room before the person arrives. If your facility provides them, obtain an admissions pack for the person. A typical admissions pack would contain a basin, a water pitcher, a drinking cup, a package of tissues, and assorted personal care items (such as toothpaste, soap, and shampoo). Preparing the room

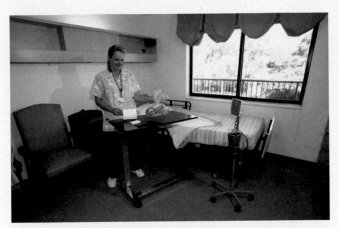

Figure 18-4 Turning the bedsheets down and opening the blinds or drapes to let the sunshine in says to a new patient or resident, "Welcome! We were expecting you!" Making sure the room is stocked with the necessary equipment and supplies, including personal toiletry items, also indicates to the new patient or resident that their arrival was planned for and expected.

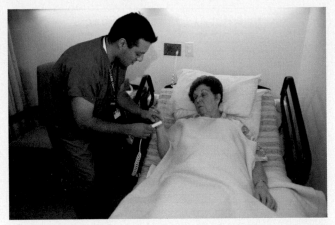

Figure 18-5 A new patient or resident must be taught how to operate the equipment in the room. Here, a nursing assistant shows a new resident how to use the call light control.

in a thoughtful manner indicates to the new patient or resident that their arrival was anticipated and planned for (Fig. 18-4).

Greet the Person Warmly and Introduce Yourself

When you meet the person and their family members for the first time, be sure to introduce yourself. Give your title and explain how you will be involved in the care of the person. A warm, courteous, professional greeting helps put people at ease and gives them confidence that they will be well taken care of by the health care team.

Help the Person Settle into Their New Home

Always take the time to give a new patient or resident a "tour" of the room. Point out the location of the bathroom. Show the person how to use the call light control, how to adjust the bed, how to adjust the lights, and how to operate any other appliances or pieces of equipment in the room (Fig. 18-5). For example, in a hospital setting, you may need to show the person how to get an outside line on the telephone, or how to turn the television on and off and adjust the volume.

You should also help the person unpack and find appropriate places for their personal belongings (Fig. 18-6). If you work in a long-term care facility, you will need to complete a resident inventory sheet as part of the unpacking process. The **resident inventory sheet** is a document that lists and briefly describes all of the resident's personal belongings (Fig. 18-7). When completing the resident inventory

sheet, make sure that you describe each item objectively. For example, when describing a resident's ring, you would write, "yellow metal ring with two blue stones" instead of "gold ring with two sapphires" because you do not know for sure that the ring is gold or the stones are sapphires. The resident inventory sheet is used to help make sure that a resident leaves the facility with all of their belongings, in the event of a transfer or discharge. It is also used to assist with tracking if belongings are misplaced or borrowed. Some long-term care facilities require each resident to write their name inside of each article of clothing to help with laundry sorting. You may need to help the resident do this if it has not been done already.

If the person has brought personal items to decorate with, let the person know that you are willing to assist in any way that you can. For example, a resident

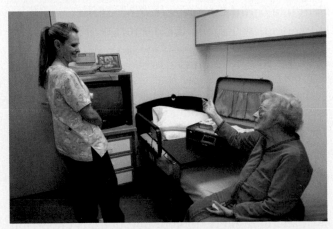

Figure 18-6 Helping the person to unpack and find suitable spots for personal items can make a new environment feel more "homelike" instantly.

Inventory of Personal Effects

Resident _____ Room _____ No. _____

Description :	
Bathrobe	Cane
Bed Jackets	Comb Brush
Belts	Crutches
Blouses	Dentures-Full Upper ( ) Lower ( )
Bras	Partial Upper ( ) Lower ( )
Coat	Furniture
Dresses	Glasses-Rimmed ( ) Rimless ( )
Girdles	Luggage
Hat	Other
Hose	Prosthesis
Nightgowns	Purse
Pajamas	Radio
Panties	Razors - Electric ( ) Safety ( )
Shirts	Rings
Shoes	Toothbrush
Skirts	Walker
Slips	Watch
Slippers	Wheelchair
Sweaters	
Ties	
Trousers	
Undershirts	
Undershorts	
Wallet	

I certify that the above is a correct list of my personal belongings.
I take full responsibility for retaining in my possession the articles listed above and any others brought to me while in this facility.

ALL ITEMS BROUGHT FOR THE PERSONAL USE OF THE RESIDENT MUST BE PROPERLY MARKED AND LISTED AS ARE THE ABOVE.   Please bring additional items to the Nurses' Station for proper handling.

Resident's washable clothing to be: _____ taken home for laundering
_____ laundered here at the center.

I understand the Management will not be responsible for any valuables, money, or clothing left in the possession of the resident._____ Date_____

Signature of Resident (or Relative) _____ Date _____
Signature of Nurse _____ Date _____

Disposition on Discharge   *Upon Discharge, all personal items are sent with resident or picked up by responsible party. Upon transfer, all personal items are to be boxed and placed in designated storage area for safekeeping.
Signature of Nurse _____   Signature of Resident/Relative _____
Date _____   Date _____

Figure 18-7 A resident inventory sheet is completed when a person is admitted to a long-term care facility. This document is used to keep track of each person's belongings.

of a long-term care facility may need your help with hanging a favorite picture on the wall or obtaining a bulletin board to display treasured cards and pieces of art.

Practice Good Communication Skills

While you are helping the person get settled, talk to them! Involving the person in conversation will indicate that you are interested in them, personally, and it will let you get to know the person a little bit better. You know your own duties better than anyone else, and questions that you ask the patient or resident will help you plan each person's care. For example, you might ask the person when they prefer to bathe, whether they like to take a nap between lunch and dinner, or whether they would prefer to take meals in the dining room or in their room. Be sure to listen to what the person is saying to you, both on their own and in response to your questions. Is the person asking questions or expressing feelings that suggest that they may be scared, worried, or upset? Answer questions about your specific responsibilities to the

best of your ability. Questions the patient or resident may have about their medical care should be directed to the nurse. Report any concerns that you may have about the person's ability to adjust to the new environment to the nurse.

TRANSFERS

A **transfer** occurs whenever a patient or resident is moved within or between health care settings. A transfer can be:

- From one room to another (for example, from a semiprivate to a private room)
- From one unit to another (for example, from the intensive care unit [ICU] to a standard care floor)
- From one health care facility to another (for example, from a long-term care facility to a hospital for the treatment of an acute illness)

Transfers can occur when a person's medical condition improves or when it worsens. Transfers can also occur when a preferred room becomes available for a person on a waiting list, or when it is necessary to move people to resolve conflicts between roommates.

As is the case with admissions, transfers can be stressful for the patient or resident, as well as their family members. The reason for the transfer may cause anxiety, especially if the person's condition has worsened or if the person is being transferred from a hospital to a long-term care facility. These transfers may not be expected or desired by either the person or their family members. They are usually the result of necessity. Even if the transfer is expected and desirable (for example, a resident in a long-term care facility is moving from one room to another because the view is better), the person being transferred may still experience some stress as a result of the change. Any type of change can be especially stressful for people with dementia.

The physical transfer can be carried out in a number of ways. The patient or resident may simply walk, or they may be transported in a wheelchair or on a stretcher. Sometimes, the person does not even need to get out of bed. The bed (with the person in it) is simply moved to another room or unit. An ambulance or wheelchair van may be used when a person is being moved from one health care facility to another. However, many people are transferred from one facility to another by their regular means of transportation, such as a private car or taxi.

Your duties related to assisting with transfers will vary according to the type of facility where you work. In a hospital or acute care setting, you will be responsible for gathering and packing the person's belongings. It is very important that you help make sure

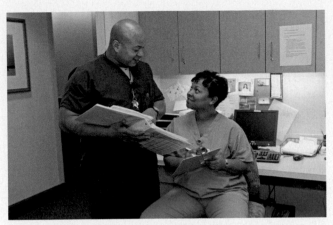

Figure 18-8 Two nursing assistants meet to discuss the personal care needs of a resident who is being transferred from one part of the facility to another.

that all of the person's belongings are packed and sent along with them, so that nothing gets lost. You may also need to assist the nurse in transporting the person to the new room or unit, or to the waiting ambulance, car, or taxi. The nurse is usually responsible for reporting information about the person's medical condition and medications or other treatments to the receiving nurse. If the transfer is taking place within the hospital, you may be asked to report information about the person's preferences and habits to the receiving nursing assistant.

In a long-term care facility, the assistance you provide will be more personal. Although the nurse will report medical information about the resident to the receiving nurse, you will be responsible for reporting personal care information about the resident to the receiving nursing assistant (Fig. 18-8). This is appropriate because you are the caregiver who is most likely to know the most about your resident's personal preferences. For example, you would know that Mr. Vasquez does not like overcooked vegetables, that he requires minimal assistance in the bathroom, and that he likes to read the paper after breakfast. By providing the new nursing assistant with this information, you are helping to ensure that your resident's transition from one caregiver to another is as seamless as possible.

DISCHARGES

A **discharge** is the official release of a patient or resident from a health care facility to their home. A patient's or resident's discharge is ordered by the doctor. Occasionally, a person will insist on leaving a health care setting without a doctor's order, or **against medical advice (AMA)**. A person who is mentally competent may choose to leave a facility if

they wish to. However, that person must sign certain documents first stating that they understand that leaving the facility without a doctor's order releases the doctor and the facility from any legal responsibility regarding their health status, since they have refused to follow the recommendations for care. If a person tells you that they are leaving the facility, you must report this to the nurse immediately. The nurse will follow the facility's policy for ensuring that a person who is leaving AMA is aware of the consequences of their actions.

Although some people initiate their own departure from a health care facility, most people wait to be officially discharged. Many times, the official discharge is a happy event, but sometimes, people have mixed emotions about leaving. As you will recall from Chapter 1, the ever-increasing costs of health care have created a situation where patients are being discharged from hospitals before they are fully recovered. Many patients are still acutely ill or need complicated treatment and care at the time of discharge. For these people and their family members, leaving behind the safe, professional care provided by the hospital staff can be a frightening experience.

To help ease the transition from a health care facility to home for patients and residents, preparations for discharge begin as soon as a person is admitted to the health care facility. **Discharge planning** is the process used by the members of the health care team to help prepare a patient or resident to leave the facility. Discharge planning helps to make sure that the person continues to receive quality care, either from a home health care agency or from family members, after the discharge. For example, as a result of discharge planning:

- A patient's family members may be taught how to change a wound dressing before the patient is sent home
- A resident and their family may receive help in planning a special diet before the resident is sent home
- Arrangements may be made to transfer a patient from the hospital to a long-term care facility for a short recovery period
- The services of a home health care agency may be obtained

The ultimate goal of discharge planning is to help the patient or resident achieve the best health status possible after they leave the health care facility (Fig. 18-9).

When a patient or resident is discharged from a health care facility, the nurse is responsible for making sure that the person and their family members have been taught what they need to know about the person's condition and how to monitor or care for it. Your

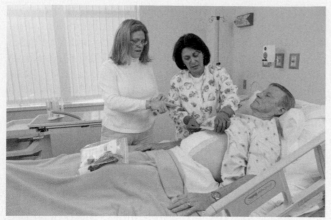

Figure 18-9 Nurses are responsible for discharge planning, a process that helps to ensure a continuation of care for people after they leave a health care facility. Here, a nurse is showing a patient's family member how to change a wound dressing.

responsibilities when a person is discharged are related more to helping the person gather and pack their belongings and say goodbye to friends and caregivers. Ask the nurse or the person about the estimated time of discharge so that you can have the person ready to leave on time, taking into account the time the person needs to pack and say their goodbyes. You may need to assist the person out of the facility or help carry their belongings.

Tell the Nurse!

The changes that accompany discharges, transfers, and admissions to health care facilities can be very stressful for a person and their family members. Often, a lot of information is communicated in a very short period of time, and the patient or resident (as well as their family members) may have trouble absorbing and understanding everything. Make sure you observe and listen carefully to your patient or resident and to their family members during these transitions. Report any of the following to the nurse immediately:

- Any questions that have to do with a person's medical condition or transfer

- Any comments that would indicate that the person or a family member does not fully understand what they have been told by a doctor or nurse

- Any signs of anxiety, such as crying, confusion, agitation, or other unexplained behavior

- Any changes in the person's vital signs or mental status

- Any mention of leaving the facility against medical advice (AMA)

SUMMARY

- Admission to a health care facility is a time of orientation. The patient or resident must learn to accept their new environment and their new status as a "patient" or "resident," and the members of the health care team must learn about their new patient or resident.

  - Assuming the role of a patient or resident can be stressful for a person. Therefore, the person's physical and emotional needs must always remain the focus of the admissions process.

  - Newly admitted patients or residents should be welcomed as if they are guests in your facility.

  - A smooth admissions process helps reduce a person's anxiety about entering the health care

facility. Many of the nursing assistant's duties revolve around making the admissions process easier for the patient or resident and their family members.

  - Nursing assistants are responsible for preparing the person's room, taking the person's vital signs and measuring height and weight, helping the person unpack, and teaching the person how to use the equipment in the room.

  - By actively listening to the comments made by the person and their family members during the admissions process, the nursing assistant can notify the nurse of any specific concerns that may need to be addressed.

- Transfers occur when a patient or resident is moved, either within a health care setting or between health care settings.
  - Transfers can occur when a person's medical condition improves or when it worsens.
  - When a person is transferred within a hospital or long-term care facility, the nursing assistant is responsible for passing vital information about the resident's care to the receiving nursing assistant.
- Although many people look forward to going home after being discharged from a health care

facility, some might wonder whether they will be able to manage on their own, or with only the help of family members.
  - Discharge planning helps to ensure that a patient or resident continues to receive quality health care, even after being released from a health care facility. Discharge planning begins at the time of admission and is the responsibility of the nurse.
  - The nursing assistant is responsible for helping a person prepare for discharge by gathering and packing all of a person's personal items.

WHAT DID YOU LEARN?

Multiple Choice

Select the single best answer for each of the following questions.

1. One of your patients is being transferred to another unit in the hospital. What would you pack for them to take along?
   a. The bed linens
   b. Their medical record
   c. Their personal belongings
   d. All of the above

2. One of your patients, Mrs. Sarandis, mentions to you that she is leaving the hospital, and her son is coming to pick her up. Before Mrs. Sarandis can be permitted to leave the premises, she must have:
   a. A nurse's order for discharge
   b. A doctor's order for discharge
   c. An admissions sheet on record
   d. A completed resident inventory sheet

3. As a nursing assistant, one of your tasks during the admission process will be to:
   a. Take and record the new patient's or resident's vital signs
   b. Assess the new patient's or resident's medical condition
   c. Hurry the new patient or resident through the admissions process to keep things running smoothly
   d. Reassure the new patient or resident by telling them that everything will be fine

4. Who writes the orders on admission for a person's diet, medications, level of activity, and type of room?
   a. The admissions clerk
   b. The patient or resident, or one of their family members
   c. The Director of Nursing
   d. The person's doctor

5. Discharge planning begins:
   a. A couple of days before the patient or resident is scheduled to be discharged
   b. When the patient or resident is admitted to the health care facility
   c. The day the patient or resident is scheduled to be discharged
   d. Before the patient or resident is admitted to the health care facility

6. The ultimate goal of discharge planning is to:
   a. Make sure that the room is clean and ready for the next patient or resident
   b. Close out the nursing care plan
   c. Help the person who is being discharged achieve their best level of health
   d. Make sure that all of the patient's or resident's belongings are accounted for

7. Who is responsible for carrying out the actions prescribed by the discharge plan (for example, teaching a patient's family member how to change a dressing)?

a. The doctor
b. The hospital social worker
c. The nurse
d. The nursing assistant

8. Mr. Singer, one of your patients, tells you that he hates the food at the hospital and feels that being hospitalized is actually doing him more harm than good. He says that he has called his wife, and she is coming that afternoon to take him home. As far as you know, Mr. Singer's discharge has not been ordered. What should you do?

a. Apply a restraint
b. Help Mr. Singer pack; it is his right to leave if he wants to
c. Tell the nurse immediately
d. Remind Mr. Singer's roommate that the door to the room must be kept shut and locked at all times

9. Why should a newly admitted patient or resident be given a warm welcome?

a. Because they represent more revenue for the facility
b. Because they will be a good roommate for another lonely patient or resident
c. Because they may be feeling scared and uncomfortable about entering a health care facility
d. You should simply just go about your duties; after all, admissions happen every day and a "business as usual" attitude is best to avoid upsetting the other patients or residents

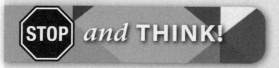

- Mr. Gardner has been a resident in your facility for several months and he has reached his maximum potential in therapy. Medicare will no longer pay for his care. Mr. Gardner's son is transferring him to an assisted-living facility for monetary reasons. Mr. Gardner tells you that he is uncomfortable and scared about the new facility, since he does not know anyone there. How can you help Mr. Gardner?
- Mrs. Becker is being admitted as a new resident to the long-term care facility where you work.

Mrs. Becker's daughter, Rhonda, has accompanied her mother to her room. Rhonda mentions to you that she is feeling "like a bad daughter" because she is unable to care for her mother in her own home. She goes on to explain that both she and her husband travel extensively for work, and there would be periods when no one would be around to help care for Mom. Describe some things that you could do to help both Mrs. Becker and Rhonda feel more comfortable about Mrs. Becker coming to live at the long-term care facility.

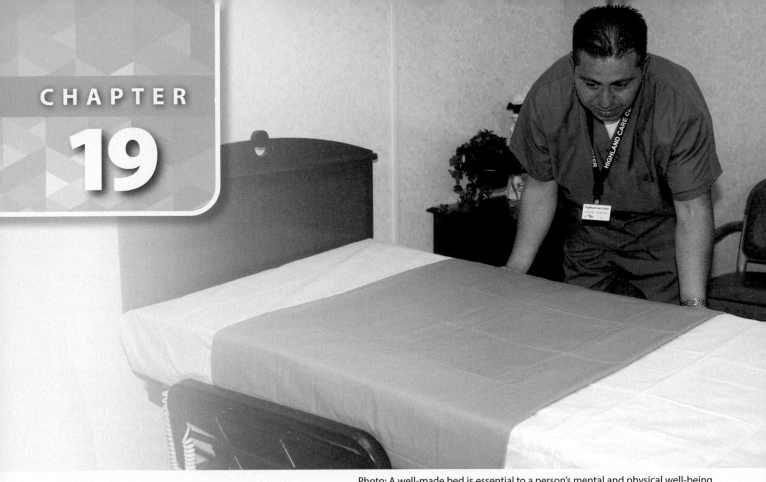

Photo: A well-made bed is essential to a person's mental and physical well-being.
Here, a nursing assistant tucks in a draw sheet.

Bedmaking

 ## WHAT WILL YOU LEARN?

For someone who is tired or ill, nothing is quite as comforting as clean, crisp linens on the bed. Clean linens are essential not only for your patient's or resident's comfort but also for infection control and the prevention of skin breakdown and pressure ulcers. A neat, well-made bed is a sign that the facility provides capable, competent care to its patients or residents. When you are finished with this chapter, you will be able to:

1. Describe how a properly made bed can increase a person's comfort and well-being.
2. List the different types of linens and their uses.
3. Demonstrate the proper way to handle and care for linens.
4. Explain the infection control measures that are used during bedmaking.
5. Demonstrate proper bedmaking techniques, including making a closed bed, opening a bed, preparing a surgical bed, and making an occupied bed.

Vocabulary

Draw sheet	Pressure-relieving	Mitered corner	Surgical bed
Lift sheet	mattress	Closed bed	Occupied bed
Bed protector	Bed cradle	Fanfolded	Toe pleat
Bath blanket	Footboard	Open bed	

LINENS AND OTHER SUPPLIES FOR BEDMAKING

Although bedmaking is a simple process for most people at home, in a health care facility, many different materials can be involved. Linens and other supplies for bedmaking all help to ensure the comfort and health of your patients and residents in different ways, and as a nursing assistant, it is important to know their types and uses.

Linens

Many types of linens are used to make a bed. On your bed at home, you probably have a mattress pad, a bottom (or fitted) sheet, a top (or flat) sheet, a pillow covered in a pillowcase, and a bedspread or comforter. If you live in a cold climate, you may add a blanket to your bed during the winter months to provide extra warmth. In a health care facility, all of these basic linens are used, and some special ones may be added, depending on the needs of the patient or resident. Linens that you may see in use in a health care facility include the following.

Mattress Pads

A mattress pad is a thick layer of padding that is placed on the mattress to help make the bed more comfortable for the patient or resident, and to protect the mattress from moisture and soiling. The mattress pad may be "fitted." In this case, it will have elasticized sides that wrap around and underneath the mattress, holding the pad securely to the mattress. Or, the mattress pad may be "flat" (nonfitted).

Often, in health care facilities, the mattress has a rubber or plastic coating that helps to keep the mattress dry. When no mattress pad is used, and a bottom sheet is placed directly on the rubberized mattress, the person may become very warm and start to sweat because the rubber retains the person's body heat. The bottom sheet becomes damp and stays damp because the rubberized mattress does not absorb the extra moisture. Lying on a damp sheet is uncomfortable for the patient or resident. In addition, lying on a damp sheet can cause the skin to become reddened and irritated, which can lead to skin breakdown and pressure

ulcers. Therefore, when a rubberized mattress is in use, a mattress pad may be used to help pull moisture away from the person's skin.

In a home environment or a long-term care facility, the person may use a standard mattress on their own bed. In this situation, a waterproof mattress pad can be used to help protect the mattress, especially if the person is incontinent (unable to control their bladder or bowels).

Many health care facilities now have mattresses that do not require the use of a mattress pad. The mattress is covered with a material that is resistant to liquid and easily cleaned but allows air to circulate so that heat does not build up underneath the person lying there. This helps to prevent skin breakdown for patients and residents (Fig. 19-1).

Bottom and Top Sheets

The sheets used to make a bed may be white or colored, plain, or printed. Regardless of their other characteristics, however, sheets need to be clean and wrinkle free. A bed is made with two sheets, a bottom sheet and a top sheet. Some facilities use flat or nonfitted sheets as bottom sheets, or the bottom sheet may be fitted. When you are using a flat sheet as the bottom sheet, it is important to tuck the sheet tightly so that movement does not cause the sheet to loosen and wrinkle underneath the person. Wrinkled sheets are uncomfortable and can create areas of pressure on a person's skin, which can lead to skin breakdown.

The top sheet is a flat sheet.

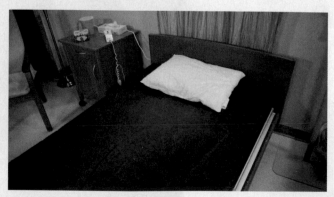

Figure 19-1 Mattress pads are not necessary for many of the more modern mattresses used in the health care setting.

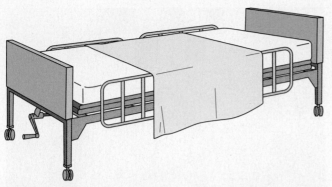

Figure 19-2 A draw sheet is a small sheet that is placed over the middle of the bottom sheet to absorb extra moisture when a mattress pad is not used. Sometimes, draw sheets are used to assist with turning or lifting a person. When a draw sheet is used for this purpose, it is called a "lift sheet."

Draw Sheets

A **draw sheet** is a small, flat sheet that is placed over the middle of the bottom sheet, covering the area of the bed from above the person's shoulders to below the buttocks (Fig. 19-2). When a rubberized mattress is in use, a draw sheet may be used instead of a mattress pad to form a protective, moisture-absorbing barrier between the person's body and the rubberized mattress. Some facilities use padded waterproof draw sheets to protect the mattress from soiling, especially if a patient or resident is incontinent. These draw sheets have a padded absorbent top and a waterproof bottom, and may be made of reusable fabric or disposable material. The sides of the draw sheet are tucked tightly under the mattress to prevent wrinkling.

A **lift sheet** (also referred to as a "friction-reducing sheet") is simply a draw sheet that is used to help lift or reposition a person who needs assistance with moving in bed (see Chapter 15). Both draw sheets and lift sheets can be made easily by folding a flat sheet in half. Make sure that the seams are folded toward the inside so that they do not rub against the person's skin. If a folded flat sheet is being used as a lift sheet, the folded edge of the sheet is positioned above the person's shoulders and the loose ends are positioned below the buttocks. When a draw sheet is to be used as a lift sheet, the sides are usually allowed to hang free although some facilities may require you to tuck the sides of the lift sheet under the mattress after lifting or repositioning the person, to reduce wrinkling.

Bed Protectors

A **bed protector** is a square of quilted absorbent fabric backed with waterproof material. The bed protector measures approximately 3 feet by 3 feet. Bed protectors may be disposable, or they may be laundered and reused.

Some facilities may call bed protectors "incontinence pads" or "soaker pads." In addition to being used for people who are incontinent, bed protectors are often used for people with draining wounds. The urine, feces, or wound drainage is pulled away from the person's body by the absorbent layers of the bed protector, and the waterproof layer keeps the liquid from soiling the rest of the linens on the bed. Sometimes, only the bed protector needs to be changed, resulting in more efficient and economical care.

Blankets

Blankets provided by a facility are usually woven cotton and should be available as requested by a person for their comfort. Residents of long-term care facilities or home health care clients may use their own blankets, which may be wool, cotton, or synthetic, depending on the person's preference and the climate. Because wool blankets can create static and sparks, they should be used with caution if the patient or resident is receiving supplemental oxygen. Electric blankets should be checked for faulty wiring or plugs and may not be safe to use if the person is incontinent or unable to adjust the controls independently (for example, if the person is very old or very young). Electric blankets are usually turned on to warm the bed and then turned off once the person gets in bed. Make sure to use electric blankets according to your facility's policy.

Bedspreads

A bedspread adds the finishing touch to a well-made bed and can add a decorative touch to a person's room. Hospitals and subacute care facilities may supply bedspreads for their patients to use. Other types of health care facilities may encourage their residents to use their own bed coverings. Allowing a person to use a bedspread from home is one way that long-term care facilities help foster a sense of independence and individuality in residents.

Pillows and Pillowcases

Pillows are used for comfort and to aid in positioning. They may be available in many sizes and are made from a variety of materials. Some pillows are covered with waterproof material or treated with a waterproofing substance to protect them from moisture and to aid with cleaning. Pillows are always covered with clean pillowcases. Care for pillows that become wet or soiled will vary according to facility.

Bath Blankets

A **bath blanket** is a lightweight cotton blanket or flannel sheet that is used to provide modesty and warmth during a bed bath or a linen change. A flat sheet may also be used for this purpose if the facility does not provide a special bath blanket. The bath blanket is not made into the bed, but because it is used during bed baths and linen changes, it is gathered along with the other linens.

Concerns for Long-Term Care

Many long-term care facilities use flannel-type sheets to provide extra warmth, especially for older residents who may feel cold in bed. Residents are encouraged to use their own bedspreads, comforters, decorative pillows, and coverlets to add a "touch of home" and promote that person's own individuality. Be sure that you handle these personal items with care when you are changing the person's bed linens.

Other Bedmaking Supplies

Occasionally, other equipment or supplies are used on a person's bed, depending on the specific needs of the patient or resident. Some of the items used include the following.

- A **pressure-relieving mattress** may be placed on top of the regular mattress to help prevent skin breakdown in patients and residents who must stay in bed for long periods of time. Thin foam pads that resemble the inside of an egg carton, called "egg crate mattresses," were used in the past to help relieve pressure but now are used only for comfort. Use of foam pads is decreasing because the foam is difficult to keep clean and dry, especially if the person is incontinent. Newer versions of pressure-relieving mattresses may be filled with air, gel, or water and are made out of a material that is easily cleaned. Special beds used to prevent skin breakdown are described in Chapter 29.
- A **bed cradle** is a metal frame that is placed between the bottom and top sheets to keep the top sheet, the blanket, and the bedspread away from the person's feet (Fig. 19-3). Bed cradles are often used for people who are recovering from burns to prevent the top sheet from touching the burned skin, which would be very painful. They are also used for people who are at risk for developing pressure ulcers on their feet.
- A **footboard** is a padded board that is placed upright at the foot of the bed (Fig. 19-4). The person's feet rest flat against the footboard, helping to keep the feet in proper alignment.

HANDLING OF LINENS

The types of linens used for bedmaking will vary, depending on the facility and the needs of the patient

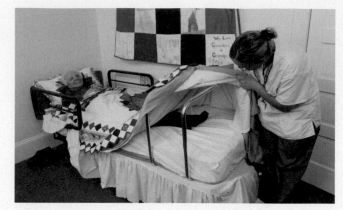

Figure 19-3   A bed cradle is used to keep the top sheet, the blanket, and the bedspread off the patient's or resident's feet. The linens are tucked in at the end of the bed and along the sides to keep the person from getting cold.

or resident. During your employee orientation, you will learn which linens to use. Additional information specific to each patient or resident will be provided on the nursing care plan.

No matter which linens are used in your facility, you should always collect the linens in the order that they will be used—mattress pad (if needed), bottom sheet, draw sheet, bed protector (if needed) top sheet, blanket, bedspread, pillowcases. Once you have collected your stack of linens, flip the stack over so that the item you will need first is on the top of the stack (Fig. 19-5). Collecting linens in the order that they will be put on the bed helps you to remember which linens you need to collect. In addition, because the linens will be arranged in order of use, you will be able to make the bed more efficiently, without searching through the stack for the proper item.

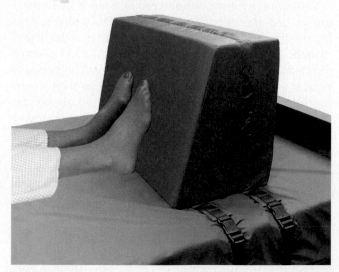

Figure 19-4   A footboard is placed against the end of the bed to keep the person's feet in proper alignment. (*Courtesy of Skil-Care Corporation, Copyright 2023.*)

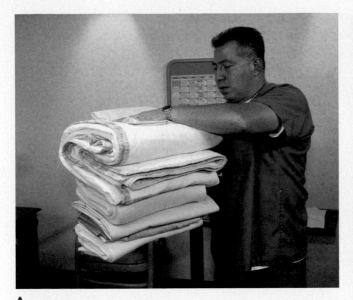

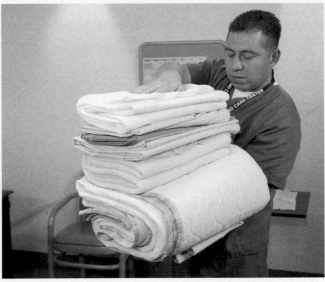

A   **B**

Figure 19-5 Handling linens. **A.** First, collect the linens in the order that they will be used. Here, the nursing assistant has gathered a mattress pad, a bottom sheet, a draw sheet, a top sheet, a blanket, a bedspread, and two pillowcases. The mattress pad is on the bottom of the stack and the pillowcases are on the top. Note that the nursing assistant is holding the linens away from their body. **B.** Next, flip the stack of linens over so that the item you will need first is on top. Now the pillowcases are on the bottom of the stack and the mattress pad is on top, ready to be put on the bed.

Always remember that linens can act as fomites, or objects capable of spreading infection. For this reason, you should always use infection control practices when handling linens. Always perform hand hygiene before collecting clean linens and avoid letting clean linens come into contact with dirty surfaces, such as your uniform or the floor. When removing used linens from the bed, wear gloves, and roll the linens toward the center of the bed (down from the top and up from the bottom) to confine any soiled areas on the inside (Fig. 19-6). To help prevent the spread of pathogens,

place the used linen in a linen hamper as it is removed from the bed. The linen hamper is then removed from the room and taken to a designated area. Do not place dirty linens on the floor, on furniture or equipment, or hold them against your uniform.

Guidelines Box 19-1 summarizes some general guidelines for the handling of linens. These guidelines apply no matter where you work.

STANDARD BEDMAKING TECHNIQUES

Routine bedmaking is usually done in the morning, before visiting hours, while your patients or residents are bathing or dressing. How often a person's linens are changed will vary according to the type of health care facility and the person's needs. For example, in a hospital, the policy may be to change each person's linens completely on a daily basis. In a long-term care setting, the policy may call for less frequent linen changes. However, a person's bed must be remade each time any of the linens become soiled or excessively wrinkled, regardless of the time of day. Soiling of the sheets can occur as a result of spilled food or drink or as a result of excessive sweating, vomit, urine, feces, wound drainage, or leakage from a feeding tube. In each of these instances, a linen change would be required. Change as many of the bed linens as necessary to ensure a clean, dry, wrinkle-free bed

Figure 19-6 Gloves are worn to remove linens from the bed because the linens may be soiled with body fluids. The soiled area is rolled toward the center of the bed.

Guidelines Box 19-1 Guidelines for Handling Linens

WHAT YOU DO	WHY YOU DO IT
Always perform proper hand hygiene before collecting clean linens.	Proper hand hygiene prevents microbes on your hands from being transferred to the clean linens.
Do not hold linens, clean or dirty, against your uniform.	If you hold clean linens against your uniform, microbes on your uniform could be transferred to the linens. If you hold dirty linens against your uniform, then microbes from the dirty linens could be transferred to your uniform.
When collecting linens, collect only those that you will need for that person's bed. For example, if a draw sheet is not needed, do not collect one.	Extra linens brought into a person's room are considered contaminated, and therefore, must not be returned to the clean linen cart or used for another person. These linens must now be laundered, which costs the facility extra money and manpower and creates additional wear on the linens, shortening their lifetime of use.
Collect linens in the order that they will be used. Once you have collected your stack of linens, flip the stack over so that the item you will need first is on the top of the stack.	Collecting linens in the order that they will be put on the bed helps you to remember which linens you need to collect. In addition, because the linens will be arranged in order of use, you will be able to make the bed more efficiently, without searching through the stack for the proper item.
Place clean linens on a clean surface in the room, such as the over-bed table or a chair. Do not place clean linens on the floor.	Clean linens can become contaminated with microbes if you place them on a "dirty" surface, such as the floor.
Wear gloves when removing used linens from a bed. Roll the linens toward the center of the bed to confine the soiled area inside.	Any item contaminated with blood or other body substances is a potential source of exposure to pathogens for the health care worker. Following the standard precautions and wearing proper personal protective equipment (PPE) will help to minimize your exposure. Confining the soiled area to the inside of the linens helps to ensure that other people, such as the people in the laundry, do not come in contact with the potentially infectious material.
If body fluids or substances leak through the linens to the mattress or bed frame, the mattress or bed frame should be wiped with an appropriate cleaning solution before placing clean linens on the bed. Remove your gloves and perform hand hygiene before handling the clean linens.	These infection control methods help to prevent the clean sheets from becoming contaminated.
After removing the dirty linens from the bed, place them in the linen hamper immediately. Your facility may require you to place dirty linens in a smaller linen bag before placing them in the linen hamper. Do not place dirty linens on the floor or on any other surface.	Placing the dirty linens in the linen hamper immediately helps to control the spread of infection.

for your patient or resident. General guidelines for bedmaking are given in Guidelines Box 19-2.

To make a bed, you will need to know how to make a **mitered corner** (Fig. 19-7). Mitering is a way of folding and tucking the sheet so that it lies flat and neat against the mattress. When a flat sheet is used as the bottom sheet, the mitered corners are made at the top of the bed to help secure the sheet to the mattress. Mitered corners are made at the foot of the bed to hold the top sheet, blanket, and bedspread in place.

Guidelines Box 19-2 Guidelines for Bedmaking

WHAT YOU DO	WHY YOU DO IT
Always place linens on the bed so that the seams of the sheets face away from the person's skin.	The seams of the sheets can rub the person's skin, causing irritation and leading to skin breakdown.
Linens must be pulled tightly to avoid wrinkling. Layering should be kept to a minimum.	The wrinkles and extra layers of linens can cause skin breakdown and contribute to the formation of pressure ulcers.
Linens should be changed whenever they become soiled or wet, regardless of the time of day.	Besides causing discomfort, soiled or wet sheets can cause skin breakdown and contribute to the formation of pressure ulcers.
Do not shake linens when placing them on the bed.	Dust is a transport mechanism for microbes. Shaking linens stirs up dust from the floor. The dust then settles on surfaces in the room and can be easily transferred onto eating utensils or into a wound, causing an infection.
When you need to change the linens on a person's bed with the person still in the bed, always be sure to explain what you are doing throughout the procedure. Talk reassuringly to the person, even if the person is unconscious and you think that the person cannot hear you. Close the door, pull the privacy curtain, and keep the person covered at all times.	Having the bed linens changed while still in the bed can be a frightening experience for a bedridden person, particularly if the person is unconscious. Even if the person is conscious, movement may cause pain and incontinence (the involuntary loss of urine or feces) that can be embarrassing, if it occurs. If the person is mentally impaired, they may become combative. Explaining what you are doing and taking care to preserve the person's modesty during the procedure will make the procedure more pleasant for the person.
Disconnect the call light control and any tubes or drains that may be connected to the bed linens before removing the linens from the bed.	Disconnecting equipment and tubes from the linens will help prevent discomfort from pulling on or possibly accidental removal of tubes and drains.
Check the bed linens for personal items before removing the linens from the bed.	Personal items, such as dentures, eyeglasses, or jewelry, may become lost in the bed linens. If these linens are removed from the bed, bundled up, and sent to the laundry, the mislaid personal items may not be discovered and they could be damaged in the wash cycle, or they may be lost altogether. Personal items may be expensive and inconvenient to replace. If they hold sentimental value, they may be irreplaceable.

Closed (Unoccupied) Beds

A **closed bed** is an empty bed (Fig. 19-8A). A bed that is unoccupied because the previous patient or resident has been discharged from the facility and a new patient or resident has yet to arrive is considered a closed bed. Similarly, a bed that is unoccupied because the patient or resident is simply not in it at the moment (and is not expected back any time soon) is also considered a closed bed. For example, many long-term care facilities make closed beds each day for residents who are not bedridden. Procedure 19-1 explains how to make a closed bed.

When the top sheet, blanket, and bedspread of a closed bed are turned back, or **fanfolded**, the closed bed becomes an **open bed**, or a bed ready to receive a patient or resident. For example, you would open a bed in preparation for a new admission, or after you have changed the linens while a patient or resident is bathing or out of the room for a diagnostic test. Because the patient or resident would be expected to return to the bed shortly, you would fanfold the linens back in anticipation of their return. Similarly, in some long-term care facilities, the linens on the beds of residents who are not bedridden are folded back in the evening, before the residents return to their rooms. To open a

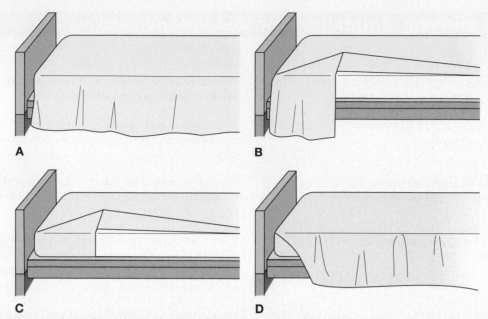

Figure 19-7 How to make a mitered corner. Here, a mitered corner is being made on a top sheet. **A.** The bottom of the sheet has been tucked under the end of the mattress. The side of the sheet is hanging over the side of the bed. **B.** Grasp the edge of the sheet about 12 inches from the foot of the bed and lift it up, forming a triangle. Lay the triangular fold on the top of the bed, and smooth the hanging portion of the sheet against the side of the mattress. **C.** Tuck the hanging portion of the sheet underneath the mattress while holding the triangular fold taut against the top of the bed. **D.** Bring the triangular fold back down over the edge of the mattress, and leave the side hanging loose.

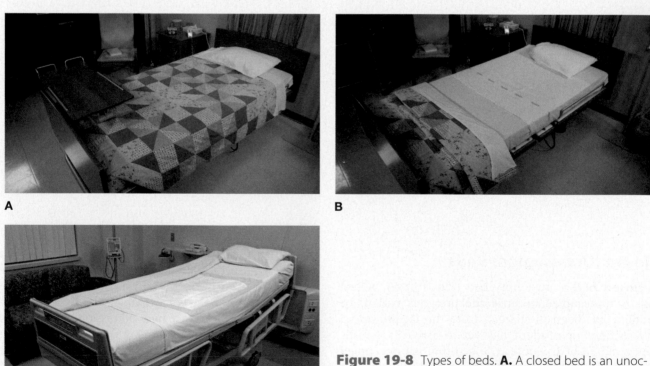

Figure 19-8 Types of beds. **A.** A closed bed is an unoccupied bed. **B.** When a closed bed is "opened," the top sheet, blanket, and bedspread are "fanfolded" to the foot of the bed. **C.** A surgical bed is a closed bed that has been "opened" to receive a person on a stretcher. The top linens are fanfolded to the side of the bed.

closed bed, you first grasp the bedspread, blanket, and top sheet and fold them back to the foot of the bed, creating a fanfold (Fig. 19-8B). Finish by making sure that the bed is in the lowest position and the bed wheels are locked. Place the call light control near the head of the bed within easy reach of the patient or resident, clipping it to the bottom sheet.

A **surgical bed** is a closed bed that has been opened to receive a patient or resident who will be arriving by stretcher. A surgical bed may be prepared for a patient who is returning to the room following surgery or a diagnostic procedure, or for one who is being transferred from another unit (such as the emergency room). When preparing a surgical bed, instead of folding the top sheet, blanket, and bedspread to the foot of the bed, you loosen these linens from the foot of the bed and fold them toward the side of the bed, leaving one side open and ready to receive the person (Fig. 19-8C). After folding the linens to the side, raise the bed so that the stretcher will be level with the bed. Make sure that the bed wheels are locked, and ensure a clear path by moving any furniture away from the bed.

Occupied Beds

> *"She went out of the room and came back with the old nurse of the early morning. Together they made the bed with me in it. That was new to me and an admirable proceeding."*
>
> —*A Farewell to Arms*, Ernest Hemingway

Some conditions make it difficult or impossible for a person to get out of bed for a linen change. When this is the case, it is necessary to change the linens while the person is still in the bed. This is called making an **occupied bed** (Procedure 19-2). In most facilities, this procedure is carried out on a routine basis after the person has been bathed. However, as always, if the linens become wet or soiled in between scheduled linen changes, then they must be changed. Because it can be frightening for a bedridden person to have the linens changed while they are still in the bed, remember to explain to the person what you are doing throughout this procedure. Keep the privacy curtain and the door closed during the procedure, to help maintain the person's modesty. If the linens you are removing from the bed may be soiled with blood or other body substances, you must wear gloves. Remember to remove the soiled gloves and put on clean ones before handling the clean linens.

Helping Hands and a Caring Heart

Focus on Humanistic Health Care

All of us can probably remember a time when we were really sick and someone came and freshened us up and changed our sheets. Think about how loved and well-cared-for you felt! That is how your patients or residents will feel when you replace their hot, wrinkled, soiled linens with cool, smooth, clean ones. When a complete linen change is not necessary, the simple act of pulling the wrinkles out of the linens and plumping up the pillow can be very comforting to a patient or resident.

SUMMARY

- A well-made bed is essential to a person's mental and physical well-being.
  - Clean, dry, wrinkle-free linens help make a person who is ill feel cared for and more comfortable.
  - Clean, dry, wrinkle-free linens help to prevent complications, such as pressure ulcers.
  - Clean, dry linens are important for odor and infection control.
- A variety of linens are used in bedmaking, depending on facility policy and the patient's or resident's particular needs.
- Special devices, such as pressure-relieving mattresses and bed cradles, are used to improve the patient's or resident's comfort and prevent complications related to spending long periods of time in bed, such as pressure ulcers.
- Because linens soiled with body fluids and substances can act as fomites, it is important to use good infection control practices when handling them.
  - Never hold dirty linens against your uniform or place them on the floor or other surface. Dirty linens must be placed in the linen hamper immediately.
  - Always perform hand hygiene before handling clean linens. Never hold clean linens against your uniform or place them on the floor. Clean linens may be placed on a clean surface in the room, such as the over-bed table.
  - Always wear gloves when you may be handling soiled linens.
- A bed is either unoccupied ("closed") or occupied. A closed bed may be "opened" in anticipation of receiving a patient or resident by fanfolding the sheets to allow easier access.

► **Procedure 19-1**

Making an Unoccupied (Closed) Bed

WHY YOU DO IT Clean, dry, wrinkle-free linens promote comfort, help to prevent complications (such as pressure ulcers), and are important for odor and infection control.

Getting Ready

1. Complete the "Getting Ready" steps.*

Supplies

- mattress pad (if necessary)
- bottom sheet
- lift (draw) sheet (if necessary)
- bed protector (if necessary)
- top sheet
- blanket
- bedspread
- pillowcase

Procedure

2. Place the linens on a clean surface close to the bed (for example, the over-bed table).

3. Make sure that the bed is positioned at a comfortable working height to promote good body mechanics (usually elbow height of the caregiver) and that the wheels are locked.

4. Lower the side rails and move the mattress to the head of the bed (it may have shifted toward the foot of the bed if the occupant of the bed had the head of the bed elevated).

   Note: The mattress pad, bottom sheet, and draw sheet are positioned and tucked in on one side of the bed before moving to the other side to complete these actions. This is most efficient in terms of energy and time.

5. Place the mattress pad on the bed and unfold it so that only one vertical crease remains. Make sure that this crease is centered on the mattress. If the mattress pad is fitted, carefully pull the corners of the near side over the corners of the mattress and smooth down the sides. If the mattress pad is flat, make sure the top of the pad is even with the head of the mattress. Open the mattress pad across the bed, taking care to keep it centered.

6. Place the bottom sheet on the bed. If the bottom sheet is fitted, carefully pull the corners of the near side over the corners of the mattress and smooth down the sides. If the bottom sheet is flat:

   a. Place the sheet so that when you unfold it, the wide hem will be at the head of the bed and the hem stitching will be against the mattress, away from the person who will be occupying the bed.

   b. Unfold the sheet so that only one vertical crease remains. Make sure that this crease is vertically centered on the mattress.

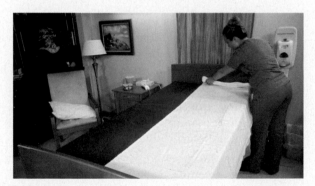

STEP 6b Unfold the sheet so that only one vertical crease remains.

   c. Open the sheet across the bed, taking care to keep it centered. The same length of sheet (approximately 12 to 18 inches) should hang over each side of the bed. Make sure that the lower edge of the sheet is even with the foot of the mattress.

(continued)

---

*It is assumed that the dirty linens have been removed from the bed, and the bed has been cleaned, as per facility policy, prior to beginning this procedure.

d. Tuck the sheet under the mattress at the head of the bed and miter the corner.

e. Tuck the near side of the sheet underneath the mattress, working from the head of the bed toward the foot. As you tuck, make sure there are no wrinkles in the sheet and that the mattress pad remains smooth and in place.

7. Place the lift sheet on the bed so that the top of the sheet is approximately 12 inches from the head of the mattress. Smooth the lift sheet across the bed and tuck the near side under the mattress.

8. Now, move to the other side of the bed and repeat the process of aligning the mattress pad, mitering the corner, and tucking in the bottom sheet and lift sheet.

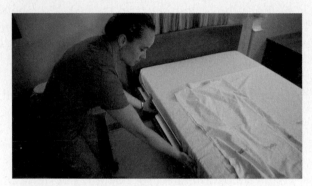

STEP 8 After mitering the corner at the head of the bed, tuck the side of the sheet underneath the mattress.

9. Place the top sheet on the bed so that when you unfold it, the wide hem will be at the head of the bed and the hem stitching will be facing upward, away from the person who will be occupying the bed.

a. Unfold the sheet so that only one vertical crease remains. Make sure that this crease is centered vertically on the mattress.

b. Open the sheet across the bed, taking care to keep it centered. The same length of sheet (approximately 12 to 18 inches) should hang over each side of the bed. Make sure that the top edge of the sheet is even with the head of the mattress. Pull the bottom of the sheet over the foot of the bed, but do not tuck it in yet (it will be tucked in with the blanket and bedspread).

10. Place the blanket on the bed and unfold it in the same manner as the sheet, keeping the center crease in the center of the bed. The same length of blanket (approximately 12 to 18 inches) should hang over each side of the bed. Make sure that the top edge of the blanket is approximately 6 to 8 inches from the head of the mattress. Pull the bottom edge of the blanket over the sheet at the foot of the bed, but do not tuck anything in yet.

11. Place the bedspread on the bed and unfold it in the same manner as the sheet, keeping the center crease in the center of the bed. The sides of the bedspread should be even and cover all of the other bed linens. Make sure that the top of the bedspread is even with the head of the mattress, unless the pillow is to be tucked under the bedspread (in which case you will need to allow more length at the top). Pull the bottom of the bedspread over the blanket and sheet at the foot of the bed.

12. Together, tuck the bedspread, the blanket, and the top sheet under the foot of the mattress. Make a mitered corner at the foot of the bed on both sides.

13. Fold the upper 6 inches of the top sheet and blanket down over the spread to make a cuff.

14. Rest the pillow on the bed. Grasping the closed end of the pillowcase, turn the pillowcase inside out over your hand and arm. Grasp the pillow through the pillowcase and pull the pillowcase down over the pillow. Make sure any tags or zippers are on the inside of the pillowcase.

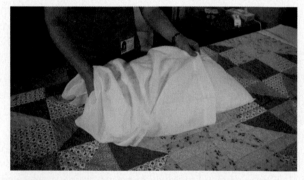

STEP 14 Grasp the pillow through the pillowcase and pull the pillowcase down over the pillow.

15. Place the pillow on the bed with the open end of the pillowcase facing away from the door.

Finishing Up

16. Complete the "Finishing Up" steps.

Procedure 19-2

Making an Occupied Bed

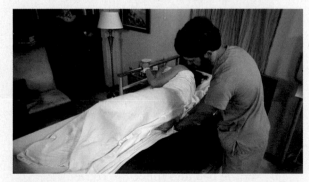

WHY YOU DO IT Clean, dry, wrinkle-free linens promote comfort, help to prevent complications (such as pressure ulcers), and are important for odor and infection control.

Getting Ready WEAVERS

1. Complete the "Getting Ready" steps.

Supplies

- gloves
- bath blanket
- mattress pad (if necessary)
- bottom sheet
- lift (draw) sheet
- bed protector (if necessary)
- top sheet
- blanket
- bedspread
- pillowcase
- linen hamper

Procedure

2. Place the linens on a clean surface close to the bed (for example, the over-bed table). Make sure to position the table holding the linens close enough to the bed that you don't have to step away from the bedside to reach it.

3. Make sure that the bed is positioned at a comfortable working height to promote good body mechanics (usually elbow height of the caregiver) and that the wheels are locked.

4. Disconnect the call light control and any tubes or drains from the bed linens. Check the bed for dentures or any other personal items.

5. Lower the head of the bed so that the bed is flat (as tolerated).

6. Put on the gloves (the linens may be wet or soiled).

7. Remove the bedspread and blanket from the bed. If they are to be reused, fold and place them on a clean surface, such as a chair.

8. Loosen the top sheet at the foot of the bed and spread a bath blanket over the top sheet (and the person).

9. If the person is able, have them hold the bath blanket. If not, tuck the corners under the person's shoulders. Remove the top sheet by

pulling it out from underneath the bath blanket, being careful not to expose the person.

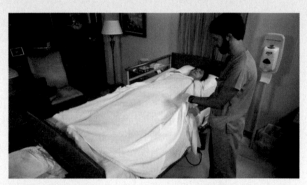

STEP 9 Remove the top sheet by pulling it out from underneath the bath blanket.

10. Place the top sheet in the linen hamper.

11. If the side rails are in use, lower the side rail on the working side of the bed. The side rail on the opposite side of the bed should remain up. Turn the person onto their side so that they are facing away from you. Reposition the pillow under the person's head, and adjust the bath blanket to keep the person covered.

12. Loosen the lift sheet, bottom sheet, and (if necessary) the mattress pad.

13. Fanfold the bottom linens toward the person's back, tucking them slightly underneath them.*

STEP 13 Fanfold the bottom linens toward the person's back.

---

*If the linens are wet or soiled, make sure you change your gloves before handling the clean linens.

(continued)

14. Straighten the mattress pad (if it is not being changed). If the mattress pad is being changed, place the clean mattress pad on the bed and unfold it so that only one vertical crease remains. Make sure that this crease is centered vertically on the mattress. If the mattress pad is fitted, carefully pull the corners of the near side over the corners of the mattress and smooth down the sides. If the mattress pad is flat, make sure the top of the pad is even with the head of the mattress. Fanfold the opposite side of the mattress pad close to the patient or resident tucking them underneath the old linens.

15. Place the clean bottom sheet on the bed. If the bottom sheet is fitted, carefully pull the corners over the corners of the mattress and smooth down the sides. If the bottom sheet is flat:

    a. Place the sheet so that when you unfold it, the wide hem will be at the head of the bed and the hem stitching will be against the mattress, away from the person who will be occupying the bed.

    b. Unfold the sheet so that only one vertical crease remains. Make sure that this crease is centered vertically on the mattress.

    c. Open the sheet across the bed, taking care to keep it centered. The same length of sheet (approximately 12 to 18 inches) should hang over each side of the bed. Make sure that the lower edge of the sheet is even with the foot of the mattress. Fanfold the opposite side of the sheet close to the patient or resident tucking it underneath the old linens.

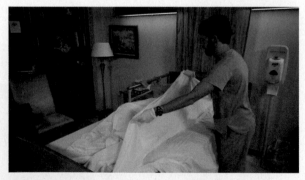

STEP 15c Open the sheet across the bed, taking care to keep it centered.

    d. Tuck the sheet under the mattress at the head of the bed and miter the corner.

    e. Tuck the near side of the sheet underneath the mattress, working from the head of the bed toward the foot. As you tuck, make sure there are no wrinkles in the sheet and that the mattress pad remains smooth and in place.

16. Place the lift sheet on the bed so that the top of the sheet is approximately 12 inches from the head of the mattress. Fanfold the opposite side of the lift sheet close to the patient or resident tucking it underneath the old linens. Smooth the lift sheet across the bed and tuck the near side under the mattress.

17. Raise the side rail on the working side of the bed. Help the person to roll toward you, over the folded linens. Reposition the pillow under the person's head and adjust the bath blanket to keep the person covered.

18. Move to the other side of the bed and lower the side rail.

19. Loosen and remove the soiled bottom linens and place them in the linen hamper. Change your gloves if they become soiled.

20. Now, repeat the process of aligning the mattress pad, mitering the corner, and tucking in the bottom sheet and lift sheet.

21. Help the person to move to the center of the bed and position them comfortably. Raise the side rail on the working side of the bed.

22. Change the pillowcase and place the pillow under the person's head.

23. Place the clean top sheet over the person (who is still covered with the bath blanket), being careful not to cover their face. The sheet should be placed so that when you unfold it, the wide hem will be at the head of the bed and the hem stitching will be facing upward, away from the person who will be occupying the bed.

    a. Unfold the sheet so that only one vertical crease remains. Make sure that this crease is centered vertically on the mattress.

    b. Open the sheet across the bed, taking care to keep it centered. The same length of sheet (approximately 12 to 18 inches) should hang over each side of the bed.

    c. If the person is able, have them hold the top sheet. If not, tuck the corners under their shoulders. Remove the bath blanket by pulling it out from underneath the top sheet, being careful not to expose the person. Place the bath blanket in the linen hamper.

24. Place the blanket and then the bedspread over the top sheet. Together, tuck the bedspread, the blanket, and the top sheet under the foot of the mattress. Make a mitered corner at the foot of the bed on both sides.

25. Make a **toe pleat** by grasping the top sheet, the blanket, and the bedspread over the person's feet and pulling the linens straight up. The toe pleat allows the person to move their feet and helps to relieve pressure on the feet from tightly tucked linens.

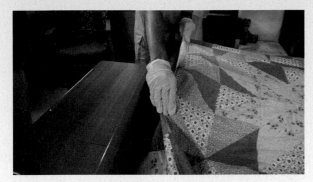

STEP 25 Make a toe pleat by pulling straight up on the top linens.

26. Lower the bed to its lowest position and make sure that the wheels are locked. Raise the head of the bed as the person requests.

27. Remove your gloves, dispose of them in a facility-approved waste container, and perform hand hygiene.

Finishing Up

28. Complete the "Finishing Up" steps.

WHAT DID YOU LEARN?

Multiple Choice

Select the single best answer for each of the following questions.

1. What is a draw sheet?
   a. A fitted bottom sheet
   b. A half-sized sheet that is placed over the middle of the bottom sheet and has varied uses, including repositioning and lifting a person in bed
   c. A half-sized sheet that is placed over the middle of the top sheet and used to make toe pleats
   d. A sheet used to add a decorative touch to the person's room

2. What is a bed that has a person in it called?
   a. An open bed
   b. A closed bed
   c. A surgical bed
   d. An occupied bed

3. A bed that has the top linens fanfolded to the side has been prepared for what type of patient?
   a. A patient who is paraplegic
   b. A patient who is incontinent
   c. A patient who will be arriving on a stretcher
   d. A patient who will be returning to bed in the evening

4. What is the purpose of a "toe pleat?"
   a. To hold the bedspread in place at the foot of the bed
   b. To relieve pressure on the feet from tightly tucked sheets
   c. To hold a person's feet in proper alignment
   d. To make a person's personal bed coverings look neat

5. When you are handling linens, always remember to:
   a. Shake the bedspread to remove dust
   b. Place the dirty linens on the floor, to get them out of your way
   c. Hold the linens away from your body
   d. All of the above

6. What do you call a metal frame that is placed between the bottom and top sheets to keep the bed linens from resting on the person's feet?
   a. A bed board
   b. A pressure-relieving mattress
   c. A bed cradle
   d. A footboard

7. What personal protective equipment (PPE) should be worn when removing used bed linens?
   a. Gloves
   b. A gown
   c. Eye goggles
   d. No PPE is necessary

8. When are bed linens changed?
   a. When they become wet or soiled
   b. According to facility policy
   c. When they become excessively wrinkled
   d. All of the above

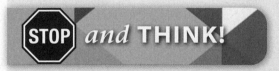

- You are making an occupied bed. There is no linen hamper in the room and you have already removed the soiled linens from the bed. What should you do with the soiled linens until you can take them to the linen room or hallway hamper? Mrs. O'Shea, the resident, is lying on her side in the bed, covered with a bath blanket.
- Barbara is a nursing assistant on 3 West. She has already changed the bed linens twice during her shift for one of her patients, Mrs. Bridges. Mrs. Bridges is receiving chemotherapy for cancer, and one of the side effects of the medication is uncontrollable diarrhea. Now Mrs. Bridges' call light is on again. When Barbara goes to check on her, she discovers that Mrs. Bridges has soiled the bed again. Barbara tells Mrs. Bridges she'll be right back and leaves to go get supplies from the linen closet. What are some items Barbara should collect, along with clean sheets?

Photo: A nursing assistant takes a resident's blood pressure.

Vital Signs, Height, and Weight

 WHAT WILL YOU LEARN?

The word "vital" means "necessary to life." This is why those in the health care field refer to certain key measurements that provide essential information about a person's health as **vital signs**. When we evaluate a person's vital signs, we look at the person's body temperature, heartbeat (pulse), breathing (respirations), and blood pressure. One of the many important duties you will perform as a nursing assistant will be to routinely measure and record your patients' or residents' vital signs. A person's height and weight, although not technically vital signs, also provide insight into a person's overall health status. Therefore, you will also be responsible for obtaining and recording these measurements (although not as frequently as the vital sign measurements). Because a change in a person's normal vital sign measurements can be a sign of illness, your ability to detect a change and report this to the nurse promptly is essential to the well-being of your patients or residents. When you are finished with this chapter, you will be able to:

1. Explain the term *vital signs* and how they reflect changes in a person's medical condition.
2. Explain the importance of accurately measuring and recording vital signs, and of reporting any changes to the nurse.
3. Define the term *body temperature* and describe the factors affecting a person's body temperature.

4. List common sites used for measuring a person's body temperature and the advantages and disadvantages of each.

5. Demonstrate the proper use of a glass thermometer, an electronic or digital thermometer, a tympanic thermometer, and a temporal thermometer.

6. Define the term *pulse* and describe factors that may affect a person's pulse.

7. List common sites used for taking a person's pulse.

8. Demonstrate the proper way to measure and record a radial pulse and an apical pulse, including using a stethoscope.

9. Explain the terms used to describe a person's respirations and the factors that may affect a person's respirations.

10. Demonstrate the proper way to measure and record a person's respirations.

11. Define the term *blood pressure* and describe factors that may affect a person's blood pressure.

12. Demonstrate the proper way to measure a person's blood pressure, including using a sphygmomanometer and listening for Korotkoff sounds.

13. Define various terms used to describe an abnormal blood pressure.

14. Discuss factors that can lead to a change in a person's weight.

15. Demonstrate the proper way to measure a person's height and weight using an upright scale, a chair scale, and when the person is in bed.

Vocabulary

Vital signs	Stethoscope	Respiratory rhythm	Systolic pressure
Body temperature	Diaphragm	Depth of respiration	Diastolic pressure
Metabolism	Bell	Eupnea	Pulse pressure
Febrile	Pulse deficit	Tachypnea	Sphygmomanometer
Pulse	Tachycardia	Bradypnea	Korotkoff sounds
Pulse rate	Bradycardia	Dyspnea	Hypertension
Pulse rhythm	Inhalation (inspiration)	Hyperventilation	Hypotension
Dysrhythmia	Exhalation (expiration)	Hypoventilation	Orthostatic hypotension
Pulse amplitude	Respiratory rate	Blood pressure	

WHAT DO VITAL SIGNS TELL US?

Vital signs reflect functions that are regulated automatically by the body, such as:

- How fast the heart beats
- The internal temperature of the body
- The rate at which a person breathes

Because the body is always trying to maintain a state of balance, "control centers" (located mostly in the brain) regulate what is going on inside the body and make adjustments as necessary to keep things within the range of normal. Therefore, a change in a vital sign may indicate that something has put the body out of balance, and the body is trying to get that balance back. Pain is often considered the "fifth vital sign" because the presence of pain is another indicator that the body is out of balance. Pain is discussed in detail in Chapter 21.

There are many factors that can cause changes in a person's vital sign measurements. A person's vital sign measurements may vary over the course of a day (for example, in response to emotional or physical stress or a change in position) while still staying within the range of "normal." However, a major or a long-lasting change in one or more of a person's vital sign measurements may be a response to illness or injury. As you read this chapter, pay attention to the ranges that are considered "normal" for each vital sign. Knowing these ranges will allow you to quickly recognize measurements that are not within the range of normal. Also remember that your definition of "normal" will vary according to the person. For example, you may come to know that Ms. Goldblum's blood pressure tends to be at the low end of the normal range while Mr. Singh's tends to be a little bit higher than average. Your knowledge of your patient or resident will allow you to know whether the vital sign measurements you have obtained are normal readings for that person.

MEASURING AND RECORDING VITAL SIGNS

Vital signs are measured and compared with normal values (as well as the values that are considered normal for the individual) under many different circumstances. For example, it is routine for vital signs to be taken each time a person visits the doctor and when a person is admitted to a hospital or long-term care facility. It may also be necessary to check a person's vital signs:

- Before and after certain medications are given
- Before, during, and after a surgical or diagnostic procedure
- In an emergency situation
- After an incident or accident, such as a fall

Patients in a hospital may have their vital signs taken every shift or every few hours while residents of a long-term care facility may have their vital signs taken only once daily or even weekly. A patient who is critically ill may be attached to machines that measure their vital signs continuously and display the results on a monitor. The nursing care plan and Kardex, the doctor's orders, or all will specify how often each of your patient's or resident's vital signs are to be measured and recorded. However, it is also within your scope of practice to take a person's vital signs if the person complains of dizziness, nausea, or pain, or if you notice that the person just is not looking or acting like they normally do. If a person has been participating in an activity that may affect their vital signs (for example, walking, drinking, eating), you should give the person a few minutes to sit and relax before taking their vital signs.

Facilities will have different policies regarding how vital signs are recorded. Some facilities will record vital sign measurements on one flow sheet for the unit, which lists the names of all of the patients or residents on a particular unit. Other facilities will use one flow sheet per patient or resident. This flow sheet may be kept in the person's medical record, or at the person's bedside. Many health care facilities are now using electronic methods of recording vital signs.

In some instances, the nursing assistant uses a computer "tablet" to record and document each person's vital sign measurements. If you take a person's vital signs and get a measurement that is abnormal (either higher or lower than normal for that particular person), you should take the measurement again for the sake of accuracy and then report your findings to the nurse immediately.

The skills you will use to measure a person's vital signs may seem difficult when you are first learning them, but practice will make you more comfortable with taking vital sign measurements. Measuring and recording vital sign measurements accurately is critical because many people rely on this information to make important decisions about the patient's or resident's care. In addition, a problem may go unnoticed if a vital sign is measured or recorded inaccurately. Always ask for assistance, either from another nursing assistant or a nurse, if you are having difficulty when checking a person's vital signs. Asking for help when you need it is not a sign of failure or an inability to do your job—rather, it demonstrates that you are responsible and committed to seeing that your patient or resident receives the best possible care. Let's take a look now at the individual vital signs, starting with body temperature.

BODY TEMPERATURE

The **body temperature** is simply how hot the body is. When we measure someone's body temperature, what we are measuring is the difference between the heat produced by the person's body and the heat lost by the person's body. The human body produces heat as a normal process of **metabolism**. Metabolism is the term for the physical and chemical changes that occur when the cells of the body convert the food that we eat into energy. Muscle movement also produces heat. This is why we become hotter when we exercise, and why we shiver when we are cold (shivering moves the muscles, producing heat). Heat loss occurs normally through the skin, through the passing of urine and feces, and through the process of breathing, and is increased by bodily responses such as sweating. The body temperature is regulated by a "control center" that is located in the brain.

Factors Affecting the Body Temperature

Although a healthy person's body temperature is usually fairly constant, small changes may occur as a result of physical or emotional stress, the environmental temperature, or even the time of day. For example, it is typical for a person's body temperature to be lower in the morning and increase slightly throughout the day, probably from an increase in activity levels. Stress causes the release of hormones that increase metabolism and the heart rate, readying the body to respond to the source of the stress. This response, called the "fight or flight" response, is discussed in detail in Chapter 35. The increase in metabolism and heart rate can lead to an increase in body temperature as well. Finally, exposure to either very hot or very cold environmental temperatures can cause changes in a person's body temperature.

A person's age and sex also play a role in determining body temperature. Very young people and very old people tend to be more sensitive to environmental temperature changes. Infants often have immature control centers, which means that their bodies are slower to adjust to changes in temperature. In addition, infants usually lose body heat through their skin more easily. An older person's body may not produce as much heat as it did in younger years, due to muscle loss as a result of normal aging. Finally, body temperature for females tends to change more frequently than that of males, because of the hormonal changes that occur with the menstrual cycle and during pregnancy and menopause.

Measuring the Body Temperature

The body temperature can be measured from several different areas of the body:

- Mouth (an *oral temperature*)
- Rectum (a *rectal temperature*)
- Armpit (an *axillary temperature*)
- Ear (a *tympanic temperature*)
- Forehead (a *temporal temperature*)

Where the body temperature is measured depends on facility policy and the needs of the patient or resident. Because the method used to measure the temperature affects the accuracy of the measurement, you should note which method was used when you record the temperature, as per your facility's policy. For example, many facilities use "O" for oral, "R" for rectal, "T" for tympanic or temporal artery, and "A" for axillary. The body temperature is measured in either degrees Fahrenheit (°F) or degrees Celsius (°C), using a clinical thermometer.

Types of Thermometers

There are many different types of thermometers in use.

Glass Thermometers

When many of us think of a thermometer, we think of a glass thermometer (Fig. 20-1). In past years, glass

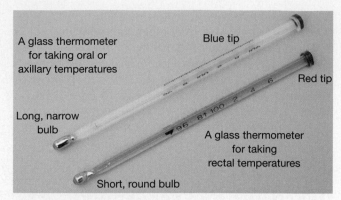

A glass thermometer for taking oral or axillary temperatures

Blue tip

Long, narrow bulb

Red tip

A glass thermometer for taking rectal temperatures

Short, round bulb

Figure 20-1 Glass thermometers may vary slightly in appearance depending on their intended use.

thermometers contained mercury, a toxic substance. Because of the dangers associated with breakage and spilled mercury, most health care settings do not use glass thermometers at all. Some settings still use glass thermometers, but have switched to using newer models, which contain a substance that behaves the same way as mercury but is less toxic. Glass thermometers consist of a glass bulb attached to a thin glass tube that is marked with a temperature scale and filled with a liquid substance. The liquid inside the thermometer expands with heat and moves up the glass tube, showing the temperature on the scale. The Fahrenheit thermometer is scaled from 94° to 108°F while the Celsius thermometer is scaled from 34° to 43°C (Fig. 20-2). Before you use a glass thermometer, the liquid must be "shaken down" to below the 94° mark on a Fahrenheit thermometer, or the 34° mark on a Celsius thermometer (Fig. 20-3). To read a glass thermometer, hold it horizontally by the stem at eye level and rotate it until the line of liquid becomes visible (Fig. 20-4). It will show up as a thin silvery or red line.

In facilities that still use glass thermometers, each patient or resident has their own thermometer, which is kept in a case at the person's bedside. Because glass thermometers are not disposable, they must be cleaned properly after each use, according to facility policy. Sometimes, a clear plastic cover called a *sheath* is used to cover the thermometer, and then the sheath is discarded. The thermometer is washed with cool water and soap (never hot water, which can cause the thermometer to shatter), rinsed with cool water, and cleaned with a disinfectant solution. If a glass thermometer breaks while you are cleaning it (or at any other time), avoid touching the liquid and the broken glass, and prevent others from doing so as well.

Glass thermometers are still sometimes used in the home health care setting and some states still require nursing assistants to learn how to use them.

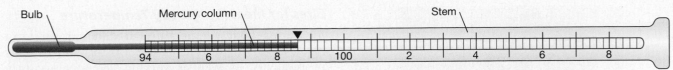

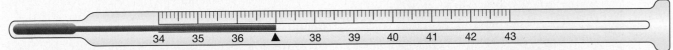

A **Fahrenheit (°F) thermometer** is scaled from 94° to 108°F. Each long line indicates 1 degree and each short line indicates $^2/_{10}$ (0.2) of a degree. This thermometer is reading 98.6°F.

A **Celsius (°C) thermometer** is scaled from 34° to 43°C. Each long line indicates 1 degree and each short line indicates $^1/_{10}$ (0.1) of a degree. This thermometer is reading 37°C.

Figure 20-2 Temperature scales on glass thermometers.

You will be taught how to use the equipment that is required by your particular state guidelines and used in the type of setting in which you will work.

Electronic Thermometers

Because of the safety risks of glass thermometers, almost all health care facilities use electronic thermometers instead (Fig. 20-5). Electronic thermometers are powered by batteries, and the temperature is displayed on a screen on the front of the instrument. A probe, covered with a disposable sheath, is placed in the patient's or resident's mouth, rectum, or armpit to measure the temperature. A blue probe is used for taking oral or axillary temperatures. A red probe is used for taking rectal temperatures. After the probe is used, the disposable sheath is discarded.

Tympanic Thermometers

A tympanic thermometer (Fig. 20-6) is an electronic thermometer used to measure the body temperature in the ear. The probe of this battery-operated instrument is inserted into the ear canal, where it

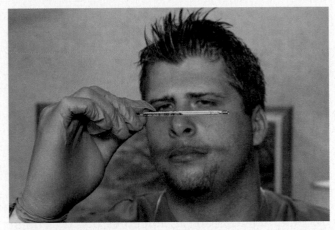

Figure 20-4 To read a glass thermometer, hold it horizontally by the stem at eye level.

rests near the eardrum (tympanic membrane). The person's temperature is displayed on a screen after a few seconds. Tympanic thermometers are often used for children because they allow a temperature to be

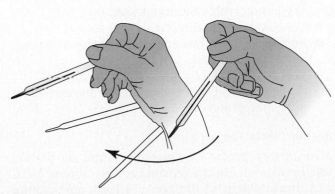

Figure 20-3 A glass thermometer is "shaken down" before use by holding the thermometer firmly by the stem and snapping your wrist downward.

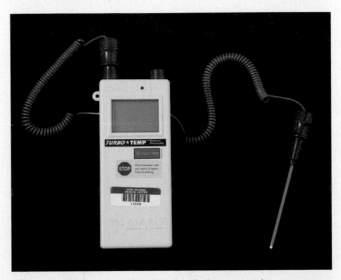

Figure 20-5 A battery-operated electronic thermometer.

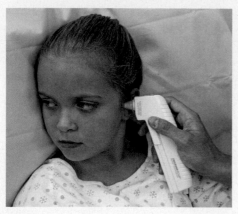

Figure 20-6 A tympanic thermometer is inserted into the ear canal.

measured in a safe, quick, and relatively painless manner.

Temporal Artery Thermometers

The temporal artery thermometer represents the latest development in thermometer technology (Fig. 20-7). Remember how a parent or caregiver used to place a cool hand on your hot forehead to check for a fever? The temporal artery thermometer is simply a "high-tech" version of this gesture. As the device is passed over a person's forehead, it detects the body temperature at numerous points. It then performs a series of calculations on the readings to arrive at the person's peak body temperature. The temporal artery thermometer is even more accurate than a tympanic thermometer, and because it does not have to be inserted into any body opening, it is considered the least invasive of all of the thermometers available.

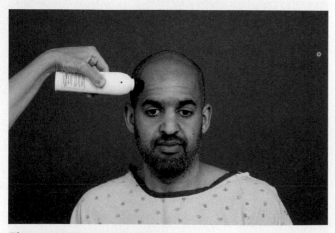

Figure 20-7 A temporal artery thermometer is placed on the middle of the person's forehead and swept toward the ear, stopping in front of the ear.

Sites for Measuring Body Temperature

Measuring body temperature at different sites can result in varying degrees of comfort for your patients or residents, as well as varying levels of accuracy in the measurement. Several factors can determine which site is best for measuring the body temperature of your patient or resident.

Mouth (Oral Temperature)

Measuring a person's body temperature by placing the thermometer into the mouth is simple and causes the person minimal discomfort. Because the thermometer is being placed in the mouth, which is not an entirely enclosed space, the temperature reading may not be as accurate as with some of the other methods. For example, measuring the temperature in the rectum or ear gives a more accurate reading, because the thermometer is placed into a tightly closed space. However, many times, the reading provided by placing the thermometer in the mouth is accurate enough. An oral temperature may be measured using a glass thermometer or an electronic thermometer (Procedure 20-1).

If a person eats, drinks, smokes, or chews gum 15 minutes before having an oral temperature taken, the measurement may not be accurate. If one of your patients or residents has done any of these things shortly before you intend to take their temperature orally, then you must either use a different method or wait for a period of time as specified by your facility's policy (usually 15 to 30 minutes).

In certain situations, an oral temperature should not be taken. For example, an oral temperature should not be taken if the patient or resident is:

- Unconscious
- Unable to keep the mouth closed (necessary in order to keep the thermometer in place)
- Unable to breathe through the nose
- Likely to bite the oral thermometer (for example, a child younger than 5 years, a disoriented person, or a person with a history of seizures)
- Coughing or sneezing
- Recovering from recent mouth surgery or an injury to the mouth
- Receiving oxygen by a face mask (because the oxygen may cause the temperature measurement to be inaccurate)

Rectum (Rectal Temperature)

Measuring a person's body temperature by placing the thermometer in the rectum provides a more accurate measurement of the person's body temperature because the thermometer is placed in an enclosed space. However, placing the thermometer rectally is also the riskiest method of taking a temperature, and it can be uncomfortable and embarrassing for the patient or resident.

A rectal temperature may be obtained using a glass thermometer or an electronic thermometer (Procedure 20-2). The thermometer must be lubricated and inserted carefully into the rectum, not more than one half inch in a child or one inch in an adult.

When you are taking a temperature rectally, it is important that you stay with the patient or resident during the entire procedure, both to hold the thermometer in place and to make sure that the person is all right. The thermometer could stimulate the vagus nerve, an important nerve that begins in the brain and sends branches to the heart, lungs, stomach, and rectum. Stimulation of the vagus nerve may temporarily decrease the person's heart rate and blood pressure, which can be dangerous. A different method of measuring the temperature should be used if the person has:

- Hemorrhoids, rectal bleeding, or a disease involving the rectum
- Diarrhea
- Certain heart conditions
- Recently had rectal surgery

Armpit (Axillary Temperature)

An axillary temperature is measured by placing the thermometer under the person's arm, directly in contact with the person's skin, and then having the person hold the arm close to their body. The axillary method provides the least reliable measurement of body temperature, but if the oral and rectal methods are not safe, and a tympanic or temporal thermometer is not available, then the axillary method can be used. The axillary temperature may be taken using a glass thermometer or an electronic thermometer (Procedure 20-3). If the person has just washed under their arms, or applied deodorant or antiperspirant, then you must wait for at least 15 minutes before taking the axillary temperature. Also, if the person has recently had chest or breast surgery, and it is necessary to take the person's temperature using the axillary method, then the thermometer should be placed on the unaffected side of the body.

Ear (Tympanic Temperature)

Because a tympanic thermometer measures the temperature of the blood in the small vessels in the eardrum, the temperature it gives is very accurate. Procedure 20-4 describes how to take a tympanic temperature. If a patient or resident has an earache or drainage from the ear, use the other ear to prevent discomfort. If the person has been sleeping with one side of the head against a pillow, use the other ear for taking their temperature. Heat may be increased on the side against the pillow, resulting in an inaccurate measurement.

Forehead (Temporal Temperature)

A person's temporal artery has branches that run very close underneath the skin across the forehead and in front of the ear. The reading is very accurate. However, if a person is sweating, the evaporation from the sweat on the skin can lower the temperature in this area and give a false low reading. A temporal artery thermometer is swept across a person's forehead to obtain a body temperature measurement. Procedure 20-5 describes how to take a temporal artery temperature. If a patient or resident has anything covering the forehead, such as hair, a wig, a hat, or bandages, they can insulate the area, making it warmer and cause an inaccurate measurement. Make sure that you measure only the side of the forehead that is uncovered.

Normal and Abnormal Findings

The normal body temperature varies slightly from person to person. In fact, a person's normal body temperature may be anywhere from 0.5° to 1°F higher or lower than the range generally considered normal. The normal range also varies according to what method is used to measure the body temperature (Table 20-1).

TABLE 20-1 Normal Temperature Ranges

METHOD USED TO OBTAIN TEMPERATURE	ADULT RANGES		PEDIATRIC RANGES	
	Fahrenheit (°F)	Celsius (°C)	Fahrenheit (°F)	Celsius (°C)
Oral	97.6–99.6	36.5–37.5	97–99	36–37
Rectal	98.6–100.6	37–38.1	98–100	37–38
Axillary	96.6–98.6	36–37	96–98	35–36
Tympanic	98.6	37	98.6	37
Temporal	99.6	37.5	99.6	37.5

Oral temperatures are not taken in children younger than 5 years.

A person who has an increased body temperature is said to have a fever, or to be **febrile**. Fever is a common finding with illness and is the body's normal response to infection. Fever may also be caused by chemicals that the body releases when tissues are injured, for example, after a heart attack, traumatic injuries, surgery, and cancer treatments. However, an older person's temperature may actually decrease, or only slightly increase, in response to illness or infection. For this reason, even a very slight change in an older person's temperature should be reported to the nurse.

PULSE

Each time the heart beats, it sends a wave, or **pulse**, of blood through the arteries. The arteries are the blood vessels that carry oxygen-containing blood away from the heart to all of the tissues of the body. The pulse, a throbbing sensation just underneath the skin, can be felt (palpated) by placing your fingers gently over an artery that runs close to the surface of the skin, such as the carotid artery in the neck or the radial artery in the wrist (Fig. 20-8). Although we can only feel the pulse in a few of the body's arteries (those that run closest to the surface of the skin), all of the arteries in the body have a pulse. The pulse tells us many things:

■ By feeling for and counting the pulse, we are able to measure the **pulse rate**, or the number of pulsations that can be felt in 1 minute. The pulse rate tells us the heart rate, or how fast the heart is beating.

■ In addition to measuring the pulse rate, we can detect the **pulse rhythm**, or the pattern of the pulsations and the pauses between them. Normally, the pulse rhythm is smooth and regular, with the same amount of time in between each pulsation. An irregular pulse rhythm is called a **dysrhythmia** (*dys*- means "bad" or "difficult").

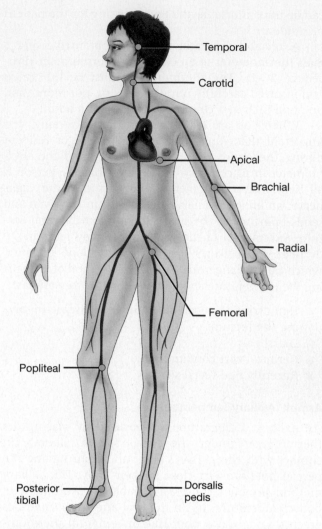

Figure 20-8 The pulse points are places where the arteries run close to the surface of the skin, allowing the pulse to be felt. When taking a person's pulse, it is common to place your fingers on the radial artery (in the wrist). An apical pulse can be taken by placing a stethoscope on the person's chest, over the apex of the heart.

■ Finally, we can evaluate the force or quality of the pulse, known as the **pulse amplitude** or the pulse character. Each pulsation should be strong and easy to feel. Pulses that are difficult to feel may be described as "weak" or "thready." A weak or thready pulse usually means that the heart is having trouble circulating blood throughout the body.

Factors Affecting the Pulse

The rate at which the heart beats is controlled automatically by the body's central nervous system. When the nervous system senses that the tissues need more oxygen and nutrients (for example, when a person is exercising), it increases the heart rate so that blood reaches the tissues faster. A person's heart rate will also increase during times of anger and anxiety, illness, pain, fever, and excitement, and when taking certain medications.

Measuring the Pulse

There are two main methods for measuring a person's pulse rate.

Radial Pulse

One common way of measuring the pulse rate is by placing the middle two or three fingers lightly over the radial artery, which is located on the inside of the wrist (see Fig. 20-8) and counting the number of pulses that occur in either 30 seconds or 1 minute. The thumb is not used to palpate the artery because the thumb has its own fairly strong pulse. Although the pulse may be taken at other pulse points, taking the pulse at the radial artery is easiest for the patient or resident. The carotid or femoral arteries may be used to assess the pulse during an emergency situation when cardiopulmonary resuscitation (CPR) is being administered. Procedure 20-6 describes how to take a radial pulse.

Apical Pulse

The apical pulse is measured by listening (auscultating) over the apex of the heart with a stethoscope. The apex of the heart (that is, the lower tip of the heart) is located slightly to the left side of the chest, between the sternum (breast bone) and the left nipple. The apical pulse is best heard approximately 2 inches below the level of the left nipple (see Fig. 20-8). An apical pulse is taken when a person has a weak or irregular pulse that may be difficult to feel in the radial artery. An apical pulse may also be used to measure heart rate in infants and in people with known heart disease.

A **stethoscope**, a device that makes sound louder and transfers it to the listener's ears, is used to take an apical pulse. The stethoscope allows you to hear, rather than feel, each beat of the person's heart. The stethoscope has the following parts (Fig. 20-9):

- Earpieces, which are placed in your ears
- A brace and binaurals, which connect the earpieces to the rubber or plastic tubing that conducts the sound
- An amplifying device, which makes the sound louder

The amplifying device, which is the part of the stethoscope that is placed against the person's skin, is usually two-sided. One side, called the **diaphragm**,

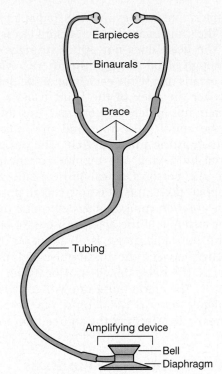

Figure 20-9 A stethoscope is used to listen to the heartbeat (when taking an apical pulse) or blood moving through the arteries (when taking a blood pressure). The sound is made louder by the amplifying device and transmitted by the rubber tubing to the earpieces, which fit snugly in the user's ear canals. The brace and binaurals, which are usually made of metal, connect the rubber or plastic tubing to the earpieces and prevent it from twisting or kinking, which could distort the sound. The rubber or plastic tubing may be single (as shown) or double.

is a large flat surface that is used to hear loud, harsh sounds like an apical pulse, blood rushing through the arteries, or respiratory sounds. The other side, called the **bell**, is a small, rounded surface that is designed to pick up softer sounds like heart murmurs or difficult-to-hear blood pressures. The bell side is also commonly used to listen to apical pulses in infants and small children. The amplifying device rotates so that the sound comes from either the diaphragm or the bell, but not both at once.

Before using a stethoscope, clean both the earpieces and the diaphragm or bell by wiping them with alcohol wipes. Place the earpieces in each ear canal. You will know that the earpieces are placed correctly when they fit snugly, yet comfortably, and block out any outside sound. Next, tap lightly on the diaphragm. You should be able to hear the tapping. If you cannot hear the tapping, rotate the amplifying device and tap again. When you can hear the tapping, you are ready to go! Procedure 20-7 describes how to take an apical pulse using a stethoscope.

The apical pulse rate and the radial pulse rate should be the same in any single person. Occasionally, however, the heart does not pump strongly enough to send enough blood through the arteries with each beat. This means that while each beat of the heart may be heard over the apex of the heart using a stethoscope, it may not be felt in the wrist. This difference between the apical pulse rate and the radial pulse rate is known as the **pulse deficit**. The pulse deficit is measured by having one member of the nursing team take the person's apical pulse while another team member takes the person's radial pulse. The two counts are then compared to determine the pulse deficit. For example, if the apical pulse is 84 beats per minute and the radial pulse is 80 beats per minute, the difference between the apical pulse and the radial pulse (that is, the pulse deficit) is 4 beats per minute (84 − 80 = 4). The apical pulse rate will always be the same or higher than the radial pulse rate because it is easier to hear a heartbeat at the source than to feel it.

Normal and Abnormal Findings

As with temperature, there is an accepted normal pulse rate. The pulse rate is faster in infants and small children and gradually slows as a person reaches adulthood. **Tachycardia** is a rapid heart rate, or a pulse rate of more than 100 beats per minute for an adult (*tachy-* means "fast" and *cardia* means "heart"). A heart rate that is slower than normal (that is, a pulse rate of less than 60 beats per minute) is called **bradycardia** (*brady-* means "slow"). Certain illnesses or conditions can cause bradycardia. Bradycardia may also be a normal finding in a young, athletic person who is very physically fit because the person's physical conditioning allows the heart to pump stronger and more effectively, which slows the heart rate. Table 20-2 lists normal pulse rate ranges for adults and children.

Tell the Nurse!

Changes in a person's pulse rate, rhythm, or amplitude can be a sign that something is wrong. Be sure to report the following observations to the nurse immediately:

● The person's pulse rate is higher than normal

● The person's pulse rate is lower than normal

● The person's pulse rhythm is irregular

● The person's pulse is weak or "thready"

● You have difficulty taking the person's pulse

TABLE 20-2 Normal Pulse Rate Ranges

AGE OF PERSON	PULSE RATE (beats/min)[a]
Adult	60–100
Adolescent (12–20 years)	60–100
School-aged child (5–12 years)	75–110
Preschooler (3–5 years)	80–120
Toddler (1–3 years)	80–140
Infant (0–1 year)	80–180

[a]The pulse rate is always measured for a full minute in children younger than 12 years.

RESPIRATION

Respiration is the process of breathing. To live, we must have oxygen. We must also get rid of waste products that are created as a result of normal cellular function (metabolism). One of these waste products is carbon dioxide (see Chapter 31).

During the **inhalation (inspiration)** phase of respiration, the chest expands (rises) as air is brought into the lungs. During the **exhalation (expiration)** phase of respiration, the chest deflates (falls) as air moves out of the lungs. When we measure a person's respirations, we look at the person's:

■ **Respiratory rate**, or the number of times the person breathes in 1 minute (one breath is both an inhalation and an exhalation).

■ **Respiratory rhythm**, or the regularity with which the person breathes.

■ **Depth of respiration**, or the quality of each breath (for example, is it deep or shallow?).

■ We also listen for any abnormal sounds, such as wheezing or congestion.

Factors Affecting Respiration

As with other vital functions, the process of breathing is controlled mainly by the central nervous system, in a part of the brain called the medulla. Control centers, called chemoreceptors, are located in the medulla and in some of the major arteries. These control centers monitor the carbon dioxide and oxygen content of the blood and adjust the rate and depth of breathing accordingly. For example, exercise increases the body's use of oxygen as well as its production of carbon dioxide, and will increase both the rate and depth of a person's respirations. Other factors that may affect respiration rate, depth, and regularity include anxiety, pain, fear, fever, infections and diseases of the heart and lungs, stroke or head injury, and certain medications.

In addition to being controlled automatically by the nervous system, breathing can also be controlled to a certain extent by the individual (for example, when we "hold our breath" while swimming). In this respect, breathing is different from the other vital signs.

Measuring Respiration

Many tests are available to evaluate a person's respiratory function. The simplest approach involves no equipment, other than a watch. The respiratory rate is easily determined by watching the rise and fall of a person's chest and counting the number of breaths that occur in either 30 seconds or 1 minute. (Remember that one breath consists of both an inhalation and an exhalation.) Usually, the rise and fall of the chest can be easily observed by standing beside the person, or by watching their back. In some situations, you may need to stand slightly behind the person while they are seated and look down at the chest to detect the movement. Or, you can actually place your hand either near the collarbone or on the person's side to feel them breathing if it is not easily seen. Most small children and some older adults use their abdominal muscles to assist with breathing. In these people, breathing can be easily seen by watching the abdomen move instead of the chest.

Because a person can consciously control their respirations if they are aware that they are being observed, a more accurate measurement may be obtained if you measure the respiratory rate right after you take the person's pulse, with your fingers still on the person's wrist as if you were still counting the pulse. It is also easy to count a person's respirations while they sleep, before you have awakened them to measure other vital signs. This is the one instance where it is acceptable to carry out a task without telling the patient or resident exactly what you are doing! Procedure 20-8 describes how to measure a person's respiratory rate.

In some facilities, you will be asked to record a patient's or resident's *pulse oximetry* measurement, which is how much oxygen is being carried by the blood cells. This procedure is discussed in Chapter 31.

Normal and Abnormal Findings

Under normal conditions, a healthy, resting adult will breathe about 12 to 20 times a minute, while infants and children may have a significantly higher respiratory rate. A normal respiratory rate is called **eupnea**. (The prefix *eu-* means "good" and the suffix *-pnea* means "breathing.") A respiratory rate that is higher than normal (greater than 24 breaths per

TABLE 20-3 Normal Respiration Rate Ranges

AGE OF PERSON	RESPIRATION RATE (breaths/min)[a]
Adult	12–20
Adolescent (12–20 years)	15–20
School-aged child (5–12 years)	15–25
Preschooler (3–5 years)	20–34
Toddler (1–3 years)	20–40
Infant (0–1 year)	30–60

[a]The respiration rate is always measured for a full minute in children younger than 12 years.

minute in an adult) is called **tachypnea** while a respiratory rate that is lower than normal (less than 10 breaths per minute) is called **bradypnea**. (Recall that *tachy-* means "fast," and *brady-* means "slow.") Table 20-3 lists the normal respiratory rates for adults and children.

Normally, the chest should rise and fall evenly, in a regular rhythm. Breathing should be quiet and easy. Labored or difficult respirations are termed **dyspnea** (recall that *dys-* means "bad" or "difficult"). Other notable respiratory patterns are **hyperventilation** (increased rate and depth of breathing) and **hypoventilation** (decreased rate and depth of breathing).

Tell the Nurse!

Changes in a person's respiratory rate, respiratory rhythm, or depth of respirations can be a sign that something is wrong. Be sure to report the following observations to the nurse immediately:

- The person's respiratory rate is greater than 24 breaths per minute
- The person's respiratory rate is less than 10 breaths per minute
- The person's respiratory rhythm is irregular
- The person's breaths are either very deep or very shallow
- The person's breathing is difficult or painful
- The person's chest does not rise equally on both sides
- The person's respirations are noisy with wheezing sounds or congestion

BLOOD PRESSURE

The force of the blood pushing against the arterial walls is known as the **blood pressure**. There are two pressure levels that are measured when taking a person's blood pressure measurement. The first, known as the **systolic pressure**, is the pressure that is caused by the blood when the heart muscle contracts, sending a wave of blood through the artery. The second, known as the **diastolic pressure**, occurs when the heart muscle relaxes. Although the heart is relaxed, there is still pressure as the blood flows through the arteries.

Blood pressure is measured in *millimeters of mercury* (mm Hg) and is recorded as a fraction. The systolic pressure, which is higher, is recorded first, followed by the diastolic pressure, which is lower. For instance, if a person's systolic measurement is 110 mm Hg and the diastolic measurement is 72 mm Hg, then the blood pressure would be recorded as 110/72 mm Hg. The difference between the systolic and diastolic pressures is known as the **pulse pressure**, which in this case would be 38 mm Hg (110 − 72 = 38).

Blood pressure is considered a vital sign because it gives us important information about a person's health and risk for disease. Adequate blood pressure is necessary to keep blood flow constant to all of the tissues of the body. A blood pressure that is too low is a bad sign because it means the tissues of the body may not be receiving enough oxygen and nutrients. On the other hand, a blood pressure that is too high forces the heart to do extra work, which, over time, damages the heart. High blood pressure also places stress on the kidneys, which can lead to kidney failure, and the blood vessels, which can lead to stroke. Blood pressure measurements allow health care workers to monitor existing problems and possibly prevent future ones.

Factors Affecting Blood Pressure

The pressure that the blood puts on the arterial walls is controlled by three factors:

- **Cardiac output.** The cardiac output is the amount of blood that the heart is able to pump in a minute. If the heart is able to pump more blood into the blood vessels with each beat, then blood flow increases, leading to an increase in blood pressure. On the other hand, if the cardiac output is lower, then blood flow decreases, leading to a decrease in blood pressure.
- **Blood volume.** The amount of blood in the vessels at any given time influences the blood pressure. If the blood volume is low, for example, as a result of hemorrhage (see Chapter 16), then

the blood pressure will decrease. Similarly, an increase in blood volume leads to an increase in blood pressure. In some people, a salty meal is enough to increase blood pressure because the salt causes the body to store water, which increases the blood volume.

- **Resistance to blood flow.** Resistance is how hard it is for the blood to flow through the vessels. If the vessels are narrowed (for example, as a result of arteriosclerosis ["hardening of the arteries"]), then the resistance will be high and so will the blood pressure. Resistance is also increased when the blood is thick, for example, if a person is dehydrated.

Blood pressure is also influenced by certain factors that we cannot do anything about, such as age, sex, and race:

- **Age.** Young people tend to have lower blood pressures than older people. Aging causes a decrease in the elasticity of the blood vessels (that is, the blood vessels' ability to stretch and bounce back as the blood pulses through). Decreased elasticity results in increased resistance and a higher blood pressure.
- **Sex.** Females tend to have lower blood pressures than males. However, females who take oral contraceptives ("birth control pills") may have a slightly increased blood pressure.
- **Race.** People of certain races (for example, African Americans) tend to have higher blood pressures than people of other races.

Measuring Blood Pressure

Measuring and recording a person's blood pressure is a routine task for nursing assistants. There are many ways to measure a person's blood pressure.

Manually Operated Sphygmomanometers

The most common method of measuring blood pressure is by using a manually operated **sphygmomanometer** and a stethoscope. *Sphygmo-* is from the Greek word for "pulse," and *-manometer* means "a flat instrument used to measure pressure." A manual sphygmomanometer consists of:

- A cuff (a flat, cloth-covered inflatable pouch)
- A bulb, which is squeezed or pumped to fill the cuff with air
- A manometer (the device that measures the air pressure in the inflatable pouch)

Cuffs come in various sizes and may be disposable or reusable. The cuff must fit the person properly, or the blood pressure measurement will not be accurate.

TABLE 20-4 Blood Pressure Cuff Sizes

ARM MEASUREMENT (cm)	NAME OF CUFF TO USE
13–20	Child
24–32	Adult
32–42	Large adult
42–50	Thigh

To find the right size to use, measure around the person's upper arm, halfway between the elbow and shoulder. Cuff sizes are given in Table 20-4.

Two tubes are attached to the pouch within the cuff—one is attached to the bulb used to inflate the pouch, and the other is attached to the manometer. The manometer may be either aneroid or mercury (Fig. 20-10). An aneroid manometer is a small, round dial with a needle that indicates the pressure. A mercury manometer is a column of mercury that may be mounted on a wall or placed on a table. The manometer measures the pressure of the air in the cuff in millimeters of mercury (mm Hg). Long dashes mark increments of 10 mm Hg and the short dashes in between mark increments of 2 mm Hg.

The most common place to measure a person's blood pressure is in the brachial artery of the upper arm. However, the popliteal artery (which can be felt at the back of the person's knee) can be used as well. Measuring a blood pressure is quite simple, once you have had some practice. The cuff is wrapped around the person's upper arm where the brachial artery is located. You can feel the brachial artery pulse in the antecubital space (the inner bend of the elbow) by straightening the person's arm and placing your fingers across the inside of the joint. After positioning the cuff, place the diaphragm of your stethoscope directly over where you felt the brachial artery in the antecubital space, and close the valve on the pumping bulb by turning it clockwise. Do not close the valve too tightly, or it will be difficult to release the air when you are ready. As you pump the bulb, air will enter the pouch in the cuff and you will see the needle (on an aneroid manometer) or the column of mercury (on a mercury manometer) move, indicating that the pressure of the air in the cuff is increasing.

Remember that you have two pressures that are measured within an artery, the systolic pressure (when the heart pumps) and the diastolic pressure (when the heart relaxes). When the pressure within the cuff becomes higher than the systolic pressure in the artery, it will essentially cut off the circulation and not allow any blood to flow through the brachial artery past the cuff. Continue pumping the bulb until the pressure in the cuff is 30 mm Hg higher than the systolic pressure. There are two ways to do this:

- Place the stethoscope over the brachial artery, and inflate the cuff slowly. After you have inflated the cuff a bit, you will start to hear the pulse through your stethoscope. Continue inflating the cuff until you hear the pulse stop (this is the person's systolic pressure) and continue inflating the cuff 30 mm Hg more.
- Or, with your fingers on the person's brachial or radial pulse, you can inflate the cuff until you no longer can feel the pulse. The reading on the manometer will indicate the person's systolic pressure. Continue inflating the cuff 30 mm Hg more.

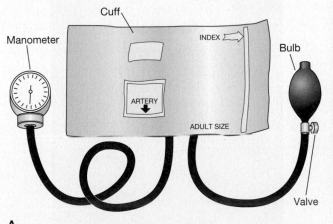
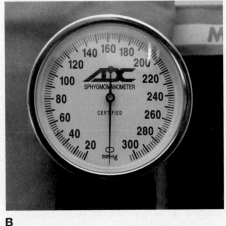
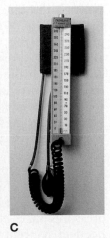

Figure 20-10 A. A manual sphygmomanometer consists of a cuff, a bulb, and a manometer. The manometer may be either aneroid or mercury. Do you know which type of manometer is shown here? The tubes attach the inflatable pouch inside the cuff to the bulb and to the manometer. **B.** An aneroid manometer. **C.** A mercury manometer.

Box 20-1 Korotkoff Sounds

In some people, you will only be able to hear the beginning and ending sounds while auscultating the blood pressure, but in others, all of these sounds will be distinct.

Phase I: Faint but clear tapping sounds that gradually become louder. The first tapping sound is the systolic pressure.

Phase II: Muffled or swishing sounds that may actually disappear if a person has significant hypertension.

Phase III: Distinct, loud tapping sounds as the blood begins to flow more freely through the artery.

Phase IV: The sound may abruptly become muffled and soft. Keep listening.[a]

Phase V: The last sound heard before a period of continuous silence. This is the diastolic pressure.

_____

[a]Occasionally, the tapping sounds of the pulse will be heard all the way down to zero. In this case, listening for the abrupt softening of phase IV will give you an approximate diastolic reading.

When the pressure in the cuff is 30 mm Hg higher than the systolic pressure, place the diaphragm of your stethoscope over the brachial artery and open the valve slightly (by turning it counter clockwise). Opening the valve slightly allows the slow release of air from the cuff, which lowers the pressure in the cuff. Under normal conditions, you may not be able to hear the brachial pulse, but under pressure, you will be able to hear the pulse through the stethoscope. As the pressure in the cuff falls (as indicated by the needle on the aneroid dial or the column of mercury) you listen for sounds, called **Korotkoff sounds** (Box 20-1), through the stethoscope. When the pressure in the cuff is equal to or slightly lower than the systolic pressure in the artery, blood will suddenly begin to flow through the brachial artery, and you will start hearing the pulse. When you hear the first sound of the pulse, note the reading on the manometer. This is your systolic pressure. Now continue to listen to the pulse. When the pressure inside the cuff is less than the lowest arterial pressure, or diastolic pressure, the sound of the pulse will stop, because the artery is no longer under pressure. The last sound that you hear is the diastolic pressure and is shown by the reading on the manometer.

Procedure 20-9 summarizes how to take a blood pressure. Guidelines for taking a blood pressure are given in Guidelines Box 20-1. Learning to take blood pressures takes time and practice. At first, you will need to concentrate on how to operate the equipment and control the rate at which the air leaves the cuff. Next, you will need to become familiar with the sounds that you hear as the cuff deflates, and learn to recognize the beginning and ending sounds. Each

person's blood pressure will sound slightly different. In some people, the blood pressure is easy to measure. In others, measuring the blood pressure will challenge even the most experienced nursing assistant. A good rule of thumb is if a person's brachial or radial pulse feels stronger in one arm over the other, you will have an easier time taking the blood pressure in the arm with the stronger pulse. Do not get discouraged if taking blood pressures is difficult at first. The more you practice, the more competent and confident you will become. As with any skill you will learn, if you have difficulty taking a person's blood pressure or if you are unsure of a reading you get, always ask for a second opinion or help from another nursing assistant or a nurse. Your responsibility to the people you care for takes priority over your pride.

Automated Sphygmomanometers and Other Means of Measuring Blood Pressure

Your facility may use automated (electronic) sphygmomanometers instead of manual ones. Some automated models feature automatic inflation and deflation of the cuff while others require the cuff to be manually inflated but will deflate it automatically. The blood pressure is displayed digitally (Fig. 20-11). If a person has an irregular heart rate, tremors, or

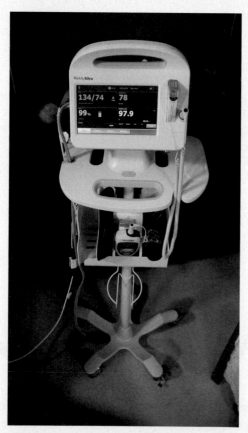

Figure 20-11 Automatic blood pressure machine being used showing digital display of the person's blood pressure.

Guidelines Box 20-1   Guidelines for Taking a Person's Blood Pressure

WHAT YOU DO	WHY YOU DO IT
Allow the person time to relax for at least 5 minutes prior to taking the blood pressure.	Recent exercise and emotions (such as fear or anxiety) can cause a blood pressure reading to be falsely elevated.
Make sure the manometer is properly calibrated (that is, it reads "0" when there is no air in the cuff).	A manometer that is not properly calibrated will not give an accurate pressure reading.
Use a cuff that is properly sized for the patient or resident.	A cuff that does not fit will not allow you to accurately measure the person's blood pressure. A cuff that is too small will result in a high reading while a cuff that is too large will result in a low reading.
Make sure the cuff fits snugly around the person's arm before inflating it.	A cuff that is too loose can cause the skin to "pinch" under the cuff when the cuff is inflated, damaging the skin.
Do not place the cuff over a person's clothing.	Clothing will distort the Korotkoff sounds.
Have the patient or resident assume a comfortable lying or sitting position with the forearm supported at the level of the heart and the palm of the hand facing upward.	If the upper arm is positioned below the level of the heart, the blood pressure measurement will read too high. If the upper arm is above the level of the heart, the measurement will read too low.
Do not take a blood pressure on an arm where an intravenous (IV) line is placed, or on an arm that is injured or in a cast.	Inflating the cuff can cause pain and swelling, and it may dislodge an IV line if one is present.
In a person who has had a mastectomy, do not take a blood pressure on the arm that is on the same side of the body as the breast that was removed.	Some people who have mastectomies also have the lymph nodes in the armpit removed, which disrupts fluid flow from the tissues in the hand and lower arm. This can lead to an inaccurate blood pressure reading.
Do not take a blood pressure on an arm that is used for hemodialysis access.	Pressure from the blood pressure cuff can cause the fistula or shunt used for dialysis to clot or be damaged.
Do not partially deflate the cuff and then reinflate it while taking a blood pressure measurement. If you make a mistake, release all of the air from the cuff and wait at least 1 minute before trying again.	Partially deflating and then reinflating the cuff is uncomfortable for the patient or resident, and it will result in an inaccurate reading.
If you are unable to hear the Korotkoff sounds, make sure the room is quiet and check your equipment: • Make sure the diaphragm of the stethoscope is active by gently tapping on it. • Make sure the diaphragm of the stethoscope is placed directly over the brachial pulse. • Make sure the earpieces of the stethoscope are seated properly in your ears.	Most difficulties with measuring blood pressure result from operator error. However, if you have checked your equipment and you still cannot hear the Korotkoff sounds, notify the nurse immediately. The person may have severe hypotension.

is unable to remain still, an electronic blood pressure device may not be able to be used. If the device detects the extra movement or pulse irregularities, it will continue to repeatedly inflate and deflate without recording a measurement. This may cause the person to experience pain and discomfort from the cuff.

A person's blood pressure can also be measured directly, by inserting a catheter into an artery, or possibly even the heart. Because this procedure is invasive (that is, something is inserted into a normally enclosed part of the person's body), it carries some risk for the person. This method of assessing blood pressure might be used when continuous blood pressure monitoring is required, such as during a surgical procedure or when a patient is critically ill.

Normal and Abnormal Findings

Normally, a person's blood pressure moves up and down within the range of normal during the course of a day. For example:

- Blood pressure readings are usually lowest in the morning and can increase by as much as 10 mm Hg later in the day.
- Blood pressure is generally slightly higher when a person is lying down, as compared to sitting or standing.
- Blood pressure readings are usually slightly higher after a meal. Wait for at least an hour after mealtime to take a routine blood pressure.
- Exercise will temporarily increase the systolic blood pressure.
- Stress, anxiety, fear, and pain will also temporarily raise a person's blood pressure.

Much medical research has been done related to blood pressure and its effects on health. Studies have shown that for any individual, there is a wide range of blood pressure readings that can be considered "normal." When you are taking a person's blood pressure, it is important to allow that person time to relax or rest for a bit so that the blood pressure reading reflects the person's normal pressure and not the changes that can occur from exertion or being emotionally upset. Also, as a nursing assistant, you must learn to recognize the range of blood pressure measurements that can be considered "normal" for each of your patients or residents, so that you will be able to recognize any changes. A person's blood pressure could rise or fall 20 to 30 mm Hg and still be within the range of what is considered normal for that person. However, a large change in a person's blood pressure should be recognized and reported immediately to the nurse. Table 20-5 lists normal blood pressure measurements for adults and children.

Tell the Nurse!

Changes in a person's blood pressure can be a sign that something is wrong. Be sure to report the following observations to the nurse immediately:

- The person's blood pressure is higher than normal
- The person's blood pressure is lower than normal
- You have difficulty measuring the person's blood pressure

TABLE 20-5 Normal Blood Pressure Measurements

AGE OF PERSON	BLOOD PRESSURE (mm Hg)
Adult	120/80
Adolescent (12–20 years)	102/80
School-aged child (5–12 years)	100/62
Preschooler (3–5 years)	95/75
Toddler (1–3 years)	90/55
Infant (0–1 year)	73/55

Accepted normal adult ranges for the systolic pressure are between 90 and 120 mm Hg, and for the diastolic pressure, between 60 and 80 mm Hg. If a person has a blood pressure that is consistently higher than 140 mm Hg (systolic) and/or 90 mm Hg (diastolic), then that person is said to have **hypertension** (high blood pressure). To diagnose a person with hypertension and start treatment for this condition, the person's blood pressure measurements must be taken and recorded over a period of time to show a pattern of constant elevation. Medications that are taken for hypertension should be taken as ordered. If the person stops taking the medication or does not take it according to the prescribed schedule, the person's hypertension will usually return. Too often, a patient or resident will tell you that "I used to take medicine for my blood pressure, but the medicine brought my pressure back to normal, so I don't need to take it anymore." Measuring that person's blood pressure will usually tell a completely different story! Hypertension is often called the "silent killer" because a person with this condition does not feel ill, yet is at great risk for complications (and possibly even death) as a result of it.

A person who has a blood pressure that is consistently lower than 90 mm Hg (systolic) and/or 60 mm Hg (diastolic) is said to have **hypotension** (low blood pressure). Some people may have **orthostatic hypotension**, which is a sudden decrease in blood pressure that occurs when a person stands up from a sitting or lying position. When a person is sitting or lying down, the heart does not need to work as hard to pump blood throughout the body and the blood vessels are relaxed, so resistance is low. However, when the person stands up, the body needs to make up for the change in position. The heart pumps harder and the vessels constrict to bring the blood pressure back up to a normal level.

Until the body manages to make up for the sudden change in position, the person may feel lightheaded and faint. Some medications and aging can increase the time the body needs to adjust. The lack of blood flow to the brain can cause the person to feel dizzy. This is why, when you are assisting a person to "dangle" (see Chapter 15), you must give the person a minute to adjust before proceeding. Always remind your patients or residents to first sit for a moment before standing up, to allow time for the body to adjust. Helping a person who experiences orthostatic hypotension to remember to take those extra few moments for the body to adjust can help prevent a fall.

For some patients or residents, you may be asked to take a sequence of blood pressures—usually first with the person lying down, then sitting, then standing. This is done to evaluate how well the person's body adapts to changes in position. Facility policy will state the order of the blood pressure measurements when a sequence of measurements is needed.

Concerns for Long-Term Care

Normal ranges for vital signs vary somewhat in healthy older adults. In older persons who have chronic health conditions or take multiple medications, vital sign measurements may vary significantly from person to person. Older adults also have an increased tendency for their pulse rates and blood pressure measurements to fluctuate in response to postural changes (moving from supine to sitting or standing) and other factors, such as physical exertion or illness.

Normal pulse rates for healthy older adults are slightly lower than for younger adults, but older adults are more likely to have irregular rhythms. Blood pressure is likely to increase, especially if the older person has arteriosclerosis. Respiratory changes in the older adult can increase the respiratory rate, especially with mild exertion or exercise. If the person has a history of cigarette smoking, their resting respiratory rate may be significantly higher.

HEIGHT AND WEIGHT

Although height and weight are not technically vital signs, these measurements are taken periodically while a person is receiving care. The relationship of a person's weight to their height can provide insight into the person's overall health and nutritional status. In addition, a person's weight is often used to calculate medication dosages. In some cases, a change in a person's weight might indicate that the person's condition is getting worse or better. For all of these reasons, it is useful to obtain a "baseline" height and weight for each patient or resident and to measure the person's weight periodically thereafter.

A person's height is measured only on admission. A person's weight is measured on admission and on transfer, or discharge. It may also be necessary to measure a person's weight at regular intervals throughout the person's stay. A person's weight is rechecked periodically for various reasons:

- Weight is an indicator of nutritional status.
- Weight is an indicator of heart and kidney function. If the heart or kidneys are not functioning well, the person may retain fluid, which will cause an increase in weight.
- Changes in weight can be a sign of disease. For example, one of the signs of some types of cancer is major, unexplained weight loss.
- Many medications are prescribed according to body weight. If a person gains or loses a great deal of weight, it may be necessary to adjust the person's medication dosages.

If a person's weight is to be measured on a regular basis, make sure to take the measurement:

- At the same time each day
- With the person wearing the same type of clothing and no shoes
- After the person has emptied their bladder

Measuring Height and Weight

Height is measured in feet (ft) and inches (in) or in centimeters (cm). Weight is measured in pounds (lb) or kilograms (kg).

The type of scale you will use to measure a person's weight will depend on the person's ability to get out of bed and stand. Common types of scales include upright scales, chair scales, and sling scales.

Scales may be mechanical or digital. If you are using a mechanical scale, you must slide weights along a bar by hand until the bar is balanced (Fig. 20-12). If you are using a digital scale, you simply turn the scale on. The digital scale measures the person's weight automatically and displays it on a screen. Digital scales are now used most often in the health care setting.

Measuring Height and Weight Using an Upright Scale

An upright scale is used to obtain height and weight measurements for a person who is able to stand on their own. Procedure 20-10 describes how to use an upright scale to measure a person's height and weight.

Measuring Weight Using a Chair Scale

A chair scale (Fig. 20-13) is used to obtain a weight measurement for a person who cannot stand independently,

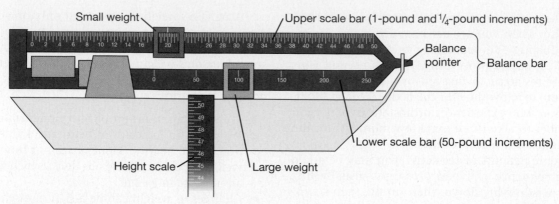

Figure 20-12 A mechanical scale. The *balance bar* has two scale bars and two weights. The *large weight* slides along the *lower scale bar*, which is marked off in 50-lb increments. The *small weight* slides along the *upper scale bar*, which is marked off in quarter-pound and pound increments. The *balance pointer* is centered between the two scale bars when the weight on the scale bars equals the person's weight.

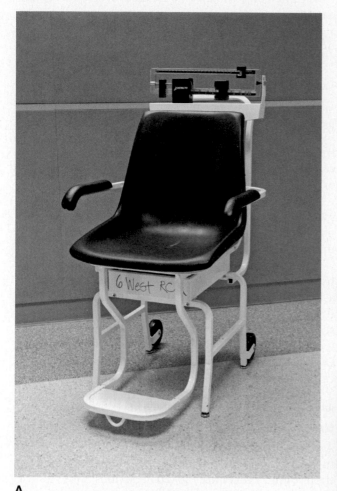

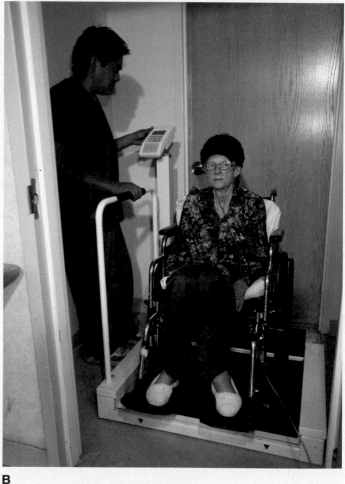

A

B

Figure 20-13 A chair scale is used to obtain weight measurements for a person who cannot stand up independently but is able to get out of bed. **A.** A chair scale. **B.** A chair scale for use with a wheelchair.

but is able to get out of bed. One type of chair scale is for use with a wheelchair. The wheelchair is first weighed without the person in it to determine its weight. Next, the wheelchair, with the person in it, is rolled onto the scale. The weight of the empty wheelchair is subtracted from the weight of the wheelchair with the person in it to determine the person's weight. The other type of chair scale is simply a chair-like device that allows the person to sit while having their weight measured. Procedure 20-11 describes how to use a chair scale.

Measuring Height and Weight Using a Tape Measure and a Sling Scale

If a person is unable to get out of bed at all, the person will have to be weighed in bed. Some acute care facilities have beds with built-in scales. If this type of bed is not available where you work, then you will have to weigh the person using a sling scale (Fig. 20-14). The person's height is measured using a tape measure. Procedure 20-12 describes how to obtain height and weight measurements using a tape measure and a

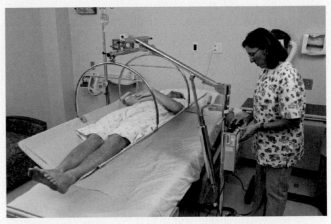

Figure 20-14 A sling scale is used to obtain weight measurements for a person who cannot get out of bed.

sling scale. Because sling scales from different manufacturers may vary greatly in their procedures for use, do not attempt to use a sling scale unless you have been trained in its use.

SUMMARY

- Vital signs provide essential information about a person's health.
  - Vital signs include body temperature, pulse, respirations, and blood pressure. A person's height and weight also provide insight into a person's overall health.
  - Measuring and recording vital signs is a routine part of a nursing assistant's daily duties.
    - Vital signs must be measured and recorded accurately because many people rely on this information to make decisions about the person's care. In addition, a change in vital signs can be an important early sign that something is wrong.
    - Nursing assistants must be familiar with accepted normal ranges for all of the vital signs, as well as what is "normal" for each of their patients or residents.
    - Learning to take vital signs confidently takes practice.

- Body temperature is a measure of how hot the body is.
  - The body temperature can be measured using a number of devices at a number of sites.
    - Types of thermometers include glass thermometers, electronic thermometers, tympanic thermometers, and temporal artery thermometers.
    - A person's temperature may be measured in the mouth, rectum, ear, armpit, or forehead.
  - An elevated temperature may be a sign of infection. Extreme changes in the environmental temperature can also affect a person's body temperature.
- The pulse reflects the rate, rhythm, and strength of the heartbeat.
  - The pulse can be measured by feeling the radial artery (in the wrist) or by listening to the apical pulse (on the chest) with a stethoscope.
  - Tachycardia is an excessively rapid heartbeat. Bradycardia is an excessively slow heartbeat.

- The respiratory rate, rhythm, and depth are a reflection of how well the person is breathing.
  - The respiratory rate is measured by counting the number of times the person inhales and exhales in 30 seconds (or 1 minute, if the respirations are irregular).
    - The chest rises with each inhalation and falls with each exhalation.
    - One respiration = one inhalation + one exhalation.
  - Dyspnea is labored breathing. Tachypnea is a respiratory rate that is too fast, and bradypnea is a respiratory rate that is too slow.
- The blood pressure reflects the force the blood exerts against the arterial walls. Cardiac output, blood volume, and resistance affect the blood pressure.
  - Blood pressure is most often measured in the brachial artery using a sphygmomanometer and a stethoscope or an electronic blood pressure device.

- Korotkoff sounds are the sounds the blood makes as it rushes through the artery.
- Hypertension, or a consistently high blood pressure, can have serious long-term consequences if not treated.
- Orthostatic hypotension, or low blood pressure on changing positions, affects many people and is the reason people are encouraged to sit for a minute before standing up from a lying position.
- Height and weight are measured when a person enters a health care facility.
  - Weight is measured periodically. Major weight loss or gain can be an early sign of disease. In addition, many medication dosages are calculated according to a person's body weight.
  - A variety of devices, including upright scales, chair scales, and sling scales, can be used to measure a person's weight, depending on the person's situation.

▶ **Procedure 20-1**

Measuring an Oral Temperature (Glass or Electronic Thermometer) ▶

WHY YOU DO IT A change in a person's normal temperature may be a sign of illness. Taking an oral temperature is fast and causes the patient or resident minimal discomfort.

Getting Ready W E A V E R S

1. Complete the "Getting Ready" steps.

Supplies

If using a glass thermometer:
- paper towels
- tissues
- thermometer sheath
- oral glass thermometer

If using an electronic thermometer:
- probe sheath
- electronic thermometer with oral (blue) probe

Procedure

2. Ask the person if they have eaten, consumed a beverage, chewed gum, or smoked within the last 15 minutes. If so, wait 15 to 30 minutes before proceeding (or follow facility policy).

3. Prepare the thermometer.

  a. Glass thermometer: Run cool water over the thermometer to rinse away the disinfectant. Dry the thermometer with a paper towel and inspect it for cracks or chips. Carefully shake down the glass thermometer so that the indicator material is below the 94° mark (if using a Fahrenheit thermometer) or the 34° mark (if using a Celsius thermometer). Cover the end of the glass thermometer with the thermometer sheath.

  b. Electronic thermometer: Cover the electronic probe with the probe sheath. Turn the thermometer on and wait until the "ready" sign appears on the display screen.

4. Ask the person to open their mouth. Slowly and carefully insert the thermometer, placing the tip under the person's tongue and to one side.

5. Ask the person to gently close their mouth around the thermometer without biting down.

If necessary, hold the thermometer in place. Ask the person to breathe through their nose.

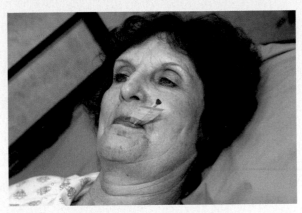

STEP 5 The person breathes through the nose while holding the thermometer in their mouth.

6. Leave the thermometer in place for the specified amount of time:

  a. Glass thermometer: 3 to 5 minutes (or follow facility policy)

  b. Electronic thermometer: until the instrument blinks or beeps (usually just a few seconds)

7. Ask the person to open their mouth. Remove the thermometer from the person's mouth.

8. Read the temperature measurement.

  a. Glass thermometer: Using a tissue, remove the thermometer sheath from the glass thermometer, being careful not to touch the bulb end of the thermometer. Dispose of the tissue and the thermometer sheath in a facility-approved waste container. Hold the thermometer horizontally by the stem at eye level while facing a light source. Rotate the thermometer until you can see the level of the indicator material. Read the temperature.

(continued)

b. Electronic thermometer: Read the temperature on the electronic thermometer's display screen. Remove the probe sheath from the probe by pushing the button on the top of the probe. Direct the probe sheath into a facility-approved waste container.

9. Prepare the thermometer for its next use.

a. Glass thermometer: Shake down the glass thermometer, clean it according to facility policy, and return it to its case.

b. Electronic thermometer: Replace the probe into the electronic thermometer. (Always read the temperature before placing the probe in the instrument because this action clears the display screen.) Turn the instrument off if it does not automatically turn itself off. Place the thermometer in its charger.

Finishing Up

10. Complete the "Finishing Up" steps.

What You Document

- The time and date
- The person's temperature
- The method—"O" for oral

Report an abnormal temperature to the nurse immediately.

▶ **Procedure 20-2**

Measuring a Rectal Temperature (Glass or Electronic Thermometer)

WHY YOU DO IT A change in a person's normal temperature may be a sign of illness. The rectal temperature measurement is a very accurate measurement of the body's temperature.

Getting Ready

1. Complete the "Getting Ready" steps.

Supplies

- gloves
- paper towels
- tissues
- lubricant jelly

If using a glass thermometer:
- thermometer sheath
- rectal glass thermometer

If using an electronic thermometer:
- probe sheath
- electronic thermometer with rectal (red) probe

Procedure

2. Make sure that the bed is positioned at a comfortable working height (to promote good body mechanics) and that the wheels are locked.

3. Prepare the thermometer.

a. Glass thermometer: Run cool water over the thermometer to rinse away the disinfectant. Dry the thermometer with a paper towel and inspect it for cracks or chips. Carefully shake down the glass thermometer so that the indicator material is below the 94° mark (if using a Fahrenheit thermometer) or the 34° mark (if using a Celsius thermometer). Cover the end of the glass thermometer with the thermometer sheath.

b. Electronic thermometer: Cover the electronic probe with the probe sheath. Turn the thermometer on and wait until the "ready" sign appears on the display screen.

4. Place the thermometer on a clean paper towel on the over-bed table. Open the lubricant package and squeeze a small amount of lubricant onto the paper towel. Lubricate the tip of the thermometer to ease insertion.

5. If the side rails are in use, lower the side rail on the working side of the bed. The side rail on the opposite side of the bed should remain up. Lower the head of the bed so that the bed is flat (as tolerated).

6. Ask the person to lie on their side, facing away from you, in Sims' position. Help the person into this position, if necessary.

7. Fanfold the top linens to below the person's buttocks. Adjust the person's hospital gown or pajama bottoms as necessary to expose the person's buttocks.

8. Perform hand hygiene and put on the gloves.

9. With one hand, raise the person's upper buttock to expose the anus. Suggest that the person take a deep breath and slowly exhale as the thermometer is inserted. Using your other hand, gently and carefully insert the lubricated end of the thermometer into the person's rectum (not more than 1 inch for adults, or ½ inch for children). Never force the thermometer into the rectum. If you are unable to insert the thermometer, stop and call the nurse.

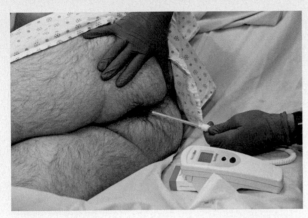

STEP 9 Gently and carefully insert the lubricated end of the thermometer into the person's rectum.

10. Hold the thermometer in place for the specified amount of time:

    a. **Glass thermometer:** 3 to 5 minutes (or follow facility policy)

    b. **Electronic thermometer:** until the instrument blinks or beeps (usually just a few seconds)

11. Remove the thermometer from the person's rectum. Wipe the person's anal area with a tissue to remove the lubricant, and adjust the person's hospital gown or pajama bottoms as necessary to cover the buttocks.

12. Read the temperature measurement.

    a. **Glass thermometer:** Using a tissue, remove the thermometer sheath from the glass thermometer, being careful not to touch the bulb end of the thermometer. Dispose of the tissue and the thermometer sheath in a facility-approved waste container. Hold the thermometer horizontally by the stem at eye level while facing a light source. Rotate the thermometer until you can see the level of the indicator material. Read the temperature.

    b. **Electronic thermometer:** Read the temperature on the electronic thermometer's display screen. Remove the probe sheath from the probe by pushing the button on the top of the probe. Direct the probe sheath into a facility-approved waste container.

13. Remove your gloves and dispose of them according to facility policy. Perform hand hygiene.

14. Help the person back into a comfortable position, straighten the bottom linens, and draw the top linens over the person. Raise the head of the bed, as the person requests.

15. Make sure that the bed is lowered to its lowest position and that the wheels are locked. If the side rails are in use, return the side rails to the raised position.

16. Prepare the thermometer for its next use.

    a. **Glass thermometer:** Shake down the glass thermometer, clean it according to facility policy, and return it to its case.

    b. **Electronic thermometer:** Replace the probe into the electronic thermometer. (Always read the temperature before placing the probe in the instrument because this action clears the display screen.) Turn the instrument off if it does not automatically turn itself off. Place the thermometer in its charger.

Finishing Up

17. Complete the "Finishing Up" steps.

What You Document

- The time and date
- The person's temperature
- The method—"R" for rectal

Report an abnormal temperature to the nurse immediately.

▶ Procedure 20-3

Measuring an Axillary Temperature (Glass or Electronic Thermometer) ▶

WHY YOU DO IT   A change in a person's normal temperature may be a sign of illness. The axillary method is used when other methods cannot be used.

Getting Ready WF GQ AV EE PR S

1. Complete the "Getting Ready" steps.

Supplies

- paper towels
- tissues

If using a glass thermometer:
- thermometer sheath
- oral glass thermometer

If using an electronic thermometer:
- probe sheath
- electronic thermometer with oral (blue) probe

Procedure

2. Ask the person if they have bathed or applied deodorant or antiperspirant within the last 15 minutes. If so, wait 15 to 30 minutes before proceeding (or follow facility policy).

3. Prepare the thermometer.

   a. Glass thermometer: Run cool water over the thermometer to rinse away the disinfectant. Dry the thermometer with a paper towel and inspect it for cracks or chips. Carefully shake down the glass thermometer so that the indicator material is below the 94° mark (if using a Fahrenheit thermometer) or the 34° mark (if using a Celsius thermometer). Cover the end of the glass thermometer with the thermometer sheath.

   b. Electronic thermometer: Cover the electronic probe with the probe sheath. Turn the thermometer on and wait until the "ready" sign appears on the display screen.

4. Assist the person with removing their arm from the sleeve of their hospital gown or pajama top in order to expose the axilla. The thermometer must be placed directly in contact with the skin.

5. Pat the axilla (underarm area) gently with a paper towel.

6. Ask the person to lift their arm slightly. Position the tip of the thermometer in the center of the axilla and ask the person to hold the thermometer in place by holding the arm

close to the body (or by grasping the arm with the opposite hand).

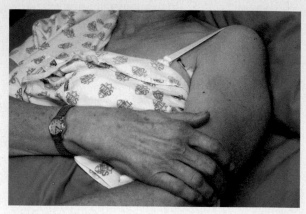

STEP 6 The person holds the thermometer in place by grasping the arm with the opposite hand.

7. Leave the thermometer in place for the specified amount of time:

   a. Glass thermometer: 10 minutes (or follow facility policy)

   b. Electronic thermometer: until the instrument blinks or beeps (usually just a few seconds)

8. Ask the person to lift their arm slightly. Remove the thermometer.

9. Read the temperature measurement.

   a. Glass thermometer: Using a tissue, remove the thermometer sheath from the glass thermometer, being careful not to touch the bulb end of the thermometer. Dispose of the tissue and the thermometer sheath in a facility-approved waste container. Hold the thermometer horizontally by the stem at eye level while facing a light source. Rotate the thermometer until you can see the level of the indicator material. Read the temperature.

   b. Electronic thermometer: Read the temperature on the electronic thermometer's display screen. Remove the probe sheath from the probe by pushing the button on the top of the probe. Direct the probe sheath into a facility-approved waste container.

10. Help the person back into their hospital gown or pajama top.

11. Prepare the thermometer for its next use:

    a. **Glass thermometer:** Shake down the glass thermometer, clean it according to facility policy, and return it to its case.

    b. **Electronic thermometer:** Replace the probe into the electronic thermometer. (Always read the temperature before placing the probe in the instrument because this action clears the display screen.) Turn the instrument off, if it does not automatically turn itself off. Place the thermometer in its charger.

Finishing Up

12. Complete the "Finishing Up" steps.

What You Document

- The time and date
- The person's temperature
- The method—"A" for axillary

Report an abnormal temperature to the nurse immediately.

 Procedure 20-4

Measuring a Tympanic Temperature (Tympanic Thermometer)

WHY YOU DO IT A change in a person's normal temperature may be a sign of illness. Taking a tympanic temperature is fast and causes the patient or resident minimal discomfort.

Getting Ready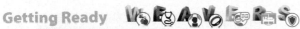

1. Complete the "Getting Ready" steps.

Supplies

- tympanic probe sheath (cover)
- tympanic thermometer

Procedure

2. If the person wears a hearing aid, remove it carefully and wait 2 minutes before taking the person's temperature. If the person has been sleeping or lying on their side with their ear against the pillow, use the ear that was not against the pillow for the temperature.

3. Inspect the ear canal for excessive cerumen (earwax). If you see excessive wax build-up in the ear canal, gently wipe the ear canal with a warm, moist washcloth.

4. Cover the cone-shaped end of the thermometer with the probe sheath. Turn the thermometer on and wait until the "ready" sign appears on the display screen.

5. Stand slightly to the front of, and facing, the person. To straighten the ear canal (which will ease insertion of the thermometer), grasp the top portion of the person's ear and gently pull:

    a. Up and back (in an adult)

    b. Straight back (in a child)

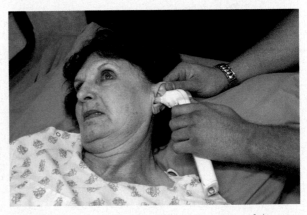

STEP 5a In an adult, grasp the top portion of the person's ear and gently pull up and back to insert the thermometer.

6. Insert the covered probe into the person's ear canal, pointing the probe down and toward the front of the ear canal (pretend that you are aiming for the person's nose). This will seal off the ear canal by seating the probe properly, leading to a more accurate temperature reading.

7. To take the temperature, press the button on the instrument. Keep the button depressed and the probe in place until the instrument blinks or beeps (usually 1 second).

8. Remove the probe and read the temperature on the display screen.

(continued)

9. Remove the probe sheath from the probe by pushing the button on the side of the instrument. Direct the probe sheath into a facility-approved waste container.

10. If your facility requires a tympanic temperature to be taken in both ears, repeat the procedure, using a clean probe cover for the other ear.

11. Turn the instrument off if it does not automatically turn itself off. Place the thermometer in its charger.

Finishing Up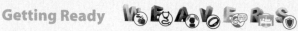

12. Complete the "Finishing Up" steps.

What You Document

- The time and date
- The person's temperature
- The method—"T" for tympanic

Report an abnormal temperature to the nurse immediately.

Procedure 20-5

Measuring a Temporal Artery Temperature

WHY YOU DO IT   A change in a person's normal temperature may be a sign of illness. Taking a temporal artery temperature is fast and accurate, and causes the patient or resident minimal discomfort.

Getting Ready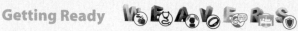

1. Complete the "Getting Ready" steps.

Supplies

- temporal artery thermometer
- probe cover (if needed)

Procedure

2. Brush the person's hair aside if it is covering the temporal artery area. Anything covering the area, such as hair, a wig, a hat, bandages, or where the person's head was resting against the pillow can result in a false high reading.

3. Apply the probe cover (if needed).

4. Hold the thermometer like a remote control device, with your thumb on the red "ON" button. Place the probe on the center of the forehead and hold the body of the thermometer sideways.

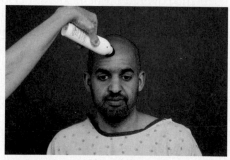

STEP 4

5. Press the ON button and keep it pressed throughout the measurement.

6. Slowly slide the thermometer straight across the forehead, midline, to the hairline. The thermometer will make a clicking noise.

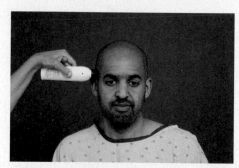

STEP 6

7. With the ON button still pressed, lift the thermometer up from the forehead and touch it to the neck, just behind the ear lobe in the little depression. This is a double check for the thermometer.

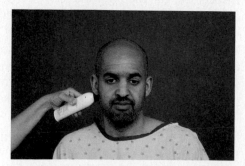

STEP 7

8. Release the ON button and read the temperature measurement.

9. Remove the probe cover (if used) by holding the thermometer over a facility-approved waste container and gently push the probe cover with your thumb.

10. Turn the thermometer off if it does not automatically turn itself off.

Finishing Up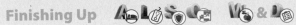

11. Complete the "Finishing Up" steps.

What You Document

- The time and date
- The person's temperature
- The method—temporal artery

Report an abnormal temperature to the nurse immediately.

 Procedure 20-6

Taking a Radial Pulse

WHY YOU DO IT A change in a person's normal pulse rate, rhythm, or amplitude may be a sign of illness. Taking the pulse at the radial artery is easiest for the patient or resident.

Getting Ready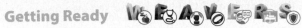

1. Complete the "Getting Ready" steps.

Supplies

- watch with second hand

Procedure

2. Rest the person's arm on the over-bed table or on the bed. Locate the radial pulse in the person's wrist using your middle two or three fingers. (TIP: The radial pulse will be on the person's "thumb" side.)

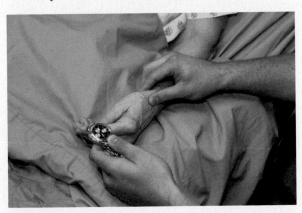

STEP 2 Locate the radial pulse in the person's wrist using your middle two or three fingers.

3. Note the strength and regularity of the pulse. Look at your watch and wait until the second hand gets to the "12" or "6." When the second hand reaches the "12" or the "6," begin counting the pulse.

   a. If the pulse rhythm is regular, count the number of pulses that occur in 30 seconds and multiply the result by 2 to arrive at the pulse rate.

   b. If the pulse rhythm is irregular, count the number of pulses that occur in 60 seconds. Counting each pulse that occurs over the course of 1 full minute is the only way to obtain a truly accurate pulse rate when the pulse is irregular.

Finishing Up

4. Complete the "Finishing Up" steps.

What You Document

- The time and date
- The pulse rate
- The pulse rhythm
- The pulse amplitude

Report an abnormal pulse rate, rhythm, or amplitude to the nurse immediately.

Procedure 20-7

Taking an Apical Pulse

WHY YOU DO IT   An apical pulse is taken when a person has a weak or irregular pulse that may be difficult to feel in the radial artery. An apical pulse may also be used to measure heart rate in infants and in people with known heart disease.

Getting Ready

1. Complete the "Getting Ready" steps.

Supplies

- alcohol wipes
- dual-sided stethoscope
- watch with second hand

Procedure

2. Help the person to a semi-sitting position by raising the head of the bed.

3. Using alcohol wipes, clean the earpieces, the diaphragm, and the bell of the stethoscope. Place the earpieces in your ears.

4. Place the diaphragm (or the bell, if the person is a child or infant) of the stethoscope under the person's clothing, on the apical pulse site (located approximately 2 inches below the person's left nipple). The diaphragm or bell must be placed directly on the person's skin because clothing will distort the sound.

5. Using two fingers, hold the diaphragm or bell firmly against the person's chest. Look at your watch and wait until the second hand gets to the "12" or "6." When the second hand reaches the "12" or the "6," begin counting the heartbeat.

6. Count the number of heartbeats that occur in 60 seconds. Each time the heart beats, you will hear two sounds, best described as a "lubb" and a "dupp." Both sounds make up one beat of the heart and should be counted as such.

7. After 60 seconds, remove the diaphragm of the stethoscope from the person's chest. Adjust the person's clothing as necessary and help the person back into a comfortable position. Lower the head of the bed, as the person requests.

8. Using alcohol wipes, clean the earpieces, the diaphragm, and the bell of the stethoscope.

Finishing Up

9. Complete the "Finishing Up" steps.

What You Document

- The time and date
- The pulse rate
- The pulse rhythm
- The pulse amplitude
- The method—"A" for apical

Report an abnormal pulse to the nurse immediately.

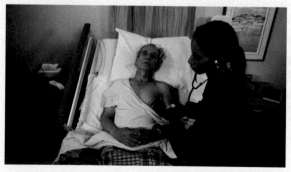

STEP 5 Hold the diaphragm or bell firmly against the person's chest.

▶ Procedure 20-8

Counting Respirations

WHY YOU DO IT A change in a person's normal respiratory rate, rhythm, or depth of breathing may be a sign of illness.

Getting Ready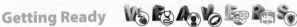

1. Complete the "Getting Ready" steps.

Supplies

- watch with second hand

Procedure

2. Look at your watch and wait until the second hand gets to the "12" or "6." When the second hand reaches the "12" or the "6," look at the person's chest (or place your hand near the person's collarbone or on their side) and begin counting each rise and fall of the chest as one breath.

   a. If the respiratory rhythm is regular, count the number of breaths that occur in 30 seconds and multiply the result by 2 to arrive at the respiratory rate.

   b. If the respiratory rhythm is irregular, count the number of breaths that occur in 60 seconds. Counting each respiration that occurs over the course of 1 full minute is the only way to obtain a truly accurate respiratory rate when the person's breathing is irregular.

Finishing Up

3. Complete the "Finishing Up" steps.

What You Document

- The time
- The respiratory rate
- The respiratory rhythm
- Any abnormal breath sounds (wheezing, congestion)

Report abnormal respirations to the nurse immediately.

▶ Procedure 20-9

Measuring Blood Pressure

WHY YOU DO IT Blood pressure measurements allow health care workers to monitor existing problems and possibly even prevent future ones.

Getting Ready

1. Complete the "Getting Ready" steps.

Supplies

- alcohol wipes
- sphygmomanometer
- stethoscope

Procedure

2. Assist the person into a sitting or lying position. Position the person's arm so that the forearm is level with the heart and the palm of the hand is facing upward. Assist the person with rolling up their sleeve so that the upper arm is exposed.

3. Using alcohol wipes, clean the earpieces, the diaphragm, and the bell of the stethoscope.

4. Stand no more than 3 feet away from the manometer. If it is not mounted on the wall, stand a mercury manometer upright on a flat surface, at eye level. Lay an aneroid manometer on a flat surface directly in front of you or leave it attached to the blood pressure cuff.

5. Squeeze the cuff to empty it of any remaining air. Turn the valve on the bulb clockwise to close it; this will cause the cuff to inflate when you pump the bulb.

(continued)

6. Locate the person's brachial artery in the antecubital space by placing your fingers at the inner aspect of the elbow.

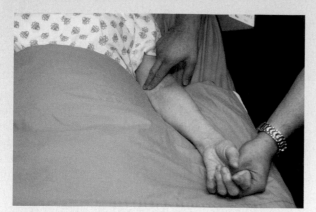

STEP 6 Locate the person's brachial artery in the antecubital space (inner aspect of the elbow).

7. Place the arrow mark on the cuff over the brachial artery. Wrap the cuff around the person's upper arm so that the bottom of the cuff is at least 1 inch above the person's elbow. The cuff must be even and snug.

8. Place the stethoscope earpieces in your ears.

9. Pump the bulb until the pressure in the cuff is 30 mm Hg higher than the systolic pressure. There are two ways to do this:

   Method "A." Hold the bulb in one hand and position the diaphragm of the stethoscope over the brachial artery with the other hand. Inflate the cuff until you hear the pulse stop and then inflate the cuff 30 mm Hg more.

   Method "B." Hold the bulb in one hand and feel for the person's brachial or radial pulse (in the wrist) with the other hand. Inflate the cuff until you are no longer able to feel the radial pulse and then inflate the cuff 30 mm Hg more.

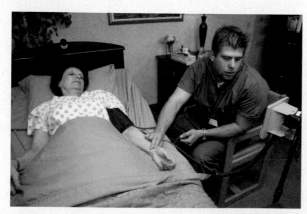

STEP 9 Hold the bulb in one hand and feel for the person's radial pulse (in the wrist) with the other hand.

10. Position the diaphragm of the stethoscope over the brachial artery (or continue to hold it there if you used method "A" to inflate the cuff).

11. Turn the valve on the bulb slightly counter-clockwise to allow air to escape from the cuff slowly.

12. Note the reading on the manometer where the first Korotkoff sound is heard. This is the systolic reading.

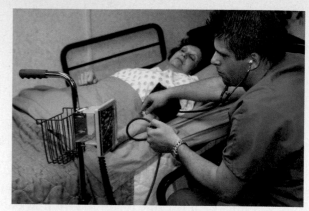

STEP 12 With the diaphragm of the stethoscope over the person's brachial artery, allow the air to leave the cuff slowly while listening for the beginning and ending sounds of the brachial pulse and watching the manometer.

13. Continue to deflate the cuff. Note the reading on the manometer where the last Korotkoff sound is heard. This is the diastolic reading.

14. Deflate the cuff completely and remove it from the person's arm. Remove the stethoscope from your ears.

15. Return the sphygmomanometer to its case or wall holder.

16. Using alcohol wipes, clean the earpieces, the diaphragm, and the bell of the stethoscope.

Finishing Up

17. Complete the "Finishing Up" steps.

What You Document

■ The time and date
■ The person's blood pressure

Report an abnormal blood pressure to the nurse immediately.

▶ Procedure 20-10

Measuring Height and Weight Using an Upright Scale ▶

WHY YOU DO IT An upright scale is used to measure the height and weight of a person who can stand independently. A person's weight is often used to calculate medication doses. In some cases, a change in a person's weight might indicate that the person's condition is getting worse or that it is getting better.

Getting Ready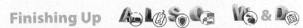

1. Complete the "Getting Ready" steps.

Supplies

■ upright scale

Procedure

2. Ask the person to urinate. If necessary, assist the person to the bathroom or offer the bedpan or urinal.

3. Move the weights all the way to the left of the balance bar.

4. Help the person onto the scale platform so that they are facing the balance bar. Once the person is on the scale platform, do not allow them to hold on to you or to the scale.

5. Move the large weight on the lower scale bar to the right to the weight closest to the person's prior weight. For example, if the person weighed 155 pounds the last time you weighed them, you would move the large weight to the "150" mark.

6. Move the small weight on the upper scale bar to the right until the balance pointer is centered between the two scale bars.

7. Read the numbers on the upper and the lower scale bars where each weight has settled and add these two numbers together. This is the person's weight.

8. Have the person carefully turn around to face away from the scale bar. Slide the height scale up so that you can pull out the height rod, which extends from the top of the height scale. Be careful not to hit the person in the head with the height rod.

9. Slide the height rod down so that it lightly touches the top of the person's head. Read the number at the point where the height rod meets the height scale. This is the person's height.

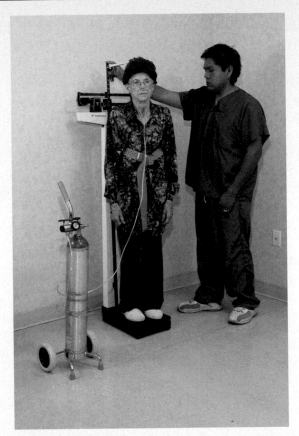

STEP 9 Slide the height rod down so that it lightly touches the top of the person's head.

10. Hold the height rod in your hand, and help the person step down from the scale.

11. Assist the person back to their room.

Finishing Up

12. Complete the "Finishing Up" steps.

What You Document

■ The time and date
■ The person's weight
■ The person's height

Report a change in the person's weight to the nurse.

▶ **Procedure 20-11**

Measuring Weight Using a Chair Scale

WHY YOU DO IT   A chair scale is used to measure the weight of a person who cannot stand independently but is able to get out of bed. A person's weight is often used to calculate medication doses. In some cases, a change in a person's weight might indicate that the person's condition is getting worse or that it is getting better.

Getting Ready

1. Complete the "Getting Ready" steps.

Supplies

- transfer belt
- wheelchair[a]

Procedure

2. Ask the person to urinate. If necessary, assist the person to the bathroom or offer the bedpan or urinal.

3. Assist or wheel the person to the scale, using a transfer belt, a wheelchair, or both.

4. Reset the scale to "0" by turning it on.

5. Help the person onto the scale.

   a. If a regular chair scale is being used, help the person to sit in the chair on the scale. Make sure the person is seated properly, with their buttocks against the back of the chair and feet on the footrests.

   b. If a wheelchair scale is being used, roll the occupied wheelchair onto the platform and lock the wheels.

6. Read the weight on the display screen. If a wheelchair scale is being used, you must subtract the weight of the unoccupied wheelchair from this figure to determine the person's weight.

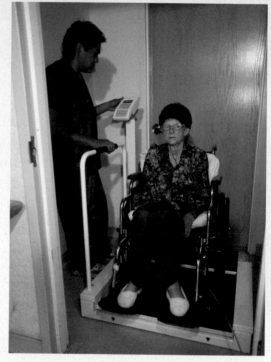

STEP 6 Read the weight on the display screen.

7. Help the person off the scale.

   a. If a regular chair scale is being used, assist the person out of the chair and back into a wheelchair if one was used for the transfer.

   b. If a wheelchair scale is being used, unlock the wheels and roll the wheelchair off the platform.

8. Assist the person back to their room.

Finishing Up

9. Complete the "Finishing Up" steps.

What You Document

- The date and time
- The person's weight

Report a change in the person's weight to the nurse.

---

[a]If you will be using a wheelchair scale to weigh the person, take the empty wheelchair to the wheelchair scale and weigh it before taking it to the person's room. Be sure to write down the weight of the empty wheelchair.

▶ Procedure 20-12

Measuring Height and Weight Using a Tape Measure and a Sling Scale

WHY YOU DO IT   A tape measure and a sling scale are used to obtain a person's height and weight when the person cannot get out of bed at all. A person's weight is often used to calculate medication doses. In some cases, change in a person's weight might indicate that the person's condition is getting worse or that it is getting better.

Getting Ready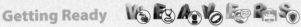

1. Complete the "Getting Ready" steps.

Supplies

- sling scale
- tape measure

Procedure

2. Ask the person to urinate. If necessary, assist the person to the bathroom or offer the bedpan or urinal.

3. Position the sling scale next to the bed. Make sure that the bed is positioned at a comfortable working height (to promote good body mechanics) and that the wheels are locked. If the side rails are in use, lower the side rail on the working side of the bed. The side rail on the opposite side of the bed should remain up.

4. Fanfold the top linens to the foot of the bed.

5. Center the sling under the person. (To get the sling under the person, move the person as if you were making an occupied bed. See Procedure 19-2.)

6. Position the person in the supine position, or according to the manufacturer's instructions.

7. Move the release valve on the sling scale to the closed position.

8. Raise the sling scale so that it can be positioned over the person.

9. Spread the legs of the sling scale to provide a solid base of support. The legs must be locked in this position, or the scale could tip over, injuring you, the person you are trying to weigh, or both.

10. Move the scale into position over the person.

11. Fasten the sling to the straps or chains of the scale. Make sure the hooks face away from the person.

12. Cross the person's arms over their chest.

13. Slowly raise the sling until the person is clear of the bed.

14. Read the weight on the display screen.

15. Gently lower the person to the bed and remove the sling by gently rolling the person first to one side, then the other.

16. Position the person in the supine position, with their arms by their sides and their legs straight.

17. Using a pencil, make a small mark on the bottom sheet at the top of the person's head. Make another small mark at their heels.

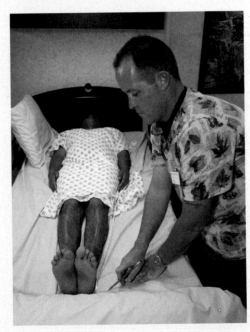

STEP 17 Using a pencil, mark the bottom sheet at the top of the person's head and at their heels.

(continued)

18. Using the tape measure, measure the distance between the pencil marks. This is the person's height.

19. Make sure that the bed is lowered to its lowest position and that the wheels are locked. If the side rails are in use, return the side rails to the raised position.

Finishing Up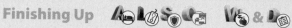

20. Complete the "Finishing Up" steps.

What You Document

■ The date and time
■ The person's weight
■ The person's height

Report a change in a person's weight to the nurse.

WHAT DID YOU LEARN?

Multiple Choice

Select the single best answer for each of the following questions.

1. A stethoscope is used to determine the:
   a. Brachial pulse rate
   b. Carotid pulse rate
   c. Apical pulse rate
   d. Popliteal pulse rate

2. Which one of the following is the pressure exerted by the blood flowing through the arteries when the heart muscle relaxes?
   a. Diastolic pressure
   b. Pulse pressure
   c. Pulse deficit
   d. Systolic pressure

3. The most common site for counting the pulse is the:
   a. Brachial artery
   b. Radial artery
   c. Carotid artery
   d. Apex of the heart

4. When counting respirations, you should:
   a. Have the person exercise first to get a true reading
   b. Count five respirations and then check your watch
   c. Count respirations for a full minute if they are irregular
   d. Have the person count respirations while you take their pulse

5. You are using a glass Fahrenheit thermometer. When you shake it down, the liquid indicator should be below the:
   a. 98.6°F mark
   b. Arrow
   c. 100°F mark
   d. 94°F mark

6. Which of the following can cause an inaccurate oral temperature reading?
   a. The person exercised vigorously 15 minutes prior to having their temperature taken
   b. The nursing assistant failed to shake down the mercury thermometer
   c. The person drank a cup of hot coffee 15 minutes prior to having their temperature taken
   d. All of the above

7. One of your patients, Ms. Jones, has a temperature of 98.8°F, a pulse rate of 80 beats per minute, and a respiratory rate of 30 breaths per minute. Which finding should be reported to the nurse immediately?
   a. Ms. Jones' respiratory rate
   b. Ms. Jones' pulse rate
   c. Ms. Jones' temperature
   d. None of these findings needs to be reported to the nurse

8. Which one of the following could cause a decreased pulse rate?
   a. Pain
   b. Anger
   c. Certain medications
   d. Fever

9. What should you observe when taking a person's pulse?
   a. The rhythm and regularity of the pulse
   b. The number of beats per minute
   c. The strength of the pulse
   d. All of the above

10. If you notice a significant change in a person's vital signs, what should you do?
   a. Record the change with a special notation to indicate that the reading was different
   b. Mention the change to the nurse at the end of your shift
   c. Tell the patient or resident about the change
   d. Report the change to a nurse immediately

11. Which instrument is used to measure blood pressure?
   a. A temporal artery thermometer
   b. A sphygmomanometer
   c. An upright scale
   d. A watch with a second hand

12. Which one of the following conditions would prevent you from taking an oral temperature?
   a. The person has diarrhea
   b. The person has just had a mastectomy
   c. The person is unconscious
   d. The person is a 10-year-old child

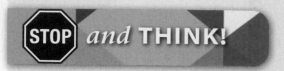

■ You are assigned to take vital signs on all the residents in the north hall of your facility. Mrs. Tito, in room 102, has a cast on her left arm and an intravenous (IV) line in her right. How are you going to take Mrs. Tito's blood pressure?

■ Vital sign measurements are routinely taken once weekly at the long-term care facility where you work. Today, as you take Mr. Hayes' pulse, you notice that it does not feel as strong as usual, and although his rate is about what it always is, the rhythm is irregular. What should you do?

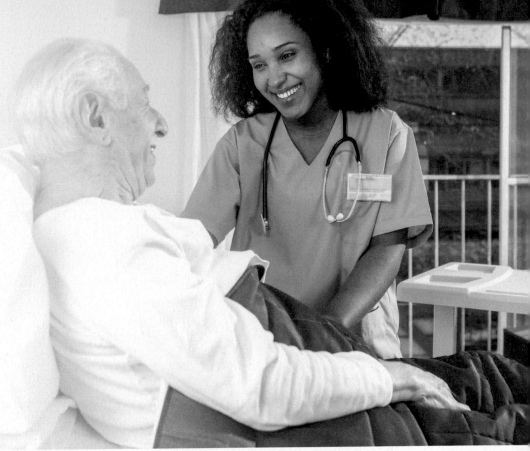

Photo: A nursing assistant helps to position a resident comfortably.

Comfort and Rest

 WHAT WILL YOU LEARN?

When we are comfortable, we feel content, without pain or distress. We are able to rest, relax, and sleep. Helping patients and residents be as comfortable as possible and promoting rest and sleep are important parts of providing holistic care. In this chapter, you will learn about rest and sleep, and why being able to get sufficient rest and sleep is so important to a person's health and well-being. You will also learn about pain, which affects many patients' and residents' comfort. When you are finished with this chapter, you will be able to:

1. Explain the importance of rest and sleep to a person's overall well-being.
2. Describe the normal sleep cycle.
3. Describe factors that can affect a person's ability to obtain a good night's sleep.
4. Describe actions a nursing assistant can take to help patients and residents get the rest and sleep that they need.
5. Define pain and the difference between acute pain and chronic pain.
6. Discuss factors that can affect a person's response to pain.
7. List nonverbal signs of pain that a person may show.
8. Describe methods a nursing assistant can use to gather more information about the nature of a person's pain.

9. Explain the importance of promptly and accurately reporting a patient's or a resident's pain.
10. Discuss the use of medications, physical therapy, and heat and cold applications to relieve pain and promote comfort.
11. Demonstrate how to safely use heat and cold applications in the health care setting.
12. Describe actions a nursing assistant can take to help a person who is experiencing pain.

Vocabulary

Insomnia	Pain	Pain tolerance
Sleep apnea	Acute pain	Radiating pain
Continuous positive airway pressure (CPAP) therapy	Chronic pain	Pain scale
	Pain threshold	Breakthrough pain

PHYSICAL AND EMOTIONAL BENEFITS OF REST AND SLEEP

Rest and sleep are basic physical needs that may be difficult to meet in a health care setting. A lack of rest and sleep can lead to many problems that can interfere with a person's ability to function at their best, including:

- **Worsened pain.** As a result of sleep loss, a person's ability to handle pain is often decreased.
- **Increased risk for illness and lengthened healing process.** A lack of sleep and rest can decrease the immune system's effectiveness (putting the person at increased risk for infections) and affect heart function (resulting in high blood pressure and an irregular heartbeat). In order for tissues to heal properly following an injury, surgery, or an acute illness, the body needs extra sleep and rest.
- **Emotional and behavioral problems.** A lack of sleep can affect a person's ability to cope with everyday challenges. The person may become irritable, or cry easily. The person may even become depressed.
- **Decreased cognition.** A person who is not getting enough sleep may have difficulty concentrating, paying attention, remembering information, and making decisions. The person may even fall asleep during routine activities. This can make it difficult for the person to learn new information and skills, which can negatively affect the person's ability to reach their goals.

- **Fatigue and decreased physical ability.** Fatigue resulting from a lack of rest and sleep can affect the person's ability to participate in self-care, physical therapy, or other activities. As a result, the person may experience a decrease in physical function, as well as emotional difficulties. Fatigue and decreased physical ability also increase the person's risk for falls and other injuries.

Normal Sleep

Sleep gives the body and brain a chance to rest and recover from the activities and stresses of everyday life. During sleep, the eyes are closed and the muscles are completely relaxed. The person's respirations and heart rate slow down. The body works to heal and repair the tissues from the wear and tear of daily activity, strengthening the immune system and refreshing and reenergizing brain cells.

There are two different types of sleep: nonrapid eye movement (NREM) sleep and rapid eye movement (REM) sleep. A complete sleep cycle consists of four stages of NREM sleep, followed by a period of REM sleep (Fig. 21-1).

- **NREM sleep:** The four stages of NREM sleep progress from a light sleep to a very deep sleep. Each stage of NREM sleep lasts from 5 to 15 minutes.
- **REM sleep:** During REM sleep, there is increased activity in the brain. The heart and respiratory rates increase, and the eyes move back and forth rapidly. Dreaming occurs during REM sleep.

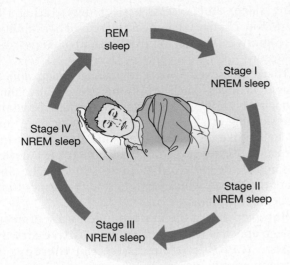

Figure 21-1 A complete sleep cycle includes four stages of nonrapid eye movement (NREM) sleep, followed by a period of rapid eye movement (REM) sleep. After REM sleep, the cycle begins again. On average, a person completes four or five sleep cycles during a night's sleep.

After completion of REM sleep, the cycle begins again. Through each cycle, REM sleep lasts a bit longer, eventually reaching approximately 1 hour. On average, a person completes four or five sleep cycles during a night's sleep.

Newborns need the greatest amount of sleep, often sleeping up to 20 hours a day. As a child becomes older, their need for sleep gradually decreases. Most adults need 7 to 8 hours of sleep per 24-hour period. Older people need this amount of sleep as well, but they often have a hard time getting this amount of uninterrupted sleep at night. Taking naps during the day may help an older person to meet the need for 7 to 8 hours of sleep per 24-hour period.

Factors That Can Affect Sleep

A number of factors can affect a person's ability to obtain a good night's sleep.

Environment

Environmental conditions, such as noise, light, and room temperature, can affect a person's ability to sleep. For people in health care facilities, environmental factors often cause problems in sleeping. There may be more noise, or strange noises. Depending on the type of health care setting, noise and activity may be constant both day and night. For example, care required by a patient in a hospital's critical care unit may require that lights remain on and procedures be carried out 24/7. Alarm noises from numerous monitors and machines can also disrupt sleep.

A lack of exposure to bright light, especially sunlight, during the day can affect a person's normal sleep/awake cycles. So can spending one's time all in one room. A patient or resident who spends most of their time in the same room with the window shades drawn may experience difficulty sleeping.

The bed may feel different from the bed the person was used to at home. The person may have to adjust to having a roommate. The person (or the roommate) may require care during the night. Although the care is necessary, the person's sleep is disturbed when staff members enter the room.

Pain and Chronic Conditions

Many people in a health care setting will experience some degree of pain or discomfort, and many have chronic health conditions. Pain and other symptoms of chronic health conditions (such as shortness of breath, coughing, or frequent urination) can make it hard for the person to fall asleep, or to stay asleep. Many medications used in the health care setting can also cause sleep disruptions.

Emotional Concerns

A person in a health care setting may have many worries regarding their health. The person may be awaiting the results of a medical test or biopsy for a diagnosis. Financial concerns, especially related to the cost of health care, or time lost from work to recover from surgery or an illness can cause emotional distress. Many people worry about family members or pets that have been left at home.

Concerns for Long-Term Care

Older people take longer to fall asleep and awaken more frequently during the night. As a person ages, they become more sensitive to noise when sleeping and will awaken more easily. This is a major concern in the long-term care setting. Because of this, an older person is more likely to need a regular daytime nap, which can help compensate for the loss of sleep at night and prevent daytime drowsiness.

An older person is also more likely to have one or more chronic health conditions that cause enough discomfort to interfere with a good night's sleep. Older people, especially males, wake up to urinate several times during the night and may have difficulty falling back asleep. Many people suffer from what is known as *restless leg syndrome*, an irresistible urge to move one's legs accompanied by unpleasant sensations in the legs. Many medications can cause a person to have difficulty with falling asleep or staying asleep.

Studies have shown that many residents in the long-term care setting seldom sleep for more than 1 hour at a time. A lack of sleep for older people can increase the risk of anxiety, delirium, and depression. Physical fatigue from lack of sleep can also make a person more likely to fall.

Sleep Disorders

Sleep disorders are medical conditions characterized by inadequate sleep, disturbed sleep, or sleep at inappropriate times. There are many different types of sleep disorders. In fact, many health care facilities have specialized units to monitor people who have sleep disorders so that the type of disorder can be diagnosed and appropriate treatment can be prescribed. Two of the most common sleep disorders are insomnia and sleep apnea.

Insomnia

Insomnia is a disorder characterized by an inability to fall asleep or to stay asleep. The person may have trouble falling asleep, wake frequently during the night, or wake up too early in the morning and then be unable to fall back asleep. The person does not get an adequate amount of sleep, and the quality of the sleep that the person does get is poor.

Be sure to tell the nurse if a patient or a resident reports experiencing insomnia. The health care team will need to assess the person to determine the cause and take actions to address it. Medications can aid in the treatment of insomnia, but these medications must be used with caution in older people. Some have side effects that cause the person to become groggy and less alert during the day, which can lead to falls and other accidents. Providing care and an environment that promotes sleep and rest without medication is preferred for older people with insomnia.

Sleep Apnea

Sleep apnea is a disorder that causes the person to stop breathing for varying periods of time during sleep. There are several forms of sleep apnea, but the most common form is obstructive sleep apnea. In this condition, the soft tissue in the back of the throat collapses, blocking the airway and causing the person to stop breathing. When the person's blood oxygen level gets low, the person wakes up and starts breathing again. Because the person's sleep is interrupted many times during the night, the quality of sleep is very poor. The person wakes up feeling tired and may have difficulty staying awake during the day.

Sleep apnea is most common in males older than 40 years and people who are overweight. Symptoms include chronic, loud snoring; gasping and choking during sleep; and excessive sleepiness during the day. Mood changes (such as increased irritability) and cognitive (mental or intellectual) changes can also occur.

There are several ways to manage sleep apnea. Lifestyle changes, such as losing weight, avoiding alcohol and smoking, and avoiding certain positions while sleeping can help. Some people may have surgery to remove or reduce the tissue that causes the obstruction. Newer surgeries involve inserting a device to stimulate the nerves that control the tongue and back of the throat, which helps to stop the tissues from obstructing the airway.

However, one of the most common ways of treating sleep apnea is with **continuous positive airway pressure (CPAP**, pronounced *see-pap*) **therapy**. In this treatment, the person wears a special CPAP mask while sleeping (Fig. 21-2). The CPAP mask forms a tight seal over the nose (and sometimes the mouth as well). The mask is attached to a machine that forces air into the airway, keeping it open during sleep. This keeps the person's blood oxygen level at an acceptable level, allowing the person to sleep through the night.

When caring for a person in a hospital setting who uses CPAP at home, they may either bring their own unit, or one may be ordered by the doctor and set up by the respiratory therapy department. If you are caring for a resident in a long-term care facility who is receiving CPAP therapy, you may need to assist the resident with applying the mask and turning on the CPAP machine. The nurse will show you how the person's mask should be applied and how the machine operates. You may also be responsible for helping the person keep the equipment clean.

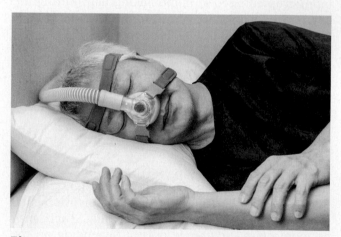

Figure 21-2 Many people who have sleep apnea will receive continuous positive airway pressure (CPAP) therapy. The special CPAP mask delivers air under pressure. The pressure keeps the airways open so that the person gets enough oxygen, allowing the person to sleep through the night. (*Chalermpon Poungpeth\Shutterstock.com*)

Tell the Nurse!

When caring for a person who is being treated with CPAP therapy for sleep apnea, be sure to report the following observations to the nurse:

- The person refuses to put on the mask or takes it off
- There is a hissing noise coming from around the seal of the mask or the tubing
- The CPAP machine is not working properly
- The mask or straps are causing irritation of the person's skin

Tell the Nurse!

As a nursing assistant, you may be the first to notice that a patient or a resident is having difficulty sleeping. A person may also mention difficulties sleeping to you. Be sure to report any of the following observations about a person's ability to sleep to the nurse right away:

- The person is awake frequently during the night
- The person lies awake for long periods before falling asleep
- The person reports wakefulness or difficulty sleeping
- The person seems sleepy during the day
- The person gets up frequently during the night to urinate
- The person tells you about, or shows signs of, pain or discomfort
- The person reports an inability to get to sleep or stay asleep as a result of something in the environment (for example, the noise in the hallway or another room; being too hot or too cold)
- The person expresses worry or anxiety about something

The Nursing Assistant's Role in Promoting Rest and Sleep

As a nursing assistant, there are many things you can do to help your patients and residents get the rest and sleep that they need.

Always respect each person's preferences with regard to times for going to bed and waking up. Some people are "early to bed, early to rise." Other people are "night owls," meaning they like to go to bed late and sleep in the morning. Disrupting these natural patterns can affect the person's quality of sleep.

Remember that a quiet, dark environment promotes rest and sleep. When working during the evening and night hours, be especially mindful of things you do that could affect a person's ability to sleep. Keep noise at a minimum, particularly at the change of shift when there is a lot of staff activity. Keep your voice low and encourage others to do the same. Avoid calling out to coworkers unless you need help in an emergency. Finally, be thoughtful about the use of lights. If you need to enter a person's room to provide care, avoid turning on bright overhead lights. Use night lights or other soft lighting, if possible. Gently awaken the person who needs care, and be sure to explain to the person who you are and what you are there to do. If more light is needed to safely complete the task, turn on only the lights you need. When you have finished providing care, make sure the person is positioned comfortably, and turn out the lights as soon as you can.

Other actions you can take are listed in Box 21-1. By being sensitive to the patient's or resident's needs, you can help provide an atmosphere that promotes rest and sleep.

PAIN

Pain is an unpleasant sensation that can range from mild discomfort to intense suffering. Many of the people whom you care for in the health care setting will have some type of pain. **Acute pain** is sharp, sudden pain, such as that which occurs with an injury or illness. Acute pain lasts a short period of time and decreases as the body's tissues repair themselves and heal. **Chronic pain** is pain that lasts beyond the usual time that it would take for the tissues to heal. Pain may be caused by many conditions, ranging anywhere from sore and stiff muscles and joints to incisional pain following surgery. Pain can make it difficult for a person to rest, relax, and sleep.

How People Respond to Pain

Pain is a totally subjective experience. Only the person who is experiencing the pain knows what it feels like. Different people do not experience pain in the same way due to differences in pain threshold and pain tolerance. A person's **pain threshold** is the point at which the person becomes aware of pain. A person

Box 21-1   Actions to Promote Rest and Sleep for Your Patients and Residents

- Encourage increased physical activity during the day. Physical activity during the day promotes better sleep at night. This is especially important for residents of a long-term care facility.
- Increase a person's exposure to daytime lighting, especially sunlight, during the day.
- Limit time for naps during the day. Although a short nap during the day can help an older person meet their sleep requirements, taking too many naps or naps that are too long can negatively affect the person's ability to sleep at night.
- Avoid giving the person beverages with caffeine (such as regular coffee, tea, or cola) in the afternoon or evening. Many people are sensitive to caffeine and find that it keeps them up at night if they have it too late in the day.
- Promote relaxation by giving the person a warm bath in the evening, or providing a massage. Finding out the person's normal bedtime routines, and following them as closely as possible, is also important for promoting relaxation and sleep.
- Offer the person a snack at bedtime.

- Assist the person with basic hygiene and elimination just before bedtime.
- Create a comfortable environment for sleeping. Straighten the bed linens and fluff the pillows. Provide a warmed blanket. Make sure items are put away and the room is neat and free of clutter. Close the blinds or draperies to darken the room, and turn off the overhead lights. (A night light may be left on for safety.) Make sure the room temperature is not too hot or too cold.
- Position the person carefully, using good body alignment.
- Turn off the television set or radio (unless the person watches television or listens to the radio to relax before bed). Many people find soft music very relaxing at bedtime. Others like to be read to from a favorite book.
- Be observant. For example, if the person seems upset or worried about something, you should report this to the nurse because stress or worry can impact the person's ability to sleep. Similarly, if the person seems to be in pain or has some other type of physical discomfort, report this to the nurse.

with a low pain threshold is very sensitive to pain, whereas a person with a high pain threshold is less sensitive to it. **Pain tolerance** is the level of pain that a person can endure before taking action to seek relief.

There are other factors that affect a person's response to pain as well. Culture and upbringing play a very large role in how people perceive and manage pain. For example, in some families, admitting to pain may be considered a sign of weakness. People who were raised in families that took a stoic approach to pain may feel that it is better to "grin and bear it" than to complain about the pain or ask for relief. Other people, however, may come from families where family members discussed every little ache and pain loudly and in great detail. People with a background like this might not hesitate to discuss or ask for relief from their own pain. A person's age and experience with pain can also affect how the person responds to pain. For example, it is quite common for older people to think that pain is just a part of aging that needs to be tolerated. As a result, some people may not mention their pain to caregivers, because they may feel that there is nothing to be done about it anyway. Some patients and residents may not mention pain because they do not want to trouble caregivers for medication, or because they do not want to worry their loved ones.

It is very important to understand that each person experiences and expresses pain differently. As caregivers, we never want to assume that a person does not have pain or that the person's pain is minimal, because the person does not complain. Nor should we ever assume that a person who complains

about pain is exaggerating their pain, even if the person's pain seems out of proportion to the injury or condition causing the pain.

Recognizing and Reporting Pain

As a nursing assistant, you may be the first to notice that one of your patients or residents is in pain. Sometimes, the person will tell you about their discomfort. Other times, your observation skills will tip you off (Fig. 21-3). Nonverbal signs of pain may include:

- Facial expressions (such as grimacing or gritting the teeth)

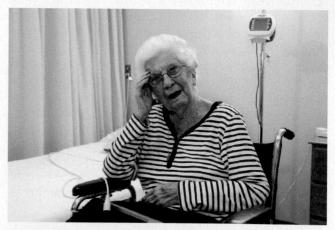

Figure 21-3 Paying close attention to nonverbal cues can help you to recognize when a patient or a resident is experiencing pain or discomfort.

- Moaning
- Crying
- Restlessness
- Calling out
- Rubbing the area of the body that is in pain
- Guarding (avoiding use of) the area of the body that is in pain
- Resisting care
- Redness or swelling in an area
- Profuse sweating
- Changes in the person's vital signs or behavior

A person who has dementia or is unable to communicate clearly due to cognitive challenges may not be able to effectively express that they are having pain. The person may simply be resistant of care or other activities that are painful. You may notice that a person who may be normally smiling and cooperative might suddenly change their behavior and be quiet and uncooperative.

When reporting a person's pain to the nurse, it is helpful to provide additional details about the pain in your report, if possible. This additional information will help the nurse assess what is happening and determine the appropriate action to take. If the patient or the resident is able to understand and answer questions, try to obtain the following information:

- **Location of the pain.** Ask whether the pain is localized (in one area) or whether it travels anywhere else. Pain that travels from one area to another is called **radiating pain.**
- **Characteristics of the pain.** Not all pain or discomfort feels the same. Identifying the characteristics of the pain the person is experiencing may help the nurse to identify the cause of the pain. Examples of words that can be used to describe pain include *aching, throbbing, stabbing, piercing, dull, sharp, cramping, burning, constant,* and *intermittent* (that is, the pain comes and goes).
- **Intensity of the pain.** The intensity of the pain is how much it hurts. As you have learned, pain is a subjective experience. Only the person experiencing the pain knows what the pain is like. **A pain scale** (a tool or guide that helps translate a person's subjective rating of their pain into an objective measurement) can be helpful in understanding the extent of a person's pain (Table 21-1).
- **Circumstances surrounding the pain.** It will be useful for the nurse to know when the pain started, what the person was doing when the pain started, whether or not the person has ever experienced a similar pain before, and whether or not there is anything that makes the pain feel better or worse.

Another important bit of information for you to report to the nurse will be the person's vital signs. Pain accompanied with fever can be a sign of infection. If the pain is new, the nurse will need to take steps to find out what is causing it. Even if the pain is familiar and the cause of it is known, there may still be something the nurse can do to help make the person more comfortable. Unrelieved pain and discomfort can lead to a significant decline in a person's condition. Pain can negatively affect a person's sleep, appetite, energy levels, ability to heal quickly, and the ability or desire to participate in self-care activities and to move. Pain also has an emotional impact and can lead to depression. All of these factors affect the person's general well-being and ability to attain or maintain their highest level of function.

Treatments for Pain

Treatments for pain include medication, physical therapy, and heat and cold applications.

Pain Medications

Over-the-counter pain medications—such as aspirin, acetaminophen (Tylenol), and ibuprofen (Advil)—can be very effective for relieving mild to moderate pain. Severe pain, such as that which often accompanies surgery, an acute illness or injury, or some types of cancer, may be controlled only by the use of narcotics, such as morphine. Many narcotic-type pain medications may make a patient or resident groggy or dizzy, increasing their risk of falling. You may need to raise the person's side rails on the bed and have them call for assistance prior to trying to get out of bed. An older person may become confused or disoriented. Narcotic pain medications can also decrease a person's respirations and lower their blood oxygen levels. Make sure to check on the person frequently.

Patients and residents with both acute and chronic pain may need regular dosing of pain medication to keep the pain under control throughout the day and night (Fig. 21-4). The nurse and the doctor will schedule the person's doses to stay ahead of the pain because if the pain is allowed to reoccur, a higher dose of medication may be necessary to relieve it. Some people may experience **breakthrough pain** (pain that occurs before the next regularly scheduled dose of pain medication). It is important to recognize and report breakthrough pain so that the person does not have to be unnecessarily uncomfortable while waiting for the next scheduled dose of pain medication. You can help the doctor and the nurse plan the patient's or the resident's medication schedule by reporting your observations about the person's pain to the nurse promptly.

TABLE 21-1 Pain Scales

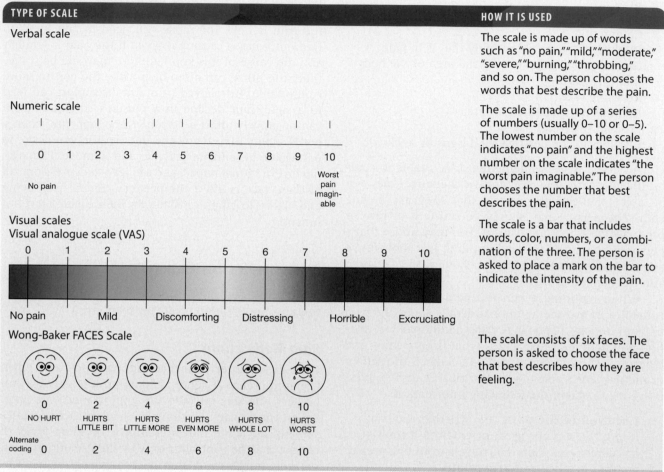

TYPE OF SCALE	HOW IT IS USED
Verbal scale	The scale is made up of words such as "no pain," "mild," "moderate," "severe," "burning," "throbbing," and so on. The person chooses the words that best describe the pain.
Numeric scale	The scale is made up of a series of numbers (usually 0–10 or 0–5). The lowest number on the scale indicates "no pain" and the highest number on the scale indicates "the worst pain imaginable." The person chooses the number that best describes the pain.
Visual scales **Visual analogue scale (VAS)**	The scale is a bar that includes words, color, numbers, or a combination of the three. The person is asked to place a mark on the bar to indicate the intensity of the pain.
Wong-Baker FACES Scale	The scale consists of six faces. The person is asked to choose the face that best describes how they are feeling.

From Hockenberry MJ, Wilson D. *Wong's Essentials of Pediatric Nursing.* 8th ed. Mosby; 2009. Used with permission. Copyright Mosby.

Some people may be concerned about becoming addicted to pain medications. Report any concerns a person may have about possible addiction or side effects to the nurse promptly. The nurse will work with the person to address those concerns.

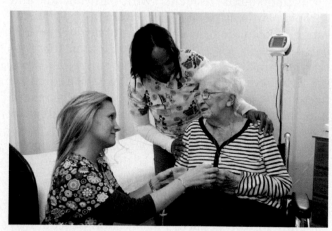

Figure 21-4 Many patients and residents will take medication for pain.

Physical Therapy

Physical therapy can be useful for relieving some types of pain. For example:

- **Exercise.** The physical therapist may assist the person with exercises that stretch and strengthen the muscles, reducing the pain and stiffness often associated with musculoskeletal disorders.
- **Ultrasound therapy.** The physical therapist uses an ultrasound device to transmit sound waves to muscle tissue and blood vessels in the painful area. The sound waves cause the tissue to relax and increase blood circulation in the area, reducing muscle tightness and spasms.
- **Transcutaneous electrical nerve stimulation (TENS).** The physical therapist uses a device to deliver electrical impulses through electrodes that are attached to the surface of the skin (Fig. 21-5). The electrical impulses help to block pain signals in the body.

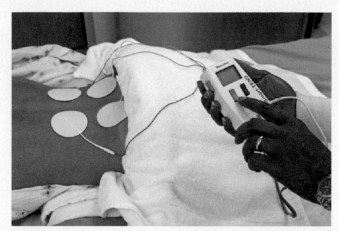

Figure 21-5 Transcutaneous electrical nerve stimulation (TENS) may be used to provide relief from some types of pain. Electrodes are attached to the skin over the painful area and a device is used to deliver electrical impulses through the electrodes. The electrical impulses help to block pain signals.

Heat and Cold Applications

Many people with musculoskeletal pain can benefit from the application of heat or cold to an affected joint or muscle, which can reduce or prevent tissue swelling, promote healing, ease pain, and promote comfort. Heat and cold have opposite effects on the body, which are summarized in Table 21-2. Because the application of heat or cold can be dangerous, these treatments require a doctor's order, and in some facilities, the application of heat or cold may be outside of the nursing assistant's scope of practice. However, even if you are not permitted to give these treatments, you will be involved with monitoring patients and residents who are receiving them.

Older people and very young children are at very high risk for injury from the application of heat or cold because their skin is very fragile and sensitive. Other factors that can increase a person's risk for injury from the application of heat or cold include:

- **Fair skin.** Fair skin tends to be more sensitive to temperature changes than darker skin.
- **Impaired sensation.** People with impaired sensation, such as those who are paralyzed or who have diabetes, are at risk for injury because they are unable to detect whether an application is too hot or too cold.
- **Impaired consciousness.** People who are disoriented or taking pain medications may be unaware that an application is too hot or too cold, or unable to communicate discomfort caused by the application to others.

People with these risk factors for injury must be monitored especially carefully during the application of heat or cold.

Heat Applications

Heat relaxes the muscles, relieves pain, and promotes blood flow to the area. When heat is applied to the skin, the blood vessels dilate (widen), allowing more blood to flow to the tissues. Increased blood flow speeds healing by bringing more oxygen, nutrients, and infection-fighting white blood cells to the area. The increased blood flow helps to reduce swelling by removing excess fluid from the tissues. In addition, heat relaxes the muscles and helps loosen stiff joints.

Heat applications can be either moist or dry (Fig. 21-6). In moist applications, moisture comes in direct contact with the skin. Moist heat penetrates tissues more quickly and deeply than dry heat. For this reason, moist heat applications are used at a lower temperature to reduce the risk of burns. Examples of moist heat applications include warm compresses and hot water soaks (see Fig. 21-6A).

Dry applications prevent moisture from coming in direct contact with the skin. Examples of dry heat applications include an electric heating pad or a hot water bottle wrapped in a towel. An Aquamatic pad (or K-pad) is a special type of heating pad (see Fig. 21-6B). The pad is connected to a heating unit that heats water to a preset temperature. The water circulates through the pad and then back into the heating device so that a constant temperature is maintained. A key is used to set the temperature, and then the key is removed, preventing the heat from being turned up or down. Because the temperature remains at a constant, preset temperature, the Aquamatic pad is much safer to use than an electric heating pad or hot water bottle. Procedure 21-1 describes how to apply a dry heat application using an Aquamatic pad.

Burns are the most common complication of heat applications. Some burns, especially on thin, delicate skin, can be very severe, resulting in blistering, tissue

TABLE 21-2 Uses of Heat and Cold Applications

HEAT	COLD
Reduces pain and swelling and promotes circulation to speed healing	Reduces pain and swelling
Relieves muscle spasms	Reduces muscle spasms
Provides warmth	Numbs sensation and controls bleeding
Accelerates the inflammatory response, promoting healing	Reduces fevers
Decreases muscle and joint stiffness	

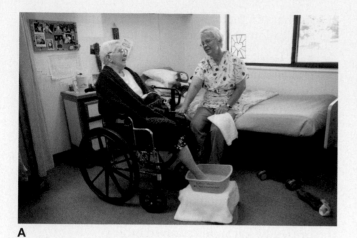

A

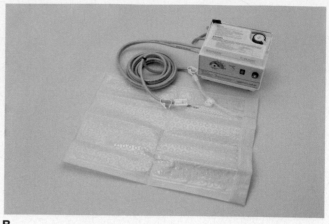

B

Figure 21-6 Heat applications are used to relax muscles, relieve pain, and promote blood flow to an area. Heat applications may be either moist or dry. **A.** A warm soak is an example of a moist heat application. Soaks are done in either a wash basin (if the area to be soaked is small) or a tub (if the area to be soaked is large). **B.** An Aquamatic pad is an example of a dry heat application. Water is heated in the heating unit. The heated water passes through the tubing and into a network of tubes inside the heating pad. The water never comes in contact with the person's skin.

loss, and the need for skin grafting. In addition to increasing the person's risk for burns, heat applications that are left in place for too long will eventually cause the blood vessels to constrict, putting the person at risk for tissue breakdown. For these reasons, heat applications should not be left in place for longer than 20 minutes. Make sure that you check the skin underneath the heat application every 5 minutes and stop the treatment immediately if you observe any evidence of burning. Warmth causes the skin to become pink or slightly reddened. Skin that is bright red or very pale could be burned. Report any observations that may indicate a burn to the nurse immediately, along with any complaints of pain, burning, or stinging.

Cold Applications

Cold applications are often used for people who have musculoskeletal injuries resulting from trauma, such as sprains and fractures. Cold applications are also frequently used on incisions following surgical procedures. Cold applications may be used for an extended period of time following orthopedic surgical procedures, such as total knee and shoulder replacement. The application of cold reduces pain and swelling and decreases bleeding by cooling the skin and underlying tissues, causing the blood vessels to constrict (narrow). Because the blood vessels are constricted, less blood is carried to the tissues, resulting in less bleeding and decreased tissue swelling. The numbing effect of the cold helps to reduce pain and allows joints to move easier. Cold applications are also used to help reduce chronic pain and for muscle spasms.

Like heat applications, cold applications can be either moist or dry (Fig. 21-7). Moist applications allow the cold to penetrate the tissues more quickly and deeply. A cold compress, made by soaking a gauze pad, towel, or washcloth in cold water, wringing it out, and then applying it with light pressure to the affected area, is an example of a moist cold application (see Fig. 21-7A). Procedure 21-2 explains how to give a moist cold application.

Dry applications are usually colder than moist applications. An ice bag is an example of a dry cold application (see Fig. 21-7B). Commercially prepared ice packs that are kept frozen until the time of use are available, or a dry cold application can be made by filling an ice bag with crushed ice and wrapping it in a towel or washcloth. Units that contain ice and water are often used to circulate cold water through a special pad, similar to an Aquamatic pad. These pads can be placed around arms or legs to administer dry cold applications after orthopedic surgery. Procedure 21-3 explains how to give a dry cold application.

When applied directly to a person's skin, cold can cause severe burns and blisters. Dry cold applications should be wrapped in a protective cloth to prevent the icy cold plastic from coming in direct contact with the person's skin. If a cold application is left in place for too long, prolonged constriction of the small blood vessels can keep oxygen and nutrients from reaching the skin, resulting in tissue death and skin breakdown. For this reason, cold applications should not be left in place for longer than 20 minutes. Make sure that you check the skin underneath the cold application every 5 minutes and stop the treatment immediately if you observe any

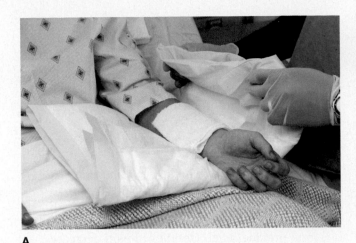

A

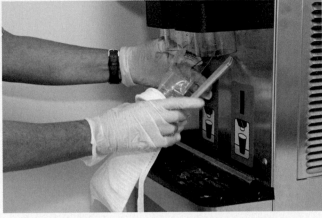

B

Figure 21-7 Cold applications are used to reduce pain and swelling. Cold applications may be either moist or dry. **A.** A cold compress is a moist cold application. **B.** An ice bag is a dry cold application.

evidence of a burn or blister. Pale skin, resulting from the constriction of the blood vessels, should return to its normal color quickly after the cold application is removed. If it does not, or if you notice a burn or blister starting to develop, inform the nurse immediately. Also, if you have questions about how to apply the cold application or for how long, please ask the nurse for help.

The Nursing Assistant's Role in Managing Pain

As a nursing assistant, there are many things you can do to help a patient or a resident who is experiencing pain and discomfort.

- **Help the person to relax.** Anxiety causes the body to become tense, which increases pain. Dim lights and a quiet environment can promote relaxation. Some people find that breathing slowly, regularly, and deeply in a calm, comfortable environment promotes relaxation and reduces pain. Have the person close their eyes and visualize a very relaxing place to be.
- **Provide distractions from the pain.** Activities such as listening to music, watching television, reading, or sharing memories can help reduce pain and discomfort by giving the person something to focus on, other than the pain.
- **Pay attention to positioning.** Positioning and supporting the body in proper alignment relieve strain on the muscles and joints and promote comfort.

- **Offer a massage.** Massage may help relieve discomfort and can be very relaxing for the person. As with any personal care procedure, always check with the nurse or read the person's care plan first to make sure that it is all right for the person to have a massage. In general, avoid massaging areas that are red, swollen, warm, and painful. The procedure for giving a back massage is found in Chapter 22.
- **Assist a person in pain slowly and gently.** Although you should be gentle with all of your patients and residents, it is important to be especially gentle when assisting those who are in pain to move because even the slightest movement may make the pain worse. In some cases, the nurse may administer pain medication before an activity to reduce the pain and make the activity more tolerable. When this is the case, wait 20 to 30 minutes until the pain medication takes effect before working with the person.

Remember that each person's response to pain, and the methods that they are most comfortable using to address it, will vary.

As the staff member who works most closely with people in a health care setting, you will play a vital role in helping to detect and manage pain. Being sensitive to what your patient or resident is feeling and taking action to provide physical comfort and emotional support are important measures you can take to help promote comfort and relieve a person's pain.

SUMMARY

- The body refreshes and repairs itself during sleep. Adequate rest and sleep are very important for a person's overall health and well-being.
  - Most adults need 7 to 8 hours of sleep per 24-hour period to function at their best. Infants and small children need more sleep.
  - Factors that can negatively affect a person's sleep include environmental conditions (such as noise, light, heat or cold), pain and other symptoms of chronic conditions, and sleep disorders (such as insomnia and sleep apnea).
  - Nursing assistants can help patients and residents to get the rest and sleep they need by ensuring a restful environment, providing for physical comfort, and minimizing noise and other disruptions when providing care during the night.

- Pain is an unpleasant sensation that can range from mild discomfort to intense suffering. Pain can be acute or chronic.
  - Each person experiences and expresses pain differently.
  - Nursing assistants play a very important role in recognizing and reporting pain. In this way, they help other members of the health care team determine the cause of the pain and provide relief. Unrelieved pain decreases a person's quality of life and can lead to a significant decline in their condition.
  - Common treatments for pain include medication, physical therapy, and heat and cold applications. In addition, there are many things nursing assistants can do independently to help patients and residents who are in pain.

Procedure 21-1

Giving a Dry Heat Application With an Aquamatic Pad

WHY YOU DO IT   Heat applications relax the muscles, relieve pain, and promote blood flow to the area.

Getting Ready

1. Complete the "Getting Ready" steps.

Supplies

- Aquamatic pad
- heating unit
- distilled water
- cloth cover or towel
- ties or tape

Procedure

2. Check the pad for leaks. Make sure that the cord is not frayed and the plug is in good condition. Check the heating unit to be sure that it is filled with water. If you need to fill it, use distilled water. Tap water contains minerals that can corrode the unit.

3. Place the heating unit so that the tubing and pad are level with the heating unit at all times. Make sure that the tubing is free of kinks. Plug the cord into an outlet.

4. Allow the water to warm to the desired temperature, as specified by the nurse or the care plan (usually not to exceed 105° to 109.4°F depending on facility policy). If the temperature is not preset, set the temperature with the key and then remove the key.

5. Place the pad in its cover. If the cover is not made of cloth, make sure to place a cloth towel in between the pad and the person's skin.

6. Make sure that the bed is positioned at a comfortable working height (to promote good body mechanics) and that the wheels are locked.

7. Help the person to a comfortable position and expose only the area to be treated.

8. Apply the pad to the treatment site.

9. Leave the pad in place for the designated amount of time, usually 15 to 20 minutes. The pad may be secured in place with ties or tape,

or the resident may assist by holding the pad in place. (Do not use pins to secure the pad. Pins can puncture the pad, causing it to leak.)

   a. Check the skin beneath the pad every 5 minutes. If the skin appears red, swollen, or blistered or if the person complains of pain, numbness, or discomfort, discontinue treatment immediately and notify the nurse.

   b. Refill the heating unit if the water level drops below the fill line.

   c. If you must leave the room, place the call light control within easy reach and ask the person to signal if they experience numbness or burning.

10. When the treatment is complete, remove the pad.

11. Straighten the bed linens and make sure the person is comfortable and in good body alignment. Draw the top linens over the person.

12. Make sure that the bed is lowered to its lowest position and that the wheels are locked.

13. Gather the soiled linens and place them in the linen hamper. Dispose of disposable items in a facility-approved waste container. Clean equipment and return it to the storage area.

Finishing Up

14. Complete the "Finishing Up" steps.

What You Document

- Date and time
- Type of heat application
- Body part treated
- Length of time treatment left in place
- Observation of skin after treatment
- Patient or resident comments: "Leg feels better," etc.

Procedure 21-2

Giving a Moist Cold Application

WHY YOU DO IT Cold applications reduce pain and swelling and decrease bleeding.

Getting Ready

1. Complete the "Getting Ready" steps.

Supplies

- bed protector
- compress (for example, 4 × 4 gauze pad or washcloth)
- bath basin
- bath towel
- ice
- rolled gauze or ties (optional)

Procedure

2. Put the ice in the bath basin and fill the basin with cold water at the sink.

3. Make sure that the bed is positioned at a comfortable working height (to promote good body mechanics) and that the wheels are locked.

4. Help the person to a comfortable position and expose only the area to be treated.

5. Position the bed protector as necessary to keep the bed linens dry.

6. Moisten the compress with the ice water as ordered. Wring out the compress and apply it to the treatment site.

7. Leave the compress in place for the designated amount of time, usually 15 to 20 minutes. The compress may be secured in place with ties or rolled gauze, or the patient or resident may assist by holding the compress in place.

   a. Keep the compress moistened with ice water.

   b. Check the skin beneath the compress every 5 minutes. If the skin appears pale or blue or if the person complains of numbness or a burning sensation, discontinue treatment immediately and notify the nurse.

   c. If you must leave the room, place the call light control within easy reach and ask the person to signal if they experience numbness or burning.

8. When the treatment is complete, remove the compress and carefully dry the skin.

9. Remove the bed protector. Straighten the bed linens and make sure the person is comfortable and in good body alignment. Draw the top linens over the person.

10. Make sure that the bed is lowered to its lowest position and that the wheels are locked.

11. Gather the soiled linens and place them in the linen hamper. Dispose of disposable items in a facility-approved waste container. Clean equipment and return it to the storage area.

Finishing Up

12. Complete the "Finishing Up" steps.

What You Document

- Date and time
- Type of cold application
- Body part treated
- Length of time treatment left in place
- Observation of skin after treatment
- Patient or resident comments

▶ **P r o c e d u r e   2 1 - 3**

Giving a Dry Cold Application

WHY YOU DO IT   Cold applications reduce pain and swelling and decrease bleeding.

Getting Ready

1. Complete the "Getting Ready" steps.

Supplies

- crushed ice
- ice bag
- towel or cloth bag cover
- rolled gauze or ties (optional)

Procedure

2. Fill the ice bag with water, close it, and turn it upside down to check for leaks. Empty the bag.

3. Fill the bag one half to two thirds full with crushed ice. Do not overfill the ice bag. Squeeze the bag to force out excess air and close the bag.

4. Dry the outside of the bag and wrap it in the towel or place it in the bag cover.

5. Make sure that the bed is positioned at a comfortable working height (to promote good body mechanics) and that the wheels are locked.

6. Help the person to a comfortable position and expose only the area to be treated.

7. Apply the ice bag to the treatment site.

8. Leave the ice bag in place for the designated amount of time, usually 15 to 20 minutes. The ice bag may be secured in place with ties or rolled gauze, or the person may assist by holding the bag in place.

   a. Check the skin beneath the ice bag every 5 minutes. If the skin appears pale or blue or if the person complains of numbness or a burning sensation, discontinue treatment immediately and notify the nurse.

   b. Refill the bag with ice as necessary.

   c. If you must leave the room, place the call light control within easy reach and ask the person to signal if they experience numbness or burning.

9. When the treatment is complete, remove the ice bag.

10. Straighten the bed linens and make sure the person is comfortable and in good body alignment. Draw the top linens over the person.

11. Make sure that the bed is lowered to its lowest position and that the wheels are locked.

12. Gather the soiled linens and place them in the linen hamper. Dispose of disposable items in a facility-approved waste container. Clean equipment and return it to the storage area.

Finishing Up

13. Complete the "Finishing Up" steps.

What You Document

- Date and time
- Type of cold application
- Body part treated
- Length of time treatment left in place
- Observation of skin after treatment
- Patient or resident comments

WHAT DID YOU LEARN?

Multiple Choice

Select the single best answer for each of the following questions.

1. Which one of the following can be used to treat and control pain?
   a. Medications, such as aspirin and morphine
   b. Back massage
   c. Heat and cold applications
   d. All of the above

2. The purpose of cold applications is usually to:
   a. Prevent heat exhaustion
   b. Speed the flow of blood to an injured area
   c. Prevent swelling
   d. Prevent the formation of scar tissue

3. What is a heat application used for?
   a. To relieve muscle and joint stiffness
   b. To reduce pain
   c. To promote circulation and speed healing
   d. All of the above

4. Dreaming occurs during which stage of sleep?
   a. Stage I NREM sleep
   b. Stage IV NREM sleep
   c. REM sleep
   d. Stage II NREM sleep

5. Mrs. Moyer likes to go to bed at 11:00 PM and sleep in late the next morning. What could happen if Mrs. Moyer is required to go to bed earlier than her preferred bedtime?
   a. Mrs. Moyer could experience a better quality of sleep
   b. Mrs. Moyer could have difficulty falling asleep, which could negatively affect her quality of sleep
   c. Mrs. Moyer could learn to become an "early bird"
   d. Mrs. Moyer could be at risk for having bad dreams

6. When might physical therapy be used for pain management?
   a. When a person is having musculoskeletal pain
   b. When a person is young
   c. When a person is in acute pain
   d. When pain medications are not effective

7. A patient or a resident who has difficulty sleeping may experience all of the following except:
   a. Difficulty remembering information
   b. Increased risk for falls
   c. Increased alertness
   d. Difficulty concentrating

8. Which of the following actions can disrupt a patient's or a resident's sleep?
   a. Darkening the room and minimizing noise
   b. Performing routine incontinence care during the night
   c. Making sure the room temperature is comfortable
   d. Increasing the person's level of activity during the day

9. Unrelieved pain can have which of the following effects?
   a. Increased sleep
   b. Depression
   c. Increased appetite
   d. Increased physical activity

10. You are assisting Mr. Levine to prepare for sleep. The nurse has informed you that Mr. Levine has sleep apnea and is receiving continuous positive airway pressure (CPAP) therapy. Which of the following should you do to ensure that Mr. Levine's treatment for this condition is being followed?
   a. Assist Mr. Levine to sleep on his back, supporting his neck in an extended position to open the airway
   b. Make sure that Mr. Levine's nasal cannula is secure and the oxygen is running at the right amount
   c. Make sure that Mr. Levine's mask is fit snugly over his nose and that no hissing sound is heard when the CPAP machine is turned on
   d. None of the above

Matching   *Match each numbered item with its appropriate lettered description.*

_____ **1.** Pain tolerance

_____ **2.** Insomnia

_____ **3.** Radiating pain

_____ **4.** Pain threshold

_____ **5.** Transcutaneous electrical nerve stimulation (TENS)

_____ **6.** Pain scale

_____ **7.** Chronic pain

_____ **8.** Breakthrough pain

a. The point at which a person becomes aware of pain

b. A tool or guide that helps to translate a person's subjective rating of their pain into an objective measurement

c. Pain that lasts beyond the usual time that it would take for the tissues to heal

d. Pain that occurs before a person's next regularly scheduled dose of pain medication

e. A treatment for pain that uses electrical impulses to block pain signals

f. The level of pain that a person can endure before taking action to seek relief

g. Pain that travels from one area to another

h. A disorder characterized by an inability to fall asleep or to stay asleep

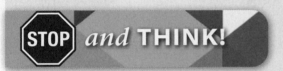

- You are caring for Mrs. Lasorda, who has debilitating rheumatoid arthritis. She has many "good" days when she is able to manage her personal care and get around pretty well. This week, however, she is having a severe flare-up of her illness. What are some measures that you may be asked to do to help Mrs. Lasorda be more comfortable?

- You are caring for Mrs. Benson during the night shift. She was just admitted to your facility from the hospital 2 weeks ago, following surgery for a broken hip. She goes to physical therapy daily. Lately, the therapy has not been going very well as she is having a hard time with the exercises. You enter the room for your first rounds around midnight and find Mrs. Benson awake. She tells you that she has not been able to fall asleep, and this is the third night this week that she has been like this. Mrs. Benson gets tearful as she talks to you, telling you that her inability to sleep makes her too tired to do what she needs to do in physical therapy. She is afraid that if she does not make progress, she will not be able to go back home. What can you do that may help Mrs. Benson?

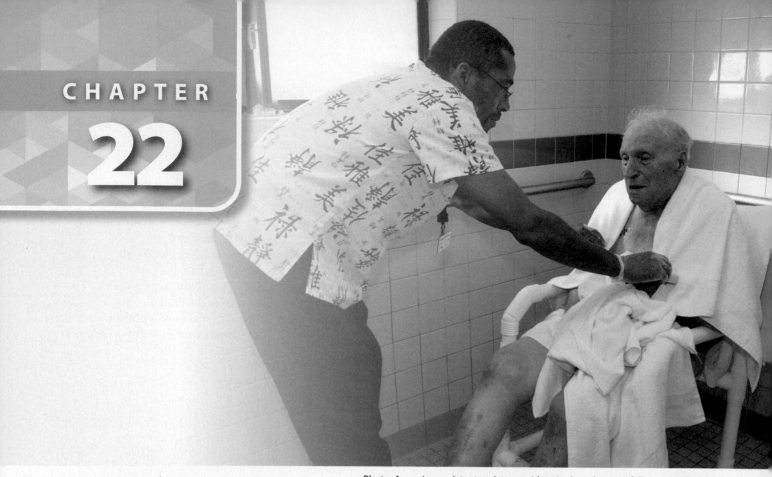

Photo: A nursing assistant assists a resident in the tub room, following a shower.

Cleanliness and Hygiene

 WHAT WILL YOU LEARN?

In this chapter, we will begin to explore the nursing assistant's role in helping people with activities of daily living (ADLs), or the routine tasks of daily life (such as bathing, eating, and grooming). Most people handle these tasks easily on their own, but people who are sick, injured, or have a disability often need help with these basic activities. You will recall the discussion in Chapter 3 about how important good personal hygiene (cleanliness) is for both physical and emotional health. In this chapter, you will learn how to assist your patients or residents with keeping their skin and mouths clean, two activities that are key to maintaining personal hygiene. When you are finished with this chapter, you will be able to:

1. Explain the importance of good hygiene for a person's physical and emotional well-being.
2. Describe the scheduling of routine personal care in the health care setting.
3. Discuss how personal and cultural preferences influence a person's hygiene practices.
4. Explain the importance of allowing residents in the long-term care setting to participate in their own self-care to the greatest extent possible.
5. Describe practices that are considered part of oral care.
6. Demonstrate proper technique for providing oral care for a person with natural teeth, for a person with dentures, and for an unconscious person.

7. Explain why perineal care is essential to daily hygiene.

8. Discuss sensitivity issues that a nursing assistant should be aware of when assisting with perineal care.

9. Demonstrate proper technique for providing perineal care for males and for females.

10. Explain how bathing and skin care benefit a person's health.

11. List the methods of bathing that a nursing assistant may be asked to assist with and demonstrate proper technique, including for bathing a person in bed and in a shower or bathtub.

12. Describe observations that a nursing assistant should make while assisting a person with bathing and skin care.

13. Explain the benefits of massage and demonstrate proper technique for giving a back massage.

Vocabulary

Early morning care
Morning (AM) care
Afternoon care
Evening (hour of sleep, hs) care

PRN (as-needed) care
Diaphoretic
Dental caries
Halitosis
Gingivitis

Periodontitis
Edentulous
Perineal care (peri-care)
Perineum
Circumcision

Foreskin
Deodorant
Antiperspirant

THE BENEFITS OF PERSONAL HYGIENE

Personal hygiene (cleanliness) helps promote both physical and emotional health. The practices associated with personal hygiene—skin care (including bathing and moisturizing) and oral care (including brushing the teeth and flossing)—keep the skin and the mucous membranes of the mouth healthy. As you will remember from Chapter 10, the skin and mucous membranes of the body act as the first line of defense against infection. Caring for the skin and the mouth helps to prevent conditions such as rashes, dry skin, and cracked lips, which interrupt the body's first line of defense by creating a portal of entry for microbes. In addition, keeping the skin and mouth clean helps reduce the number of microbes on these surfaces, which also helps to minimize the risk of infection.

In addition to promoting physical health, good personal hygiene promotes emotional health by helping a person to feel relaxed and well cared for. A person who feels relaxed and comfortable is able to rest better. Being clean and refreshed also helps a person meet their need for self-esteem (see Chapter 6) by preventing body and breath odors and making the person feel attractive to others.

SCHEDULING OF ROUTINE CARE

In many health care facilities, routine activities associated with personal hygiene are carried out at specific times throughout the day:

- **Early morning care** is provided after a person wakes up to prepare them for breakfast or early diagnostic testing or treatment. The person is assisted with using the toilet, washing the face and hands, and mouth care. Dentures may need to be inserted prior to eating. Many people will want to have their hair brushed or combed. Residents of long-term care facilities may need help with dressing, in preparation for breakfast in the dining room.
- **Morning (am) care** is when the morning personal hygiene routine is completed, to prepare the person for the day. During morning care, patients and residents are assisted with using the toilet, bathing, oral care, shaving, hair care, dressing, and putting on make-up. The

amount of assistance each patient or resident will need in carrying out these activities will vary. In some facilities, the morning bath is followed by a back massage. General housekeeping duties, such as tidying the person's room and changing the bed linens, are also performed during morning care. Facility policies differ regarding the frequency of bathing and linen changes.

■ **Afternoon care** is care that is provided before and after lunch and dinner. Many people rest or receive visitors in the early afternoon. A general "freshening up" involves assistance with using the toilet, washing of the hands and face, and oral care.

■ **Evening (hour of sleep, hs) care** is provided in preparation for sleep. During evening care, patients or residents are assisted with washing their hands and face, brushing their teeth, changing into sleepwear, and using the toilet. Other bedtime preparations include straightening the bed linens and fluffing the pillows. Many residents in long-term care facilities may prefer to bathe in the evening instead of in the morning. "Extras," such as a bath, soft music, a back massage, or reading in bed for a while before turning out the light can help a person fall into a restful sleep. Allowing for these "extras" when providing evening care shows a caring and compassionate attitude because you are considering the person's preferences and honoring these wishes whenever possible.

The scheduling of routine personal care promotes efficiency and allows the nursing staff to plan these activities around others, such as meals, treatments, visiting hours, and social events. Sometimes, however, it is necessary to break from the schedule in order to accommodate a person's needs. **PRN (as-needed) care** is personal hygiene care that is provided whenever a patient or resident needs it, throughout the day or night. For example, a person in a coma needs frequent mouth care because they tend to breathe through their mouth and cannot take food or liquids orally, situations that put the person at risk for a dry mouth. An incontinent person requires perineal care (peri-care), or cleansing of the genital and anal region, each time they lose control of their bowel or bladder. If their clothing or bedding is wet or soiled, these items will need to be changed as well. A person who is **diaphoretic** (sweating heavily) may need partial sponge baths, fresh linens, and a change of clothes frequently throughout the day. Any situation or condition that causes wetness or soiling of the skin, clothing, or bedding needs immediate attention.

Helping Hands and a Caring Heart

Focus on Humanistic Health Care

Care is provided according to the facility's or agency's schedule, but adjustments can be made to take into account the patient's or resident's personal preferences. For example, many long-term care facilities schedule baths as a routine part of the morning care, but some residents may prefer a bath later in the day or in the evening. Whenever possible, grant the resident's request. If you had always bathed in the evening, and then after entering a nursing home were told you had to bathe in the morning, how would you feel? Patients and residents may be required to change their normal routines to a certain extent to conform to the policies of the hospital or long-term care facility, but you can look for ways to accommodate your patient's or resident's personal preferences, while still following facility rules. For example, asking a person whether they prefer to bathe in the morning or in the evening, allowing them to choose either bar soap or liquid soap, and permitting them to use the type of deodorant they prefer shows that you care about the person as an individual. These actions will also help the person maintain a sense of familiarity in an otherwise changed life. Certain cultural and religious beliefs may discourage bathing during certain times or may promote ritualistic bathing as part of a ceremony or spiritual service. Whenever possible, you should make an effort to accommodate these preferences as well.

Concerns for Long-Term Care

When assisting a resident in the long-term care setting with personal care, it is important to allow the resident to do as much for themselves as possible, even if it takes longer to complete the task. Provide assistance, as needed, to fill in for what the resident is not able to do. Participating in self-care helps the resident attain or maintain their highest level of function and well-being. This is important for the resident's self-esteem and also for meeting OBRA requirements.

As a result of the culture change movement that is happening in long-term care right now, many facilities are changing their policies to allow residents to have more control over their daily lives. Upon admission, residents are asked about their preferences for care, and these preferences are accommodated as much as possible within the daily routines of the facility.

ASSISTING WITH ORAL CARE

Keeping the mouth and teeth clean and healthy is an important part of personal hygiene. A clean, healthy mouth feels good and makes food taste better, and contributes to overall health. **Dental caries** (cavities) and **halitosis** (bad breath that does not go away) are caused by poor oral hygiene. Poor oral hygiene can also cause **gingivitis** (inflammation of the gums), which can lead to **periodontitis** (infection and inflammation of the soft tissue and bones that support the teeth). Periodontitis is the main cause of tooth loss in people older than 35 years, and it may be associated with other serious health problems as well, such as atherosclerosis ("hardening of the arteries"). Assisting your patients or residents with regular oral care is an important responsibility because healthy teeth and gums are important for a person's overall health and well-being.

A person who has lost one or more natural teeth may have dental implants (prosthetic teeth that are surgically placed in the bone), dentures (prosthetic teeth that can be taken in and out), or a combination of these. A person may have a partial denture or a full denture. Partial dentures are used when only some teeth are missing and may or may not be removable. Full dentures are used when a person is missing all of the top teeth or all of the bottom teeth. A person who has no teeth at all is said to be **edentulous** (without teeth).

Oral care is usually provided on awakening, after meals, and before bed. People who are unable or not allowed to take food or fluids by mouth will need oral care as often as every 1 or 2 hours to keep their mouths fresh and moist. Most people can manage their own oral care, with assistance as needed. A person who is not allowed out of bed may still be able to brush and floss their own teeth if you provide the necessary supplies. Occasionally a person will be too ill or weak to provide oral care for themselves, and you will need to provide this care for them. Because the gums sometimes bleed as a result of routine oral care, it is important to practice standard precautions when assisting with brushing and flossing the teeth or cleaning dentures. Droplet precautions should be taken if the patient or resident is known to have an infection that can be

Tell the Nurse!

While assisting a person with oral care, pay attention to the following:

- Dry, red, cracked, or bleeding lips, gums, or mucous membranes
- Cold sores on the lips or mucous membranes
- Red, irritated, swollen, or bleeding gums
- Cracked, chipped, or broken teeth; loose teeth; blackened teeth
- Chipped, cracked, or poorly fitting full or partial dentures
- Red sores or canker sores inside the mouth; white spots inside the mouth; any areas of pus or infection
- Bad breath that does not improve after oral care
- Fruity-smelling breath (possibly a sign of diabetes mellitus)
- A red or swollen tongue or a white coating on the tongue
- Complaints of pain or sensitivity

transmitted by exposure to droplets released from the mouth or nose.

Helping your patients or residents with oral care presents many opportunities for observation.

Providing Oral Care for a Person With Natural Teeth

Natural teeth are best cleaned with a toothbrush and toothpaste, followed by flossing. Because bacteria in the mouth do the most damage to the teeth and gums after eating, the best time to brush is after meals. Brushing alone is not enough to remove food that lodges between the teeth, so flossing once a day is recommended as part of good oral hygiene. Many people like to use a mouthwash after brushing to complete their oral care routine. The use of mouthwash can further reduce harmful bacteria in the mouth.

Toothbrushes should have soft bristles and be small enough to reach all of the teeth. Electric toothbrushes are simple to use and effective, especially for people who have limited strength or use of their hands.

Procedure 22-1 describes how to assist a person with brushing and flossing the teeth.

Providing Oral Care for a Person With Dentures

Dentures take the place of a person's natural teeth, allowing the person to chew their food properly. Dentures that do not fit properly or that hurt the mouth when worn are not very useful for chewing. Proper care of the gums and dentures helps to keep the dentures fitting properly and comfortably.

Some people wear their dentures all of the time. Others may leave their dentures out at night or only wear them for meals. Personal preference for wearing dentures is to be respected. Remember that people are more likely to wear their dentures if they are kept clean.

A denture brush (or a toothbrush) and denture cleaner are used to clean all surfaces of the denture. The use of regular toothpaste on dentures is not recommended because the abrasives in the toothpaste can scratch and damage the denture surfaces. Some people use a denture adhesive to help keep the denture in place better. Be sure to remove all of the adhesive material when cleaning the denture.

Rinse the denture with lukewarm water. Hot water should not be used because it can damage the dentures.

A person who wears dentures still needs to clean their gums and mouth to keep them healthy. Brushing the gums and tongue with a soft toothbrush with a small amount of toothpaste, mouthwash, or saline (salt water) solution will help to remove food particles and bacteria. For people who still have a few natural teeth and wear a partial denture, the natural teeth need to be brushed and flossed routinely.

General guidelines for providing oral care for a person with dentures are given in Guidelines Box 22-1. Procedure 22-2 describes how to provide oral care for a person who wears dentures.

Providing Oral Care for an Unconscious Person

A person who is unconscious needs frequent mouth care to keep the mucous membranes of the mouth

---

Guidelines Box 22-1   Guidelines for Providing Oral Care for a Person With Dentures

WHAT YOU DO	WHY YOU DO IT
Handle a person's dentures with care.	Dentures are expensive and difficult to replace.
When a person is not wearing their dentures, store them in a denture cup filled with lukewarm water or a denture solution.	The water or solution prevents the dentures from drying out and warping. If the dentures warp, they will not fit properly.
When cleaning dentures, use lukewarm (not hot) water.	Hot water can damage the dentures.
When cleaning dentures, line the sink with a washcloth or paper towels.	The washcloth or towels help to prevent breaking or chipping of the denture if you accidentally drop it into the sink.
Have the person rinse their dentures after eating.	Rinsing the dentures after eating removes food trapped between the gums and dentures. Trapped food can cause discomfort and promotes the growth of bacteria.
Before placing the dentures in the person's mouth, allow the person to rinse with water or mouthwash or use a soft-bristled toothbrush or a moist, foam-tipped applicator to clean the surfaces inside the person's mouth. Wet the dentures before placing them in the person's mouth.	Placing dentures inside the mouth is more difficult when the mouth and dentures are dry. In addition, the moisture helps to create the suction that is needed to hold the dentures in place.
Label the person's denture cup with the person's name and room number.	Putting the person's name and room number on the denture cup helps prevent the dentures from being misplaced.

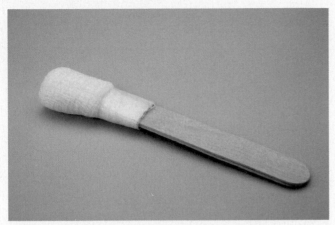

Figure 22-1 It may be necessary to use a padded tongue blade to keep an unconscious person's mouth open while providing oral care. A padded tongue blade is made by folding a gauze square around two wooden tongue blades and taping the gauze in place.

moist and healthy. An unconscious person breathes with the mouth open, which causes secretions to thicken and dry on the lips and in the mouth. These dried secretions, along with the intake of air through the mouth, can lead to cracking of the lips and tongue. Cracked, dry lips are very uncomfortable and they create a portal of entry for microbes.

Natural teeth are gently brushed with either a small amount of toothpaste or saline. If the person is edentulous, the gums, tongue, and inside of the cheeks are cleaned using a soft-bristled toothbrush or a sponge-tipped swab moistened with saline or mouthwash. The mouth can be rinsed with a small amount of saline or water to clean out dried secretions. You may need to place a padded tongue blade between the upper and lower back teeth to keep the mouth open during oral care (Fig. 22-1). General guidelines for providing oral care for a person who is unconscious are given in Guidelines Box 22-2. Procedure 22-3 describes how to provide oral care for a person who is unconscious.

ASSISTING WITH PERINEAL CARE

Perineal care (peri-care) is the cleaning of the **perineum** and associated structures (Fig. 22-2). In females, the perineum extends from the bottom of the vagina to the anus. In males, the perineum extends from the root of the penis to the anus. When nurses talk about "providing perineal care," they mean cleaning the perineum and anus, as well as the vulva (in females) and the penis (in males).

Making sure that the perineum, the vulva, and the penis are clean is important for two main reasons:

- **Prevention of infection.** Because many microbes live in our digestive tracts and are passed from the body in the feces, there are always large numbers of microbes in and around the anus. The perineal area provides the perfect environment to support the growth of these microbes because it is warm, dark, and moist. Because the perineum is close to the

---

Guidelines Box 22-2   Guidelines for Providing Oral Care for a Person Who Is Unconscious

WHAT YOU DO	WHY YOU DO IT
Turn the person on their side with their head tilted forward so that fluids run out of the mouth, not back toward the throat.	Turning the person onto their side helps to prevent aspiration (the accidental inhalation of foreign material into the airway). Aspiration can lead to complications such as choking or pneumonia.
Never place your fingers in the person's mouth.	An unconscious person may bite down involuntarily and without warning.
Explain what you are doing throughout the procedure, even though the person may not seem to be able to hear you or respond to you.	The person may be aware on some level that someone is doing something to them. Telling the person what you are doing reassures the person and helps the person to feel safe.
Apply lip lubricant to the person's lips as needed.	This helps to prevent drying and cracking of the lips, which is uncomfortable for the person and can lead to infection.

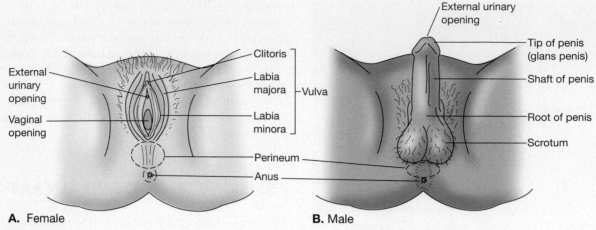

Figure 22-2 Perineal care refers to care of the perineum and associated structures. **A.** The female perineum and associated structures. **B.** The male perineum and associated structures.

vulva (in females) and the penis (in males), these microbes can easily enter the vagina or urethra, causing infection. Therefore, inadequate hygiene in the perineal area puts the person at risk for infection.

■ **Prevention of skin breakdown and odor.** The perineum, vulva, and penis are delicate, with many folds of skin. Feces, urine, and other body fluids, such as menstrual blood, can become trapped in these folds, leading to skin irritation and odor if they are not properly removed.

Perineal care is routinely performed at least once daily, as part of the bath. People with diarrhea or who are incontinent of urine or feces will need perineal care performed more frequently. For these patients or residents, a barrier cream or ointment may be applied after perineal care to help protect the skin from contact with urine or feces. Females

with vaginal bleeding (from surgery, childbirth, or menses) or vaginal discharge will also need more frequent perineal care. Any person who can manage their own perineal care should be encouraged to do so to the best of their ability. A person who is unable to provide for their own self-care will need your help. When helping your patients and residents with perineal care, be aware of signs and symptoms that could indicate a health problem.

When you are providing perineal care for a person, you must have the person's consent for the procedure before beginning. For example, while helping a person with a bath, you may explain what you are about to do and ask the person's permission to go further. Make sure to explain the procedure completely using professional yet understandable words (such as "crotch," "privates," "bottom," or "the area between your legs"). When there is a language barrier, stop and think. You may need an interpreter.

For many reasons (such as cultural or religious beliefs, or a history of physical abuse), some people may object strongly to being touched by a person of another sex, or even by a person of the same sex. Please respect your patient's or resident's wishes and work to find a suitable compromise, if at all possible. Perineal care can be embarrassing, both for the person receiving it and for the person providing it. Very few people are comfortable exposing their most private body parts to strangers or seeing the private body parts of strangers. Draping the person's body with a bath blanket so that only the area to be cleaned is exposed helps preserve the person's sense of modesty (Fig. 22-3). Another potential source of embarrassment for both the patient or resident and the nursing assistant is the fact that male patients or residents may become aroused during perineal care, simply from stimulation of the penis

Tell the Nurse!

Tell the nurse immediately if you observe any of the following signs when providing perineal care for one of your patients or residents:

● Any unusual redness, inflammation, or skin rashes in the perineal area

● Any unusual discharge from the vagina or penis

● Any bleeding from the vagina (especially in a post-menopausal patient or resident) or the anus

● Any abnormal odor

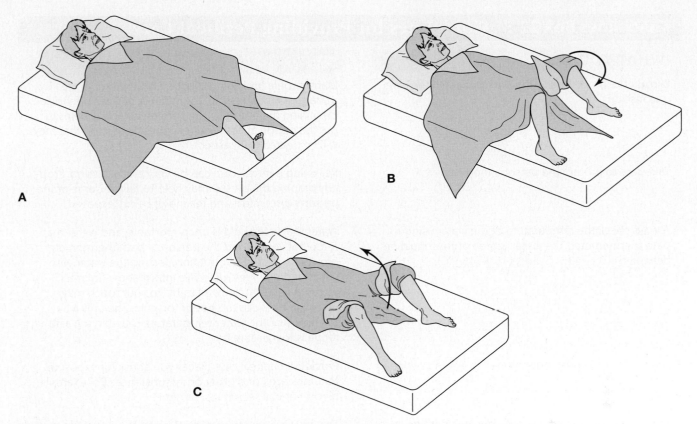

Figure 22-3 A bath blanket is used to preserve the person's modesty during perineal care. **A.** The bath blanket is placed over the person's body so that one corner is pointing toward the person's head and the other is between the person's legs, covering the perineum. The other two corners are to the right and to the left, respectively. **B.** The right corner is brought under and around the person's right leg, and then the same is done on the left. **C.** The top corner is lifted up to expose only the perineal area.

during washing. Acting in a professional, competent manner and using a gentle touch will help to ease embarrassment on the part of the patient or resident. Guidelines for providing perineal care are given in Guidelines Box 22-3.

Helping Hands and a Caring Heart

Focus on Humanistic Health Care

Helping another person with perineal care may seem very unpleasant or embarrassing to you. But think of it this way—what if you were sick or injured to the point that you had wet yourself or had a bowel movement in the bed? Think of how wonderful it would feel to have someone clean you up, help you change your clothes, and give you fresh bed linens. You would feel clean and cared for.

Providing Perineal Care for Female Patients and Residents

Procedure 22-4 describes how to assist a female patient or resident with perineal care.

Providing Perineal Care for Male Patients and Residents

Male patients or residents may be circumcised or uncircumcised (Fig. 22-4). **Circumcision** is a procedure involving the removal of the **foreskin**, the fold of loose skin that covers the head of the penis. Male infants are often circumcised for religious or cultural reasons. When you are assisting an uncircumcised male with perineal care, it is important to pull the foreskin back so that the head of the penis can be cleaned thoroughly. After cleaning and rinsing the penis, always remember to pull the foreskin back up over the head of the penis. If the foreskin is not pulled back into place, it can create a band around the penis, causing pain and possible tissue damage.

Guidelines Box 22-3 Guidelines for Providing Perineal Care

WHAT YOU DO	WHY YOU DO IT
Explain the procedure to the person, even if they are unconscious.	Many people find being touched in an intimate area by a stranger embarrassing, frightening, or even offensive. Explaining the procedure in a professional way helps to put the person at ease and reassures the person that they will be treated with respect.
Take care to protect the person's modesty.	Receiving perineal care can be very embarrassing. Properly draping the person may help to relieve some of the person's discomfort and feeling of being "exposed."
Always check the temperature of the water using a bath thermometer. The water temperature should be between 110°F (43.3°C) and 115°F (46.1°C).[a]	Water that is too cold is uncomfortable, and water that is too hot could scald the person. A bath thermometer provides *objective* information. Testing the water with your hand provides *subjective* information. (In other words, water that "feels all right" to your touch may, in reality, be much too hot or too cold. The only way to know that the water temperature is within the safe range is to measure it.)
Follow standard precautions when providing perineal care.	Providing perineal care places you at risk for exposure to urine, feces, and other body substances (for example, blood, vaginal secretions, semen).
Perineal care is the last part of a person's bathing routine. Washcloths, towels, and the water in the wash basin (if a bed bath is being given) are discarded and not used on any other body parts after the perineal care is completed.	The anus is a source of microbes and the perineum provides an environment that supports their growth. To prevent spread of these microbes to other parts of the body, where they may gain access and cause infection, the perineal area is washed last.
The vulva (in females) or the penis (in males) is cleaned before the perineum.	Because the anus opens onto the perineum, the perineum is often contaminated with microbes from the digestive tract. Therefore, this area is washed last to prevent microbes from the digestive tract from being introduced into the vagina or urethra, where they can cause infection.
Rinse the skin thoroughly to remove all soap.	The skin of the perineum and surrounding structures is delicate. If the person is incontinent and requires frequent cleaning, do not use soap. Instead, use a soap-free cleanser specifically for the perineal area. Soap is drying and can irritate the skin if not rinsed away.
Gently pat the skin dry. Do not rub vigorously. Dry the skin thoroughly.	The skin of the perineum and surrounding structures is delicate. Vigorously rubbing the skin with a towel is uncomfortable for the person and can create friction, which in turn can cause skin breakdown. Moisture in areas where skin comes in contact with skin can also lead to skin breakdown.
Remove your gloves and perform hand hygiene before touching clean clothing or linens.	Gloves worn while providing perineal care are considered contaminated.

[a]The water in the basin can be slightly hotter (110°F [43.3°C]) than the water in a tub or shower (105°F [40.5°C]) because it cools off quickly and the person will not be immersed in it.

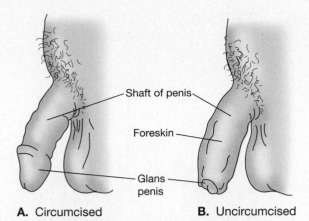

A. Circumcised   B. Uncircumcised

Figure 22-4 Male patients or residents may have a circumcised or uncircumcised penis. **A.** A circumcised penis. **B.** An uncircumcised penis.

Procedure 22-5 describes how to assist a male patient or resident with perineal care.

ASSISTING WITH SKIN CARE

Skin care, including bathing and moisturizing, are important for maintaining good hygiene and overall health and well-being.

Bathing

Bathing serves many purposes. The act of bathing:

- Helps a person feel relaxed and refreshed
- Cleans the skin and eliminates body odors
- Exercises muscles that might otherwise not be used
- Stimulates blood flow to the skin (through touching and massaging of the skin), which helps to prevent skin breakdown
- Helps the patient or resident meet the needs of love and belonging and self-esteem
- Gives the nursing assistant an opportunity to observe for skin problems and to communicate and bond with the patient or resident

The frequency and method of bathing are determined by many factors, including:

- Personal choice
- The person's state of health
- The weather
- The person's level of activity
- The person's ability to care for themselves
- The policies and procedures of the facility
- Cultural or religious beliefs

For example, people may bathe more often during the warmer months or when they are most active,

and less often during the winter months or periods of physical inactivity. Hospital policy may state that patients receive daily baths, while the policy of a long-term care facility may call for residents to receive complete baths or showers two or three times weekly with partial baths on days in between.

Some patients or residents may refuse a bath, and they do have the right to refuse. For example, a resident may ask to skip their bath for many reasons: "I'm tired and I want to sleep." "I feel a cold coming on," "I don't feel up to it today." You could insist that the person bathe, creating tension and causing the person to feel unappreciated and disrespected. Or, you could offer to help the person "just freshen up a bit instead" and actually achieve the goal of bathing in a different manner. For example, you could assist the person with a partial bath at the sink instead of a complete bath in a tub or shower. With this approach, the person is clean but was allowed to refuse their bath (so to speak), and you have fulfilled your responsibility while also respecting the person's wishes.

For some patients and residents, such as those who have dementia or are confused, bath time can be very frightening. People who are confused simply do not understand what you intend to do to them and they cannot remember what bathing is all about. Extra help from your coworkers and a calm, efficient attitude will help. Sometimes, singing to a confused person or playing soothing music will help to calm the person a bit. If a person refuses personal hygienic care consistently, report this to the nurse. If a person is unable to understand the consequences that can result from a lack of bathing or skin care, the decision may be made to bathe the person against their wishes out of respect for the person's health.

Supplies for Bathing

Various supplies are used for bathing and skin care, many of which you are already familiar with:

- **Soap,** available in liquid or cake form, is used to clean the skin. The lather lifts away dirt, oil, microbes, and sweat. Because soap is drying to the skin, it is important to rinse it away completely. For people with dry, fragile skin (such as older people), it may be better to use a soap-free, no-rinse cleanser or just plain water.
- **No-rinse cleansers.** Often, these products are supplied on premoistened disposable cloths. Other products come in the form of soft, dry disposable cloths that create lather when placed in water. Liquid no-rinse cleansers are usually added to a basin of water. Be sure that you add the correct amount of cleanser to the water according to the product directions. No-rinse cleansers do not need to be rinsed away. These

products clean, moisturize, and protect the skin. Some of these products are for use specifically in the perineal area.

- **Bath oils** are added to the bath water to scent and moisten the skin. Because bath oils make the surface of the bathtub slippery, these products should be used with caution.
- **Lotions** and **creams,** which may be perfumed or unscented, are applied to skin that is still slightly damp to create a moisture barrier that helps to prevent drying and chapping. Lotions and creams are an especially important part of skin care for older people, because with aging, the skin secretes a reduced amount of natural oil, resulting in dryness and a loss of elasticity.
- **Body powder** can help absorb moisture and sweat and reduces friction between skin surfaces that touch. Powder should only be applied to skin that has been dried thoroughly. When using powder, sprinkle a small amount into the palm of your hand, and then gently pat it onto the person's skin. Avoid big clouds of powder—too much powder can irritate the skin, and if the person inhales it, then it can irritate the airways too. In addition, powder spilled on the floor can be very slippery.
- **Deodorants** and **antiperspirants** are often applied after bathing to help prevent body odor. **Deodorants** are products that cover or mask odor. **Antiperspirants** contain ingredients that stop or slow sweating. Most antiperspirant products also contain a deodorant. Application of an antiperspirant or deodorant should be included as part of a person's hygiene routine if the person requests it.

Most people are particular about the skin care products they use. Some people are sensitive or allergic to ingredients commonly used in skin care products. If you notice that one of your patients or residents develops itching, redness, or a rash after using a skin care product, please report this observation to the nurse and stop use of that particular product until the source of the skin irritation has been determined. Always ask new patients or residents if they have particular preferences in skin care products or if there are any products that cause problems for them.

In addition to skin care products, a variety of linens are used for bathing. Bath blankets are used to preserve a person's modesty during a bed bath or when providing perineal care. A washcloth is wrapped around the hand to form a "mitt" for cleansing the body (Fig. 22-5). A towel is used to dry the body and can also be used to help preserve the person's modesty. A clean gown, pajamas, or change of clothes should be available for the patient or resident to put on after the bath.

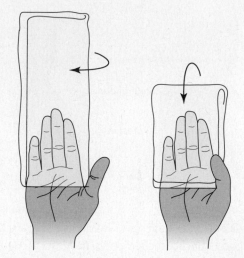

Figure 22-5 Making a bath mitt from a washcloth.

Standard Bathing Techniques

A complete bath, or one that involves the entire body, is not always necessary. In some cases, a complete bath may not be allowed for medical reasons. For example, a person who has just had surgery may not be able to take a complete bath until their incision has healed. When a complete bath is not possible, a partial bath will provide many of the same health benefits and achieve the same goals of odor and infection control. During a partial bath, only the face, hands, axillae (armpits), back, buttocks, and perineal area are washed. A partial bath can be done at the sink or, if the person cannot get out of bed, at the bedside. In long-term care facilities, a partial bath is often part of the morning care on days that the resident is not scheduled to have a complete bath. A partial bath can also be provided anytime a person needs to "freshen up."

The amount of assistance each resident or patient will need to bathe will vary according to the person's degree of disability. For people who can bathe themselves, you will only need to see that they have bathing supplies and clean clothes. Some people will only need your help cleaning hard-to-reach areas, such as the back or feet. Others will need your help throughout the bath. You should encourage your patients or residents to do as much for themselves as possible. Doing so encourages their feelings of independence and self-worth and provides a form of exercise, increasing the person's muscle tone, mobility, and circulation. General guidelines for assisting patients and residents with bathing are given in Guidelines Box 22-4.

Assisting your patients or residents with bathing provides an excellent opportunity for you to observe the patient's or resident's skin and body for any changes in condition that should be reported to the nurse. Because you will be caring for the person regularly, you will be more likely to notice changes that might go unnoticed by others.

Guidelines Box 22-4 Guidelines for Bathing

WHAT YOU DO	WHY YOU DO IT
Follow the doctor's orders or the nursing care plan when determining what type of bath the person is to receive.	A person's medical condition may dictate the type of bath they can have. For example, a person with a spinal injury may not be permitted to have a whirlpool bath, while for a person with poor skin circulation, a whirlpool bath may be considered a type of therapy.
Before beginning the bath, explain to the person how the bathing procedure will be carried out (and how the person can assist in the process). In addition, explain the benefits of bathing (such as comfort, healthy skin).	Explaining the details of the bathing process may help to relieve the person's fears (for example, about potential exposure) and will help the person to see how they can participate in the process. Explaining the procedure is particularly important for people with memory problems, who may find the bathing experience frightening because they cannot remember what bathing is or why it is important.
Collect all necessary equipment, linens, bath products, and clothing before beginning the bath. If the person will be taking a tub bath, check the tub room for cleanliness and prepare the tub before bringing the person into the room.	Being prepared and having all necessary supplies and equipment at hand will allow the bath to proceed efficiently. Efficiency is necessary to protect the person's modesty and to prevent chills.
Close all doors and windows in the room, and make sure the blinds are down or the curtains are drawn.	Closing doors and windows eliminates drafts in the room, which could cause the person to become chilled. In addition, closing doors and covering the windows protect the person's modesty and privacy.
If nonskid strips are not in place, make sure to place a nonskid mat in the bathtub or on the shower floor. Encourage the person to use handrails. Provide a shower chair for people who are weak or unsteady. Make sure that the wheels are locked on the shower chair so that it does not move when the person is using it.	These measures help to protect the person from falling.
Never lock the bathroom door.	Because you should never leave a person alone in the bathtub or shower, if you need help for any reason, you will have to call for someone to come to you. This person will need to be able to access the bathroom without your help.
Always check the temperature of the water using a bath thermometer. The water temperature should be at 105°F (40.5°C). Older people may require a slightly cooler water temperature, especially in a whirlpool tub. Make sure you check for specific temperatures in the person's care plan.	Water that is too cold is uncomfortable, and water that is too hot could scald the person. A bath thermometer provides *objective* information. Testing the water with your hand provides *subjective* information. (In other words, water that "feels all right" to your touch may, in reality, be much too hot or too cold. The only way to know that the water temperature is within the safe range is to measure it.)
When assisting a person to and from the tub room, always make sure that they are adequately covered.	The person's privacy and modesty must be protected at all times.
Always help the person into and out of the bathtub or shower.	A wet bathroom floor can be slippery and can place the person at risk for falling.

(continued)

Guidelines Box 22-4   Guidelines for Bathing (*continued*)

WHAT YOU DO	WHY YOU DO IT
Follow standard precautions when bathing a person.	Bathing a person places you at risk for coming into contact with nonintact skin or body fluids.
Wash from the cleanest to the dirtiest areas.	This approach prevents contamination of clean areas.
Touch the person's body gently yet deliberately, using long, firm strokes.	A gentle yet firm touch conveys to the person that this is a routine procedure being carried out by a professional, ensures that the skin is properly cleaned, and stimulates skin circulation.
Rinse the skin thoroughly to remove all soap.	Soap is drying and can irritate the skin if not rinsed away.
Gently pat the skin dry. Do not rub vigorously. Dry the skin thoroughly, especially in areas where skin touches skin (for example, underneath the breasts, between the legs).	The skin, especially that of elderly people, is fragile. Vigorously rubbing the skin with a towel is uncomfortable for the person and can create friction, which in turn can cause skin breakdown. Moisture in areas where skin comes in contact with skin can also lead to skin breakdown.

Tell the Nurse!

Tell the nurse immediately if you observe any of the following signs or symptoms while assisting a person with their bath:

- New rashes, bruises, broken skin, bleeding, or unusual odors

- Areas that are red, pale, or have a bluish cast (cyanosis)

- Areas that are swollen or tender

- Any complaints of burning or itching

- New hair loss (anywhere on the body, not just on the head)

- A flaking, itchy, or sore scalp or the presence of nits (head lice)

- Redness or yellow discoloration of the sclera (that is, the whites of the eyes)

- Yellowing or thickening of the fingernails or toenails

- Changes in mental status and alertness (for example, disorientation, confusion)

Shower or Tub Baths

A shower or tub bath is the preferred method of bathing because it allows for thorough cleaning and rinsing of the skin. Showers in many facilities have stalls that are large enough for a shower chair to fit inside,

allowing a weak or unsteady person to sit down while taking a shower (Fig. 22-6). Most long-term facilities have whirlpool tubs that stimulate blood flow and relax muscles by the action of the water (Fig. 22-7). These tubs usually have chair-lift devices to allow for easy and safe transfer of residents into and out of the tub. The lift devices also allow people who are in a coma or who have severe physical disabilities to

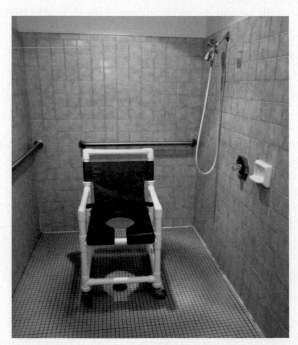

Figure 22-6 Shower stalls in health care facilities are usually wide enough to accommodate a shower chair. Use of a shower chair helps to reduce the risk of falling.

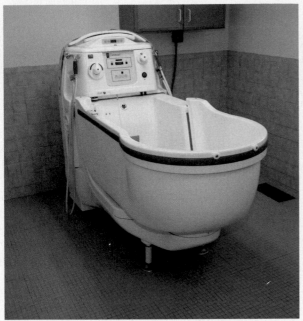
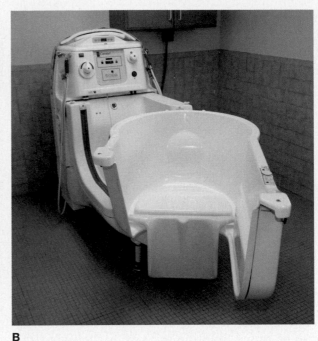

A   **B**

Figure 22-7 **A.** Many long-term care facilities have whirlpool tubs, which help to stimulate circulation and massage the skin. **B.** On this model, the front of the tub swings open to make it easier for the patient or resident to get into and out of the tub.

receive the comfort and benefit of a whirlpool bath. Most tubs have a shower attachment so that hair can be washed during the bath. Many modern tub and shower units also have controls that preset the water temperature, ensuring that it is not too hot or too cold.

Procedure 22-6 describes how to assist with a tub bath or shower. After each use, the tub or shower stall (and the shower chair, if one was used) is disinfected. This is important to prevent the spread of infection. Facility policy will state who is responsible for cleaning and disinfecting the bathing equipment.

Bed Baths

Some patients and residents are simply too weak or ill to take a shower or tub bath. In this situation, bath supplies and a basin of warm water are brought to the bedside, and the person is assisted with bathing in bed (Fig. 22-8). A complete or partial bed bath is given, depending on the needs of the patient or resident (Procedures 22-7 and 22-8, respectively).

An alternative to the traditional bed bath is the use of a "bag bath." "Bag baths" are very comfortable and refreshing for a patient or resident, and they are efficient and effective for the nursing staff. A "bag bath" can be accomplished in a few different ways. Commercial bag baths are available (Fig. 22-9), or you can make your own by placing 8 to 10 washcloths soaked in a soap-free cleanser in a plastic bag. The commercial bag bath or the plastic bag containing the washcloths is heated in the microwave or commercial

heated storage cabinet, and then a different cloth is used to clean each main body part. Because the microwave can heat items unevenly, always check the temperature of the cloths before using them on

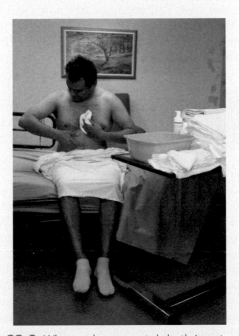

Figure 22-8 When a shower or tub bath is not possible, a bed bath can be given. Some patients or residents, like the person shown here, will be able to bathe themselves with minimal assistance, while others will require a great deal of assistance.

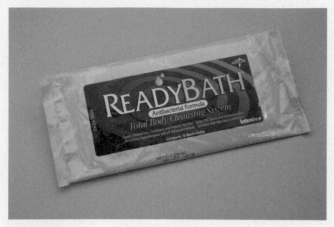

Figure 22-9 Many facilities use "bag baths" as a quick and efficient alternative to a traditional bed bath.

the patient or the resident. Some commercial products are available as dry disposable cloths that produce lather when placed in water. The cleanser does not need to be rinsed from the skin and is allowed to air dry or is patted dry with a towel.

Another way of giving a bath is to moisten a fanfolded bath blanket and two washcloths with a solution of warm water and soap-free cleanser. The moistened bath blanket is placed over the patient or resident while they are in bed and then covered with a dry bath blanket. The person's body is massaged through the blanket layers to clean the skin. The washcloths are used to cleanse the person's face and the perineal area. You will need to check the temperature of the bath blanket and washcloths before using them on the patient or resident to make sure that they are not too hot or too cold.

Helping Hands and a Caring Heart

Focus on Humanistic Health Care

When assisting a patient or resident with bathing, think about how you would feel if you were in that person's situation. You might feel embarrassed because you have to rely on someone else to help you with one of life's most basic tasks. You might also feel exposed because another person is seeing and touching your body. Acknowledge your patient's or resident's feelings by providing as much privacy as possible during the procedure and by maintaining a professional attitude at all times.

Massage

Illness, disability that results in loss of mobility, and aging all contribute to a decrease in blood flow (circulation) to the skin. A person who sits in a chair or wheelchair for long periods of time or who must remain in bed is at an increased risk for developing pressure ulcers (see Chapter 29) as a result of that lack of blood flow. Massaging the skin regularly helps to stimulate the circulation. It is also very relaxing for the patient or resident. A back massage is usually performed after a person's bath while rubbing lotion or cream into the skin, when repositioning a helpless person, or as a part of evening care to promote relaxation and sleep. Some studies have shown that slow, gentle massage can calm sick babies and confused or older people with dementia who become agitated easily.

An effective back massage takes approximately 4 to 6 minutes to complete and can be performed with the person in either the prone or the lateral position. The extra minutes spent massaging a patient's or resident's back are well worth the effort and are beneficial for both physical and emotional health. While performing a back massage, you have an excellent opportunity to observe the person's skin for potential problems.

Tell the Nurse!

Skin breakdown can lead to pressure ulcers. Tell the nurse immediately if you observe any of the following early signs of skin breakdown:

- Reddened skin, especially over a bony area, that does not return to its normal color after pressure is relieved
- Pale, white, or shiny skin over a bony area
- Areas of skin that are hot to the touch
- Areas of skin that are painful or tender

As with any personal care procedure, always check with a nurse or read the person's nursing care plan before beginning—a back massage should not be performed on a person with fractured ribs or a back injury, nor should it be performed on a person who has recently had back surgery. Procedure 22-9 describes how to give a back massage.

SUMMARY

- Cleanliness of the body is essential for a person's physical and emotional well-being.
  - Healthy skin and mucous membranes help protect the body from infection-causing microbes.
  - Feeling clean also increases a person's self-esteem and comfort.
- Allowing people to participate in their own self-care helps maintain independence, but assisting as necessary helps ensure thorough hygiene. Assisting a person with personal hygiene activities also provides opportunities for observation.
- Personal hygiene activities are usually carried out at scheduled times.
  - When possible, adjustments are made to accommodate personal preferences (for example, bathing in the evening vs. the morning).
  - Assistance with personal hygiene is provided any time that a patient's or resident's condition warrants it. Wet or soiled skin, clothing, or bedding requires immediate attention.
- Oral care involves caring for the teeth, gums, lips, and mucous membranes of the mouth. A clean, healthy mouth makes food taste better, defends against infection, and allows a person to chew their food properly.
  - Natural teeth should be brushed and flossed daily.
  - Dentures must be handled with care because they are expensive.
  - Standard precautions should be taken when providing oral care because contact with body fluids is possible. Droplet precautions should be taken if the patient or resident has an infection that can be transmitted by droplets released from the mouth or nose.
- Perineal care involves cleansing of the perineum, the anus, the vulva (in females), and the penis (in males).
  - Inadequate hygiene in the perineal area places a person at risk for infection and skin breakdown, and can lead to unpleasant odors.
  - Because receiving assistance with perineal care is embarrassing for most people, take extra care to preserve the person's modesty. Having a professional attitude when assisting demonstrates competence and helps to ease embarrassment on the part of the patient or resident.
  - Standard precautions should be taken when providing perineal care because contact with body fluids is likely.
  - Always wash toward the anus, away from the urethra. This helps to prevent the spread of microbes from the anus and perineum into the urethra or vagina, where they could cause infection.
- Skin care involves keeping the skin clean and moisturized, and may also involve massage to enhance blood flow to the skin.
  - Bathing may be accomplished in a bathtub or shower, at the sink, or in bed.
  - During a partial bath, only the face, hands, axillae, back, buttocks, and perineum are washed.
  - A back massage is relaxing for the patient or resident and helps prevent the development of pressure ulcers.

Procedure 22-1

Brushing and Flossing the Teeth

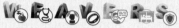

WHY YOU DO IT Brushing and flossing the teeth helps to keep the teeth and gums healthy, makes the mouth feel better and food taste better, and prevents bad breath.

Getting Ready

1. Complete the "Getting Ready" steps.

Supplies

- gloves
- paper towels
- straw (optional)
- cup of cool water
- emesis basin
- toothbrush
- toothpaste
- dental floss
- lip lubricant (optional)
- mouthwash (optional)
- towel and washcloth

Procedure

2. Clean the surface of the over-bed table and cover with paper towels. Place the oral care supplies on the over-bed table.

3. Make sure that the bed is positioned at a comfortable working height (to promote good body mechanics) and that the wheels are locked.

4. If the side rails are in use, lower the side rail on the working side of the bed. The side rail on the opposite side of the bed should remain up.

5. Raise the head of the bed as tolerated. Place a towel across the person's chest.

6. Perform hand hygiene and put on the gloves.

7. Wet the toothbrush. Put a small amount of toothpaste on the toothbrush.

8. Brush the person's teeth as follows:

   a. Position the toothbrush at a 45-degree angle to the gums, against the outer surface of the top teeth. Starting at the back of the mouth, brush the outer surface of each tooth using a gentle circular motion. Repeat for the lower teeth. Allow the person to spit toothpaste into the emesis basin as necessary.

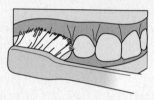

STEP 8a Clean the outer surfaces of the teeth.

   b. Position the toothbrush at a 45-degree angle to the gums, against the inner surface of the top teeth. Starting at the back of the mouth, brush the inner surface of each tooth using a gentle circular motion. Repeat for the lower teeth.

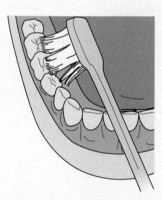

STEP 8b Clean the inner surfaces of the teeth.

   c. Brush the chewing surfaces of the upper and lower teeth using a gentle circular motion.

   d. Brush the tongue.

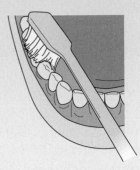

STEP 8c Clean the chewing surfaces of the teeth.

9. Offer the person the cup of water (and a straw, if desired) and ask them to rinse their mouth completely. Hold the emesis basin underneath the person's chin so that they can spit the water into the basin.

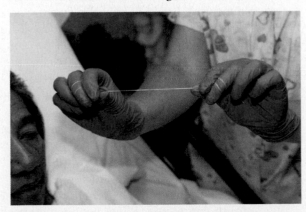

STEP 9 Hold the emesis basin underneath the person's chin so that they can spit.

10. Place the emesis basin on the over-bed table and dry the person's mouth and chin thoroughly using the washcloth.

11. Cut a piece of dental floss measuring about 18 inches. Wrap the dental floss around the middle finger of each hand. Hold the dental floss between your thumb and index finger on each hand and stretch it tight.

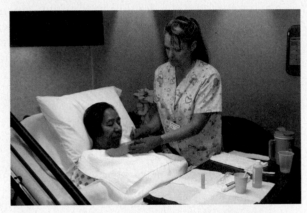

STEP 11 Hold the dental floss between your thumb and index finger on each hand and stretch it tight.

12. Insert a segment of dental floss between two teeth, starting with the back upper teeth. Move the floss up and down gently, and then remove the dental floss from the person's mouth. Advance the floss a bit by releasing it from one middle finger and wrapping it around the other, and move on to the next two teeth. Use a new strand of dental floss as necessary. Offer the person the cup of water (and the straw, if desired) to rinse as necessary. Floss all of the person's teeth.

13. Offer the person the cup of water (and the straw, if desired) and ask them to rinse their mouth completely. Hold the emesis basin underneath the person's chin so that they can spit the water into the basin.

14. Place the emesis basin on the over-bed table and dry the person's mouth and chin thoroughly using the washcloth.

15. Pour a small amount of mouthwash (approximately ¼ cup) into the cup and help the person to rinse, as the person requests.

16. Apply lip lubricant to the lips, as the person requests. Remove your gloves, perform hand hygiene, and put on a clean pair of gloves.

17. If the side rails are in use, return the side rails to the raised position. Lower the head of the bed as the person requests. Make sure that the bed is lowered to its lowest position and that the wheels are locked.

18. Gather the soiled linens and place them in the linen hamper or linen bag. Dispose of disposable items in a facility-approved waste container. Clean the over-bed table per facility policy. Clean equipment and return it to the storage area.

19. Remove your gloves, dispose of them in a facility-approved waste container, and perform hand hygiene.

Finishing Up

20. Complete the "Finishing Up" steps.

What You Document

■ The date and time
■ Level of assistance needed
■ Any unusual observations

▶ Procedure 22-2

Providing Oral Care for a Person With Dentures ▶

WHY YOU DO IT Proper care of the gums and dentures helps to keep the mouth healthy and the dentures fitting properly and comfortably. It also makes the mouth feel better and food taste better and prevents bad breath.

Getting Ready WEAVERS

1. Complete the "Getting Ready" steps.

Supplies

- gloves
- paper towels
- gauze squares (4" × 4")
- straw (optional)
- toothpaste and dental floss (if person has any natural teeth)
- soft-bristled tooth-brush or foam-tipped applicators
- emesis basin
- cup with cool water
- denture cup
- denture brush or toothbrush
- denture cleaner
- denture solution (optional)
- mouthwash (optional)
- lip lubricant (optional)
- towel
- washcloth

Procedure

2. Clean the surface of the over-bed table and cover with paper towels. Place the oral care supplies on the over-bed table.

3. Make sure that the bed is positioned at a comfortable working height (to promote good body mechanics) and that the wheels are locked. Raise the head of the bed as tolerated. Place a towel over the person's chest.

4. Perform hand hygiene and put on the gloves.

5. Ask the person to remove their dentures and place them in the emesis basin. If the person needs assistance with removing their dentures:

   a. Ask the person to open their mouth.

   b. Holding a gauze square between your thumb and index finger, grasp the upper denture, moving it up and down slightly to break the seal. Ease the denture down, forward, and out of the mouth. Place the denture in the emesis basin.

   c. Holding a gauze square between your thumb and index finger, grasp the lower denture. Turn the denture slightly, lifting it out of the mouth. Place the denture in the emesis basin.

6. Take the emesis basin, the washcloth, the denture cup, the denture brush or toothbrush, and the denture cleaner to the sink. Line the sink with the washcloth to provide extra cushioning. Fill the sink partially with lukewarm water. Do not place the dentures in the sink.

7. Wet the denture brush or the toothbrush. Put a small amount of denture cleaner on the denture brush or toothbrush. Working with one denture at a time, hold the denture in the palm of your hand and brush it on all surfaces until it is clean. Rinse the denture thoroughly under lukewarm running water and place it in the denture cup. Repeat with the other denture.

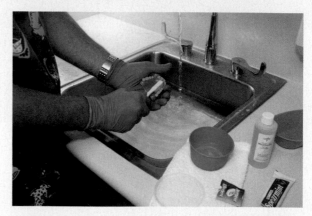

STEP 7 Hold the denture in the palm of your hand, and brush it on all surfaces until it is clean.

8. If the dentures are to be stored, fill the denture cup with lukewarm water, a mixture of one part mouthwash to one part lukewarm water, or a denture solution so that the dentures are covered. Put the lid on the denture cup. Return the denture cup to the person's bedside table, making sure that it is within easy reach.

9. If the dentures are to be reinserted in the person's mouth, take the emesis basin and the denture cup to the over-bed table. If the side rails are in use, lower the side rail on the working side of the bed. The side rail on the opposite side of the bed should remain up.

   a. Offer the person the cup of water (and a straw, if desired) and ask them to rinse their mouth completely. Some people may wish to use mouthwash instead of water. Hold the emesis basin underneath the person's chin so that they can spit the water or mouthwash into the basin.

b. Place the emesis basin on the over-bed table and dry the person's mouth and chin thoroughly using a face towel.

c. Gently clean the person's gums and tongue and the insides of the cheeks with the toothbrush or a foam-tipped applicator moistened with water or mouthwash. Use fresh applicators as needed. If the person has any remaining natural teeth, assist with brushing and flossing those teeth.

d. Ask the person to insert their dentures. If the person needs assistance with inserting their dentures:

- Ask the person to open their mouth.
- Gently lift the person's upper lip up. Grasp the upper denture between your thumb and index finger and insert it in the person's mouth. Press gently on the denture to be sure that it is seated properly.
- Gently pull the person's lower lip down. Grasp the lower denture between your thumb and index finger and insert it in the person's mouth.

e. Return the denture cup to the person's bedside table, making sure that it is within easy reach.

10. Dry the person's mouth and chin thoroughly using a towel. Apply lip lubricant to the lips, as the person requests. Remove your gloves, perform hand hygiene, and put on a clean pair of gloves.

11. Reposition the person comfortably and lower the head of the bed if necessary. If the side rails are in use, return the side rails to the raised position. Make sure that the bed is lowered to its lowest position and that the wheels are locked.

12. Gather the soiled linens and place them in the linen hamper or linen bag. Dispose of disposable items in a facility-approved waste container. Clean the over-bed table per facility policy. Clean equipment and return it to the storage area.

13. Remove your gloves, dispose of them in a facility-approved waste container, and perform hand hygiene.

Finishing Up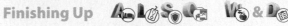

14. Complete the "Finishing Up" steps.

What You Document

- Date and time
- Amount of assistance needed
- Any unusual observations

▶ Procedure 22-3

Providing Oral Care for an Unconscious Person

WHY YOU DO IT   An unconscious person breathes through the mouth, causing the lips and mucous membranes to dry out. Frequent mouth care keeps the mucous membranes of the mouth moist and healthy and promotes comfort.

Getting Ready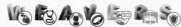

1. Complete the "Getting Ready" steps.

Supplies

- gloves
- paper towels
- sponge-tipped applicators or soft-bristled toothbrush
- padded tongue blade
- cup with appropriate solution (cool water, saline, mouthwash)
- emesis basin
- toothbrush and toothpaste (if the person has natural teeth)
- lip lubricant
- towel and washcloth

Procedure

2. Clean the surface of the over-bed table and cover it with paper towels. Place the oral care supplies on the over-bed table.

3. Make sure that the bed is positioned at a comfortable working height (to promote good body mechanics) and that the wheels are locked. If the side rails are in use, lower the side rail on the working side of the bed. The side rail on the opposite side of the bed should remain up.

4. Position the person onto their side, with the head tilted forward.

(continued)

5. Place a towel across the pillow underneath the person's face and spread it across their chest. Position the emesis basin on the towel underneath the person's chin.

6. Perform hand hygiene and put on the gloves.

7. Open the person's mouth by gently applying pressure to the lower jaw in front of the mouth. Be gentle; do not force the mouth open. Insert the tongue blade between the upper and lower teeth at the back of the mouth to hold the person's mouth open.

8. Clean the inside of the mouth:

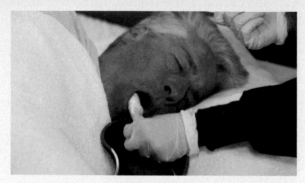

STEP 8 Clean the inside of the person's mouth, using a padded tongue blade to keep the mouth open.

a. If the person has natural teeth, they should be gently brushed as described in Procedure 22-1.

b. If the person is edentulous, gently clean the person's gums and tongue and the insides of the cheeks with the toothbrush or a foam-tipped applicator moistened with water,

saline, or mouthwash. Use fresh applicators as needed.

Note: Do not use a foam-tipped applicator for people who may bite it. Pieces can be aspirated by the person if they remain in the mouth.

9. Dry the person's mouth and chin thoroughly using a washcloth. Apply lip lubricant to the lips. Remove your gloves, perform hand hygiene, and put on a clean pair of gloves. Reposition the person comfortably.

10. If the side rails are in use, return the side rails to the raised position. Make sure that the bed is lowered to its lowest position and that the wheels are locked.

11. Gather the soiled linens and place them in the linen hamper or linen bag. Dispose of disposable items in a facility-approved waste container. Clean the over-bed table per facility policy. Clean equipment and return it to the storage area.

12. Remove your gloves, dispose of them in a facility-approved waste container, and perform hand hygiene.

Finishing Up

13. Complete the "Finishing Up" steps.

What You Document

- Date and time
- Type of care given (teeth brushed, mouth swabbed, etc.)
- Any unusual observations

▶ Procedure 22-4

Providing Female Perineal Care   ▶

WHY YOU DO IT Proper perineal care helps to prevent skin breakdown (which can lead to pressure ulcers), infection, and odor.

Getting Ready

1. Complete the "Getting Ready" steps.

Supplies

- gloves
- paper towels
- bed protector
- bath thermometer
- wash basin
- bedpan
- soap, no-rinse cleansing solution, or commercially packaged disposable cleaning cloths
- bath blanket
- washcloths
- towel
- clean clothing
- clean linens (if necessary)

Procedure

2. Clean the surface of the over-bed table and cover with paper towels. Place the wash basin, cleansing solution or soap, washcloths, towels, and bed protector on the over-bed table. Other clean linens and clothing (if needed) can be placed on a nearby clean bedside table or chair.

3. Make sure that the bed is positioned at a comfortable working height (to promote good body mechanics) and that the wheels are locked.

4. Perform hand hygiene and put on the gloves.

5. Because bathing often stimulates the urge to urinate, offer the bedpan. If the person uses the bedpan, empty and clean it before proceeding with the perineal care. Remove your gloves and dispose of them in a facility-approved waste container. Perform hand hygiene and put on a clean pair of gloves.

6. Lower the head of the bed to a flat position (as tolerated).

7. Fill the wash basin with warm water (110°F [43.3°C] to 115°F [46.1°C] on the bath thermometer). If using a liquid no-rinse cleansing solution that is added to water, add the proper amount of the cleanser to the basin of water. Place the basin on the over-bed table. If using commercially packaged no-rinse disposable products, you will not need a basin of water unless the disposable cloths need to be placed in water to activate them.

8. If the side rails are in use, lower the side rail on the working side. The side rail on the opposite side of the bed should remain up.

9. Spread the bath blanket over the top linens (and the person). If the person is able, have them hold the bath blanket. If not, tuck the corners under the person's shoulders. Fanfold the top linens to the foot of the bed.

10. Assist the person with undressing.

11. Ask the person to open their legs and bend their knees, if possible. If they are not able to bend their knees, help them spread their legs as much as possible. (If a person is unable to spread their legs enough to expose the perineal area, you may position them onto their side with their knees bent forward to expose the perineum for cleaning.)

12. Position the bath blanket over the person so that one corner can be wrapped under and around each leg.

13. Position the bed protector under the person's buttocks to keep the bed linens dry.

14. Lift the corner of the bath blanket that is between the person's legs upward, exposing only the perineal area.

15. Wash and rinse the groin area.

16. Form a mitt around your hand with one of the washcloths. Wet the mitt with warm, clean water and apply soap or no-rinse cleansing solution. If you are using the prepackaged disposable cleaning cloths, the steps of the procedure will remain the same. You will use a clean disposable cloth for each area you clean.

17. Using the other hand, separate the labia. Clean the vulva by placing your washcloth-covered hand at the top of the vulva and stroking downward toward the anus. Use a different part of the washcloth for each stroke. Repeat until the area is clean.

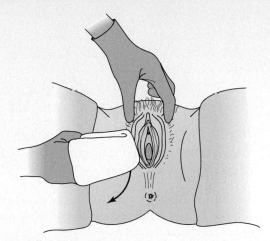

STEP 17 Clean the vulva by placing your washcloth-covered hand at the top of the vulva and stroking downward toward the anus.

18. Rinse the vulva and perineum thoroughly (if using a no-rinse product, omit this step):

   Form a mitt around your hand with a clean, wet washcloth. Using the other hand, separate the labia. Rinse the vulva by placing your washcloth-covered hand at the top of the vulva and stroking downward toward the anus. Use a different part of the washcloth for each stroke. Repeat until the area is free of soap.

19. Dry the perineal area thoroughly using a towel.

20. Turn the person onto their side so that they are facing away from you. Help the person toward the working side of the bed so that their buttocks are within easy reach. Adjust the bath blanket to keep the person covered.

21. Form a mitt around your hand with one of the washcloths. Wet the mitt with warm, clean water and apply soap or no-rinse cleansing solution.

(continued)

22. Using the other hand, separate the buttocks. Place your washcloth-covered hand at the front of the anal area and stroke toward the back. First clean one side, then the other side, and finally the middle, using a different part of the washcloth each time, until the anal area is clean.

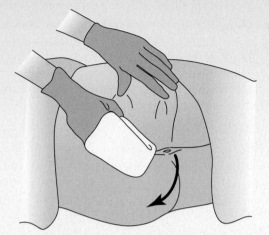

STEP 22 Clean the anal area by placing your washcloth-covered hand at the front of the body and stroking toward the back.

23. Rinse (if necessary) and dry the anal area thoroughly. Remove the bed protector from underneath the person.

24. Remove your gloves and dispose of them in a facility-approved waste container. Perform hand hygiene and put on a clean pair of gloves.

25. Assist the person into the supine position. Reposition the pillow under their head. Remove the bath blanket and help the person into the clean clothing.

26. If the bedding is wet or soiled, change the bed linens.

27. If the side rails are in use, return the side rail to the raised position. Raise the head of the bed as the person requests. Make sure that the bed is lowered to its lowest position and that the wheels are locked.

28. Gather the soiled linens and place them in the linen hamper or linen bag. Dispose of disposable items in a facility-approved waste container. Clean the over-bed table per facility policy. Clean equipment and return it to the storage area.

29. Remove your gloves, dispose of them in a facility-approved waste container, and perform hand hygiene.

Finishing Up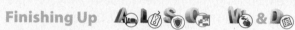

30. Complete the "Finishing Up" steps.

What You Document

- Date and time
- Presence of urine or stool
- Level of assistance needed
- Condition of skin

▶ Procedure 22-5

Providing Male Perineal Care ▶

WHY YOU DO IT Proper perineal care helps to prevent skin breakdown (which can lead to pressure ulcers), infection, and odor.

Getting Ready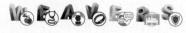

1. Complete the "Getting Ready" steps.

Supplies

- gloves
- paper towels
- bed protector
- bath thermometer
- wash basin
- bedpan or urinal
- soap, no-rinse cleansing solution, or commercially packaged
- disposable cleansing cloths
- bath blanket
- washcloths
- towel
- clean clothing
- clean linens (if necessary)

Procedure

2. Clean the surface of the over-bed table and cover with paper towels. Place the wash basin, toiletries, clean clothing, and clean linens on the over-bed table.

3. Make sure that the bed is positioned at a comfortable working height (to promote good body mechanics) and that the wheels are locked.

4. Perform hand hygiene and put on the gloves.

5. Because bathing often stimulates the urge to urinate, offer the bedpan or urinal. If the person uses the bedpan or urinal, empty and clean it before proceeding with the perineal care.

Remove your gloves and dispose of them in a facility-approved waste container. Perform hand hygiene and put on a clean pair of gloves.

6. Lower the head of the bed to a flat position (as tolerated).

7. Fill the wash basin with warm water (110°F [43.3°C] to 115°F [46.1°C] on the bath thermometer). If using a no-rinse cleansing solution, add the appropriate amount to the water in the basin. Place the basin on the over-bed table. If using commercially packaged no-rinse disposable products, you will not need a basin of water unless the disposable cloths need to be placed in water to activate them.

8. If the side rails are in use, lower the side rail on the working side. The side rail on the opposite side of the bed should remain up.

9. Spread the bath blanket over the top linens (and the person). If the person is able, have them hold the bath blanket. If not, tuck the corners under the person's shoulders. Fanfold the top linens to the foot of the bed.

10. Assist the person with undressing.

11. Ask the person to open their legs and bend their knees, if possible. If they are not able to bend their knees, help them spread their legs as much as possible.

12. Position the bath blanket over the person so that one corner can be wrapped under and around each leg.

13. Position the bed protector under the person's buttocks to keep the bed linens dry.

14. Lift the corner of the bath blanket that is between the person's legs upward, exposing only the perineal area.

15. Wash and rinse the groin area.

16. Form a mitt around your hand with one of the washcloths. Wet the mitt with warm, clean water and apply soap or the no-rinse cleansing solution. If you are using the prepackaged disposable cleaning cloths, the steps of the procedure will remain the same. You will use a clean disposable cloth for each area you clean.

17. Using the other hand, hold the penis slightly away from the body.

   a. If the person is circumcised: Place your washcloth-covered hand at the tip of the penis and wash in a circular motion, downward to the base of the penis. Repeat, using a different part of the washcloth each time, until the area is clean. Rinse and dry the tip and the shaft of the penis thoroughly (if using a no-rinse cleansing solution, omit the rinse):

Form a mitt around your hand with a clean, wet washcloth. Using the other hand, hold the penis slightly away from the body. Place your washcloth-covered hand at the tip of the penis and wipe in a circular motion, downward to the base of the penis. Repeat, using a different part of the washcloth each time, until the area is rinsed. Dry the penis thoroughly.

   b. If the person is uncircumcised: Retract the foreskin by gently pushing the skin toward the base of the penis. Place your washcloth-covered hand at the tip of the penis and wash in a circular motion, downward to the base of the penis. Repeat using a different part of the washcloth each time until the area is clean. Rinse and dry the tip and shaft of the penis thoroughly before gently pulling the foreskin back into its normal position.

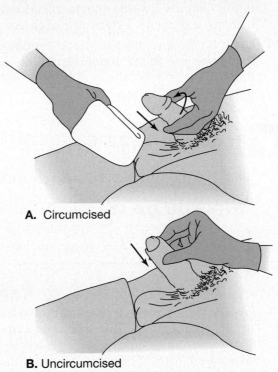

A. Circumcised

B. Uncircumcised

STEP 17 To wash the penis, pass the washcloth in a circular motion, moving from the tip of the penis to the base. (**A**) circumcised penis; (**B**) uncircumcised penis.

18. Form a mitt around your hand with one of the washcloths. Wet the mitt with warm, clean water and apply soap or no-rinse cleansing solution. Wash the scrotum and perineum. Rinse (if necessary) and dry the scrotum and perineum thoroughly.

(continued)

19. Turn the person onto their side so that they are facing away from you. Help the person toward the working side of the bed so that their buttocks are within easy reach. Adjust the bath blanket to keep the person covered.

20. Form a mitt around your hand with one of the washcloths. Wet the mitt with warm, clean water and apply soap or no-rinse cleaning solution.

21. Using the other hand, separate the buttocks. Place your washcloth-covered hand at the front of the body and stroke toward the back. First clean one side, then the other side, and finally the middle, using a different part of the washcloth each time, until the anal area is clean.

22. Rinse (if necessary) and dry the anal area thoroughly. Remove the bed protector from underneath the person.

23. Remove your gloves and dispose of them in a facility-approved waste container. Perform hand hygiene and put on a clean pair of gloves.

24. Assist the person into the supine position. Reposition the pillow under the person's head. Remove the bath blanket and help the person into the clean clothing.

25. If the bedding is wet or soiled, change the bed linens.

26. If the side rails are in use, return the side rail to the raised position. Make sure that the bed is lowered to its lowest position and that the wheels are locked.

27. Gather the soiled linens and place them in the linen hamper or linen bag. Dispose of disposable items in a facility-approved waste container. Clean the over-bed table per facility policy. Clean equipment and return it to the storage area.

28. Remove your gloves, dispose of them in a facility-approved waste container, and perform hand hygiene.

Finishing Up

29. Complete the "Finishing Up" steps.

What You Document

- Date and time
- Presence of urine or feces
- Level of assistance needed
- Condition of skin

▶ Procedure 22-6

Assisting With a Tub Bath or Shower ▶

WHY YOU DO IT   Cleansing of the skin helps to prevent skin breakdown (which can lead to pressure ulcers), infection, and odor. A shower or tub bath allows for thorough cleaning and rinsing of the skin.

Getting Ready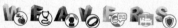

1. Prepare the tub room. If permanent nonskid strips are not present, place a nonskid mat on the floor of the tub or shower. If the person will be taking a tub bath, fill the tub halfway with warm water (105°F [40.5°C] on the bath thermometer) or as indicated on the person's care plan. Obtain a shower chair if necessary and place it in the shower. Place a towel on the chair in the tub room where the person will sit while drying off.

2. Complete the "Getting Ready" steps.

Supplies

- gloves
- bath thermometer
- soap or no-rinse cleansing solution
- washcloths
- towels
- lotion (optional)
- powder (optional)
- deodorant or antiperspirant (optional)
- clean clothing

Procedure

3. Ask the person if they need to use the bathroom before bathing.

4. Assist the person to the tub room.

5. If the person will be taking a tub bath, check the temperature of the water and make sure the nonskid mat is secure. If the person will be taking a shower, turn on the water and adjust the temperature until the water is comfortable.

6. Assist the person with undressing. Assist the person into the bathtub or shower.

7. If the person is able to bathe themselves, either partially or completely:

   a. Place bathing supplies within easy reach.

   b. Many facilities require you to remain in the room while the person bathes or showers. If facility policy permits you to leave the room, explain how to use the call light control and ask the person to signal when bathing is complete or when they have done as much as they can on their own and need help completing the bath. Stay nearby and check on the person every 5 minutes. The person should not remain in the bathtub or shower for longer than 20 minutes. Return when the person signals. Remember to knock before entering.

8. If the person is unable to bathe themselves or requires assistance:

   a. Perform hand hygiene and put on the gloves. Form a mitt around your hand with one of the washcloths.

   b. If necessary, ask the person what parts of the body were not washed. Assist the person as needed with completing the bath. Wash the cleanest areas first and the dirtiest areas last:

    ■ **Eyes.** Wet the mitt with warm, clean water. Do not use soap around the eyes. Ask the person to close their eyes. Place your washcloth-covered hand at the inner corner of the eye and stroke gently outward, toward the outer corner. Use a different part of the washcloth for each eye.

    ■ **Face, neck, and ears.** Ask the person if you should use soap on the face. Rinse the washcloth and apply soap, if requested. Wash the face, neck, and ears, moving from the top of the head to the bottom (so that the nose and mouth are washed last). Rinse thoroughly.

    ■ **Arms and axillae (armpits).** Rinse the washcloth and apply soap. Place your washcloth-covered hand at the shoulder and stroke downward, toward the hand, using long, firm strokes. Wash the hand. If necessary, assist the person with raising their arm so that you can wash the axilla. Repeat for the other arm and axilla.

    ■ **Chest and abdomen.** Using long, firm strokes, wash the person's chest and abdomen.

    ■ **Legs and feet.** Place your washcloth-covered hand at the top of the thigh and stroke downward, toward the foot, using long, firm strokes. Wash the foot. Repeat for the other leg.

    ■ **Back and buttocks:** Wash the person's back and buttocks, moving from top to bottom and using long, firm strokes.

    ■ **Perineal area:** Complete perineal care.

9. Make sure that soap is thoroughly rinsed from all parts of the body.

10. Remove your gloves and dispose of them in a facility-approved waste container. Perform hand hygiene and put on a clean pair of gloves.

11. If the person is taking a tub bath, drain the water and carefully assist the person out of the tub and into the towel-covered chair. If the person is taking a shower, turn the water off and assist the person into the towel-covered chair.

12. Wrap a towel around the person. Using another bath towel, help the person to dry off, patting the skin dry. Take care to ensure that areas where "skin meets skin" are dried thoroughly (for example, in between the toes and underneath the breasts).

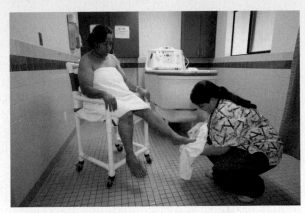

STEP 12 Help the person to dry off, taking extra care to dry areas where "skin meets skin."

13. Help the person to apply lotion, powder, deodorant, antiperspirant, or other personal care products as the person requests.

14. Help the person into the clean clothing. If the person is wearing nightwear, help them into a robe. Help the person into their slippers.

15. Remove your gloves, dispose of them in a facility-approved waste container, and perform hand hygiene.

16. Assist the person back to their room.

Finishing Up

17. Complete the "Finishing Up" steps.

18. Gather the soiled linens and place them in the linen hamper. Dispose of disposable items in a facility-approved waste container. Clean equipment and return it to the storage area.

19. Clean the tub room and shower chair (if used), if housekeeping is not responsible for this task at your facility.

What You Document

- Date and time
- Type of bath/shower given
- Level of assistance needed
- Any unusual observations

▶ Procedure 22-7

Giving a Complete Bed Bath

WHY YOU DO IT   Cleansing of the skin helps to prevent skin breakdown (which can lead to pressure ulcers), infection, and odor. A bed bath is given when a person is too weak or ill to take a shower or tub bath.

Getting Ready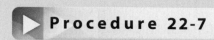

1. Complete the "Getting Ready" steps.

Supplies

- gloves
- paper towels
- bed protectors
- oral hygiene supplies (see Procedures 22-1 through 22-3)
- bath thermometer
- wash basin
- bedpan or urinal
- soap, no-rinse cleansing solution, or commercially prepared disposable cleansing cloths
- lotion (optional)
- powder (optional)
- deodorant or antiperspirant (optional)
- washcloths
- towels
- bath blanket
- clean clothing
- clean linens (if necessary)

Procedure

2. Clean the surface of the over-bed table and cover with paper towels. Place the wash basin, toiletries, bed protectors, washcloths, and towels on the over-bed table. Place additional linens and clean clothing on a nearby clean bedside table or chair.

3. Make sure that the bed is positioned at a comfortable working height (to promote good body mechanics) and that the wheels are locked.

4. Perform hand hygiene and put on the gloves.

5. Because bathing often stimulates the urge to urinate, offer the bedpan or urinal. If the person uses the bedpan or urinal, empty and clean it before proceeding with the bath. Remove your gloves and dispose of them in a facility-approved waste container. Perform hand hygiene and put on a clean pair of gloves.

6. Assist the person with oral care.

7. Remove the bedspread and blanket from the bed. If they are to be reused, fold them and place them on a clean surface, such as the chair.

8. Spread the bath blanket over the top linens (and the person). If the person is able, have them hold the bath blanket. If not, tuck the corners under the person's shoulders. Fanfold the top linens to the foot of the bed.

9. Assist the person with undressing.

10. Lower the head of the bed so that the bed is flat (as tolerated). Position the pillow under the person's head.

11. Fill the wash basin with warm water (110°F [43.3°C] to 115°F [46.1°C] on the bath thermometer). If using a no-rinse cleansing solution, add the appropriate amount to the water in the basin. Place the basin on the over-bed table. If using commercially packaged no-rinse disposable products, you will not need a basin of water unless the disposable cloths need to be placed in water to activate them.

12. If the side rails are in use, lower the side rail on the working side of the bed. The side rail on the opposite side of the bed should remain up.

13. Place a towel over the person's chest to keep the bath blanket dry.

14. To keep the bath water from becoming soapy too quickly, you can use two washcloths—one with soap, for washing; and one without soap, for rinsing. If using the commercially prepared disposable cleansing cloths, the steps of the procedure will remain the same. You will use a new cloth for each area and will omit the rinsing step. Form a mitt around your hand with one of the washcloths. Wet the mitt with warm, clean water. Ask the person to close their eyes. Place your washcloth-covered hand at the inner corner of the eye and stroke gently outward, toward the outer corner. Use a different part of the washcloth for each eye. Using a towel, dry the person's eyes.

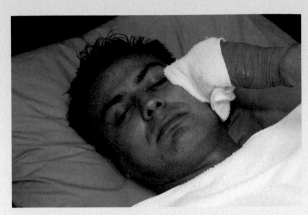

STEP 14 Wash the person's eyes, moving from the inside corner toward the outer corner.

15. Ask the person if you should use soap on the face. Rinse the washcloth and apply soap, if requested. Wash the face, neck, and ears, moving from the top of the head to the bottom (so that the nose and mouth are washed last). Using the clean washcloth, rinse thoroughly (if necessary), and pat the person's face, neck, and ears dry with a towel.

16. Place a bed protector under the person's far arm, to keep the linens dry. Form a mitt around your hand with the washcloth. Wet the mitt and apply soap. Place your washcloth-covered hand at the shoulder and stroke downward, toward the hand, using long, firm strokes. Wash the hand by placing it in the basin of water to soak for a moment. If necessary, assist the person with raising their arm so that you can wash the axilla. Rinse thoroughly (if necessary), and pat the person's arm, hand, and axilla dry with a towel. Remove the bed protector from underneath the person's arm.

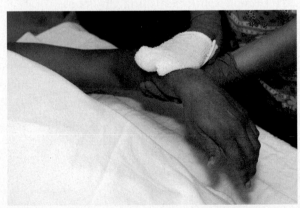

STEP 16 Wash the person's arm, moving from the shoulder to the wrist.

17. Repeat for the other arm.

18. Place a towel horizontally across the person's chest. (The person is now covered with both a bath blanket and a towel.) With the towel in place, fold the bath blanket down to the person's waist. Wet the mitt and apply soap. Reach under the towel and wash the person's chest, using long, firm strokes. Using the clean washcloth, rinse thoroughly (if necessary), and pat the person's chest dry with a towel.

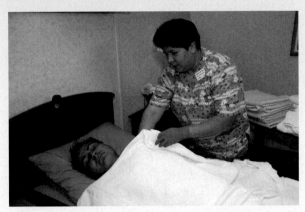

STEP 18 Reach under the towel and wash the person's chest.

19. With the towel still in place, fold the bath blanket down to the pubic area. Form a mitt around your hand with the washcloth. Wet the mitt and apply soap. Reach under the towel and wash the person's abdomen, using long, firm strokes. Rinse thoroughly (if necessary) and pat the person's abdomen dry with a towel.

20. Replace the bath blanket by unfolding it back over the towel and the person's body. Slide the towel out from underneath the bath blanket.

21. Change the water in the wash basin if it is cool or soapy. (If the side rails are in use, raise the side rails before leaving the bedside.)

22. Fold the bath blanket so that the far leg is completely exposed. Place a bed protector under the person's far leg to keep the linens dry. Wet the mitt and apply soap. Place your washcloth-covered hand at the top of the thigh and stroke downward, toward the foot, using long, firm strokes. Rinse thoroughly (if necessary) and pat the person's leg dry with a bath towel.

23. Put the wash basin on the bed protector and place the person's foot in the basin. Wash the entire foot, including between the toes, with the soapy washcloth. Rinse thoroughly (if necessary) and pat the person's foot dry with a towel. Be sure to dry between the toes. Remove

(continued)

the wash basin. Remove the bed protector from underneath the person's leg.

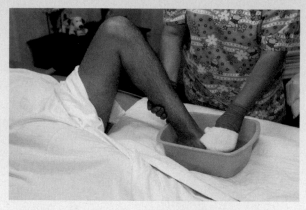

STEP 23 Put the wash basin on the bed protector and place the person's foot in the basin.

24. Repeat for the other leg and foot.

25. Change the water in the wash basin. (If the side rails are in use, raise the side rails before leaving the bedside.)

26. Turn the person onto their side so that they are facing away from you. Help the person toward the working side of the bed so that their back is within easy reach. Adjust the bath blanket to keep the front of the person covered (exposing only the back and buttocks). Place a bed protector on the bed alongside the person's back to keep the linens dry.

27. Form a mitt around your hand with the washcloth. Wet the mitt and apply soap. Wash the person's back first and then the buttocks, moving from top to bottom and using long, firm strokes. Rinse thoroughly (if necessary) and pat the person's back and buttocks dry using a bath towel. At this point, a back massage may be given.

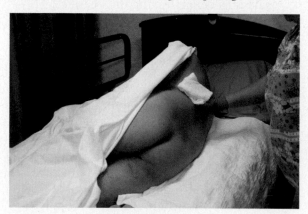

STEP 27 Wash the person's back and buttocks using long, firm strokes.

28. If the person is able to perform perineal care, assist the person into Fowler's position and adjust the over-bed table so that the bathing supplies are within easy reach. Place the call light control within easy reach and ask the person to signal when perineal care is complete. If the person is unable to perform perineal care, assist the person onto their back and complete perineal care.

29. Remove your gloves and dispose of them in a facility-approved waste container. Perform hand hygiene and put on a clean pair of gloves.

30. Help the person to apply lotion, powder, deodorant, antiperspirant, or other personal care products as the person requests.

31. Help the person into the clean clothing.

32. If the bedding is wet or soiled, change the bed linens.

33. Carry out range-of-motion exercises as ordered.

34. If the side rails are in use, return the side rails to the raised position. Raise or lower the head of the bed as the person requests. Make sure that the bed is lowered to its lowest position and that the wheels are locked.

35. Gather the soiled linens and place them in the linen hamper or linen bag. Dispose of disposable items in a facility-approved waste container. Clean the over-bed table per facility policy. Clean equipment and return it to the storage area.

36. Remove your gloves, dispose of them in a facility-approved waste container, and perform hand hygiene.

Finishing Up

37. Complete the "Finishing Up" steps.

What You Document

- Date and time
- Bathing products used (bag bath, no-rinse cleanser, etc.)
- Level of assistance needed
- Condition of skin, especially over pressure points

> ## Procedure 22-8

Giving a Partial Bed Bath

WHY YOU DO IT Cleansing of the skin helps to prevent skin breakdown (which can lead to pressure ulcers), infection, and odor. A partial bed bath is given when a complete bath or shower is not allowed for medical reasons, or when a patient or resident does not feel up to a complete bath or shower.

Getting Ready WGASERS

1. Complete the "Getting Ready" steps.

Supplies

- gloves
- paper towels
- bed protectors
- oral hygiene supplies (see Procedures 22-1 through 22-3)
- bath thermometer
- wash basin
- bedpan or urinal
- soap, no-rinse cleansing solution, or commercially prepared disposable cleansing cloths
- lotion (optional)
- powder (optional)
- deodorant/antiperspirant (optional)
- washcloths
- towels
- bath blanket
- clean clothing
- clean linens (if necessary)

Procedure

2. Clean the over-bed table and cover with paper towels. Place the wash basin, toiletries, washcloths, and towels on the over-bed table. Place additional linens and clean clothing on a clean bedside table or chair. Perform hand hygiene and put on the gloves.

3. Because bathing often stimulates the urge to urinate, offer the bedpan or urinal. If the person uses the bedpan or urinal, empty and clean it before proceeding with the bath. Remove your gloves and dispose of them in a facility-approved waste container. Perform hand hygiene and put on a clean pair of gloves.

4. Assist the person with oral hygiene. Remove your gloves and dispose of them in a facility-approved waste container. Perform hand hygiene.

5. Fill the wash basin with warm water (110°F [43.3°C] to 115°F [46.1°C] on the bath thermometer). If using a no-rinse cleansing solution

that is added to water, add the appropriate amount to the basin. Place the basin on the over-bed table. If using commercially packaged no-rinse disposable products, you will not need a basin of water unless the disposable cloths need to be placed in water to activate them.

6. If the person will be bathing independently, make sure that the bed is lowered to its lowest position and that the wheels are locked. If you will be assisting the person with bathing, make sure that the bed is positioned at a comfortable working height (to promote good body mechanics) and that the wheels are locked. If the side rails are in use, lower the side rail on the working side. The side rails on the opposite side of the bed should remain up.

7. The bath may either be carried out with the person in Fowler's position, or the person can be assisted to sit on the edge of the bed. Help the person to undress as necessary.

8. If the person is able to bathe themselves, either partially or completely:

   a. Place bathing supplies within easy reach.

   b. Many facilities require you to remain in the room while the person bathes. If facility policy permits you to leave the room, explain how to use the call light control and ask the person to signal when bathing is complete or when they have done as much as they can on their own and need help completing the bath. Stay nearby and check on the person every 5 minutes. Return when the person signals. Remember to knock before entering.

9. If the person is unable to bathe themselves, or requires assistance:

   a. Put on the gloves and form a mitt around your hand with one of the washcloths. If commercially prepared disposable cloths or no-rinse cleansing solutions are being used, the steps of the procedure remain the same, just omit the rinsing.

(continued)

b. If necessary, ask the person what parts of the body were not washed. Assist the person as needed with completing the bath. Wash the cleanest areas first and the dirtiest areas last:

■ **Face, neck, and ears.** Ask the person if you should use soap on the face. Rinse the washcloth and apply soap, if requested. Wash the face, neck, and ears, moving from the top of the head to the bottom (so that the nose and mouth are washed last). Rinse thoroughly (if necessary), and pat the person's face, neck, and ears dry with a towel.

■ **Hands.** Wash the hand. Rinse thoroughly (if necessary), and pat the hand dry with a towel. Repeat for the other hand.

■ **Axillae (armpits).** If necessary, assist the person with raising their arm so that you can wash the axilla. Rinse thoroughly (if necessary), and pat the axilla dry with a towel. Repeat for the other axilla.

■ **Back and buttocks.** Rinse the washcloth and apply soap. Wash the person's back first and then the buttocks, moving from top to bottom and using long, firm strokes. Rinse thoroughly (if necessary), and pat the back and buttocks dry with a towel.

■ **Perineal area.** Complete male or female perineal care.

10. Remove your gloves and dispose of them in a facility-approved waste container. Perform hand hygiene and put on a clean pair of gloves.

11. Help the person to apply lotion, powder, deodorant, antiperspirant, or other personal care products as the person requests.

12. Help the person into the clean clothing.

13. If the bedding is wet or soiled, change the bed linens.

14. Carry out range-of-motion exercises as ordered.

15. If the side rails are in use, return the side rails to the raised position. Raise or lower the head of the bed as the person requests. Make sure that the bed is lowered to its lowest position and that the wheels are locked.

16. Gather the soiled linens and place them in the linen hamper or linen bag. Dispose of disposable items in a facility-approved waste container. Clean the over-bed table per facility policy. Clean equipment and return it to the storage area.

17. Remove your gloves, dispose of them in a facility-approved waste container, and perform hand hygiene.

Finishing Up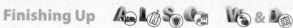

18. Complete the "Finishing Up" steps.

What You Document

■ Date and time
■ Bathing products used (bag bath, no-rinse cleanser, etc.)
■ Level of assistance needed
■ Condition of skin, especially over pressure points

▶ Procedure 22-9

Giving a Back Massage

WHY YOU DO IT   A back massage promotes comfort and relaxation. Massage also stimulates blood flow to the skin, which helps to prevent pressure ulcers.

Getting Ready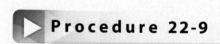

1. Complete the "Getting Ready" steps.

Supplies

■ gloves (if contact with broken skin is likely)
■ wash basin
■ lotion
■ bath blanket
■ towel

Procedure

2. Fill the wash basin with warm water. Place the bottle of lotion in the basin of warm water to warm it.

3. Make sure that the bed is positioned at a comfortable working height (to promote good body mechanics) and that the wheels are locked.

4. Lower the head of the bed so that the bed is flat (as tolerated). If the side rails are in use, lower the side rail on the working side of the bed. The side rail on the opposite side of the bed should remain up.

5. Help the person into the prone position, or turn the person onto their side so that they are facing away from you.

6. Reposition the pillow under the person's head and adjust the bath blanket to keep the person covered, exposing only the back and buttocks.

7. Perform hand hygiene and put on the gloves if contact with broken skin is likely.

8. Pour some lotion into your cupped palm and rub your hands together to distribute the lotion onto both palms.

9. Apply the lotion to the person's back with the palms of your hands. Massage the lotion into the person's skin, using long, gliding strokes (effleurage), moving up the center of the back from the buttocks to the shoulders, and then back down along the outside of the back. Do not directly rub any reddened areas. Repeat four times.

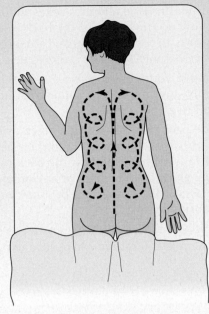

STEP 10 For the next set of strokes, massage the person's shoulders and back using a small circular motion on the downstroke.

11. For the next set of strokes, move up the center of the back from the buttocks to the shoulders, and then back down along the outside of the back. On the downstroke, massage the person's shoulders, back, and buttocks using a small circular motion, paying special attention to the area at the base of the spine. Repeat four times.

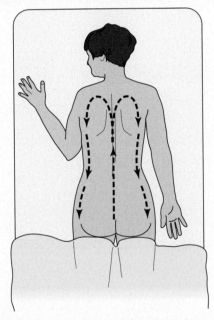

STEP 9 Move up the center of the back from the buttocks to the shoulders, and then back down along the outside of the back.

10. For the next set of strokes, move up the center of the back from the buttocks to the shoulders and then back down along the outside of the back. On the downstroke, massage the person's shoulders and back using a small circular motion. Repeat four times.

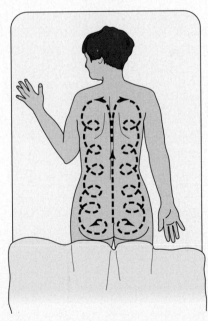

STEP 11 For the final set of strokes, massage the person's shoulders, back, and buttocks using a small circular motion on the downstroke.

(continued)

12. Finish with long, gliding strokes (effleurage), moving up the center of the back from the buttocks to the shoulders and then back down along the outside of the back. Repeat four times.

13. Remove your gloves, dispose of them in a facility-approved waste container, and perform hand hygiene.

14. If the back massage is being given as part of a bath, assist the person onto their back and continue with the bath. If the back massage is being given before bed or at any other time, help the person back into their pajamas, nightgown, or hospital gown.

15. If the side rails are in use, return the side rails to the raised position. Make sure that the bed is lowered to its lowest position and that the wheels are locked.

16. Gather the soiled linens and place them in the linen hamper or linen bag. Dispose of disposable items in a facility-approved waste container. Clean equipment and return it to the storage area.

Finishing Up

17. Complete the "Finishing Up" steps.

What You Document

■ Date and time

■ Condition of skin, especially at pressure points

WHAT DID YOU LEARN?

Multiple Choice

Select the single best answer for each of the following questions.

1. As a safety measure, when you give mouth care to an unconscious person, you should position the person in which position?
   a. Lateral with the head tilted forward
   b. Supine position
   c. Fowler's position
   d. Prone position

2. Why do you line the sink with a washcloth when cleaning a person's dentures?
   a. To ensure that you always have a wet washcloth handy when you need one
   b. To protect the sink from scratches
   c. To guard against breaking the dentures
   d. To prevent contamination of the dentures

3. Which one of the following is within the range of appropriate temperatures for bath water?
   a. 98°F (36.6°C)
   b. 212°F (100°C)
   c. 120°F (48.9°C)
   d. 105°F (40.5°C)

4. When giving a complete bed bath, you should:
   a. Position yourself on one side of the bed and stay there
   b. Use the same water throughout the bath to minimize trips to the sink
   c. Avoid washing the person's perineal area because the person may be embarrassed
   d. Keep the person covered as much as possible

5. When assisting a male patient or resident with perineal care, you should always:
   a. Hold the penis at a 90-degree angle to the body
   b. Wash from the base of the penis toward the tip
   c. Retract the foreskin if the man is uncircumcised
   d. Clean the scrotum first

6. When assisting a person with a shower, you should:
   a. Use a bath blanket to prevent falls
   b. Run the water until the temperature reaches 125°F (51.6°C)
   c. Wear waterproof personal protective equipment (PPE) to protect yourself from getting wet
   d. Use a shower chair if the person is weak or unsteady

7. Which one of the following actions must be taken to keep the skin healthy?
   a. Use strong soap to kill all the germs on the skin
   b. Rinse the skin well and dry it thoroughly, especially in areas where "skin meets skin"
   c. Apply generous amounts of powder after the bath
   d. Rub the skin vigorously with the washcloth

8. How are natural teeth brushed?
   a. Using a circular motion
   b. For at least 10 minutes on each side
   c. Using an "up and down" motion
   d. All of the above

9. When assisting a female patient or resident with perineal care, you should always:
   a. Gently yet thoroughly dry the perineal area and vulva
   b. Clean the rectal area last
   c. Move the washcloth in a downward direction, from front to back
   d. All of the above

10. What is the first thing you should do before assisting a person with a tub bath?
   a. Gather the necessary supplies
   b. Make sure the tub is clean
   c. Check the temperature of the water
   d. Check the nursing care plan to make sure the person is allowed to have a tub bath

11. Which of the following observations made while assisting with mouth care would you report to the nurse?
   a. Lips that are dry, cracked, swollen, or blistered
   b. Irritations, sores, or white patches in the mouth or on the tongue
   c. Bleeding, swelling, or redness of the gums
   d. All of the above

12. How long should a back massage last?
   a. 2 minutes
   b. 1 minute
   c. 4 to 6 minutes
   d. 15 minutes

Matching *Match each numbered item with its appropriate lettered description.*

_____ **1.** Perineal care (peri-care)

_____ **2.** Activities of daily living (ADLs)

_____ **3.** Evening (hour of sleep, hs) care

_____ **4.** Gingivitis

_____ **5.** PRN (as-needed) care

_____ **6.** Antiperspirant

_____ **7.** Edentulous

a. Without teeth

b. Routine tasks of daily life, such as bathing, eating, and grooming

c. Care that is provided at any time of the day or night, when the person's condition warrants it

d. Inflammation of the gums, caused by poor oral hygiene

e. Stops or slows secretion of sweat

f. Care that is routinely provided at bedtime

g. Cleaning of the perineum, the anus, and the vulva or penis

STOP *and* THINK!

- Mrs. Davis is a resident at your facility, which specializes in caring for people with Alzheimer disease. As Mrs. Davis' disease has progressed, she has become progressively more lax about matters related to personal hygiene. She dislikes bathing, and if you do not remove her soiled clothes from her room she will continue to wear them every day. Today Mrs. Davis is scheduled to have a shower, and as you might have predicted, she tells you that she "will not take a shower today." What should you do?

- Jaxon is a 15-year-old who was recently admitted to your rehabilitation unit following an accident. The doctor ordered complete bed rest for Jaxon until his condition stabilizes. You need to give Jaxon a bed bath, and you can tell that he is very embarrassed at the prospect. What can you do to make the situation more comfortable for Jaxon?

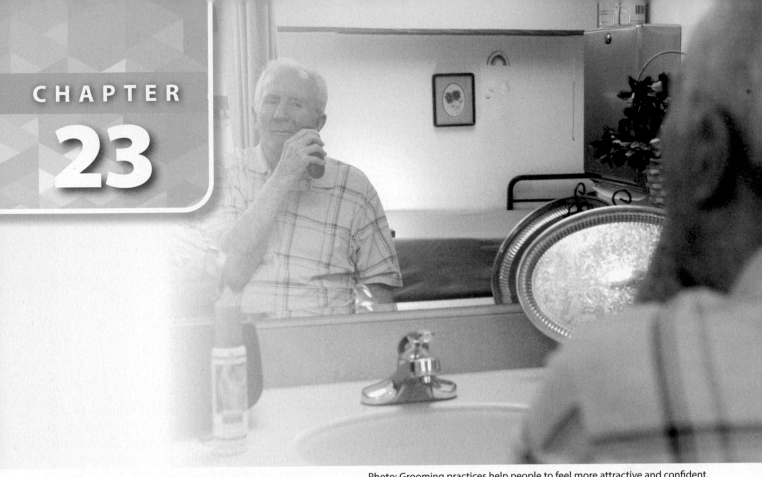

Photo: Grooming practices help people to feel more attractive and confident.

Grooming

 WHAT WILL YOU LEARN?

In the previous chapter, you learned how to help people with the most basic aspects of personal care related to keeping the body clean and healthy. **Grooming**, or activities related to maintaining a neat and attractive appearance, goes beyond basic personal hygiene. The routine care of the hands and feet (including the nails), shampooing and styling of the hair, the application of makeup, and shaving are all grooming practices that play a role in maintaining both physical and emotional health. Helping your patients and residents with "putting their best face forward," the subject of this chapter, is part of providing holistic care. When you are finished with this chapter, you will be able to:

1. Describe factors that influence a person's grooming habits and ability to perform their grooming routine.
2. Explain the importance of proper hand and foot care.
3. List changes that occur in a person's feet as a result of aging or illness.
4. Demonstrate proper technique for assisting with hand and foot care.
5. Demonstrate proper technique for helping a person to dress and undress.
6. Discuss disorders a nursing assistant may observe when assisting with hair care.

7. Describe the different methods used to assist a person with shampooing and styling their hair, including for a patient who is bedridden.

8. Describe the tools and supplies used for shaving.

9. Demonstrate how to safely shave a person's face and other body areas.

10. Explain how the use of makeup can affect a person's sense of well-being.

Vocabulary

Grooming	Podiatrist	Alopecia
Cuticle	Dandruff	Pediculosis capitis
Hangnails	Tinea capitis	Nits
Tinea pedis	Seborrheic dermatitis (cradle cap)	

A person's grooming practices may be very simple (for example, washing and combing the hair and applying a bit of moisturizing lotion to the skin). Or they may be very complex (for example, styling the hair with a blow dryer and curlers, applying makeup, wearing perfume or cologne, and polishing the nails). Think for a moment about the routine grooming practices that you perform each day before you leave home to face the world. Have you ever overslept and had to go to school or work without your grooming routine accomplished? How did you feel? Did it affect your self-esteem?

Patients and residents have personal grooming routines, just as you do. Like yours, their personal grooming practices are influenced by cultural and religious beliefs, upbringing, current fashion, and their feelings about their own gender and sexuality. However, illness or disability can affect a person's ability to complete their own personal grooming practices, causing the person to feel unattractive and "not quite themselves."

Many patients or residents can use assistive devices to complete grooming tasks independently. However, some patients or residents will need your help to complete their grooming routine. As with any aspect of care, check with the nurse or check the person's nursing care plan to find out about any limitations or specifics related to grooming.

Helping Hands and a Caring Heart

Focus on Humanistic Health Care

As a nursing assistant, you must provide humanistic, holistic care for your patients and residents. Helping a person to complete their routine grooming practices meets many of the person's emotional needs, as well as some physical ones. When you take the time and make the effort to style a person's hair attractively, polish their nails, or help apply makeup as part of morning care, you make that person feel extra special. Your actions help the person to meet the needs of love and belonging, because they feel cared for as the unique individual that they are. You also help the person meet their need for self-esteem. Not only are they clean and comfortable, but they feel attractive too.

ASSISTING WITH HAND AND FOOT CARE

Many people consider hair care, shaving, and applying makeup and perfume or cologne to be important aspects of one's grooming routine. However, the care of the hands and feet are also important parts of a grooming routine that are very beneficial.

Care of the Hands

Soft, smooth skin and trimmed, filed fingernails feel wonderful and are important for overall health and comfort. Dryness and chapping of the skin on the hands is uncomfortable and creates a portal of entry for microbes. Poorly cared for fingernails can become long and rough, placing the person at risk for accidentally scratching themselves. For example, a person who is disoriented can hurt themselves if their fingernails are not kept short and smooth. For people who

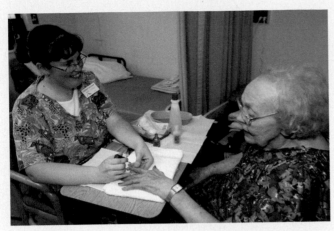

Figure 23-1 Giving a person a manicure gives you the opportunity to spend "quality time" with a patient or resident.

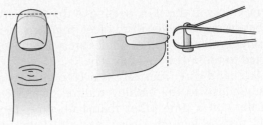

Figure 23-2 Nails are cut using nail clippers. Cut the nails straight across, being careful not to cut too close to the skin. Always make sure that it is within your scope of practice to trim a patient's or resident's fingernails or toenails. In many facilities, this task must be performed by a nurse.

are alert and oriented, fingernail length is a personal choice, but the edges should be kept smooth.

A simple care routine is used to keep the skin of the hands healthy and the fingernails neat (Procedure 23-1). Even if the person can care for their own hands and fingernails, getting a manicure from someone else can really lift the person's spirits, especially if the person is not feeling their best (Fig. 23-1). In addition to making the person feel cared for, helping a patient or resident with hand and nail care gives you the chance to observe for signs of health. In a healthy person, the nail bed is pink. There is no gap between the nail and the nail bed. When viewed from the side, the nail is convex (it curves slightly). The **cuticle** (the skin along the edges of the nail) is smooth and unbroken.

Nail care is usually easiest to perform on nails that have been soaked for a short time in warm water. During or immediately following a bath is an ideal time to perform nail care, because the water makes the nails soft and flexible. When nail care is to be provided at a time other than bath time, the nails can be softened by soaking the ends of the fingers for a short time in a small basin of warm water.

Fingernails are trimmed with clippers, not scissors, to a length no shorter than even with the ends of the fingers (Fig. 23-2). In some states and facilities, trimming a patient's or resident's fingernails is outside of the scope of practice for nursing assistants, so be sure to follow the policy at the facility where you work. After trimming, the nails are filed into an oval shape using an emery board (nail file). Pain or tenderness can result from **hangnails** (broken pieces of cuticle). Hangnails may need to be trimmed using cuticle scissors so that they do not rub or snag on clothing or linens. Torn hangnails can cause bleeding and inflammation of the cuticle.

The blunt end of an orange stick or the edge of a washcloth is used to gently push the cuticles back, and then the orange stick is used to clean underneath the tips of the nails.

Some people like to use nail polish. If nail polish is not used, then the surfaces of the nails can be lightly buffed to give them shine. Applying hand cream helps to seal in moisture and prevent dryness of the skin and cuticles.

Care of the Feet

Care of the feet is essential for good grooming as well as for good health. The feet tend to sweat, especially when slippers or shoes and socks are worn, leading to odors and a warm, moist environment that encourages the growth of microbes. For example, the disorder commonly known as "athlete's foot" (**tinea pedis**) is a fungal infection of the skin and nails. ("Pedis" comes from the Latin word for foot, *pedalis*.) Toenails that are allowed to grow too long can make wearing footwear uncomfortable, and the nails may become ingrown (a condition where the nail curves down and back into the skin, causing injury and pain). Finally, the feet are at risk for injury—how many times have you had your foot stepped on, stubbed your toes against a piece of furniture, or developed a blister as a result of shoes that did not fit properly?

Injuries such as cuts and blisters are painful for a person with normal blood flow to the feet and toes. For a person with poor blood flow (for example, as a result of the normal aging process, a heart problem, or diabetes mellitus), a cut or a blister might develop into a life-threatening condition. Because the wounded area is not receiving the normal amount of blood flow, the area receives less oxygen and nutrients and fewer infection-fighting white blood cells. Healing is delayed, and the risk of infection is increased. In addition, people with poor blood flow often have reduced sensation as well. While you would certainly notice if a new pair of shoes made a blister on your heel, a person with reduced blood flow and sensation might not be aware of the blister, and a small blister could quickly become a dangerous infection. Helping a person with foot care allows you to observe the person's feet for small blisters, cracks in the skin, peeling of the skin between the toes or on the soles of the feet, ingrown toenails, and other problems. Red or tender areas should also be reported to the nurse immediately.

Like hand care, foot care is a grooming task that is easily added to the bathing routine. If foot care is to be done at a time other than bath time, the feet should first be bathed, rinsed, and dried thoroughly (especially between the toes). Prolonged soaking is not recommended. In most facilities, nursing assistants are not allowed to trim the toenails of patients or residents, because a small injury could cause a life-threatening infection. This task is usually performed by a nurse or a **podiatrist**, a doctor who specializes in the care of the feet. The attention of a podiatrist is especially necessary when the toenails are thick and difficult to trim (as a result of aging or poor blood flow; Fig. 23-3). If you are allowed to trim your patients' or residents' toenails, use clippers and cut the toenails straight across. Never try to trim or file corns or calluses.

After the toenails are trimmed, they are filed to remove rough edges. Applying foot powder or lotion to dry feet is refreshing and comforting. Cotton socks help to keep the feet warm and will absorb sweat. (Be careful when helping an older person put on socks—roll the cuff of the sock down before putting it on the person's foot and take care not to accidentally scratch the person with your fingernails or jewelry when pulling the sock up over the heel.) Encourage your patients or residents to wear appropriate footwear. Well-fitting, supportive shoes with nonskid soles help protect the feet and make walking safer by helping to prevent falls and slipping. Procedure 23-2 describes how to assist a patient or resident with foot care.

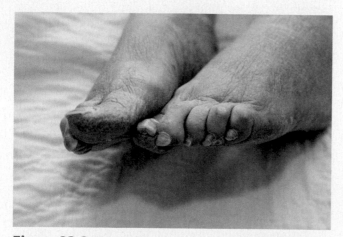

Figure 23-3 Many older people have thick, yellowed toenails as a result of age or poor circulation. Because thickened toenails may be difficult to trim and an accidental injury can have serious consequences, many health care facilities require that a nurse or a podiatrist trim patients' or residents' toenails.

Tell the Nurse!

While providing hand and foot care, always be aware of potential signs and symptoms of illness or infection. Tell the nurse if you observe any of the following:

- Nail beds that are either very pale or blue, or bruised
- Nails that are unusually yellow or white
- Nails that are unusually thick
- Nails that are broken or have been cut too short (especially if there is also bleeding or tenderness)
- Nails that are ingrown
- Cuticles that are torn, red, or swollen
- Skin that is blistered, red, or tender (especially on the feet)
- Any unusual rashes or odors

ASSISTING WITH DRESSING AND UNDRESSING

As a nursing assistant, you will be responsible for helping your patients or residents to change their clothes, possibly several times a day. Dressing is usually a routine part of morning and evening care. However, clothing should be changed any time that it becomes wet or soiled. The type of clothing worn by people receiving health care services differs according to the type of facility and the abilities of the person. If a resident of a long-term care facility is able to be out of bed during the day, they may wear street clothes during the day and a hospital gown, a nightgown, or pajamas at night. Procedure 23-3 describes how to assist a person with dressing in street clothes and nightwear. A patient in a hospital or acute care setting or a resident who has a specific physical disability or medical condition may wear a hospital gown or nightwear day and night. Procedure 23-4 describes how to change a hospital gown.

As with other personal care routines, the amount of help that each person needs for dressing will vary. Some people will need no assistance, except perhaps for some help tying their shoes or zipping a back zipper. Others may need a lot of assistance with every part of the process, from selecting clothes to putting them on. Allowing a person to choose the clothing they prefer to wear is a top priority when assisting with dressing (Fig. 23-4). When a person is unable to choose their own clothes, use good taste and common sense when choosing items for the person to wear.

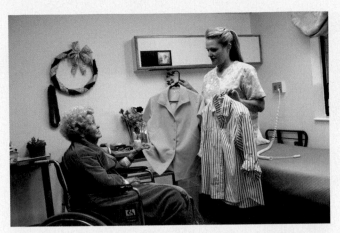

Figure 23-4 Whenever possible, a person should be permitted to choose which articles of clothing they prefer to wear.

Dressing appropriately for the day's activities and with consideration for the season and environment will help residents and patients stay comfortable. If a person chooses an item of clothing that is not appropriate for the weather or the day's planned activities, gently suggest a more appropriate choice. Remember that some older or ill people may chill more easily than others and may need a sweater or jacket to remain warm, especially if there is air conditioning.

Some patients or residents will need your help with dressing and undressing. For example, consider the following situations:

- A person has an extremity (an arm or a leg) that is weak, paralyzed, in a cast, or splinted.
- A person has recently had surgery on an arm or a leg.
- A person has an intravenous (IV) line (Fig. 23-5).

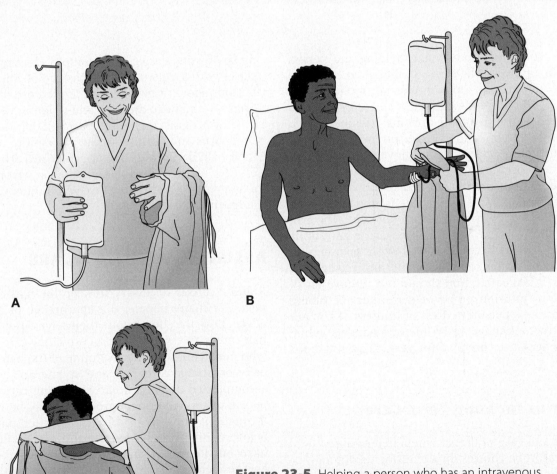

A

B

C

Figure 23-5 Helping a person who has an intravenous (IV) line in place get dressed is not as difficult as it may seem. **A.** Put the IV bag and tubing through the sleeve of the gown first, and place the IV bag on the hook. **B.** Gently thread the sleeve down the tubing and gently bring the person's arm through the sleeve of the gown. **C.** Bring the gown across the person's chest and guide the other arm through the other sleeve.

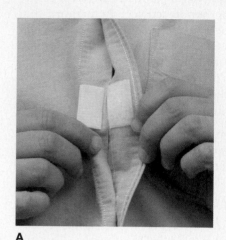

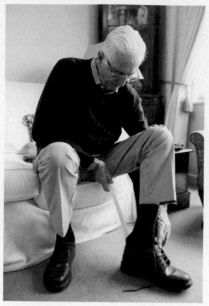

A

B

Figure 23-6 Assistive devices are available to help people with disabilities dress themselves independently. **A.** Velcro fasteners on this shirt replace buttons or a zipper, which require more use of the fingers to manage. **B.** A shoehorn makes it easier to put on shoes. (*A, Courtesy of Sammons Preston Rolyan, Bolingbrook, IL. B, Daisy Daisy/Shutterstock.com*)

These conditions may make helping the person to dress or undress a bit more challenging, but good planning on your part can simplify the situation. For example, if you place the garment's sleeve or leg onto the affected extremity first, dressing becomes much easier for both you and the person being dressed. (When the time comes to remove the garment, reverse the procedure—work with the strong arm or leg first and undress the affected extremity last.) If the person has an IV line, bring the IV bag and tubing through the sleeve first and then follow with the arm (see Fig. 23-5). Some hospitals and acute care units may have special hospital gowns with openings in the shoulder that make dressing and undressing with IV lines in place easier. You should not remove an IV line from an infusion pump or disconnect IV tubing when assisting a person to dress or undress. If you are unsure how to manage an IV line or a bandage while helping a person to dress or undress, ask a nurse for assistance.

Concerns for Long-Term Care

Comfort and ease of dressing help determine many wardrobe choices for the residents of long-term care facilities. Many residents undergo rehabilitation following an accident or a disabling illness, such as a stroke. The goal of rehabilitation is to return the person to the highest level of independent functioning as possible. In addition to selecting clothes that are easy to take on and off, a weak or disabled person may use one or more of the many assistive devices that are available to make dressing easier. For example, clothing that closes with a Velcro fastener instead of zippers or buttons allows a person with limited use of their fingers to manage dressing and toileting with little or no assistance (Fig. 23-6A). Long-handled shoehorns and graspers allow a person to put on their own socks and shoes (Fig. 23-6B). The use of these assistive devices can allow a person with a disability to maintain a large amount of personal independence.

ASSISTING WITH HAIR CARE

Routine care is necessary to keep the hair clean and neat. For many people, the appearance of their hair affects how they feel about themselves. Helping with hair care is an essential part of providing care for those who need you. Routine grooming of the hair involves daily brushing, combing, and styling and is usually accomplished as part of early morning care, when a person arises. Additional grooming may be necessary throughout the day, for example, after napping or before visiting times. Many health care facilities now have on-site salons and barbershops where patients and residents can have their hair cut, washed, and professionally styled (Fig. 23-7).

The texture and length of the hair affect how a person cares for it. Hair that is straight and fine can require as much maintenance as hair that is curly and coarse. The hair of older people tends to be fragile. Personal preferences regarding hairstyle and the products used when grooming the hair vary and should be respected whenever possible. Asking a person

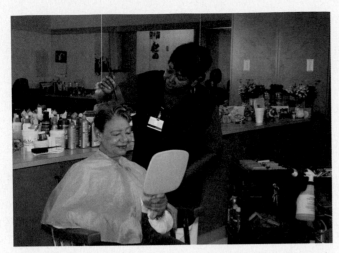

Figure 23-7 Many facilities now have on-site salons and barbershops for the convenience of residents.

about their usual hair care routine and preferred products will provide you with much useful information. Patients and residents should be encouraged to participate in caring for their own hair to their fullest ability. For example, a person with a paralyzed or injured arm can be encouraged to brush their hair on their "strong" side, and then you can complete the job on the other side (Fig. 23-8).

When assisting with grooming of the hair, it is important to observe the hair and scalp for any abnormalities. Common conditions of the hair and scalp that you may see in your patients or residents include the following:

- **Dandruff** is itching and flaking of the scalp. Daily brushing and using a medicated shampoo may be all that is needed to control dandruff.
- **Tinea capitis**, a fungal infection of the scalp, may also cause itching and flaking of the scalp.

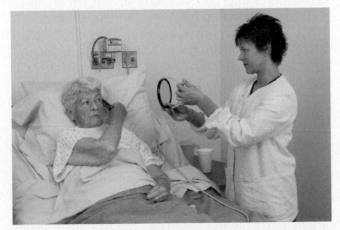

Figure 23-8 To foster independence and self-esteem, encourage your patients or residents to do as much as possible for themselves, while you stand by ready to offer assistance as needed.

("Capitis" comes from the Latin word for head, *caput*.) An antifungal medication will be needed to treat this infection.

- **Seborrheic dermatitis** (commonly referred to as **"cradle cap"** when it occurs in infants) causes severe scaling of the scalp. Thick, yellow, crusty patches are seen. The nurse may ask you to help shampoo the person daily with a medicated shampoo until the scaling is cleared up.
- **Alopecia**, or baldness, can be caused by many conditions. Alopecia is most commonly the result of an inherited trait in males and is rarely seen in females, although females may experience thinning of the hair with aging. Medications used to treat cancer (chemotherapy) and certain forms of radiation treatment can cause total baldness in both males and females. Stress, illness, and poor nutrition can also cause the hair to thin.
- **Pediculosis capitis**, or head lice, is particularly common in children. Lice, as you will recall from Chapter 10, are very small parasitic insects that feed on the blood of the host, or the person who is infected. The insects lay their eggs (called **nits**) on the hair shaft, near the root. The nits look like dandruff flakes or small pieces of lint, but they cannot be brushed or shaken off the hair. Head lice are transmitted from person to person by direct contact with an infected person's hair. They may also be transmitted indirectly, through contact with clothing, bed linens, brushes and combs, and cloth-covered furniture (for example, the back of a sofa or chair where an infected person has rested their head). Pediculosis is treated with medicated creams and shampoos. The person's clothing and bed linens must be washed in very hot water to prevent reinfection.

Tell the Nurse!

When providing hair care, it is important to observe the condition of the person's hair and scalp. Make sure to report any of the following findings to the nurse immediately:

- Flaking, crusting, or scaling of the scalp
- Redness, itching, or tenderness of the scalp
- Unusual hair loss, especially if it is occurring in patches
- A foul smell
- Severely matted or tangled hair
- Nits ("flakes" that cannot be brushed or shaken off the hair)

Shampooing the Hair

Hair should be washed as often as is necessary to keep it clean. The frequency of shampooing will vary according to personal preference and health status. People who are feverish or who have been sweating from an illness or from physical activity may welcome a nonscheduled shampoo to help them feel fresh and clean. Other people may only need their hair washed once or twice a week.

Many people in health care facilities can shampoo their own hair when they bathe. Others will need help. There are several ways to help a person shampoo their hair. Many bathtubs and showers have handheld showerheads that make it easy to shampoo the hair during a person's bath. The hair can also be shampooed in a sink, either by having the person sit with their back to the sink and tilt the head backward, or by having the person face the sink and bend the head forward. However, remember that for many older people, shampooing at the sink is either uncomfortable or impossible because it is more difficult for an older person to bend their neck to the degree required. When a person cannot get out of bed, a shampoo trough is used to wash the hair (Procedure 23-5), or a shampoo cap containing a dry shampoo product may be used instead (Fig. 23-9).

As any trip down a drugstore or grocery store aisle will reveal, there are many different types of shampoos and conditioners to choose from. (Conditioners are used by many people to improve the hair's texture and reduce tangles.) Respecting personal preference in products is important. Before shampooing a patient's or resident's hair, always check with the nurse or check the person's nursing care plan to find out necessary details, such as the frequency of shampooing, the method used, and the products preferred.

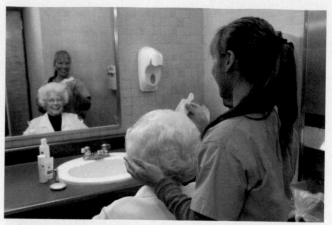

Figure 23-10 After shampooing, some people may like to have their hair dried and styled.

Styling the Hair

After the hair has been washed and towel dried, the hair is dried and styled according to the person's wishes (Fig. 23-10). Many people with shorter hair may prefer to allow their hair to air dry. Others may want to have their hair styled and dried with a blow dryer, or they may want their hair rolled on curlers and dried under a salon-style dryer. If you are using electric appliances to dry and style a person's hair, be sure to follow the safety precautions related to the use of electrical items as described in Chapter 13—for example, check for frayed cords, and never use an electrical appliance near water. Be very careful not to burn the person's scalp with the dryer or curling iron. It is best to use a low-heat setting.

Preventing Tangles

Regular brushing and combing of the hair help to keep hair soft and tangle free. The scalp produces oil that keeps the hair shiny and soft. Brushing distributes this oil throughout the hair. Hair that is long or curly may need to be braided after it is brushed to help prevent tangling (Fig. 23-11). Many African American people have curly hair and a very dry scalp. The hair of African American patients or residents may require braiding and the application of a moisturizing product to keep the hair soft and pliable. The use of barrettes, headbands, and clips can be both functional (by keeping hair out of the face) and decorative.

Sometimes the hair becomes tangled, especially if the person has been restricted to bed for a period of time. To remove tangles from the hair, use a wide-tooth comb and start at the ends of the hair, one section at a time, gently working up toward the scalp (Procedure 23-6). Hair that is very tangled or matted may need to be cut, but the nurse must first obtain

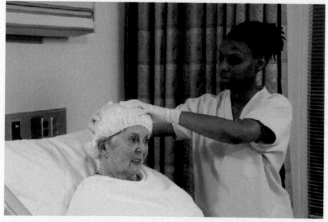

Figure 23-9 Shampoo caps contain a product that cleans the hair and scalp without water.

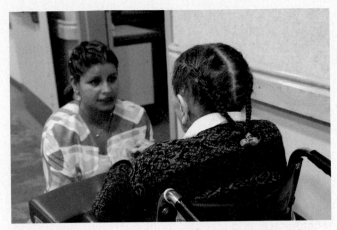

Figure 23-11 Braiding helps to prevent tangles in hair that is long or curly.

permission from the person or their legal guardian to cut the hair.

ASSISTING WITH SHAVING

Shaving is part of routine grooming for many people. This practice includes facial shaving as well as shaving of other areas of the body. Shaving practices vary among individuals depending on factors such as personal preference and cultural influence.

Facial Shaving

Shaving a person's face should be a part of either morning or evening care, depending on the person's preference (some people prefer to shave before going to bed). Prior to shaving, the face should be cleaned

and the beard softened, making bath time an ideal time to complete the shave. The frequency of shaving depends on how fast and thick the beard grows and on personal preference.

The type of shaving tool used also varies (Fig. 23-12). Many people prefer to use a safety razor, which may be disposable or have a changeable blade unit. Blades that are dull pull at the beard and do not cut the hair smoothly and should be changed. Disposable razors are used once and then discarded. Used blades and disposable razors should always be disposed of in a sharps container, not in a wastebasket. When using a safety razor, the beard is softened with warm water and a shaving cream or gel is applied to retain the moisture and reduce the friction of the blade against the skin. Some people may prefer to use shaving soap instead of a shaving cream or gel. In this case, a shaving brush is used to lather the soap and apply it to the beard. Procedure 23-7 describes how to shave a person's face using a blade razor and shaving cream, gel, or soap.

Other people prefer to use electric razors. People who are taking medications that decrease the blood's ability to form a clot should always use an electric razor, because electric razors are less likely to cut or nick the skin. If an electric razor is being used, a preshave lotion is applied to soften the beard and allow the razor to glide smoothly across the face. The usual safety precautions that are taken with all electrical appliances should be taken when using an electric razor. The electric razor is cleaned after each use.

If a person is able, they should be encouraged to do their own shaving. You should provide whatever assistance is necessary, which may range from placing a chair and a mirror near the sink or bringing supplies and water to the bedside, to completing the shave in

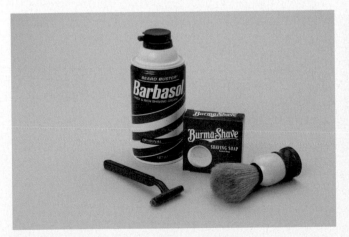

A

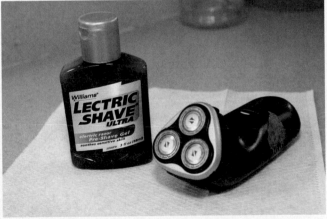

B

Figure 23-12 Shaving supplies. **A.** A safety razor is used with shaving cream or gel or shaving soap. **B.** An electric razor is used with a preshave lotion. An electric razor carries less risk of cuts or nicks, and therefore is preferred for a person who is taking medications that affect the blood's ability to clot.

full. When shaving a person, always remember to wear gloves because a cut or a nick will put you at risk for exposure to bloodborne pathogens. Always ask the nurse or check the nursing care plan to determine if there are any limitations or special instructions for a person's shave.

A person may prefer to have a beard or mustache instead of being clean shaven. Beards and mustaches need routine grooming care also. They must be kept clean and free of food and drink and will need to be combed or brushed and trimmed regularly. It is important to know that in addition to personal preference, some people maintain a beard as part of cultural or religious practice. For both these reasons, never shave off a person's beard or mustache unless the person requests that you do so. Be careful when shaving near the mustache or beard to avoid accidentally shaving part of the facial hair off.

Shaving Other Areas

Shaving the legs, underarms, or other areas of the body are also common practice. Many of the same principles used when assisting with shaving facial hair apply to shaving other parts of the body as well. The hair should be softened with warm water first, making bath time the ideal time to shave. A safety razor or an electric razor may be used. If a safety razor is used, shaving cream or gel should be applied first. When shaving the armpits, chest, or groin area, it is best to move in the direction of hair growth. When shaving the legs, start at the ankle and move upward, against the direction of hair growth. Many people prefer to shave their legs only below the knee, while others may shave the thigh as well.

ASSISTING WITH THE APPLICATION OF MAKEUP

Many people wear makeup because it helps them to feel more confident and attractive. A person's culture, religion, age, and feelings about their own gender and sexuality all contribute to that person's feelings about, and use of, makeup. Many times, the types of makeup and cosmetics a person likes and the way they apply them are influenced by the time in that person's life when they felt most attractive.

Helping a person to continue with their normal personal grooming routine has an enormous impact on the person's continued well-being. For some people, wearing makeup increases their self-esteem and feelings of self-worth. When you help a person who likes to wear makeup complete this part of their grooming routine, the person will feel that you take special care of them and that you value them as the unique human being that they are. This idea is at the heart of humanistic care.

SUMMARY

- Caring for the hands and feet (especially the nails), selecting an outfit to wear, shampooing and styling the hair, shaving, and applying makeup are grooming practices that people may engage in to make themselves feel more attractive and confident.

  - Grooming practices differ from hygiene practices in that they are performed mainly for the sake of appearance. Therefore, good grooming is more essential for emotional health than for physical health. However, grooming practices do benefit physical health as well.

  - Personal grooming practices vary and are influenced by many factors, including culture, religion, upbringing, current fashion, and a person's feelings about their own gender and sexuality. Respecting your patient's or resident's personal preferences is an important part of providing holistic care.

- Care of the hands and feet focuses on keeping the skin and nails clean and healthy.

  - Assisting with hand and foot care gives the nursing assistant the chance to observe for potential health problems, including poor blood flow and fungal infections.

  - Poor blood flow to the feet is associated with many health problems, including decreased sensation and an increased risk for a life-threatening infection. Poor blood flow may be caused by heart disease, diabetes mellitus, or the normal aging process.

  - Trimming a person's toenails is usually beyond the nursing assistant's scope of practice. Instead, this task is performed by a nurse or a podiatrist.

- Dressing daily is necessary for warmth and modesty, and it gives people a sense of purpose.

- For many people, dressing is a way of expressing themselves. A person's preferences should be followed whenever possible. Sometimes, due to disability or illness, a person will be required to wear a hospital gown or nightwear during the day.

  - Wet or soiled garments must be exchanged for dry, clean ones as often as necessary.

  - Assistive devices, such as Velcro fasteners, shoehorns, and graspers, increase a disabled person's independence and therefore their self-esteem.

  - Certain conditions (for example, a weak, paralyzed, or injured arm or leg or an IV line) can make dressing more challenging.

- Most people feel best when their hair is clean, free of tangles, and styled in a familiar style.

  - Assisting with hair care gives the nursing assistant a chance to observe for conditions of the scalp and hair, including dandruff, tinea capitis, seborrheic dermatitis (cradle cap), alopecia, and pediculosis capitis (head lice).

  - Hair may be shampooed as part of a tub or shower bath, at the sink, or in bed, using a shampoo trough or a shampoo cap.

  - Styling tools include blow dryers, curling irons, curlers, and salon-style hairdryers. Caution must be used when operating these electrical appliances.

  - Regular brushing and combing keep the hair shiny and tangle free.

- Many people shave their facial hair daily, either completely or partially. Many people shave their legs, their underarms, or other parts of their bodies.

- Many people consider the application of makeup and other cosmetics to be an essential grooming activity.

Procedure 23-1

Assisting With Hand Care

WHY YOU DO IT Soft, smooth skin and trimmed, filed fingernails are important for overall health and comfort.

Getting Ready

1. Complete the "Getting Ready" steps.

Supplies

- gloves (if contact with broken skin is likely)
- paper towels
- orange stick
- nail clippers
- emery board (nail file)
- bath thermometer
- emesis basin
- soap
- lotion
- nail polish remover (optional)
- nail polish (optional)
- cotton balls (optional)
- washcloth
- towel

Procedure

2. Make sure that the bed is lowered to its lowest position and that the wheels are locked.

3. Clean the top of the over-bed table and cover it with paper towels. Pour some liquid soap into the emesis basin and fill the basin with warm water (100°F [37.7°C] to 115°F [46.1°C] on the bath thermometer). Place the emesis basin on the over-bed table, along with the nail care supplies and clean linens.

4. If the side rails are in use, lower the side rail on the working side of the bed. The side rail on the opposite side of the bed should remain up.

5. Help the person to transfer from the bed to a bedside chair, assist the person to sit on the edge of the bed, or raise the head of the bed as tolerated.

6. Perform hand hygiene and put on the gloves if contact with broken skin is likely.

7. If the person is wearing nail polish and wants it removed, remove the nail polish by putting a small amount of nail polish remover on a cotton ball and gently rubbing each nail.

8. Help the person to position the tips of their fingers in the basin to soak. Let the person soak their fingers for about 5 minutes.

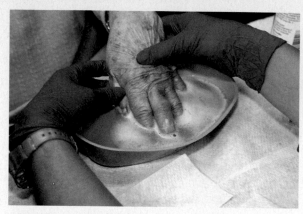

STEP 8 Soak the nails to soften them.

9. Working with one hand at a time, lift the person's hand out of the basin and wash the entire hand, including between the fingers, with the soapy washcloth. Use the orange stick to gently clean underneath the person's fingernails. Rinse thoroughly and pat the person's hand dry with a towel. Be sure to dry between the fingers. Repeat with the other hand.

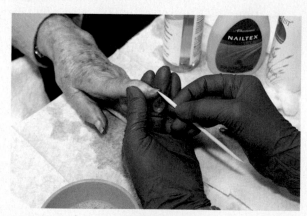

STEP 9 Clean under the person's nails using the orange stick.

10. If facility policy allows it, gently push the cuticles back with the orange stick.

11. If facility policy allows it, use the nail clippers to cut the person's fingernails. If the person's nails need to be trimmed but this task is outside of your scope of practice, report this need to the nurse.

12. Use the emery board to file the fingernails into an oval shape and smooth the rough edges.

13. Apply lotion to the person's hands and gently massage it into the skin.

14. Apply nail polish as the person requests.

15. If necessary, help the person return to bed. If the side rails are in use, return the side rails to the raised position. Lower the head of the bed as the person requests.

16. Gather the soiled linens and place them in the linen hamper or linen bag. Dispose of disposable items in a facility-approved waste container. Clean equipment and return it to the storage area. Clean the over-bed table according to facility policy.

17. Remove your gloves, dispose of them in a facility-approved waste container, and perform hand hygiene.

Finishing Up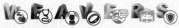

18. Complete the "Finishing Up" steps.

What You Document

- Date and time
- Type of care provided (trimming nails, filing, etc.)
- Any unusual observations (rashes, hangnails, discolored nails)

▶ Procedure 23-2

Assisting With Foot Care

WHY YOU DO IT Soft, smooth skin and trimmed, filed toenails are important for overall health and comfort.

Getting Ready

1. Complete the "Getting Ready" steps.

Supplies

- gloves (if contact with broken skin is likely)
- paper towels
- bed protector
- orange stick
- nailbrush
- nail clippers
- emery board (nail file)
- wash basin
- bath thermometer
- soap
- lotion
- nail polish remover (optional)
- nail polish (optional)
- cotton balls (optional)
- washcloth
- towels
- bath blanket (if remaining in the bed)

Procedure

2. Make sure that the bed is lowered to its lowest position and that the wheels are locked.

3. Clean the top of the over-bed table and cover it with paper towels. Pour some liquid soap into the wash basin and fill the basin with warm water (100°F [37.7°C] to 115°F [46.1°C] on the bath thermometer). Place the wash basin on the over-bed table, along with the nail care supplies and clean linens.

4. If the side rails are in use, lower the side rail on the working side of the bed. The side rail on the opposite side of the bed should remain up.

5. If the person is able to get out of bed, help the person to transfer from the bed to a bedside chair. If the person is not able to get out of bed, raise the head of the bed as tolerated. Fanfold the top linens to the foot of the bed. Cover the person with a bath blanket for warmth and modesty, leaving the feet exposed.

6. Perform hand hygiene and put on the gloves if contact with broken skin is likely.

7. If the person is wearing nail polish and wants it removed, remove the nail polish by putting a small amount of nail polish remover on a cotton ball and gently rubbing each nail.

8. Place a bed protector on the floor in front of the chair (if the person is out of bed) or on the bottom sheet (if the person is in bed). Place the wash basin on the bed protector.

9. Help the person to position their feet in the basin to soak. Let the person soak their feet for about 5 minutes.

10. Working with one foot at a time, lift the person's foot out of the basin and wash the entire

(continued)

foot, including between the toes, with the soapy washcloth. Apply soap to the nailbrush and gently scrub any rough areas. Use the orange stick to gently clean underneath the person's toenails. Rinse thoroughly and pat the person's foot dry with a towel. Be sure to dry between the toes. Repeat with the other foot.

11. If facility policy allows it, use the nail clippers to cut the person's toenails. If the person's nails need to be trimmed but this task is outside of your scope of practice, report this need to the nurse.

12. Use the emery board to smooth the rough edges of the toenails.

13. Apply lotion to the person's feet and gently massage it into the skin.

14. Apply nail polish as the person requests.

15. If necessary, help the person return to bed. If the side rails are in use, return the side rails to the raised position. Lower the head of the bed as the person requests.

16. Gather the soiled linens and place them in the linen hamper or linen bag. Dispose of disposable items in a facility-approved waste container. Clean the over-bed table according to facility policy. Clean equipment and return it to the storage area.

17. Remove your gloves, dispose of them in a facility-approved waste container, and perform hand hygiene.

Finishing Up

18. Complete the "Finishing Up" steps.

What You Document

- Date and time
- Type of care provided
- Condition of skin and nails
- Presence of broken skin or rashes

▶ Procedure 23-3

Assisting a Person With Dressing ▶

WHY YOU DO IT People who are able to be out of bed during the day usually wear regular clothing during the day and pajamas or nightgowns at night. Getting dressed in the morning helps people to feel better about themselves. Clothing must be changed every time it becomes wet or soiled.

Getting Ready

1. Complete the "Getting Ready" steps.

Supplies

- gloves (if contact with broken skin is likely)
- bath blanket
- clean clothing

Procedure

2. Make sure that the bed is positioned at a comfortable working height (to promote good body mechanics) and that the wheels are locked.

3. Lower the head of the bed so that the bed is flat (as tolerated). If the side rails are in use, lower the side rail on the working side of the bed. The side rail on the opposite side of the bed should remain up.

4. Perform hand hygiene and put on the gloves if contact with broken skin is likely.

5. Spread the bath blanket over the top linens (and the person). If the person is able, have them hold the bath blanket. If not, tuck the corners under the person's shoulders. Fanfold the top linens to the foot of the bed.

6. Assist the person with undressing:

   a. Garments that fasten in the back. Undo any fasteners, such as buttons, zippers, snaps, or ties. Gently lift the person's head and shoulders and gather the garment around the person's neck. Working with the person's strongest side first, gently remove the arm from the garment by sliding the garment down the arm. Repeat with the other arm. (If it is not possible to lift the person's head and shoulders, roll the person onto their side facing away from you. Working with the person's strongest side first, gently remove the arm from the garment. Roll the person onto their other side, facing you and remove the other arm from the garment.) Remove the garment completely by lifting it over the person's head.

b. Garments that fasten in the front. Undo any fasteners, such as buttons, zippers, snaps, or ties. To remove the top, gently lift the person's head and shoulders. Working with the person's strongest side first, gently remove the arm from the garment by sliding the garment over the shoulder and down the arm. Gather the garment behind the person and remove the garment completely by sliding the other sleeve over the weak shoulder and arm. To remove the bottoms, undo any fasteners, such as buttons, zippers, or snaps. Ask the person to lift their buttocks off the bed and gently slide the pants down to the ankles and over the feet. (If the person cannot raise their buttocks off the bed, help the person to roll first to their weak side, allowing you to pull the bottoms down on the strong side. Then roll the person to their strong side and finish pulling the bottoms down.)

7. Assist the person with putting on their undergarments:

a. Underpants. Facing the foot of the bed, gather the underpants together at the leg opening and at the waistband. Working with one foot at a time, slip first one foot and then the other through the waistband and into the leg openings. Slide the underpants up the person's legs as far as they will go, and then ask the person to lift their buttocks off the bed. Gently slide the underpants up over the buttocks. (If the person cannot raise their buttocks off the bed, help the person to roll first to their strong side, allowing you to pull the underpants up on the weak side. Then roll the person to their weak side and finish pulling the underpants up.) Adjust the underpants so that they fit comfortably.

b. Bra. Working with the person's weak side first, slip the arms through the straps and position the straps on the shoulders so that the front of the bra is covering the person's chest. Adjust the cups of the bra over the person's breasts. Raise the person's head and shoulders and help the person to lean forward so that you can fasten the bra in the back.

c. Undershirt. Facing the head of the bed, gather the top and the bottom of the undershirt together at the neck opening. Place the undershirt over the person's head. Working with the person's weak side first, slip the arms through the arm openings. Raise the person's head and shoulders and help the person to lean forward so that you can pull the undershirt down, smoothing out any wrinkles.

8. Assist the person with putting on their outerwear:

a. Pants. Assist the person with putting on their pants by following the same procedure as that used for putting on underpants (see step 7a). Fasten any buttons, zippers, snaps, or ties.

b. Shirts and sweaters that fasten in the front. Facing the head of the bed, place your hand and arm through the wristband of the garment. Working with the person's weak side first, grasp the person's hand and slip the garment off of your hand and arm, gently guiding the person's arm into the sleeve. Pull the sleeve up, adjusting it at the shoulder. Raise the person's head and shoulders and help the person to lean forward so that you can bring the other side of the garment around the back of the person's body. Guide the person's strong arm into the sleeve of the garment. Fasten any buttons, zippers, snaps, or ties.

c. Sweatshirts and pullover sweaters. Assist the person with putting on a sweatshirt or pullover sweater by following the same procedure as that used for putting on an undershirt (see step 7c). Fasten any buttons, zippers, snaps, or ties.

d. Blouses that fasten in the back. Facing the head of the bed, place your hand and arm through the wristband of the garment. Working with the person's weak side first, grasp the person's hand and slip the garment off of your hand and arm, gently guiding the person's arm into the sleeve. Pull the sleeve up, adjusting it at the shoulder. Repeat for the other side. Raise the person's head and shoulders and help the person to lean forward so that you can bring the sides of the garment around to the back. Fasten any buttons, zippers, snaps, or ties.

9. Assist the person with putting on footwear:

a. Socks or knee-high stockings. Gather the sock or stocking, bringing the toe area and the opening together. With the toe area facing up, slip the sock or stocking over the person's foot. Smooth the heel of the sock or

(continued)

stocking over the person's heel, and pull the sock or stocking up into position. Adjust the sock or stocking so that it fits comfortably. Repeat for the other foot.

b. **Shoes or slippers.** If the shoe has laces, loosen them completely to make it easier to slip the shoe onto the foot. Guide the person's foot into the shoe or slipper. A shoe-horn may be used to help ease the person's heel into the shoe. Make sure that the foot is seated properly in the shoe. Socks or stockings should not be bunched at the toe. If necessary, tie the shoe or fasten the Velcro fasteners securely.

10. If the person will be remaining in bed and the side rails are in use, return the side rails to the raised position. Raise the head of the bed as the person requests.

11. Gather the soiled garments and place them in the linen hamper or linen bag.

12. Remove your gloves, dispose of them in a facility-approved waste container, and perform hand hygiene.

Finishing Up

13. Complete the "Finishing Up" steps.

What You Document

- Date and time
- Type of clothing applied
- Any abnormal observations

 Procedure 23-4

Changing a Hospital Gown

WHY YOU DO IT   People who are too ill to get out of bed may wear a hospital gown. The gown must be changed every time it becomes wet or soiled.

Getting Ready

1. Complete the "Getting Ready" steps.

Supplies

- gloves (if contact with broken skin is likely)
- clean hospital gown

Procedure

2. Make sure that the bed is positioned at a comfortable working height (to promote good body mechanics) and that the wheels are locked.

3. Lower the head of the bed so that the bed is flat (as tolerated). If the side rails are in use, lower them on the working side of the bed. The side rails on the opposite side of the bed should remain up.

4. Perform hand hygiene and put on the gloves if contact with broken skin is likely.

5. Fanfold the bed linens toward the foot of the bed.

6. Have the person turn onto their side facing away from you so that you can untie the gown at the neck and waist. Assist the person back into the supine position.

7. Loosen the gown from around the person's body.

8. Unfold the clean gown and lay it over the person's chest.

9. Working with the person's strongest side first, remove one sleeve at a time, leaving the old gown draped over the person's body.

10. Working with the person's weakest side first, slide the arm through the sleeve of the clean gown. Repeat for the other arm.

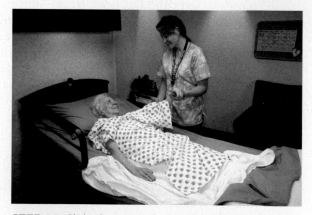

STEP 10 Slide the person's arm through the sleeve of the clean gown.

11. Remove the soiled gown from underneath the clean gown and place it in the linen hamper or linen bag.

12. Have the person turn onto their side, facing away from you, so that you can tie the gown at the neck and waist. Adjust the gown so that it fits comfortably and does not have wrinkles underneath the person.

13. Pull the bed covers back up over the person.

14. If the side rails are in use, return the side rails to the raised position. Raise the head of the bed as the person requests.

15. Remove your gloves, dispose of them in a facility-approved waste container, and perform hand hygiene.

Finishing Up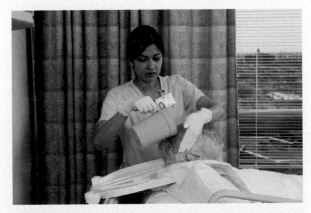

16. Complete the "Finishing Up" steps.

What You Document

- Date and time
- Any abnormal observations

 ## Procedure 23-5

Shampooing a Person's Hair in Bed

WHY YOU DO IT   Clean hair helps a person to look and feel attractive and is important for a person's self-esteem.

Getting Ready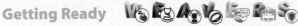

1. Complete the "Getting Ready" steps.

Supplies

- gloves (if contact with broken skin is likely)
- paper towels
- bed protector
- wash basin
- water pitcher
- bath thermometer
- shampoo trough
- comb
- brush
- blow dryer (optional)
- shampoo
- conditioner (optional)
- washcloth
- towels

Procedure

2. Make sure that the bed is positioned at a comfortable working height (to promote good body mechanics) and that the wheels are locked.

3. Fill the water pitcher with warm water (100°F [37.7°C] to 115°F [46.1°C] on the bath thermometer).

4. Clean the top of the over-bed table and cover it with paper towels. Place the hair care supplies and clean linens on the over-bed table.

5. Raise the head of the bed as tolerated. Comb the person's hair to remove snarls and tangles.

6. Lower the head of the bed so that the bed is flat (as tolerated). If the side rails are in use, lower the side rail on the working side of the bed. The side rail on the opposite side of the bed should remain up.

7. Perform hand hygiene and put on the gloves if contact with broken skin is likely.

8. Gently lift the person's head and shoulders and reposition the pillow under the person's shoulders. Cover the head of the bed and the pillow with the bed protector and place the shampoo trough on the bed protector. Help the person to rest their head on the shampoo trough. Place a towel across the person's shoulders and chest.

9. Place the wash basin on the floor beside the bed to catch the water as it drains from the shampoo trough.

10. Ask the person to hold the washcloth over their eyes.

11. Holding the water pitcher in one hand, slowly pour water over the person's hair until the hair is completely wet. Use your other hand to help direct the flow of water away from the person's eyes and ears.

STEP 11 Wet the person's hair, being careful to keep the water out of their eyes.

(continued)

12. Apply a small amount of shampoo to the wet hair. Lather the hair and massage the scalp to help stimulate the circulation.

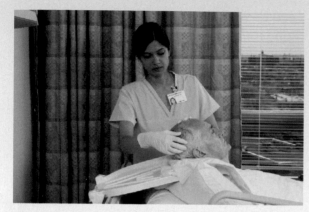

STEP 12 Apply a small amount of shampoo and work it into a lather.

13. Using the water pitcher, rinse the hair thoroughly.

14. Apply conditioner, as the person requests. Rinse the hair thoroughly.

15. Gently lift the person's head and shoulders and remove the shampoo trough and bed protector. Wrap the person's hair in a towel.

16. Raise the head of the bed as tolerated. Gently pat the person's face, neck, and ears dry and finish towel drying the hair.

17. Replace any wet or soiled linens. (If the side rails are in use, raise the side rails before leaving the bedside to get the necessary replacement linens.)

18. If wearing gloves, remove them and perform hand hygiene. Put on a clean pair of gloves.

19. Comb the person's hair to remove snarls and tangles.

20. Dry and style the hair with the brush and blow dryer, as the person requests. Use the cool setting and take care not to burn the person's scalp or face.

21. Reposition the pillow under the person's head and straighten the bed linens. If the side rails are in use, return the side rails to the raised position. Lower the head of the bed as the person requests.

22. Gather the soiled linens and place them in the linen hamper or linen bag. Dispose of disposable items in a facility-approved waste container. Clean the over-bed table according to facility policy. Clean equipment and return it to the storage area.

23. Remove your gloves, dispose of them in a facility-approved waste container, and perform hand hygiene.

Finishing Up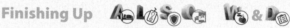

24. Complete the "Finishing Up" steps.

What You Document

- Date and time
- Type of care provided
- Any unusual observations of the hair or scalp

 Procedure 23-6

Combing a Person's Hair

WHY YOU DO IT   Combing the hair helps to prevent tangles and gives the hair a neat appearance.

Getting Ready

1. Complete the "Getting Ready" steps.

Supplies

- paper towels
- wide-tooth comb or pick
- brush
- mirror
- hair accessories (optional)
- detangler or leave-in conditioner (optional)
- towels

Procedure

2. Make sure that the bed is positioned at a comfortable working height (to promote good body mechanics) and that the wheels are locked.

3. Clean the top of the over-bed table and cover it with paper towels. Place the hair care supplies and clean linens on the over-bed table.

4. Raise the head of the bed as tolerated. Gently lift the person's head and shoulders and cover the pillow with a towel. Drape another towel across the person's back and shoulders.

5. If the side rails are in use, lower the side rail on the working side of the bed. The side rail on the opposite side of the bed should remain up.

6. If the hair is tangled, work on the tangles first. Put a small amount of detangler or leave-in conditioner on the tangled hair. Begin at the ends of the hair and work toward the scalp. Hold the lock of hair just above the tangle (closest to the scalp) and use the wide-tooth comb to gently work through the tangle.

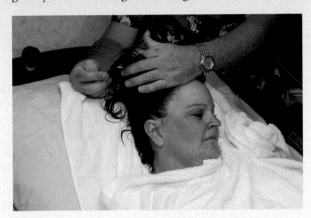

STEP 6 Hold the lock of hair just above the tangle.

7. Using the brush and working with one 2-inch section at a time, gently brush the hair, moving from the roots of the hair toward the ends.

8. Secure the hair using barrettes, clips, or pins or braid the hair, as the person requests. Make sure that the hair accessories are not positioned where the person will be lying on them. Offer the person the mirror to check their appearance when you are finished.

9. Remove the towels and reposition the pillow under the person's head and straighten the bed linens. If the side rails are in use, return the side rails to the raised position. Lower the head of the bed as the person requests.

10. Gather the soiled linens and place them in the linen hamper or linen bag. Dispose of disposable items in a facility-approved waste container. Clean the over-bed table according to facility policy. Clean equipment and return it to the storage area.

Finishing Up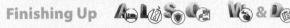

11. Complete the "Finishing Up" steps.

What You Document

■ Date and time
■ Type of care provided
■ Presence of excessive tangling or any unusual observations of the hair or scalp

  Procedure 23-7

Shaving a Person's Face

WHY YOU DO IT Shaving removes unwanted hair and is a routine grooming practice for many patients and residents.

Getting Ready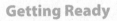

1. Complete the "Getting Ready" steps.

Supplies

■ gloves
■ paper towels
■ safety razor
■ shaving cream/gel/soap
■ shaving brush (if using shaving soap)
■ aftershave lotion (optional)
■ wash basin
■ bath thermometer
■ mirror
■ washcloth
■ towels

Procedure

2. Make sure that the bed is lowered to its lowest position and that the wheels are locked.

3. Fill the wash basin with warm water (100°F [37.7°C] to 115°F [46.1°C] on the bath thermometer).

4. Clean the top of the over-bed table and cover it with paper towels. Place the wash basin, shaving supplies, and clean linens on the over-bed table.

5. If the side rails are in use, lower the side rail on the working side of the bed. The side rail on the opposite side of the bed should remain up.

(continued)

6. Help the person to transfer from the bed to a bed-side chair, assist the person to sit on the edge of the bed, or raise the head of the bed as tolerated.

7. Place a towel across the person's shoulders and chest.

8. Perform hand hygiene and put on the gloves.

9. Wet the washcloth with warm, clean water. Soften the beard by holding the washcloth against the person's face for 2 to 3 minutes.

10. Apply shaving cream, gel, or soap to the beard.

11. Shave the person's cheeks:

   a. Stand facing the person.

   b. Gently pull the skin tight and shave downward, in the direction of hair growth (that is, toward the chin). Use short, even strokes, rinsing the razor frequently in the wash basin. Repeat until all of the lather on the cheek has been removed.

   c. Repeat for the other cheek.

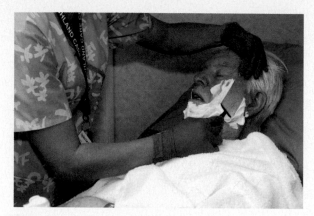

STEP 11 Shave downward, in the direction of hair growth.

12. Shave the person's chin:

   a. Ask the person to "tighten the chin" by drawing the lower lip over the teeth.

   b. Shave the chin using short, even, downward strokes. Repeat until all of the lather on the chin has been removed, rinsing the razor frequently in the wash basin.

13. Shave the person's neck:

   a. Ask the person to tip their head back.

   b. Gently pull the skin tight and shave upward, in the direction of hair growth (that is,

toward the chin). Use short, even strokes, rinsing the razor frequently in the wash basin. Repeat until all of the lather on the neck has been removed.

14. Shave the area between the person's nose and upper lip:

   a. Ask the person to "tighten their upper lip" by drawing the upper lip over the teeth.

   b. Shave the area between the nose and the upper lip using short, even downward strokes. Repeat until all of the lather has been removed, rinsing the razor frequently in the wash basin.

15. Change the water in the wash basin. (If the side rails are in use, raise the side rails before leaving the bedside.) Form a mitt around your hand with the washcloth and wet the mitt with warm, clean water. Wash the person's face and neck. Rinse thoroughly and pat the person's face, neck, and ears dry with the face towel.

16. Apply aftershave lotion, as the person requests.

17. If you have accidentally nicked the skin and the person is bleeding, apply direct pressure with a tissue until the bleeding stops. Report the incident to the nurse.

18. If necessary, help the person return to bed. If the side rails are in use, return the side rails to the raised position.

19. Gather the soiled linens and place them in the linen hamper or linen bag. Dispose of disposable items in a facility-approved waste container. Clean equipment and return it to the storage area.

20. Remove your gloves, dispose of them in a facility-approved waste container, and perform hand hygiene.

Finishing Up

21. Complete the "Finishing Up" steps.

What You Document

- Date and time
- Type of razor used
- Occurrence of cuts or nicks in skin
- Unusual observations of skin

WHAT DID YOU LEARN?

Multiple Choice

Select the single best answer for each of the following questions.

1. You are a nursing assistant in a long-term care facility. Which one of the following procedures may be beyond your scope of practice?
   a. Assisting a resident with bathing
   b. Polishing a resident's fingernails
   c. Trimming the toenails of a resident with diabetes
   d. Assisting a resident with oral hygiene

2. When helping a person to dress, which item of clothing would you put on first?
   a. Underpants
   b. Socks
   c. Slacks
   d. Sweater

3. Mrs. Romero, one of your residents, had a stroke that caused her left side to become weak. You are helping Mrs. Romero put on a cardigan sweater. Which arm should you put in the sleeve first?
   a. The left arm
   b. The right arm
   c. Either arm; it makes no difference
   d. Neither arm; Mrs. Romero should wear a hospital gown

4. Mr. Joyce has just been admitted to the long-term care facility where you work. You are telling him about the facility's policies. One of these policies is that residents are bathed on Monday, Wednesday, and Friday mornings. Mr. Joyce looks worried and says that he always bathes and shaves before he goes to bed, and he likes to do this every night. How do you react to this?
   a. You tell Mr. Joyce that you're sorry, but he has to follow facility policy
   b. You tell Mr. Joyce "OK" but then schedule him for a bath every Monday, Wednesday, and Friday morning, just like everyone else
   c. You respect Mr. Joyce's choice and ask the nurse if you can schedule him for a bath and a shave as part of evening care, every evening
   d. You report Mr. Joyce to the nurse because he is being difficult

5. Brushing the hair is important to:
   a. Make it grow faster
   b. Make it soft and shiny and prevent tangles
   c. Keep it clean
   d. Keep it free from lice

6. When shaving a person's face with a safety razor and shaving cream, you should:
   a. Soften the beard with warm water before applying the shaving cream
   b. Apply lotion after the shave is complete, if the person requests it
   c. Give the person a mirror so that they can check their appearance when you are finished
   d. All of the above

7. When shaving a person's face, you should:
   a. Apply shaving cream sparingly
   b. Use upward strokes when shaving the cheeks
   c. Apply an antiseptic to any cuts or nicks
   d. Use downward strokes to shave the chin

8. Which one of the following statements about nail care is true?
   a. Scissors are used to trim the nails
   b. Older people do not need nail care because their nails do not grow as fast
   c. Providing nail care allows you to examine the hands and feet for signs of health and disease
   d. Nail care is an activity that can be skipped if there is not enough time

9. Which one of the following benefits does a patient or resident enjoy when you shampoo their hair?
   a. Improved circulation (blood flow) to the scalp
   b. A clean, neat appearance
   c. Increased feelings of well-being
   d. All of the above

10. Which one of the following statements about helping a resident to dress is true?
   a. Residents like staff members to decide what they are going to wear
   b. Residents are used to being dressed in front of others
   c. Residents care about how they look
   d. Residents who are disabled do not need to dress in street clothes

11. One of your residents, Mrs. Ament, has diabetes. Why is providing foot care an important part of caring for Mrs. Ament?
   a. The circulation to her feet is likely to be poor, which puts her at risk for infection and other complications
   b. Diabetes makes the toenails grow faster
   c. People with diabetes usually do not take good care of their feet
   d. All of the above

12. You must remove a soiled gown from a patient who has an intravenous (IV) line. What is the best way to do this?
   a. Remove the gown from the arm with the IV first
   b. Ask the nurse to disconnect the bag and tubing before beginning
   c. Disconnect the bag and tubing before beginning
   d. Remove the opposite arm from the gown first

Matching *Match each numbered item with its appropriate lettered description.*

_____ **1.** Pediculosis

_____ **2.** Alopecia

_____ **3.** Podiatrist

_____ **4.** Tinea pedis

_____ **5.** Tinea capitis

   a. A fungal infection of the scalp
   b. Loss of hair
   c. A fungal infection of the feet
   d. Head lice
   e. A doctor who specializes in the care of the feet

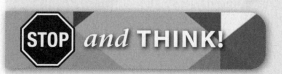

STOP *and* **THINK!**

Today, you are helping Mrs. Sayed get dressed. She is especially excited this morning because it is Saturday and her son is coming to visit. Since her son's favorite color is blue, Mrs. Sayed has picked out a lightweight blue blouse to wear. You know that Mrs. Sayed tends to chill easily, and you don't think she is going to be comfortable wearing the blouse that she has picked out. You suggest a different blouse, but Mrs. Sayed tells you that she would rather wear the blouse that she picked out originally. How can you provide Mrs. Sayed with her choice of clothing and still make sure that she is warm enough? What other grooming tasks can you help Mrs. Sayed with so that she feels presentable for her son's visit?

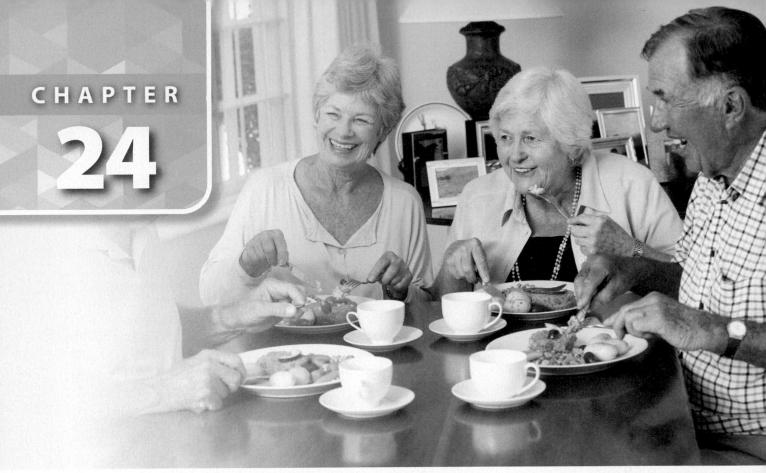

Photo: Meal time is as much about socializing as it is about eating. (Punchstock) (Monkey Business Images\Shutterstock.com)

Basic Nutrition

WHAT WILL YOU LEARN?

Few things are more satisfying than a good meal—you know, one that is made up of your favorite foods, all cooked to perfection, just like Mom's home cooking. Eating meets many needs for people, both emotionally and physically. In this chapter, you will learn about what we need to eat to keep our bodies healthy. You will also learn how to help your patients and residents meet their own nutritional needs. When you are finished with this chapter, you will be able to:

1. Define the term *nutrition* and explain why our bodies need adequate nutrition.
2. List the general types of nutrients and describe how the body uses them.
3. Discuss how the *2020–2025 Dietary Guidelines for Americans* recommendations can be used to help plan and provide better nutrition for a person.
4. Explain factors that influence a person's food preferences.
5. List and describe common special diets.
6. Explain the steps to take to assist a person before and during meal time, including for feeding a person who cannot feed themselves.
7. Describe how the amount of solid food eaten is recorded.

8. Discuss other ways of providing nutrition for people who are unable to take food by mouth.

9. Explain the fluid needs of the body and factors that affect the body's fluid balance.

10. Demonstrate methods used to measure and record fluid intake and output.

Vocabulary

Nutrients	Water-soluble	Nasogastric tube	Fluid balance
Nutrition	Obese	Nasointestinal tube	Dehydration
Ingestion	Appetite	Gastrostomy tube	Edema
Digestion	Anorexia	Jejunostomy tube	NPO status
Absorption	Dysphagia	Percutaneous endoscopic	Intake and output (I&O)
Calories	Nutritional supplements	gastrostomy (PEG) tube	flow sheet
Glucose	Dietitian	Total parenteral	Graduate
Amino acids	Intravenous (IV) therapy	nutrition (TPN,	
Fat-soluble	Enteral nutrition	hyperalimentation)	

FOOD AND HOW OUR BODIES USE IT

All living things eat. The food that we take into our bodies is broken down into essential elements, called **nutrients**. The body uses these nutrients to grow, repair itself, and carry out essential processes. **Nutrition**, or the process of taking in and using food, involves the following steps:

- **Ingestion**, the intake of food
- **Digestion**, the breakdown of food into simple elements (nutrients)
- **Absorption**, the transfer of these nutrients from the digestive tract into the bloodstream
- **Metabolism**, the conversion of nutrients into energy (occurs in cells)

To function, the body needs a continuous supply of energy, which it gets from the metabolism of food. You know that your body uses energy when you run to catch a bus, reposition a patient or resident, or climb a flight of stairs. But did you also know that your body uses energy even when you are sitting perfectly still? Every time you blink, or your heart beats, or your lungs expand to take in air, you are using energy. The energy to power our bodies comes from food, especially food that is high in carbohydrates, protein, or fat. Energy is measured in units called kilocalories, more commonly known as **calories**.

In addition to providing us with energy, food provides us with other substances our bodies need to function properly. These beneficial substances include vitamins and minerals, fiber, and water:

- **Vitamins** and **minerals** are small molecules that help regulate body processes and form structures within the body. For example, vitamin K helps the blood to clot, and calcium, a mineral, helps to build strong bones. Table 24-1 lists some of the common vitamins and minerals and describes how they benefit the body.
- **Fiber** is found in fruits, vegetables, and whole-grain cereals and breads. Fiber may be soluble, which means that it can be broken down (digested). Or it may be insoluble, which means that it cannot be digested. Insoluble fiber helps prevent problems with bowel movements by adding bulk to the feces.
- **Water,** which will be discussed in more detail later in this chapter, plays many important roles in maintaining body function.

Types of Nutrients

There are six general types of nutrients. Three of these nutrient types (carbohydrates, proteins, and fat) supply energy. The remaining three (minerals, vitamins, and water) regulate body processes.

Carbohydrates

Foods containing carbohydrates form the basis of many diets throughout the world because they tend to be plentiful and inexpensive. Carbohydrates are found in bread, cereal, fruit, vegetables, and sugar.

TABLE 24-1 Vitamins and Minerals

NUTRIENT	SOURCES	FUNCTION
VITAMINS		
Vitamin A	Liver, carrots, egg yolks, fortified milk	Helps us to see in dim light Keeps skin and mucous membranes healthy
Vitamin B_1 (thiamin)	Pork, liver, whole and enriched grains, legumes	Helps produce energy from glucose Assists with nerve function
Vitamin B_2 (riboflavin)	Milk, organ meats (for example, brain, kidneys, liver), enriched grains, green vegetables	Assists with the metabolism of carbohydrates, protein, and fat
Vitamin B_3 (niacin)	Kidneys, grains, lean meats, nuts	Assists with the metabolism of carbohydrates, protein, and fat
Vitamin B_{12}	Meat (including organ meats), eggs, milk, cheese	Assists with the formation of hemoglobin (the molecule that carries oxygen throughout the body) and red blood cells
Folic acid	Green leafy vegetables, meats, and whole grains	Assists with protein metabolism and the formation of red blood cells
Vitamin C (ascorbic acid)	Citrus fruits, broccoli, green peppers, strawberries, green leafy vegetables	Assists with tissue healing, building red blood cells, and iron absorption
Vitamin D	Sunlight, fortified milk, fish liver oils	Assists with the absorption of calcium and phosphorus to strengthen bones
Vitamin E	Vegetable oils, wheat germ, whole grains	Assists with the formation of red blood cells Assists with the reproductive system
Vitamin K	Vegetable oils, wheat germ, whole grains, liver, green leafy vegetables, eggs	Assists with metabolism of the proteins necessary for normal blood clotting
MINERALS		
Calcium	Milk, cheese, canned fish with bones, green leafy vegetables	Keeps the teeth and bones strong Assists with blood clotting Assists with nerve function and contraction of the heart and skeletal muscles
Phosphorus	Milk, meat, nuts, peas, beans	Keeps the teeth and bones strong Assists with the metabolism of carbohydrates, protein, and fat
Iron	Liver, lean meats, enriched and whole-grain breads, cheese, green leafy vegetables	Used to produce hemoglobin (the molecule that carries oxygen throughout the body)
Iodine	Table salt and seafood	Used by the thyroid gland to produce hormones for cell metabolism
Sodium	Table salt	Assists with fluid balance, nerve function, and contraction of the heart and skeletal muscles
Potassium	Whole grains, fruits, green leafy vegetables	Assists with fluid balance, nerve function, and contraction of the heart and skeletal muscles
Magnesium	Green leafy vegetables, nuts, beans, grains	Assists with bone and tooth formation, protein synthesis, and carbohydrate metabolism

Carbohydrates are the source of the body's most basic type of fuel, **glucose.** Glucose, sometimes called "blood sugar," is carried in the blood and rapidly absorbed by every cell in the body. The cells use the glucose to "run," much like your car uses gas. Glucose is a simple carbohydrate, or sugar, which means that it passes quickly from the digestive tract into the bloodstream. Other carbohydrates, known as complex carbohydrates, or starches, must be broken down into simple sugars before the body can use them. Extra carbohydrates that are not used immediately as fuel are either stored in the liver or converted to fat and stored elsewhere in the body. Each gram of carbohydrate provides the body with 4 calories, or energy units.

Protein

Protein is found in foods such as milk and cheese, meat, poultry, fish, eggs, nuts, and dried peas and beans. Proteins contain **amino acids**, small molecules that are the "building blocks" of all of the body's cells. Therefore, foods containing protein help the body to rebuild tissue that breaks down from normal use and to grow new tissue after illness or injury. In addition to providing amino acids, protein is a source of fuel. Like carbohydrates, protein provides the body with 4 calories per gram.

Fats (Lipids)

Fats are found in butter, cooking oils, whole milk, cheese, meat, egg yolks, nuts, shortening, and lard. Fats make food taste better and satisfy the appetite longer because they take longer to digest than most other food sources. Although a "low-fat" diet is recommended for most people to maintain health, not all fats are bad. In fact, the body requires a certain amount of dietary fat to function properly. For example, some vitamins will dissolve only in fat, not water (that is, they are **fat-soluble**). This means that fat must be present in order for the body to use the vitamins. Fat also protects our organs and helps us to stay warm. Finally, fats are the most concentrated source of energy, providing 9 calories per gram.

Vitamins

Vitamins, as described earlier and in Table 24-1, play a key role in many body processes. Vitamins are classified as water-soluble or fat-soluble. **Water-soluble** vitamins dissolve in water. Water-soluble vitamins (vitamin C and the B-complex vitamins) are absorbed directly from the digestive tract into the bloodstream. The body cannot store water-soluble vitamins. Instead, any extra amounts of these vitamins are passed from the body in the urine. This means that water-soluble vitamins must be replenished daily for use by the body.

Fat-soluble vitamins (vitamins A, D, E, and K) are absorbed and stored in the body's fat, where they can be used as needed. Unlike water-soluble vitamins, fat-soluble vitamins are not easily passed from the body. For this reason, consuming too much of a fat-soluble vitamin can be as harmful as not consuming enough because the vitamin builds up in the body. In some cases, this build-up may actually be harmful.

Minerals

Minerals help provide structure within the body. For example, fluoride strengthens the teeth and calcium strengthens the bones. Minerals also regulate body processes. For example, red blood cells need iron to do their job of carrying oxygen to all of the cells in the body. Some of the key minerals that the body needs to function properly are summarized in Table 24-1.

Water

Water is provided in the diet in the form of beverages, such as juice, soda, milk, coffee, tea, and, of course, water! Water is also found in many foods, such as fruits and vegetables. Water provides no calories or nutrition, but it may be more essential to life than food. You can live for quite a long time without food, but only for 3 to 7 days without water. Every cell in your body contains water, which is why water accounts for approximately 50% to 60% of your body weight! Water does the following things for our bodies:

- Water forms the basis for the fluid that dissolves and circulates nutrients throughout the body.
- Water transports waste products out of the body, by way of the urine and feces.
- Water keeps us cool when it evaporates from our skin in the form of sweat.
- Water keeps the mucous membranes moist.
- Water forms the basis of the fluid that helps our joints move smoothly.

A Balanced Diet

For the best health, you must follow a diet that provides your body with a balanced amount of the essential nutrients. Two tools are available to help you achieve this goal—MyPlate and the nutrition labels on food.

MyPlate

In the United States, the number of children and adults whose Body Mass Index (BMI) falls into the overweight and/or **obese** ranges (25.0 or above) is increasing every year. About two thirds of adults have a BMI of 25.0 or higher, and of these, nearly one third has a BMI of 30.0 or higher. For children between the ages of 2 and 19, approximately 32% have a BMI of 25.0 or higher. Unhealthy eating habits, combined with a lack of physical activity, are the primary reasons we are seeing an increase in obesity. As a result, we are also seeing a significant increase in related health problems, such as cardiovascular disease and diabetes.

The best way to get the nutrients you need is to eat a variety of healthy food every day. Some foods contain many nutrients that our bodies need to remain healthy, but other foods have little or no nutritional value. To help Americans plan a healthy diet, the U.S. Department of Agriculture (USDA) developed MyPlate. MyPlate uses a place setting to illustrate the five food groups in the proportion they should appear on a person's plate (Fig. 24-1). MyPlate was part of a 2015 initiative based on the *Dietary Guidelines for Americans,* which are updated every 5 years.

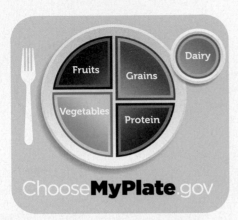

Figure 24-1 MyPlate was developed by the U.S. Department of Agriculture to remind people to eat healthfully.

The updated *2020–2025 Dietary Guidelines for Americans* state that more than half of the U.S. population meets or exceeds total protein and grain recommendations, but consumption of vegetables, fruit, and dairy remains too low to meet nutritional requirements. The following suggestions, found at www.ChooseMyPlate.gov and DietaryGuidelines.gov, are intended to help people make healthier food choices and maintain a healthy weight:

- **Build a healthy plate**
  - Make half your plate fruits and vegetables, especially vegetables that are red, orange, and dark green
    - Focus on whole fruits
    - Vary your veggies
  - Switch to low-fat and fat-free milk or yogurt
  - Make at least half your grains whole; check the ingredients list on your food packages to make sure they contain whole grains
  - Vary your protein food choices by eating seafood twice a week, adding beans as a protein source, and keeping meat and protein portions small and lean
- **Cut back on foods high in solid fats, added sugars, and salt**
  - Choose foods and drinks with little or no added sugar by drinking water instead of sugary drinks and selecting fruit instead of sugary desserts
  - Look out for salt (sodium) in the foods you buy by comparing packaging labels and choosing foods with lower numbers
  - Eat fewer foods that are high in solid fats and select lean cuts of meats or poultry and low-fat milk, yogurt, and cheese
- **Eat the right amount of calories for you**
  - Enjoy your food, but eat less
  - Cook more often at home, where you are in control of what's in your food

- When eating out, choose lower calorie menu options
- Write down what you eat to keep track of how much you eat
- **Be physically active your way**
  - Pick activities that you like and start by doing what you can, at least 10 minutes at a time

In addition, the new dietary guidelines in the *2020–2025 Dietary Guidelines for Americans*, referred to as "make every bite count," include recommendations for each life stage, from birth through older adulthood. As a whole, it is recommended that Americans focus on following these four guidelines:

1. **Follow a healthy dietary pattern at every life stage.**
   - Infants and young children have an increased need for calories and iron because they are growing rapidly.
   - Teenagers experiencing "growth spurts" have increased caloric and nutritional needs.
   - People who are pregnant and/or breast-feeding need more protein and calcium.
   - People who are recovering from physical trauma, such as that caused by burns or surgery, have different nutritional requirements than healthy people. Similarly, some illnesses change the nutritional requirements of the body, including chronic conditions such as diabetes, kidney disease, or alcoholism.
2. **Customize and enjoy nutrient-dense food and beverage choices to reflect personal preferences, cultural traditions, and budgetary considerations.**
3. **Focus on meeting food group needs with nutrient-dense foods and beverages, and stay within calorie limits.**
4. **Limit foods and beverages higher in added sugars, saturated fat, and sodium, and limit alcoholic beverages.**

Concerns for Long-Term Care

Older people have different nutritional requirements due to the physical changes that occur with aging. Older people do not need as many calories as younger people because they experience a slowdown in metabolism and are usually less physically active. Although the need for calories decreases as we age, the need for other nutrients, especially protein, increases or remains the same. Older people also may not feel thirsty as often, although the need for water and other fluids increases with age. This age-related decline in thirst can increase the person's risk of

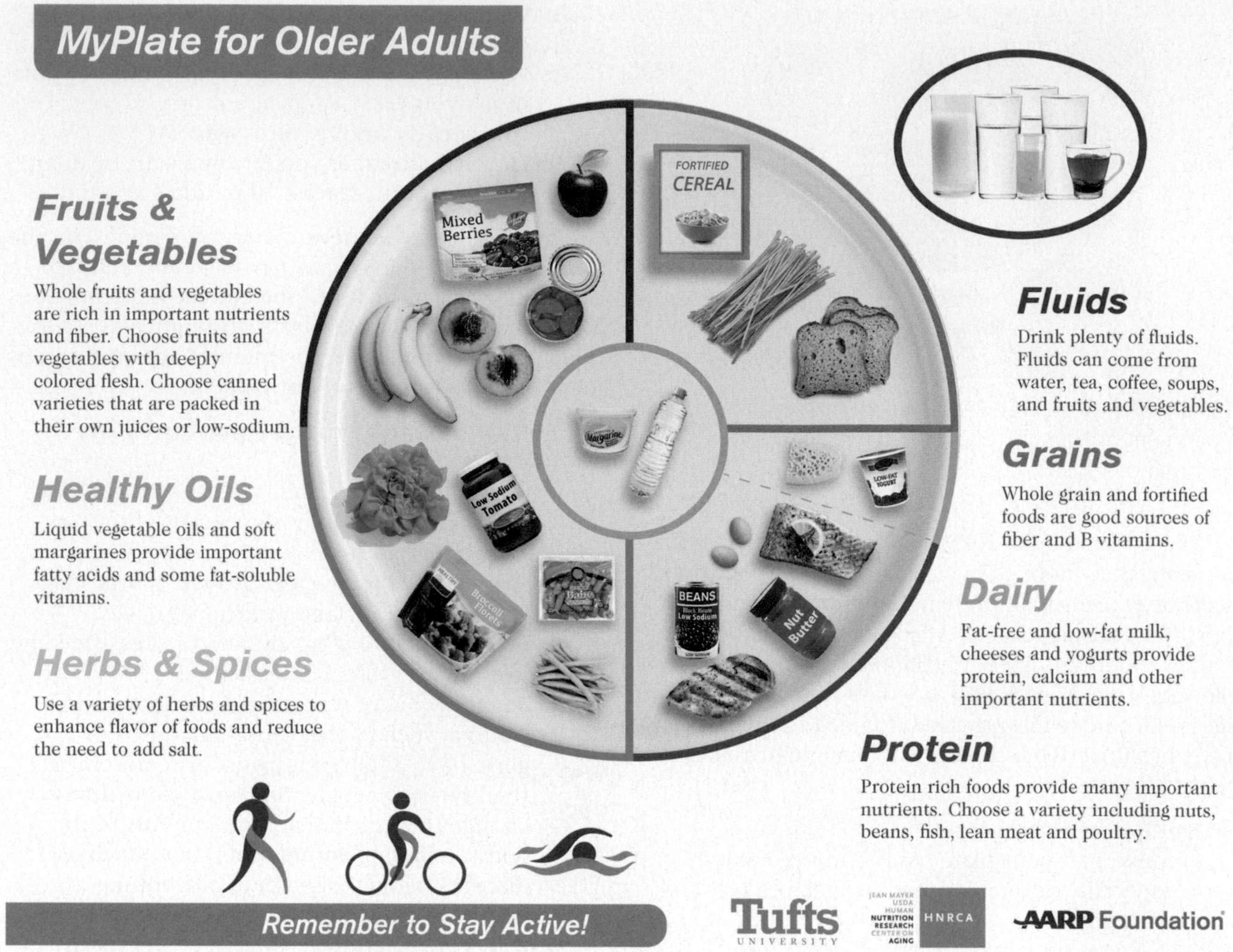

MyPlate for Older Adults

Fruits & Vegetables

Whole fruits and vegetables are rich in important nutrients and fiber. Choose fruits and vegetables with deeply colored flesh. Choose canned varieties that are packed in their own juices or low-sodium.

Healthy Oils

Liquid vegetable oils and soft margarines provide important fatty acids and some fat-soluble vitamins.

Herbs & Spices

Use a variety of herbs and spices to enhance flavor of foods and reduce the need to add salt.

Fluids

Drink plenty of fluids. Fluids can come from water, tea, coffee, soups, and fruits and vegetables.

Grains

Whole grain and fortified foods are good sources of fiber and B vitamins.

Dairy

Fat-free and low-fat milk, cheeses and yogurts provide protein, calcium and other important nutrients.

Protein

Protein rich foods provide many important nutrients. Choose a variety including nuts, beans, fish, lean meat and poultry.

Remember to Stay Active!

Tufts UNIVERSITY   JEAN MAYER USDA HUMAN NUTRITION RESEARCH CENTER ON AGING HNRCA   AARP Foundation

Figure 24-2 MyPlate for Older Adults. (*"My Plate for Older Adults"* Copyright 2016 Tufts University, all rights reserved. *"My Plate for Older Adults"* graphic and accompanying website were developed with support from the AARP Foundation. *"Tufts University"* and *"AARP Foundation"* are registered trademarks and may not be reproduced apart from their inclusion in the *"My Plate for Older Adults"* graphic without express permission from their respective owners.)

dehydration, especially during illness or periods of hot weather.

MyPlate for Older Adults was introduced in 2011 by the USDA Human Nutrition Research Center on Aging. It was updated along with the *2020–2025 Dietary Guidelines for Americans.* MyPlate for Older Adults addresses the unique nutritional and physical needs associated with people 70 years and older. MyPlate for Older Adults (Fig. 24-2) contains drawings of examples of different forms of foods for each food group that are convenient, affordable, and readily available. The MyPlate for Older Adults diagram focuses on the importance of eating several servings of bright- and deep-colored fruits and vegetables each day. Icons representing frozen, dried, and low-sodium/low-sugar–canned options are also added because fruits and vegetables in these forms

contain as many nutrients as the fresh and are easier to prepare and more affordable. An increase in the consumption of whole grains and low-fat protein and dairy is also highly recommended. Other icons on the diagram emphasize adequate fluid intake and regular physical activity, both of which are a particular concern for older people.

Long-term care facilities that receive government funding must follow Omnibus Budget Reconciliation Act (OBRA) regulations pertaining to meals (Box 24-1). These regulations ensure that each resident's rights are respected. They help to ensure that mealtime is as enjoyable as possible for the resident. However, even if you work in a facility that is not required to follow OBRA regulations, you must make an effort to make mealtime as pleasant as possible for your patients or residents.

Box 24-1	Aspects of the Resident's Dining Experience Regulated by the Omnibus Budget Reconciliation Act	

- Meals must meet the individual nutritional needs of each resident.
- Food must be served at the proper temperature.
- Food must be appealing to look at and seasoned to the individual resident's preference.
- Special diets, such as those followed for religious reasons, must be provided.

- Dining in the company of other residents is recommended.
- Residents in rehabilitation who are learning how to eat independently again must have a private area in which to eat.

Food Labels

There is a second tool available to help you plan a balanced diet—the nutrition labels that appear on most foods offered for sale at the grocery store. Education about proper nutrition and diet planning is one of the most effective ways of promoting health and helping to prevent some illnesses. In recognition of this fact, the U.S. Congress passed the Nutritional Labeling and Education Act in 1990, which requires that the labels of all packaged foods include information about the food's nutritional value, approximate serving size, and any related health claims (Fig. 24-3). By reading the

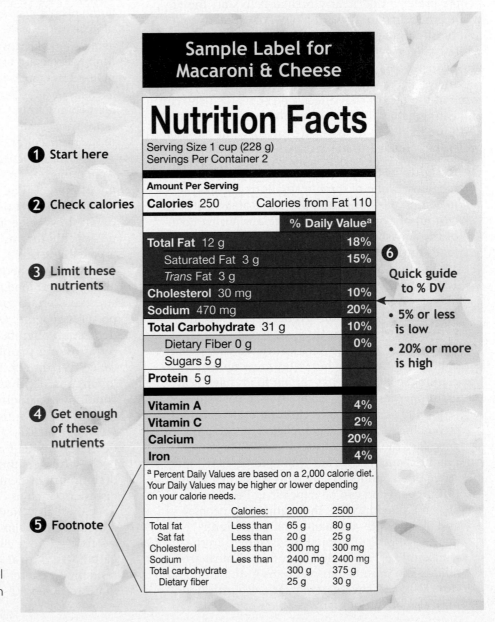

Figure 24-3 The law requires all packaged foods to have a nutrition label like this one.

nutrition label, you can see how the food can help you to achieve your nutrition goals for the day. Look at the label to see how big a serving size is and how many calories are contained in a serving size. The % daily value (DV) shows the percentage that each nutrient meets based on a 2,000 calorie/day diet. Try to choose foods that contain lower calories, saturated fat, trans fat, and sodium.

FACTORS THAT AFFECT FOOD CHOICES AND EATING HABITS

MyPlate guidelines and food labels help us make wise food choices. However, factors other than the nutritional content of a food often affect the choices we make about what we eat and when we eat it. Some people prefer a hot, hearty breakfast to start the day while others may only want a bowl of cereal or coffee and toast. Some people like a light meal at lunchtime while others eat their main meal at mid-day. Dinner may consist of a light snack for some while others routinely have a seven-course meal. Listed below are some of the factors that affect a person's food choices and eating habits. Think about your own eating habits and food likes and dislikes. Are any of your personal preferences related to the factors listed here?

- **Religion.** Dietary restrictions are a part of many religions. Some of these restrictions are specific to certain days (for example, the Roman Catholic custom of avoiding meat on Fridays during Lent, or the Jewish tradition of avoiding flour-based foods during Passover). Other dietary restrictions are in effect all of the time (for example, some Jewish people keep a kosher kitchen). A person may decide to confirm to all dietary guidelines of their particular religion or only parts of them.
- **Culture and geography.** People often like certain foods because they are associated with their culture, or the area where they grew up. Some cultural beliefs hold that certain foods have healing properties or help maintain balance, both physically and spiritually. Cultural preferences are a combination of heritage, religion, geography, and all of the characteristics that make a person unique. Some people are willing to try new foods, while others prefer to stay with what they know.
- **Finances.** Food can be expensive. People who are on a fixed income, including older people and people with a disability, may find it difficult to afford nutritional foods. Often, fresh fruits and vegetables and lean cuts of meat are among the most expensive items in the grocery cart. Milk and cheese, which are also nutritious, may also be out of many people's price range.

Instead, people who do not have higher levels of income often rely on cheaper foods that are high in calories and carbohydrates, but low in many nutrients. Fortunately, a small food budget does not necessarily make it impossible to eat healthy foods. Many frozen, dried, and canned foods contain as many, if not more, nutrients as fresh foods and are both less expensive and more convenient than fresh alternatives. With information and planning, it is possible to afford nutritionally sound food, even on a fixed income.

- **Kitchen skills.** People who do not know how to cook, do not like to cook, or do not have time to cook may choose to eat in restaurants or pick up "fast food" more often. They may also rely on convenience foods and frozen meals high in sodium.
- **Individual taste.** Some people find certain foods delicious while others can barely swallow a bite. Some people may not like a certain food because of its texture, or the degree of spiciness. Others will avoid a food because of the way it looks or smells. Many people are unable to eat certain foods, no matter how much they love them, because of food allergies or other physical reactions. As you certainly know from your own experience, individual tastes vary greatly, even among people who belong to the same culture (or the same family)!
- **Appetite.** Appetite is simply the desire for food. Appetite is both physically driven (by the feeling of hunger) and emotionally driven. It is not uncommon for a person who is ill or under emotional stress to be physically hungry, but have no appetite for any food. This loss of appetite is called **anorexia.** However, the opposite can be true as well because some people will actually eat more food when they are emotionally stressed. Certain medications can also affect a person's appetite. Older people who suffer from depression often become malnourished.
- **Swallowing problems.** Difficulty swallowing is called **dysphagia.** Difficulty chewing and swallowing can occur as a result of many different conditions, including disorders that affect the function of the muscles of the mouth and throat (such as a stroke, the result of a facial injury, or from treatment of cancers of the mouth and neck), disorders that affect the brain (such as brain injury or dementia), and developmental disorders (such as cerebral palsy). People who have difficulty chewing or swallowing may need a modified diet that makes it easier to chew and swallow without choking. A speech–language pathologist may also work with the patient or resident on exercises and positioning techniques that can help with controlling food in the mouth and swallowing.

- **Disability.** Many people in the health care setting have temporary or permanent disabilities that may affect their ability to eat. A patient or resident may have an injury to a hand or arm and have to wear a cast or splint for several weeks. The person may have had a stroke that resulted in paralysis or muscle weakness. Depending on the severity of the disability, the person may be totally unable to feed themselves and either need to use assistive devices or be fed by another person.
- **Impaired cognitive function.** People who have dementia, certain developmental disabilities, or brain injury may not know how to or have forgotten how to feed themselves.

Helping Hands and a Caring Heart

Focus on Humanistic Health Care

Meal times can be difficult for people who are receiving health care. The person may miss their family members. Foods that the person used to love may no longer be in the person's diet. Pain, anxiety, illness, and medication side effects can cause the person to have little or no appetite. Part of providing humanistic care is encouraging your patients and residents to eat adequate amounts of food, even when they have no appetite. Actions such as making sure the food is served at the appropriate temperature, providing pleasant conversation, and assisting the person to be physically comfortable help the person to relax and enjoy the meal.

SPECIAL DIETS

Meals prepared for people in health care facilities are specific to each person's individual needs. Personal preferences are taken into account when planning meals. To find out as much as possible about the patient's or resident's eating habits and food likes and dislikes, a nurse completes a dietary assessment as part of the admissions process. During the assessment, the nurse asks the person (or their family members, if the person cannot answer for themselves) about eating habits, cultural and religious preferences and restrictions, favorite foods, and foods that should be avoided. This information is shared with the **dietitian**, a person who has a degree in nutrition. The dietitian uses the information from the dietary assessment, as well as their knowledge of nutrition, to plan a diet for the person that they will enjoy eating and that will keep them healthy.

The type of diet that is ordered for a person in a health care setting is determined by many factors. People with illnesses such as diabetes, heart disease, or kidney disease require special diets. People who are recovering from surgery or trauma may require liquid or high-calorie diets for a period of time. Just the normal changes in the digestive system that accompany aging may require foods that are easier to chew, easier to digest, and have added fiber to help prevent constipation. Specific diets are ordered by a doctor and prepared by a dietitian.

Brief descriptions of some of the special diets that you may see ordered in a health care facility are provided in Box 24-2. It is important for you to familiarize yourself with your facility's specific diets and the foods that they include. That way, if a mistake is made in the kitchen and the wrong meal is delivered for one of your patients or residents, you will be able to recognize that an error has been made.

Some of your patients or residents will have **nutritional supplements** that are either offered with the meal or as an in-between meal snack. These nutritional supplements, which can be used to supply extra calories or protein, often take the form of a flavored shake or drink. These drinks are convenient and easy to serve. People with diabetes mellitus may require snacks in between meals to keep their blood sugar levels stable. The dietitian will plan for the nutritional supplements. It is usually the nursing assistant's responsibility to serve these nutritional supplements at specific times throughout the day and record that the supplements have been consumed. If your patient or resident refuses to eat an ordered supplement, report this to a nurse.

As you can see, the people you care for could be placed on any number of special diets for a variety of reasons. Take the time to learn about a person's medical condition and the reason a particular diet was ordered for that person. For example, you could ask the nurse if they know of any articles you could read about the person's condition, or you could search for information online. This additional information will give you the insight you need to make good observations about a person's dietary habits. Your patients or residents will benefit, and so will you because you will become a more effective member of the health care team.

MEAL TIME

A tasty meal, good company, and a relaxed dining atmosphere satisfy physical needs (hunger) as well as emotional ones (the need for love and belonging). In most cultures, eating is a social event. We

Box 24-2   Types of Special Diets

Regular ("house") diet. This is simply a well-balanced diet. There are no restrictions on specific foods or condiments (for example, salt, pepper, ketchup, salad dressing). There are many variations to the regular diet. For example, a high- or low-calorie version may be ordered to promote weight gain or weight loss. A low-residue or high-fiber version may be ordered to either decrease or increase dietary fiber for people with certain digestive problems. A bland diet contains foods that are easy to digest and will not irritate the digestive tract.

Mechanical diet. A mechanical diet is a diet that has been changed slightly to remove foods that are hard to chew or digest. The texture of the foods is altered to make them easier to eat, and fried or high-fiber foods may be eliminated or very limited. A *mechanical chopped* diet provides foods cut in small pieces to make them easier to chew. Some people need only chopped meats. Others may also need vegetables chopped, depending on the vegetable. A *mechanical soft* diet includes foods that are ground up. For example, a sirloin steak would be put through a meat grinder to make a sirloin patty. Vegetables and other foods may also need to be altered to make them easier to chew.

Pureed diet. For a pureed diet, the food is blended to a smooth consistency, similar to that of pudding or very moist mashed potatoes. Some people may require a *drinkable puree*. To create a drinkable puree, the food is blended to a liquid, milk shake–like consistency. Pureed and drinkable puree diets are often prepared for those who have very poor dentition, have dysphagia, are very frail, or who have end-stage disease. Pureed food may not be very appealing to you, but it is important not to voice or show that opinion while serving or feeding this diet to others!

Carbohydrate (CHO)-controlled diet. This diet, which contains limited amounts of carbohydrates, is ordered for people who have diabetes. The person's specific energy and nutritional requirements determine the amounts of fat, protein, and carbohydrates that are permitted. Because these amounts vary among individuals, this diet is different for each person. The amount of carbohydrates that should be eaten daily is calculated by the dietitian. This amount is then spaced out throughout the day between the three main meals and snacks. This helps to maintain steady blood glucose levels throughout the day. Carbohydrate intake needs to be balanced with any medications that the person may be taking to lower blood glucose levels. When caring for a person with diabetes, you must make special note of the amount of food the person eats at each meal.

Clear-liquid diet. Clear liquids are substances that can be poured at room or body temperature and that you can see through. Foods that are considered clear liquids include water, gelatin, fat-free broth or bouillon, popsicles, clear juices (for example, apple, cranberry, grape), clear carbonated sodas, and coffee and tea (without cream). Some medical tests require a person to be placed on a clear-liquid diet for a short period of time. A person who is nauseous or vomiting, or who has just had surgery or is recovering from an acute illness or trauma, may be given a clear-liquid diet initially. Clear liquids do not contain enough nutrients to maintain health for very long, so a person is usually progressed into a more nutritious diet as soon as the body can tolerate it.

Full-liquid diet. A full-liquid diet is the clear-liquid diet, plus any food that can be poured at room or body temperature. For example, milk, plain frozen desserts (such as popsicles, ice cream, or frozen yogurt), pasteurized eggs (egg custard or eggnog), cereal gruels, and strained soups and juices are all considered full liquids. Full liquids contain more nutrition than clear liquids, but a high-calorie, high-protein liquid dietary supplement may be added if the person must be on a full-liquid diet for more than 3 days.

Sodium-restricted diet. Sodium restriction is helpful for the treatment of certain types of heart disease, hypertension (high blood pressure), and kidney disease. A person on a sodium-restricted diet may be allowed to have a small amount of salt, or none at all. For example, some people may be able to eat foods that have some salt in them, but they will not be allowed to add extra salt at the table or eat very salty foods, such as pickles. Other people may have severe restrictions placed on their salt intakes. For these people, food will be prepared without any salt at all, and of course, the person will not be able to add salt to the food at the table. Some people on sodium-restricted diets may use salt substitutes. If you have a patient or a resident who has been placed on a sodium-restricted diet, make sure you know whether they are allowed to use a little bit of salt or salt substitute, or none at all.

Low-cholesterol diet. Following a diet that is low in saturated fats and cholesterol is good advice for everybody, but it is especially good advice for a person with heart disease. Foods are chosen that are lower in animal fat and prepared in ways that do not add additional fats. The addition of butter, shortening, and margarine to foods is avoided, and foods such as fruits and vegetables, whole grains, and skim milk are encouraged.

---

eat at parties and celebrations, we eat on dates, we eat certain foods on certain holidays, and we look forward to catching up with family members and friends over the dinner table (Fig. 24-4). Now imagine that you have just moved into a long-term care facility or been admitted to the hospital. Who will you share your meals with? Would you miss one special dish that your family always has for Sunday dinner? You might find yourself feeling a little lonely and homesick.

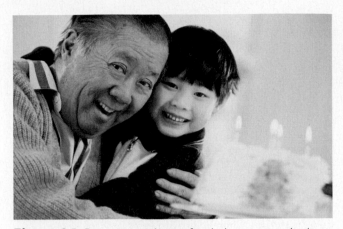

Figure 24-4 In most cultures, food plays a central role at social events.

Meal time for people in a health care setting can be difficult for many reasons:

- The person may miss family members or familiar foods.
- Food choices may be limited or the food may not be prepared the way the person likes it.
- Meals are usually served at specific times, not just when the person feels like eating.
- Meal time can be lonely, especially if the person must stay in their room to eat.
- Physical problems (such as pain or nausea) and emotional problems (such as anxiety) can affect a person's appetite.
- The person may be embarrassed if they need help to eat.

By providing companionship and assistance as needed, you can help to make sure that meal time remains a pleasant part of your patient's or resident's daily routine. Food should be presented in a way that will stimulate the appetite. Offering small portions of favorite foods frequently throughout the day can help increase a person's desire to eat. A clean, fresh mouth makes food taste better. A comfortable position, whether the person is using an over-bed table in bed or is seated at a regular table in the dining room, keeps the person focused on the food. If the person uses glasses or a hearing aid, make sure that these aids are in place. Provide pleasant conversation. All of these measures help to set a relaxed overall atmosphere and stimulate the appetite.

Preparing for Meal Time

Be sure to give your patients or residents enough time to prepare for meals. Allowing time to prepare is especially important before breakfast because early morning care must be completed before the meal. In a long-term care facility, the residents are assisted to the dining room to eat. In a hospital, the patients usually take their meals in their rooms. The assistance you provide will vary, depending on the person you are helping. Some people only need to be reminded that it is "almost time for lunch" and they will prepare themselves to eat. Others will need your help to get ready for the meal. The following actions help prepare a person for meal time:

- Assist the person with toileting. Help them to the bathroom or offer the bedpan or urinal.
- Assist the person with basic hygiene. Help them to wash their hands and face and brush their teeth. If the person wears dentures, glasses, or a hearing aid, make sure these items are clean and in place.
- Position the person for eating. Residents in long-term care facilities are walked to the dining room or taken in a wheelchair. In many facilities, the resident is helped from the wheelchair into a standard dining chair for the meal. If the person will be eating their meal in bed, smooth the bed linens and position the bed in a high-Fowler's position if permitted. Clear the over-bed table of clutter and wipe down the surface if necessary.
- Provide a pleasant environment. Remove any offensive or odorous items, such as bedpans or emesis basins, from the room. Adjust the lighting for comfort and turn on the radio or television if the person asks you to. Many people like to listen to music or watch a favorite program while they eat.

Assisting the Person to Eat

Once these preparations are completed, it is time to eat! Meals should be served as soon as they are delivered from the kitchen. Check that the name on the meal tray matches the name of the resident or patient who will be receiving it (Fig. 24-5). Also make sure that the diet noted on the tray matches the diet noted on the person's medical chart or nursing care plan. If the meal is not as

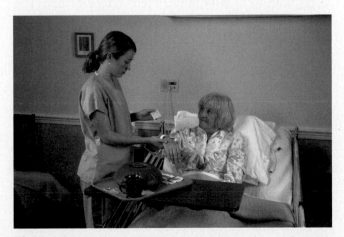

Figure 24-5 Always make sure that the right meal tray is being delivered to the right person.

ordered, ask a nurse to confirm that a mistake has been made, and then return the meal to the kitchen. The kitchen will replace the meal with the correct one.

Box 24-1 states that food should be served at the appropriate temperature. It is important to keep "hot foods hot and cold foods cold." The USDA requires that hot foods be cooked to a safe internal temperature and be kept at least 140°F until being served. Bacteria that may be in the food can multiply rapidly at temperatures between 40° and 140°F. If a person eats food that has been allowed to cool and sit for a while, they can become sick with a foodborne illness, commonly known as food poisoning. Make sure that you serve food trays promptly when they arrive on the unit or are ready in the dining room. If a person's meal needs to be reheated in the microwave, make sure that it reaches at least 165°F.

It is also important that you wear gloves if it is necessary for you to touch a person's food with your hands. Gloves are not necessary if you are only opening juice or milk cartons or holding a spoon when feeding a patient or resident. Just make sure you only touch the person's eating utensils by the handles and not the part that touches the food or goes into the mouth. As always, perform hand hygiene after assisting one person, before going to assist someone else.

In many facilities, especially long-term care facilities, a cloth or paper clothing protector is used. This protector is placed over the person's chest to prevent the clothing from being soiled with food during the meal. Wearing a clothing protector is a matter of personal choice, so always ask the resident if it is all right for you to put the clothing protector on them before the meal. Please do not refer to the clothing protector as a "bib." An adult, especially one who is already feeling self-conscious because they need help eating, will not appreciate being treated like a helpless baby!

Help the person to eat as necessary. Encourage your patients or residents to do as much for themselves as possible to help promote their independence. The nursing care plan will have basic information about the type of assistance the person needs, or you can ask the nurse. First, remove the cover from the tray and tell the person what foods are on the tray. No one likes "mystery meat" for dinner! Depending on the situation, you may also need to help the person with opening milk cartons or removing silverware from its wrapper, buttering bread, or cutting up meat (Fig. 24-6). If the person needs help seasoning the food, make sure that you add salt, pepper, and condiments according to the patient's or resident's tastes, not your own. If the person has limited vision, you will need to tell them where items are on the tray. Describe the food and help the person to find it on the plate by referencing a clock face (Fig. 24-7). For example, you might say, "Okay, Mr. Diaz—your pork chop is

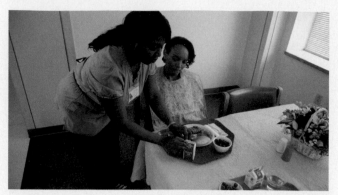

Figure 24-6 Some people will be able to eat on their own if you give them a little bit of assistance.

at 12 o'clock. The potatoes are at 3 o'clock, the green beans are at 6 o'clock, and the corn is at 9 o'clock. Your milk is on the upper right corner of the tray and your roll is on a bread plate to the left of your dinner plate."

Special forks, knives, spoons, plates, and cups can help people with physical disabilities that limit their ability to feed themselves to regain their independence. For example, many people who have had a stroke may have limited use of their hands and arms. They may be able to make big, sweeping movements, but small, delicate movements, such as those needed to hold and use regular silverware, are difficult. Specially made eating utensils, like those shown in Figure 24-8, allow the person to overcome these difficulties and feed themselves. A person who has lost the use of one hand will have to learn to eat using only the other hand. In this situation, a plate with a raised rim is very helpful. The rim is used to help guide food, much as you would use a knife to guide peas onto your fork. Special holders that fit around drinking glasses make it easier to hold the glass. All of these assistive devices help a person with a disability to regain independence, which is important for self-esteem.

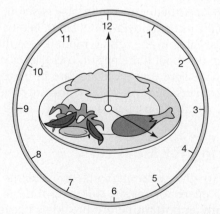

Figure 24-7 You can help a person with limited vision locate food on the plate by describing its location in terms of a clock face.

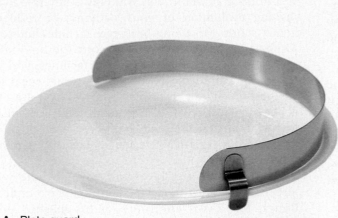

A. Plate guard

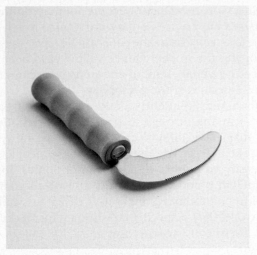

B. Knife with a rounded blade

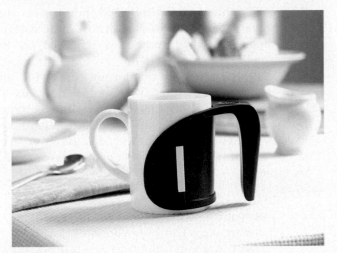

C. Cup holder

Figure 24-8 Assistive eating utensils help people with physical disabilities feed themselves. **A.** Plate guards help to keep food on the plate and provide an "extra hand" for pushing food onto the fork. **B.** A knife with a rounded blade can be rocked back and forth to cut food. This knife prevents the food from sliding on the plate. **C.** A cup holder fits around a drinking glass, giving the person a firmer grip. (*Courtesy of CaregiverProducts.com.*)

Feeding Patients and Residents Who Need Complete Assistance

Some people may not be able to feed themselves at all (Fig. 24-9). Even though these patients and residents will depend on you to do most of the work, it is very important that you involve them as much as possible in the process of eating. For example, you might ask the patient or resident to help you by holding their own napkin. Remember that meal time is a very social time in a person's day. It is important to talk to the person you are feeding, even if the person does not answer you. Hearing your voice and knowing that you care about them will increase the person's appetite and aid digestion.

The types of food served will differ according to the person's chewing and swallowing abilities. Some people may be able to eat solid food while others will require semisolid or liquid food. When feeding another person, always use a spoon, not a fork, because the blunt edge of the spoon is safer than the sharp tines of the fork. Fill the spoon only about one third full for each bite, and offer the bites slowly to prevent choking. Never rush the person through eating. Be sure to tell the person what foods you are offering. If the person is alert and able to respond, ask them in what order they would like to try the food on the plate.

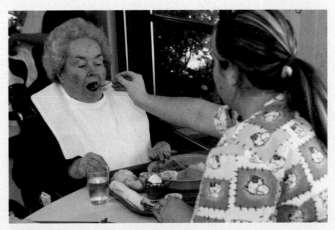

Figure 24-9 Some people may not be able to feed themselves.

Make sure you have seasoned the food according to the person's preference. If they are unable to tell you their preference, season the food mildly. Give the person enough time to chew and swallow each bite. You may need to gently remind the person to chew and swallow, especially if the person has dementia.

Offer liquids frequently, between bites. Some people find drinking through a straw to be easiest. Some people may have difficulty swallowing as the result of a stroke, injury, or dementia. These people can choke easily on liquids, so always offer liquids slowly. Sometimes the doctor orders the use of an additive that thickens the liquid, making it easier to swallow. The doctor orders a specific consistency for thickened liquids. These consistencies are:

- **Nectar.** A nectar consistency can be poured very easily. When poured, the stream has a ribbon-like appearance. The consistency can be compared to fruit nectar, such as apricot or pear.
- **Honey.** A honey consistency is thicker than a nectar consistency and is not as easily poured. When poured, the stream looks like a solid column, or it drizzles.
- **Pudding.** A pudding consistency "plops" rather than pours from a cup. Although it is a thickened liquid, this consistency is eaten with a spoon.

The nurse or therapist will show you how to use a thickener to thicken liquids if this is necessary for one of your patients or residents. Guidelines for providing thickened liquids are given in Guidelines Box 24-1. Some patients or residents may find the consistency of thickened liquids very unpleasant and refuse them. Providing other foods with high liquid content will be necessary to prevent possible dehydration. Procedure 24-1 gives the steps for feeding a patient or a resident who needs complete assistance with eating.

Helping Hands and a Caring Heart

Focus on Humanistic Health Care

Think for a moment—when you are hungry, you sit down and eat. You cut your juicy steak, butter your hot rolls, and never give the act of eating a second thought. How would it feel to have to rely on another person to feed you, or cut up your food? Would you feel like a small child again, or a burden, or just useless? Be sensitive to your patients' or residents' feelings as you assist them with meals. Realize how much they would like to be able to perform routine activities like eating without a second thought, just like you do.

Measuring and Recording Food Intake

As a nursing assistant, you will play a key role in the ongoing evaluation of your patients' or residents' dietary status. Most long-term care facilities and some hospitals will require you to record the amount of food that the person eats. In some facilities, you will just have to note the portion of the total meal that was consumed (for example, Mrs. Vellinga ate 60% of her breakfast, 80% of her lunch, and 30% of her dinner). Many facilities will want you to tell the nurse if one of your patients or residents eats less than 70% of their meal.

In other facilities, you will have to note what percentage of *each* food was eaten (for example, at dinner, Mr. Zakos ate 100% of his mashed potatoes, 50% of his salad, and 75% of his chicken breast). The nurse or dietitian will then convert the percentages that you provide into "total calories consumed," and this number is recorded on the person's chart.

Of all the nursing team members, you will have the most contact with your patients or residents during meal times. You will see which foods are eaten readily and which are left on the tray. When you notice that a food has not been eaten, you might talk to the person about it. For example:

Nursing assistant: Hi, Mr. Wheeling! How was your lunch? (*Noticing that the dessert has not been eaten*) Oh! I see you didn't eat your dessert. Are you full, or do you just not like vanilla tapioca?

Mr. Wheeling: Well, actually, I am pretty full, so I decided to skip the tapioca today. It's not my favorite anyway. (*Wrinkling nose*) I don't like the lumps.

Nursing assistant: Well, I'm glad you told me! We ought to be able to avoid "lumpy" desserts in the future ... maybe vanilla pudding or ice cream would be better instead?

Mr. Wheeling (*smiling*): Thanks, Nancy. That would be great. I do look forward to dessert!

Using good communication skills and asking questions that encourage the person to talk, instead of just answering yes or no, will help give you better information. Talking with the person about why a food was not eaten serves two purposes. First, it allows you to give the nurse information that they and the dietitian can use to plan future meals for the person. Second, when you notice that a food has gone untouched and take the time to ask the person about it, you let the person know that you care about them as an individual (Fig. 24-10).

Guidelines Box 24-1   Guidelines for Providing Thickened Liquids

WHAT YOU DO	WHY YOU DO IT
If thickened liquids have been ordered for a person, thicken all of the liquids on the person's tray, including soup.	Thickened liquids have been ordered for the patient or the resident because the person has difficulty swallowing. Providing any liquid without the thickener puts the person at risk for choking.
Carefully read and follow the instructions on the thickener to prepare the desired consistency.	There are several thickeners available, and the product used in the facility can change on the basis of availability or pricing. There may be some variation in the amount of product needed to produce a particular consistency.
When adding a thickener to a liquid, use a "sprinkle and stir" technique, rather than a "plop and stir" technique.	It is better to add the thickener gradually. "Plopping" a spoonful of the thickener into the liquid makes it more difficult to dissolve the thickener in the liquid. You do not want the resident to taste gritty particles of thickener when drinking. Also, plopping the thickener into the liquid often results in the liquid becoming too thick. If the liquid becomes too thick, then the consistency will need to be adjusted by adding more liquid.
Allow the liquid to sit for a minute or two before serving to make sure it is the right consistency.	It takes a few minutes for the full effect of the thickener to take place. If you think the liquid is the right consistency and serve it right away, the liquid will continue to thicken and in a few minutes it will no longer be the consistency ordered for the person. If the liquid becomes too thick, then the consistency will need to be adjusted by adding more liquid.
Add all condiments (for example, creamer, lemon juice) to the liquid before adding the thickening product.	Adding anything to a prepared thickened liquid can change the consistency.
Do not add ice to thickened liquids.	As the ice melts, it thins down the liquid.
Check the person's hot beverages periodically for changes in consistency.	Hot beverages thicken as they cool. Some additional hot liquid may need to be added to return the beverage to the correct consistency.
Do not give the person any food item that melts at room temperature (such as gelatin or ice cream).	These kinds of foods melt in the mouth and may become too thin for the person to swallow without choking.
Do not provide the resident with a bedside water pitcher.	Water must be thickened before drinking. Leaving unthickened liquid at the bedside puts the person at risk for choking. You cannot thicken the water ahead of time to leave at the bedside because the water continues to thicken as it sits.
Offer thickened beverages throughout the day.	Like all patients and residents, those on thickened liquids need to drink throughout the day to maintain adequate hydration. Because the person must depend on the staff to prepare all liquids, they cannot drink whenever they want to, so it is important to offer beverages frequently throughout the day.

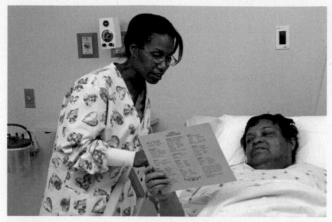

Figure 24-10 Respecting a person's preferences when it comes to food lets the person know that you care about them as an individual.

OTHER WAYS OF PROVIDING FLUIDS AND NUTRITION

Drinking water and chewing, swallowing, and digesting food are the best ways to obtain fluids and nutrients; however, sometimes these methods are simply not possible. For people who have problems chewing, swallowing, or digesting their food, fluids and nutrients must be provided another way. Three alternate methods of providing fluids and nutrition include intravenous (IV) therapy, enteral nutrition, and total parenteral nutrition (TPN, hyperalimentation).

Intravenous (IV) Therapy

In **intravenous (IV) therapy**, fluids are given through a small catheter (tube) that is inserted into a vein (*intra* = in; *venous* = vein). The IV tubing (sometimes called an "IV line") is connected to a bag that contains the IV fluid (Fig. 24-11). The fluid slowly drips through the tubing and into the vein. Usually the IV line, which is thin, is inserted into one of the small veins in the arm or the back of the hand.

IV therapy is not a source of complete nutrition, but it is useful when a person needs fluids. In addition to water, the IV fluid usually contains glucose, vitamins, and minerals. Drugs, such as pain medications or antibiotics, may also be added to the IV fluid. Sometimes, blood is given through an IV line.

You will not be responsible for managing IV therapy, but you may care for many people who have an IV line in place.

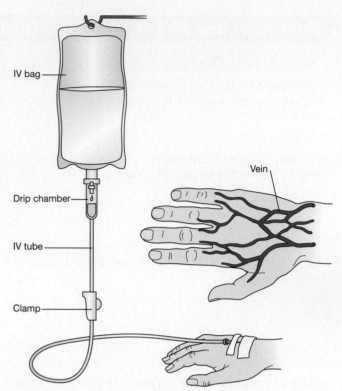

Figure 24-11 Intravenous (IV) therapy is used to give fluids. The IV fluid drips from the bag, into the tubing, and into the person's vein. The nurse uses the clamp to control the rate of flow.

Labels: IV bag, Drip chamber, IV tube, Clamp, Vein

Taking It to the Next Level:
Advanced Skills

More in-depth information related to advanced skills used when caring for a person receiving intravenous therapy can be found in *Lippincott Acute Care Skills for Advanced Nursing Assistants*. Visit thePoint® at thepoint.lww.com for access to the ebook.

Tell the Nurse!

When caring for a person with an IV line, report any of the following observations to the nurse immediately:

● The tubing has become disconnected

● The fluid bag is empty

● The IV fluid is not dripping into the drip chamber

● Blood has backed up into the IV tubing

● The person complains of pain at the IV site

● There is swelling or redness at the IV site

Enteral Nutrition

The word "enteral" comes from the Greek word for "intestines," *enteron*. **Enteral nutrition** involves placing food directly into the stomach or intestines, which eliminates the need for the person to chew or swallow. For example, a person who is in a coma is not able to chew and swallow. Certain injuries to the head and neck may prevent a person from chewing and swallowing, as might certain cancers. Sometimes people in the advanced stages of dementia "forget" how to swallow. All of these people may require enteral nutrition.

Enteral nutrition is sometimes called "tube feeding" because food, in the form of a formula-like fluid, is delivered through a tube that has been passed into the digestive tract. There are several ways to access the digestive tract with the feeding tube (Fig. 24-12):

- A **nasogastric tube** is inserted through the nose (*naso-*), down the throat, and into the stomach (*gastric*).
- A **nasointestinal tube** is inserted through the nose (*naso-*), down the throat, and into the small intestine (*intestinal*).
- A **gastrostomy tube** is inserted into the stomach (*gastro-*) through a surgical incision (*stoma*). The incision is made in the abdomen.
- A **jejunostomy tube** is inserted into the jejunum (part of the small intestine) through a surgical incision (*stoma*). The incision is made in the abdomen.
- A **percutaneous endoscopic gastrostomy (PEG) tube** is a special type of gastrostomy tube that is inserted into the stomach with the aid of an *endoscope*, a lighted, flexible tool that allows the doctor to see inside the body. The endoscope is passed through the mouth, down the throat, and into the stomach to help the doctor determine where to make the incision for the PEG tube. Placement of a PEG tube is faster, cheaper, and less risky for the patient than placement of a regular gastrostomy tube because abdominal surgery is not needed.

When a person needs enteral nutrition for only a short time, a nasogastric or nasointestinal tube is usually used. These tubes do not require a surgical incision for placement. However, they can cause irritation of the nose and the back of the throat and may be difficult for the person to tolerate. The tube can be easily displaced, especially if the person vomits, coughs, or pulls on the tube. Because it is possible for the tube to become displaced during feeding, nurses are responsible for feeding people with nasogastric or nasointestinal tubes.

When a person needs enteral nutrition for more than a few days, a gastrostomy, jejunostomy, or PEG

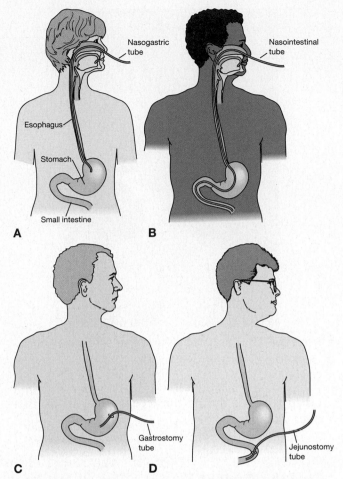

Figure 24-12 Enteral feeding tubes are inserted directly into the stomach or intestines. **A.** A nasogastric tube is passed through the nose, down the throat, and into the stomach. **B.** A nasointestinal tube is passed through the nose, down the throat, and into the small intestine. **C.** A gastrostomy tube is inserted into the stomach through a surgical incision. **D.** A jejunostomy tube is inserted into the small intestine through a surgical incision.

tube is used. These tubes are inserted through an incision in the abdomen, so irritation of the nose and throat is not a problem. Gastrostomy, jejunostomy, and PEG tubes are not as easily dislodged from their position as nasogastric or nasointestinal tubes are. However, they can come loose when a person moves or is repositioned. People who are disoriented or confused may also pull them out by accident.

Enteral feedings may be given at scheduled times or continuously by an infusion pump (Fig. 24-13). A person who is receiving nourishment through an enteral tube is at high risk for aspiration (inhalation of foreign material into the lungs). Aspiration can occur if the person regurgitates (vomits) the feeding formula and it goes down the windpipe and into the lungs. To help avoid regurgitation and aspiration, the head of

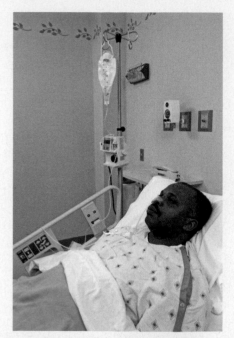

Figure 24-13 This patient is receiving enteral nutrition through a continuous infusion pump.

the bed is raised during the feeding and for at least 1 hour afterwards.

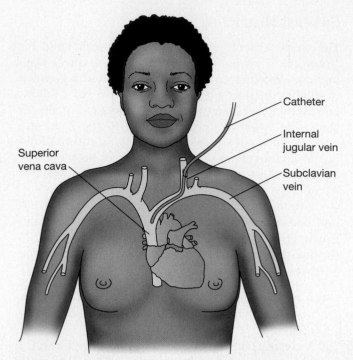

Figure 24-14 Total parenteral nutrition (TPN) delivers nutrients directly to the bloodstream. A large catheter (or "central line") is inserted into a large vein near the heart.

Tell the Nurse!

Notify the nurse if you suspect that a person who is receiving enteral nutrition has regurgitated or aspirated the feeding or if you think that the feeding tube has become displaced. (Remember that only nurses can reconnect tubing that has been displaced.) Signs and symptoms of problems with enteral feeding devices include:

- Nausea, bloating, or pain during the feeding
- Coughing, gagging, or vomiting during the feeding
- Abdominal distention (a swollen abdomen)
- Diarrhea
- Drainage from around the tube insertion site
- Disconnected tubing

Total Parenteral Nutrition (TPN, Hyperalimentation)

People who are very ill, injured, or recovering from surgery, especially gastrointestinal surgery, may not be able to tolerate food in the digestive tract. For these people, nourishment is delivered directly into the bloodstream through a large catheter (tube) inserted into a large vein near the heart (Fig. 24-14). This method of nutrient delivery is called **total parenteral nutrition (TPN) or hyperalimentation**. *Parenteral* means "by some way other than through the digestive tract." And *hyperalimentation* means "above (*hyper*) the alimentary (or digestive) tract." So you can see that both terms refer to a method of feeding that does not involve the digestive tract.

As you will recall from the beginning of the chapter, the digestive tract breaks food down into nutrients, and then these nutrients are absorbed into the bloodstream. If a person is receiving TPN, then the nutrients must be delivered to the bloodstream in their smallest form because digestion does not occur. Water, glucose, vitamins, and minerals are small molecules. But proteins and fats are bigger. This is why a large catheter is used for TPN, instead of an IV line. The large catheter used for TPN is wider and allows the bigger fat and protein molecules to pass through. An IV line is smaller and only allows smaller molecules, such as water, glucose, vitamins, minerals, and medications to pass. The ability to administer fats and proteins, as well as the other four classes of nutrients, is where the "total" comes from in the term *total parenteral nutrition*.

As a nursing assistant, you will not be responsible for giving TPN feedings, but you may care for people receiving them.

Taking It to the Next Level:

Advanced Skills

More in-depth information related to advanced skills used when caring for a person receiving enteral or total parental nutrition can be found in *Lippincott Acute Care Skills for Advanced Nursing Assistants.* Visit thePoint® at thepoint.lww.com for access to the ebook.

FLUIDS AND HYDRATION

As you learned earlier, water is just as necessary to life as food, if not more so. A healthy adult needs to drink between 1.5 and 3 quarts (48 and 96 ounces) of fluid each day just to keep up with the fluid that normally leaves the body in urine, feces, sweat, and the air we exhale. Most of these fluid needs are met by drinking water, juice, milk, and other beverages. However, certain foods, such as cucumbers, watermelon, grapes, and soup, have high water contents as well and provide for some of the fluid the body needs.

Fluid Balance

When the amount of fluid taken into the body equals the amount of fluid that leaves the body, a state of **fluid balance** occurs. Fluid balance is important for health. **Dehydration** occurs when there is too little fluid in the tissues of the body. Causes of dehydration include diarrhea, vomiting, hemorrhage, severe burns, diaphoresis (excessive sweating), and simply not drinking enough fluids. In all of these situations, the amount of fluid that leaves the body is greater than the amount of fluid taken in. Older people are often at risk for dehydration because they do not feel thirsty as often as younger people do. People in comas and people with dementia are also at risk for dehydration because they may not be able to ask for a drink.

The opposite of dehydration, **edema**, occurs when there is too much fluid in the tissues of the body. Kidney disease and certain types of heart disease can make it hard for the body to get rid of extra water, resulting in edema. In these situations, the amount of fluid that leaves the body is less than the amount of fluid taken in. For a person with edema, the doctor may restrict the person's fluid intake or order certain medications to help the body rid itself of the excess fluid.

Offering Fluids

Nursing assistants are responsible for providing fresh drinking water and other fluids to patients and

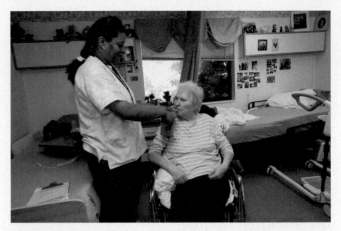

Figure 24-15 Water is essential to life.

residents. Many of your patients or residents will be allowed to have as much water as they like and should be encouraged to drink (Fig. 24-15). If a person is allowed to have ice water, make sure that the water pitcher is filled with fresh, cold water. Replace the water when the ice melts or when the pitcher is almost empty. People are more likely to drink fluids that taste good and are served at the appropriate temperature. Remember to also offer a drink regularly to people who are older, restricted to bed, confused, or taking pain medications. These people might not remember to drink fluids often enough, or they may feel that they are being a burden to you by asking for a drink.

Sometimes, the doctor may either increase or restrict a person's fluid intake. An order to encourage fluids means that the person should increase their fluid intake. The nurse will give you information about the amount and type of fluids to offer. Most people do not like having to drink a large amount of liquid all at once. Offering small amounts of a drink that the person likes frequently throughout the day is a better approach. Make sure that the fluids you offer are cold or hot, and fresh. Not many people like room temperature water, flat soda, or lukewarm tea.

Offering small amounts of fluids at regular times throughout the day is also a good approach when the doctor has restricted a person's fluid intake. This approach spreads out a person's fluid intake over the course of the day and helps to make sure they are never too thirsty.

Some patients or residents will not be allowed to have any fluids at all in preparation for surgery or a diagnostic procedure. A person who is not allowed to have any fluids at all is said to be on **"NPO status."** *NPO* stands for *nils per os,* or "nothing by mouth" in Latin. NPO means exactly what it stands for—no fluids (not even water or ice chips), no food, no hard candy, no gum. If one of your patients or residents has been placed on NPO status, empty their water pitcher and store it out of sight. You might also want to gently remind visitors that the person is not allowed to have anything to eat or drink and suggest that they enjoy their own snacks and beverages in another room. Being on NPO status can be extremely uncomfortable, since being thirsty and unable able to drink is difficult.

For a patient or resident whose fluid intake has been restricted or who is on NPO status, frequent oral care helps to relieve some of the discomfort and prevent "dry mouth" until the person is allowed to have fluids again.

Measuring and Recording Intake and Output

Certain medical conditions can make monitoring a person's fluid balance very important. Recording fluid intake is an important part of your duties when you are either encouraging or restricting fluids for a person. For those people, an order to "maintain intake and output measurements" will be followed. All of the fluids that enter and leave the body are measured and recorded on an **intake and output (I&O) flow sheet.** In health care facilities, fluids are measured and recorded in milliliters (mL). One fluid ounce is equal to 30 mL.

Each time the person takes in fluids, or fluids leave the body, the amount is recorded. The amounts are totaled at the end of the shift and again at the end of the 24–hour reporting period. The amount of intake can then be compared with the amount of output to monitor the person's fluid balance.

Measuring Fluid Intake

Fluid intake includes all of the fluids that a person drinks, including those foods that are liquid at room or body temperature (such as gelatin, ice cream, pudding, and popsicles). Other fluids that are considered as part of a person's total intake include enteral or TPN feedings and IV fluids, but the nurse will be responsible for recording these amounts. The health care facility where you work will have a listing of the amount of fluid in common servings, and you will need to become familiar with the amount of fluid contained by the cups, glasses, and bowls used in your facility. Remember that 30 mL is equal to 1 fluid ounce, so an 8-oz (ounce) carton of milk would equal 240 mL (8 × 30 = 240). But what if the person did not drink the entire carton of milk? In this case, you can estimate how much fluid was taken in. For example, if the person drank half of the carton of milk, then half of 8 oz is 4, so 4 × 30 would be 120 mL.

Sometimes it is necessary to calculate intake exactly. In this situation, you would calculate how many fluids were offered to the person before they started to eat. For example, let's say a person's meal tray contained 150 mL of orange juice, 240 mL of milk,

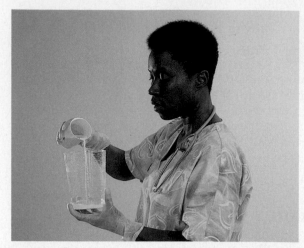

Figure 24-16 A graduate is a measuring device that is used to measure fluids. The graduate is marked with lines that indicate milliliters (mL) on the left and ounces (oz) on the right. (*Copyright B. Proud.*)

and 90 mL of water at the beginning of the meal. This would mean that 480 mL of fluid were offered (150 + 240 + 90 = 480). After the person has finished with the meal, you would take all of the fluids left in the glasses and pour them into a **graduate** (a measuring device) to measure the amount left (Fig. 24-16). Let's say that

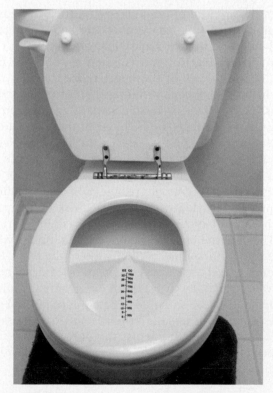

Figure 24-17 A collection device (sometimes called a "commode hat") is placed over the toilet seat before the person urinates, to contain and measure the amount of urine. (*Rob Byron\Shutterstock.com*)

40 mL of fluid are left. You would subtract the amount left (40 mL) from the total amount offered (480 mL) and record the total consumed as 440 mL. When using a graduate to measure fluids, make sure to place it on a flat surface so your measurements are accurate.

Measuring Fluid Output

Fluids that are considered output are urine, vomit, blood, wound drainage, and diarrhea. Output is measured and recorded the same way that intake is. A person who has a doctor's order for all of their intake and output to be recorded is said to be on I&O status and will need to be reminded to urinate into a measuring device. The urine cannot be discarded until you have measured and recorded the amount. Urine collection devices are available that can be used on a regular toilet or with a bedside commode (Fig. 24-17). Urinals have measurements marked on the side so that you can easily see the amount that they contain. Urine from a bedpan or a urinary catheter drainage bag is poured into a graduate for measurement. (Urinary catheters are discussed in detail in Chapter 25.)

If a person vomits, the amount can be measured using the markings on the emesis basin. If the person vomited somewhere other than in the emesis basin (for example, on the floor or bed linens), then the nurse will estimate the amount of vomit. Blood and wound drainage is either estimated by the nurse or measured in a graduate if it is collected into a drainage device. Diarrhea is estimated for amount also.

Always remember to wear gloves when measuring output.

SUMMARY

- Food and fluids are necessary for life.
  - Food provides us with energy and nutrients that our bodies need to work properly.
  - The six types of nutrients are carbohydrates, proteins, fats, vitamins, minerals, and water.
    - Carbohydrates, proteins, and fat provide energy.
    - Vitamins, minerals, and water regulate body processes.
- We need to eat a variety of nutritious foods every day.
  - Not all foods are equally nutritious.
  - Nutrients work best in combination with other nutrients.
  - MyPlate guidelines and nutrition labels can be used to plan a healthy diet.
  - MyPlate for Older Adults contains dietary suggestions directed specifically for people over 70 years of age.
  - People in health care settings often have special nutritional needs.
- Factors that influence a person's eating habits include religion, culture, geography, finances, kitchen skills, food likes and dislikes, and appetite.
- Difficulties with eating, such as dysphagia, disability, and impaired cognitive function, also influence a person's eating habits.
- Meals prepared for people in health care facilities are specific to each person's individual needs.
- The type of diet that is ordered for a person in a health care setting is determined by many factors.
- Eating helps us to meet both physical and emotional needs.
  - Helping a person to prepare for meal time and serving meals promptly contribute to comfort and a relaxed atmosphere.
  - Respecting the individual's preferences is important when it comes to food.
  - Talking with the person as you assist with the meal is important, even if the person cannot answer you.
  - Ensuring that meal time is pleasant can help improve a person's appetite.
- Nursing assistants assist people with meals as necessary.
  - Patients and residents are encouraged to do as much as they can for themselves.
  - Assistive devices are available to help people with physical limitations to eat on their own.
  - Some people will need to be fed.
- When a person cannot take food or fluids by mouth, nutrition and fluids are provided in other ways.
  - Intravenous (IV) therapy provides fluids, glucose, vitamins, and minerals through a small catheter inserted into one of the small veins of the arm or hand. IV therapy does not provide complete nutrition.

- Enteral nutrition is provided by a tube that is placed directly into the stomach or intestines.
  - Nasogastric tubes, nasointestinal tubes, gastrostomy tubes, jejunostomy tubes, and PEG tubes are used for enteral feeding.
  - Formula-like food is usually delivered through an infusion device, either continuously or at specified times.
  - Total parenteral nutrition (TPN, hyperalimentation) involves the delivery of all six classes of nutrients through a catheter inserted into a large vein near the heart.
- Maintaining proper fluid balance is important for health.
  - The amount of fluids taken into the body should equal the amount of fluids that leave the body.
  - If the amount of fluid leaving the body is greater than the amount taken in, dehydration can occur.
  - If the amount of fluid leaving the body is less than the amount taken in, edema can occur.
- A doctor may order a person's fluid intake to be increased or restricted. People who have no fluid restrictions should be encouraged to drink frequently.
- A person's fluid balance is monitored by measuring and recording fluid intake and output. One fluid ounce = 30 milliliters (mL).

▶ Procedure 24-1

Feeding a Patient or Resident Who Needs Complete Assistance ▶

WHY YOU DO IT A person who cannot feed themselves will need to be fed to ensure that they receive proper nutrition. Providing companionship during the meal is just as important as providing assistance with the task of eating.

Getting Ready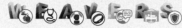

1. Complete the "Getting Ready" steps.

Supplies

- gloves
- paper towels
- clothing protector
- oral hygiene supplies
- wash basin
- bedpan or urinal
- towel
- washcloth

Procedure

2. Clean the surface of the over-bed table and cover it with paper towels. Place the oral hygiene supplies on the over-bed table. Fill the wash basin with warm water (110°F [37.7°C] to 115°F [46.1°C] on the bath thermometer). Place the basin on the over-bed table.

3. If the side rails are in use, lower the side rail on the working side of the bed. The side rail on the opposite side of the bed should remain up. Raise the head of the bed. Make sure that the bed is positioned at a comfortable working height (to promote good body mechanics) and that the wheels are locked.

4. Perform hand hygiene and put on the gloves.

5. Assist the person with oral hygiene.

6. Offer the bedpan or urinal. If the person uses the bedpan or urinal, empty and clean it before proceeding with the meal. Remove your gloves and dispose of them in a facility-approved waste container. Perform hand hygiene.

7. Wash the person's hands and face.

8. Clear the over-bed table, wipe the surface with a facility-approved cleaning solution, and position it over the bed at the proper height for the person.

9. Perform hand hygiene and get the meal tray from the dietary cart. (If the side rails are in use, raise the side rails before leaving the bedside.) Check the meal tray to make sure that it has the person's name on it and that it contains the correct diet for the person. Place the meal tray on the over-bed table.

10. Ask the person if they would like to use a clothing protector. Put the clothing protector on the person, if desired.

11. Uncover the meal tray, and prepare the food for eating (for example, cut the meat, butter the bread, open any containers). Remember to put on gloves if you will be touching any of the food with your hands. Tell the person what is on the tray.

12. Take a seat.

13. Allow the person to choose what they would like to taste first. Using a spoon, offer a small bite to the person (fill the spoon no more than one third full). Allow the person enough time to swallow the food.

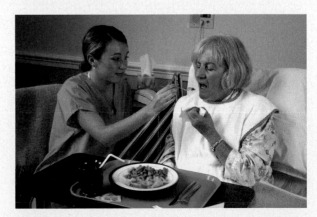

STEP 13 Using a spoon, offer a small bite to the person.

(continued)

14. Offer the person something to drink every few bites. Use the napkin to wipe the person's mouth and chin as often as necessary. Allow the person to assist with the eating process to the best of their ability.

15. Continue in this manner until the person is finished. Encourage the person to finish the food on the tray, but do not force the person to eat.

16. Remove the tray and the clothing protector when the person has finished eating.

17. Perform hand hygiene and put on a clean pair of gloves. Assist the person with oral hygiene.

18. If the side rails are in use, return the side rails to the raised position. Lower the head of the bed as the person requests. Make sure that the bed is lowered to its lowest position and that the wheels are locked.

19. Gather the soiled linens and place them in the linen hamper or linen bag. Dispose of disposable items in a facility-approved waste container. Clean equipment and return it to the storage area.

20. Remove your gloves, dispose of them in a facility-approved waste container, and perform hand hygiene.

Finishing Up

21. Complete the "Finishing Up" steps.

What You Document

- Date and time
- Percentage of food eaten
- Fluid intake
- Report an abnormal appetite or if person consumes less than 70% of meal to the nurse

WHAT DID YOU LEARN?

Multiple Choice

Select the single best answer for each of the following questions.

1. When assisting a person with eating, one of the first things you should do is:
   a. Provide the person with privacy
   b. Butter the person's bread
   c. Wash your hands and the person's hands
   d. Cut the food into large pieces

2. Mrs. Wellington is blind. Which one of the following should she have during meal time?
   a. A soft diet
   b. Help identifying the location of the food on the plate
   c. A large spoon
   d. A cup holder

3. Mr. Zakos is 98 years old and has no food restrictions on his diet. However, he is missing several teeth. Which one of the following menus would be the best choice for Mr. Zakos?
   a. Spare ribs, macaroni and cheese, coleslaw, and fruit cocktail
   b. Hamburger, french fries, corn on the cob, and ice cream
   c. Baked fish, mashed potatoes, spinach soufflé, and tapioca
   d. Fried chicken, baked potato, green beans, and chocolate chip cookies

4. Which one of the following lists only items that would be included in fluid intake?
   a. Orange juice, soft boiled egg, toast
   b. Milk, soup, gelatin
   c. Water, mashed potatoes, egg custard
   d. Milk, ham sandwich, ice cream bar

5. Miss Lee drank one third of an 8-oz glass of iced tea. How many milliliters of fluid did Miss Lee drink?
   a. 60 mL
   b. 80 mL
   c. 100 mL
   d. 240 mL

6. Which one of the following lists foods that are good sources of protein?
   a. Steak, chicken, fish
   b. Spinach, carrots, beets
   c. Bread, cereal, rice
   d. Apples, oranges, bananas

7. Which one of the following nutrients accounts for 50% to 60% of our total body weight?
   a. Vitamin A
   b. Glucose
   c. Water
   d. Calcium

8. At the beginning of your shift, you give Mr. Gibson a water pitcher containing 270 mL of water. At the end of your shift, you note that 35 mL of water are left in the pitcher. How much water did Mr. Gibson drink?
   a. 35 mL
   b. 175 mL
   c. 235 mL
   d. 140 mL

9. Which of the following lists foods that are good sources of carbohydrates?
   a. Liver, fish, chicken
   b. Cereal, fruit, bread
   c. Milk, beans, cheese
   d. Water, soda, butter

10. Which one of the following can be harmful if too much is consumed?
   a. Folic acid
   b. Water-soluble vitamins (for example, vitamins C and B12)
   c. Fat-soluble vitamins (for example, vitamins A, D, E, and K)
   d. None of the above

11. Which health care professional is specially trained to plan for the patient's or resident's nutritional needs and teach about good nutrition?
a. The nurse
b. The dietitian
c. The nursing assistant
d. The doctor

12. Which one of the following can affect a person's food likes and dislikes?
a. The person's religious beliefs
b. The person's culture
c. Where the person lives
d. All of the above

13. Hot foods must be kept at or above what temperature to avoid pathogen growth?
a. 100°F
b. 100°C
c. 40°C
d. 140°F

Matching *Match the amount of fluid in milliliters (mL) with the same amount in ounces (oz).*

_____ **1.** 240 mL

_____ **2.** 180 mL

_____ **3.** 300 mL

_____ **4.** 30 mL

_____ **5.** 120 mL

_____ **6.** 150 mL

a. 10 oz
b. 5 oz
c. 8 oz
d. 4 oz
e. 1 oz
f. 6 oz

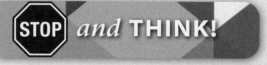

■ Mrs. Giovanni was recently admitted to your long-term care facility. Her body weight falls in the underweight range, and her doctor wants her to consume more calories each day. The problem is Mrs. Giovanni will only eat about half of her meal at mealtime. She says, "I just get full quickly." What are some ways you may be able to help Mrs. Giovanni improve her nutritional intake?

■ You work in an assisted-living facility, and one of your residents, Mr. Wayne, has severe arthritis in his hands. The arthritis makes it hard for Mr. Wayne to use his silverware, but he refuses to let you help him eat. He says that he'll let you feed him "if and when they cut off both of my hands!" Lately, the arthritis has gotten much worse and Mr. Wayne is having more and more difficulty eating. Most of the food winds up beside the plate, instead of in his mouth, and what little food makes it to his mouth is cold by the time it gets there. You know that Mr. Wayne has to eat to maintain his health. What can you do to assist Mr. Wayne in feeding himself? What member of the staff could you ask to assist you?

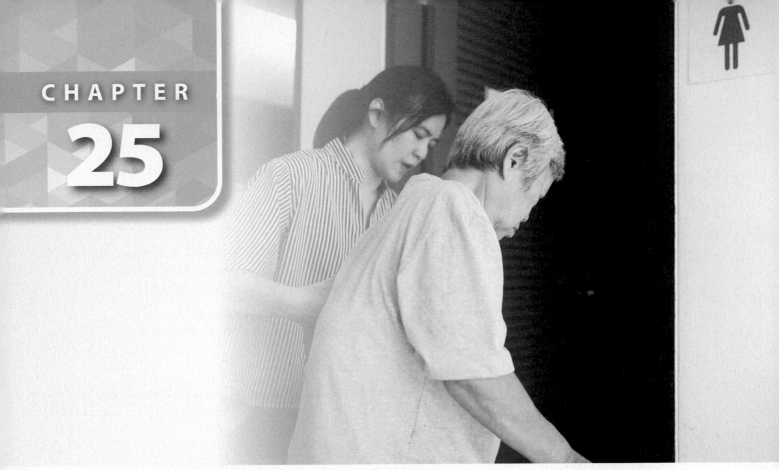

Photo: Nursing assistants help their patients or residents to meet their elimination needs by providing assistance as necessary.

25

Assisting With Urinary and Bowel Elimination

 WHAT WILL YOU LEARN?

In Chapter 24, you learned about how we take in food and convert it to energy in a process called *metabolism*. During this conversion process, waste materials (or by-products) are created. These waste products must be removed from our bodies, or we will become sick. Wastes are eliminated from the body in various forms. The urinary system rids the body of waste products that have been filtered from the bloodstream, along with excess fluid, in the form of urine. The digestive system rids the body of the solid waste that is left over from the foods that we eat, in the form of feces, or bowel movements. Although there are other ways the body rids itself of waste, urinary and bowel elimination—and assisting your patients or residents with both as needed—is the subject of this chapter. When you are finished with this chapter, you will be able to:

1. Describe two methods the body uses to eliminate waste products.
2. Discuss attitudes that people may have regarding the processes of urinary or bowel elimination.
3. Explain why normal urinary and bowel elimination is essential to health and actions the nursing assistant can take to promote normal elimination.

457

4. List normal characteristics of urine and describe observations that a nursing assistant may make when assisting a person with urinary elimination that should be reported to the nurse.

5. Demonstrate methods used to measure and record urinary output.

6. Describe the use of urinary catheters and demonstrate how to provide routine catheter care.

7. Describe five types of urinary incontinence and methods the nursing assistant uses to assist people who are incontinent of urine.

8. Discuss the process of bowel elimination and characteristics of normal stool.

9. Define problems with bowel elimination that are often seen in the health care setting.

10. List the types of enemas and discuss reasons why a person may require an enema.

11. Demonstrate proper technique for assisting with urinary and bowel elimination, obtaining urine and stool samples, providing catheter care, and administering enemas.

12. Demonstrate how to provide routine stoma care.

Vocabulary

Bedside commode	Frequency	Catheter care	Laxative
Bedpan	Urgency	Urinary incontinence	Stool softeners
Fracture pan	Nocturia	Urinary retention	Fiber supplements
Urinal	Dysuria	Condom catheter	Fecal impaction
Urinalysis	Oliguria	Chyme	Digital examination
Midstream ("clean catch") urine specimen	Polyuria	Peristalsis	Flatulence
	Diuresis	Feces	Fecal (bowel) incontinence
Urination	Anuria	Defecate	
Voiding	Catheter	Stool	Enema
Micturition	Straight catheter	Flatus	Ostomy
Hematuria	Indwelling catheter	Diarrhea	Ileostomy
Occult	Suprapubic catheter	Constipation	Colostomy

ASSISTING WITH ELIMINATION

Your patients or residents may have physical or cognitive difficulties that affect their ability to manage urinary or bowel elimination, or both. As a nursing assistant, you will need to assist your patients or residents with elimination as necessary.

Elimination Equipment

Many of your patients or residents will need no more assistance with elimination than a steady arm to lean on during the trip to the bathroom. The bathrooms in many health care facilities have special features that make them easier for people with physical disabilities to use (Fig. 25-1A). For example, hand rails attached to the walls alongside the toilet or onto the toilet itself make it easier for the person to sit down and get back up. Some toilets have higher seats, so the person does not have to bend their knees as much to sit down and get back up. Modifications like these allow many patients or residents to use the toilet in the bathroom with very little assistance from you. However, some of your patients or residents may not be able to get out of bed at all, or they may be too weak or ill to walk to the bathroom. These people will need more help with elimination, and special equipment.

Bedside Commodes

For a person who is able to get out of bed, but who is not able to walk to the bathroom, a bedside

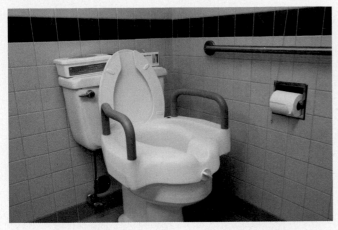

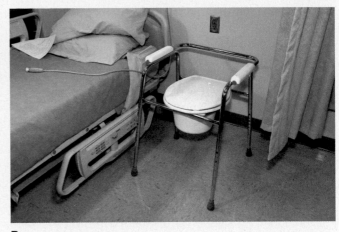

A   **B**

Figure 25-1 A. Many toilets in health care facilities have special modifications that make them easier to use. **B.** A bedside commode can be used if a person can get out of bed but is not capable of walking the distance to the bathroom.

commode can make toileting easier (see Fig. 25-1B). The **bedside commode** is a chair frame with a toilet seat and a removable collection bucket. Bedside commodes are available in different sizes that can accommodate very small or very large patients or residents. If the person is weak or unsteady, you will need to help them get out of bed and over to the bedside commode.

Bedpans

A **bedpan** is used for elimination when a person is unable to get out of bed at all (Fig. 25-2A). A female patient or resident who cannot get out of bed uses a bedpan to urinate, and for bowel movements. A male patient or resident who cannot get out of bed uses a bedpan for bowel movements, and a urinal to urinate (see next section).

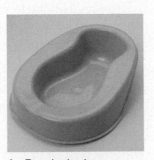

A. Regular bedpan

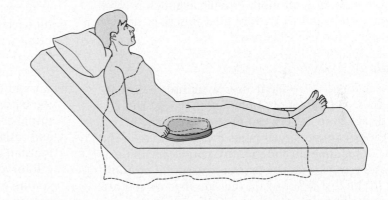

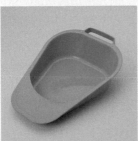

B. Fracture pan

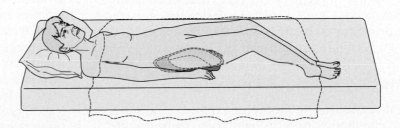

Figure 25-2 Bedpans are used for females who cannot get out of bed to urinate or have a bowel movement. A male also uses a bedpan for bowel movements. **A.** A standard bedpan. Position a standard bedpan like a regular toilet seat—the buttocks are placed on the wide, rounded shelf, with the open end pointed toward the foot of the bed. **B.** A fracture pan. Position a fracture pan with the thin edge toward the head of the bed.

Bedpans, while sometimes necessary, must be used with extreme care. It is very easy to bruise or tear the fragile skin of an older person or a person with a disability. In addition to causing immediate pain to the person, an injury like this can also lead to the formation of a pressure ulcer later on. Arthritis can make using a bedpan very painful, as can fractures of the back or legs. If a person has an injury or disability that makes it too uncomfortable or dangerous to use a regular bedpan, a special, wedge-shaped bedpan called a **fracture pan** is placed underneath the person's buttocks, with the thin edge toward the person's back (Fig. 25-2B). The fracture bedpan is usually easier to use and more comfortable for very thin or much older people.

Using a bedpan is uncomfortable, which alone can cause the person to have difficulty using it. Many facilities use disposable bedpans that are made from molded plastic. However, some facilities still use bedpans made from stainless steel. If the facility where you work uses metal bedpans, be sure to warm the bedpan before offering it to the patient or resident. You can do this by wrapping the bedpan in a warm towel, or running warm water over the seat area and then drying it before use. Rubbing a small amount of powder on the rim of the bedpan can make it easier to slide under the person. If the person's condition allows, raise the head of the bed to promote a more natural elimination position. Provide as much privacy as safely as possible. Procedure 25-1 describes how to help a person to use a bedpan.

Urinals

A male patient or resident uses a **urinal** to urinate when they cannot get out of bed (Fig. 25-3). The urinal is designed to fit between the person's legs. To urinate, the person puts their penis in the opening of the urinal. Depending on the person's condition, the urinal may be used with the person in a sitting position, either in the bed or sitting on the side. The person can also use the urinal by standing and leaning against the side of the bed. If the person is very weak or disabled, you may need to place their penis inside the opening of the urinal for them. Procedure 25-2 describes how to help a person to use a urinal.

Promoting Normal Elimination

Being in a health care facility can change a person's normal elimination patterns, which can cause health problems. The most effective method of treating urinary and bowel problems is to prevent them from happening in the first place. As a nursing assistant, you can help promote normal urinary and bowel function for your patients or residents. The following tips are simple, but effective.

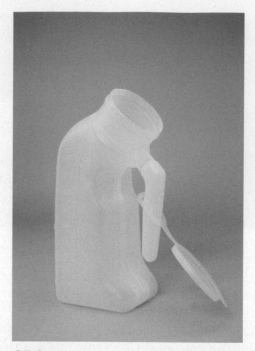

Figure 25-3 Males who cannot get out of bed to urinate can use a urinal.

- Encourage plenty of fluids, unless a person has a medical condition that requires fluid restriction. Drinking plenty of fluids helps the kidneys work properly, and regular urination flushes harmful bacteria from the bladder, helping to prevent urinary tract infections. In addition, drinking enough fluids helps to keep the feces soft, making bowel movements easier.
- Answer call lights promptly and take people to the bathroom or provide them with a bedpan or urinal as soon as they ask you to. Many patients and residents do not want to "bother" the nursing staff and will wait until the last minute to call for assistance with the bedpan or for help getting to the bathroom. If the person must wait too long for help to arrive, they may have an accident. Many falls that occur in long-term care facilities are the result of a resident rushing to make it to the bathroom.
- Encourage your patients or residents to call when they first feel the urge to void. This can help prevent accidents. In addition, "holding" urine or feces is not only uncomfortable, it can lead to problems such as constipation.
- Offer people the chance to eliminate frequently, especially if they must remain in bed or in a wheelchair, have dementia, or require assistance. Some people may find it easier to accept an offer of assistance than to ask for help.
- Provide privacy and comfort. A person is able to urinate or have a bowel movement much more

easily if they are warm enough, in a comfortable position, and have as much privacy as possible. Most females urinate and have bowel movements in a sitting or squatting position. Help a female patient or resident to sit upright by elevating the head of the bed (if they are using a bedpan), or have them lean forward a bit while seated on the toilet or bedside commode. Most males stand up to urinate and sit down to have a bowel movement. Some have no difficulty using a urinal while lying down, but others will need to sit up or even to stand. In this case, you may need to help the person to sit or stand up.

If a person is having difficulty urinating, there are some things you can do to help. For example, try turning on the faucet and allowing water to run into the sink. The sound of running water, which accompanied many of our early toilet training lessons, can help a person relax enough to start the urine stream. The sound of the running water also helps to cover up the sounds of urination, which may put some people more at ease. Putting the person's fingers in a basin of warm water can also help stimulate urination.

If a person is having difficulty moving their bowels, make sure that the person does not feel rushed. Many people like to read while having a bowel movement. Some people find that drinking warm fluids (such as coffee, tea, or warm water with lemon) helps stimulate the bowels to empty. Finally, regular exercise and foods that contain insoluble fiber help to promote regular bowel movements.

General guidelines for assisting a person with elimination are given in Guidelines Box 25-1.

Obtaining Urine and Stool Specimens

Because the contents of a person's urine or feces can provide a doctor with clues about the person's overall health status, you may be asked to obtain a urine or stool specimen (sample) for laboratory study. When assisting with specimen collection, it is very important to make sure that the specimen container is properly labeled with the person's name and room number. Otherwise, a person may be diagnosed with, and receive treatment for, a condition they do not have! Most health care settings now use computer-generated

Helping Hands and a Caring Heart

Focus on Humanistic Health Care

Everyone urinates and has bowel movements. However, most people consider elimination a private activity and would prefer not to discuss it with others. In a health care facility, people may be forced to think about and discuss elimination much more than they would normally care to! Think about how it would affect you to be a patient or a resident in a health care facility. Nurses and nursing assistants ask you about your bathroom patterns. They want to know if you have had a bowel movement today, how big it was, and what it looked like. They want you to urinate into a cup and then carry the sample to the nurses' station in full view of everyone. You may have to share a bathroom, or worse yet, use a bedpan while being separated from other people in the room by only a curtain! Elimination, especially when it must take place in a fairly public way, is very embarrassing for many people.

A patient or a resident in a health care facility may have difficulty with elimination, especially if elimination must occur under conditions that are not as private as the person would like. Regardless of the amount of assistance that your patients or residents need, privacy and consideration for individual preferences are essential. Provide privacy to the extent possible with regard to

the safety of the person. Close the bathroom door, or close the privacy curtains and the door to the room, if the person cannot use the regular toilet. If there are visitors present, ask them to step outside the room for a few minutes. Always make sure the call light is in reach so that the person can call you when they are ready for assistance. Some people are too weak or unsteady to be left alone while they urinate or have a bowel movement. In fact, some people will actually need for you to help hold them in the correct position during elimination. Being professional, kind, and straightforward about the "business at hand" will help ease your patient's or resident's embarrassment.

Similarly, it is important to help your patients or residents keep their sense of dignity. Feelings of embarrassment and shame are made worse when patients or residents accidentally soil themselves, their bed linens, or their clothing with urine or feces. This is a fairly common occurrence in health care facilities. The effects of medications, being in a strange place, reluctance to ask for help, and physical or mental disabilities can all lead to accidents. Again, kindness, empathy, and a professional attitude can go a long way toward easing the patient's or resident's embarrassment.

Guidelines Box 25-1 Guidelines for Assisting With Elimination

WHAT YOU DO	WHY YOU DO IT
Always honor a person's request for assistance with elimination as quickly as possible.	Answering call lights quickly builds trust and prevents accidents. If a person who is bed bound must wait too long for assistance, they could have an accident in the bed. A weak or unsteady person may try to walk to the bathroom on their own, rather than waiting for help to arrive. This puts the person at risk for a fall. Finally, it is very uncomfortable to "hold" urine or feces for a long time, and doing so can change the normal elimination patterns, causing health problems.
Always provide the person with as much privacy as safety considerations will allow.	Regular elimination is essential to health, so it is important to make this process as normal as possible for your patients or residents. Many people have difficulty urinating or having a bowel movement if they think that someone else can hear them, or if someone else is in the bathroom with them.
If you leave the person alone, always make sure that the call light control is within easy reach of the person.	The person will need the call light control to let you know when they are finished, or needs help.
Make sure the toilet paper is within easy reach of the person. If the person is unable to wipe themselves, assist with this task.	Wiping promotes comfort and helps to prevent irritation, odors, and infection.
Be sure to provide good perineal care as necessary, especially after bowel movements (see Chapter 22).	Good perineal care promotes comfort and helps to prevent irritation, odors, and infection.
Provide the person with the chance to wash their hands after elimination. This can be accomplished by stopping by the sink if the person is in the bathroom, or by providing a warm, wet washcloth or moist hand wipes after assisting the person from the bedside commode or removing the bedpan or urinal.	Most people prefer to wash their hands after using the toilet. Allowing people to follow their normal routines whenever possible is important, especially when other aspects of the routine need to be altered. In addition, handwashing is important for hygiene.
Always wear gloves when assisting a person with elimination, or when handling a bedpan, bedside commode bucket, or urinal that contains waste.	Urine and feces are considered body fluids and may contain pathogens.
When wearing gloves while assisting a person with elimination, be sure to remove at least one glove prior to touching side rails, door knobs, or other objects in the person's room. You may need to change gloves several times while assisting a person with elimination.	Gloves that are possibly contaminated with urine or fecal material will spread germs to other objects and surfaces that you touch.
Before disposing of waste, observe the feces or urine for amount and any unusual characteristics. Report and record your observations.	Abnormalities in the urine or feces could indicate a health problem.

Guidelines Box 25-1 Guidelines for Assisting With Elimination (*continued*)

WHAT YOU DO	WHY YOU DO IT
Never place a bedpan or urinal on an over-bed table or bedside table, even if the bedpan or urinal is clean. Dirty bedpans and urinals are taken to the bathroom immediately after use and cleaned and disinfected according to facility policy. If a bedpan or urinal must be set down while you help wipe the person or pull up clothing, bed linens, or the side rail, place it on a chair that is covered with paper towels. Clean bedpans are either stored in a cabinet underneath the bedside table or returned to the equipment room. Clean urinals may be hung over the side rail, stored in a cabinet, or returned to the equipment room.	The over-bed table and bedside table are considered "clean" areas. Even if the bedpan or urinal is clean, most people do not want items associated with elimination placed on surfaces where they eat or have personal items displayed.
If there are odors in the room as a result of elimination, use an air freshener.	Most people will appreciate the use of an air freshener to make the air in the room smell fresher. Just be professional in any remarks you may make about the odor.
Disinfect equipment used for elimination carefully, according to facility policy.	Bedpans, urinals, and bedside commode buckets can act as fomites (that is, nonliving objects that can transmit pathogens and cause infection) if they are not properly disinfected.

labels for specimen containers. Please be sure that you have the label for the correct patient or resident when preparing to collect a specimen.

It is also important to make sure that the specimen is handled correctly after you obtain it. For example, in certain situations, the specimen may need to be delivered to the laboratory while it is still warm, or placed in a special plastic transport bag. If a specimen is not being delivered to the laboratory right away, then it needs to be stored properly until the scheduled pick-up time. Before collecting *any* specimen—of urine, feces, or any other body fluid—always ask yourself the following questions:

- Do I have the right person?
- Do I have the right laboratory requisition slip? (The laboratory requisition slip states the person's name, the date, and the type of test to be done. It is filled out by the nurse and sent with the specimen to the laboratory.)
- What method is to be used to collect the specimen?
- Do I have the right type of specimen container?
- Is the specimen container properly labeled?
- What is the correct date and time?
- What storage and delivery method must I use?

Finally, always remember to wear gloves when assisting with specimen collection and when handling the specimen containers. Specimen containers

that are sent to a lab for analysis should always be placed in a sealed specimen bag. Be careful not to contaminate the outside of the bag with your gloved hands.

Obtaining a Urine Specimen

Urinalysis, or examination of the urine under a microscope and by chemical means, is a commonly used diagnostic tool in the health care setting. Substances found in urine during urinalysis can help doctors diagnose kidney disease, certain metabolic diseases, and infections. The collection and analysis of urine over the course of 24 hours allows for evaluation of kidney function.

Depending on the situation, the method of collecting a urine specimen may vary. For routine urinalysis, no special collection procedures are necessary. The person is asked to urinate directly into the specimen cup, if possible. If this is difficult for the person, they can urinate into a specimen collection device ("commode hat"; see Chapter 24, Fig. 24-17), or into a bedpan or urinal. The person must not have a bowel movement at the same time the urine is being collected, or place toilet paper in the collection device, because these actions will change the urinalysis results. The urine is then poured from the collection device, bedpan, or urinal into the specimen cup. The procedure for obtaining a routine urine sample is described in Procedure 25-3.

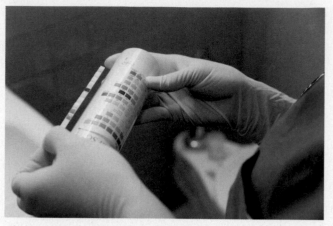

Figure 25-4 Chemically treated reagent strips are used to test urine for some substances. Your facility may train you to do this type of urinalysis.

In some situations, it may be necessary to obtain a **midstream ("clean catch") urine specimen** using a sterile specimen container. This method of collecting urine prevents contamination of the urine by the bacteria that normally live in and around the urethra. A midstream ("clean catch") urine specimen is usually ordered when the doctor suspects a urinary tract infection. This way, if any bacteria are found in the urine sample, the doctor knows that they are the ones most likely responsible for the infection. When a midstream ("clean catch") urine specimen is requested, the person is asked to clean the area around the urethral opening with a special cleansing wipe. The urine flow is started, then stopped, then started again. The urine sample is collected from the restarted flow. Procedure 25-4 describes how to assist a person with obtaining a midstream ("clean catch") urine specimen.

Your facility or agency may train you to do a type of routine urine testing that involves dipping chemically treated paper strips into a urine sample. Chemicals on the paper react with certain substances that may be found in the urine, causing the chemical blocks on the paper to change color if these substances are present in the urine. The paper is then compared with a color chart that comes with the strips (Fig. 25-4), and the results are recorded in the person's chart and reported to the nurse.

Obtaining a Stool Sample

Stool can be analyzed for the presence of blood, pathogens (such as parasites or bacteria), fat, and other things that are not normally found in feces. Because people do not have bowel movements as often as they urinate, if a stool sample is needed, the person should be notified well in advance so that the specimen can be collected when it becomes

available. Ask the nurse if there are any particular collection methods that should be used. Stool can be collected in a bedpan, bedside commode, or in a collection device placed onto a regular toilet. The person must not urinate at the same time the stool sample is being collected, or place toilet paper in the collection device, because these actions will change the test results. The procedure for collecting a stool sample is given in Procedure 25-5.

URINARY ELIMINATION

The urinary system, which is discussed in more detail in Chapter 37, is made up of the kidneys, ureters, urinary bladder, and urethra (Fig. 25-5). Blood passes through the kidneys, which remove waste products and excess fluid, forming urine. It takes the kidneys approximately one half hour to process the body's total blood volume. As it forms, the urine flows from the kidneys through the ureters and is stored in the urinary bladder. As the

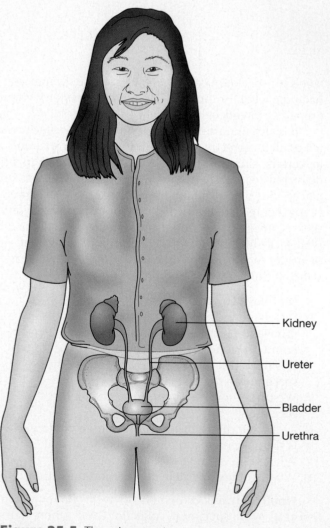

Kidney

Ureter

Bladder

Urethra

Figure 25-5 The urinary system.

bladder fills, we begin to feel the urge to urinate. Urine leaves the body through the urethra.

The process of passing urine from the body is known by several terms, including **urination, voiding**, and **micturition**. Many of your patients or residents will have their own terms for urinating, such as "peeing" or "passing water." When talking about urination with a patient or resident, you should use words that the person is familiar with. This is especially important when talking with children.

In healthy people, urine is clear, without cloudiness or particles. Sometimes urine that has been in a container for a while will become cloudy as it cools. Healthy urine is pale yellow, straw-colored, or dark gold (amber) in color, with a slight odor. A slight red tinge to the urine may indicate **hematuria**, or the presence of blood in the urine. This is an abnormal finding. Sometimes hematuria is **occult** (that is, hidden) and must be detected using urinalysis. Some foods and medications can also affect the color and odor of urine. When you are helping a patient or resident with urination, observe the urine and report any abnormalities to the nurse. Urine with an unusual odor or appearance could be a sign of illness or infection.

The frequency of voiding, and the amount of urine voided each time, will differ from person to person. Many factors influence a person's urination habits, including the amount of fluids the person drinks, the types of medications the person takes, the person's age, and the person's lifelong tendencies. For example, some people void quite frequently, at the first urge, while others may hold their urine for as long as possible, even if a bathroom is readily available. You will soon become aware of the urination habits that are normal for each person in your care. This knowledge will allow you to recognize any changes that may occur. For example, **frequency** is the term used to describe voiding that occurs more often than usual. Frequency is often accompanied by a feeling of **urgency**, or the need to urinate immediately. A person with a urinary tract infection may experience frequency and urgency. **Nocturia** is the need to get up more than once or twice during the night to urinate, to the point where sleep is disrupted. Nocturia can be a sign of pain or depression, a prostate or bladder disorder, or heart failure.

Urination should not cause discomfort. **Dysuria** is difficulty voiding that may or may not be associated with pain. Some people describe the discomfort they feel during urination as a "burning" or "cramping" sensation. Dysuria is often associated with bladder infections, prostate problems, and some sexually transmitted infections (STIs).

Tell the Nurse!

Changes in the quality of a person's urine or urination habits can be a sign that something is wrong. Be sure to report the following observations to the nurse immediately:

- The urine is cloudy or contains particles, has an abnormal color, or has an abnormal odor

- The person complains that the urine is difficult or painful to pass (that is, the person has dysuria)

- The person is experiencing frequency, urgency, or both

- The person needs to get up more frequently than usual to use the bathroom during the night

- The person is having incontinence accidents, or more frequent incontinence accidents

Measuring Urine Output

As you learned in Chapter 24, urine output is a key indicator of fluid balance. In a person who is maintaining a good fluid balance, urine output is neither too high nor too low.

- **Oliguria** is the state of voiding a very small amount of urine over a given period of time (for example, voiding only 100 to 400 mL of urine over 24 hours). *Olig-* means "few" and *-uria* means "urine." A person who is dehydrated might become oliguric (that is, have a urine output that is well below normal).

- **Polyuria** (*poly-* means "many") is excessive urine output. Polyuria, also known as **diuresis**, can be a sign of a health problem. For example, polyuria can be a symptom of poorly controlled diabetes. Or, polyuria may be the desired effect of a medication. For example, a person who is retaining excessive amounts of fluid (for example, as the result of a heart disorder) may be put on a medication called a diuretic to help rid the body of the extra fluid. The polyuria that results is a sign that the medication is having the desired effect.

Evaluating a person's urine output is also a good way to determine how well a person's kidneys are working. **Anuria** (*an-* means "none") is defined as the state of voiding less than 100 mL of urine over the course of 24 hours. Anuria usually indicates that a person is in kidney failure.

Not all of the people you care for will need to have their urine output measured and recorded, but people who have illnesses or take medications that may alter their body's ability to maintain a healthy fluid balance will need to have their urine output measured regularly. Some people who are critically ill will have their urine output measured and recorded every hour, but most people in the health care setting have routine orders for their urine output to be measured and recorded each shift.

If a person uses a regular toilet, you will need to remind the person to void into a specimen collection device ("commode hat") and call you after they have finished voiding so that you can measure and record the amount of urine. Specimen collection devices, urinals, and the drainage bags used with urinary catheters often have markings that make measuring urine output easy. If they do not, then the urine output can be measured by pouring it into a graduate. A graduate is also used to measure urine output if a person voids into a bedpan or bedside commode bucket. Remember to place the graduate on a flat surface and view it at eye level when measuring urine so that your measurements are accurate.

If the urine output of one of your residents or patients is being monitored, you will need to keep a record of the amount of urine passed at each voiding. Some intake and output (I&O) flow sheets will have spaces to record the amount of each individual voiding, while others may only have a space to record the end-of-shift amount. To obtain the end-of-shift amount, simply add the individual amounts together and record the total in the appropriate space.

Urinary Catheterization

Sometimes a person is unable to urinate using a toilet, bedpan, urinal, or bedside commode, due to disability or illness. In these situations, a urinary catheter is used. A **catheter** is a tube that is inserted into the body for the purpose of administering or removing fluids. A urinary catheter is inserted into the bladder through the urethra (or through an incision made in the abdominal wall) to allow the urine in the bladder to drain out. A urinary catheter is used in many different situations, including:

- To drain the bladder before or during a surgical procedure, during recovery from a serious illness or injury, or to collect urine for testing
- For a person who is incontinent of urine, if the person has wounds or pressure ulcers that would be made worse by contact with urine
- When a person is unable to urinate because of an obstruction in the urethra

Usually, inserting a urinary catheter is beyond the scope of practice for a nursing assistant, although in some facilities, nursing assistants are provided with additional training that allows them to catheterize

residents or patients. Inserting a catheter is a procedure that requires sterile technique because it involves putting a foreign object (that is, the catheter) into a person's body. If sterile technique is not used, the catheter can introduce infection-causing bacteria into the bladder. Regardless of whether or not you are trained to actually insert urinary catheters, caring for people who have urinary catheters in place will almost certainly be a part of your daily duties.

Taking It to the Next Level:
Advanced Skills

More in-depth information related to advanced skills used when caring for a person with a urinary catheter can be found in *Lippincott Acute Care Skills for Advanced Nursing Assistants*. Visit thePoint® at thepoint.lww.com for access to the ebook.

Types of Urinary Catheters

You will see many different types of urinary catheters in use.

Straight Catheters

A **straight catheter**, also known as a Robinson, Rob-Nel, or Red Rubber catheter, is used when the catheter is to be inserted and removed immediately. The catheter is introduced into the bladder, the urine is allowed to drain out, and the catheter is removed (Fig. 25-6A). This type of catheterization may be used to obtain a sterile urine specimen from a female, before or after surgery, after a vaginal delivery, or when a person needs to empty their bladder but cannot as a result of pain or swelling that is temporary. New guidelines issued by the CDC state that urinary catheters should not be used to obtain urine samples from a person who is able to void voluntarily because of the increased risk of infection.

Indwelling Catheters

An **indwelling catheter**, also known as a retention or Foley catheter, is left inside the bladder to provide continuous urine drainage. An indwelling catheter has a soft balloon that is inflated inside the bladder to keep the catheter from sliding out of the urethra (see Fig. 25-6B). Urine collects in a drainage bag, which is attached to the indwelling catheter by a length of tubing.

An indwelling catheter may have two lumens or three lumens (Fig. 25-7). A double-lumen indwelling catheter has two lumens. One lumen, which connects to the catheter tubing, is for urine drainage. The other is used to inflate the balloon that holds the catheter

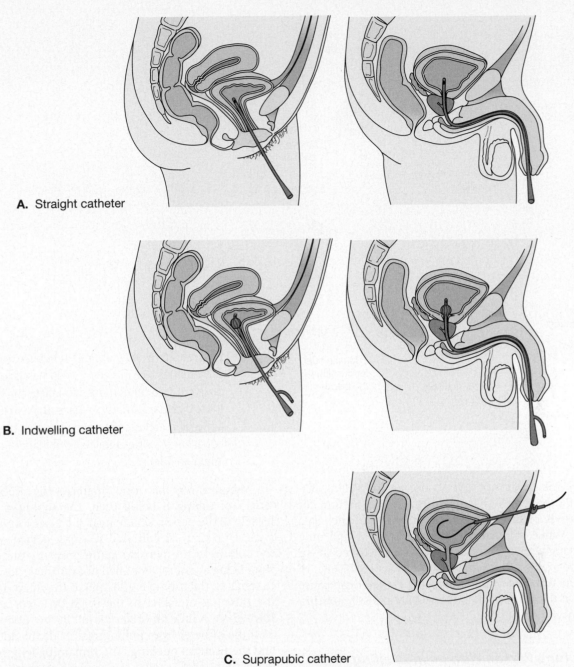

A. Straight catheter

B. Indwelling catheter

C. Suprapubic catheter

Figure 25-6 Types of catheters. **A.** A straight catheter is inserted into the bladder, the urine is drained, and then the catheter is removed. **B.** An indwelling catheter, also known as a Foley catheter or a retention catheter, remains in the body and urine drains continuously into a drainage bag. **C.** A suprapubic catheter is inserted into the bladder through a surgical incision made above the pubic bone (*supra-* means "above"). A suprapubic catheter is a bit less likely to promote urinary infections because its location keeps the opening away from the contaminated perineal area.

in place. A triple-lumen indwelling catheter has three lumens. The extra lumen is used to flush the bladder with irrigation fluid. Regular flushing of the bladder with irrigation fluid helps to keep blood clots from forming inside the bladder. This is important in certain situations, such as when a person has just had prostate surgery.

Suprapubic Catheters

A **suprapubic catheter** is a type of indwelling catheter. The suprapubic catheter is inserted into the bladder through a surgical incision made in the abdominal wall, right above the pubic bone (see Fig. 25-6C). This type of catheter is most often used for people with blocked urethras, after some gynecologic surgeries, and for males.

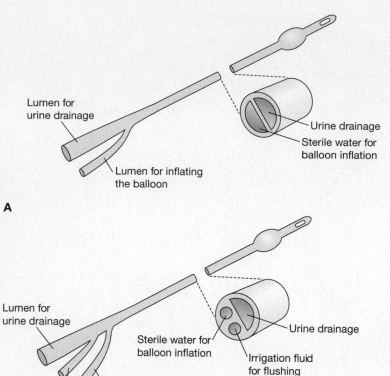

A

Lumen for
urine drainage

Lumen for inflating
the balloon

Urine drainage

Sterile water for
balloon inflation

B

Lumen for
urine drainage

Sterile water for
balloon inflation

Lumen for flushing
the bladder

Lumen for inflating
the balloon

Urine drainage

Irrigation fluid
for flushing
the bladder

Figure 25-7 A. A double-lumen indwelling catheter has two lumens. One lumen is for urine drainage. The other is used to inflate the balloon that holds the catheter in place. **B.** A triple-lumen indwelling catheter has three lumens. The additional lumen is used to flush the bladder with irrigation fluid.

Typically, males are not able to use an indwelling urinary catheter that is inserted through the urethra for long periods of time due to the anatomy of the male urethra. While a female's urethra is straight and only about 2 inches long, a male's urethra is curved in an "S" shape and is about 6 inches long (see Fig. 25-6B). In males, the pressure of the indwelling catheter can cause erosion of the mucous membrane that lines the urethra in the curved areas.

Caring for a Person With an Indwelling Urinary Catheter

Indwelling urinary catheters are connected by a length of tubing to a urine drainage bag. Urine drains continuously from the bladder, through the catheter, down the tubing, and into the drainage bag (Fig. 25-8). There are several different types of urine drainage bags that you will see in the health care setting. Some urine drainage bags have a long length of tubing that allows them to be carried or secured to a bed frame or the back of a wheelchair. Other urine drainage bags, called "leg bags," are connected to the catheter by a short length of tubing and secured to the person's thigh with straps. Leg bags are useful because they can be concealed underneath a person's clothing and they allow the person to move around freely.

When a regular urine drainage bag with a long length of tubing is being used, the tubing is secured loosely to the person's body near the insertion site using a catheter strap or adhesive securing device. Securing the tubing to the person's body prevents the catheter from being accidentally pulled out during repositioning. In females, the tubing is attached to the thigh. In males, the tubing is attached to the thigh or lower abdomen (Fig. 25-9). A little bit of slack is left in the tubing to prevent the catheter from pulling against the bladder outlet and the urethral opening. The remaining length of tubing is then gently coiled and secured to the bed linens using a plastic clip (Fig. 25-10). Coiling the tubing prevents the tubing from becoming bent or kinked, which would stop the free flow of urine into the drainage bag. Coiling the tubing and securing it to the bed linens also keeps the weight of the tubing from pulling against the person's body. The drainage bag is then secured to the bed frame or the back of the person's wheelchair, at a level lower than the person's bladder (Fig. 25-11). If the drainage bag and tubing are higher than the person's bladder, then gravity could cause old, contaminated urine to run back down the tubing and into the person's bladder, causing an infection.

All urine drainage bags have a connection adapter (where the catheter tubing attaches) and an emptying spout that is opened to allow urine to drain from the

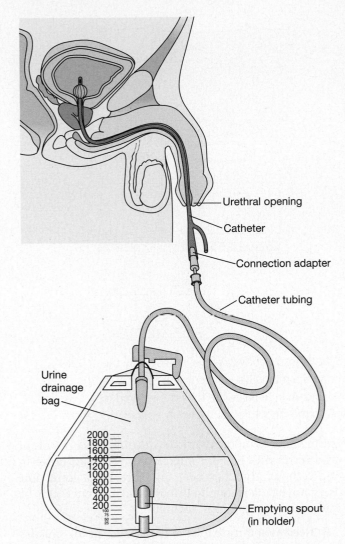

- Urethral opening
- Catheter
- Connection adapter
- Catheter tubing
- Urine drainage bag
- Emptying spout (in holder)

2000
1800
1600
1400
1200
1000
800
600
400
200
100
75
50
25

Figure 25-8 The indwelling urinary catheter drainage system consists of a catheter that is connected to a urine drainage bag by way of a length of tubing. The urine drainage bag has a connection adapter, where the tubing attaches, and an emptying spout, which is unclamped to allow the urine to drain from the bag. When not in use, the emptying spout is stored in a holder that is part of the bag.

bag. Because the inside of the catheter and tubing is sterile, it is safer for the person if the bag is not disconnected from the tubing once the catheter is in place. Disconnecting the bag from the tubing can allow harmful bacteria to enter the catheter. Occasionally, the tubing has to be disconnected from the bag (for example, to change the bag if it is leaking, to replace a regular drainage bag with a leg bag, or to perform certain procedures). If you must disconnect the tubing from the bag, be sure to prevent the end of the tubing from touching anything, and wipe the exposed tubing with an antibacterial wipe before reconnecting the drainage bag. General guidelines for caring for a person with an indwelling catheter are given in Guidelines Box 25-2.

Providing Catheter Care

Although you may not be permitted to catheterize your patients or residents, you will most likely be responsible for providing catheter care. **Catheter care** involves thorough cleaning of the perineal area (especially around the urethra) and the catheter tubing that extends outside of the body, to prevent infection. Providing good catheter care is important because the catheter provides a pathway for bacteria to travel up from the perineum into the bladder, where they can cause infection. In addition, having a catheter in place eliminates the "flushing" action of normal urination, which helps to remove bacteria from the urinary tract naturally. Because bacteria can be introduced into the body both when a urinary catheter is inserted and after it is in place, urinary tract infections in catheterized people are among the most common health care–associated infections (HAIs). (Remember that HAIs are acquired in the health care setting.)

In an effort to reduce the risk of HAIs in people who are catheterized, many facilities require catheter care to be provided routinely (for example, once or twice daily), and again whenever the perineal area becomes soiled (such as when a person is incontinent of feces). Soap and water or a special cleanser should be used when providing catheter care. The procedure for providing catheter care is given in Procedure 25-6.

Emptying Urine Drainage Bags

Urine drainage bags are routinely emptied and the urine measured at the end of each shift unless ordered otherwise. Urine drainage bags should also be emptied if they become too full. Leg bags need to be emptied frequently because they are smaller and hold less urine. The procedure for emptying a urine drainage bag is given in Procedure 25-7.

Tell the Nurse!

When caring for a catheterized person, make sure you report any of the following observations to the nurse immediately:

- Changes in the color, clarity, or odor of the urine
- Failure of urine to flow freely through the tubing (make sure that the tubing is not kinked or bent)
- The person complains of pain or discomfort as a result of the catheter
- Redness, swelling, or discharge from the catheter insertion site
- Leaking of urine around the catheter insertion site

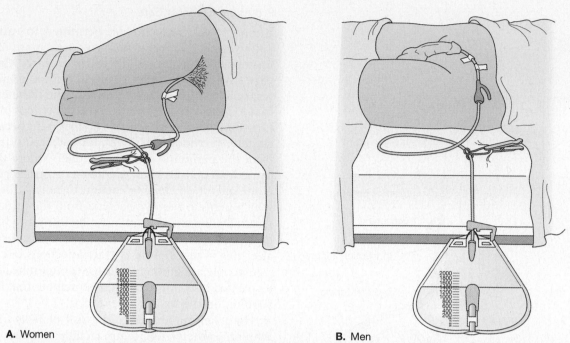

A. Women

B. Men

Figure 25-9 The catheter tubing is secured loosely to the person's body to prevent tension on the tubing and catheter, which could cause discomfort. Securing the tubing also prevents the catheter from accidentally being pulled out of the body during repositioning. **A.** In females, the tubing is secured to the inner thigh. **B.** In males, the tubing is connected either to the inner thigh or the lower abdomen.

Urinary Incontinence

Urinary incontinence is the inability to hold one's urine, or the involuntary loss of urine from the bladder. Urinary incontinence may be temporary or permanent. Temporary urinary incontinence can occur as a result of a bladder infection, or after an indwelling catheter that has been in place for a long time is removed. Permanent urinary incontinence can be caused by many things, including:

■ Decreased muscle tone in the bladder or the muscles that support the bladder, such as occurs after childbirth or from obesity

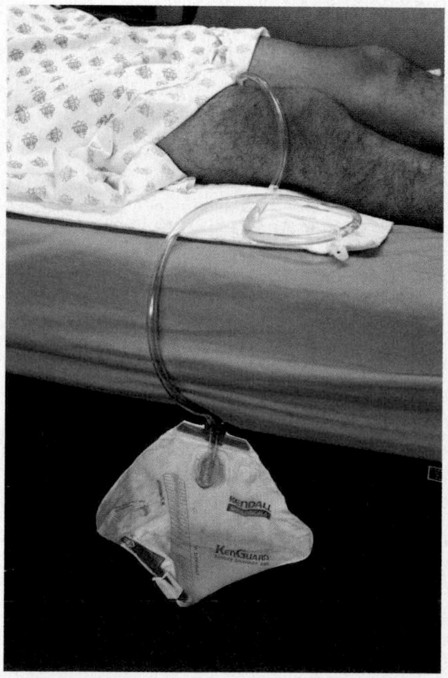

Figure 25-10 The catheter tubing is gently coiled (to prevent it from kinking) and secured to the bed linens with a plastic clip.

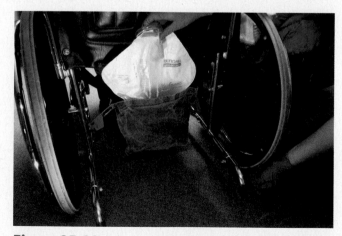

Figure 25-11 When a person with an indwelling urinary catheter is in a wheelchair, the urine drainage bag is attached to the back of the person's wheelchair, away from the wheels and at a level that is lower than the person's bladder. When the person is in bed, the urine drainage bag is attached to the bed frame (see Fig. 25-10).

Guidelines Box 25-2 Guidelines for Caring for People With Indwelling Catheters

WHAT YOU DO	WHY YOU DO IT
Loosely secure the catheter tubing to the person near the insertion site, using a catheter strap or adhesive device.	Securing the catheter tubing helps to prevent the catheter from being pulled out during repositioning. Allowing a little bit of slack helps to prevent the catheter from pulling against the bladder outlet and the urethral opening.
Gently coil the remaining length of tubing and secure it to the bed linens using a plastic clip.	Coiling the tubing helps to prevent kinking, which could stop the free flow of urine into the drainage bag. It also keeps the weight of the tubing from pulling against the area where the tubing is secured to the person's body.
When repositioning a person who has an indwelling catheter, always make sure to unclip the coiled tubing from the linens before beginning the procedure. When you are finished with the procedure, secure the coiled tubing to the linens again.	The person needs to be able to move freely during procedures such as repositioning. If you try to move a person in the direction opposite from the length of tubing, and the length of tubing is still attached to the bed linens, then the catheter could be pulled out of the person's body.
Make sure that the person is not lying on the coiled tubing.	This would be uncomfortable for the person. In addition, the weight of the person's body on the tubing could stop the free flow of urine into the drainage bag.
Always make sure the urine drainage bag is placed at a level lower than that of the person's bladder.	Raising the urine drainage bag up higher than the bladder can cause old, contaminated urine to run back into the bladder, which can lead to infection.
Never attach a urine drainage bag to a side rail. Instead, attach the drainage bag to the bed frame.	Raising the side rail would raise the drainage bag to a level that is higher than the person's bladder. The bed frame does not move; therefore, the level of the drainage bag cannot change.
Keep the drainage bag off the floor. When emptying the drainage bag, be sure that the open emptying spout does not touch anything.	Bacteria can enter the closed drainage system in this manner. The presence of bacteria in the system can lead to health care–associated urinary tract infections in people with indwelling catheters.
Always wear gloves when emptying the urine drainage bag.	Urine is a body fluid and may contain pathogens.
Empty the collecting bag using a separate graduate for each patient or resident.	Using a separate graduate for each person helps to prevent the transfer of harmful bacteria from one person to another.

- Injuries or illnesses that affect the spinal cord, the brain, or the nerves that control bladder function
- Dementia

Urinary incontinence can be emotionally devastating for both the incontinent person and the person's caregivers. For the person who is incontinent, having wet clothes or smelling like urine can be very embarrassing. In addition, being incontinent of urine places a person at risk for developing skin problems (such as rashes and pressure ulcers) and for falling (as the person rushes to the bathroom to avoid having an accident). For the caregiver, caring for a person who is incontinent of urine can be frustrating and emotionally draining. It is not uncommon to change a person's clothes or bedding, only to have the person wet themselves all over again. Because caring for an incontinent person can be so emotionally trying and time consuming, incontinence is the factor that most often leads family members to have a relative admitted to a long-term care facility. In fact, studies have shown that in the long-term care setting, as many as 90% of the residents who have dementia are incontinent of urine.

Types of Urinary Incontinence

There are many types of urinary incontinence.

- **Stress incontinence** is probably the most common type of urinary incontinence. In stress incontinence, urine leaks from the bladder when the person coughs, sneezes, or exerts themselves. Stress incontinence can also occur if a person delays voiding and the bladder becomes too full. Childbirth, obesity, and loss of muscle tone as a result of aging are all factors that can contribute to stress incontinence. Stress incontinence can also occur after prostate surgery. Stress incontinence can often be corrected with exercises or surgery.

- **Urge incontinence** is the involuntary release of urine right after feeling an urge to void. This type of incontinence is common in people with urinary tract infections because irritation of the bladder causes the bladder muscle to spasm, expelling the contents of the bladder with little warning. Other conditions that decrease the ability of the bladder to hold urine, such as an enlarged prostate gland or increased intake of caffeinated beverages or alcohol, can also cause urge incontinence.

- **Functional incontinence** occurs in the absence of physical or nervous system problems affecting the urinary tract. The person just cannot make it to the bathroom in enough time, or wait until a bedpan or urinal is provided. It is thought that being in a strange environment (as a hospital or long-term care facility would be to someone who has just been admitted) contributes to functional incontinence. Confusion, disorientation, and loss of mobility are also contributing factors.

- **Overflow incontinence** occurs when the bladder is too full of urine. Overflow incontinence is associated with **urinary retention**, which is the inability of the bladder to empty either completely during urination, or at all. Urinary retention can result from blockage of the bladder outlet (such as occurs with an enlarged prostate gland or from swelling of the urethra during labor or childbirth), or from pain following a surgical procedure. Some injuries that involve the spinal cord can also keep the bladder from emptying fully, leading to urinary retention. Because the bladder does not empty completely when the person voids, it refills with urine quickly, and the urine simply overflows. A person with overflow incontinence may "dribble" urine in between visits to the bathroom. If a person cannot empty their bladder completely, it may be necessary to insert a catheter (either temporarily or permanently) to allow urine to drain from the bladder and prevent urinary retention and overflow incontinence from occurring.

- **Reflex incontinence** (also known as *neurogenic incontinence*) occurs when there is damage to the nerves that enable the person to control urination. The bladder fills, but the person does not feel the urge to urinate. When the bladder is completely full, it empties reflexively (that is, automatically). Some people with certain disorders of the nervous system, such as paralysis from a spinal cord injury, will catheterize themselves with a straight catheter on a regular basis to prevent reflex urinary incontinence.

Managing Urinary Incontinence

Many products are available to help manage urinary incontinence. Techniques such as bladder training may also be used to help a person overcome certain types of incontinence. For some people, temporary or permanent catheterization may be necessary to manage the incontinence.

Incontinence Pads and Briefs

Incontinence pads and briefs are specially made to help prevent soiling of clothes and furniture by absorbing urine and holding it away from the person's skin (Fig. 25-12). Incontinence pads are placed inside the person's underpants to prevent wetting of the clothes and to draw the moisture away from the person's body. Incontinence briefs are worn instead of

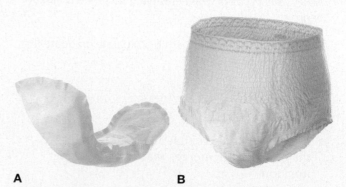

A   B

Figure 25-12 Incontinence pads and briefs are worn under clothing to absorb moisture and keep it away from the body. **A.** DEPEND Guards for Males. **B.** DEPEND Underwear for Females. (*Photographs courtesy of Kimberly-Clark Worldwide, Inc., Neenah, WI.*)

underpants. Keeping the skin dry helps to reduce the skin problems that can occur from prolonged contact with urine. In addition, incontinence pads and briefs are very useful for active people.

For a person with incontinence who is lying in bed, special bed protectors are used to help keep the bed linens and mattress dry and to wick or draw urine away from the person's skin. Many facilities have policies that specify that incontinence briefs are to be used only when the person is out of bed, and that bed protectors are to be used when the person is sleeping. Incontinence briefs tend to fit closely, which makes it difficult for air to reach the skin. Switching between briefs and bed protectors helps to prevent skin breakdown by allowing the skin to be exposed to the air at night. As a nursing assistant, you must make sure that these incontinence products are changed frequently, and that urine is cleaned from the skin whenever the change occurs. (See Chapter 22 for a discussion of providing perineal care, which is especially important in people who are incontinent of urine, feces, or both.)

Female External Catheters

The female external catheter is a device used for female patients or residents who are incontinent of urine and are experiencing skin irritation. One system, called the "PureWick™ System," uses a soft wicking device that fits up against the female vulva and is attached by tubing to a suction device. The suction pulls the urine away from the person and collects it in a collection canister (Fig. 25-13). This system is only used when a person must remain in bed, or at night, when the person is sleeping. Frequent perineal

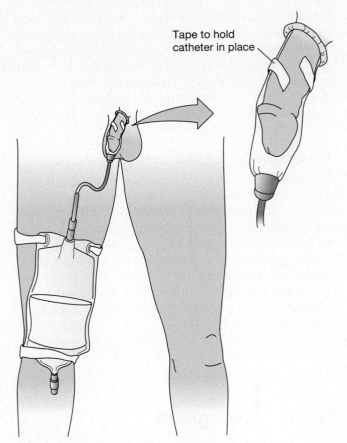

Figure 25-14 A condom catheter can be used to manage urinary incontinence in males. If tape is used to secure the condom catheter to the penis, it should be applied in a spiral fashion, not a circular fashion.

care must be performed to prevent skin irritation and breakdown.

Condom Catheters

A **condom catheter** can be used to manage incontinence in males. A condom catheter is not a true catheter because it is not placed inside the body. It consists of a soft plastic or rubber sheath, tubing, and a collection bag for the urine (Fig. 25-14). The sheath is placed over the penis and the collection bag is attached to the leg. The urine flows through the tubing into the collection bag, allowing the person to urinate at will.

The condom must fit the penis. It should be fastened securely enough to prevent leaking, but not so snugly that it restricts circulation. Many condom catheters have adhesive material on the inside of the condom that allows for a good seal. Others must be secured with elastic tape. The tape strip is applied in a spiral fashion to allow for changes in the size of the penis (see Fig. 25-14). Applying the tape in an overlapping, circular fashion would compromise blood flow if the person had an erection, possibly causing permanent damage to the penis.

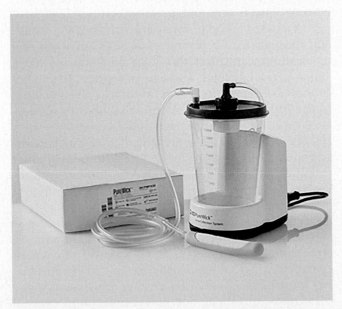

Figure 25-13 A female external catheter can be used to manage urinary incontinence in females.

Use of a condom catheter requires good skin care. The penis must be cleaned, and the condom apparatus changed, daily. Using a skin protectant product underneath a self-adhesive condom catheter can help decrease the risk of skin irritation from the adhesive and moisture. The skin protector also helps to increase the adhesive's ability to adhere to the skin, decreasing the chance of leakage of urine.

Bladder Training

Bladder training is commonly used to help people relearn how to control their urinary elimination. For example, a person may be encouraged to use the bedpan, urinal, or commode at scheduled times. Scheduling helps promote regular emptying of the bladder. The primary goal is for the person to be able to control involuntary urination. If this is not possible, then the person may still at least be able to get to the bathroom in time to avoid accidents, because they will know when voiding is due to occur. The person's care plan will note any special bladder training techniques that are being used and the nurse will instruct you on any specific duties you will be assigned as part of that training.

BOWEL ELIMINATION

The digestive tract, which is discussed in more detail in Chapter 36, consists of the mouth, esophagus, stomach, small intestine, large intestine, rectum, and anus (Fig. 25-15). The rectum is actually part of the large intestine, and together, the large and small intestines are sometimes referred to as "bowels." Essentially, the digestive tract is a long, hollow tube. The food and fluids that we take in are broken down into smaller pieces and mixed together in the stomach, forming a partially digested food and fluid mixture known as **chyme**. From the stomach, the chyme passes slowly into the small intestine, where more digestion occurs and nutrients and fluid are absorbed, and then into the large intestine. Wave-like muscular movements, called **peristalsis**, move the chyme through the intestines. Finally, the chyme reaches the last part of the large intestine, called the rectum. At this point, all of the nutrients have been removed, and what remains is a semi-solid waste material, called **feces**. The presence of feces in the rectum stimulates the urge to **defecate** (that is, have a bowel movement), and the feces leave the body through the anus, the very end of the digestive tract. Sometimes fecal material is referred to as "**stool**" after it leaves the body.

Flatus (or gas) is a natural byproduct of digestion, just as feces are. Eating certain foods, such as beans, broccoli, cabbage, cauliflower, and onions, can lead to the formation of excess flatus. The passing of flatus may be quite noisy and depending on what was eaten,

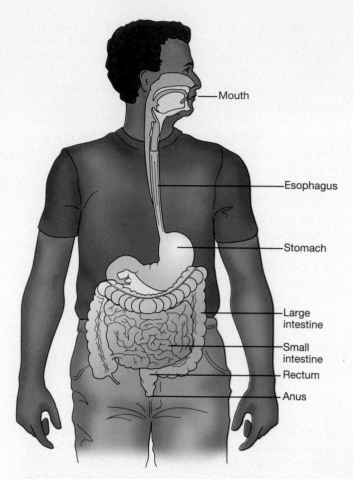

Figure 25-15 The digestive tract consists of the mouth, esophagus, stomach, small intestine, large intestine, rectum, and anus.

the flatus may have a foul odor. For some people, passing flatus is very embarrassing.

In healthy people, feces are soft, brown, moist, and formed, with a distinct odor. Certain foods and medications can affect the color and odor of feces. When you are helping a patient or resident with defecation, observe the feces and report any abnormalities to the nurse. Feces with an unusual odor or appearance could be a sign of illness or infection.

The frequency of a person's bowel movements, and the amount of feces passed each time, will differ from person to person. Many factors influence a person's bowel elimination pattern, including the amount of fluid the person drinks, the type of food they eat, the types of medications they take, and the person's age, level of activity, and lifelong elimination habits. For example, some people have a bowel movement every morning. Other people are not so predictable. For some people, one or two bowel movements a day is normal. For others, one bowel movement every 2 or 3 days is normal. You will soon become aware of the bowel elimination pattern that is normal for each person in your care. This knowledge will allow you to recognize any changes that may occur.

Problems With Bowel Elimination

Problems with bowel elimination that are often seen in the health care setting include diarrhea, constipation, fecal impaction, flatulence, and fecal incontinence.

Diarrhea

Diarrhea is the passage of liquid, unformed stool. Diarrhea may occur frequently and can be accompanied by abdominal cramping. If diarrhea is frequent or excessive, the loss of fluid from the body can quickly cause dehydration, especially in young children or older adults. When caring for a person with diarrhea:

- Practice good infection control techniques. A common cause of diarrhea is a bacterial or viral infection. Because the pathogen that caused the diarrhea will be present in the feces, it is important to use good infection control techniques when caring for a person with diarrhea.
- Answer the call light quickly to provide access to the toilet, bedside commode, or bedpan. A normally continent person can have temporary fecal incontinence from diarrhea, which can be very humiliating. Being quick to respond, compassionate, and supportive can help the person to feel better.
- Provide gentle, thorough skin care and apply a barrier ointment or cream after each bowel movement to prevent skin breakdown.
- Make sure to record and report the frequency and amount of each incident of diarrhea.

Constipation

The opposite of diarrhea is constipation. **Constipation** occurs when the feces remain in the intestines for too long. The delay allows too much fluid to be reabsorbed by the intestines, resulting in hard, dry feces that are difficult to pass. Constipation is fairly common among patients and residents. Risk factors for developing constipation include:

- Taking medications that slow peristalsis (for example, pain medications)
- Lack of dietary fiber or fluids
- Lack of exercise
- Delaying a bowel movement after the urge occurs
- Lack of privacy

As you learned earlier in this chapter, a nursing assistant can do many things to help a patient or resident maintain normal bowel function and prevent constipation. For example, encouraging patients or residents to eat fiber-rich foods, drink plenty of fluids, and exercise regularly can help keep bowel function regular. However, if a person is constipated and all other methods of promoting normal bowel function have failed, the doctor may order a laxative, stool softener, or fiber supplement.

- A **laxative** is a medication that chemically stimulates peristalsis so that material inside the intestines moves through at a faster pace. The resulting bowel movement is soft (or possibly liquid) and occurs within a few hours of taking the laxative, or overnight. Laxatives are acceptable for occasional use, but should not be used regularly, because they cause the chyme to pass through the intestines too quickly for nutrients and fluids to be absorbed. This can result in poor nutrition and dehydration. The intestines also become used to being chemically stimulated to move and can become dependent on the laxative.
- **Stool softeners** help to keep fluid in the feces and are used to help prevent constipation for some people. Unlike laxatives, stool softeners do not chemically stimulate the intestines to cause a bowel movement.
- **Fiber supplements**, in the form of tablets or drink additives, can add bulk to the feces, causing it to hold fluid and preventing constipation.

Fecal Impaction

A **fecal impaction** occurs when constipation is not relieved. The feces build up in the rectum and become harder and harder as more and more fluid is absorbed. Eventually, it becomes almost impossible to pass the feces normally. The impaction blocks the passage of normal stool, but liquid stool may go around the impacted mass. A person with an impaction is usually very uncomfortable, and may complain of abdominal or rectal pain or of liquid feces "seeping" out of the anus. The person's abdomen may be swollen. The person may also have a decreased appetite, nausea, or vomiting.

If a person is thought to have a fecal impaction, a **digital examination** is done (Fig. 25-16). During the digital examination, a finger is inserted into the person's rectum to feel for the impacted mass (*digital* means "finger"). The impaction is then removed by using the finger to break the impacted feces apart and scoop it out of the rectum piece by piece. The doctor may also order the use of an oil retention enema or medication to help remove the impaction. Digital removal of a fecal impaction is very uncomfortable and embarrassing for most patients and residents.

Many facilities require that a nurse remove an impaction. Nursing assistants are usually responsible for assisting the nurse during the procedure by supporting the person in the proper position, providing reassurance, and monitoring the person for signs of distress

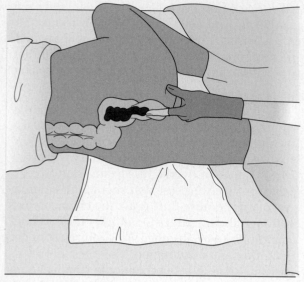

Figure 25-16 Digital examination. A finger is inserted into the person's rectum to check for a fecal impaction.

(because the nurse will not be able to see the person's face). Rectal procedures can stimulate the vagus nerve, which can affect the person's heart rate and blood pressure. Be alert for a change in the person's color, shortness of breath, or loss of consciousness. If you are allowed to remove an impaction, make sure you have been adequately trained for the procedure and that it is part of your job description.

Flatulence

Flatulence is the presence of excessive amounts of flatus (gas) in the intestines, causing abdominal distention (swelling) and discomfort. Sometimes people have difficulty passing flatus because of a lack of activity or a recent surgical procedure. Getting out of bed and walking might be all that is needed to help the person to expel the gas. If walking is not allowed, positioning the person on their left side may help.

Fecal Incontinence

Fecal (bowel) incontinence is the inability to hold one's feces, or the involuntary loss of feces from the bowel. Like urinary incontinence, fecal incontinence can be temporary or permanent. Temporary fecal incontinence can occur with a severe case of diarrhea, simply because the person might not be able to get to the bathroom quickly enough. Some people experience temporary fecal incontinence if the call light is not answered soon enough. Diseases or injuries that affect the nervous system can also result in temporary or permanent fecal incontinence. A person who is unconscious will be incontinent of feces. A person who has dementia will develop fecal incontinence as the disease progresses.

Bowel training is very similar to bladder training and works to promote regular, controlled bowel movements. Offering the commode or bedpan at regular scheduled intervals is a common method of bowel training. Bowel training is often started by keeping track of when an incontinent person usually has a bowel movement, then making sure to provide the appropriate toilet facilities during that time period.

Tell the Nurse!

Changes in the quality of a person's feces or pattern of defecation can be a sign that something is wrong. Be sure to report the following observations to the nurse immediately:

- The person has diarrhea or is constipated
- There is blood or mucus in the stool
- The stool is black or dark green
- The stool is foul-smelling
- The person complains that the feces are painful or difficult to pass
- There is bleeding from the anus during or after a bowel movement
- The person has a swollen abdomen or complains of abdominal pain
- The person complains of liquid feces "seeping" from the anus
- The person has excessive flatus (gas)

Concerns for Long-Term Care

The normal effects of aging can cause the older adult to experience difficulty with bowel elimination. Slower peristalsis, inactivity, decreased food and fluid intake, certain medications, and a diet low in fiber can dramatically increase the person's risk for constipation. Aging also causes a decrease in person's sensory perception, which decreases the feeling of the urge to have a bowel movement. Constipation, if not prevented and treated, can lead to fecal impaction.

Fecal impaction is considered a *sentinel event* (that is, a condition that should rarely, if ever, be seen in a resident of a long-term care facility). If a resident develops a fecal impaction, the government survey team will be observing the care that is provided to all residents to maintain regular bowel elimination. The surveyors will also check documentation to make sure that proper care was provided to the resident who developed the fecal impaction. As a nursing assistant, you play a very important role in helping to prevent your residents from developing fecal impactions. To help prevent fecal impactions:

- Find out from the nurse how much fluid you need to provide to ensure that the resident takes in enough fluid to maintain effective bowel elimination and prevent dehydration. Be sure to tell the nurse immediately if you cannot get the resident to take the needed amount.
- Offer the resident fluids at every opportunity (unless the resident has orders for fluid restriction).
- If the resident does not find water or other beverages appealing, try offering snacks that count as fluid (such as ice cream, popsicles, and gelatin).
- If the resident needs help drinking or eating, provide the necessary assistance.
- Report to the nurse any problems you have getting the resident to take fluids.
- Know what bowel habits are normal for the resident, and report changes in bowel habits to the nurse immediately. Promptly reporting changes, such as hard stool, difficulty passing stool, or more than 2 days without a bowel movement, can allow the nurse to take quick action and possibly prevent a fecal impaction from occurring.

Enemas

An **enema** is the introduction of fluid into the large intestine by way of the anus for the purpose of removing stool from the rectum. There are several reasons a person would be given an enema. Enemas are used to relieve constipation and fecal impactions and to empty the intestine of fecal material before surgery or certain diagnostic tests. Sometimes enemas are used as part of a bowel training program.

Types of Enemas

Several types of enemas are used in the health care setting (Fig. 25-17). Some are prepared by the nurse or nursing assistant, and others come prepackaged. The solution that is placed into the rectum varies according to the reason the enema was ordered.

- **Cleansing enemas**. Cleansing enemas, sometimes called "large-volume enemas," contain from 500 to 1,000 mL of solution and are primarily used to remove feces from the lower large intestine. **Tap water enemas** and **saline (salt water) enemas** help soften the stool and stimulate peristalsis. Enemas containing these solutions should not be given repeatedly because the intestine can absorb the solution, causing a fluid imbalance in the body. **Soapsuds enemas** consist of water and a small amount of a very gentle soap called *castile soap*. The soap solution irritates the lining of the bowel, stimulating peristalsis.

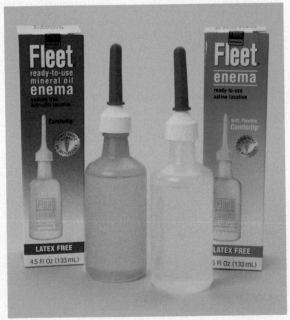

A

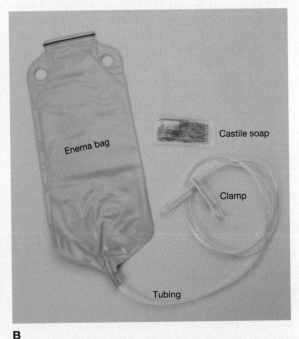

B

Figure 25-17 There are many different types of enema solutions. **A.** Commercially prepared enema solutions. **B.** A soapsuds enema is prepared using castile soap and water (not shown) and administered using an enema bag.

These, too, must be used with caution because too much soap can cause damage to the lining of the intestines.

■ **Oil retention enemas.** An oil retention enema contains mineral, olive, or cottonseed oil. The oil lubricates the inside of the intestine and any stool that is present, making the stool easier to pass or remove. Oil retention enemas are useful for helping to remove fecal impactions.

■ **Commercial enemas.** Commercially prepared and packaged enemas, also called "small-volume enemas," usually contain 70 to 130 mL of a solution that irritates the intestinal mucosa to promote peristalsis. Some commercial enemas contain a solution that is absorbed into the stool to make it softer and easier to pass.

Administering Enemas

Enemas are ordered by a doctor and usually given by a nurse. Some facilities allow nursing assistants to administer enemas after adequate training. Make sure you are familiar with your facility's policies on the administration of enemas. If you are permitted to give enemas, be sure to follow proper procedure and the doctor's orders closely. Make sure the solution is correct for the person, that you have the correct amount of solution, and that the solution is at the proper temperature. Enema solutions that are too cool can cause abdominal cramping and pain, while solutions that are too hot can cause serious injury and possibly even death. When you are assisting with the administration of an enema, make sure that a bed protector and bedpan are in place, or that the path to the bathroom is clear. When it comes time for the person to expel the enema, they will need immediate access to toilet facilities.

An enema is given with the person on their left side in Sims' position. When a person is lying on the left side in Sims' position, the intestine is positioned to take the best advantage of gravity. The solution will flow downward to clean a longer segment of bowel (Fig. 25-18). Having the person lie on their right side in Sims' position is not as effective because the enema solution flows only as far as the rectum and does not clean as much of the bowel. After the enema has been administered, the person is asked to hold the solution in the bowel for the specified amount of time, and then to expel the solution. The doctor may order a cleansing enema to be administered "until clear," which means that enemas are to be given until the enema returning from the person does not contain any fecal material. If you are responsible for giving a cleansing enema, make sure to ask the nurse how many enemas are allowed to be given during a particular session.

Receiving an enema can be uncomfortable and embarrassing. To make the procedure easier for the

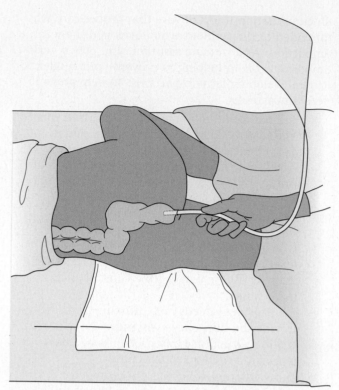

Figure 25-18 The left Sims' position is used when a person is to receive an enema. This position exposes the greatest amount of the bowel to the enema solution.

person, keep the person covered as much as possible and ensure that they have as much privacy as possible. Having the person take a few slow, deep breaths as the enema tubing is inserted into the rectum may help to relax the person and make insertion easier. The procedure for administering an enema is given in Procedure 25-8.

Rectal Suppositories

A **rectal suppository** is a small, wax-like cone or oval that is inserted into the anus. The wax-like substance dissolves at body temperature, stimulating peristalsis or lubricating and softening the stool. Glycerin rectal suppositories are often used to help with bowel elimination before resorting to an enema. Some rectal suppositories also contain medication. These should only be inserted by a nurse.

CARING FOR A PERSON WITH AN OSTOMY

As a nursing assistant, you may care for people with ostomies. For example, a person with a tumor in the large intestine may have surgery to remove the diseased part of the intestine. Depending on the location of the tumor and the length of the segment of the intestine that has to be removed, the person may need an alternate way of eliminating feces from the body following the surgery. In this case, the person may have an **ostomy**. An artificial opening, called a *stoma*, is made in the abdominal wall and the remaining portion of the intestine is connected to it (Fig. 25-19). Feces pass through the stoma and into a pouch (called

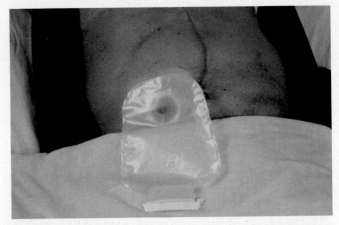

Figure 25-20 An ostomy appliance is worn over the stoma to collect the feces.

an ostomy appliance) that is worn over the stoma (Fig. 25-20).

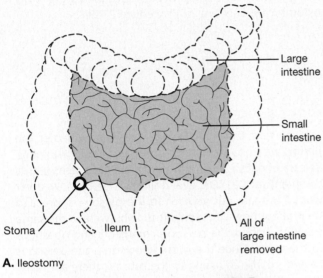

A. Ileostomy

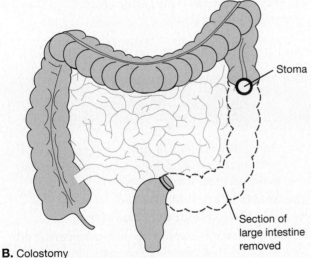

B. Colostomy

Figure 25-19 Some of the people you will care for may have had surgery to remove all or part of the large intestine. Such a surgery may be necessary because of cancer, a bowel obstruction, or trauma. **A.** Ileostomy. The entire large intestine is removed. A stoma is made in the abdominal wall, and the end of the small intestine (the ileum) is sewn into place. **B.** Colostomy. Part of the large intestine is removed. A colostomy can be done at any point along the large intestine; here, a section of the descending colon was removed. A stoma is made in the abdominal wall, and the healthy end of the remaining large intestine is sewn into place.

- An **ileostomy** is created if the entire large intestine must be removed. The end of the small intestine (that is, the ileum) is attached to the abdominal wall. Because the chyme does not have the chance to travel through the large intestine (where water is reabsorbed), the person's feces are very liquid and may flow fairly continuously. For this reason, a person with an ileostomy is quite prone to dehydration.

- A **colostomy** is created if part of the large intestine is still present. After the diseased part of the large intestine is removed, the healthy end is attached to the abdominal wall. Among people with colostomies, the feces vary in consistency. If the portion of the intestine that was removed was near the beginning of the large intestine, then the feces will be more liquid because the chyme will spend less time in the large intestine. On the other hand, if the portion of the intestine that was removed was near the end of the large intestine, then the feces will be more solid and formed.

Cancer is not the only reason a person might have to have an ostomy procedure. Bowel trauma and disease such as diverticulitis (an inflammatory disease of the bowel) are other common reasons that ostomies are performed. Sometimes, a temporary ostomy is done to allow a portion of the bowel to "rest." Later, the ends of the bowel are re-attached and normal bowel elimination resumes.

In some states and facilities, helping patients or residents to care for an ostomy is within the nursing assistant's scope of practice. Ostomies, like the people who have them, are very individual. Ostomies can be located in many different places on the abdomen. In addition, abdomens vary from person to person. For these reasons, the supplies used for ostomies vary greatly. Some ostomy appliances consist of a bag with an adhesive opening that adheres to the skin around the stoma. Other ostomy appliances have two pieces—a ring of flexible rubber that is applied to the skin around the stoma and a bag that is snapped onto the ring. Some appliances are used only once and then discarded, whereas others are emptied, cleaned, and used again. If you are permitted to provide ostomy care, make sure that you are familiar with the different types of ostomy appliances used in your facility and ask the nurse for help with any that are new to you.

No matter what type of ostomy appliance is used, certain principles of ostomy care remain the same for every patient or resident with an ostomy. Because the skin around the ostomy comes into contact with feces, it must be kept clean to prevent irritation. The ostomy appliance can be changed with the person sitting or standing in the bathroom, or while the person is in bed. If the ostomy appliance is being changed while the person is in bed, the person should either sit upright or lie flat. The procedure for providing routine ostomy care is given in Procedure 25-9.

Helping Hands and a Caring Heart

Focus on Humanistic Health Care

For many people, having an ostomy is very difficult, emotionally. First, the person must cope with having an illness or injury serious enough to require major surgery. Second, many people consider elimination, especially bowel elimination, a very private activity. Having to wear a bag to collect feces on the outside of the body can be very embarrassing.

Especially in the beginning, it may be very hard for a person to accept the ostomy. If you are caring for someone who is getting used to the idea of having an ostomy, take the time to listen carefully whether the person wants to talk about their fears or uncertainties. Be careful not to brush off the person's concerns with a comment such as "Oh, everything will be OK now; don't worry." Instead, put yourself in the person's shoes and think about how you would feel if you were in the same situation. Report the person's comments and questions to the nurse. Once the nurse knows that the person is having trouble adjusting to the ostomy, there are many things they can do to help the person adjust.

SUMMARY

- The elimination of waste from the body is a basic physical need.
  - Elimination is natural, but many people are not comfortable discussing it or doing it in front of others. A person's culture and upbringing influence their comfort level with the bodily processes involved in elimination.
  - Normal urinary and bowel elimination can be promoted by encouraging fluids, answering the call light promptly, and providing for the person's privacy and comfort.
  - Incontinence is the inability to hold one's urine, feces, or both until a suitable receptacle (for example, a toilet, bedside commode, or bedpan) is made available. Incontinence has many causes and may be temporary or permanent.
    - Incontinence is difficult emotionally for both the person who is incontinent and that person's caregiver.

  - Being incontinent of urine or feces places a person at risk for skin breakdown. Providing good perineal care is essential.
- The urinary system rids the body of waste that has been filtered from the bloodstream.
  - Normal urine is clear, pale yellow to dark gold in color, with a characteristic odor. Individual urinary patterns vary. Abnormal observations should be reported to the nurse.
  - A person who is having difficulty urinating may need a urinary catheter.
    - Urinary catheters may be left in place for a period of time or inserted and then removed as soon as the bladder has been drained.
    - The use of urinary catheters is the leading cause of HAIs. Good catheter care is essential.

- The digestive system rids the body of waste left over from digestion.
  - Normal stool is soft, brown, moist, formed, and has a distinct odor. Individual bowel elimination patterns vary. Abnormal observations should be reported to the nurse.
    - Diarrhea is the passage of liquid, unformed stool. Diarrhea can lead to dehydration.
    - Constipation occurs when feces remain in the intestine too long and excess fluid is absorbed, leaving the stool hard and difficult to pass. Fecal impaction can result if constipation is not relieved.
  - An enema is the introduction of solution into the large intestine. An enema is sometimes ordered by a doctor to treat or prevent bowel elimination problems.
    - The type of enema solution used is determined by the reason for the enema.
    - Enemas are usually given by a nurse. However, in some facilities, enema administration is within the scope of practice of the nursing assistant. Enemas must be administered correctly, with special attention paid to the position of the person.
- An ostomy is an alternative way of removing feces from the body.
  - For many people, having an ostomy is emotionally difficult.
  - Proper care of the ostomy site is necessary to keep the skin clean and healthy.

Procedure 25-1

Assisting a Person With Using a Bedpan

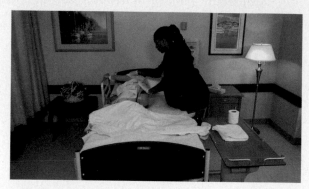

WHY YOU DO IT Bedpans are used for females who cannot get out of bed to urinate or have a bowel movement and for males who cannot get out of bed to have a bowel movement.

Getting Ready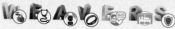

1. Complete the "Getting Ready" steps.

Supplies

- gloves
- bed protector
- toilet paper
- bedpan
- bedpan cover (or paper towels)
- perineal care supplies
- washcloth
- towel

Procedure

2. Make sure that the bed is positioned at a comfortable working height (to promote good body mechanics) and that the wheels are locked. If the side rails are in use, lower the side rail on the working side of the bed. The side rail on the opposite side of the bed should remain up. If necessary, lower the head of the bed so that the bed is flat (as tolerated).

3. Perform hand hygiene and put on the gloves.

4. Fanfold the top linens just far enough down to place the bedpan. Place the bed protector on the bed. Adjust the person's hospital gown or pajama bottoms as necessary to expose the person's buttocks.

5. Place the bedpan underneath the person's buttocks. This can be accomplished by either helping the person to lie on their side, facing away from you, or by asking the person to bend their knees, press their heels into the mattress, and lift their buttocks. Slide the bedpan underneath the person (if the person is holding their buttocks away from the bed by bending their knees) or place the bedpan against their buttocks and help them to roll back onto it while you press the bedpan firmly down against the mattress.

   a. A standard bedpan is positioned like a regular toilet seat.

   b. A fracture pan is positioned with the narrow end pointed toward the head of the bed.

STEP 5 Place the bedpan against the person's buttocks and help the person to roll back onto it.

6. Raise the head of the bed as tolerated. Draw the top linens over the person for modesty and warmth.

7. Make sure that the toilet paper and the call light control are within reach. If the side rails are in use, return the side rails to the raised position.

8. Remove your gloves and perform hand hygiene.

9. If safety permits, leave the room and ask the person to call you when they have finished. Remember to close the door on your way out.

10. Return when the person signals. Remember to knock before entering.

11. If the side rails are in use, lower the side rail on the working side of the bed. Lower the head of the bed so that the bed is flat (as tolerated).

12. Perform hand hygiene and put on a clean pair of gloves.

13. Fanfold the top linens to the foot of the bed.

14. Ask the person to bend their knees, press their heels into the mattress, and lift their buttocks so that you can remove the bedpan and bed protector. (Or help the person to roll onto their

side, facing away from you, while you hold the bedpan securely in place against the mattress to prevent the contents from spilling. Remove the bedpan and bed protector and then help the person to roll back.) If necessary, help the person to use the toilet paper.

15. Cover the bedpan with the bedpan cover or paper towels. Remove one of your gloves if you need to raise the side rails or open a door using a doorknob. Take the bedpan to the bathroom. (If the side rails are in use, raise them before leaving the bedside.)

16. Remove your gloves and dispose of them in a facility-approved waste container. Perform hand hygiene.

17. Return to the bedside. Put on a clean pair of gloves. Give the person a wet washcloth or moist hand wipes and help the person to wash their hands. Make sure the person's perineum is clean and dry. If necessary, provide perineal care. Remove your gloves and perform hand hygiene.

18. Adjust the person's hospital gown or pajama bottoms as necessary to cover the buttocks. Help the person back into a comfortable position, straighten the bottom linens, and draw the top linens over the person. Raise the head of the bed, as the person requests. Make sure that the bed is lowered to its lowest position and that the wheels are locked.

19. Return to the bathroom. Put on a clean pair of gloves. If the person is on intake and output (I&O) status, measure the urine. Note the color, amount, and quality of the urine or feces before emptying the contents of the bedpan into the toilet. (If anything unusual is observed, do not empty the bedpan until a nurse has had a chance to look at its contents.) Clean and disinfect the bedpan according to your facility policy.

20. Gather the soiled linens and place them in the linen hamper or linen bag. Dispose of disposable items in a facility-approved waste container. Clean equipment and return it to the storage area.

21. Remove your gloves, dispose of them in a facility-approved waste container, and perform hand hygiene.

Finishing Up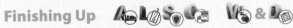

22. Complete the "Finishing Up" steps.

What You Document

- Date and time
- Color, amount, and quality of urine or feces
- Any abnormal observations; and if present, that a nurse was notified

---

▶ **Procedure 25-2**

Assisting a Person With Using a Urinal ▶

WHY YOU DO IT Urinals are used for males who cannot get out of bed to urinate.

Getting Ready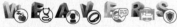

1. Complete the "Getting Ready" steps.

Supplies

- gloves
- toilet paper
- urinal
- washcloth
- towel

Procedure

2. Ask the person what position they prefer—lying, sitting, or standing. If necessary, raise the head of the bed as tolerated. If the person would prefer to stand, help them sit on the edge of the bed and then stand up.

3. Perform hand hygiene and put on the gloves.

4. Hand the person the urinal. If necessary, assist with positioning it correctly.

5. Remove your gloves and perform hand hygiene.

6. Make sure that the toilet paper and the call light control are within reach.

7. If safety permits, leave the room and ask the person to call you when finished. Remember to close the door on your way out.

8. Return when the person signals. Remember to knock before entering.

9. Perform hand hygiene and put on a clean pair of gloves. Have the person hand you the urinal, or remove it if they are unable to hand it to you. Put the lid on the urinal and hang it on the

(continued)

side rail while you assist the person with hand-washing and perineal care as needed. Remove your gloves and perform hand hygiene. Lower the head of the bed as the person requests.

10. Put on a clean pair of gloves. Take the urinal to the bathroom. If the person is on intake and output (I&O) status, measure the urine. Note the color, amount, and quality of the urine before emptying the contents of the urinal into the toilet. (If anything unusual is observed, do not empty the urinal until a nurse has had a chance to look at its contents.) Clean and disinfect the urinal according to your facility policy.

11. Gather the soiled linens and place them in the linen hamper or linen bag. Dispose of disposable items in a facility-approved waste container. Clean equipment and return it to the storage area.

12. Remove your gloves, dispose of them in a facility-approved waste container, and perform hand hygiene.

Finishing Up

13. Complete the "Finishing Up" steps.

What You Document

- Date and time
- Amount, color, and quality of urine
- Any abnormal observations; and if present, that a nurse was notified

---

▶ Procedure 25-3

Collecting a Routine Urine Specimen

WHY YOU DO IT A routine urine specimen is often requested for urinalysis. Proper collection and handling of the urine specimen helps to ensure that the urinalysis results are accurate.

Getting Ready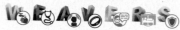

1. Complete the "Getting Ready" steps.

Supplies

- gloves
- paper towel
- toilet paper
- specimen container and label
- plastic transport bag (if required at your facility)
- plastic bag or waste container
- specimen collection device ("commode hat"), bedpan, or urinal

Procedure

2. Complete the label with the person's name, room number, and other identifying information. If your facility uses computer-generated printed labels for specimens, make sure it is correct for the person. Put the completed label on the specimen container. Take the specimen container to the bathroom. Place a paper towel on the counter. Open the specimen container and place the lid on the paper towel, with the inside of the lid facing up.

3. If the person will be using a regular toilet or bedside commode, fit the specimen collection device underneath the toilet or commode seat. Otherwise, provide the person with a bedpan or urinal, as applicable.

4. Assist the person with urination as necessary. Before leaving the room, remind the person not to have a bowel movement or place toilet paper into the specimen collection device, bedpan, or urinal. Provide a plastic bag or waste container for the used toilet paper.

5. Return when the person signals. Remember to knock before entering.

6. Perform hand hygiene and put on the gloves.

7. If the person used a regular toilet or bedside commode, assist the person with handwashing and perineal care as necessary and then help the person to return to bed. If the person used a bedpan or urinal, cover and remove the bedpan or urinal and assist the person with handwashing and perineal care as necessary.

8. Take the covered bedpan, urinal, or specimen collection device (if the person used a bedside commode) to the bathroom. (If the side rails are in use, raise the side rails before leaving the bedside.)

9. If the person is on intake and output (I&O) status, measure the urine. Note the color, amount, and quality of the urine.

10. Raise the toilet seat. While holding the specimen container over the toilet, carefully fill it about three quarters full with urine from the specimen collection device, bedpan, or urinal. Discard the rest of the urine into the toilet.

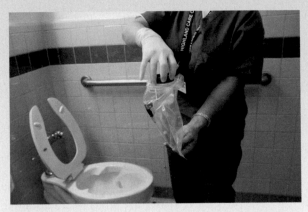

STEP 12 Place the specimen container into the transport bag with your gloved hand.

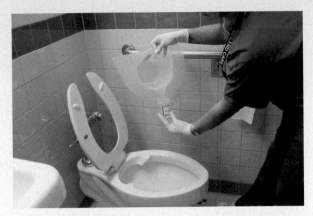

STEP 10 Hold the specimen container over the toilet and fill it about three quarters full with urine.

11. Put the lid on the specimen container. Make sure that the lid is tight. Put the specimen container on the paper towel on the counter.

12. Remove one glove and dispose of it in a facility-approved waste container. Holding the plastic transport bag in your ungloved hand, place the specimen container into the transport bag with your gloved hand. Avoid touching the outside of the transport bag with your glove.

13. Remove the other glove, dispose of it in a facility-approved waste container, and perform hand hygiene. Put on a clean pair of gloves.

14. Gather the soiled linens and place them in the linen hamper or linen bag. Dispose of disposable items in a facility-approved waste container. Clean equipment and return it to the storage area. Remove your gloves and perform hand hygiene.

15. Take the specimen container to the designated location.

Finishing Up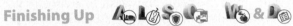

16. Complete the "Finishing Up" steps.

What You Document

- Date and time specimen was collected
- Where the specimen was taken or stored for pickup

▶ **Procedure 25-4**

Collecting a Midstream ("Clean Catch") Urine Specimen

WHY YOU DO IT A midstream ("clean catch") urine specimen is often requested for urinalysis when the doctor suspects a urinary tract infection. Proper collection and handling of the urine specimen helps to ensure that the urinalysis results are accurate.

Getting Ready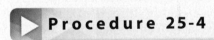

1. Complete the "Getting Ready" steps.

Supplies

- gloves
- paper towel
- toilet paper
- specimen container and label
- "clean catch" kit
- plastic transport bag (if required at your facility)
- bedpan or urinal (if necessary)

Procedure

2. Complete the label with the person's name, room number, and other identifying information. If your facility uses computer-generated

(continued)

printed labels for specimens, make sure it is correct for the person. Put the completed label on the specimen container.

3. If the person will be using a regular toilet or bedside commode, help the person to the bathroom or bedside commode. Otherwise, provide the person with a bedpan or urinal, as applicable.

4. Perform hand hygiene and put on the gloves.

5. Place a paper towel on the counter (if the person is in the bathroom) or on the over-bed table (if the person is using a bedside commode, bedpan, or urinal). Open the specimen container and place the lid on the paper towel, with the inside of the lid facing up.

6. Open the "clean catch" kit. Have the person clean their perineum using the wipes in the kit. Assist as necessary:

   a. **If the person is female:** Use one hand to separate the labia. Hold the wipe in the other hand. Place your wipe-covered hand at the top of the vulva and stroke downward to the anus.

   b. **If the person is a circumcised male:** Use one hand to hold the penis slightly away from the body. Hold the wipe in the other hand. Place your wipe-covered hand at the tip of the penis and wash in a circular motion, downward to the base of the penis.

   c. **If the person is an uncircumcised male:** Retract the foreskin by gently pushing the skin toward the base of the penis. Place your wipe-covered hand at the tip of the penis and wash in a circular motion, downward to the base of the penis.

7. Assist the person with urination as necessary. Before leaving the room, remove your gloves and perform hand hygiene. Then:

   a. Make sure that the toilet paper, call light control, and specimen container are within reach.

   b. Remind the person that they must start the stream of urine, then stop it, then restart it.

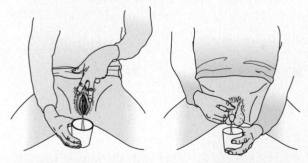

STEP 7b Females must hold the labia open while voiding to prevent contamination of the urine sample. Uncircumcised males must keep the foreskin pulled back.

The urine sample is to be collected from the restarted flow. If the person is female, they must hold the labia open until the specimen is collected. If the person is an uncircumcised male, they must keep the foreskin pulled back until the specimen is collected.

8. Return when the person signals. Remember to knock before entering.

9. Perform hand hygiene and put on a clean pair of gloves.

10. If the person used a regular toilet or bedside commode, assist the person with handwashing and perineal care as necessary and then help the person to return to bed. If the person used a bedpan or urinal, remove the bedpan or urinal and assist the person with handwashing and perineal care as necessary.

11. Remove your gloves and perform hand hygiene. Put on a clean pair of gloves.

12. Put the lid on the specimen container, being careful not to touch the inside of the lid or container. Make sure that the lid is tight. Put the specimen container on the paper towel on the counter or over-bed table.

13. Remove one glove and dispose of it in a facility-approved waste container. Holding the plastic transport bag in your ungloved hand, place the specimen container into the transport bag with your gloved hand. Avoid touching the outside of the transport bag with your glove.

14. Remove the other glove, dispose of it in a facility-approved waste container, and perform hand hygiene. Put on a clean pair of gloves.

15. Gather the soiled linens and place them in the linen hamper or linen bag. Dispose of disposable items in a facility-approved waste container. Clean equipment and return it to the storage area. Remove your gloves and perform hand hygiene.

16. Take the specimen container to the designated location.

Finishing Up

17. Complete the "Finishing Up" steps.

What You Document

- Date and time specimen was collected
- Amount of assistance needed
- Where the specimen was taken or stored for pickup

▶ Procedure 25-5

Collecting a Stool Specimen

WHY YOU DO IT   A stool sample is often requested for analysis. Proper collection and handling of the stool sample helps to ensure that the test results are accurate.

Getting Ready

1. Complete the "Getting Ready" steps.

Supplies

- gloves
- paper towel
- tongue depressor
- toilet paper
- specimen container and label
- plastic transport bag (if required at your facility)
- plastic bag or waste container
- specimen collection device ("commode hat") or bedpan

Procedure

2. Complete the label with the person's name, room number, and other identifying information. If your facility uses computer-generated printed labels for specimens, make sure it is correct for the person. Put the completed label on the specimen container. Take the specimen container to the bathroom. Place a paper towel on the counter. Open the specimen container and place the lid on the paper towel with the inside of the lid facing up.

3. Perform hand hygiene and put on gloves. If the person will be using a regular toilet or bedside commode, fit the specimen collection device underneath the toilet or commode seat. Otherwise, provide the person with a bedpan.

4. Assist the person with defecation as necessary. Remove your gloves and perform hand hygiene. Before leaving the room, remind the person not to urinate or place toilet paper into the specimen collection device or bedpan. Provide a plastic bag or waste container for the used toilet paper.

5. Return when the person signals. Remember to knock before entering.

6. Perform hand hygiene and put on the gloves.

7. If the person used a regular toilet or bedside commode, assist the person with handwashing and then help the person to return to bed. Provide perineal care as necessary. If the person used a bedpan, cover and remove the bedpan and assist the person with handwashing and perineal care as necessary.

8. Take the covered bedpan or specimen collection device (if the person used a bedside commode) to the bathroom. (If the side rails are in use, raise the side rails before leaving the bedside, making sure you remove your gloves and perform hand hygiene before touching the side rails or other items.)

9. Put on a clean pair of gloves. Note the color, amount, and quality of the feces. Using the tongue depressor, take about 1 inch of feces from the bedpan or specimen collection device and put it into the specimen container. Dispose of the tongue depressor in a facility-approved waste container. Empty the remaining contents of the bedpan or specimen collection device into the toilet.

10. Put the lid on the specimen cup. Make sure that the lid is tight. Put the specimen container on the paper towel on the counter.

11. Remove one glove and dispose of it in a facility-approved waste container. Holding the plastic transport bag in your ungloved hand, place the specimen container into the transport bag with your gloved hand. Avoid touching the outside of the transport bag with your glove.

12. Remove the other glove, dispose of it in a facility-approved waste container, and perform hand hygiene.

13. Put on a clean pair of gloves. Gather the soiled linens and place them in the linen hamper or linen bag. Dispose of disposable items in a facility-approved waste container. Clean equipment and return it to the storage area. Remove your gloves and perform hand hygiene.

14. Take the specimen container to the designated location.

Finishing Up

15. Complete the "Finishing Up" steps.

What You Document

- Date and time specimen was collected
- Color, amount, and quality of feces
- Where the specimen was taken or stored for pickup

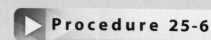

Procedure 25-6

Providing Catheter Care

WHY YOU DO IT Providing proper catheter care helps to prevent the person from getting a urinary tract infection.

Getting Ready

1. Complete the "Getting Ready" steps.

Supplies

- gloves
- paper towels
- bed protector
- bath thermometer
- wash basin
- soap or no-rinse cleanser
- bath blanket
- washcloths
- towels
- clean clothing

Procedure

2. Clean the over-bed table and cover it with paper towels.

3. Lower the head of the bed so that the bed is flat (as tolerated). Make sure that the bed is positioned at a comfortable working height (to promote good body mechanics) and that the wheels are locked.

4. Fill the wash basin with warm water (110°F [43.3°C] to 115°F [46.1°C] on the bath thermometer). Place the wash basin, soap, towels, and washcloths on the over-bed table.

5. If the side rails are in use, lower the side rail on the working side of the bed. The side rail on the opposite side of the bed should remain up.

6. Perform hand hygiene and put on the gloves.

7. Spread the bath blanket over the top linens (and the person). If the person is able, have them hold the bath blanket. If not, tuck the corners under the person's shoulders. Fanfold the top linens to the foot of the bed.

8. Adjust the person's hospital gown or pajama bottoms as necessary to expose the person's perineum.

9. Ask the person to open their legs and bend their knees, if possible. If the person is not able to bend their knees, help the person to spread their legs as much as possible.

10. Position the bath blanket over the person so that one corner can be wrapped under and around each leg.

11. Position a bed protector under the person's buttocks to keep the bed linens dry.

12. Lift the corner of the bath blanket that is between the person's legs upward, exposing only the perineal area.

13. Form a mitt around your hand with one of the washcloths. Wet the mitt with warm, clean water and apply soap or the no-rinse cleanser.

    a. **If the person is female:** Using the other hand, separate the labia. Place your washcloth-covered hand at the top of the vulva and stroke downward to the anus. Repeat, using a different part of the wash-cloth each time, until the area is clean. Rinse and dry the vulva and perineum thoroughly.

    b. **If the person is a circumcised male:** Place your washcloth-covered hand at the tip of the penis and wash in a circular motion, downward to the base of the penis. Repeat, using a different part of the washcloth each time, until the area is clean. Rinse and dry the tip and the shaft of the penis thoroughly.

    c. **If the person is an uncircumcised male:** Retract the foreskin by gently pushing the skin toward the base of the penis. Place your washcloth-covered hand at the tip of the penis and wash in a circular motion, downward to the base of the penis. Repeat, using a different part of the washcloth each time, until the area is clean. Rinse and dry the tip and the shaft of the penis thoroughly before gently pulling the foreskin back into its normal position.

14. Using a clean washcloth, apply soap or use no-rinse cleanser and clean the catheter tubing, starting at the body and moving outward from the body about 4 inches. Hold the catheter near the opening of the urethra. This will help to prevent tugging on the catheter as you clean it.

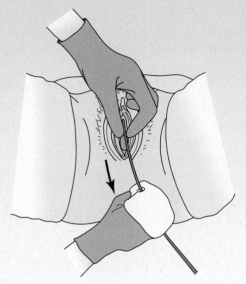

STEP 14 Clean the catheter tubing, starting at the body and moving outward.

15. Rinse the catheter tubing, if necessary, using a clean washcloth. Dry the perineal area thoroughly using a towel.

16. Check that the catheter tubing is free from kinks. Make sure that it is secured to the person's leg.

17. Remove your gloves and perform hand hygiene.

18. Assist the person into the supine position. Remove the bath blanket, and help the person into the clean clothing.

19. If the side rails are in use, return the side rails to the raised position. Raise the head of the bed as the person requests. Make sure that the bed is lowered to its lowest position and that the wheels are locked.

20. Put on a clean pair of gloves. Gather the soiled linens and place them in the linen hamper or linen bag. Dispose of disposable items in a facility-approved waste container. Clean the over-bed table according to facility policy. Clean equipment and return it to the storage area.

Finishing Up

21. Complete the "Finishing Up" steps.

What You Document

- Date and time
- Type of care given
- Condition of skin
- Any abnormal observations; and if present, that they were reported to the nurse

▶ **Procedure 25-7**

Emptying a Urine Drainage Bag

WHY YOU DO IT   Urine drainage bags must be emptied whenever they are full and at the end of every shift (or as ordered).

Getting Ready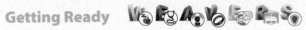

1. Complete the "Getting Ready" steps.

Supplies

- gloves
- paper towels
- alcohol wipes (optional)
- graduate (each person should have their own graduate)

Procedure

2. Perform hand hygiene and put on the gloves.

3. Place a paper towel on the floor, underneath the urine drainage bag. Unhook the drainage bag emptying spout from its holder on the urine drainage bag. Position the graduate on the paper towel underneath the emptying spout.

4. Unclamp the emptying spout on the urine drainage bag and allow all of the urine to drain into the graduate. Avoid touching the tip of the emptying spout with your hands or the side of the graduate.

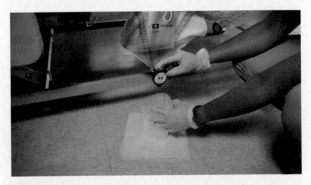

STEP 4 Unclamp the emptying spout on the urine drainage bag and allow the urine to drain into the graduate.

(continued)

5. After the urine has drained into the graduate, wipe the emptying spout with an alcohol wipe (or follow facility policy). Reclamp the emptying spout and return it to its holder.

6. If the person is on intake and output (I&O) status, measure the urine. Note the color, amount, and quality of the urine before emptying the contents of the graduate into the toilet. (If anything unusual is observed, do not empty the graduate until a nurse has had a chance to look at its contents.)

7. Dispose of disposable items in a facility-approved waste container. Clean equipment and return it to the storage area.

8. Remove your gloves, dispose of them in a facility-approved waste container, and perform hand hygiene.

Finishing Up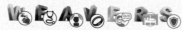

9. Complete the "Finishing Up" steps.

What You Document

- Date and time
- Amount, color, and quality of urine
- Any unusual observations

 Procedure 25-8

Administering a Soapsuds (Large-Volume) Enema

WHY YOU DO IT   A soapsuds enema may be ordered to remove feces from the large intestine prior to surgery or a diagnostic procedure. Proper administration of the enema is important to protect the person's safety and privacy during the procedure and to ensure that the enema is effective.

Getting Ready

1. Complete the "Getting Ready" steps.

Supplies

- gloves
- paper towel
- toilet paper
- bed protector
- lubricant jelly
- 5-mL packet of castile soap
- bedpan or bedside commode
- bedpan cover (if needed)
- enema bag with tubing and clamp
- IV pole
- bath thermometer
- bath blanket
- perineal care supplies

Procedure

2. Make sure that the bed is positioned at a comfortable working height (to promote good body mechanics) and that the wheels are locked.

3. Prepare the enema solution in the bathroom or utility room. Clamp the tubing and then fill the enema bag with warm water (105°F [40.5°C] on the bath thermometer) in the specified amount (usually from 500 to 1,000 mL). Add the castile soap packet and mix by gently rotating the enema bag. Do not shake the solution vigorously.

4. Release the clamp on the tubing and allow a little water to run through the tubing into the sink or bedpan. This will remove all of the air from the tubing. Reclamp the tubing.

5. Hang the enema bag on the IV pole and bring it to the person's bedside. Adjust the height of the IV pole so that the enema bag is hanging no more than 18 inches above the person's anus.

6. If the side rails are in use, lower the side rail on the working side of the bed. The side rail on the opposite side of the bed should remain up. Lower the head of the bed so that the bed is flat (as tolerated).

7. Spread the bath blanket over the top linens (and the person). If the person is able, have them hold the bath blanket. If not, tuck the corners under their shoulders. Fanfold the top linens to the foot of the bed.

8. Ask the person to lie on their left side, facing away from you, in Sims' position. Help them into this position, if necessary.

9. Perform hand hygiene and put on the gloves.

10. Adjust the bath blanket and the person's hospital gown or pajama bottoms as necessary to expose the person's buttocks. Position the bed protector under the person's buttocks to keep the bed linens dry.

11. Open the lubricant package and squeeze a small amount of lubricant onto a paper towel. Lubricate the tip of the enema tubing to ease insertion.

12. Suggest that the person take a deep breath and slowly exhale as the enema tubing is inserted. With one hand, raise the person's upper buttock to expose the anus. Using your other hand, gently and carefully insert the lubricated tip of the tubing into the person's rectum (not more than 3 to 4 inches for adults). Direct the tube upward toward the umbilicus, not the bladder. Never force the tubing into the rectum. If you are unable to insert the tubing, stop and call the nurse.

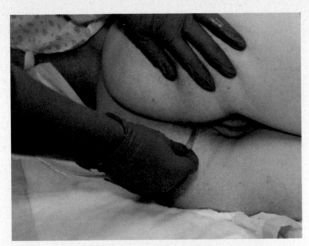

STEP 12 Gently insert the top of the tubing into the person's rectum.

13. Unclamp the tubing and allow the solution to begin running slowly. Allow 5 to 10 minutes for all of the solution to be instilled. Hold the enema tubing firmly with one hand so that it does not slip out of the rectum. If the person complains of pain or cramping, slow down the rate of flow by tightening the clamp a bit. If the pain or cramping does not stop after slowing the rate of flow, stop the procedure and call the nurse.

14. When the fluid level reaches the bottom of the bag, clamp the tubing to avoid injecting air into the person's rectum.

15. Remove the tubing from the person's rectum and place it inside the enema bag. Gently place several thicknesses of toilet paper against the person's anus to absorb any fluid.

16. Ask the person to retain the enema solution for the specific amount of time.

17. Dispose of the enema bag, tubing, and other items. Remove your gloves and perform hand hygiene before touching any items that are clean, such as the side rails of the bed.

18. Perform hand hygiene and put on gloves. Assist the person with expelling the enema as necessary, using the bedpan, bedside commode, or toilet. If the person is using a regular toilet, ask them not to flush the toilet after expelling the enema.

19. If the person used a regular toilet or bedside commode, assist them with handwashing and then help them to return to bed. Provide perineal care as necessary. If the person used a bedpan, cover and remove the bedpan and assist with handwashing and perineal care as necessary.

20. Remove your gloves and perform hand hygiene.

21. Raise the head of the bed as the person requests. Make sure that the bed is lowered to its lowest position and that the wheels are locked. (If the side rails are in use, raise the side rails before leaving the bedside.)

22. Put on gloves. Take the covered bedpan or commode bucket (if the person used a bedside commode) to the bathroom.

23. Note the color, amount, and quality of feces before emptying the contents of the bedpan or commode bucket into the toilet. (If anything unusual is observed, do not empty the bedpan or commode bucket until a nurse has had a chance to look at its contents.)

24. Gather the soiled linens and place them in the linen hamper. Dispose of disposable items in a facility-approved waste container. Clean equipment and return it to the storage area.

25. Remove your gloves, dispose of them in a facility-approved waste container, and perform hand hygiene.

Finishing Up

26. Complete the "Finishing Up" steps.

What You Document

- Date and time
- Type of enema given
- Amount of fluid instilled
- How long patient or resident "held" the enema fluid
- Complaints of pain or cramping
- Color, amount, and quality of feces and enema fluid expelled
- Any abnormal observations; and if present, that they were reported to the nurse

▶ **Procedure 25-9**

Providing Routine Ostomy Care

▶

WHY YOU DO IT   Because the skin around the stoma comes in contact with feces, it must be kept clean to prevent irritation.

Getting Ready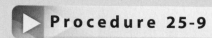

1. Complete the "Getting Ready" steps.

Supplies

- gloves
- paper towels
- bed protector
- toilet paper
- 4 × 4 gauze pad
- clean ostomy appliance
- skin barrier
- bedpan
- bedpan cover (or paper towels)
- wash basin
- mild soap (or other cleansing agent, per facility policy)
- adhesive remover (optional)
- washcloths
- towel
- graduate container

Procedure

2. Clean the surface of the over-bed table and cover it with paper towels. Place the ostomy supplies and clean linens on the over-bed table.

3. Make sure that the bed is positioned at a comfortable working height (to promote good body mechanics) and that the wheels are locked.

4. If the side rails are in use, lower the side rail on the working side of the bed. The side rail on the opposite side of the bed should remain up. If necessary, lower the head of the bed so that the bed is flat (as tolerated).

5. Fanfold the top linens to below the person's waist.

6. Position the bed protector on the bed alongside the person to keep the bed linens dry. Adjust the person's clothing as necessary to expose the person's stoma.

7. Perform hand hygiene and put on the gloves.

8. Remove the clamp from the end of the ostomy bag and fold the end of the pouch upward like a cuff. Empty the contents of the ostomy bag into the graduate container.

9. Wipe the lower 2 inches of the ostomy bag with toilet tissue and uncuff the pouch. Reapply the closure clip.

10. Take the graduate container to the bathroom. If you must raise the side rails on the bed or touch the door handle, remove one of your gloves.

11. Remove your gloves and perform hand hygiene.

12. Put on a clean pair of gloves. Disconnect the ostomy appliance from the ostomy belt if one is used. Remove the belt. If the ostomy belt is soiled, dispose of it in a facility-approved waste container (if it is disposable), or place it in the linen hamper or linen bag (if it is not disposable).

13. Remove the ostomy appliance by holding the skin taut and gently pushing the skin away from the appliance, starting at the top. If the adhesive is making removal difficult, use warm water or the adhesive solvent to soften the adhesive. Place the ostomy appliance in the bedpan.

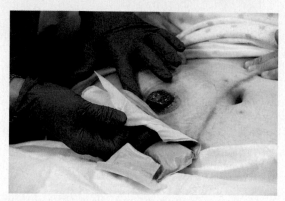

STEP 13 Hold the skin taut and gently push the skin away from the appliance.

14. Gently wipe the stoma with toilet paper to remove any feces or drainage. Place the toilet paper in the bedpan. Cover the stoma with the gauze pad to absorb any drainage that may occur until the new appliance is in place.

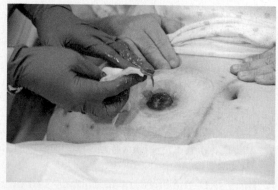

STEP 14 Gently wipe the stoma with toilet tissue to remove drainage.

15. Cover the bedpan with the bedpan cover or paper towels. Take the bedpan to the bathroom. (If the side rails are in use, remove one glove and raise them before leaving the bedside.)

16. Note the color, amount, and quality of the feces before emptying the contents of the ostomy appliance and the bedpan into the toilet. (If anything unusual is observed, do not empty the ostomy appliance until a nurse has had a chance to look at its contents.)

17. Dispose of the ostomy appliance in a facility-approved waste container.

18. Remove your gloves and perform hand hygiene.

19. Fill the wash basin with warm water (110°F [43.3°C] to 115°F [46.1°C] on the bath thermometer). Return to the bedside. Place the basin on the over-bed table. If the side rails are in use, lower the side rail on the working side of the bed.

20. Perform hand hygiene and put on a clean pair of gloves.

21. Form a mitt around your hand with one of the washcloths. Wet the mitt with warm, clean water and apply mild soap (or other cleansing agent, per facility policy). Remove the gauze pad from the stoma and dispose of it in a facility-approved waste container. Clean the skin around the stoma. Rinse and dry the skin around the stoma thoroughly.

22. Apply the skin barrier if needed, according to the manufacturer's directions.

23. Put the clean ostomy belt on the person if an ostomy belt is used.

24. Make sure that the opening on the ostomy appliance is the correct size. Remove the adhesive backing on the ostomy appliance.

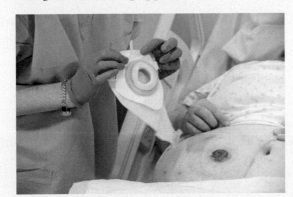

STEP 24 Make sure the opening on the ostomy appliance is the correct size.

25. Center the appliance over the stoma, making sure that the drain or the end of the bag is

pointed down. Gently press around the edges to seal the ostomy appliance to the skin.

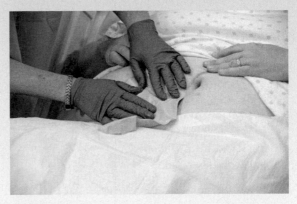

STEP 25 Gently press the edges to seal the ostomy appliance to the skin.

26. Connect the ostomy appliance to the ostomy belt, if one is used.

27. Remove the bed protector.

28. Remove your gloves and perform hand hygiene.

29. Adjust the person's clothing as necessary to cover the ostomy appliance. If the bedding is wet or soiled, change the bed linens. Help the person back into a comfortable position, straighten the bottom linens, and draw the top linens over the person. Raise the head of the bed, as the person requests.

30. If the side rails are in use, return the side rail to the raised position. Make sure that the bed is lowered to its lowest position and that the wheels are locked.

31. Put on gloves and gather the soiled linens and place them in the linen hamper or linen bag. Dispose of disposable items in a facility-approved waste container. Clean the over-bed table according to facility policy. Clean equipment and return it to the storage area. Remove your gloves and perform hand hygiene.

Finishing Up

32. Complete the "Finishing Up" steps.

What You Document

■ Date and time
■ Type of care given
■ Type of ostomy appliance used
■ Condition of skin around ostomy
■ Amount, color, and character of feces
■ Any abnormal observations; and if present, that they were reported to the nurse

WHAT DID YOU LEARN?

Multiple Choice

Select the single best answer for each of the following questions.

1. The perineum (perineal area) is cleaned with a special cleansing wipe before collecting a:
a. 24-hour urine specimen
b. Clean catch urine specimen
c. Random urine specimen
d. Stool specimen

2. The most comfortable position for using a bedpan is:
a. Fowler's position
b. Sims' position
c. Prone position
d. Supine position

3. How far is an enema tube inserted into the rectum in an adult?
a. 3 to 4 inches
b. 5 to 6 inches
c. 7 to 8 inches
d. 12 to 16 inches

4. One of your residents needs to have an enema administered. How should you position the resident in preparation for the enema?
a. Left Sims' position
b. Fowler's position
c. Supine position
d. Right Sims' position

5. In a person with an indwelling urinary catheter, why must the urine drainage bag be kept lower than the person's bladder?
a. Keeping the drainage bag below bladder level will prevent a bedridden person from seeing the bag, which they may find embarrassing
b. Keeping the drainage bag below bladder level will keep the person comfortable in bed
c. Keeping the drainage bag below bladder level will prevent urine from returning to the bladder, where it could cause infection
d. Keeping the drainage bag below bladder level will prevent the urine from leaking out

6. Which one of the following describes normal urine?
a. Cloudy with a strong odor
b. Well-formed
c. Red-tinged
d. Clear, light yellow, or golden with a slight odor

7. A healthy person's feces will be:
a. Black and tarry
b. Soft, brown, formed, and moist with a distinct odor
c. Hard and pellet-like
d. Long and stringy

8. To help your residents or patients to maintain healthy bowel function, it is important to:
a. Answer call lights promptly
b. Encourage them to eat a well-balanced diet and drink plenty of fluids
c. Assist them with exercise
d. All of the above

9. When caring for a person who is incontinent of urine or feces, it is important to:
a. Provide good perineal care
b. Let the person know that their behavior is inappropriate, so it will stop
c. Take the person to the bathroom once daily
d. Restrict fluids to reduce the chance of an accident

10. When caring for a person with an indwelling catheter, always remember to:
a. Leave the drainage bag above the level of the bladder, while the person is in bed
b. Tape any leaks at the connection site
c. Wear gloves when providing daily catheter care
d. Tape the drainage tube under the leg

11. Mr. Pak has an ileostomy and you assist him with stoma care. What would you expect his feces to be like?
a. Very liquid, continuously flowing
b. Hard, dry pellets
c. Soft, brown, moist, and formed
d. Firm

12. What is the artificial opening for a colostomy called?
a. Rectum
b. Stoma
c. Anus
d. Diverticulum

Matching   *Match each numbered item with its appropriate lettered description.*

_____ **1.** Hematuria

_____ **2.** Peristalsis

_____ **3.** Micturition

_____ **4.** Defecation

_____ **5.** Nocturia

_____ **6.** Dysuria

_____ **7.** Urinalysis

_____ **8.** Anuria

_____ **9.** Oliguria

_____ **10.** Polyuria

a. Excessive urine production
b. Excessive urination at night
c. Difficulty urinating
d. No urine production
e. Urination
f. Passing of feces
g. Routine urine test
h. Inadequate urine production
i. Blood in the urine
j. Wave-like muscular movement of the intestines

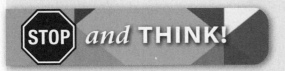

STOP *and* THINK!

- You are a nursing assistant in a hospital. One of your patients, Mrs. Dimitri, must use a bedpan because she is confined to bed, but she is having a hard time relaxing enough to urinate "in bed." What sorts of things could you do to help make using a bedpan easier for Mrs. Dimitri?

- You are caring for Miss Ahn, who has an indwelling catheter. When you are making your end-of-shift rounds, you note that Miss Ahn's urinary drainage bag has very little urine in it. You know that the drainage bag was emptied right before you started your shift. That was almost 8 hours ago. What should you do?

Respect

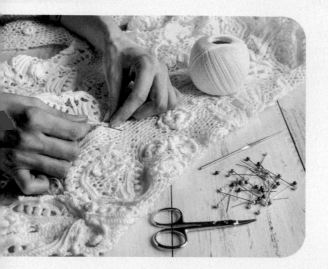

People often take an active interest in their own personal heritage. We ask, Who am I? Where do my ancestors come from? How can I express my heritage? My fingers shook as I opened the results of my DNA profile that I had submitted to a genealogy company. All I knew was that my parents were of mixed Asian and European ancestry, but no one really discussed our family's history. Now I would know.

My interest in finding out about my heritage started with listening to one of my residents at the long-term care facility where I work. Miss O'Meary's mother had immigrated to the United States from Ireland as a young girl. Miss O'Meary would sit in her rocking chair and crochet the most beautiful pieces of lace. She said her mother had taught her, and as she worked the lace, she would tell me the stories her mother had told of coming to this country in a large ship. She said the passage was really hard and many people got sick along the way. Some even died before making it to their new homeland.

Miss O'Meary said her mother never tired of telling about finally approaching the harbor in New York and seeing the Statue of Liberty for the first time. That was the first time during the long voyage that she had felt a sense of safety and calm. She always got teary-eyed when she talked about how sad her mother had been to leave Ireland, but still the excitement of a new life ahead kept her hopeful.

Miss O'Meary said that she had visited Ireland once and had seen Lady Liberty several times. She said that she was proud to be an American, but loved her Irish heritage. She loved to decorate her room in the facility with pieces of the lace she made and even had a few pieces that her mother had brought with her from Ireland. Miss O'Meary said that the lace brought back such beautiful memories of her mother and her own childhood. Since knowing her, she has shared recipes, tales of Ireland, and of course, a piece of that beautiful Irish lace with me. She has helped me learn to respect our different heritages and how our family histories are so important to who we are today.

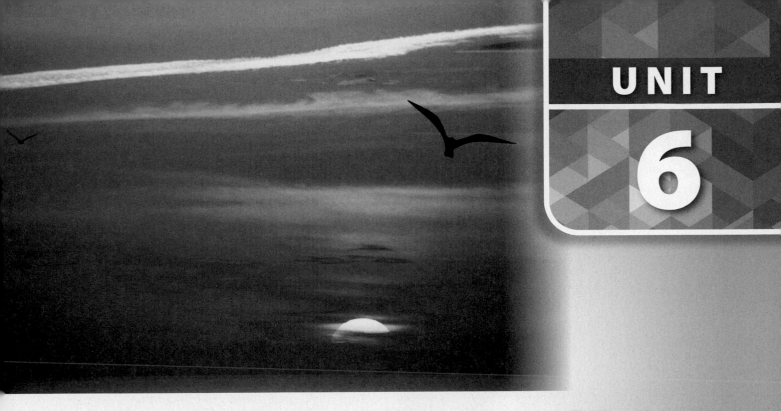

Death and Dying

Do not go gentle into that good night,
Old age should burn and rave at close of day
Rage, rage against the dying of the light.
—From *Do Not Go Gentle Into That Good Night*
by Dylan Thomas

IN THIS POEM BY THE WELSH POET DYLAN THOMAS (1914–1953), the speaker begs his father to fight, rather than accept, death. Although everyone who lives must die, accepting the certainty of our own death, or the death of someone we care about, is rarely easy. In Unit 6, we will look at the final stages of life, and the role the nursing assistant plays in providing compassionate care to those who are dying and their families.

Photo: Sunset over the ocean. (Gabriele Maltinti\Shutterstock.com)

497

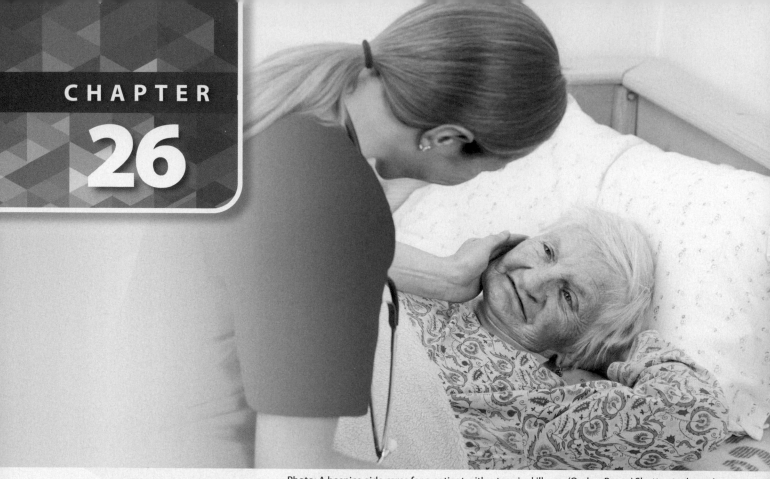

Photo: A hospice aide cares for a patient with a terminal illness. (Ocskay Bence\Shutterstock.com)

CHAPTER

26

Caring for People Who Are Terminally Ill

 WHAT WILL YOU LEARN?

This chapter focuses on caring for people with a terminal illness (an illness that will end in death). You will learn about the stages of grief a dying person experiences, and the role health care workers play in caring for a dying person. You will also learn about care considerations for the family of a person with a terminal illness, and the effects of caring for terminally ill people on the caregiver. When you are finished with this chapter, you will be able to:

1. Define the term *terminal illness* and give examples of specific illnesses that are considered terminal.
2. List the stages of grief and discuss their effects on a person with a terminal illness.
3. Describe the effects of a terminal illness on the person's family.
4. Describe care concerns when providing for the needs of a person with a terminal illness.
5. Define the terms *supportive care* and *palliative care*, and explain how these types of care can be used to maintain a person's quality of life during the end-of-life period.
6. Discuss the role of hospice in the care of a person with a terminal illness.
7. Explain how caring for terminally ill people can affect the nursing assistant.

Vocabulary

Grief	Bargaining	Will	No-code or do-not-
Denial	Depression	Life-sustaining treatment	resuscitate (DNR) order
Anger	Acceptance	Supportive care	Palliative care

People die from many different causes and at many different ages. Some people die suddenly of accidents or acute illnesses; others die simply as a result of the natural aging process. Still others die from a *terminal illness*, an illness or condition for which there is no cure. There are many types of terminal illnesses. Alzheimer disease, as well as certain cancers, heart conditions, chronic respiratory disorders, kidney disorders, and liver disorders are all examples of conditions that can become terminal.

Some of you will have experienced life events, such as the death of someone close to you, that inspired you to enter the health care industry. However, many of you are entering the nursing assisting profession with little or no exposure to death and the process of grieving. Caring for a person with a terminal illness can be very rewarding, but it can also be emotionally draining. To become emotionally secure enough to be supportive of a person with a terminal illness and their family, you will need to explore your own feelings and emotions regarding death and dying. However, you must also remember that everyone has their own beliefs and ideas about death and that these beliefs and ideas are just as important and meaningful to that person as yours are to you. (See Chapter 27, "Caring for People Who Are Dying," for a more detailed discussion of beliefs and practices related to death and dying across various religions and cultures.)

When you are caring for people who are dying, you should be aware of the power of listening and touch. In many cases, it is not necessary to say anything at all—your presence will be noticed and will be reassuring for the dying person. Listen to whatever the person needs to say, without imposing your own opinions or beliefs. Remember that this is your patient's or resident's grief, and they must work through it on their own terms.

STAGES OF GRIEF

Anyone experiencing any type of loss, be it the loss of health, loss of a relationship, loss of a loved one, or the impending loss of their own life, will experience grief. **Grief** is defined as mental anguish, specifically associated with loss. Dr. Elisabeth Kübler-Ross (1926–2004), a Swiss-born doctor who came to the United States in the 1950s, is the author of a well-known book called *On Death and Dying*. Dr. Kübler-Ross, a psychiatrist, chose to work with people who are terminally ill. During her conversations with her patients, they expressed to her their feelings about what they were going through. These conversations formed the basis for many of the ideas in *On Death and Dying*. One key idea Dr. Kübler-Ross outlined is that dying people experience distinct stages of grief. These same stages are also seen to some degree in people who are diagnosed with chronic illnesses, especially those illnesses that will greatly affect the person's way of living. For example, a person who has recently been told they have diabetes, heart disease, or hypertension may go through the same stages of grief as a person who has been told they are dying. The stages of grief that Dr. Kübler-Ross identified are denial, anger, bargaining, depression, and acceptance.

Denial, the first stage of grief, occurs when a person is told that they have a terminal illness. The person refuses to accept the diagnosis or feels that a mistake has been made (Fig. 26-1). They may ask for a second opinion, or act as if nothing is wrong and avoid returning to the doctor for a period of time. Denial helps to protect a person emotionally from overwhelming grief. This stage of grief can last only a few minutes, or it may last until the person actually dies. As a nursing assistant, it is not your place to convince the person that their illness exists, or to argue with the person about treatment or care issues. Instead, recognize that denial is a normal part of the grieving process, respond to the person in an honest yet

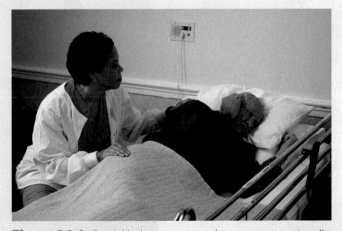

Figure 26-1 Denial helps to protect the person emotionally from overwhelming grief.

TABLE 26-1   Stages of Grief

STAGE	SAMPLE DIALOGUE	APPROPRIATE RESPONSE FROM NURSING ASSISTANT
Denial	**Patient:** "They don't know what they're talking about. I can't possibly have an incurable brain tumor." **Nursing assistant:** "I'm sorry; it must have been very hard for you to learn the results of the MRI."	Acknowledges what the person is saying by responding in an honest, yet neutral way.
Anger	**Patient:** "If you medical people weren't so incompetent, I wouldn't be so sick!" **Nursing assistant:** "Mr. Santos, you seem so angry."	Acknowledges the person's anger and allows them to talk about it; by practicing empathy, avoids feeling defensive or taking the person's anger personally.
Bargaining	**Patient:** "If I could just hang on until my sister arrives…" **Nursing assistant:** "We'll do all we can to help you do that. But until then, I'll be with you."	Offers support that they can realistically provide and reassures the person that they will be cared for.
Depression	**Patient:** "I don't want to die…. I'm so sad." **Nursing assistant** (sitting quietly and holding the patient's hand): "I'm here for you."	Offers comfort in the form of touch and silence; does not attempt to "cheer the person up"; if the person is refusing food or not sleeping, could offer to obtain whatever foods appeal to the person's appetite or to talk to the nurse about arranging for medication to aid sleep.
Acceptance	**Patient:** "It won't be long until I'm going on to my reward." **Nursing assistant:** "You're going on to your reward?"	Uses communication techniques that encourage the person to talk, such as rephrasing the person's statement as an open-ended question.

neutral way, and communicate your observations to the nurse (Table 26-1). Be sure to tell the nurse if the person refuses medication or other medical treatment.

Anger occurs when the person realizes that they are actually going to die (Fig. 26-2). People may feel angry for different reasons, and each person handles anger differently. Some people may be angry with themselves for not seeking help sooner, or for making a lifestyle choice that contributed to the illness, such as smoking. People express anger differently. Some people become moody and withdrawn, or uncooperative and hostile. Others may yell or throw objects. If the person is religious, they may lose faith. Some people take their anger out on family members. Others may direct their anger toward health care professionals, feeling that the people they have placed so much trust in have somehow failed them. You must not take the anger personally—doing so can hurt your emotional well-being, as well as your ability to care for the person.

Bargaining is typically done on a very private basis by a person with a terminal illness. The person wants to "make a deal" with someone they feel has control over their fate, such as God or a health care provider (Fig. 26-3). The person may want to live long enough to accomplish a goal, or to witness a specific event, such as the birth of a child, a wedding, or an anniversary celebration. The will to live can be a very powerful force and may, in fact, extend the person's life by a few months. As a nursing assistant, it is important for you to allow the terminally ill person to experience the feeling of hope that accompanies this stage of grieving.

Depression is the stage in which the person fully realizes that death will be the end result of the illness (Fig. 26-4). The person will be sad and may have regrets about things they were not able to accomplish during their lifetime. Some people are quite withdrawn and may say little, while others may want to openly mourn for their loss. Recognize that depression is a normal part of the grieving process, and be supportive. Let the person know that it is all right for them to be feeling the way they are feeling. Tell the nurse if a grieving person's depression causes the person to cry constantly, refuse food, or fail to sleep. Some people will require medical intervention to treat their depression.

Acceptance occurs when a terminally ill person comes to terms with the reality of their own death and is finally at peace with this knowledge (Fig. 26-5).

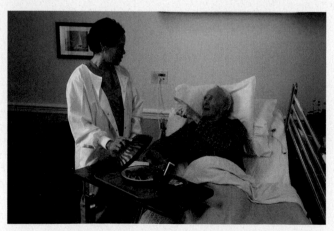

Figure 26-2 Many people who are grieving pass through a period of anger.

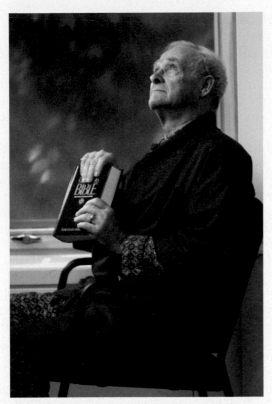

Figure 26-3 The bargaining stage is usually accompanied by a feeling of hope.

Typically, people who have reached the acceptance stage will demonstrate their acceptance by completing unfinished business and saying their goodbyes. Many will plan their funeral service or write a poem or letter to be read after they are gone. Often, they will want to talk about their death, in an effort to help family members accept it also. The acceptance stage does not necessarily occur when death is near; some people gain acceptance months or even years prior to their eventual death from the illness.

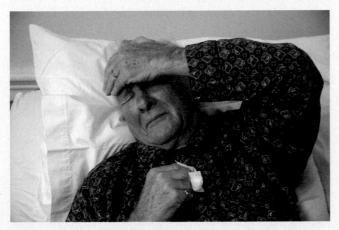

Figure 26-4 During the depression phase, the person realizes the full impact of their illness.

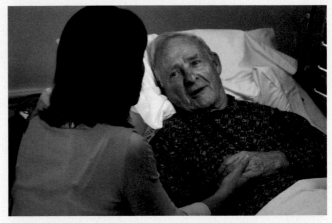

Figure 26-5 During the acceptance phase, the grieving person comes to terms with their death and begins to make plans for the future.

Terminally ill people may not pass through all the stages of grief, and they may not pass through them in order. Many people work through the first five stages of grief, only to "relapse" and experience some of the earlier stages again. Throughout the grieving process, the one thing that usually persists is hope. Even the most realistic and accepting people hold onto the hope that a new drug will be developed, or that a new research project will yield a cure. Hope is what helps a terminally ill person face another day or another painful treatment. It is what drives the person to keep up with normal activities, such as eating and praying, when they might otherwise feel like giving up entirely. As a nursing assistant, you must be responsive to, and nurture, a person's hope, without being unrealistic.

One factor that influences how a person handles the grieving process is where the person is in their life in terms of responsibilities, commitments, accomplishments, hopes, and dreams. For example, a mother with young children will have different concerns than a grandmother whose children are grown and independent. A terminally ill person who is able to view their life with a feeling of satisfaction may act very differently from a person who has regrets about choices made, opportunities lost, or goals unmet. A child will handle a terminal illness very differently from an adult (often, children reach the acceptance stage faster than adults). It is important for you to recognize the stages of grief and understand that although these stages have been identified, each person will experience and react to them differently. Being able to recognize the stages of grief will enable you to provide better care to your patients or residents because you will have a better understanding of what they are going through. This understanding will help you to be more effective in determining what your patients or residents need from you.

The family and loved ones of a terminally ill person will also go through the stages of grief as they prepare

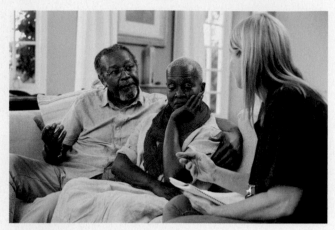

Figure 26-6 Grief counseling may be a comfort to the patient and the family. (*Monkey Business Images\Shutterstock.com.*)

for their loss. Remembering this will help you understand behavior that may not seem fair or appropriate. For example, a family member of a terminally ill person may direct their anger at you, but the family member is not necessarily angry with you—they are angry that they are losing someone they love. Like the dying person, the family members will each pass through the stages of grief individually and at their own order and pace. Sometimes there is emotional upset and conflict within a family when the members of the family (including the person who is ill) are at different stages of the grieving process. Reporting your observations of this turmoil to the nurse will be helpful. Arranging for the assistance of a religious leader or other professionals experienced in grief counseling may be of great comfort to the person and the family (Fig. 26-6).

Tell the Nurse!

When caring for a terminally ill person, pay attention to the person's emotional well-being, as well as their physical well-being. Report any of the following observations to the nurse immediately:

- The person refuses medications, or other medical treatment
- The person cries constantly, refuses food, or cannot sleep
- There is tension and disagreement within the family
- The person or a family member requests the assistance of a religious leader or grief counselor
- The person expresses interest in making or changing legal documents related to end-of-life care, such as advance directives or a will.

Concerns for Long-Term Care

Many of your residents are entering the last phase of their lives when they come to live in a long-term care facility. Some of your residents will simply die as the result of advanced age. Others will die as the result of an acute illness such as cancer, stroke, or pneumonia. Many of your residents will have one or more chronic conditions associated with aging (such as heart conditions, chronic respiratory disorders, or dementia). These conditions usually worsen over time. Eventually, there is nothing more that can be done to treat the disorder. When this occurs, the person is said to have *end-stage disease*, and death is usually expected within a relatively short period of time.

Many of your residents will pass through the stages of grief over a period of many years. As a result, you may not actually see all of the stages of grief in a resident who is coming to terms with their own impending death. This is especially true of residents who have chronic conditions that they have struggled with for many years. These residents may have been hospitalized many times, when worsening symptoms put their overall health in danger. Each time such a health crisis occurred, the possibility of death loomed overhead. As a result, these residents may have worked through the various stages of grief over the course of many years as their condition worsened. Many live in a state of acceptance, recognizing and accepting that death could come at any time.

WILLS

A **will** is a legal statement that expresses a person's wishes for the management of their affairs after death. For a will to be valid, the person must be deemed competent, or "of sound mind," at the time the will is made or changed. If a patient or resident expresses a desire to make or change a will, you should relay this information to the nurse so that arrangements can be made for the person to talk with someone who is qualified to assist with preparing a will. Many health care facilities have people on site who are able to provide this kind of assistance. Or, the patient or resident may prefer to have the will prepared by their personal lawyer. As a nursing assistant, you may be asked to sign a will as a witness. When you sign as a witness, your signature means that you saw the person sign the document and that, to the best of your knowledge, the document accurately expresses that person's wishes. You should never sign a will as a witness if you have been named as a benefactor of the will. A benefactor is a person who will receive money or other items belonging to the person who has died when the will is read.

DYING WITH DIGNITY

All people have the right to die in a way that is as peaceful and dignified as possible. Advance directives and hospice care can help to ensure a person's comfort and dignity during the end-of-life period.

Advance Directives

In Chapter 4, you learned that advance directives are documents that allow a person to make their wishes regarding health care known to family members and health care workers, in case the time comes when they are no longer able to make those wishes known themselves. You will recall that a person's advance directive could include a living will, the naming of a durable power of attorney for health care (also known as a health care agent), or both.

Many people arrange for living wills, durable powers of attorney, or both as a way of ensuring that their wishes regarding their end-of-life care are known and honored (Fig. 26-7). Many people specify in their advance directives that they would like to avoid **life-sustaining treatments** (treatments that will prolong life) if by having these treatments, their quality of

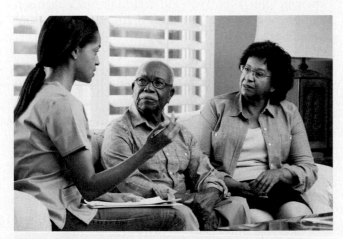

Figure 26-7 Having a living will, a durable power of attorney, or both helps to ensure that a person's wishes regarding their health care are known and honored in case the person is not able to make these wishes known themselves. Many people seek a lawyer's assistance in completing these documents, just so they have them in case they ever need them. Health care facilities also have staff members who are able to assist patients or residents with writing a living will or durable power of attorney. (*Monkey Business Images\Shutterstock.com*)

life will be compromised. Examples of life-sustaining treatments include respiratory ventilation, cardiopulmonary resuscitation (CPR), and the placement of a feeding tube or intravenous (IV) line for the provision of nutrition. Instead, the person may specify that only supportive care should be provided. **Supportive care** includes treatments that will not prolong life but will make the person more comfortable, such as oxygen therapy, nutritional supplementation, pain medication, range-of-motion exercises, grooming and hygiene, and positioning assistance. A person who has made the decision to receive only supportive care at the end of life will have a **no-code or do-not-resuscitate (DNR) order** written in their medical record. This means that the usual efforts to save the person's life will not be made. Some facilities use the term "allow natural death (AND)" instead of DNR. The entire health care team should be aware of this order so that the person will be allowed to die with the compassion and dignity they have requested.

Hospice Care

Hospice organizations have the mission of offering the terminally ill person the best quality of life possible and ensuring their comfort and dignity as death approaches. Hospice care is provided by a multidisciplinary team (made up of nurses, nursing assistants, religious leaders, social workers, doctors, mental health providers, and other professionals). The team seeks to meet the physical, emotional, and spiritual needs of the terminally ill person and their family. After the person's death, hospice provides grief counseling and other types of assistance for the family. Hospice care is available to patients and families 24 hours a day, 7 days a week, and can be provided to a terminally ill person in their home, a long-term care facility, or the hospital. In addition, some facilities specialize in providing hospice care. People become eligible for hospice care when their doctors tell them they have approximately 6 months left to live.

The first hospice program, St. Christopher's Hospice in London, was opened in 1974 to provide supportive care and palliative care to terminally ill people. **Palliative care** focuses on relieving uncomfortable symptoms, not on curing the problem that is causing the symptoms (Fig. 26-8). Examples of palliative treatments include the administration of medications to control pain, the use of chemotherapy or radiation to shrink a tumor (thereby making a person more comfortable), and the use of oxygen therapy to help keep a person with breathing problems comfortable. Surgical procedures can also be of a palliative nature. For example, surgery to remove a tumor that is blocking the intestines may be done primarily to increase the person's comfort, not to cure the cancer. Although

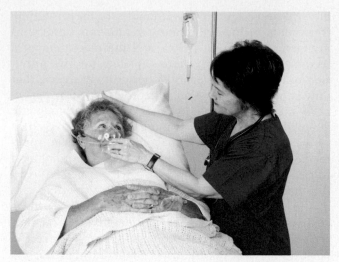

Figure 26-8 Hospice organizations can provide palliative care. Here, a nurse administers oxygen to help the patient breathe more comfortably. (*Lisa F. Young\Shutterstock.com*)

hospice care focuses on pain and symptom control and not curative measures, it in no way asks that a terminally ill person give up hope for recovery or a cure from their illness.

Palliative care also involves eliminating certain routine procedures or treatments when they no longer offer any benefit to the person. For example:

- Medications that no longer serve a purpose may be discontinued.
- A therapeutic diet may be eliminated, and instead food and fluids are provided according to desire and tolerance.
- Routine weight measurements may be eliminated (unless they are needed for calculating medication dosages).
- Blood draws for laboratory tests may be eliminated (unless they are needed to monitor medication therapy).

In addition to providing palliative and supportive care, hospice organizations can assist with having special equipment (such as a hospital bed or bedside commode) brought into a person's home. This special equipment often makes it easier for family and other caregivers to meet the person's physical needs.

The primary focus of the hospice team's efforts is to honor the wishes of the terminally ill person and the family. If a person wishes to die at home or at the hospital, the hospice organization will make every effort to honor these wishes. The person can take much comfort in knowing that their wishes for living life and experiencing a dignified and peaceful death will be honored and that hospice is there to offer support and comfort to the family.

EFFECTS OF CARING FOR THE TERMINALLY ILL ON THE CAREGIVER

Caring for a terminally ill person will affect you. As we work with patients and residents, we become part of their lives and they become part of ours. When one of our patients or residents is diagnosed with a terminal illness, we go through a grief process very similar to that experienced by the person and the family. In addition, because members of the health care profession feel a great need to be able to help others, we often feel inadequate when we must watch others suffer and grieve, and there is little we can do to relieve their pain. We may even question our professional calling. Regardless of how long you work in the medical profession, terminal illness and death will impact you emotionally.

Taking time for yourself is very important. Doing this will help you keep your feelings and emotions in perspective and allow you to continue to give of yourself to others. Talking to your supervisor, a religious leader, or a mental health counselor about questions and fears you have about death can help you to clarify your feelings about death and dying (Fig. 26-9). In addition, you might find seeking advice from an expert helpful when you are trying to work through feelings concerning a specific situation with a patient or resident.

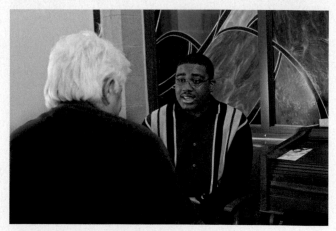

Figure 26-9 Clarifying your beliefs and confronting your fears about death and dying can help you to care for your patients and residents more effectively.

SUMMARY

- As health care providers, we must strive to meet the physical, spiritual, and emotional needs of the terminally ill people who trust us to care for them.

- Caring for people with a terminal illness requires understanding the ways in which people grieve.

  - Dr. Elisabeth Kübler-Ross identified five stages of grief that a person who is dying from a terminal illness experiences: denial, anger, bargaining, depression, and acceptance.

  - Understanding these stages and what the person is feeling during each enables us to be more compassionate and understanding toward both the person and the family.

- Advance directives and hospice care seek to preserve the terminally ill person's right to die in as peaceful and dignified a manner as possible.

- Caring for a terminally ill person and their family can be very rewarding. It can also be very difficult, emotionally.

  - Exploring your own feelings about death (with the help of a professional, if necessary) can help prepare you for the loss of a patient or resident.

  - When caring for a terminally ill person, recognize that you will also go through the grieving process as part of caring for the person, and make allowance for this.

WHAT DID YOU LEARN?

Multiple Choice

Select the single best answer for each of the following questions.

1. Denial is:
   a. The stage of the grieving process in which the person becomes very depressed
   b. A form of bargaining with God for more time
   c. The final step of the grieving process
   d. The time during the grieving process when the person may believe that the diagnosis is incorrect

2. An organization that cares only for people who are dying is a:
   a. Skilled facility
   b. Subacute care unit
   c. Long-term care facility
   d. Hospice organization

3. The stage of grief when a person begins to say goodbye and make arrangements for their death is the:
   a. Bargaining stage
   b. Anger stage
   c. Denial stage
   d. Acceptance stage

4. Hospice care is designed to:
   a. Keep the person comfortable
   b. Prolong the person's life
   c. Treat the person aggressively
   d. All of the above

5. A patient with terminal cancer says they plan to live long enough to walk their daughter, who is getting married, down the aisle. This is an example of:
   a. Acceptance
   b. Depression
   c. Bargaining
   d. Denial

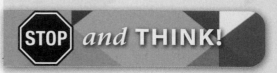

Mrs. Decartez, a resident in your long-term care facility, has a heart condition that is terminal. You have been caring for Mrs. Decartez for a year or so now and have observed her working through the stages of grief as her condition has worsened. She seems to be in acceptance about her impending death and often talks about her funeral. The trouble is with Mrs. Decartez's son. He used to visit quite often and was always friendly and courteous to the staff. Over the last few months, however, he has been visiting less often. When he has visited, he has been critical of you and the other caregivers, and once or twice he has even snapped at you. And just yesterday, you overheard him angrily telling his mother that he didn't want to hear anything else about a funeral! Why do you think Mrs. Decartez's son is acting this way, and how can you help?

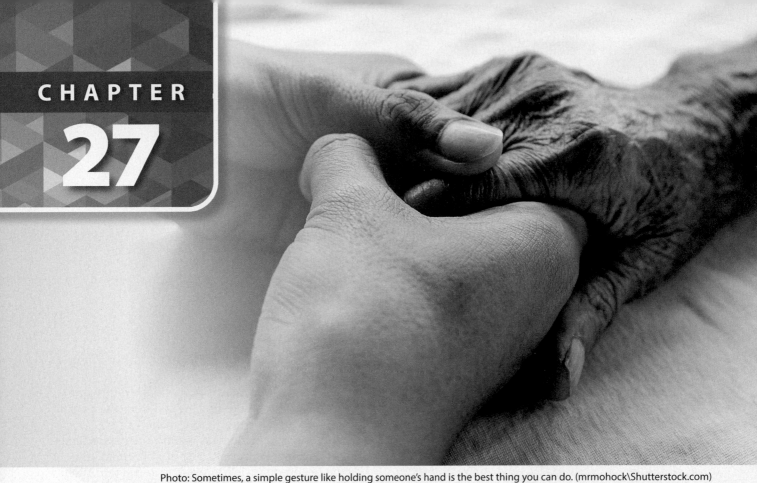

CHAPTER

27

Photo: Sometimes, a simple gesture like holding someone's hand is the best thing you can do. (mrmohock\Shutterstock.com)

Caring for People Who Are Dying

Each person is born to one possession which outvalues all the others—his last breath.
—Mark Twain

 WHAT WILL YOU LEARN?

Most of us give little, if any, thought to what our "last breath" will be like. Sure, we read death notices in the newspaper and hear stories on the evening news about murders and fatal accidents, but do we ever really think about what the person who died experienced during their last moments alive? Was the person in pain, were they lonely, did someone hold their hand, was someone there to hear the person's last words? In the quote above, the American writer Mark Twain (1835–1910) suggests that the very end of life is an important life experience, just like all of the experiences leading up to that moment. As a nursing assistant, you will find yourself in the position of caring for a patient or resident who is dying. In this chapter, you will learn how you can help the dying person, and their family, in the time leading up to the person's "last breath," so that when the time comes, it is as peaceful as possible. You will also learn how to care for a person's body after death occurs. When you are finished with this chapter, you will be able to:

1. **Describe the physical signs that frequently signal impending death.**
2. **Discuss how a nursing assistant's own feelings about death can affect the care they give to a dying patient or resident.**
3. **Describe ways in which the nursing assistant can provide comfort for the dying person.**

507

4. **Discuss how cultural and religious influences can affect how the dying person views death.**

5. **Describe the different ways in which family members may show grief.**

6. **Describe ways that a nursing assistant can help the family of a dying person.**

7. **Discuss the responsibilities that a nursing assistant may have following the death of a patient or resident.**

Vocabulary

Cyanotic	Afterlife	Postmortem care	Autopsy
Cheyne–Stokes respiration	Reincarnation	Rigor mortis	Shroud

SIGNS OF APPROACHING DEATH

Usually, we consider a person "dead" when the heart stops beating and cannot be started again.

Many people die suddenly. However, often there is some warning of approaching death. As death draws near, a person may show certain characteristic physical signs, caused as the body begins to "shut down." These signs may appear over the course of a few hours or a few days, or within the space of a few minutes. Some people may not show these signs. However, recognizing these physical signs and understanding why they occur will help you to know what type of care to give the dying person. Family members may also notice these signs and become concerned. In this case, you will need to reassure them that these signs are normal signs of dying. (Any specific questions regarding the person's condition should be directed to the nurse.) Physical signs of impending death include the following:

- As circulation fails, the blood pressure drops and the pulse becomes rapid and weak. The skin feels cool and clammy, even though the body temperature is rising. The person may perspire heavily and the skin may appear mottled (blotchy), very pale, **cyanotic** (blue-tinged), or grayish. Although you may be tempted to cover the person warmly, they will need only light bed coverings.
- The respiratory pattern changes. The person may take very irregular, shallow breaths, in an alternating fast–slow pattern. This pattern of breathing is called **Cheyne–Stokes respiration**. As the person weakens, fluid or mucus may collect in the air passages, causing the noisy, rattling breathing that is often known as the "death rattle."
- The digestive system slows down. The person may experience nausea, vomiting, abdominal swelling, fecal impaction, or bowel incontinence. The person may not want food or water. Offering ice chips and providing frequent oral care help to keep the mouth moist.
- Urine output decreases as the kidneys respond to the lack of blood flow. In addition, the person may become incontinent of urine.
- Nervous system changes result in decreased muscle tone and sensation. The muscles relax and the person may be too weak to reposition themselves. Some people lose the ability to speak or swallow. The person may lose sensation in their arms or legs, and pain may decrease. Vision may become blurred. (You may notice that the person will turn toward a light in an effort to see better.) Hearing, however, usually remains normal until the moment of death.
- Consciousness may be altered. Some dying people lose consciousness and become comatose as death approaches. As consciousness decreases, pain usually does too. Some people remain conscious and oriented until the moment of death. It is common for a person who has drifted into and out of a semi-comatose state to become alert and oriented right before they die.

When you are caring for a person who is dying, take note of any physical changes that you observe. Report these changes to the nurse and record them in the person's medical chart, per facility policy.

CARING FOR A DYING PERSON

Dying people, like everyone else, have physical and emotional needs. These needs may change dramatically as the time of death approaches and will vary greatly depending on the person. A holistic approach to care is taken with a dying person, just as with any other person (Fig. 27-1). Further, every person has the right to die peacefully and with dignity (Box 27-1). As

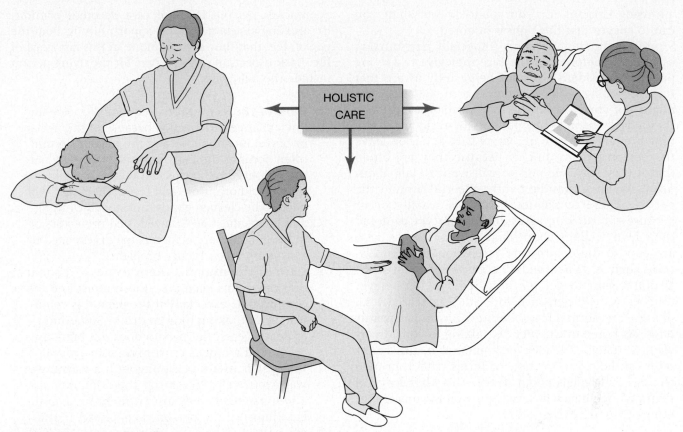

Figure 27-1 The nursing assistant provides for the dying person's physical and emotional comfort. Examples of physical comfort measures include providing frequent oral care and back massages. Examples of emotional comfort measures include caring for the family, helping the person to meet spiritual needs (for example, by reading aloud from a book that has special meaning for the person), and simply spending quiet time with the person.

Box 27-1 The Dying Person's Bill of Rights

I have the right to be treated as a living human being until I die.

I have the right to maintain a sense of hopefulness, however changing its focus may be.

I have the right to be cared for by those who can maintain a sense of hopefulness, however changing this might be.

I have the right to express my feelings and emotions about my approaching death in my own way.

I have the right to participate in decisions concerning my care.

I have the right to expect continuing medical and nursing attention even though "cure" goals must be changed to "comfort" goals.

I have the right not to die alone.

I have the right to be free from pain.

I have the right to have my questions answered honestly.

I have the right not to be deceived.

I have the right to have help from and for my family in accepting my death.

I have the right to die in peace and dignity.

I have a right to retain my individuality and not be judged for my decisions, which may be contrary to beliefs of others.

I have the right to discuss and enlarge my religious and/ or spiritual experiences, whatever these may mean to others.

I have the right to expect that the sanctity of the human body will be respected after death.

I have the right to be cared for by caring, sensitive, knowledgeable people who will attempt to understand my needs and will be able to gain some satisfaction in helping me face my death.

(Created at the workshop *The Terminally Ill Patient and the Helping Person,* in Lansing, Michigan, sponsored by the Southwestern Michigan Inservice Education Council and conducted by Amelia J. Barbus, Associate Professor of Nursing, Wayne State University, Detroit.)

a nursing assistant, it is your job to do everything you can to ensure that this right is honored.

Many nursing assistants (especially new nursing assistants) compromise the care they give to a dying patient or resident, without being fully aware that they are doing so. For example, a nursing assistant might not check in on the dying person as often as they check in on other patients or residents. They may provide only the necessary care and then leave the person's room quickly because they are afraid that if they stay, the person will want to talk about death. Or they may be overly cheerful around the person. These avoidance behaviors usually occur because the nursing assistant has not yet explored their own feelings about death. Many people who are new to the health care profession express concerns such as, "I'm afraid I'll cry if my resident dies," "I don't want to get too attached," or "I've never touched a dead person before and I'm scared." All of these are normal fears that new nursing assistants have. As noted in Chapter 26, talking to your supervisor, a religious leader, or a mental health counselor can help you to come to terms with your own feelings and beliefs about death. This knowledge of your own feelings will serve you well as you care for others who are dying.

Concerns for Long-Term Care

In older adults, death is usually associated with a combination of chronic illnesses and the aging process. As a whole, society tends to view the death of an older person as "just a part of life." Interestingly, the American Geriatrics Society (AGS) states that "birth and death give definition to life as the period in between." For many older adults, having a "good death" is just a part of the process of living and is strongly influenced by that person's cultural and spiritual beliefs.

Facing the death of a resident never gets any easier. You will become very attached to your residents. Although the relationship you have with the resident can make providing end-of-life care very emotionally difficult for you, it is this relationship that will allow you to provide the holistic care that the dying person needs so much.

Meeting the Dying Person's Physical Needs

A dying person becomes more and more dependent on others for basic physical care as the time of death approaches. As the focus of care becomes comfort, the nursing assistant has the opportunity to help the person feel that they are not alone in this last stage of life. Basic aspects of physical care for the dying person include the following:

- **Care of the skin.** More frequent skin care and linen changes are needed because of the urinary or bowel incontinence and the moist skin that often occur as the person nears death. The person will need to be checked regularly for incontinence of both urine and feces. Their skin will need to be cleaned gently, and soiled clothing and linens must be changed. Bed protectors or indwelling urinary catheters may be needed to assist with incontinence problems.
- **Care of the mucous membranes.** Frequent oral care helps keep the mouth moist and more comfortable, especially if the person is comatose or not taking food or drink. Sometimes as death nears, the person does not blink as often, and a mucus crust may form around the eyelids. Gentle cleaning with a warm, wet washcloth helps to remove the dried mucus. The nurse may apply an ointment to keep the eyes moist. If the person is comatose, moist eye pads may be used for protection. Medical equipment, such as oxygen cannulas and nasogastric tubes, may cause irritation and crusting of mucus around the nostrils. Gently removing the mucus crust with a warm, wet washcloth and applying a lubricant can help to keep the person comfortable.
- **Positioning.** As the person's condition worsens, they may not be able to reposition themselves without assistance. Frequent, regular position changes help to prevent pressure ulcers and promote comfort. However, if the process of repositioning the person causes severe pain, the decision may be made to allow the person to remain in the most comfortable position. The use of pillows or other positioning devices helps to maintain the body in proper alignment. If the person is in pain, you will need to be extra gentle and slow with position changes. Always tell the nurse if the person seems to be in pain so that necessary medications can be administered. A person who is having difficulty breathing will probably be more comfortable positioned with their head elevated.
- **Other comfort measures.** Receiving a back massage, listening to soft music, or being read to are all activities that can help a person to rest and feel better. Enemas may be necessary

to assist with bowel elimination. Secretions may collect in the person's airways, making breathing difficult. If you notice that a person is having difficulty breathing, report this to the nurse. The nurse will provide suctioning and oxygen therapy, measures that can make breathing easier and more comfortable for the person. Keep the room well lit and ventilated. Remove soiled linens, bedpans, or emesis basins and use air freshener to help eliminate unpleasant odors.

As death nears, there may be changes in the dying person's ability to communicate with others. Therefore, when caring for a dying person, you must be very observant of the person's physical needs. As the person's ability to communicate pain, thirst, or other physical needs decreases, they will rely more and more on the nursing team to notice those needs and take care of them. In addition, you must take measures to make communication easier:

- Remember that as death approaches, the person's vision may become blurry. Keep the room well lit to help the person to see better. Also, make sure you introduce yourself when entering the room and encourage family members to do the same.
- Speaking may become difficult for the person. In this case, asking simple "yes or no" questions will make communication more effective.
- Hearing usually remains quite sharp up until the time of death, even if the person is comatose. Always talk to the person as if they are able to hear you, even if they cannot respond. Explain procedures to the person and offer reassurance that you are there and will return soon when you leave the room. Gently remind family members that the person may still be able to hear their conversations and encourage them to talk to the person. Hearing the voices of family can be comforting for the dying person. However, family members should be advised that potentially upsetting topics should be discussed elsewhere, out of earshot of the dying person.

A person's family may wish to assist in providing physical care. If a family member says that they would like to be involved in caring for the dying person, encourage this by suggesting ways that they can help. For example, you might ask the family member if they would be willing to help you out by giving the person sips of water or ice chips, and then show them how to do this (Fig. 27-2). Family members often feel useless or helpless when it becomes clear that there is nothing

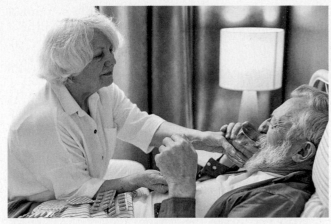

Figure 27-2 Sometimes, family members want to assist in meeting a dying person's physical needs. Here, a family member offers the dying person sips of water. (*Roman Chazov\Shutterstock.com*)

left to do except wait for death to arrive. Participating in the care of a dying loved one can help a family member feel that they are making a positive impact on their loved one's comfort.

Meeting the Dying Person's Emotional Needs

Emotionally, people prepare for death very individually. People may have many fears regarding death, such as a fear of the unknown or a fear of losing dignity and self-control. Some may fear that death will be painful, or worry about the effects of their death on the people left behind. Some people have concerns about unfinished business. Another concern that many dying people have is a fear of facing death alone (Fig. 27-3). Some people are

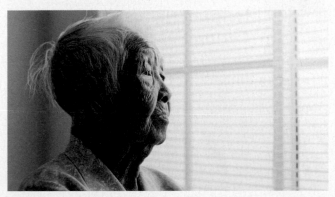

Figure 27-3 Many people have fears related to death, such as a fear of dying alone or of dying in pain. As a nursing assistant, you can help to relieve some of these fears. (*Nattakorn_Maneerat\Shutterstock.com*)

able to speak of their fears, while others remain silent, afraid to even speak of what frightens them the most.

Being a Good Listener

A nursing assistant can help meet a dying person's emotional needs by being a good listener. A dying person may want to talk about their fears related to dying, or what they expect the afterlife to be like. Or, the person might just want to remember significant events in their life and share those memories with you now. If you sense that a person wants to talk, use the communication techniques you learned in Chapter 5 to encourage the person and let them know that you are there to listen. Even though you may be uncomfortable at first when a patient or resident brings up the subject of death, do not change the subject, make yourself "busy," or simply pat the person on the hand and say, "Oh, don't worry, honey; you've got lots of time left." Many dying people are very aware of their situation and they may tell you that their time here is very short. Do not avoid spending time with a dying person because you are afraid that the person will bring up a subject and you will not know what to say in response. You do not need to say anything—you just need to listen to what the person wants to tell you.

Other dying people do not want to talk and can become annoyed at your attempts to make small talk. Use your observation skills to note when a person would prefer not to talk. Although the person may not want to have a conversation, they will still want to know that you are nearby and watching out for them. Check on the person frequently and remind them that you are close by if they need anything.

Helping Hands and a Caring Heart

Focus on Humanistic Health Care

Many dying people genuinely appreciate it when someone takes the time to sit near them quietly. Touch can convey so much more than words can in a situation like this. Gently hold the person's hand or touch their shoulder when you are speaking to them. Gently smooth the person's hair after you have finished straightening the bed linens or repositioning the pillow, or comfort the person with a back massage. All of these actions let a person know that they are cared for and not alone.

Culture, Religion, and Spirituality

As you learned in Chapter 6, a person's culture and religion often influence how the person responds to illness and other life experiences, including death. Cultural and religious beliefs influence how a person feels about death and prepares for it. For example, some people may not feel comfortable talking about dying because in their culture, death is considered a very private matter. On the other hand, some people may seem very accepting of death because their culture or religion has taught them that death is not to be feared. Some examples of death rituals that vary across cultures are shown in Box 27-2.

Many dying people find peace and comfort in their religious beliefs. They may wish to visit with religious leaders, surround themselves with religious items, or spend time alone praying, meditating, or reading religious texts. Some people may ask you to read to them. Although you may not share the person's beliefs, you should honor this request. For the dying person, hearing familiar words that reflect their deepest beliefs can bring great comfort. You must respect the beliefs of your patients or residents, even if you do not share them; remember that they are just as important to them as yours are to you.

A dying person may request that you call a religious leader to administer religious blessings or "last rites." If such a request is made, report it immediately to the nurse so that the necessary arrangements can be made. When the religious leader arrives, make sure that there is a place for them to sit, and ensure privacy. As part of preparing for death, people often want to confess to a religious leader, and they will want privacy to do this.

Religion is but one aspect of spirituality and many people are very spiritual without belonging to any particular religious group. Most people who consider themselves "spiritual" believe that a higher being or spirit offers hope and peace although this higher being may not necessarily be one that is recognized by the world's organized religions. Spirituality gives a person inner strength to face life's challenges. It gives meaning to a person's life. Many people exhibit their inner spirituality by listening to music, reading poetry, or spending time in nature.

When cultural and religious or spiritual beliefs provide an explanation for what happens to a person after death, they can be a source of comfort for the dying person (as well as for the person's family). For example, many people believe in an **afterlife**, a state of being where the dead meet again with loved ones who have passed on before them. Other people believe in **reincarnation**, the idea that a person's

Box 27-2   Common Death Rituals That May Differ Among Cultural Groups

Remember that culture, religion, and spirituality strongly influence how people view and respond to death. Death rituals that your patients or residents and their families practice will vary based on these influences. As a nursing assistant, you must always use your skills of observation and communication to assess how to appropriately support your patients or residents and their families in their need to practice different rituals during and immediately after the time of death.

Aspect of Ritual	Death Ritual	Intervention
Grief and Mourning	Responding to news of death of a loved one with sudden collapse, paralysis, inability to see or speak, or hyperkinetic and seizure-like activity to release strong emotions.	Recognize that this is not an emergency medical condition and treatment is usually not necessary; remain with the person, provide support, and involve family with assistance, if possible.
Religious and Spiritual Beliefs and Practices	Belief that a dying person should not be left alone.	Make accommodations for family members to be present at all times.
	A wake-like "sitting up" during the night may be performed for seriously ill and dying family members.	Arrange for privacy and accommodate family members staying overnight.
	A large gathering of relatives and friends may attend the dying person and may place religious artifacts or candles around the person.	Arrange for a gathering place close to the dying person; find electric candles if open flames are not allowed; summon religious leaders for religious rituals; do not move religious items.
	A Muslim patient may wish for the bed to be turned to face the holy city of Mecca; family may recite prayers from the Qur'an.	Facilitate positioning of the bed whenever possible; provide privacy for prayers.
	Flowers may be avoided during illness in cultures where they are usually reserved for rites of the dead.	Ask permission from the patient or family before placing flowers in a room.
Family and Gender Roles and Relationships	Death may be perceived as a time of crisis; the head of the family (that is, usually the oldest daughter or son) may be responsible for receiving the news of death; eldest son may have particular responsibilities at time of death.	Allow time for family to view, touch, and stay with the body before it is removed; ask if the family wants a religious leader called. Notify eldest son of pending death, or identify lines of communication if eldest son is not available.
	Priest and eldest son may perform death rites, with all male relatives assisting, depending on custom.	Make accommodations for privacy, encourage family to bring in religious objects, allow families to participate in postmortem care if they desire to do so.
	All family members may try to gather at the bedside at the time of death and pray or cry uncontrollably.	
Communication	It is taboo in some cultures, such as Navajo culture, to talk about a fatal disease or dying; the issue may need to be discussed in the third person, as if it is occurring in someone else.	Avoid suggesting that a member of the Navajo tribe is dying because this may be interpreted as a wish that the person be dead.

Source: Purnell, L. D. (2009). *Culturally competent health care.* F. A. Davis.

spirit or soul will live again on Earth in the form of an animal or human being yet to be born.

CARE OF THE FAMILY

Knowing that a loved one will die soon can be difficult for the person's family. Family members must cope with their own grief and possibly that of other family members as well. Remember that the stress and grief experienced by the family can cause them to act in ways that may seem strange to you. For example, some people may treat you rudely or snap at you in anger. Be polite and do not take offensive actions or words personally. Usually, these offensive behaviors are just a result of the person's grief. If a family member seems to be getting overly agitated or angry, or if arguing or aggression between family members occurs, notify the nurse immediately.

As a nursing assistant, you may feel overwhelmed at the thought of caring for the family as well as for the patient or resident. However, there are many simple things you can do to comfort the family (Fig. 27-4).

- **Ensure good communication between the family and the health care team.** Often, family members will have worries or fears related to the person's care or condition, and they may want to discuss these with you or another member of the health care team. If a family member asks you a question that you do not know the answer to or are not qualified to answer, make sure to relay this request for information to the nurse so that the family member's concerns can be addressed.

- **Allow family to stay with the dying person, and to participate in the person's care if they want to.** When a person is dying, many families wish to remain close by. Visiting hours are usually relaxed, allowing family to stay with the dying person for as long as they like. Encourage family members to talk to the dying person and to help with the person's care. However, do not push family members to do this if they seem hesitant. Although you have responsibilities to the family, your first responsibility is to your patient or resident. When providing physical care to the dying person, please ask the family to step outside for a moment (unless they have chosen to help you) and close the curtains to help maintain the person's dignity. Also, too many visitors for too long a period of time can be tiring for some patients or residents. If you suspect that the number of visitors or the length of time that they are staying is causing your patient or resident to become overly tired, report your observations to the nurse.

- **Ensure that the family members' basic needs are met.** Make sure that there are enough chairs in the room, so that everyone can sit down. Encourage family members to rest and take meals as necessary. Show them how to find the restrooms, public telephones, vending machines, and cafeteria. If a family member is showing signs of weariness, offer to stay at the dying person's side

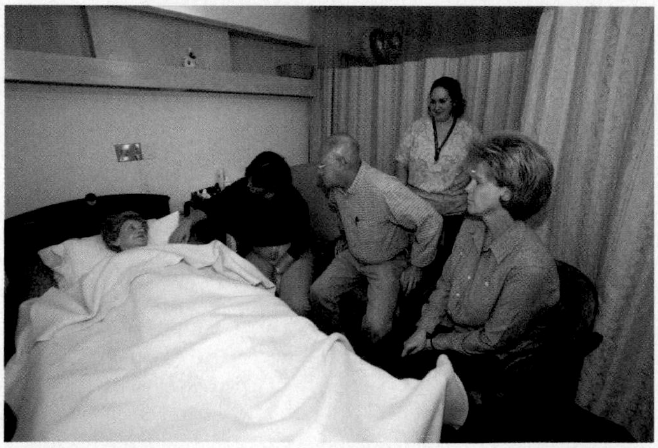

Figure 27-4 Family members will often seek reassurance and comfort from the nursing staff. As a nursing assistant, there are many simple kindnesses you can extend to the family that will help make this ordeal easier for them. Here, a nursing assistant has brought in an extra chair for a family member who has just arrived at the bedside.

Tell the Nurse!

When you are caring for a person who is dying, be sure to report the following to the nurse immediately:

- The person seems to be in pain
- The person is having trouble breathing
- The person asks to see a religious leader
- The person seems overwhelmed by the number of visitors or the length of time that they are staying
- A family member has a question about the person's care or condition that you are not qualified to answer
- The person has died

while the family member takes a short walk outside or down the hall to grab a cup of coffee.

- **Be readily available to provide needed care to the patient or resident without being intrusive of the family's privacy.** Often, the most comforting thing to family members is knowing that their loved one is receiving competent, compassionate care.

POSTMORTEM CARE

If you are present when one of your patients or residents dies, you must notify the nurse that the person has died, and note the time. You may need to document the absence of vital signs. A doctor may be called to legally pronounce the person dead. In some health care settings, the nurse may legally pronounce the person dead. The time of death is recorded on the person's death certificate. After the person has been pronounced dead, you may be required to assist the nurse in giving postmortem care, depending on the policy at the facility or agency where you work.

Postmortem care is the care of a person's body after the person's death. Cultural and religious beliefs often dictate how the body is to be cared for after death (and by whom). In some cultures, family members help to clean and prepare the body for whatever lies ahead, in accordance with cultural and religious traditions.

Postmortem care is necessary to keep the body in proper alignment and to prevent skin damage and discoloration. The skin is cleaned of any mucus, urine, feces, or other fluids. Standard precautions are followed when performing postmortem care because bodily fluids are still potentially infectious, even after death. The body is placed in proper alignment before rigor mortis occurs. **Rigor mortis** is the stiffening of the muscles that usually develops within 2 to 4 hours of death. Once rigor mortis occurs, it is difficult to reposition the body. It is not uncommon for air that has been trapped in the lungs or the digestive tract to be released from the body when the body is repositioned as part of postmortem care. It may sound like the person has sighed or moaned. This natural occurrence may frighten you, unless you are aware of its cause.

In some cases, an autopsy may be required to confirm or identify the cause of the person's death. An **autopsy** is an examination of the person's organs and tissues after the person has died. In most cases, the doctor is responsible for obtaining a family member's permission to perform an autopsy. If an autopsy is to be performed, medical devices such as tubes, drains, catheters, and intravenous (IV) lines are not

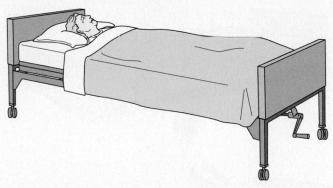

Figure 27-5 The body is placed in the supine position for viewing by the family. A pillow is placed under the person's head and shoulders.

removed as part of postmortem care. If an autopsy is not necessary, the nurse will usually remove these medical devices as part of the postmortem care procedure.

Many facilities only prepare the person's body for the family to view before sending it to the morgue or funeral home, where the funeral director completes the postmortem care procedure. In this case, the bed linens are straightened (or changed, if they are soiled). The body is cleaned, dressed in a clean gown or pajamas, and positioned in a natural position on the bed (Fig. 27-5). Draw the top sheet up to the person's shoulders and cuff it neatly. (Do not cover the person's face with the sheet. This can be very disturbing for family.) Make sure that the room is neat, and adjust the lights so that they are not too bright. As always, provide for privacy. You will need to help collect the person's personal belongings to be sent with the family. Dentures are either placed in the person's mouth, or labeled and sent with the body to the funeral home.

After the family has viewed the body and left, the body may be wrapped in a **shroud** (a covering used to wrap the body of a person who has died) for transport to the morgue or funeral home. A shroud is contained in the preassembled postmortem kits used by many facilities. The shroud may be a plastic sheet that is secured with pins, tapes, or ties (Fig. 27-6), or it may be zip closed. The procedure for postmortem care is given in Procedure 27-1. You show your respect for the person and their family by working quietly and preserving the person's privacy, even after death.

Providing postmortem care can be emotionally difficult. Health care workers often become very attached to their patients or residents and grieve when they die. It is not uncommon to feel frustrated at death when the focus of health care seems to be mostly on curing disease. It is perfectly acceptable to feel sad and cry at the passing of a patient or resident.

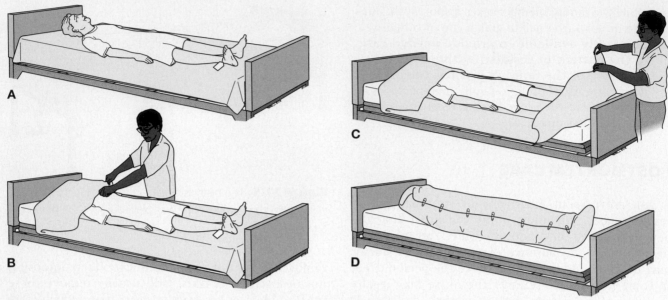

Figure 27-6 A shroud may be placed on the body after the family has left and before the body is taken to the morgue or funeral home. **A.** The shroud is unfolded on the bed, and the body is placed on the shroud. **B.** The top of the shroud is brought over the person's head. **C.** The bottom of the shroud is brought over the person's feet. **D.** The sides of the shroud are folded over the person's body and pinned, taped, or tied together. An identification tag is secured to the outside of the shroud.

You might be surprised to know that even the most experienced health care workers often seek a "shoulder to cry on." Talking about your feelings with a coworker, supervisor, religious leader, or counselor can help you work through your own grief. Allow yourself to be human and feel emotions. It might also help to think of providing postmortem care as a way of paying your last respects to the dead person. In this way, the ritual of providing this care becomes a way of coping with your grief.

SUMMARY

- Providing holistic care is as important at the end of life as it is at any other time. Nursing assistants must take steps to prevent their own discomfort with the subject of death from compromising their ability to care for dying people.
  - A dying person becomes very dependent on others for basic physical care. Recognizing the physical signs of impending death helps the nursing assistant provide the necessary care.
  - A dying person will need assistance to meet emotional and spiritual needs as well.
    - Emotionally, people prepare for death in their own ways. Cultural and religious beliefs and traditions greatly influence a person's response to illness and death.
    - Often, the best thing a nursing assistant can do is listen if the person wants to talk, or

spend quiet time with the person if they do not want to talk.
- Family members of a dying person require support as well.
  - Being respectful, thoughtful, and kind can do much to make family members feel better.
  - Some family members react poorly to grief and stress and may take out their frustrations on nursing assistants or other members of the health care team.
- Postmortem care is done to prepare the body for the morgue or funeral home. In some facilities, the body is prepared for immediate viewing by the family, and then postmortem care is done at the morgue or funeral home.

▶ **Procedure 27-1**

Providing Postmortem Care

▶

WHY YOU DO IT Postmortem care keeps the body in proper alignment and prevents skin damage and discoloration.

Getting Ready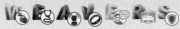

1. Complete the "Getting Ready" steps.

Supplies

- gloves
- paper towels
- cotton balls
- bed protector
- postmortem kit[a]
- wash basin
- soap or no-rinse cleanser
- comb
- bath blanket
- washcloth
- towel
- clean gown or pajamas
- clean linens (if necessary)

Procedure

2. Cover the over-bed table with paper towels. Place your supplies on the over-bed table.

3. Make sure that the bed is positioned at a comfortable working height (to promote good body mechanics) and that the wheels are locked. Lower the head of the bed so that the bed is flat. Fanfold the top linens to the foot of the bed.

4. Put on the gloves.

5. If instructed to by the nurse, remove or turn off any medical equipment.

6. Place the body in the supine position. Position the pillow under the person's head and shoulders. Undress the body and cover it with the bath blanket.

7. Close the eyes. Put a moistened cotton ball on each eyelid if the eyes do not stay closed. If the person has an artificial eye, this should be in place, unless you are instructed otherwise.

8. Replace the person's dentures, unless you are instructed otherwise. Close the mouth and, if necessary, gently support the jaw with the chin strap, a light bandage, or a rolled hand towel.

9. Remove any jewelry and place it in a plastic bag or envelope for the family. List each piece of jewelry as you remove it. Do not remove engagement or wedding rings, unless it is your facility's policy to do so.

10. Fill the wash basin with warm water. Place the basin on the over-bed table. Wash the body, place an absorbent pad under the buttocks, and comb the hair. (In some cultures, the body is washed by a family member as part of a ritual.)

11. If the family is to view the body, dress the body in a clean gown or pajamas. If the bedding is wet or soiled, change the bed linens. Draw the top linens over the person, forming a cuff at the shoulders. (Do not cover the person's face.) Remove your gloves and perform hand hygiene. Straighten the room, lower the lights, and provide for the family's privacy.

12. After the family leaves, collect all of the person's belongings, noting each item on your list.

13. Fill out three identification tags:

    a. Attach one to the right great toe or the right ankle.

    b. Attach one to the person's belongings.

    c. Save the last to be attached to the outside of the shroud (if used).

14. If a shroud is to be used, put on a clean pair of gloves, apply it now and attach the third identification tag to the outside of the shroud.

15. Gather the soiled linens and place them in the linen hamper. Dispose of disposable items in a facility-approved waste container. Clean equipment and return it to the storage area.

16. Remove your gloves, dispose of them in a facility-approved waste container, and perform hand hygiene.

[a]The contents of the postmortem kit vary, but most contain a shroud, something for securing the shroud, ties, gauze pads, a chin strap, identification tags, and a plastic bag or envelope for the person's belongings.

(continued)

17. Transfer the body from the bed to a stretcher for transport to the morgue, if appropriate. If the family has made funeral arrangements, leave the body in the room with the door or curtain closed.

18. Report the time the body was transported and the location of the person's belongings to the nurse.

Finishing Up

19. Complete the "Finishing Up" steps.

What You Document

- Date and time
- Care given
- Description of items removed from the body—for example: jewelry, dentures
- Who received the removed items and other personal belongings
- Time body is taken to morgue or funeral home

WHAT DID YOU LEARN?

Multiple Choice

Select the single best answer for each of the following questions.

1. When caring for a person who is dying, you should:
   a. Keep family members away from the dying person
   b. Keep the room dark
   c. Provide for the person's physical and emotional needs
   d. Change the subject if the person starts to talk about death or dying

2. A common sign of approaching death is:
   a. Severe pain that gets worse
   b. Normal or increased vital signs
   c. Cool, moist skin
   d. Increased appetite

3. Postmortem care is done:
   a. Right before the person dies
   b. After the doctor pronounces the person dead
   c. After rigor mortis sets in
   d. If there is time

4. As death approaches, the last sense to be lost is usually:
   a. Sight
   b. Hearing
   c. Smell
   d. Taste

5. Which one of the following is a true statement about providing postmortem care?
   a. Standard precautions are used because the body fluids may be infectious
   b. Dentures are removed from the mouth and given to the family to take home

   c. There is no need for privacy because the person is dead
   d. All of the above

6. In caring for the dying person, the nursing assistant also needs to care for the family. Which of the following can the nursing assistant do to support the family?
   a. Allow family members to stay with the dying person
   b. Be respectful of the family
   c. Provide the family with privacy
   d. All of the above

7. You are helping to care for Mrs. Wong, who has a terminal illness. One day when you are in Mrs. Wong's room, she tells you that during difficult times she has always found comfort in reading poems by her favorite poets. What is this an example of?
   a. Culture
   b. Spirituality
   c. Religion
   d. Reincarnation

8. Which of the following meets a dying person's physical needs?
   a. Providing frequent skin care
   b. Listening if the person wants to talk
   c. Preventing rigor mortis
   d. All of the above

Matching *Match each numbered item with its appropriate lettered description.*

_____ **1.** Reincarnation

_____ **2.** Cheyne–Stokes respiration

_____ **3.** Rigor mortis

_____ **4.** Postmortem care

_____ **5.** Autopsy

a. Examination of a person's tissues and organs after death
b. Stiffening of the muscles that occurs 2 to 4 hours after death
c. Care of a body after death
d. The belief that the soul of a dead person returns to Earth in the form of another human being or animal yet to be born
e. Pattern of rapid–slow respirations

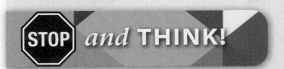
STOP *and* **THINK!**

You have been caring for Mr. Cortez, who is dying. Now it appears that the time of death is rapidly approaching. Even though Mr. Cortez is having trouble talking, he does manage to say to you, "I don't want to die alone." What can you do to help Mr. Cortez?

Respect

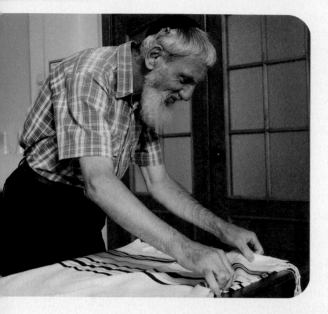

I am a nursing assistant who works in a long-term care facility. I recently moved here from a different part of the country and am learning so much about our lovely residents. Having grown up in a small farming community, I have not been exposed to many different types of people and cultures.

One of our residents, Mr. Alperstein, had become very near and dear to my heart. He was Jewish, and never tired of telling me about his faith, his family, and their customs. I learned about his dietary practices, and he shared with me some of the ritual foods that his family would bring in honor of their holy days and celebrations. He explained what each of the candles symbolizes on the menorah during Hanukkah, and that the colors blue and white are the colors of Israel. This was all very different from the Christmas traditions I grew up sharing with my own family.

Sadly, Mr. Alperstein had a terminal illness, which made him weaker as he got closer to the end of his time. He sat in his chair more, near the window, often wrapped in his prayer shawl. If you stopped by his door, you could often hear him speaking softly in Yiddish. He said his prayers give him great comfort as he faced death.

One beautiful October morning, the doctor said that Mr. Alperstein's time was very close, and that the family needed to be called in. As they arrived, I made sure that there were plenty of chairs for their comfort and that they could call on me if they needed anything. During the next few hours, I quietly came and went as I provided for Mr. Alperstein's physical needs. And then he passed away quietly.

I gently asked Mrs. Alperstein how she and their family wished to follow Mr. Alperstein's passing. According to custom, the family stayed with Mr. Alperstein's body until the funeral director arrived to take him. It was all very special for me to assist Mr. Alperstein and his family during this time. Mr. Alperstein had been so kind and patient, and he had taught me so much about learning what makes everyone so uniquely themselves. He certainly opened my eyes to learning to respect people whose beliefs were different from my own, and how to offer comfort when they need it most.

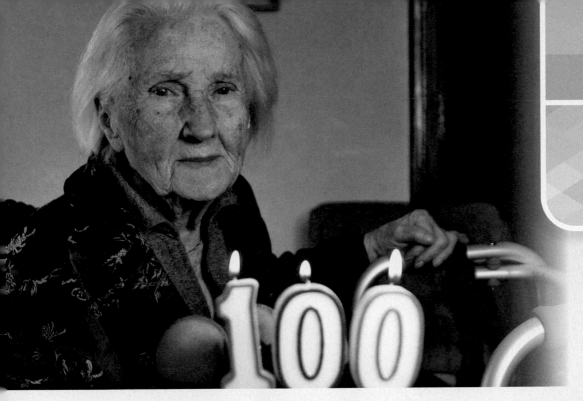

Body Systems: Normal Function and the Effects of Aging and Disease

THE HUMAN BODY HAS AMAZING CAPABILITIES. Our bodies allow us to fully experience the world around us, to move, to think, to create. Perhaps even more amazing than what our bodies allow us to do is what our bodies do for us automatically. For example, think about how many times a day your heart beats or your lungs inhale and exhale. What would it be like if you had to remember to do this on your own? Or think about the last time you had a cold or the flu, and your body fought off the infection. The human body is truly remarkable in its ability to maintain health and to heal from disease.

In this unit, we will explore how each organ system functions normally, as well as how disease or injury affects the function of each organ system. The process of normal aging has an impact on each organ system too, even in the healthy older adult. We will also explore the measures that are taken to help the body return to its best level of functioning after injury or illness. Knowing how the body works when it is healthy helps us to understand how to help the body heal and function more effectively during illness.

Photo: The human body has amazing capabilities. This resident is celebrating her 100th birthday. (Dan Negureanu\Shutterstock.com)

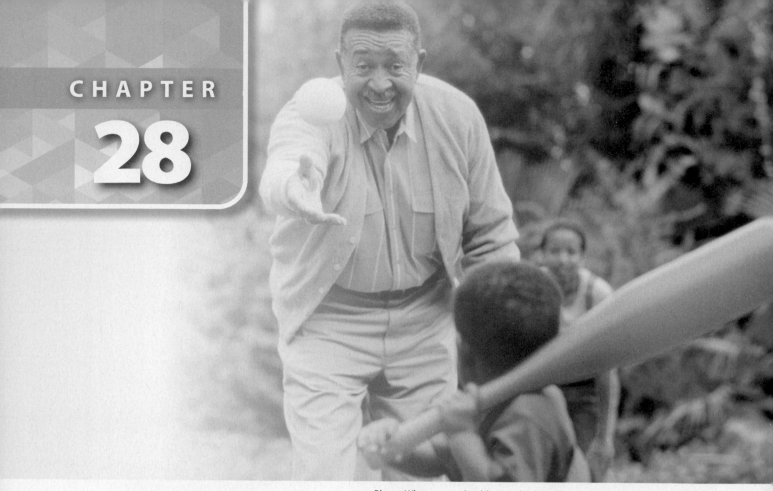

CHAPTER
28

Photo: When we are healthy, our bodies allow us to do the things we like to do.

Basic Body Structure and Function

 WHAT WILL YOU LEARN?

The human body is a wonder of design. In a healthy person, all of the body's parts work together effortlessly, like those of a highly efficient machine. To understand how a machine works, a mechanic studies the machine's parts and how they work together. The same is true of people who want to know how the human body works. **Anatomy** is the study of what body parts look like, where they are located, how big they are, and how they connect to other body parts. **Physiology** is the study of how the body parts work. In this chapter, we will take a look at the body as a whole, functioning unit. You will learn about how changes in a person's normal anatomy or physiology can lead to disease or disabilities and about the body's remarkable ability to correct small problems before they become large ones. When you are finished with this chapter, you will be able to:

1. Define the terms *anatomy* and *physiology*.
2. List and describe the basic levels of organization of the body.
3. Define the term *homeostasis* and give examples of how the body maintains the balance necessary for life.
4. Discuss how the body's inability to maintain homeostasis affects a person's health.
5. Describe the categories of disease and list some factors that may put a person at risk for developing a certain disease.

522

Vocabulary

Anatomy	Organelles	Tissue	Homeostasis
Physiology	Cytoplasm	Organ	Disease
Organism	Nucleus	Organ system	
Cell	Plasma membrane		

HOW IS THE BODY ORGANIZED?

All living things, from a jellyfish that washes up on the beach to the largest elephant roaming the plains of Africa, share the same general organization. The basic unit of life is the cell. Cells group together to form tissues. Tissues group together to form organs, and organs group together to form organ systems. These levels of organization are shared by every living thing, or **organism**, whether it is an animal or a plant (Fig. 28-1). The reason not all living things look alike or function alike is because at each level, there are variations specific to the type of organism. Let's take a closer look now at the levels of organization that make up each organism—cells, tissues, organs, and organ systems.

Cells

A **cell** is the basic unit of life. A cell is so small that it can only be seen with a microscope. A single cell, as small as it is, has all of the characteristics of life. It is capable of organization, which means that it can join with other similar cells to perform a common function. It is capable of metabolism, which means that it takes in "raw materials" and converts them into the energy it needs to stay alive. It is capable of growth, which means that it changes in size over time. And finally, it is capable of reproduction, which means that it can make a copy of itself. Organization, metabolism, growth, and reproduction are basic qualities that make a living thing different from a nonliving thing.

The human body is made up of millions of cells, of all different shapes, sizes, and functions. Each type of cell has a specific duty. Our overall health depends on the ability of the body's cells to do their jobs.

To function properly, cells require oxygen, water, nutrition, and the ability to eliminate waste products. Structures inside of the cell, called **organelles**, help the cell to make the energy it needs to stay alive and to rid itself of waste products (Fig. 28-2). The organelles float in a jelly-like substance called **cytoplasm**. In addition to organelles and cytoplasm, the cell contains a nucleus. The **nucleus** of the cell is like the cell's "brain." It contains all of the information the cell needs to do its job, grow, and reproduce. A **plasma membrane** surrounds the cytoplasm and gives the cell its shape.

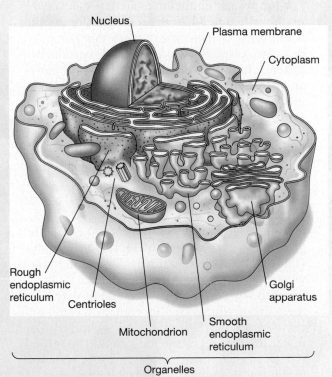

Figure 28-2 A cell contains organelles and a nucleus, which float in a jelly-like substance called cytoplasm. A plasma membrane surrounds the cytoplasm and gives the cell its shape.

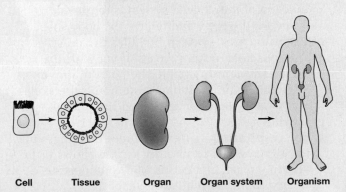

Cell   Tissue   Organ   Organ system   Organism

Figure 28-1 All living things (organisms) share the same basic levels of organization. Cells form tissues, tissues form organs, and organs form organ systems.

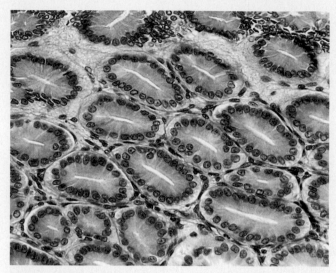

Figure 28-3 Cells join together to form tissues. (*Ocskay Bence\Shutterstock.com*)

Tissues

When cells that are similar in structure and specialized to perform a specific function join together, they form **tissue** (Fig. 28-3). There are four main types of tissue in the human body:

- **Epithelial tissue** covers the outside of the body, lines its internal structures, and forms glands. The purpose of epithelial tissue is protection. Epithelial tissue forms the outer part of the skin. It forms the mucous membranes that line our digestive, respiratory, urinary, and reproductive systems. It also covers organs such as the lungs and heart, and lines the inside of the blood vessels, abdominal cavity, and chest cavity.
- **Connective tissue** does what its name suggests— it connects other tissues together. Connective tissue supports and forms the framework for all of the parts of the body. Examples of connective tissue include bone, cartilage, ligaments, tendons, and fatty tissues. Blood is also considered a form of connective tissue.
- **Muscle tissue** produces movement. There are three types of muscle tissue found in the body (Table 28-1). Skeletal muscle allows you to move your arms, legs, and other parts of the body. Because you can decide when and how to move the parts of your body that contain skeletal muscle, skeletal muscle is said to be "voluntary," or under the control of the individual. The second type of muscle tissue, smooth muscle, is found in the walls of organs such as the intestines, the stomach, and the blood vessels. The movement provided by smooth muscle is involuntary, or out of your control. For example, it is the smooth muscle in the walls of the intestines that produces peristalsis (the wave-like movements that pass digested food through the intestines). You do not need to think about moving food through your intestines. Instead, this action occurs automatically. The third type of muscle tissue, cardiac muscle, is found in the heart. Contraction and relaxation of the cardiac muscle pumps blood throughout the body. Like smooth muscle, cardiac muscle is involuntary.
- **Nervous tissue** conducts information. The brain, spinal cord, and nerves are made of nervous tissue. Nervous tissue allows one part of the body to "talk" to another part. For example, nerves carry information to the brain to be processed and interpreted. In addition, the brain sends commands to other parts of the body through the nerves.

Organs

A group of tissues functioning together for a similar purpose form an **organ**. For example, the heart is made of all four tissue types, and its main function is to pump blood throughout the body. Other examples of organs include the stomach, liver, kidneys, and lungs. An organ may have one specific function, or it may have several.

Organ Systems

An **organ system** is a group of organs that work together to perform a specific function for the body. For the organ system to work properly, each organ within the system must function well. Human beings have 10 main organ systems (Fig. 28-4):

- The **integumentary system** includes the skin and its glands, the hair, and the nails. The main function of the integumentary system is to protect the body.
- The **skeletal system** includes the bones. The function of the skeletal system is to provide a frame for the body and to give the body shape.
- The **muscular system** includes the muscles. The muscular system works along with the skeletal system to enable the body to move. Sometimes the muscular system and the skeletal system together are called the musculoskeletal system.
- The **respiratory system** includes the lungs and the airways. The respiratory system allows us to take in oxygen and get rid of carbon dioxide, a waste product of cellular metabolism.
- The **cardiovascular system** is made up of the blood, the heart, and the blood vessels. The cardiovascular system transports nutrients and

TABLE 28-1 Types of Muscle Tissue

TYPE	FUNCTION	CONTROL
 Skeletal muscle	Attaches to the bones and allows for movement of the various parts of the body	Voluntary
 Smooth muscle	Found in the walls of the blood vessels, stomach, intestines, bladder, and other hollow organs	Involuntary
 Cardiac muscle	Forms the heart; contraction and relaxation of this muscle pumps blood throughout the body	Involuntary

oxygen to the cells of the body and carries waste products away.

■ The **nervous system** includes the brain, spinal cord, and nerves. The nervous system controls the functioning of other organ systems. It also allows us to interact with our environment through the **special senses** (sight, hearing, smell, taste, and touch).

■ The **endocrine system** is made up of glands found in specific locations throughout the body. These glands secrete chemical substances called hormones, which work with the nervous system to control other organ systems.

■ The **digestive system** includes the teeth, salivary glands, tongue, esophagus, stomach, small intestine, large intestine, liver, pancreas, and gallbladder. The digestive system allows us to take in food and water, digest the food into nutrients, and absorb the nutrients into the bloodstream. The digestive system also removes solid waste from the body in the form of feces.

■ The **urinary system** includes the kidneys, the bladder, the ureters, and the urethra. The urinary system removes liquid waste from the body in the form of urine.

■ The **reproductive system** allows the human body to produce new life. Without a means of reproduction, human life would cease to exist.

As you can see, organ systems do not work alone. They work together to maintain the life of the organism.

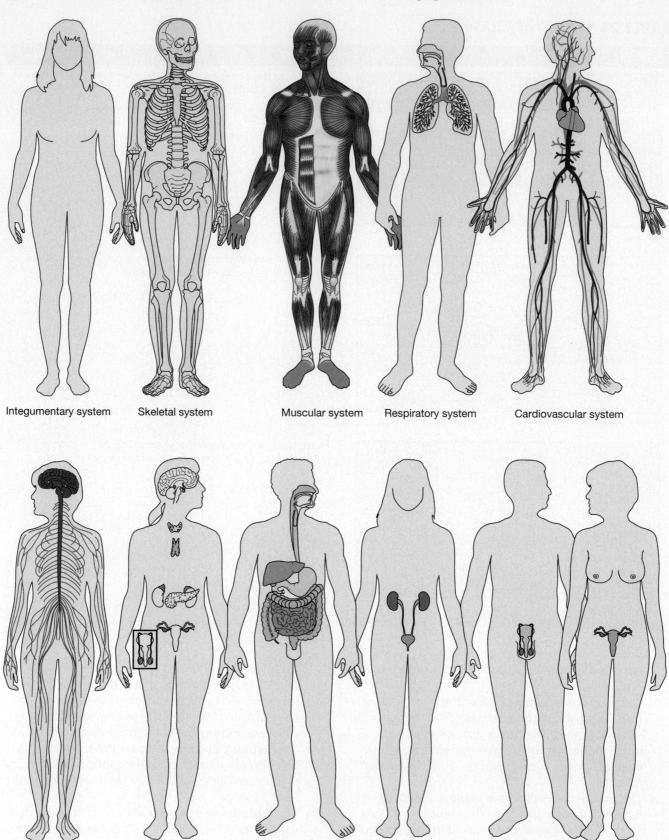

| Integumentary system | Skeletal system | Muscular system | Respiratory system | Cardiovascular system |
| Nervous system | Endocrine system | Digestive system | Urinary system | Reproductive system |

Figure 28-4 There are 10 organ systems in the human body.

HEALTH AND DISEASE

All of the organ systems work together to maintain **homeostasis**, or balance. Homeostasis is a basic concept in physiology. The word comes from the Greek words *homoios*, which means "similar," and *stasis*, which means "standing." So homeostasis means "staying similar." For an organism to stay alive, certain conditions within the body must remain relatively constant, within a range of normal limits. You were introduced to this idea in Chapter 20, when we discussed vital signs. For example, the body temperature must remain within a certain range. The blood pressure must remain within a certain range. The fluids that keep our cells healthy must not be too acidic or too basic. Our blood must contain the right amount of oxygen, carbon dioxide, and salts at all times.

All of the organ systems are constantly working together to maintain a state of balance. When the external or internal environment changes, the organ systems must make adjustments to compensate for the change. For example, imagine that you are playing basketball at the park with your friends on a very hot day. You begin to sweat. This is your body working to cool you down. As you continue to play and sweat, you begin to get thirsty. This is your body telling you that it needs more water. As you run back and forth on the court, you breathe harder, and your heart rate increases as your respiratory and circulatory systems work to send extra oxygen to your tissues. Your tissues need the extra oxygen because they use it to help produce the energy that allows you to keep playing.

Most of the time, you are not even aware of the adjustments your body is making to keep everything within the normal ranges. Even when you are sitting perfectly still, little adjustments are being made to keep the internal environment stable. Perhaps you are wondering how your body "knows" that an adjustment is needed. The answer is, through a feedback mechanism. Although all of the organ systems play a role in maintaining homeostasis, most of these feedback mechanisms are controlled by the nervous and endocrine systems.

The body's ability to maintain balance is an indicator of good health. There are times when the body's ability to maintain homeostasis is altered. This imbalance is usually the result of a disease. A **disease** (or a "disorder") occurs when the structure or function of an organ or an organ system is abnormal. Diseases can be acute (temporary) or chronic (long-term). They can be mild or severe. Sometimes, the same disease may be severe in one person but mild in another. Some diseases result in *disability*, which is impaired physical or emotional function.

Categories of Disease

There are several common categories of disease. A disease may belong to more than one of these categories. Common categories of disease include:

- **Infectious.** An infectious disease is caused by pathogens (germs). Infections are believed to play a role in approximately half of all illnesses.
- **Degenerative.** To degenerate means to "break down." Degenerative diseases occur when the tissues of the body wear out or break down. Arthritis, muscular dystrophy, osteoporosis, and Alzheimer disease are examples of degenerative diseases. These diseases can be inherited, or they can be caused by infection, injury, or aging. Sometimes there is no known cause.
- **Nutritional.** These disorders occur when a person's diet lacks certain nutrients. Consuming too much of any one nutrient (for example, vitamins) or too many calories can also cause nutritional disorders. For example, obesity is a nutritional disorder.
- **Metabolic (endocrine).** Metabolic disorders, such as diabetes, occur when the body is unable to metabolize or absorb certain nutrients. Metabolic disorders often occur when the body secretes either too much of one type of hormone, or not enough. Because the hormone is responsible for controlling the function of a particular organ, the organ does not function properly and an imbalance in homeostasis occurs.
- **Immune.** These disorders change the way the immune system behaves. Sometimes, as in acquired immunodeficiency syndrome (AIDS), the disease reduces the immune system's ability to fight off infection. Other times, the disease causes the immune system to start attacking the body's own tissues.
- **Neoplastic.** The word neoplasm means "new growth." Many people use the word "cancer" or "tumor" when they are talking about neoplastic disease. Neoplasms cause problems by invading otherwise healthy tissues. The presence of the new growth prevents the tissues from functioning properly.
- **Psychiatric.** Mental disorders that affect a person's ability to function normally, such as depression, are also considered diseases.

Risk Factors for Disease

Why do some people get certain diseases and others do not? Why does a certain disease affect one person very mildly but totally destroy the health of another person? As a nursing assistant, one of your many responsibilities will be to help improve or maintain the health of your patients or residents. To do that, you need to know about the factors that can put a person at risk for disease, or negatively affect their ability to recover from the disease. Some of these factors include the following:

- **Age.** Some disorders are more likely to occur in certain age groups. For example, chickenpox, a viral infection, is more common in children. Age can also influence how a person reacts to the disease. For example, when an adult gets the chickenpox, the infection is usually much more severe. In general, older people are more at risk for certain diseases because the process of aging causes a lot of wear and tear on the body's tissues and organs.
- **Sex.** A person's sex can increase their risk for certain diseases. For instance, breast cancer is much more common in females than in males. However, males are more likely to have heart disease.
- **Heredity.** The genes that we inherit from our parents may put us at risk for developing certain diseases. For example, scientists now know that some types of cancer, diabetes, and heart disease are inherited.
- **Lifestyle.** A person's living conditions and health habits play a major role in the person's overall health status. For example, a person who is experiencing homelessness is more likely to get sick than a person who has shelter from the weather. A person who gets too little rest and has poor nutritional habits is more likely to become ill than a person who gets enough sleep and eats well. A person who smokes is more likely to develop cancer, lung disease, or heart disease than a person who does not. A person who likes a deep, dark tan in the summer is more at risk for developing skin cancer than a person who uses sunscreen. These are just examples of the many ways in which lifestyle influences health.
- **Occupation.** Many jobs put a person at risk for certain diseases. For example, constant exposure to coal dust puts coal miners at risk for developing "black lung disease." Health care workers who do not take care to protect themselves are at risk for certain infections, such as hepatitis.
- **Chronic disease.** A person who has a chronic disease, such as diabetes or high blood pressure, is at increased risk for developing another disease. For example, a person who does not manage their diabetes well is likely to develop heart disease, blindness, or kidney failure. In addition, a person who has a chronic disease is often more

likely to experience more severe problems from something that would not really affect a healthy person. For example, an ingrown toenail will cause discomfort and inconvenience in a healthy person. However, in a person with diabetes, the ingrown toenail could cause a severe infection because diabetes changes the internal environment of the body, placing the person more at risk for infection.

- **Emotional health.** A person's emotional health can directly affect their physical health. Emotional stress can create physical problems such as headaches, digestive disorders, and muscle strain. In addition, stress makes the body more at risk for infection. If you remember from Chapter 6, just becoming a patient or resident of a health care facility can significantly increase a person's level of emotional stress and make coping with physical illness or disability more difficult.

Awareness of the factors that can put your patients or residents at risk for disease will help you to better meet their individual needs. When you meet your patient's or resident's specific needs, or observe and report signs that indicate that the person's body is struggling to return to a balanced state, you are making a very important contribution to the person's health.

Helping Hands and a Caring Heart

Focus on Humanistic Health Care

There is a fine line between our physical health and our emotional health. When we feel good physically, it is easier to be in a good mood, and it is easier to handle the day's tasks and activities. Now think about a person who is living with a chronic disease. The disease impacts the person's physical health every day. What if every day you did not feel 100% physically well? Many of the people you will be caring for are in this situation. Some people are able to adapt and will resolve themselves to "make the best of a bad situation." Others may have difficulty adjusting emotionally to the effects the illness has on their lives, and they may have problems with mood and behavior as a result. When you provide emotional support in addition to caring for your patients' and residents' physical needs, you play a very important role in helping those you care for find a sense of "balance."

SUMMARY

- Understanding how the healthy body works helps us to understand and treat disease.
- All living things share the same levels of organization.
  - A cell is the basic unit of life.
  - A group of cells that is similar in structure and specialized for a specific function forms tissue.
  - A group of tissues functioning together for a similar purpose forms an organ.
  - A group of organs functioning together for a similar purpose forms an organ system.
  - A group of organ systems working together for the purpose of maintaining life forms an organism.
- All of the organ systems work together to maintain a state of homeostasis, or balance.
  - When the body's ability to maintain homeostasis is altered, disease or illness can result.
    - There are several common categories of disease. These categories often overlap.
    - Certain factors put some people more at risk for disease than others.
- A nursing assistant who understands the factors that put a person at risk for disease and each individual's needs is able to provide better care for their patients or residents.

WHAT DID YOU LEARN?

Multiple Choice

Select the single best answer for each of the following questions.

1. Which of the following is a factor that might put a person at risk for disease?
   a. Age
   b. Heredity
   c. Sex
   d. All of the above

2. What is the purpose of epithelial tissue?
   a. To provide a frame for, and give shape to, the body
   b. To connect other types of tissue together
   c. To cover the body and line its cavities
   d. To conduct nerve impulses

3. To function properly, cells need water, nutrients, and the ability to eliminate _____.
   a. Cytoplasm
   b. Organelles
   c. Disease
   d. Waste

4. Which type of muscle tissue is found in the intestines and allows for the involuntary movement of food through the passages?
   a. Skeletal
   b. Smooth
   c. Cardiac
   d. Voluntary

Matching *Match each numbered item with its appropriate lettered description.*

_____ **1.** Anatomy

_____ **2.** Organ

_____ **3.** Cell

_____ **4.** Tissue

_____ **5.** Physiology

_____ **6.** Homeostasis

_____ **7.** Organ system

_____ **8.** Organism

a. Study of how the body parts work

b. Basic unit of life

c. Study of what body parts look like, where they are located, how big they are, and how they connect to other body parts

d. A group of organs that work together to perform a specific function for the body

e. A state of balance

f. A living thing, formed by a group of organ systems working together for the purpose of maintaining life

g. A group of tissues functioning together for a similar purpose

h. Formed when cells that are similar in structure and specialized to perform a specific function join together

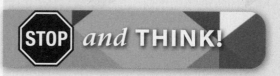

Mr. Simmons is a new patient who has just been admitted to your unit. He is 86 years old, has smoked for more than 50 years, and has diabetes. Tomorrow, he is scheduled to have knee surgery. Based on your knowledge of the factors that make a person more susceptible to illness, list the factors that could affect Mr. Simmons and describe why they increase his risk for complications.

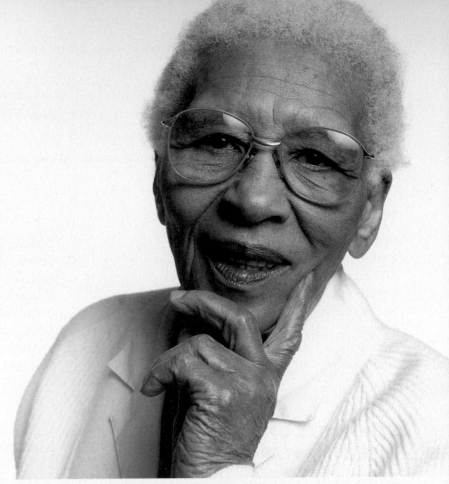

Photo: Your integumentary system includes your skin, hair, and nails.

The Integumentary System

 WHAT WILL YOU LEARN?

What is the largest organ in your body? Your skin! Just think—your body is covered in about 22 square feet of skin, and your skin alone weighs between 8 and 10 pounds. You already know that a major function of this very large organ is to cover and protect your body. But did you also know that the skin gives us clues about what is going on inside of a person's body? In this chapter, you will learn about the skin and the other organs that make up the integumentary system. You will learn about the importance of observing this organ system for changes that may indicate illness and about actions you can take to help keep the skin (and its wearer!) healthy. When you are finished with this chapter, you will be able to:

1. List the layers of the skin.
2. Describe the accessory structures of the skin.
3. Discuss the major functions of the integumentary system.
4. Describe how normal aging processes affect the integumentary system.
5. Explain how pressure ulcers are formed and what conditions may increase a patient's or resident's risk of developing a pressure ulcer.
6. Describe how the nursing assistant helps to prevent residents and patients from developing pressure ulcers.

7. Describe the different types of wounds that a patient or resident might have.

8. Discuss the nursing assistant's duties regarding wound care.

9. Define terms used to describe skin lesions.

Vocabulary

Epidermis	Pallor	Unintentional wound	Papule
Keratin	Flushing	Lesion	Vesicle
Melanin	Cyanosis	Rash	Pustule
Dermis	Bony prominences	Shingles (herpes zoster)	Excoriation
Subcutaneous tissue	Necrosis	Dermatitis	Fissure
Sebum	Pressure points	Eczema	Ulcer
Collagen	Wound	Erythema	
Jaundice	Intentional wound	Macule	

STRUCTURE OF THE INTEGUMENTARY SYSTEM

The integumentary system gets its name from the Latin word *integumentum,* which means "a covering." The integumentary system is made up of the skin, which covers the body, and the structures that develop from it, called *accessory structures* or *appendages.* The accessory structures of the skin are the nails, the hair, the sebaceous glands (which secrete oils to keep the skin moist), and the sweat glands.

Skin

The skin is made up of two layers, the epidermis and the dermis (Fig. 29-1).

Epidermis

The **epidermis** is the outer layer of the skin. The epidermis is thickest on the soles of the feet and the palms of the hands, and very thin in areas such as the eyelids.

If you look at Figure 29-1, you will notice that the epidermis contains no blood vessels. You will also notice that it has two sublayers, a deep layer and a surface layer. New cells are produced in the deep layer of the epidermis. As the cells age, they work their way up, toward the surface of the body. As the maturing cells move toward the surface, they move further away from the blood vessels, which are located in the dermis. This means that as the cells age, they move further away from their supply of oxygen and nutrients. They also produce **keratin**, a substance that causes them to

thicken and become resistant to water. When the cells reach the surface of the body, they die and are shed. This process takes approximately 29 days—so, each month, you get a "new skin!"

In addition to continually producing new cells, the deep layer of the epidermis produces a substance called melanin. **Melanin**, from the Greek word *melas* ("black"), is a dark pigment that gives our skin, hair, and eyes color. People with pale skin have less melanin than those with dark skin. Melanin helps to protect the skin from exposure to sunlight. In fact, continued exposure to sunlight causes the epidermis to produce

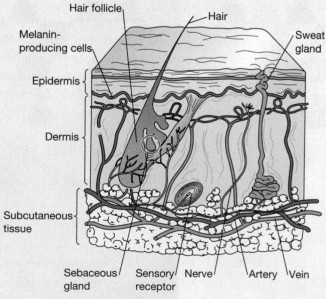

Figure 29-1 The skin has two layers, the dermis and epidermis. The skin rests on a layer of subcutaneous tissue.

more melanin, resulting in a tan. Sometimes melanin is deposited throughout the epidermis in an uneven pattern, resulting in freckles.

Dermis

The **dermis** is the deepest layer of the skin (see Fig. 29-1). The dermis consists of elastic connective tissue that allows it to stretch and move without damage. The dermis rests on a layer of fat called the **subcutaneous tissue**. Cutaneous is another word for "skin," and sub means "below." Therefore, *subcutaneous* means "below the skin." The blood vessels and nerves that supply the skin start in the subcutaneous tissue and send branches into the dermis. Looking at Figure 29-1, you can see that the sensory receptors that allow us to feel pressure, pain, and temperature are located in the dermis. (The sense of touch will be discussed in more detail in Chapter 34.) The sebaceous glands, the sweat glands, and the hair follicles are also found in the dermis.

Accessory Structures (Appendages)

The skin's accessory structures include the sebaceous glands, the sweat glands, the hair, and the nails.

Sebaceous (Oil) Glands

The sebaceous glands secrete **sebum**, an oily substance that lubricates the skin and helps to prevent it from drying out. The sebum is also slightly acidic. This acidity helps to protect the skin from harmful bacteria that may be present on its surface. The sebaceous glands open into the hair follicles, and the sebum passes along the hair and onto the surface of the skin (see Fig. 29-1).

Sweat Glands

There are two types of sweat glands: eccrine glands and apocrine glands. Eccrine glands are found in the skin that covers most parts of our bodies. Eccrine glands produce a thin, watery liquid that contains salt and small amounts of other bodily wastes. The purpose of the eccrine glands is to help cool the body through the process of evaporation. As the watery sweat leaves the surface of the skin, it takes heat with it, cooling the body down. Therefore, when you "work up a sweat," you are experiencing your eccrine glands at work! Another time you may experience your eccrine glands at work is when you notice your palms beginning to sweat as a result of being nervous. Many people sweat when they are nervous, and the palms of the hands contain a very large number of eccrine glands—hence, "sweaty palm syndrome."

The other type of sweat gland is the apocrine gland. Apocrine glands are found mostly in the skin of the armpits (axillae) and the perineum. The apocrine glands produce a thicker substance. When the bacteria that normally live on our skin mix with this substance, they produce what we know as "body odor." Apocrine glands become active when a person reaches puberty. As we age, the apocrine glands become less active.

Hair

Hair covers the skin of the entire body, except for the soles of the feet and the palms of the hands. Hair, especially that covering the scalp, helps to keep us warm. Most of the hair that covers the body is soft and fine, although in males, body hair tends to be thicker and more noticeable because of the action of certain hormones. In all people, the hair covering the scalp, armpits, and pubic area is thicker and coarser than the hair on the rest of the body.

Hair develops in the dermis of the skin from a sheath called a follicle (see Fig. 29-1). The part of the hair that we can see consists of dead cells that have been hardened by keratin. The living cells that produce new hair cells, causing the hair to grow, are found at the bottom of the follicle or hair root. Melanin gives the hair its color. Blonde hair contains a small amount of melanin, while brown or black hair contains much more.

Nails

Nails are made of special skin cells that have been hardened by the presence of keratin. Nail growth occurs from the nail root, the area where the nail emerges from the skin. Nails help to protect the ends of our fingers and toes.

FUNCTION OF THE INTEGUMENTARY SYSTEM

The integumentary system helps to maintain the body's homeostasis in three important ways. First, it offers a physical form of protection against microbes, chemicals, and other agents that could harm the body if they gained access to the delicate organs inside. Second, the skin, which is water resistant, helps to maintain the body's fluid balance by preventing excessive loss or absorption of water. Finally, the integumentary system helps to regulate the temperature of the body, ensuring that the temperature stays within a tolerable range.

Protection

As you learned in Chapter 10, the body's first line of defense against the invasion of harmful microbes is intact skin. The skin is a physical barrier that prevents microbes from entering the body. The skin also offers us some protection against harmful substances, such as chemicals, that may be encountered in the environment.

Maintenance of Fluid Balance

Imagine what would happen if your skin were not resistant to water! Every time it rained or you took a shower, you would soak up the water like a sponge. And every time you went out in the sun, you would run the risk of having all of your internal organs dry out. Needless to say, without your water-resistant skin, maintaining the proper fluid balance would be a constant struggle. Fortunately, the keratin-rich cells of the epidermis, combined with the oils secreted by the sebaceous glands, work very well to form a water-resistant protective barrier between your internal organs and the outside world.

Regulation of Body Temperature

The skin plays an important role in regulating the body temperature. When a person gets warm—for example, after working outside in the sun—the blood vessels in the dermis of the skin dilate (widen), allowing more blood to flow close to the surface of the skin. As the blood passes just beneath the surface of the skin, the heat the blood contains radiates out from the body, lowering the temperature of the blood. The cooled blood then travels, carrying its coolness, back to the central areas of the body, thus lowering the body temperature. Sweating enhances this process. If sweat is allowed to evaporate, it carries heat away with it, further cooling the skin and thus the blood. Wiping away sweat prevents it from cooling the body! In essence, these processes are the body's way of "opening the windows" to allow a cool breeze to circulate through the house (Fig. 29-2A).

The reverse is true when a person gets cold, for example, following exposure to cold air. The blood vessels in the skin constrict (become narrower), limiting the amount of blood that passes close to the surface of the skin. By keeping the blood in the warmer, central areas of the body, the amount of heat that is lost to the outside environment is kept to a minimum. You have seen how your skin becomes pale or bluish when you have been outside in the cold air. Your body is essentially "closing the windows" to stop the breeze from cooling the house too much (see Fig. 29-2B).

Sensation

The skin contains millions of sensory receptors, special structures that allow us to detect pain, pressure,

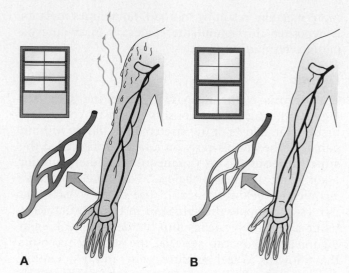

Figure 29-2 The skin plays an important role in maintaining the body's temperature within the proper range. **A.** When the internal temperature is too high, the blood vessels in the skin dilate, causing more blood to pass near the surface of the skin and allowing heat to escape into the environment. Sweat evaporating from the surface of the skin also carries heat away from the body, contributing to the cooling process. **B.** When the internal temperature is too low, the blood vessels in the skin constrict, causing less blood to pass near the surface of the skin and keeping the heat inside the body.

temperature, and touch. The sensory receptors and the role they play in sensation are discussed in detail in Chapter 34.

Vitamin D Production

As you remember from Chapter 24, vitamin D is a nutrient that helps our bodies absorb and use calcium, a mineral that keeps our bones healthy. The skin produces vitamin D when it is exposed to the sun. In fact, sun exposure is our main source of this important vitamin! Vitamin D is also obtained by eating foods such as fish and vitamin D–supplemented milk. People who live in northern regions where there is a lack of sunlight in winter months tend to rely on dietary forms of vitamin D during this time of year.

Elimination and Absorption

The skin is an active organ that is capable of both removing substances from the body and taking substances into it. For example, sweat contains small amounts of waste materials, which leave the body when the sweat evaporates. The skin can also absorb some substances, such as chemicals. We use the ability of the skin to absorb chemicals when we give medications using a "patch." An adhesive patch containing the medicine is stuck to the skin, and the medicine is slowly absorbed through the skin and into the blood vessels. You may be familiar with patches that prevent motion sickness, provide birth control, or help a person to stop smoking. In all of these cases, the medication on the patch is absorbed through the skin.

THE EFFECTS OF AGING ON THE INTEGUMENTARY SYSTEM

As we age, changes occur in all of our organ systems. These changes are not related to illness. Rather, they are normal changes that occur in everyone who reaches a certain age. These changes may just affect the person's appearance, or they may actually affect the way the person's body functions. Because there is a good chance that many of the people you will be caring for will be elderly, it is important for you to know about the changes that normally occur in each body system with aging. This knowledge will allow you to recognize age-related changes as normal. It will also allow you to provide better care for your older patients or residents because you will be aware of their unique needs.

Changes in Physical Appearance

Perhaps because the integumentary system is the most visible organ system, we have come to associate "getting older" with many of the physical changes that occur in the integumentary system as we age. Wrinkles, gray hair, and "age spots" are all visible signs of aging (Fig. 29-3). Wrinkles form due to the loss of **collagen**, a protein that supports connective tissue, such as that found in the dermis. In addition, the adipose (fatty) tissue in the subcutaneous layer that supports the dermis thins with age, making the subcutaneous layer less supportive of the dermis. As a result, the skin loses elasticity, leading to the formation of wrinkles. Melanin also is responsible for many of the changes typically associated with aging. Gray hair is caused by the loss of melanin from the hair. "Age spots" (sometimes called "liver spots") are caused by deposits of melanin in certain areas, such as the backs of the hands or the face. Whether or not a person's skin shows these signs of aging depends on many factors, such as heredity; the amount of time the person spends in the sun; the person's use of tobacco, drugs, or alcohol; and the person's overall state of health. Think about all of the people you know. Do any look much younger than their actual age, or much older? What factors do you think might be responsible for the person's remarkably youthful appearance, or unusually old appearance?

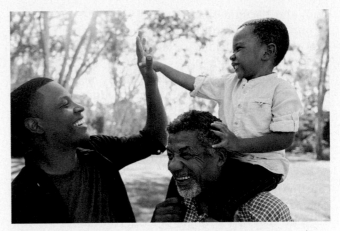

Figure 29-3 Wrinkles, gray hair, and "age spots" result from changes to the integumentary system that occur with aging. Many people view these normal signs of aging as signs of a life well-lived! The man in the center is pictured with his son and grandson. You can see how the skin changes in appearance over time. (*Monkey Business Images\Shutterstock.com*)

Fragile, Dry Skin

There are many changes that occur to the integumentary system with aging that affect more than just our appearance. As collagen is lost from the dermis and the subcutaneous layer thins, the skin becomes thinner, more fragile, and more prone to injury (Fig. 29-4). Blood flow to the dermis decreases, and the cells of the epidermis do not replace themselves as rapidly. These changes mean that when an injury occurs, the skin takes longer to heal itself, and the person is more at risk for developing an infection.

The number of sebaceous glands decreases, and as a result, so does the output of sebum. This leads to drying of the skin, which increases the risk for skin tears and injuries. In addition, with less sebum on the

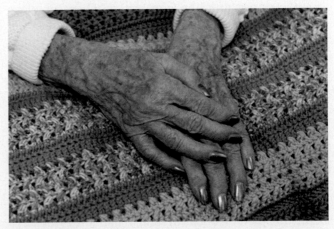

Figure 29-4 As the skin ages, it becomes more delicate and prone to injury.

skin, the bacteria that normally live on the surface of our skin have more of a chance to cause trouble. (Recall that the acidity of sebum helps to keep these bacteria in check.)

When caring for an older person, keep the delicate nature of older skin in mind. Actions that would not cause harm in a younger person, such as gripping the person's arm to help them stand or accidentally grazing their skin with your fingernails while helping them put on their socks, can cause injury in an older person. It is very easy to tear an older person's skin, causing it to bleed. In addition, the skin of an older person is more sensitive to the drying effects of bathing than that of a younger person. In Chapter 22, you learned about some of the things that you can do to increase comfort and help to keep an older person's skin healthy, such as applying lotion after a bath to keep the skin soft and pliant.

Thickening of the Nails

As we age, our nails thicken and become yellow. This is especially true of the toenails. Because the nails are so tough, they are difficult to cut, and the person may be injured during the process. As you learned in Chapter 23, a nurse or a podiatrist is usually responsible for trimming an older person's toenails. The nurse or podiatrist may use a tool that looks like a sander to accomplish this task safely.

Less Efficient Temperature Regulation

Changes to the integumentary system that occur with aging also affect the older person's ability to adjust to changes in the environmental temperature. The production of sweat decreases, making an older person more vulnerable to overheating. In addition, the decreased blood flow to the skin interferes with the skin's ability to participate in temperature regulation. These changes must be considered when an older person is outside on a hot day because they affect the ability of the body to cool itself and put the person at increased risk for heat-related problems, such as heat stroke. The age-related thinning of the subcutaneous fat layer decreases a person's "insulation" causing the person to feel colder and need an extra sweater or cover in order to stay warm.

DISORDERS OF THE INTEGUMENTARY SYSTEM

Of all the body's organ systems, the integumentary system is the most easily observed. Healthy skin is glowing and vibrant, and may range in color from very light to very dark. A change in a person's normal skin color can indicate a serious health problem and should be reported to the nurse immediately. For example:

- **Jaundice** is a yellow discoloration of the skin and the whites of the eyes. Jaundice is usually associated with liver disorders.
- **Pallor** is paleness, and **flushing** is redness. Some people appear pale or flushed most of the time. In these people, pallor or flushing would be considered "normal." However, if you notice pallor or flushing in a person who is not normally pale or flushed, you should report this finding to the nurse.
- **Cyanosis** is a blue or gray discoloration of the skin, lips, and nail beds. Cyanosis develops when the tissues are not receiving enough oxygen-rich blood. Cyanosis can be a sign of a respiratory or circulatory disorder.

As you learned in Chapter 23, the condition of a person's hair and nails can also provide clues to the person's overall health. The hair should be shiny and soft, not brittle and dry, and the scalp should not be flaky or crusty. The nail beds of healthy nails are pink. The nails are flush with the nail bed and, when viewed from the side, the nails are slightly rounded.

Tell the Nurse!

The skin gives us many clues to a person's general health. Tell the nurse immediately if you observe any of the following:

- The person's skin looks abnormally pale or flushed, or has a bluish or yellowish hue.
- The person has a new rash, or changes in an existing rash.
- The person has a mole that has changed in appearance.

Many people in your care will have a disorder of the integumentary system. Sometimes, this disorder is the reason the person is in the health care facility. For example, this might be the case for a person who has suffered severe burns or trauma. Other times, the disorder develops after the person is already in the health care facility. For example, a person might develop a rash or a pressure ulcer, or they might have surgery that results in a surgical wound that must heal. As a nursing assistant, you will play an important role in observing signs and symptoms of skin disorders, preventing the development of skin disorders, and helping people with skin disorders to heal.

Pressure Ulcers

Pressure ulcers, also known as *decubitus ulcers* or *bed sores*, form when a part of the body presses against a surface such as a mattress or chair for a long period of time. Lying on wrinkled bed linens or an object in the bed, sitting on a bedpan for a long period of time, or wearing a splint or brace that presses against the skin can also start the process of skin breakdown that leads to the formation of pressure ulcers.

Pressure ulcers are particularly likely to form over **bony prominences**, or parts of the body where there is very little fat between the bone and the skin. The weight of the person's body squeezes the soft tissue between the bony prominence and the surface the person is resting on, disrupting the flow of blood to the tissue. Lack of blood flow to the tissue deprives the tissue of oxygen and nutrients, causing it to die. Tissue death as a result of a lack of oxygen is called **necrosis**. The necrotic (dead) skin and underlying tissues peel off or break open, creating an open sore (Fig. 29-5). The sore is very painful and creates an opening for microbes to enter the body. Pressure ulcers may be very deep, extending all the way down to the bone. They are very difficult to heal once they have occurred.

You will remember from Chapter 15 that some patients and residents are not able to change position easily, due to weakness, disability, or illness. This

inability to change position without help places the person at high risk for developing a pressure ulcer. Common sites for an excess of pressure to occur are on the heels, ankles, knees, hips, toes, elbows, shoulder blades, ears, the back of the head, and along the spine (Fig. 29-6). These particular areas can be described as **pressure points**. For instance, a person who spends too much time lying on their back could develop pressure ulcers over the sacrum (lower back) and coccyx (tailbone), whereas the iliac crest and greater trochanter of the lateral hip are common sites of ulcer development for people lying on their side.

The constant application of pressure on pressure points as a result of immobility is the basic cause of all pressure ulcers. Unfortunately, many people with limited mobility also have other risk factors for developing a pressure ulcer. The presence of any one of the following risk factors in a person with limited mobility makes it even more likely that they will develop a pressure ulcer:

- **Advanced age.** As described earlier in this chapter, the normal aging process causes changes in a person's skin. The skin of an older person is fragile and thin, with less circulation. While a younger person may be able to tolerate staying in one position for 2 hours, an older person may need much more frequent position changes.
- **Poor nutrition and hydration.** For skin to remain healthy, good nutrition and proper hydration are essential. People who are not receiving adequate nutrition or fluids because of illness, depression, or other conditions are more likely to develop pressure ulcers. Poor nutrition will also delay the healing of any pressure ulcers that have already formed.
- **Moisture.** Prolonged contact with water, urine, feces, or sweat causes the epidermis to soften and break down. Areas where skin touches skin (such as between the thighs, the folds of the abdomen, the armpits, and under the breasts) are places where sweat or bath water may become trapped on the skin, leading to skin breakdown. In addition to moisture, sweat, urine, and feces contain irritants such as salt, ammonia, and bacteria, which further contribute to the breakdown of the skin. Patients and residents with obesity are at an increased risk of skin breakdown because of their skin folds. Once skin breakdown begins, the door is wide open for a pressure ulcer to form.
- **Cardiovascular and respiratory problems.** A person with a heart or lung disorder often has problems getting adequate oxygen and nutrients to the tissues. In a person with a respiratory disorder, the blood that is delivered to the tissues may not contain enough oxygen. The heart of a

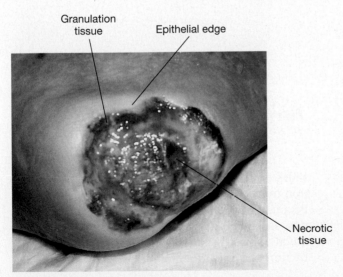

Granulation tissue

Epithelial edge

Necrotic tissue

Figure 29-5 Pressure ulcers are painful, difficult to treat, and potentially fatal. (Used with permission from Taylor, C., Lillis, C., LeMone, P., & Lynn, P. [2008]. *Fundamentals of nursing: The art and science of nursing care* [6th ed., p. 1023]. Lippincott Williams & Wilkins.)

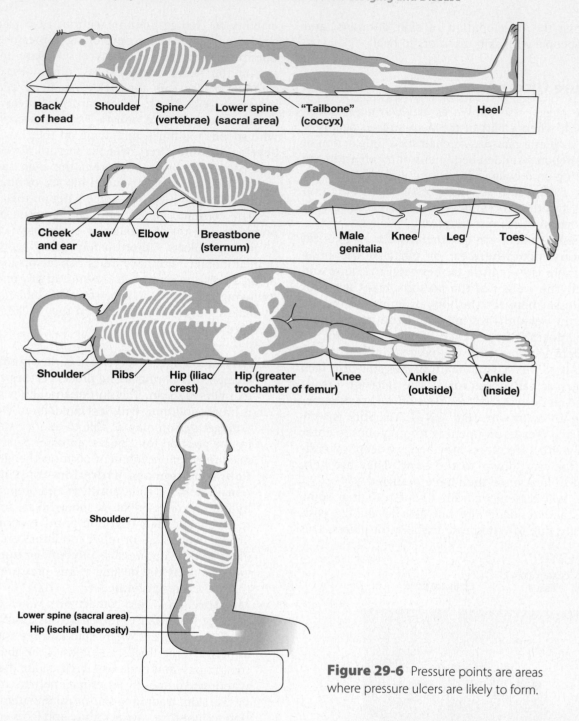

Figure 29-6 Pressure points are areas where pressure ulcers are likely to form.

person with a cardiovascular disorder may not be strong enough to deliver the blood to the tissues, even if it contains enough oxygen. Therefore, people with circulatory or respiratory problems are at even greater risk for developing pressure ulcers because their tissues are already deprived of oxygen and nutrients.

■ **Friction and shearing injuries.** In Chapter 15, you learned about how friction (rubbing) and shearing (pulling) forces can injure the skin and lead to skin breakdown. For example, shearing occurs when a person who is sitting up in bed

slides down against the sheets. Shearing and friction injuries can also occur during repositioning. People who have disorders that cause continuous, spastic movements of their arms and/or legs are at an increased risk for skin breakdown from friction and shearing.

Stages of Pressure Ulcers

Pressure ulcers develop in stages (Fig. 29-7):

■ **Stage 1.** Have you ever sat with your legs crossed for a long period of time? When you

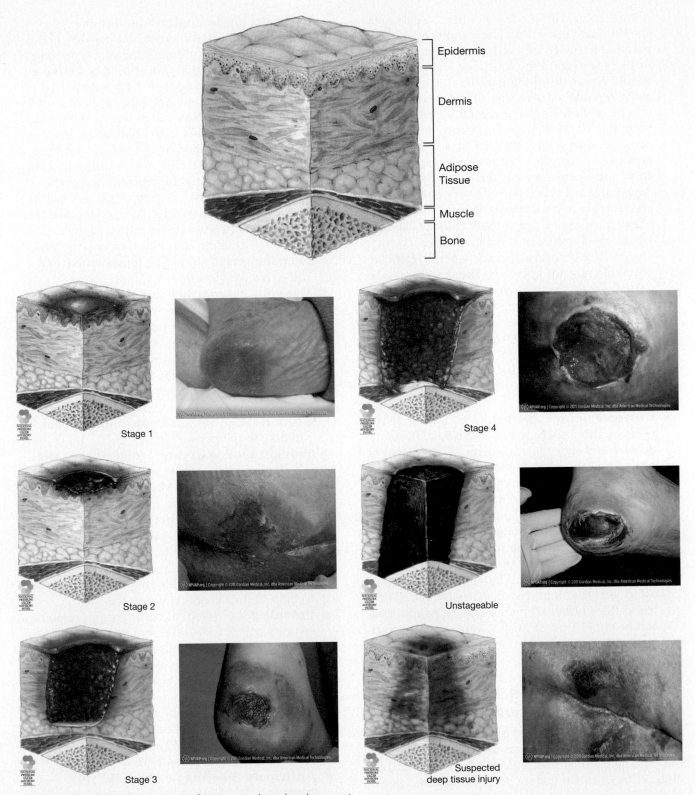

Epidermis

Dermis

Adipose Tissue

Muscle

Bone

Stage 1

Stage 4

Stage 2

Unstageable

Stage 3

Suspected deep tissue injury

Figure 29-7 The four stages of pressure ulcer development.

uncrossed your legs, the leg that had been on the bottom probably had a pale or reddened area caused by the pressure of the leg that had been on top. There may even have been a slight "dent" in the skin. After a few minutes, the paleness or red area disappeared and the skin looked normal again. Every time you reposition a patient or resident, you should look carefully for pale or reddened areas. If the person's circulation is normal, the skin will return to its normal color within a few minutes. A pale area should turn pink within a few minutes after the pressure has been relieved. If the skin stays pale or red, feels hot to the touch, or is painful, you should report this finding to the nurse immediately. A reddened area that turns white means that blood flow has been compromised to the point that tissue damage has occurred. A stage 1 pressure ulcer is characterized by a reddened area of skin that does not return to the normal color after the pressure is removed. The reddened area may then become very pale or white and develop a shiny appearance.

- **Stage 2.** A stage 2 pressure ulcer looks like a blister, an abrasion, or a shallow crater. The epidermis peels away or cracks open, creating a portal of entry for microbes. The dermis may be partially worn away as well.

- **Stage 3.** In a stage 3 pressure ulcer, the epidermis and dermis are gone, and the subcutaneous fat may be visible in the crater. There may be drainage from the wound.

- **Stage 4.** The crater of damaged tissue extends all the way through the tissues to the muscle or bone.

- **Unstageable/unclassified.** In an unstageable pressure ulcer, there is loss of the epidermis, dermis, and subcutaneous tissue. The full extent or depth of the ulcer is covered by *slough* (soft, moist, light-colored dead tissue) or *eschar* (tough, dry, leathery, dark-colored dead tissue). The ulcer will need to be cleaned and dead tissue removed to determine the true stage.

- **Suspected deep tissue injury.** This injury, resulting from pressure or shearing that has caused damage to the underlying tissue, has intact skin that is purple or maroon-colored or a blood-filled blister. The area may be painful and can be either firm or mushy, warm or cool. This type of injury may be difficult to detect in people with dark skin.

The Nursing Assistant's Role in Preventing Pressure Ulcers

As you have already learned in previous chapters, the prevention of pressure ulcers is a major concern of the nursing team. Pressure ulcers are very painful and difficult to treat. Ultimately, they can cause a person to die. For these reasons, every effort must be made to prevent a pressure ulcer from forming in the first place. As a nursing assistant, there are many things that you can do to help keep a person's skin healthy (Fig. 29-8).

- **Avoid allowing a person to remain in one position for a long period of time.** To prevent a pressure ulcer from forming, you must prevent any one part of a person's body from being under pressure for a long period of time. This means that you should not leave a person sitting on a bedpan for a long period of time because the bedpan places a lot of pressure on the person's lower spine, one of the pressure points. It also means that a patient or resident who must stay in bed be repositioned at least every 2 hours. A person who is sitting in a chair or wheelchair should be repositioned every hour. A person who has additional risk factors for developing a pressure ulcer, as described earlier, may need to be repositioned even more often. The nursing care plan will specify how often the person should be repositioned, and the sequence of positions.

- **Use your observation skills.** Look carefully at the skin of your patients or residents each and every time you provide care. After repositioning a person, move clothing and linens aside to check for pale or reddened areas on the side of the body that had been bearing the person's weight. When assisting a person with bathing, changing wet or soiled linens, or giving a person a back massage, take that opportunity to look carefully at the person's skin.

- **Provide good skin care.** When assisting with a bath, clean skin gently and thoroughly and rinse off the soap well. Make sure the skin is dried well and use lotion to keep the skin's surface healthy and soft. Thoroughly clean and dry areas where skin touches skin, such as under the breasts or other skin folds, and apply a light dusting of a powder containing corn starch to help keep the skin dry. Provide frequent back massage to help stimulate circulation in the skin.

- **Provide good perineal care.** Prompt removal of urine or feces from the skin is essential for the prevention of pressure ulcers. Good perineal care is especially important if a person is incontinent of urine or feces. Clean any urine or feces from the skin each time the person is incontinent. If the person is incontinent, the nurse may ask you to apply a product to the perineal area that helps to protect the skin from wetness, after the perineal area has been cleaned and dried.

- **Anticipate toileting needs.** Assist your patients or residents to the bathroom (or provide a bedpan or urinal) frequently, to prevent soiling of the person's clothing or bed linens. If a person is incontinent, check on them every hour or so. This will allow you to detect and change wet, soiled linens promptly.

- **Encourage mobility.** Some patients or residents will sit in a chair or wheelchair all day

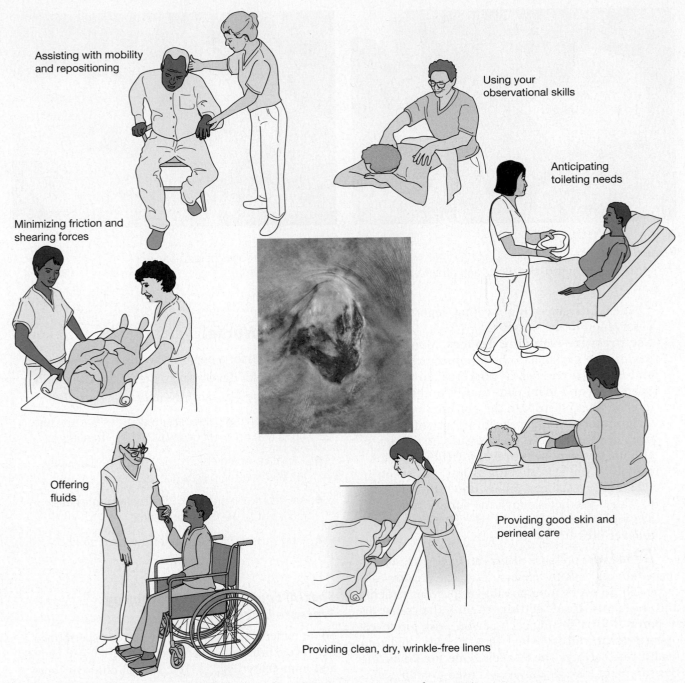

Assisting with mobility and repositioning

Using your observational skills

Anticipating toileting needs

Minimizing friction and shearing forces

Offering fluids

Providing good skin and perineal care

Providing clean, dry, wrinkle-free linens

Figure 29-8 There are many things you can do to help prevent a person from getting a pressure ulcer. (*Photograph Elena Kitch\Shutterstock.com*)

long if you do not actively encourage them to get up and move around. Ask the patient or resident to take a walk with you every hour, if they are able. The exercise helps to stimulate circulation and keeps the person from sitting in the same position for long periods of time. If a person is paralyzed, remind them to change positions in their chair or have them move between the chair and the bed to prevent skin breakdown.

- **Minimize skin injury caused by friction or shearing.** Use lift devices and lift sheets when moving and repositioning people to prevent injuries caused by friction and shearing. To help prevent shearing caused by the person sliding down in bed, do not elevate the head of the bed more than 30 degrees.
- **Encourage good nutrition and hydration.** Offer refreshing drinks frequently. Encourage your patients and residents to eat well. If

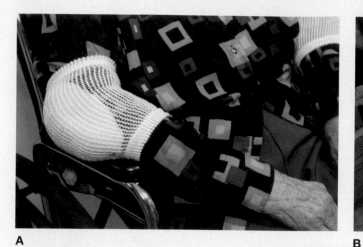

A

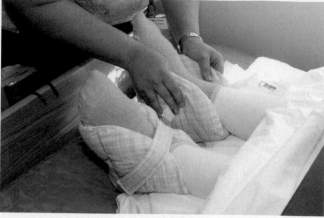

B

Figure 29-9 Pressure-reducing devices such as (**A**) elbow pads and (**B**) heel booties help to prevent the skin from rubbing against sheets and other surfaces.

a patient or resident is not eating, report this observation to the nurse.

■ **Use pressure-reducing devices.** Many devices are available to help reduce pressure and minimize the risk of skin breakdown. Special gel and foam pads that fit on beds or in chairs help distribute the person's body weight more evenly, preventing any one area from bearing most of the pressure. Elbow pads and booties may help prevent friction injuries caused by the skin rubbing against the sheets (Fig. 29-9). Placing a pillow under the calves to "float" the heels above the surface of the bed when the person is in the supine position relieves pressure on the heels.

Because pressure ulcers can have such serious consequences, OBRA expects that the health care team will do everything possible to prevent patients and residents from getting them. The nurse is responsible for assessing each person's risk for developing pressure ulcers when they are admitted to a health care facility. The Braden Scale for Predicting Pressure Sore Risk (Fig. 29-10) is used to help evaluate this risk. The nurse also documents any existing pressure ulcers. If a pressure ulcer occurs, OBRA expects the health care team to maintain or improve the person's condition. This means that the health care team works to heal existing pressure ulcers and takes measures to prevent new ones from forming. Many residents of long-term care facilities develop pressure ulcers while being treated in the hospital for an acute illness or injury and return to the long-term care facility with a pressure ulcer *and* the other condition to recover from. Nursing assistants help the health care team to achieve the patient's recovery goals by carefully following the patient's or the resident's care plan.

Tell the Nurse!

When caring for a person who has a pressure ulcer or is at risk for developing a pressure ulcer, report the following observations immediately:

● The person has paleness or redness over a pressure point that does not go away within 5 minutes.

● An area over a pressure point that was previously red has become pale, white, or shiny.

● An area over a pressure point that was previously red is hot to the touch or painful.

● A pressure ulcer has changed in size or depth.

Special Equipment for Preventing Pressure Ulcers

Some patients or residents may need a special bed to help avoid problems associated with prolonged bed rest and immobility (Fig. 29-11). Several different types of specialty beds are available:

■ An *air-fluidized bed* supports the person on a fabric-covered layer of tiny ceramic beads (see Fig. 29-11A). The beads are kept constantly in motion by a current of air. The moving beads create a fluid-like effect, much like a waterbed but without the water, that helps to prevent pressure ulcers by relieving pressure on bony prominences. In addition, the circulating air keeps the person's skin dry. If the person soils the bed, some fluids will pass through the sheet and collect in the beads. The use of a bed protector helps to greatly reduce the amount of fluid that passes through the sheet into the beads. The

BRADEN SCALE FOR PREDICTING PRESSURE SORE RISK

Patient's Name _____ Evaluator's Name _____ Date of Assessment

SENSORY PERCEPTION ability to respond meaningfully to pressure-related discomfort	**1. Completely Limited** Unresponsive (does not moan, flinch, or grasp) to painful stimuli, due to diminished level of consciousness or sedation OR limited ability to feel pain over most of body.	**2. Very Limited** Responds only to painful stimuli. Cannot communicate discomfort except by moaning or restlessness OR has a sensory impairment which limits the ability to feel pain or discomfort over ½ of body.	**3. Slightly Limited** Responds to verbal commands, but cannot always communicate discomfort or the need to be turned OR has some sensory impairment which limits ability to feel pain or discomfort in 1 or 2 extremities.	**4. No Impairment** Responds to verbal commands. Has no sensory deficit which would limit ability to feel or voice pain or discomfort.				
MOISTURE degree to which skin is exposed to moisture	**1. Constantly Moist** Skin is kept moist almost constantly by perspiration, urine, etc. Dampness is detected every time patient is moved or turned.	**2. Very Moist** Skin is often, but not always moist. Linen must be changed at least once a shift.	**3. Occasionally Moist** Skin is occasionally moist, requiring an extra linen change approximately once a day.	**4. Rarely Moist** Skin is usually dry, linen only requires changing at routine intervals.				
ACTIVITY degree of physical activity	**1. Bedfast** Confined to bed.	**2. Chairfast** Ability to walk severely limited or non-existent. Cannot bear own weight and/or must be assisted into chair or wheelchair.	**3. Walks Occasionally** Walks occasionally during day, but for very short distances, with or without assistance. Spends majority of each shift in bed or chair.	**4. Walks Frequently** Walks outside room at least twice a day and inside room at least once every two hours during waking hours.				
MOBILITY ability to change and control body position	**1. Completely Immobile** Does not make even slight changes in body or extremity position without assistance.	**2. Very Limited** Makes occasional slight changes in body or extremity position but unable to make frequent or significant changes independently.	**3. Slightly Limited** Makes frequent though slight changes in body or extremity position independently.	**4. No Limitation** Makes major and frequent changes in position without assistance.				
NUTRITION usual food intake pattern	**1. Very Poor** Never eats a complete meal. Rarely eats more than ⅓ of any food offered. Eats 2 servings or less of protein (meat or dairy products) per day. Takes fluids poorly. Does not take a liquid dietary supplement OR is NPO and/or maintained on clear liquids or IVs for more than 5 days.	**2. Probably Inadequate** Rarely eats a complete meal and generally eats only about ½ of any food offered. Protein intake includes only 3 servings of meat or dairy products per day. Occasionally will take a dietary supplement OR receives less than optimum amount of liquid diet or tube feeding.	**3. Adequate** Eats over half of most meals. Eats a total of 4 servings of protein (meat, dairy products) per day. Occasionally will refuse a meal, but will usually take a supplement when offered OR is on a tube feeding or TPN regimen which probably meets most of nutritional needs.	**4. Excellent** Eats most of every meal. Never refuses a meal. Usually eats a total of 4 or more servings of meat and dairy products. Occasionally eats between meals. Does not require supplementation.				
FRICTION & SHEAR	**1. Problem** Requires moderate to maximum assistance in moving. Complete lifting without sliding against sheets is impossible. Frequently slides down in bed or chair, requiring frequent repositioning with maximum assistance. Spasticity, contractures or agitation leads to almost constant friction.	**2. Potential Problem** Moves feebly or requires minimum assistance. During a move skin probably slides to some extent against sheets, chair, restraints or other devices. Maintains relatively good position in chair or bed most of the time but occasionally slides down.	**3. No Apparent Problem** Moves in bed and in chair independently and has sufficient muscle strength to lift up completely during move. Maintains good position in bed or chair.					
				Total Score				

Figure 29-10 The Braden Scale for Predicting Pressure Sore Risk is a tool that is used to help evaluate a person's risk for developing pressure ulcers.

beads are removed from the bed and decontaminated on a regular basis by a service technician. Airflow beds are particularly useful for critically ill patients with chronic watery diarrhea or weeping wounds.

■ An *alternating pressure bed* supports the person on a series of compartments that fill with air and then deflate on a rotating basis (see Fig. 29-11B). The shifting areas of inflation shift the areas of pressure from place to place, helping to improve blood flow to the skin and underlying tissues and helping to prevent pressure ulcers. These beds have protective covers, which can be wiped clean when soiled. The care of these beds is specific to type. If these beds are used in your facility, you will receive training in their care and use.

■ The *XPRT Pulmonary Therapy Surface* (see Fig. 29-11C) offers rotational, percussion, and vibration therapies. These beds help to prevent pressure ulcers and pulmonary complications by automatically repositioning people who may be difficult to reposition often, such as people with traumatic injuries.

Wounds

A **wound** is an injury that results in a break in the skin (and usually the underlying tissues as well). Although this discussion focuses on wounds that occur as a result of surgery or trauma, pressure ulcers and burns (also discussed in this chapter) are technically considered "wounds" too.

Types of Wounds

An **intentional wound** is a wound that is the result of a planned surgical or medical intervention (Fig. 29-12). For example, a patient who has delivered a baby via cesarean section or a person who is recovering from open-heart surgery will have intentional wounds caused by their surgeries. Intentional wounds also occur when intravenous (IV) lines, percutaneous

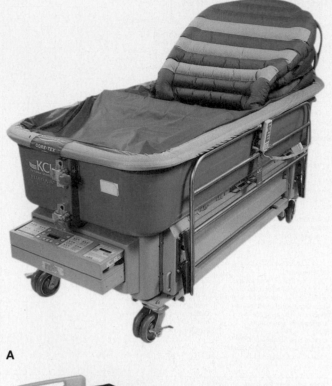

A

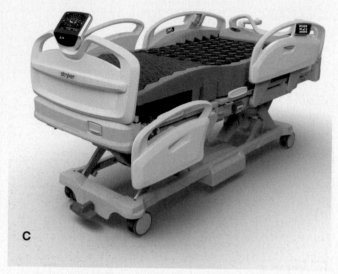

C

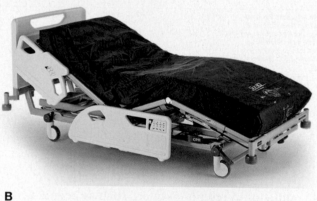

B

Figure 29-11 Specialty beds help to prevent problems related to prolonged bed rest and immobility. **A.** The FluidAir Elite airflow bed. **B.** The TheraPulse ATP alternating pressure bed. **C.** Isolibrium Pressure Injury Prevention Surface. (*A and B Courtesy of Arjo AB, Malmö Sweden. C, used with permission of Stryker Corporation.*)

endoscopic gastrostomy (PEG) tubes, or other medical devices are inserted into the body through a "man-made" opening. Intentional wounds are usually created under controlled conditions. Precautions are taken to minimize the risk of infection. The edges of the wound are usually clean and even and held together with stitches (sutures) or staples.

A **unintentional wound** is an unexpected injury that usually results from some type of trauma. Falls, car accidents, and gun and knife violence can result in unintentional wounds (Fig. 29-13). Unintentional wounds can be *open*, which means that the surface of the skin is broken. The risk of infection is high with open wounds because the open skin creates a portal of entry for microbes. In addition, the uneven wound edges and amount of tissue damage may make closing the wound difficult. A *closed* wound is one where the skin is not broken, but there is damage to the underlying tissues. The deep tissue damage associated with a closed wound can be considerable, even though the only signs of injury may be redness, swelling, or bruising of the overlying skin.

Wound Healing

The human body is quite efficient at healing wounds, especially when it is otherwise healthy. However, having multiple, severe injuries, a chronic illness, or an impaired immune system can limit a person's ability to heal on their own. A person who is very young or very old may also have a limited ability to heal, or may heal more slowly. The same is true of a person who is malnourished or dehydrated.

For a wound to heal properly, there must be increased blood flow to the injured area. The smallest blood vessels (capillaries) also become quite leaky, allowing cells and fluid to enter the damaged tissue. These changes are

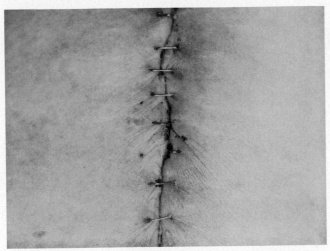

Figure 29-12 A surgical incision is an example of an intentional wound. Intentional wounds are usually created under controlled conditions, minimizing the risk of infection. The edges of the wound are usually brought together and secured with stitches or staples (shown here) to promote healing and minimize scarring. (Used with permission from Craven, R. F. [2007]. *Fundamentals of nursing: Human health and function* [5th ed., p. 1032]. Lippincott Williams & Wilkins.)

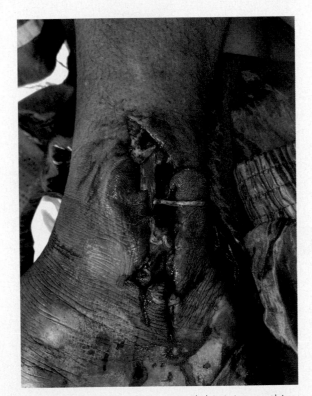

Figure 29-13 An accident caused this injury to this man's ankle. This is an example of an open unintentional wound. Open unintentional wounds carry a high risk of infection because they are often contaminated with dirt and microbes. The edges of the wound are often jagged and underlying structures, such as tendons and bones, may also be damaged. (*Worapol RESCUE\Shutterstock.com*)

responsible for the inflammation that is usually seen around an injury. Inflammation is characterized by redness, swelling, heat, and pain. It is a sign that the body is working to heal itself. Healing tissues also need good hydration and nutrition. Recall from Chapter 24 that adequate protein intake is especially important when the body is trying to rebuild injured tissues.

In the health care setting, we do many things to help support the wound healing process. Some of the measures the health care team takes to support the wound healing process include closing the wound, inserting drains, and applying dressings. As a nursing assistant, your duties related to wound care will vary, depending on your employer and the state where you work. Usually, nursing assistants are asked to assist the nurse with wound care. However, some facilities may train you to perform specific duties related to wound care on your own. As always, if you are asked to perform a task that is new to you, make sure that the task is covered by your job description and that you have received the training you will need to perform the skill properly. No matter where you work, the most important role you will play with regard to wound care is that of "observer." As a nursing assistant, you will have the best opportunity to notice and report signs that might indicate that a wound is not healing properly or has become infected.

Taking It to the Next Level:
Advanced Skills

More in-depth information related to advanced skills used when providing wound care can be found in *Lippincott Acute Care Skills for Advanced Nursing Assistants*.

Visit thePoint° at thepoint.lww.com for access to the ebook.

Wound Closure

The wound must be closed to prevent infection. If a wound is kept clean but otherwise left alone, eventually the tissue will repair itself and the wound will close on its own. However, this can take a long time, it increases the risk of infection, and it often results in a larger scar. To speed up this process, minimize the risk of infection, and reduce the amount of scarring, the doctor may decide to close the wound using sutures or staples. The timing for, and approach to, wound closure varies depending on the situation:

- **First-intention wound healing (primary wound closure).** In first-intention wound healing, open wounds are closed surgically with sutures or staples. Pulling the edges of the skin and underlying tissues together and holding them closed help speed up the healing process and minimize scarring.

- **Second-intention wound healing.** If the edges of the wound cannot be easily brought together or there is evidence of contamination or infection, the wound may be cleaned and rinsed and left open to heal from the inside out. This is called *second-intention wound healing.* Second-intention wound healing results in a wider, more noticeable scar after the wound has healed, but it prevents an unresolved infection from delaying the wound healing process.
- **Third-intention wound healing.** Sometimes it is necessary to leave a wound open, especially

a traumatic wound, for a period of time to make sure that an infection is not going to occur. Then the wound edges are cleaned and closed with sutures or staples to speed the healing process. This is called *third-intention wound healing.*

Wound Drains

As part of the healing process, some wounds will produce a lot of fluid, or drainage. A wound that is infected or bleeding will also often produce a lot of drainage. Fluid that is allowed to collect in a wound can promote infection, delaying the healing process. Therefore, wound drains are often used to allow blood and other fluids to flow out of the wound (Fig. 29-14).

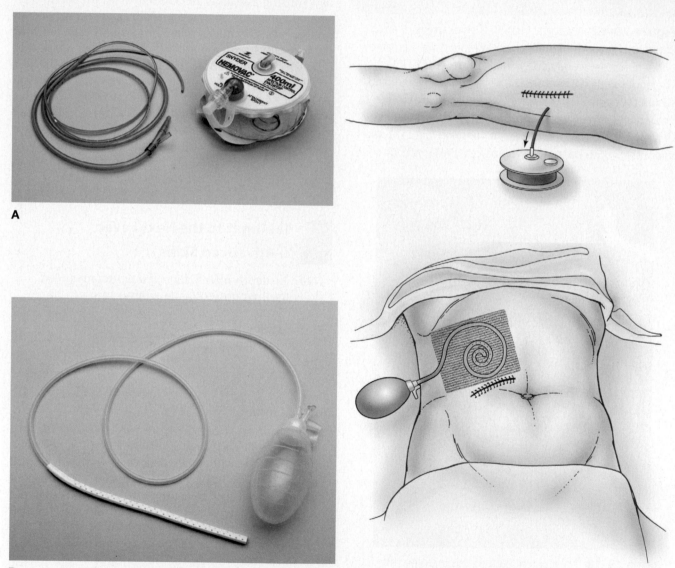

A

B

Figure 29-14 When drainage from a wound is significant, a drain may be placed. The drainage tube is placed in the wound and attached to a suction device, which draws the fluid out of the wound. Many types of drains are available. **A.** A Hemovac drain. **B.** A Jackson–Pratt or "grenade" drain. (*A and B* used with permission from Taylor, C., Lillis, C., & Lynn, P. [2014]. *Fundamentals of nursing: The art and science of nursing care* [8th ed.]. Lippincott Williams & Wilkins.)

Some drains allow fluid to collect in the wound dressing (the bandage covering the wound). Others are connected to a collection device. If a person you are caring for has a drain, take note of the characteristics of the drainage every time you check the dressing or the collection device. Is there more drainage than you expected? Does it have a foul odor that it did not have before? Has the appearance of the drainage changed? Report any unusual observations to the nurse.

When repositioning a person with a drain, take care not to pull on the drain tubing. Pulling on the drain tubing could pull the drain out of the wound. The loss of the drain will allow fluid to collect in the wound until the doctor can replace the drain. Fluid in the wound puts the person at risk for infection.

Wound Dressings

Sometimes dressings are applied to wounds to prevent microbes from gaining access to the body, to keep the wound edges moist, to keep the wound dry during procedures such as bathing, or to absorb drainage from the wound. The type of dressing used depends on several factors, including:

- The type of wound
- The location of the wound
- The amount of drainage associated with the wound
- Whether or not the wound is infected
- Whether or not the wound must be kept moist or dry
- How often the dressing must be changed

The doctor or the nurse determines which type of dressing is used.

Some dressings are made of a clear, plastic material (Fig. 29-15A). These dressings keep the wound clean and free from microbes and moisture, while allowing air to circulate freely. Some dressings are simply pieces of gauze held in place with tape (see Fig. 29-15B). Wounds that drain will have thick, absorbent dressings. There are many specialized dressings available now that are used to help promote healing on complicated or chronic wounds.

Many dressings are secured with tape. The type of tape used depends on the location of the wound and the needs of the person. For example, adhesive tape may irritate a person's skin, so a plastic or paper tape would be used instead. Elastic tape is stretchy and may be used when the wound is on a part of the body that must bend, such as the knee or elbow. Most often, dressings on extremities are held in place with rolled, stretchy gauze or elastic (ACE) bandages.

When a wound is draining heavily and the dressing must be changed often, a Montgomery tie may be used instead of tape. A Montgomery tie consists of

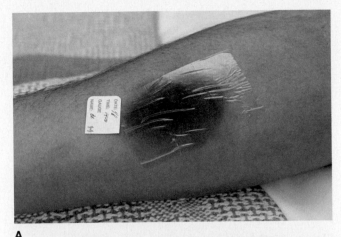

A

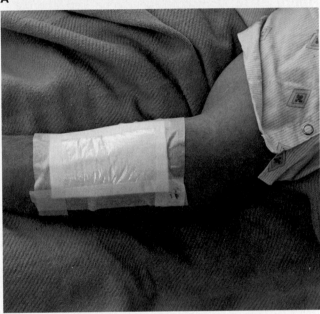

B

Figure 29-15 Various types of wound dressings and tapes are available. **A.** Here, a wound is covered with a clear dressing that keeps moisture and microbes out of the wound, but allows air to reach the wound to promote healing. This type of dressing does not absorb drainage, but it does allow members of the health care team to look at the wound without removing the dressing. **B.** This dressing is not waterproof, so it will need to be changed if it gets wet. The gauze prevents microbes from entering the wound, and it also absorbs drainage.

a strip of adhesive that is attached to a cloth tie. The dressing is placed on the wound. Then, the adhesive strip of the Montgomery tie is applied to the person's skin alongside the dressing. Another Montgomery tie is placed in the same way on the other side of the dressing. Then the ties are tied together over the dressing, to hold it in place (Fig. 29-16). When it is time to change the dressing, the ties are untied, the dressing is replaced, and then the ties are retied. Because there

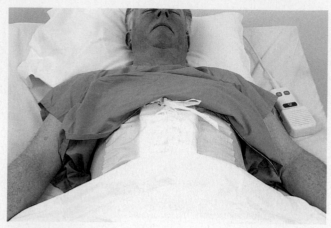

Figure 29-16 Montgomery ties can be used to secure a dressing that needs to be changed often. The adhesive is applied and then left in place. The ties secure the dressing and can be easily untied when a new dressing is needed. (© B. Proud.)

is no need to remove the adhesive tape to change the dressing, Montgomery ties help to protect the person's skin from damage caused by the frequent removal and reapplication of tape.

You may be asked to assist the nurse with dressing changes. Doing so accomplishes two things. First, it minimizes the chance that the nurse's hands or other surfaces will become contaminated by the drainage on the soiled dressing. Second, it helps to ensure that the new dressing remains free of microbes that could contaminate the wound.

Procedure 29-1 explains how to help the nurse with a dressing change.

Vacuum-Assisted Closure Therapy

Vacuum-assisted closure (VAC) therapy may be used to help promote healing of complicated or chronic wounds. In VAC therapy, the wound is covered with a foam-like dressing. Tubing is embedded in the foam. Then, the foam, the tubing, and a margin of healthy skin are covered with transparent adhesive film, forming a seal. The end of the tubing is connected to a vacuum pump. When the pump is turned on, it creates suction. The suction removes wound drainage from the surface of the wound, stimulates blood flow to the wound, and stimulates the growth of new tissue (Fig. 29-17). When caring for a patient or a resident with a wound that is being treated with VAC therapy, it is important to make sure the system is functioning properly. Tell the nurse right away if the tubing is kinked, the vacuum pump is not functioning (there is no suction), or the dressing has become loose. An increase in bright red drainage in the collection device should also be reported right away.

Burns

Burns are injuries to the skin and underlying tissues caused by contact with extreme heat (thermal burns), chemicals (chemical burns), or electricity (electrical burns). Burns can be minor, causing only slight redness and pain, or they can be very severe, extending down through the layers of the skin and possibly even involving the muscles and bones. Burns are classified according to the depth of the damage:

■ **Superficial (first-degree) burns** cause injury to the outermost layer of the skin, the epidermis. Most sunburns are superficial burns. Minor household accidents, such as touching a hot stove or leaving a heating pad that is too warm in place for too long, can also result in superficial burns. The redness and pain usually go away after a few days.

■ **Superficial partial-thickness (second-degree) burns** penetrate into the upper part of the dermis of the skin. Superficial partial-thickness burns are often associated with blisters. These burns are very painful, and the loss of the epidermis increases the risk of infection.

■ **Deep partial-thickness (third-degree) burns** affect the deeper dermis as well. They are dry, pale in color, and less painful than superficial partial-thickness burns because the pain receptors have been destroyed. They take a long time to heal and result in scarring.

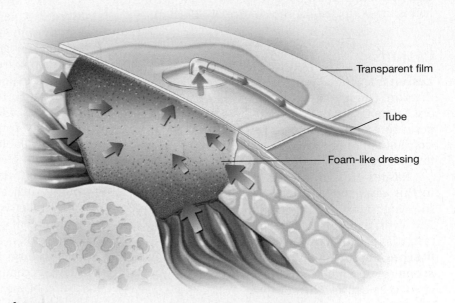

Transparent film

Tube

Foam-like dressing

A

Figure 29-17 Vacuum-assisted closure (VAC) therapy is often used to promote healing of complicated or chronic wounds. **A.** The wound is filled with a foam-like dressing. A tube is inserted into the foam, and then the area is sealed with a transparent film. When the pump is turned on, it creates suction, which draws fluid out of the wound and stimulates blood flow and the growth of new tissue. **B.** The V.A.C. ATS Therapy System. (*A and B Courtesy of KCI, an Acelity Company.*)

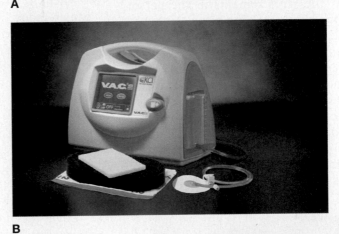

B

- **Full-thickness (fourth-, fifth-, or sixth-degree) burns** involve the epidermis and dermis, the subcutaneous layer, and often the underlying muscles and bones as well (Fig. 29-18). People with full-thickness burns need surgery and skin grafts to heal. These burns are associated with very high infection rates because the skin has been destroyed. In addition, the scarring that results from severe burns can cause severe disfigurement and contractures of the extremities.

People with deep partial-thickness and full-thickness burns often require months or even years of rehabilitation, and they must have multiple surgical procedures. These people need very special care. Because of the risk of infection, they may be placed in reverse (protective) isolation. Caregivers must often wear sterile gloves and gowns when providing care,

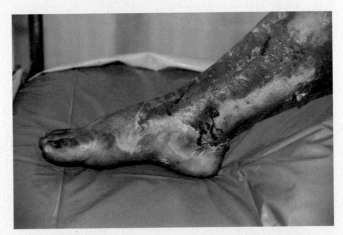

Figure 29-18 People with severe burns, such as the burns shown here, require special care to promote healing and prevent complications such as infection. (*Tewan Banditrukkanka\Shutterstock.com*)

and bed linens may need to be sterilized before the bed is made, to reduce the chance of infection.

Lesions

Lesion is a general term used to describe any break in the skin. Often you will see the term *lesion* used when discussing rashes or other skin disorders. Lesions often occur in groups, forming a **rash**. Rashes can be *localized* (limited to one area) or *systemic* (occurring all over the body).

Rashes may be caused by a systemic infection. In this case, the skin itself is not infected, but it is showing signs of an infection inside of the body. The rash seen in shingles is a good example of a rash that is caused by a systemic infection. **Shingles (herpes zoster)**, a disorder most commonly seen in people older than 65 years, is caused by the same virus that causes chicken pox. Following a case of the chicken pox, the virus remains in the person's body, but in an inactive state. The virus can become active again if the person's resistance to infection is lowered, which often happens with age. The virus causes a red rash of small, fluid-filled blisters (Fig. 29-19). Because the virus lives in the nerve cells, the rash usually follows the path of a nerve and is often accompanied by itching, stinging, or burning pain. For many people, the pain is severe, and it can last for weeks or months. Even the touch of clothing against the area may be very painful. Because shingles is most common in older people,

you may care for a patient or a resident with this disorder. A person with shingles should be cared for only by someone who has already been exposed to the chicken pox virus because it is possible to get chicken pox from a person with shingles if you have not been exposed to the virus before. It is also very important to follow your facility's infection control procedures when giving care to prevent others in the facility from being exposed to the virus. A vaccine is available to help protect an older person from getting shingles.

Rashes may also be caused by contact with an irritant, such as poison ivy. In people with sensitive skin, contact with substances like bath soap or laundry detergent can cause a rash called *contact dermatitis*. **Dermatitis** is a general term for inflammation of the skin. **Eczema** is a type of chronic dermatitis that is usually accompanied by severe itching, scaling, and crusting of the surface of the skin.

Itching, burning, or redness of the skin accompanies many skin lesions. The redness of the skin that often accompanies these lesions is known as **erythema**. Dermatologists (doctors who specialize in knowledge of the skin) look at the characteristics of the lesions on the skin, as well as the location of the lesions and the person's other signs and symptoms, to find clues to their cause. There are many different types of skin lesions (Table 29-1):

- A **macule** is a small, flat, reddened lesion. Macules form the rash that is seen in measles.
- A **papule** is a small, raised, firm lesion. Papules can be easily felt by passing your fingers lightly over the affected area.
- A **vesicle** is a small, blister-like lesion that contains watery, clear fluid. Vesicles form the rash that is seen in chickenpox or shingles.
- A **pustule** is a vesicle that contains pus, a thick, yellowish fluid that is a sign of infection. Pustules are seen in acne.
- An **excoriation** is an abrasion, or a scraping away of the surface of the skin. Excoriations can be caused by trauma, chemicals, or burns (including friction burns from sliding a person's skin across a sheet). Urine or feces, if left on the skin for too long, can cause a chemical excoriation.
- A **fissure** is a crack in the skin. Fissures can be caused by extreme dryness. Fungal infections, such as tinea pedis (athlete's foot), can also cause fissures.
- An **ulcer** is a shallow crater that is formed when the tissue dies. The dead tissue is shed, leaving a crater behind. Venous stasis ulcers, a common type of ulcer, develop as a result of poor blood flow through the veins in the legs.

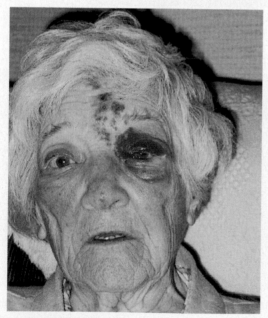

Figure 29-19 The shingles rash is a painful rash made up of fluid-filled blisters (vesicles). It is usually localized to one area or one side of the body, often in a stripe pattern.

TABLE 29-1 Types of Skin Lesions

LESION	DESCRIPTION
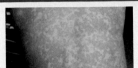 Macule (*DonyaHHI\Shutterstock.com*)	Small, flat, red lesions
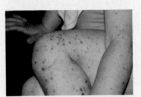 Papule (*Ressormat\Shutterstock.com*)	Small, raised, firm bumps
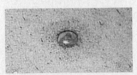 Vesicle	Small, fluid-filled, blister-like lesions
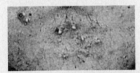 Pustule	Small, pus-filled, blister-like lesions
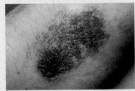 Excoriation (*Kondor83\Shutterstock.com*)	Abrasion (wearing away of the surface of the skin)
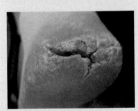 Fissure	A crack in the skin
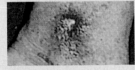 Ulcer	A crater-like open sore

Because skin lesions disrupt the skin's protective barrier, they place the person at increased risk for infection. Secondary bacterial infection of the skin is especially common when the lesion is itchy and the person scratches it excessively. *Secondary* means that the infection is occurring on top of the original problem. This is similar to what happens when you have a mosquito bite that you cannot stop scratching—eventually, you scratch it raw, it gets infected, and suddenly it takes much longer for the bite to heal than it would have if you had just left it alone.

When you are caring for a person with skin lesions, there are several things that you can do to increase the person's comfort and promote healing of the skin:

- Make sure that you are aware of any adjustments to the normal bathing and skin care routine that may be necessary. For example, you may need to use a special soap or lotion as part of the person's skin care. The nurse will be able to tell you about any necessary changes to the routine, or you can check the nursing care plan.
- Help the person to choose clothing that does not rub or irritate the skin lesion.
- Discourage the person from scratching itchy or irritated skin. Although scratching may bring temporary relief, it causes additional skin injury and puts the person at risk for infection. Soft mitt restraints or gloves may be necessary to prevent a small child or confused adult from scratching the lesions.
- Observe the lesions for changes in color, or for bleeding or drainage. Report any changes to the nurse immediately. Also note whether the lesions seem to be getting larger or spreading to other parts of the body.

SUMMARY

- The integumentary system consists of the skin and its accessory structures (hair, nails, sweat glands, and sebaceous glands).
- The integumentary system has three major functions that help maintain homeostasis.
  - The skin protects us from microbes, chemicals, and other harmful agents.
  - The skin helps maintain internal fluid balance.
  - The integumentary system helps regulate temperature. Narrowing and widening of the blood vessels in the skin help our bodies to maintain or release heat, respectively. Sweat glands help cool our bodies through evaporation. Hair on our scalps and bodies helps keep us warm.
- Like all organ systems, the integumentary system changes as we age.
  - Changes that affect appearance include wrinkles, gray hair, and "age spots."
  - The skin becomes more fragile and more prone to injury with age. The number and output of the sebaceous glands decrease, making the skin dry. Circulation to the skin decreases.
  - The output of the sweat glands decrease. This change, along with the changes in the skin, makes it harder for the older person to adjust to changes in the environmental temperature.
  - The nails become tough and yellow, making them difficult to trim.
- As the body's most visible organ system, the integumentary system can provide clues to a person's overall health. Changes in a person's skin tone or the development of a rash may signal an internal problem, such as liver disease, a heart or lung problem, or an infection.
- Pressure ulcers are a major concern in the health care setting.
  - Pressure ulcers develop when soft tissues are squeezed between the bone and a surface, such as a mattress or chair. The weight of the body disrupts the flow of oxygen-rich blood to the tissues, causing the tissues to die and leading to the formation of a pressure ulcer.
  - Immobility is the underlying cause of all pressure ulcers. Several factors, including old age, poor nutrition, and moisture trapped in the folds of the skin, can increase an immobile person's risk of developing a pressure ulcer.

- Warning signs of pressure ulcers include:
  - A reddened or pale area that does not return to its normal color after the pressure is relieved
  - A previously reddened area that is hot to the touch or painful
  - An area that is pale, white, or shiny
- Prevention of pressure ulcers is very important because pressure ulcers are extremely painful, difficult to treat, and potentially fatal.
- The nursing assistant does many things to prevent patients and residents from developing pressure ulcers, including repositioning, observing, providing good skin and perineal care, changing wet and soiled linens promptly, and encouraging exercise.
- A wound is a break in the skin. The underlying tissues are usually affected as well.
  - A wound can be intentional or unintentional.
  - A break in the skin puts the person at risk for infection. Therefore, the health care team does many things to help wounds to heal quickly and with minimal complications. Sutures, dressings, and drains are commonly used.
  - Nursing assistants are in an excellent position to notice and report signs and symptoms that suggest that the wound has become infected or is not healing well, such as a foul-smelling drainage or bleeding.
- Burns are injuries caused by heat, chemicals, or electricity. People with burn wounds require special care because of the very high risk of infection.
- Lesions are breaks in the skin.
  - Many different types of skin lesions can form rashes.
    - The type of lesion is often a clue to the cause of the rash.
    - Rashes can be localized (limited to one area) or systemic (occurring all over the body).
  - Skin lesions can be caused by infections inside the body, infections of the skin itself, or irritation of the skin.
  - Nursing assistants are often the first to notice an unusual lesion on a patient or resident.

> **Procedure 29-1**

Assisting the Nurse With a Dressing Change

WHY YOU DO IT   Helping the nurse with a dressing change minimizes the chance that the nurse's hands or other surfaces will become contaminated by the drainage on the soiled dressing. It also helps to ensure that the new dressing remains free of pathogens that could contaminate the wound.

Getting Ready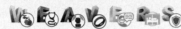

1. Complete the "Getting Ready" steps.

Supplies

- gloves
- gown (if necessary)
- mask (if necessary)
- paper towels or a bed protector
- plastic bag
- tape or Montgomery ties
- dressing material
- scissors

Procedure

2. Clean the over-bed table and cover it with paper towels or the bed protector. Place the dressing supplies on the over-bed table. Fold the top edges of the plastic bag down to make a cuff. Place the cuffed bag on the over-bed table.

3. Make sure that the bed is positioned at a comfortable working height (to promote good body mechanics) and that the wheels are locked. If the side rails are in use, lower the side rail on the working side of the bed. The side rail on the opposite side of the bed should remain up.

4. Help the person to a comfortable position that allows access to the wound.

5. Fanfold the top linens to the foot of the bed. Adjust the person's hospital gown or pajamas as necessary to expose the wound.

6. Put on the mask, gown, or both, if necessary. Perform hand hygiene and put on the gloves.

7. The nurse will remove the old dressing. The nurse may ask you to take the old dressing and place it in the cuffed plastic bag. Be careful to keep the soiled side of the dressing out of the person's sight. Do not let the dressing touch the outside of the plastic bag.

8. Remove your gloves, dispose of them in a facility-approved waste container, and perform hand hygiene.

9. Wait while the nurse inspects the wound and measures it, if necessary.

10. Put on a clean pair of gloves.

11. Assist as the nurse applies a new dressing.

    a. Open the wrapper containing the dressing and hold it open so that the nurse can remove the dressing. Do not touch the dressing. Dispose of the wrapper in a facility-approved waste container.

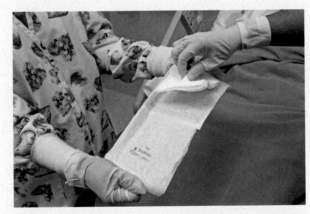

STEP 11a Hold the wrapper open so that the nurse can remove the dressing.

    b. If the dressing will be secured with tape, cut four pieces of tape for securing the dressing. For a 4 × 4 dressing, each piece of tape should measure 8 inches long. Hang the tape from the edge of the over-bed table.

(continued)

c. If the nurse asks you to, use the tape strips to secure the dressing by placing one piece of tape along each side of the dressing. Center each piece of tape equally over the dressing and the person's skin.

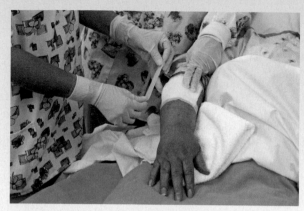

STEP 11c The dressing is secured by placing one piece of tape along each side.

12. Remove your gloves (and gown and mask, if using) and dispose of them in a facility-approved waste container. Perform hand hygiene.

13. Re-cover the wound with the hospital gown or pajamas. Help the person back into a comfortable position, straighten the bottom linens, and draw the top linens over the person.

14. Make sure that the bed is lowered to its lowest position and that the wheels are locked. If the side rails are in use, return the side rail to the raised position on the working side of the bed.

15. Dispose of disposable items in a facility-approved waste container. Clean equipment and return it to the storage area.

Finishing Up

16. Complete the "Finishing Up" steps.

What You Document

- Date and time
- Appearance of the wound
- Amount, color, and characteristics of any wound drainage
- Type of dressing applied

WHAT DID YOU LEARN?

Multiple Choice

Select the single best answer for each of the following questions.

1. Which of the following are areas that are considered pressure points in relation to pressure ulcers?
   a. The heels, ankles, and toes
   b. The elbows and shoulder blades
   c. The spine
   d. All of the above

2. Why is it important to prevent pressure ulcers from forming?
   a. Pressure ulcers are disgusting to see.
   b. People who have pressure ulcers require more care than people who do not, and this is expensive for the facility.
   c. Pressure ulcers are difficult to treat and can lead to a person's death.
   d. Pressure ulcers interfere with the skin's ability to make vitamin D.

3. What is the underlying cause of all pressure ulcers?
   a. Continuous pressure applied to one area
   b. Poor nutrition
   c. Incontinence
   d. All of the above

4. Which of the following factors can increase a person's risk of getting a pressure ulcer?
   a. Advanced age
   b. Incontinence
   c. Poor nutrition
   d. All of the above

5. Mr. Underwood has developed a white, shiny area on his left hip about the size of a quarter. Yesterday, this same area was red and hot to the touch. If you were Mr. Underwood's nursing assistant, what would be your biggest concern?
   a. That Mr. Underwood has the chickenpox
   b. That Mr. Underwood has a stage 1 pressure ulcer
   c. That Mr. Underwood's wound is not healing properly
   d. That Mr. Underwood has jaundice

6. You are caring for Mrs. Patel, a 93-year-old grandmother who has limited mobility following a stroke. What should you do to minimize Mrs. Patel's chances of developing a pressure ulcer?
   a. Dry Mrs. Patel's skin thoroughly after each bath
   b. Reposition Mrs. Patel regularly, according to the nursing care plan
   c. Encourage Mrs. Patel to eat well
   d. All of the above

7. Which one of the following is an example of an intentional wound?
   a. A gunshot wound
   b. A surgical incision
   c. A lesion
   d. A burn

8. An assessment tool that is useful in helping to predict a patient's or resident's risk for developing pressure ulcers is the:
   a. Braden Scale
   b. NPUAP scale
   c. Apgar score
   d. Miller test

9. Shingles is a skin disorder caused by the virus that is responsible for causing:
   a. Whooping cough
   b. Measles
   c. Chicken pox
   d. Fever blisters

Matching   *Match each numbered item with its appropriate lettered description.*

_____ **1.** Macules

_____ **2.** Melanin

_____ **3.** Dermatitis

_____ **4.** Vesicles

_____ **5.** Erythema

_____ **6.** Papules

_____ **7.** Pustules

_____ **8.** Excoriation

_____ **9.** Fissure

_____ **10.** Age spot

a. Redness of the skin that often accompanies rashes

b. Often seen on the backs of the hands; caused by melanin deposits

c. Cracks in the skin, such as those seen in athlete's foot

d. Abrasion or wearing away of the top layer of skin; caused by trauma, chemicals, or burns

e. Filled with pus, a thick yellow fluid associated with infection

f. Blister-like lesions that contain watery fluid, such as those seen in chickenpox

g. Flat, reddened lesions, such as those seen in measles

h. Firm, raised bumps

i. General term for inflammation of the skin

j. Gives the skin its color

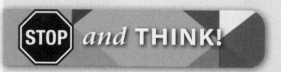

- You have been assigned to help Ms. Lazdins with her morning care. While you are helping Ms. Lazdins to put on her socks, you accidentally scratch Ms. Lazdins' ankle, causing her to bleed. What should you do? What are some steps you can take to avoid scratching a person's skin when you are providing care?

- Amir is providing care to Mr. O'Meara, who has just been transferred to Willow Wood Care Center. Mr. O'Meara is confined to a wheelchair. While giving Mr. O'Meara a back massage as part of evening care, Amir notices a reddened area at the base of Mr. O'Meara's spine. What are the possible explanations for this finding? What should Amir do?

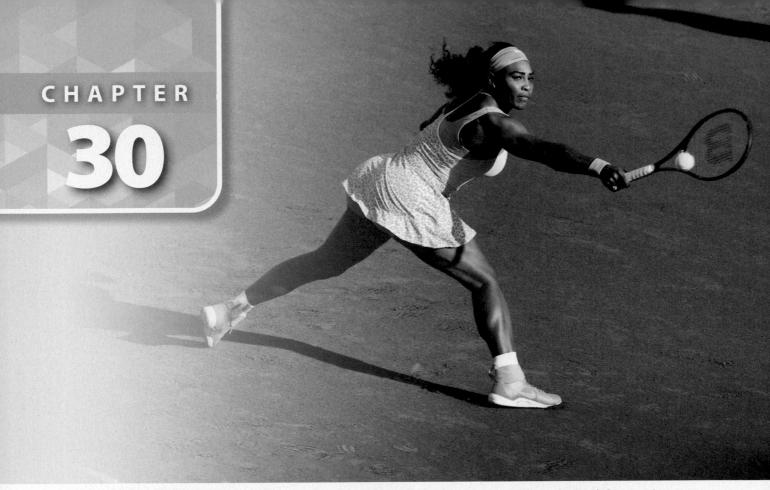

Photo: Serena Williams goes after the ball during the French Open tennis tournament.
(Leonard Zhukovsky\Shutterstock.com)

The Musculoskeletal System

 WHAT WILL YOU LEARN?

Think about everything you have done so far today. Before you even left the house this morning, you did a number of different tasks requiring the services of your musculoskeletal system—getting out of bed, brushing your teeth, eating breakfast, and taking the dog for a walk or feeding the cat, just to name a few. Think about all of the individual movements that each of these small tasks requires, and you will get a sense of how very important the musculoskeletal system is to our daily functioning.

The muscular system and the skeletal system work together to enable us to move. As you learned in Chapter 28, sometimes these two organ systems are referred to together as the *musculoskeletal system* because they work so closely together. In this chapter, you will learn about the structure and function of the musculoskeletal system and about how it is affected by aging and illness. You will also learn about how nursing assistants help residents and patients to maintain proper function of the musculoskeletal system. When you are finished with this chapter, you will be able to:

1. List the major parts of the musculoskeletal system.
2. List and describe the four types of bones found in the skeletal system.
3. Define terms used to describe joint movement.
4. List and describe the three types of muscles found in the body.

5. Discuss the main functions of the musculoskeletal system.

6. Describe how normal aging processes affect the musculoskeletal system.

7. Describe some of the disorders that can affect the musculoskeletal system.

8. Define normal range of motion and describe methods used to maintain joint function in the health care setting.

9. Demonstrate how to help a person to perform range-of-motion exercises.

Vocabulary

Skeleton	Tendons	Muscular dystrophy	Trapeze bar
Joints	Muscle tone	Fracture	Amputation
Range of motion	Atrophy	Reduction	Stump
Cartilage	Osteoporosis	Fixation	Phantom pain
Ligaments	Arthritis	Traction	

STRUCTURE OF THE MUSCULOSKELETAL SYSTEM

The musculoskeletal system consists of the skeletal system and the muscular system.

The Skeletal System

The skeletal system consists of the bones. The 206 bones in the human body form a framework called the **skeleton** (Fig. 30-1). The skeleton gives structure and shape to the body and protects key vital organs, such as the heart and the brain, from injury.

The bones of the skeleton vary in size and shape. Bones are classified according to their shape (Fig. 30-2):

- **Long bones.** When we think of a "bone," what we often picture in our mind is an example of a long bone. The long bones are found in the arms and the legs. Long bones consist of a shaft and two rounded ends.
- **Short bones.** Short bones are round or cube-shaped. Short bones are found in the wrists and ankles.
- **Flat bones** are relatively thin and may be curved. Examples of flat bones include the ribs and the bones that form the skull.
- **Irregular bones** are oddly shaped bones that are not flat. Irregular bones are found in the spinal column and face.

Bones must be strong enough to support and protect the body, yet light enough to allow us to move. Can you imagine how heavy a large bone like the bone in your thigh would be if it were solid? Instead, bones have two layers. The outer layer of compact bone is hard and solid. The inside of the bone is sponge-like and airy. Thin strands of bone form a net-like structure, and the spaces in between the thin strands of bone are filled with bone marrow (Fig. 30-3). This combination of a solid, hard outside and a sponge-like inside results in bones that are very strong and able to resist a great amount of force, yet lightweight. The tissue that forms the bones is constantly broken down and replaced with new tissue throughout a person's lifetime. A complex network of blood vessels supplies the bone cells with the oxygen and nutrients they need.

The areas where two bones join together are called **joints**. Joints allow us to move. The **range of motion** of a joint is the complete extent of movement that the joint is normally capable of without causing pain. Joints can be classified according to the amount of movement they allow (Fig. 30-4):

- **Fixed joints** do not permit any movement at all. The joints between the bones of the skull are examples of fixed joints.
- **Slightly movable joints** allow for limited movement. Slightly movable joints are found between the vertebrae in the spine, and where the ribs attach to the sternum (breastbone). **Cartilage**, a tough, fibrous substance, fills in the space between the bones in the slightly movable joint. The cartilage permits limited movement and acts as a "shock absorber" between the bones.

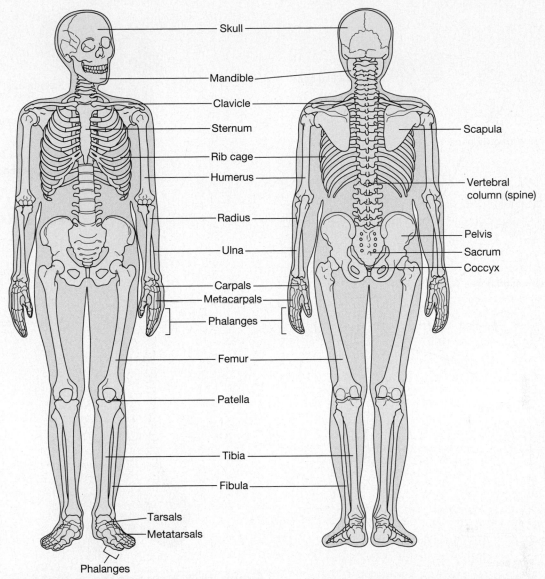

Figure 30-1 The human skeleton contains approximately 206 bones. Some of the major bones are labeled here.

■ **Freely movable joints** allow for a wide range of movement. Examples of freely movable joints include the knees, shoulders, elbows, finger and toe joints, and hip joints. Some of the ways in which freely movable joints move are shown and defined in Table 30-1. The ends of the bones that form the freely movable joint are covered with cartilage, which provides a smooth surface for the other bones to move against. A capsule formed of connective tissue encloses the ends of the bones, forming a joint cavity. The lining of the capsule secretes a thick fluid called *synovial fluid* into the joint cavity. The synovial fluid lubricates the joint, which helps the joint to move smoothly. **Ligaments**, which are very strong bands of fibrous tissue, cross over the joint capsule, attaching one bone to another and stabilizing the joint. If the ligament is torn or weak, the joint may be able to move too much in any one direction.

The Muscular System

The muscular system consists of the muscles. As you learned in Chapter 28, there are three types of muscle tissue found in the body (see Chapter 28, Table 28-1). Of the three types, skeletal muscle is the type of muscle tissue found in the musculoskeletal system. Skeletal muscle is said to be *striated* because the muscle fibers make the muscles look like they have stripes. (*Striations* is another word for "stripes.")

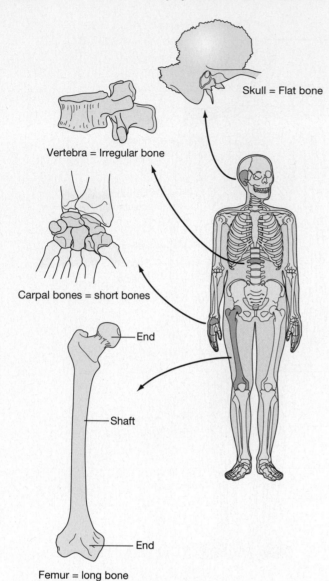

Skull = Flat bone

Vertebra = Irregular bone

Carpal bones = short bones

End

Shaft

End

Femur = long bone

Figure 30-2 *Bones can be categorized by their shape. General types of bones include long bones, short bones, flat bones, and irregular bones.*

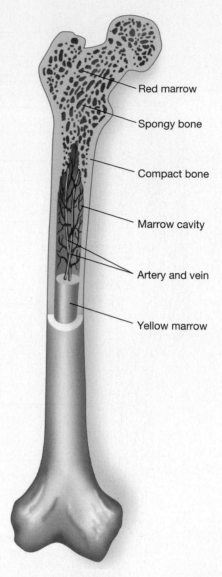

Red marrow

Spongy bone

Compact bone

Marrow cavity

Artery and vein

Yellow marrow

Figure 30-3 *Bones have two layers, a solid outside and a net-like inside. As a result, bones are very strong, yet light-weight.*

There are almost 700 individual skeletal muscles in the body (Fig. 30-5). These muscles account for about 40% of your total body weight. Skeletal muscles vary in shape. Some are long, thick, and band-like. Others are flat or fan-like. Muscles are named according to their location, their shape, or their function.

The skeletal muscles are attached to the bones by bands of connective tissue called **tendons**. Occasionally, skeletal muscles are attached to other muscles by a broad, flat sheet of tendon called an *aponeurosis*.

FUNCTION OF THE MUSCULOSKELETAL SYSTEM

The musculoskeletal system has several vital functions.

Protection

The bones of the skeletal system protect delicate internal organs. For example, the skull bones surround and protect the brain, and the rib cage surrounds and protects the lungs and heart.

Support

The bones of the skeleton form a framework that supports and gives shape to the body. **Muscle tone**, or the steady contraction of the skeletal muscles, helps us to maintain an upright posture, such as sitting or standing. The muscles of the back, neck, shoulders, and abdomen are responsible for maintaining posture.

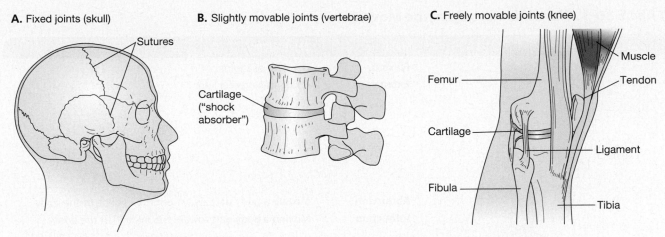

A. Fixed joints (skull)

Sutures

B. Slightly movable joints (vertebrae)

Cartilage ("shock absorber")

C. Freely movable joints (knee)

Muscle

Tendon

Femur

Cartilage

Ligament

Fibula

Tibia

Figure 30-4 Joints are often categorized by the amount of motion they permit. **A.** Fixed joints, such as the joints that join the bones of the skull, do not allow for any movement. **B.** Slightly movable joints, such as those between the vertebrae in the spinal column, permit some movement. **C.** Freely movable joints, such as the knee joints, allow for a wide range of movement.

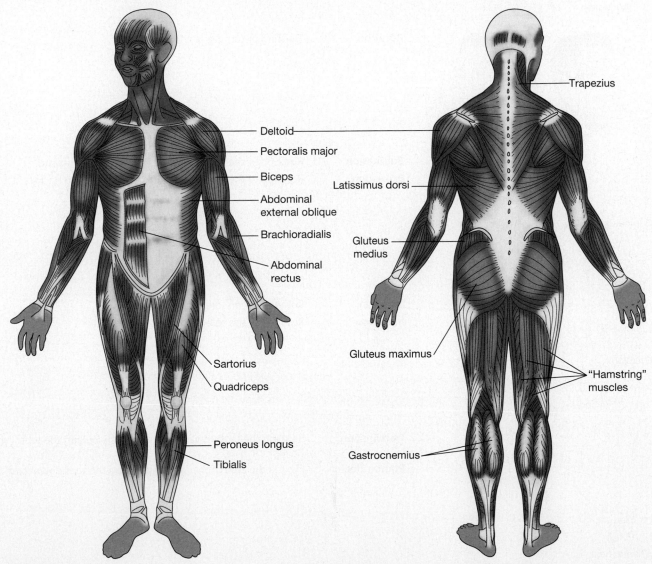

Deltoid

Pectoralis major

Biceps

Abdominal external oblique

Brachioradialis

Abdominal rectus

Sartorius

Quadriceps

Peroneus longus

Tibialis

Trapezius

Latissimus dorsi

Gluteus medius

Gluteus maximus

"Hamstring" muscles

Gastrocnemius

Figure 30-5 There are about 700 skeletal muscles in the body! Some of the more familiar ones are labeled here.

TABLE 30-1 Words Used to Describe Movement

	WORD	DEFINITION
	Flexion	Bending of a joint
	Extension	Straightening of a joint
	Abduction	Moving a body part away from the midline of the body
	Adduction	Moving a body part toward the midline of the body
	Rotation	Twisting or turning of a joint
	Supination	Rotation of the palm so that it is facing up or forward
	Pronation	Rotation of the palm so that it is facing down or backward
	Eversion	Rotation of the sole of the foot outward
	Inversion	Rotation of the sole of the foot inward
	Dorsiflexion	Bending the foot upward at the ankle by pulling the toes toward the head
	Plantar flexion	Flexing the arch of the foot by pointing the toes downward

Movement

Voluntary movement occurs when a skeletal muscle contracts (shortens) or relaxes (lengthens) across a freely movable joint. In freely movable joints, each skeletal muscle attaches to the bone in two places, the origin and the insertion. The origin and the insertion points are on opposite sides of the joint. So, when the muscle contracts, the muscle shortens and the origin and insertion points are drawn closer to each other, causing the part of the body to move (Fig. 30-6).

Skeletal muscles usually work in groups to provide body movement. For example, your biceps muscle is located on the front of your upper arm. When you contract your biceps muscle, your lower arm is drawn toward your body. When you are lifting a heavy object, the brachioradialis muscle, which is also located in your upper arm, also contracts, helping to stabilize the elbow and assisting the biceps muscle with lifting. When it is time to straighten the arm again, the biceps muscle relaxes and the triceps muscle, located on the back of the

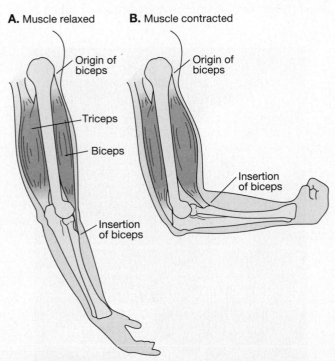

Figure 30-6 The muscular and the skeletal systems work together to produce movement. The muscle attaches to the bone in two places, the origin and the insertion. **A.** Shown here are the attachments of the biceps muscle, the muscle in your upper arm that bulges when you "make a muscle." **B.** When you contract your biceps muscle, the origin and insertion points are drawn closer together. As the muscle shortens, it pulls on the bone, bringing your lower arm toward your body.

upper arm, contracts, pulling the lower arm back into a straight position.

Heat Production

Contraction of the skeletal muscles produces heat and helps to maintain a constant body temperature. This is why we feel warmer when we move back and forth and stamp our feet while waiting outside on a cold day for a bus or train. The movement of the muscles produces heat, which makes us feel warmer. This is also why, when it is very cold, we may start to shiver. Shivering occurs when the skeletal muscles contract weakly but rapidly. The involuntary contractions help to increase the heat output of the muscles, raising the body temperature and making us feel warmer.

Calcium Storage

Calcium is an important mineral that is necessary for the proper functioning of skeletal and cardiac muscles. Calcium is also what makes the bone tissue hard and strong. Most of the calcium we need to function on a daily basis is obtained from calcium-rich foods and beverages, such as milk, cheese, yogurt, broccoli, leafy greens, tofu, and calcium-fortified orange juice. However, if we do not take in enough calcium through our diets, then calcium is released from the bones as it is needed. This is why it is important to obtain enough calcium through the diet, especially when a person is young.

Consuming enough calcium early on in life builds up the calcium stores in the bones. As we grow older, our intestines become less effective at absorbing the calcium that we eat, so calcium may be released from the bones to keep the levels in our bloodstream constant. If the amount of calcium stored in the bones is not adequate, the bones become brittle and weak as the body draws on the calcium stored there and does not replace it.

Production of Blood Cells

In addition to storing calcium, the bones also function as a factory for the production of blood cells. There are many different types of blood cells, with many different functions. For example, some blood cells play a role in the immune response and help us to fight off infection. Other blood cells carry oxygen to the tissues of the body. Blood cells form in red bone marrow, which is found in flat bones and the ends of the long bones. In young children, the shaft of the long bones also contains red bone marrow, but that red bone marrow is gradually replaced by yellow bone marrow as the person grows older. Yellow bone marrow is made up mostly of fatty tissue.

THE EFFECTS OF AGING ON THE MUSCULOSKELETAL SYSTEM

The normal processes of aging cause significant changes in the musculoskeletal system. It is the rare older person who does not have some degree of disability or discomfort related to the functioning of their musculoskeletal system! Aches, pains, and stiffness often accompany these changes. Occasionally, the person loses the ability to move one or more parts of their body. Age-related changes affecting the musculoskeletal system are the leading cause of disability in older adults.

It is now known that participating in regular physical exercise and eating properly are measures that can delay or decrease the effects of aging on the musculoskeletal system. Engaging in some form of weight-bearing exercise, such as brisk walking, aerobics, or moderate weight training, has been shown to have many positive effects, even in very old people (Fig. 30-7). Weight-bearing exercise helps to maintain bone strength by stimulating the body to store extra calcium in the bones. It improves blood flow, allowing more oxygen and nutrients to be carried to the tissues of the musculoskeletal system. Continued use of the muscles helps to retain strength. Flexibility of the joints is improved with regular exercise, which leads to fewer aches and pains.

People typically begin to experience age-related changes to the musculoskeletal system after the age of 40 years, although the onset of these changes may be significantly delayed in people who exercise regularly and are relatively healthy. The normal age-related changes that affect the musculoskeletal system include loss of bone tissue, loss of muscle mass, and wear and tear on the joints.

Loss of Bone Tissue

Aging decreases the body's ability to absorb calcium, a critical nutrient. When the body cannot get the amount of calcium it needs from the diet alone, it begins to draw on the calcium stored in the bones. Some people begin drawing on their calcium stores at a relatively young age, for example, when they are in their 40s. The continuous, gradual loss of calcium causes the bones to lose their strength and hardness, making them more fragile and prone to breaking. If other conditions, such as poor nutrition, poor circulation, or a lack of physical activity are present, the loss of strong bone tissue occurs much more rapidly.

Loss of Muscle Mass

The number of muscle cells also starts to gradually decrease when a person is in their 40s, resulting in a decrease in the size and strength of each individual muscle. The loss of muscle size and strength is called muscle **atrophy** (Fig. 30-8). If a person is poorly nourished, is not physically active, or has a chronic medical condition, muscle atrophy progresses at a much faster rate. If you have ever had a broken bone

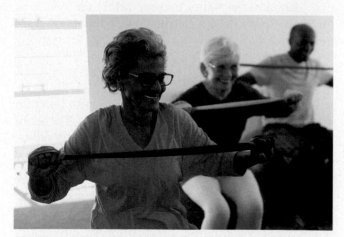

Figure 30-7 It is never too late to begin exercising! Regular exercise strengthens the muscles, helps to build bone mass, and lessens joint pain and stiffness. (*wavebreakmedia\Shutterstock.com*)

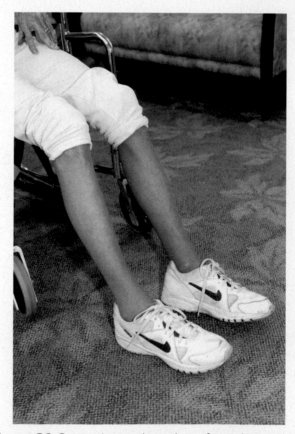

Figure 30-8 Muscle atrophy, or loss of muscle mass, is a normal age-related change. Immobility can make muscle atrophy much more severe.

that required a cast, you probably noticed that after the cast was removed, the affected limb was smaller and weaker than the other one. What you noticed was muscle atrophy as a result of not being able to use the muscle during the time that the limb was in the cast!

Significant loss of muscle tissue can leave a person too weak to walk or carry out routine activities of daily living (ADLs). Loss of muscle tissue also affects the body's ability to produce heat. This is one reason why an older person might feel chilly in a room that a younger person would consider warm or even hot.

Wear and Tear on the Joints

As we age, we lose the proteins that make the ligaments, tendons, and cartilage elastic and flexible, which can lead to stiffness and pain in the joints. The normal demands of daily life also cause a lot of wear and tear on the joints, which can, over time, lead to stiffness and pain. Overuse or injury of a joint, or having a Body Mass Index (BMI) that falls in the overweight range, can place extra strain on certain joints and make the normal changes associated with aging more severe. Joint pain and stiffness can make simple activities, such as walking or getting out of a chair, difficult. Joint stiffness can also make a person more likely to fall.

DISORDERS OF THE MUSCULOSKELETAL SYSTEM

It is likely that many of the people in your care will have some degree of musculoskeletal disability, simply as a result of their age. You may also care for people who have musculoskeletal disability as a result of disease or trauma. Examples of diseases that affect the bones, joints, and muscles include osteoporosis, arthritis, and muscular dystrophy. Fractures (broken bones) are usually caused by trauma. Amputation (the loss of a limb) may be necessary because of trauma or complications of a disease, such as diabetes.

Osteoporosis

Osteoporosis is the excessive loss of bone tissue. Although everyone experiences some loss of bone tissue as a normal part of aging, people with osteoporosis lose excessive amounts of bone tissue, causing the bones to become crumbly and very fragile. The bones most commonly affected by osteoporosis are the bones of the spine, the pelvis, and the long bones in the arms and legs. Because of the hormone changes that occur with menopause, osteoporosis is more common in older females than in older males. This is because estrogen, a hormone that is present in the bodies of females who are still having menstrual periods, helps to prevent bone loss. However, when a female goes through menopause, their body stops producing estrogen, and this puts them more at risk for bone loss. Other risk factors for the development of osteoporosis include:

- Underweight
- Smoking
- Inactivity or immobility
- Diseases of the thyroid and adrenal glands
- A diet lacking in calcium, vitamin D (necessary for the absorption of calcium), and protein
- Certain medications, such as steroids

Osteoporosis causes bones to break more easily, and physical activity becomes very difficult. Sometimes bones are so brittle that a person can break them just by bumping into a piece of furniture. Bones that have been fractured are difficult to repair and heal slowly. Crumbling of the bones of the spinal column causes the upper back to curve into the deformity known as *kyphosis* (see Fig. 30-9). These spinal column fractures are very painful and debilitating.

Some treatments for osteoporosis are available. A medication that helps to slow the progression of osteoporosis has been developed. In addition, the use of calcium and vitamin D supplements can also help in the treatment of osteoporosis. Resistance training (lifting weights) slows the progression of the disease by helping to promote bone strength. However, as with most things, prevention is the best medicine! Osteoporosis can be prevented in many cases by exercising regularly and eating a diet rich in calcium, protein, and vitamin D, starting early in life.

When caring for a person with osteoporosis, remember to be gentle when helping the person with transfers. Encourage exercise by having the person take frequent walks with you. Carefully observe and document the types of foods and liquids the person eats and drinks, and encourage snacks that are high in calcium, such as milk, yogurt, ice cream, and cheese. Be especially observant of loss of function, swelling, or complaints of pain. These signs and symptoms may indicate a new fracture in a fragile bone.

Arthritis

Arthritis is inflammation of the joints, usually associated with pain and stiffness. Arthritis is the most common disorder of the musculoskeletal system, affecting people of all ages. There are more than 20 different types of arthritis. Three of the most common types are osteoarthritis, rheumatoid arthritis, and gout.

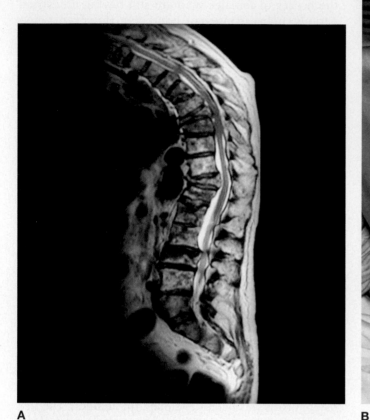

A

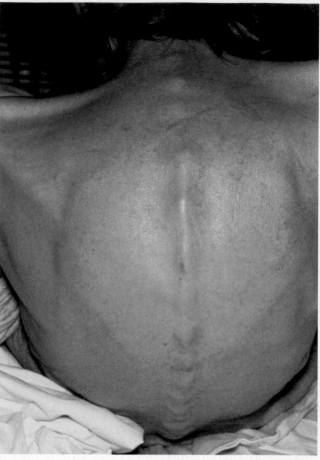

B

Figure 30-9 Osteoporosis. **A.** A magnetic resonance imaging (MRI) scan of the spine of a 60-year-old patient with osteoporosis. This is a side view (the patient is standing, facing the left). The vertebrae (*brown*) enclose the spinal cord (*pink*). Some of the vertebrae (*orange*) have collapsed as a result of osteoporosis, causing the spine to curve. **B.** This person has kyphosis as a result of osteoporosis of the spine. The deformity occurs when the fragile bones of the spine crumble. (*A, © ZEPHYR/Science Source; B, © John Radcliffe Hospital/Science Source.*)

Osteoarthritis

Osteoarthritis is the leading cause of physical disability among older people. In osteoarthritis, the cartilage that covers the ends of the bones wears away, making movement of the joint difficult and painful. Osteoarthritis appears to be the result of normal wear and tear on the joint, which is why it is seen most often in older people. However, obesity, previous joint injury, or a family history of the disease may increase a person's risk of developing osteoarthritis earlier in life and more severely.

Osteoarthritis usually affects weight-bearing joints, such as the knees, hips, and joints of the spinal column. Osteoarthritis begins when the smooth cartilage on the ends of the bones becomes rough, due to normal use of the joint. The rough area then becomes inflamed, and bony deposits build up. These bony deposits rub against the cartilage, causing even more damage. This cycle repeats until the cartilage has been worn down to the point where bone is actually rubbing against bone as the joint moves. The joint becomes swollen, stiff, and very painful.

A person with osteoarthritis may take medications to decrease both the pain and swelling. Heat and cold applications, discussed in Chapter 21, can also increase a person's level of comfort. Mild exercise that places the affected joints through their range of motion helps to diminish stiffness and maintain joint function. People who have very severe osteoarthritis may need surgery to replace the joint. Hips and knees are the joints most commonly replaced, but replacement of shoulder, elbow, wrist, and hand joints is also possible. Joint replacement surgery, also called total joint replacement, involves removing the ends of the bones in the affected joint and replacing them with parts made from metal and plastic (Fig. 30-10).

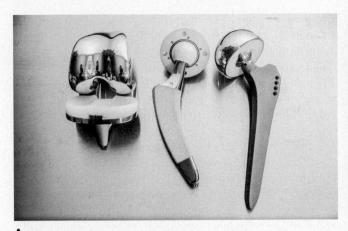

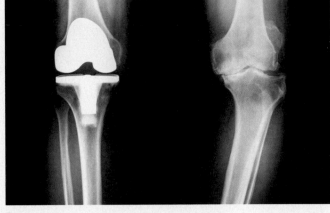

A   **B**

Figure 30-10 In joint replacement surgery, a damaged joint is replaced with an artificial (prosthetic) joint. **A.** Artificial knee and hip joint replacement components. **B.** X-ray of an artificial knee joint in place. (*A, Denis Simonov\Shutterstock.com; B, Puwadol Jaturawutthichai\Shutterstock.com*)

As a nursing assistant, you may be responsible for caring for a person who is recovering from joint replacement surgery. People who have had a joint replaced may not be allowed to bear weight on the affected joint for a period of time after the surgery, so you will need to help them with transfers. In addition, people who have had a hip joint replaced have several special care requirements during the recovery period:

- Following the surgery, the muscles and ligaments that normally hold the hip joint in place are weak, making it very easy for the head of the femur (the thigh bone) to dislocate, or pop out of joint. To prevent this from happening, the person's legs must be spread apart (abducted) when the person is in the supine or lateral position. Some people who have had hip replacement surgery will have a special wedge-shaped pillow, called an *abduction pillow*, which goes between the legs and attaches to each leg with Velcro fasteners (Fig. 30-11). The abduction pillow helps to keep the legs spread. If an abduction pillow is not available, a regular pillow can be used instead.
- When sitting, a person who has had hip replacement surgery must use a straight-backed chair. The person's hips must be flexed no more than 90 degrees, and their feet must rest flat on the floor. This is true when the person is using the toilet as well. A special device may be used to raise the height of the toilet seat to prevent flexion in excess of 90 degrees when the person is using the toilet.
- A physical therapist will work with the person after surgery. If possible, you should be present while the therapist is working with the person.

That way, you can see the specific ambulation and transfer techniques that are being used with your patient or resident.

As always, you should ask the nurse about any instructions or restrictions that are specific to your patient or resident.

Rheumatoid Arthritis

Rheumatoid arthritis is a condition that can cause severe joint deformities (Fig. 30-12). Unlike osteoarthritis, rheumatoid arthritis affects people much younger in life, most often between the ages of 20 and 40 years. This disease is more common in females than in males.

Researchers believe that rheumatoid arthritis is an autoimmune disorder. In autoimmune disorders,

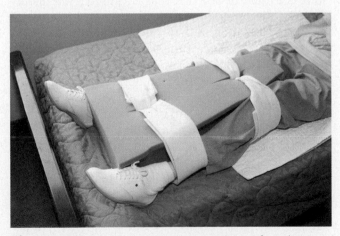

Figure 30-11 When a person is recovering from hip joint replacement surgery, an abduction pillow is used to help prevent the hip joint from becoming dislocated during the recovery period.

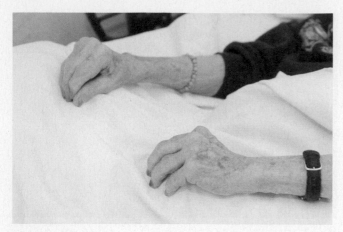

Figure 30-12 This person has rheumatoid arthritis in the joints of their hands.

the body's immune system begins to attack the body's own tissues. So, for example, in rheumatoid arthritis, the immune system attacks and destroys the cartilage that covers the ends of the bones. Scar tissue develops within the joints, causing them to become stiff and useless. For many months, a person's rheumatoid arthritis may seem to be under control, but then the person will experience an acute flare-up of the disease. During the acute phases of the disease, the person may experience pain, swelling, redness, and heat in the joints, as well as fever and general weakness. Bed rest may be necessary, and splints can help decrease joint deformity. New medications have been useful in helping to slow progression of rheumatoid arthritis. The gentle use of active and active–assistive range-of-motion exercises (discussed later in this chapter) helps to maintain joint mobility.

Gout

Gout is a type of arthritis that is caused by a disturbance in the body's metabolism. Uric acid is a waste product of metabolism that is usually eliminated from the body in the urine. If the body produces too much uric acid or the kidneys are unable to properly process the uric acid, the uric acid builds up in the body, forming crystals that are deposited within the joints. These uric acid crystals are extremely irritating to the tissues in the joint, and, as a result, the joint becomes inflamed and painful. While gout can affect any joint, the big toe is most commonly affected. Males past middle age are more commonly affected than females. Gout may be treated with a combination of diet modifications and medications.

Muscular Dystrophy

Muscular dystrophy is a general term for a group of disorders that cause the skeletal muscles to become progressively weaker over time. These disorders are inherited. The types of muscular dystrophy vary according to the muscles that are affected, the age of the person typically affected, and the rate at which the disease progresses. Some people with muscular dystrophy experience only moderate disability, whereas others may die from the disease.

Muscular dystrophy is a common reason why a younger person may become a resident of a long-term care facility. Duchenne muscular dystrophy, the most common form of muscular dystrophy, develops during childhood and usually causes death before the age of 30 years. As muscle weakness progresses and affects more of the person's body, the person becomes totally dependent on others for care. The person dies because the muscles that allow them to breathe eventually become too weak to perform this vital function.

The most common form of muscular dystrophy that begins in adulthood is myotonic muscular dystrophy. A person with myotonic muscular dystrophy has difficulty relaxing the muscles after contracting them, and the muscles may spasm. In addition, the person experiences weakness and shrinking of the muscle tissue. People with myotonic muscular dystrophy also often have heart problems, endocrine disorders, and cataracts (yellowing and hardening of the lens of the eye). A resident with muscular dystrophy will need your assistance with range-of-motion exercises, walking, positioning, and ADLs. Eventually, when the disease begins to affect the muscles that control swallowing, you will also have to help the person with eating.

Fractures

A **fracture** is a broken bone. Fractures are usually caused by trauma, such as a fall or a car accident. However, some fractures are caused when a bone is put under constant and repeated stress. For example, you may have heard of a distance runner being diagnosed with a "stress fracture" in the small bones of the foot. Think about how many times a runner's foot pounds against the pavement, and the force behind each step, and you will understand how a stress fracture can occur! Other fractures, called *pathologic fractures*, occur in bones that have been weakened by a disease process, such as osteoporosis or bone cancer.

Older people are especially at risk for fractures because the bones become more fragile with age. Older people are also more likely to have diseases that put them at risk for fractures, such as osteoporosis or bone cancer. Weak, brittle bones can fracture easily, often from a seemingly minor fall or stumble. For example, hip fractures are quite common in older females who have fallen just a short distance, such as from a standing position to the floor or sidewalk. Not only do the bones of an older person fracture more

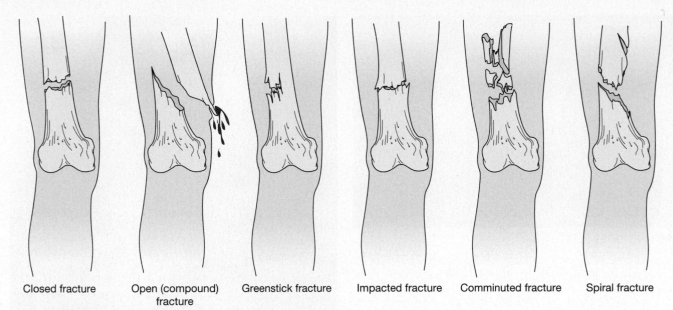

Closed fracture Open (compound) fracture Greenstick fracture   Impacted fracture Comminuted fracture Spiral fracture

Figure 30-13 There are many different types of fractures.

easily, they take longer to heal and they may heal improperly. Delayed or improper healing may cause prolonged difficulty with mobility.

Types of Fractures

Fractures can occur in almost any bone in the body and are classified in the following manner (Fig. 30-13):

- **Closed fracture.** The bone is broken, but the broken ends do not protrude through the overlying skin.
- **Open (compound) fracture.** The bone is broken, and the sharp ends of the broken bone have broken through the skin. Because the skin is broken, open fractures carry a very high risk of infection.
- **Greenstick fracture.** Have you ever tried to snap a young, green twig? Unlike a dry, brown stick, a green twig will bend and splinter, but it will not break all the way through. In a greenstick fracture, the same thing occurs—the bone bends and splinters, but it does not break all the way through. Greenstick fractures occur most commonly in children because their bones are still quite flexible.
- **Impacted fracture.** The bone is broken all of the way through, and the broken ends of the bone are jammed into each other. These fractures are often seen in people who have jumped or fallen from a height, for example, off of a roof or ladder.
- **Comminuted fracture.** The bone is splintered into several little pieces. This type of fracture is common when a bone has been crushed by a lot of force, such as what can occur during an

automobile accident. The surrounding tissues, such as muscle and skin, may be seriously injured as well.
- **Spiral fracture.** The break circles around the bone in a winding fashion. Spiral fractures are common when the bone has been subjected to a twisting force.

Treatments for Fractures

For a fractured bone to heal properly, the broken ends of the bone must be brought together (aligned) and then held in that position until the fracture heals.

Reduction and Fixation

Reduction is the word used to describe the process of bringing the broken ends of the bone into alignment. **Fixation** is the word used to describe the process of holding the bone in one position until the fracture heals. There are many ways to accomplish reduction and fixation. The method used depends on the type and location of the fracture.

In a *closed reduction*, the doctor lines up the broken ends of the bone by simply pushing or pulling them back into place. In a closed reduction, it is not necessary to create a surgical incision to access the broken bone. Following a closed reduction, a cast (made of fiberglass or plaster of Paris) or splint is applied to keep the bone in the proper alignment until healing occurs (Fig. 30-14A). First, a thin layer of cotton is placed on the skin to protect it. Then, the casting material is soaked in water and wrapped around the limb. As the casting material dries, it hardens, preventing movement of the broken bone. A cast is a method of *external fixation*, or fixation that is achieved without surgery.

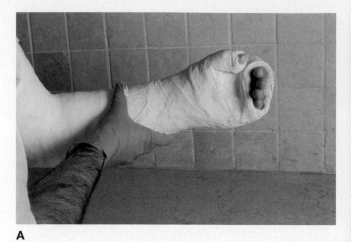

A

B

Figure 30-14 With any fracture, the broken ends of the bone need to be brought back together (reduction) and held in place (fixation). **A.** Fixation can be accomplished externally, with a cast, or **(B)** it can be accomplished internally, with devices such as plates, screws, pins, or wires. (*dnaveh\Shutterstock.com*)

General guidelines for caring for a person with a cast are given in Guidelines Box 30-1.

Sometimes it is necessary to surgically expose the bone to line up the broken ends of the bone. This is called an *open reduction*. Often, open reduction is followed by *internal fixation*. Internal fixation involves the use of metal plates, screws, rods, pins, or wires to hold the broken ends of the bone in place until the bone is healed (see Fig. 30-14B). You may see the notation "ORIF" on a person's chart. This means that the person has had surgery to achieve an "**O**pen **R**eduction, **I**nternal **F**ixation."

Traction

Some fractured bones cannot be repaired surgically for a period of time, especially if the person's overall medical condition is unstable. In these cases, traction is used to keep the broken ends of the bone in alignment until the fracture can be permanently repaired by surgery or casting. In **traction**, the ends of the bones are placed in the proper alignment and then weight is applied to exert a constant pull and keep the bone in alignment. In skin traction, weight is suspended from a traction unit that is attached to the person's skin (Fig. 30-15A). In skeletal traction, weight is suspended from pins that are driven through the bone (see Fig. 30-15B). A **trapeze bar** may be attached to

the overhead frame of the person's bed. The person grasps the trapeze bar to assist with movement.

A person in traction has several special care needs, many of which arise from the person's limited ability to move or change position:

- You may be asked to assist the person with range-of-motion exercises to work the unaffected joints and keep them limber.
- The person will have to use a fracture bedpan (see Chapter 25, Figure 25-2B), which is easier to slide under the buttocks.
- Pressure ulcers are always a concern, so it is important to keep the person's skin clean and dry, and to monitor for signs of skin breakdown.
- Two people usually work together to change the bed linens, and the linens are changed from the top of the bed (working down), instead of from side to side. If you need to do this, the nurse will show you how.

When you are working with a person who is in traction, be very careful not to disturb or remove the weights attached to the traction unit. When you lower the person's bed height, check to make sure the weights are not resting on the floor. They must hang freely to apply the correct amount of tension to the affected limb.

Guidelines Box 30-1 Guidelines for Caring for a Person With a Cast

WHAT YOU DO	WHY YOU DO IT
Do not cover the cast or place it on a plastic-covered pillow until it has dried completely.	The casting material produces heat as it dries. Covering the cast can cause the person's skin underneath the cast to burn.
Do not touch the cast with your fingertips until it is totally dry. If you must handle the cast, use the palms of your hands.	Touching the cast can cause it to dent, creating pressure spots against the person's skin.
Keep the casted body part elevated on a pillow for several days.	Elevating the casted body part helps prevent and reduce swelling around the fracture site.
Because the skin underneath the cast can start to itch, the person may try to slide an object between the cast and the skin to scratch the itchy area. Advise the person that placing objects inside of the cast should be avoided.	Sliding an object between the cast and the skin may injure the skin, which puts the person at risk for infection.
Make sure the person's toes (or fingers, if the cast is on the arm) are pink, warm, and moving. Report any complaints of increased pain, numbness, or tingling. Report any observations of cyanosis, increased swelling, cold toes or fingers, increased drainage on the cast, or a foul odor immediately.	Cyanosis; increased swelling; increased pain, numbness, or tingling; or cold fingers or toes may indicate that swelling inside the cast is interfering with blood flow. If the tissues do not receive enough oxygen and nutrients, tissue death and skin breakdown may occur. Increased drainage or a foul odor may indicate infection.
Keep the cast clean and dry.	Plaster cast material becomes soft again when it becomes wet.
Do not allow the person to place pressure or weight on the cast unless they have been specifically instructed to do so.	Placing too much pressure or weight on the cast can cause the cast to break.
Regularly inspect the condition of the cast and the skin around the edges of the cast.	A crack in the cast can cause the cast to become loose or break, which could delay healing of the bone. Rough edges on the cast can irritate or break the skin, putting the person at risk for infection and other problems.

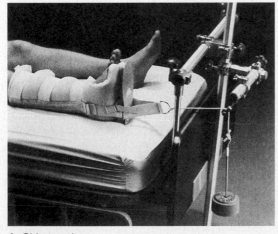

A. Skin traction

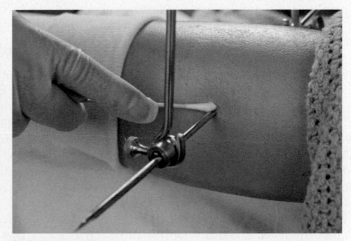

B. Skeletal traction

Figure 30-15 Traction is used to hold the broken ends of a bone in alignment until the fracture can be repaired permanently. **A.** In skin traction, a device is attached to the person's skin, and weight is suspended from it. **B.** In skeletal traction, pins are driven through the bone to support the weight.

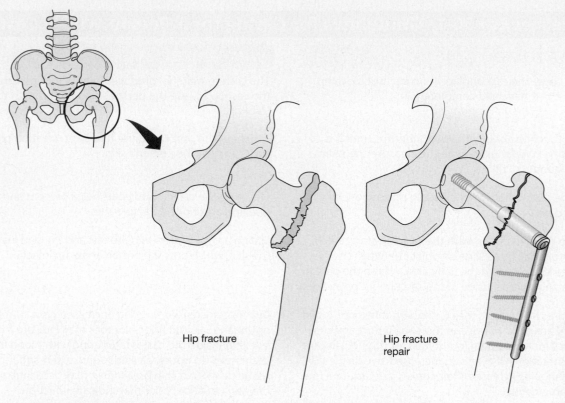

Figure 30-16 A hip fracture is a fracture that occurs at the top of the femur (the thigh bone). The fracture is often repaired using plates, pins, and screws.

Hip fracture

Hip fracture repair

Hip Fractures

As a nursing assistant, especially if you work in a long-term care facility, it is very likely that you will care for people who are recovering from hip fractures. A *hip fracture* is a fracture that occurs at the top of the femur (thigh bone) (Fig. 30-16). The two factors that put a person at high risk for a hip fracture are a tendency to fall and fragile bones (as a result of the normal aging process or a disease process, such as osteoporosis). For these reasons, hip fractures are common in older people, especially older females.

A significant number of older people die within a year of experiencing a hip fracture. In addition, a person who has experienced one hip fracture is at increased risk for falling and experiencing another fracture in the future. Most of the time, a fractured hip requires surgery. However, surgery may not be an option for an older person who is frail or has numerous medical problems. Even when surgical repair is possible, the person is still at risk for serious complications resulting from the immobility that occurs during and after treatment. Infection (either of the surgical wound or a pressure ulcer, if one develops) is also a concern.

Most hip fractures are surgically reduced and stabilized with the use of plates, screws, or pins. Some people may also require joint replacement with an artificial (prosthetic) joint. During the recovery period, the person will need extensive rehabilitation to help regain strength and mobility. A person who is recovering from a hip fracture will have very specific orders regarding mobility status. It is important for you to know what these orders are and to follow them closely. The person will most likely have limitations for positioning, mobility, and weight-bearing. As the person gains strength and mobility through rehabilitation, weight-bearing and mobility will gradually be increased.

Amputations

The removal of all or part of an arm or a leg is called an **amputation**. For example, a person may lose just a toe, or the leg from the knee down, or the entire leg. Accidents are a common cause of amputation. For example, the body part may be severed from the body during the accident. Or, the body part may be so seriously damaged during the accident that the only treatment option is to surgically remove it.

Amputation may also be necessary as a result of disease. For example, some types of cancer are treated by amputation of the affected limb. Diseases that interfere with blood flow to all or part of an extremity can also eventually result in the need for amputation. For example, as you learned in Chapter 23, people with diabetes tend to have circulatory problems, and often,

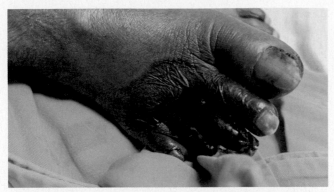

Figure 30-17 Impaired blood flow causes death of the tissues (gangrene). Once gangrene develops, the only treatment option may be amputation of the affected part. (*Casa nayafana\Shutterstock.com*)

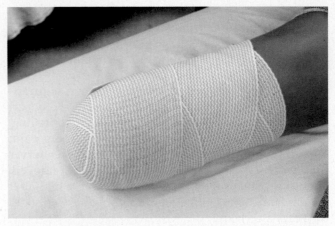

Figure 30-19 Wrapping the stump in bandages helps to shape it properly.

blood flow to their feet is poor. The poor blood flow to the feet is usually associated with poor sensation as well as an increased risk for infection. If a person with diabetes gets a foot infection, it may go unnoticed for a long time, and when it finally is noticed, it may be very difficult to treat. Eventually, death of the tissue (gangrene) occurs because the tissue is deprived of oxygen and nutrients (Fig. 30-17). Once gangrene develops, the only treatment option may be to remove the damaged part through amputation.

The loss of a body part, especially an arm or leg, is very emotionally traumatic for a person. The person's mobility, appearance, and sometimes even their ability to earn a living or enjoy a hobby they used to love can be affected by an amputation. For some people who have had a body part either partially or completely amputated, a prosthetic (false) part may allow the person to regain mobility, function, and a more normal appearance (Fig. 30-18).

For a prosthetic device to be fitted, the **stump**, or the end of the amputated limb that is left after surgery, must be cared for properly. Positioning is used to keep the muscles and tendons from shortening, and nearby joints are put through range-of-motion exercises to help maintain normal joint function and mobility. Wrapping the end of the stump with elastic bandages helps to shrink and shape the stump properly (Fig. 30-19). When assisting with caring for a person's stump, make sure to follow the nurse's or physical therapist's instructions exactly, as always. Finally, as you assist with the

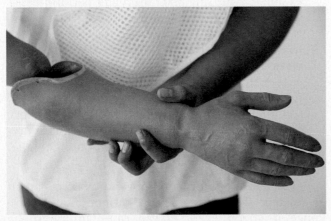

Figure 30-18 A person with a prosthetic arm is shown here. Many times, it is hard to tell a false limb from a real one when the prosthesis is being worn. A prosthetic body part can help a person who has had an amputation regain function and mobility. (*Gee363\Shutterstock.com*)

Tell the Nurse!

There are many signs and symptoms that may accompany disorders of the musculoskeletal system. As a nursing assistant, you have the opportunity to become very familiar with each of your patients' or residents' physical abilities and limitations. Report any of the following observations to the nurse immediately:

- The person has fallen
- An area has become swollen, red, bruised, tender, or painful to the touch
- The person complains of pain when moving a joint
- The person's usual range of motion of a joint has decreased
- The person limps or has pain while walking, or makes excuses to avoid walking
- The person guards or rubs a joint, even when not moving
- The person has decreased muscle strength

general care needs of your patient or resident, you will have numerous opportunities to observe the stump for any drainage, bleeding, or pain. These findings could be signs of poor tissue healing or infection and must be reported to the nurse immediately.

Many people experience what is known as **phantom pain**, or the feeling that the amputated body part is still present, after an amputation. Aching, itching, and other sensations are all types of phantom pain. The sensations are caused by the healing of the nerves that were cut when the body part was removed. Phantom pain usually goes away a short while after surgery, but some people report having these episodes for years afterward.

GENERAL CARE MEASURES

As a nursing assistant, you may be asked to assist a patient or resident with range-of-motion exercises, the application of heat or cold (Chapter 21), or physical therapy. These techniques are used to prevent complications of immobility, relieve musculoskeletal discomfort, and maintain or restore musculoskeletal function.

Range-of-Motion Exercises

As you learned earlier, the range of motion of a joint is the complete extent of movement that the joint is normally capable of without causing pain. Normal activities—such as dressing, grooming, walking, and eating—usually put all of our joints through their complete range of motion several times throughout the day. However, some of the people you will be caring for will have conditions that prevent them from doing the activities that would normally exercise their joints and muscles.

As you know from this chapter and previous ones, immobility can have a serious impact on the musculoskeletal system. Muscle atrophy, loss of bone strength, and stiffness of the joints can quickly lead to permanent muscle weakness, brittle bones, and even contractures (Fig. 30-20). As a nursing assistant, you will play a key role in preventing these complications by helping your patients or residents with range-of-motion exercises as ordered.

Range-of-motion exercises—movements that put each joint through its complete range of motion—are done to preserve joint and muscle function in a person who has limited use of their musculoskeletal system. It is very important that range-of-motion exercises be started as soon as possible. It has been shown that body changes can occur after only 3 days of immobility.

Range-of-motion exercises are usually performed at least twice a day, often along with other personal

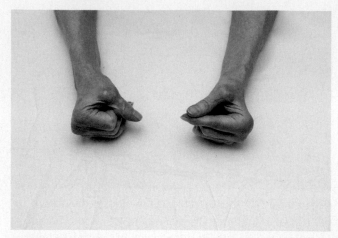

Figure 30-20 Contractures can occur when a joint is not exercised regularly. Use of the joint can be permanently lost. (*Gabdrakipova Dilyara\Shutterstock.com*)

care activities, such as bathing or dressing. The exercises can be done while the person is in bed or sitting down. Depending on the situation, range-of-motion exercises may be performed for only one, some, or all of the joints. Sometimes, the patient or resident will be able to perform the exercises on their own, and your role will be to provide guidance and encouragement. Other times, you will need to help the person to perform the exercises.

- In **active range-of-motion exercises,** the patient or resident performs the exercises independently, with verbal guidance from the nursing assistant or nurse.
- In **passive range-of-motion exercises,** the nursing assistant or nurse moves the patient's or resident's joints through the exercises, without active involvement on the part of the person. For example, a nursing assistant might perform passive range-of-motion exercises for a person who is unconscious.
- In **active–assistive range-of-motion exercises,** the patient or resident performs the exercises with some hands-on assistance from the nursing assistant or nurse. For example, a person may be able to lift their arm out to the side, but will need help from the nursing assistant or nurse to complete the movement of bringing the arm up near the head.

Procedure 30-1 explains how to assist a patient or resident with passive range-of-motion exercises. Range-of-motion exercises can cause injury to the joints if they are not performed properly. Usually a physical therapist or nurse will evaluate the person and determine which joints should be exercised. When assisting a person with range-of-motion exercises, always follow the care plan (or the nurse's or physical therapist's instructions) exactly. This is important for two reasons:

1. There may be some exercises that the person is not allowed to do.
2. The physical therapist or nurse will most likely change the care plan as the person's condition either improves or worsens.

In addition to checking the care plan, you should make sure that helping the person with the ordered exercises is within your scope of practice. For example, in some facilities, nursing assistants are not allowed to assist people with range-of-motion exercises involving the neck. General guidelines for assisting a person with range-of-motion exercises are given in Guidelines Box 30-2.

Guidelines Box 30-2   Guidelines for Assisting With Range-of-Motion Exercises

WHAT YOU DO	WHY YOU DO IT
Use good body mechanics.	Using good body mechanics saves energy and prevents muscle strain and injury.
Remove pillows and other positioning devices.	Pillows and positioning devices can prevent a person from achieving full range of motion of the joint.
Position the person so that each joint can be moved through all of the usual positions.	Positioning the person in a position that will allow each joint to be moved through all of its usual positions saves time (because the person will not have to be repositioned in between exercises) and helps to ensure that all of the exercises will be completed.
Move through the exercises in a systematic way (for example, from the head down).	Developing a routine helps to ensure that no exercise will be forgotten.
Unless instructed otherwise, perform the same exercise on each corresponding body part (for example, do the same thing for the right arm that you do for the left).	Exercising corresponding joints equally ensures that both sides of the body remain equally strong and flexible.
Support each joint as you exercise it.	Support reduces discomfort and strain on the joint.
Do not push a joint past its point of resistance.	Each joint has a limit to its range of motion. Attempting to exceed this limit can lead to joint pain and injury.
Watch the person's face for signs of pain or discomfort.	A person may not be able to tell you if what you are doing hurts. Therefore, it is important to watch the person's face for nonverbal cues, such as grimacing or wincing.
Avoid exercising a painful joint.	Exercising a painful joint can cause additional injury.
If you notice sudden, continuous contractions of the related muscles (spasticity), take a break or move the limb more slowly to allow the muscles to recover. Applying gentle pressure to the muscle can also relieve spasticity.	Spasticity is a sign that the muscles are working too hard. It may also indicate that the person is in pain, or that the joint's range of motion has been exceeded.
Expect the person's respiratory rate and heart rate to increase during the exercise. If these vital signs do not return to their normal resting rates after the activity ends, report this to the nurse immediately.	During activity, the tissues require more oxygen and nutrients, so the heart and lungs work harder to supply the tissues. However, once the activity ends, the heart rate and respiratory rate should return to normal because the tissues' demand for oxygen and nutrients will be less.
Encourage the person to help with the exercises as much as possible.	Active participation increases the person's sense of independence and improves function.

SUMMARY

- The musculoskeletal system consists of the bones, skeletal muscles, and joints.
  - The primary function of the musculoskeletal system is movement.
    - Joints are the areas where two bones meet. Most movement occurs at freely movable joints.
    - The skeletal muscles attach to the bones. When the muscle contracts, it pulls against the bone, causing the body part to move.
  - Other functions include protection, support, heat production, calcium storage, and blood cell production.
- As we age, we lose bone tissue and muscle mass, and our joints begin to show the effects. Consuming a diet rich in calcium, vitamin D, and protein and exercising regularly throughout life can help to delay or decrease the effects of aging.
- Disorders of the musculoskeletal system can make mobility very difficult.
  - Osteoporosis is the excessive loss of bone tissue, resulting in bones that break very easily.
  - Arthritis is inflammation of the joints.
    - Osteoarthritis typically affects older people. The cartilage that covers the ends of bones is worn away through normal use of the joint. Many people have joint replacement surgery to correct the condition.
    - Rheumatoid arthritis is a type of arthritis that affects younger people and can cause severe joint deformities. It is thought to be an autoimmune disorder.
    - Gout is a type of arthritis that results from the buildup of uric acid in the joints.
  - Muscular dystrophy is a general term for a group of disorders that cause the skeletal muscles to weaken over time. Muscular dystrophy is a genetic (inherited) disorder.
- Fractures are broken bones.
  - Older people are especially at risk for fractures because of the normal loss of bone tissue that is a part of aging. Fractures may take longer to heal in an older person.
  - Fractures may be treated by casting or by surgical placement of plates, screws, pins, or wires. Traction may be necessary to hold the ends of the broken bone in alignment.
  - Hip fractures are common in older people, especially older females.
- Amputation is the removal of a limb or part of a limb.
  - Amputation may be necessary because of trauma or complications related to a medical condition, such as diabetes.
  - Proper care of the stump increases the likelihood that a person can be fitted with a prosthetic limb.
- Range-of-motion exercises, the application of heat or cold, and rehabilitation measures prevent complications of immobility, relieve musculoskeletal discomfort, and maintain or restore musculoskeletal function.
  - Range-of-motion exercises preserve joint and muscle function in people who have limited use of the musculoskeletal system.
    - Active range-of-motion exercises are performed by the patient or resident.
    - Passive range-of-motion exercises are performed by the nursing assistant or nurse on behalf of the patient or resident.
    - Active–assistive range-of-motion exercises are performed by the patient or resident with some help from the nursing assistant or nurse.

> **Procedure 30-1**

Assisting a Person With Passive Range-of-Motion Exercises

WHY YOU DO IT Range-of-motion exercises help to keep the joints and muscles healthy in people who have a limited ability to move.

Getting Ready WEAVERS

1. Complete the "Getting Ready" steps.

Supplies

- bath blanket

Procedure

2. Make sure that the bed is positioned at a comfortable working height (to promote good body mechanics) and that the wheels are locked. If the side rails are in use, lower the side rail on the working side of the bed. The side rail on the opposite side of the bed should remain up. Raise or lower the head of the bed to a horizontal or semi-Fowler's position.

3. Assist the person into the supine position.

4. Spread the bath blanket over the top linens (and the person). If the person is able, have them hold the bath blanket. If not, tuck the corners under the shoulders. Fanfold the top linens to the foot of the bed.

5. Perform each range-of-motion exercise in steps 6 through 13 according to the person's care plan, being careful to expose only the part of the body that is being exercised. Repeat each exercise three to five times as written in the care plan.

6. If your facility permits, exercise the person's neck:

   a. **Forward and backward flexion and extension (neck).** Support the person's head by putting one hand under the chin and the other on the back of the head. Gently bring the head forward, as if to touch the chin to the chest, and then bring it backward, chin pointing to the sky.

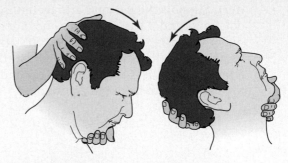

STEP 6a Gently bring the head forward, then backward.

   b. **Side-to-side flexion (neck).** Support the person's head by putting one hand under the chin and the other near the opposite temple. Gently tilt the head toward the right shoulder and then toward the left.

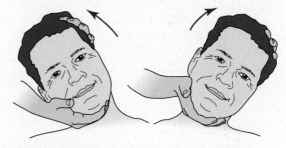

STEP 6b Gently tilt the head toward the right shoulder, then the left.

   c. **Rotation (neck).** Support the person's head by putting one hand under the chin and the other on the back of the head. Gently move the head from side to side, as if the person were shaking their head "no."

(continued)

577

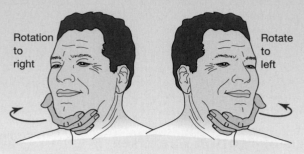

STEP 6c Gently move the head from side to side.

7. Exercise the person's shoulder:

   a. **Forward flexion and extension (shoulder).** Support the person's arm by putting one hand under the elbow and the other under the wrist. Keeping the person's arm straight with the palm facing down, lift the arm up so that it is alongside the ear and then return it to its original position.

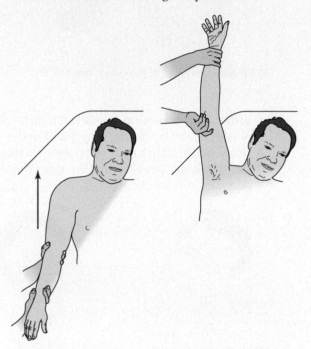

STEP 7a Lift the arm up so that it is alongside the person's ear, then return it to its original position.

   b. **Abduction and adduction (shoulder).** Support the person's arm by putting one hand under the elbow and the other under the wrist. Keeping the person's arm straight with the palm facing up, move the arm away from the side of the body and then return it to its original position.

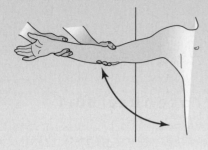

STEP 7b Move the arm away from the person's side, then return it to its original position.

   c. **Horizontal abduction and adduction (shoulder).** Support the person's arm by putting one hand under the elbow and the other under the wrist. Keeping the person's arm straight with the palm facing up, move the arm away from the side of the body. Gently bending the person's elbow, touch the hand to the opposite shoulder, then straighten the elbow and bring the arm back out to the side.

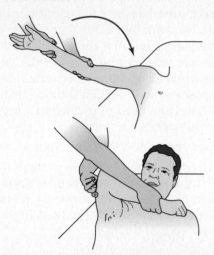

STEP 7c Move the arm away from the person's side, then touch the person's hand to the opposite shoulder.

   d. **Rotation (shoulder).** Support the person's arm by putting one hand under the elbow and the other under the wrist. Move the person's arm away from the side of the body and bend the arm at the elbow. Gently move the person's forearm up so that it forms a right angle with the mattress and then back down. This movement is similar to the motion a police officer makes when they are signaling someone to stop.

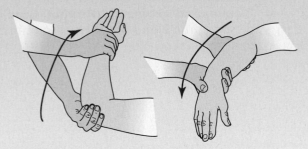

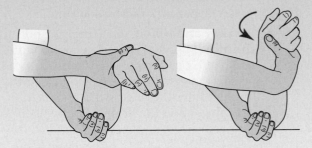

STEP 7d Move the person's forearm up, then back down.

8. Exercise the person's elbow.

   a. **Flexion and extension (elbow).** Support the person's arm by putting one hand under the elbow and the other under the wrist. Starting with the person's arm straight and with the palm facing up, bend the elbow so that the hand moves toward the shoulder. Then, straighten out the elbow, returning the person's hand to its original position.

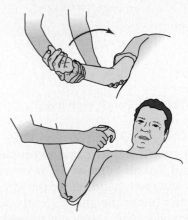

STEP 8a Bend the arm so that the hand moves toward the shoulder, then return it to its original position.

   b. **Pronation and supination (elbow).** Support the person's arm by putting one hand under the elbow and the other under the wrist. Move the person's arm away from the side of the body and slightly bend the arm at the elbow. Gently move the person's forearm up so that it forms a right angle with the mattress. Gently turn the person's hand so that the palm is facing the end of the bed. Then turn the hand the other way so that the palm is facing the head of the bed.

STEP 8b Turn the hand so that the palm is facing the end of the bed, then turn the hand the other way so that the palm is facing the head of the bed.

9. Exercise the person's wrist.

   a. **Flexion and extension (wrist).** Support the person's wrist with one hand. Use the other hand to gently bend the person's hand down and then back.

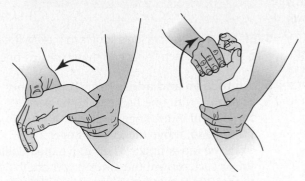

STEP 9a Gently bend the person's hand down, then back.

   b. **Radial and ulnar flexion (wrist).** Support the person's wrist with one hand. Use the other hand to gently turn the person's hand toward the thumb. Then turn the hand the other way toward the little finger.

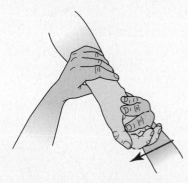

STEP 9b Gently turn the person's hand one way, then the other.

(continued)

10. Exercise the person's fingers and thumb.

   a. **Flexion and extension (fingers and thumb).** Support the person's wrist with one hand. Using your other hand, flex the person's fingers to make a fist, tucking the thumb under the fingers. Then straighten each finger and the thumb one by one.

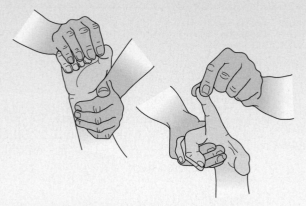

STEP 10a Flex the person's fingers to make a fist, then straighten each finger and thumb one by one.

   b. **Abduction and adduction (fingers and thumb).** With one hand, hold the person's thumb and index finger together. With the other hand, move the middle finger away from the index finger. Then move the middle finger back toward the index finger and hold the middle finger, index finger, and thumb together. Next, move the ring finger away from the other two fingers and thumb, then move it back toward the group. Do the same with the little finger. Finally, reverse the process. Hold the little finger and the ring finger together and move the middle finger away and back. Complete with the index finger and thumb.

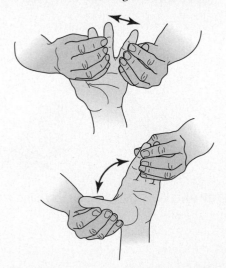

STEP 10b Spread the fingers away from each other, then back together again.

   c. **Flexion and extension (thumb).** Bend the person's thumb into the palm, then return it to its original position.

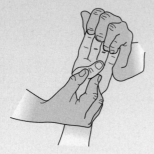

STEP 10c Bend the thumb into the palm, then return it to its original position.

   d. **Opposition.** Touch each fingertip to the thumb.

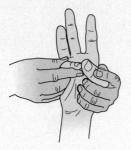

STEP 10d Touch each fingertip to the thumb.

11. Exercise the person's hip and knee.

   a. **Forward flexion and extension (hip and knee).** Support the person's leg by putting one hand under the knee and the other under the ankle. Gently bend the person's knee, moving it toward the head. Then straighten the person's knee and gently lower the leg to the bed.

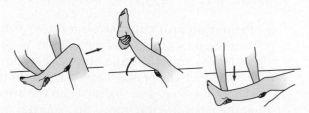

STEP 11a Gently bend the knee, moving it toward the head. Then straighten the leg and lower it to the bed.

b. Abduction and adduction (hip). Support the person's leg by putting one hand under the knee and the other under the ankle. Keeping the person's leg straight, move the leg away from the side of the body and then return it to its original position.

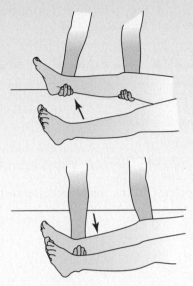

STEP 11b Move the leg away from the person's side, then return it to its original position.

c. Rotation (hip). Support the person's leg by putting one hand under the knee and the other under the ankle. Keeping the person's leg straight, gently turn the leg inward and then outward.

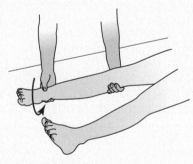

STEP 11c Gently turn the leg inward, then outward.

12. Exercise the person's ankle and foot.

a. Dorsiflexion and plantar flexion (ankle and foot). Support the person's ankle with one hand. Use the other hand to gently bend the person's foot up toward the head and then back.

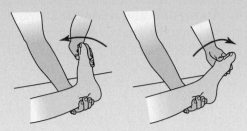

STEP 12a Gently bend the foot toward the head, then back.

b. Inversion and eversion (ankle and foot). Support the person's ankle with one hand. Use the other hand to gently turn the inside of the foot inward and then outward.

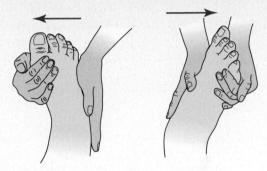

STEP 12b Gently bend the foot inward, then outward.

13. Exercise the person's toes.

a. Flexion and extension (toes). Put one hand under the person's foot. Put the other hand over the person's toes. Curl the toes downward and then straighten them.

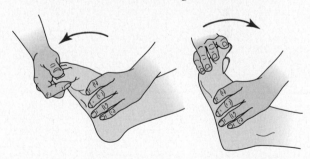

STEP 13a Curl the toes downward, then straighten them.

(continued)

b. Abduction and adduction (toes). Spread each toe the same way you spread each finger in step 10b.

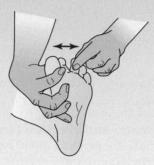

STEP 13b Spread the toes away from each other, then back together again.

14. Straighten the bed linens and make sure the person is comfortable and in good body alignment. Draw the top linens over the person and remove the bath blanket.

15. If the side rails are in use, raise the side rail on the working side of the bed. Make sure that the bed is lowered to its lowest position and that the wheels are locked.

Finishing Up

16. Complete the "Finishing Up" steps.

What You Document

- Date and time
- Body parts exercised
- Complaints of pain
- Any decrease in the person's usual range of motion

WHAT DID YOU LEARN?

Multiple Choice

Select the single best answer for each of the following questions.

1. When a muscle atrophies, it:
   a. Becomes larger and stronger
   b. Becomes thinner and weaker
   c. Becomes stiffer
   d. Becomes more flexible

2. Which musculoskeletal disorder causes severe joint deformities and often affects younger people?
   a. Osteoarthritis
   b. Rheumatoid arthritis
   c. Multiple sclerosis
   d. Muscular dystrophy

3. What is the term for a fracture where the broken ends of the bone do not penetrate the skin?
   a. Impacted fracture
   b. Comminuted fracture
   c. Spiral fracture
   d. Closed fracture

4. Excessive loss of bone tissue is:
   a. Osteoarthritis
   b. Osteoporosis
   c. A normal effect of aging
   d. Gout

5. What does the skeletal system do?
   a. It acts as a storage site for calcium.
   b. It works with the muscles to produce movement.
   c. It produces blood cells.
   d. All of the above.

6. Ms. Chen broke her leg while skiing. Surgery is required to align the broken bone, and then the bone fragments are held together with metal plates and screws. What is the name of the procedure Ms. Chen has had?
   a. Open fracture, internal fixation
   b. Open reduction, internal fixation
   c. Open reduction, external fixation
   d. Traction

7. What does the muscular system do?
   a. It produces heat.
   b. It helps to maintain posture.
   c. It works with bones to produce movement.
   d. All of the above.

8. Mr. Owen has severe osteoarthritis in his hips. You are caring for Mr. Owen following his hip replacement surgery. What do you need to remember?
   a. Mr. Owen's legs must always be kept together (adducted).
   b. When assisting Mr. Owen with range-of-motion exercises, make sure to flex the hips beyond 90 degrees to maintain flexibility in the joint.
   c. Mr. Owen should use an abduction pillow to keep his legs spread apart when he is in a supine or lateral position.
   d. Mr. Owen should be encouraged to learn to rely on a wheelchair because walking will be too difficult.

9. Ms. Curtis has just had a cast put on her leg following a horseback riding accident. What should you remember when you are helping Ms. Curtis?
   a. Ms. Curtis's leg should not be elevated.
   b. You should check Ms. Curtis's toes frequently to make sure that the cast is not too tight.
   c. Ms. Curtis should be reminded that if the skin underneath the cast begins to itch, she can slide a tongue depressor inside the cast to scratch the itchy area.
   d. Ms. Curtis should be encouraged to get out of bed and take a shower as soon as the cast dries.

10. Mr. Tanaka has poorly controlled diabetes. He injured his toe, resulting in a severe infection. Now his toes are completely black as a result of gangrene. What is the most likely treatment for Mr. Tanaka's toe?
   a. Open reduction, internal fixation (ORIF)
   b. Amputation of the toe
   c. Casting of the foot
   d. Application of heat

Matching *Match each numbered item with its appropriate lettered description.*

_____ **1.** Flexion/extension

_____ **2.** Supination/pronation

_____ **3.** Dorsiflexion/plantar flexion

_____ **4.** Rotation

_____ **5.** Abduction/adduction

_____ **6.** Inversion/eversion

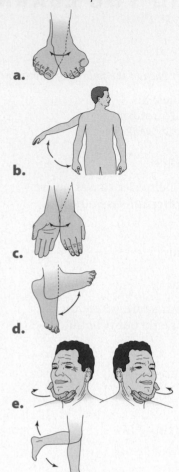

a.

b.

c.

d.

e.

f.

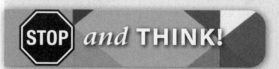

STOP *and* **THINK!**

■ You are assigned to care for Mr. Serrano. Mr. Serrano is 85 years old and fairly healthy, but he does have arthritis. One of your responsibilities is to assist Mr. Serrano to the dining room for meals. Today, while you are walking Mr. Serrano to breakfast, you notice that he is limping a bit and trying not to put weight on his left leg. You ask him if he is in pain, and he says, "I'm fine; it's just old age." What should you do?

■ You are caring for Mrs. Lasorda, who has crippling rheumatoid arthritis. She has many "good" days when she is able to manage her personal care and get around pretty well. This week, however, she is having a severe flare-up of her illness. What are some measures that you may be asked to do to help Mrs. Lasorda be more comfortable and prevent the loss of joint mobility?

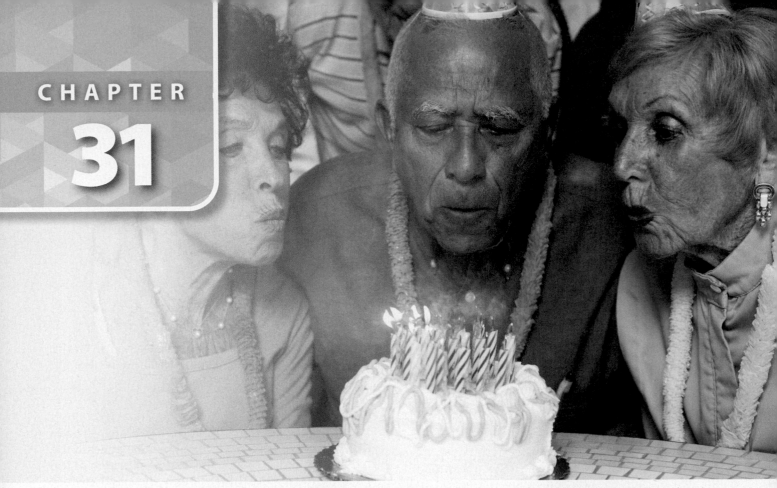

Photo: A resident of a retirement community celebrates his birthday by blowing out the candles on his cake. Regular physical exercise and avoidance of tobacco smoke and other pollutants help to keep the respiratory system functioning well into old age. (Blend Images\Shutterstock.com)

The Respiratory System

 WHAT WILL YOU LEARN?

Have you ever heard the phrase, "It's as natural as breathing?" Breathing is certainly something that many of us take for granted because we don't have to think about it. Air enters and leaves our lungs without any conscious effort on our part. With each breath, life-giving oxygen is delivered to the body, and carbon dioxide, a waste product of cellular metabolism, is removed from the body. Breathing is the function of the respiratory system, the subject of this chapter. When you are finished with this chapter, you will be able to:

1. List and describe the main parts of the respiratory system.
2. Discuss the main functions of the respiratory system.
3. Describe how normal aging processes affect the respiratory system.
4. Describe some of the disorders that can affect the respiratory system.
5. Describe how oxygen therapy is used to assist a person with respiration.
6. Describe the guidelines that a nursing assistant should follow when caring for patients or residents receiving oxygen therapy.
7. Discuss other methods used to help a person who is having trouble with respiration.

Vocabulary

Mucous membrane	Bronchioles	Asthma	Facemask
Mucus	Alveoli (alveolus)	Chronic obstructive	Nasopharyngeal airway
Nasal cavity	Gas exchange	pulmonary disease	Oropharyngeal airway
Pharyngitis	Pleura	(COPD)	Mechanical ventilation
Pharynx	Diaphragm	Emphysema	Endotracheal tube
Larynx	Pneumonia	Chronic bronchitis	Tracheostomy
Laryngitis	Sputum	Pneumothorax	Suctioning
Trachea	Hemoptysis	Hemothorax	Hypoxic
Bronchi (bronchus)	Pleurisy	Respiratory therapy	
Lungs	Bronchitis	Flow meter	
Respiration	Influenza	Nasal cannula	

STRUCTURE OF THE RESPIRATORY SYSTEM

The respiratory system consists of the lungs and a series of passages, collectively referred to as the *airway* (Fig. 31-1). You may hear people refer to the "upper respiratory tract" and the "lower respiratory tract." The upper respiratory tract consists of the structures located outside of the chest cavity (the nasal cavity, pharynx, and larynx). The lower respiratory tract consists of the structures located inside the chest cavity (the trachea, bronchi, bronchioles, and lungs).

Airway

The purpose of the airway is to move air from the outside of the body to the lungs, and from the lungs to the outside of the body. The airway consists of a series of passages that become smaller in diameter as they approach the lungs. These passages are lined with a **mucous membrane**, a sheet of epithelial tissue that is supported by an underlying layer of connective tissue. These flexible, moist membranes line many of the tubes and cavities in the body. The surface of the membrane is kept moist by **mucus**, a slippery, sticky substance that is secreted by special cells.

Nasal Cavity

Air enters the body through the nostrils and passes into the **nasal cavity**, which is lined by a mucous membrane and coarse hairs. The coarse hairs and the mucous membrane help to trap dirt, dust, microbes, and other foreign particles, preventing these substances from entering the delicate lungs. The plentiful blood vessels in the mucous membrane transfer body heat to the air, warming it up to a comfortable temperature. In addition, the air picks up some of the

moisture from the warm, moist nasal cavity. Warm, moist air is less likely than cold, dry air to damage the delicate lung tissue.

Pharynx

When you have a "sore throat," the part of your body that hurts is your pharynx. (You may have heard the term **pharyngitis**, which means inflammation of the pharynx, or a sore throat.) Both the nasal cavities and the oral cavity open into the **pharynx**, or throat region (see Fig. 31-1). This means that air passes through the pharynx on its way to the lungs, and food and fluids pass through the pharynx on their way to the stomach. This sharing of space is convenient when you have a stuffy nose because it means that you have another way to get air into your body (that is, through your mouth). However, this sharing of space can also lead to complications, such as choking, which occurs when you try to breathe and swallow at the same time. The pharynx is divided into three sections: the nasopharynx (located right behind the nasal cavities), the oropharynx (located behind the mouth), and the laryngeal pharynx (located above the larynx).

Larynx

From the pharynx, air passes into the **larynx**. The opening of the larynx is covered by a flap of cartilage called the epiglottis, which shuts when you swallow, closing off the opening and preventing food from passing into the lower respiratory tract.

In addition to serving as part of the airway, the larynx is the organ responsible for speech. The larynx, often referred to as the "voice box," contains the vocal cords. When air flows over the vocal cords, it causes them to vibrate, producing sound. Humans and other animals make recognizable sounds by controlling the flow of air over the vocal cords. An inflammation of

Figure 31-1 The respiratory system consists of the lungs and a series of passages collectively referred to as the "airway." The structures that form the airway include the nasal cavity, pharynx, larynx, trachea, bronchi, and bronchioles. Disorders of the respiratory tract are often said to affect either the "upper respiratory tract" or the "lower respiratory tract." The upper respiratory tract consists of those structures located outside the chest cavity, while the lower respiratory tract consists of those structures located inside the chest cavity.

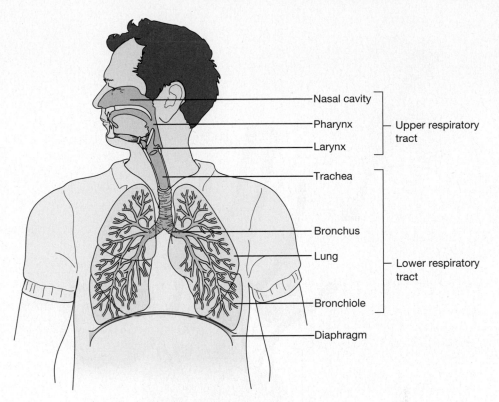

Nasal cavity
Pharynx — Upper respiratory tract
Larynx

Trachea

Bronchus

Lung — Lower respiratory tract

Bronchiole

Diaphragm

the larynx, or **laryngitis**, usually affects a person's ability to talk.

Trachea and Bronchi

The **trachea**, also called the "windpipe," is the passage that carries air from the larynx down into the chest toward the lungs. "C"-shaped rings of cartilage give the trachea its characteristic ridged appearance (see Fig. 31-1). These cartilage rings support the trachea and keep it open. At its lower end, the trachea divides into two separate passages called the **bronchi** (singular, **bronchus**). One bronchus goes to the right lung and the other goes to the left lung.

The mucous membrane lining of the trachea and bronchi contains millions of tiny hair-like structures called *cilia*. The cilia constantly move in a waving or beating fashion, moving mucus upward toward the pharynx so that it can be coughed up and removed from the respiratory tract along with any trapped particles or microbes.

Lungs

The **lungs** are the main organs of **respiration**, the process the body uses to obtain oxygen from the environment and remove carbon dioxide from the body. Once inside the lungs, the bronchi divide into smaller and smaller branches called **bronchioles** (Fig. 31-2). There are more than a million bronchioles in each

lung! At the end of each bronchiole, there is a grape-like cluster of tiny air sacs called **alveoli** (singular, **alveolus**). Each alveolus is surrounded by a network of tiny blood vessels (Fig. 31-3). The transfer of oxygen into the blood, and carbon dioxide out of it, occurs in

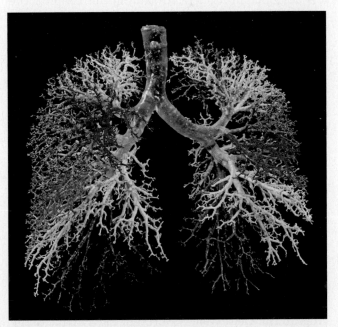

Figure 31-2 A resin cast of human lungs clearly shows the trachea, bronchi, and bronchioles. (*Ralph T. Hutchings\Science Source.*)

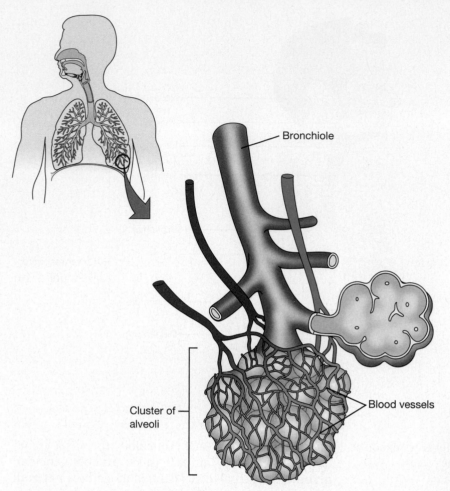

Bronchiole

Cluster of alveoli

Blood vessels

Figure 31-3 A cluster of air sacs, called alveoli, is found at the end of each bronchiole. The alveoli are surrounded by tiny blood vessels, which make gas exchange between the blood and the lungs possible.

the alveoli. This process is called **gas exchange**, and it is described in more detail later in this chapter. The tissue of healthy lungs is elastic (stretchy) and sponge-like because of all of the air-filled alveoli. The many blood vessels that surround the alveoli give healthy lung tissue its brilliant pink color.

The lungs are divided into sections called lobes. The right lung has three lobes and the left lung has only two. The left lung is slightly smaller than the right lung because of the position of the heart in the chest cavity.

The lungs are located in the chest cavity. The inside of the chest cavity is lined with a membrane called the **pleura**. A second layer of the pleura covers the outside of the lungs. The space between the two pleural layers is called the *pleural space*. A very thin layer of fluid normally fills this space. Try putting a wet glass on a table to better understand the purpose of this fluid. The glass sticks to the table, but you can slide it around. In a similar way, the pleural fluid keeps the two pleural layers together, anchoring the lungs to the chest wall. As a result, movements of the chest wall change the volume of the lungs during the process of breathing, and the lungs can slide against the chest wall.

FUNCTION OF THE RESPIRATORY SYSTEM

The main purpose of the respiratory system is respiration. Respiration is accomplished through the processes of ventilation and gas exchange.

Ventilation

Ventilation is the mechanical process of moving air in and out of the lungs (breathing). Ventilation has two phases: inhalation and exhalation. The **diaphragm** is a strong, dome-shaped muscle that separates the chest cavity from the abdominal cavity (see Fig. 31-1). When we inhale, the diaphragm contracts, moving downward and making the chest cavity bigger. Air flows into the lungs, filling the alveoli. When we exhale, the diaphragm relaxes, moving upward and pushing the air in the alveoli out of the lungs. Another group of muscles, called the intercostal muscles, helps with the respiratory effort as well by expanding the size of the chest cavity. The intercostal muscles are located between the ribs.

The rate and depth of breathing is controlled mainly by the central nervous system, in the part of the brain called the medulla. Special cells, called chemoreceptors, are located in the medulla and in some of the major arteries. If you are more active, your cells need more oxygen and produce more carbon dioxide. The chemoreceptors monitor the amount of carbon dioxide and, to a lesser extent, oxygen in the blood, and adjust the rate and depth of breathing as necessary. For example, if you are resting quietly, your body does not need to produce much carbon dioxide (or need much oxygen) and the amount of air inhaled and exhaled is minimal. But, if you are exercising, your body produces much more carbon dioxide (and needs much more oxygen), and ventilation increases as well. Although the brain ensures that breathing occurs automatically, the individual also has some control over breathing (for example, when you hold your breath while swimming).

Gas Exchange

So, we now know how air moves in and out of the lungs. But just moving air in and out of the lungs is not enough. How does oxygen get from the air into the blood? How does the carbon dioxide in the blood get into the air we exhale? This is where the second phase of respiration—gas exchange—comes into play.

Gas exchange occurs in the alveoli (Fig. 31-4). The walls of the alveoli are very thin—just one cell thick. Each alveolus is surrounded by a network of tiny blood vessels. The walls of the blood vessels are very thin too. As the blood passes through the blood vessels, it is brought very close to the air in the alveolus.

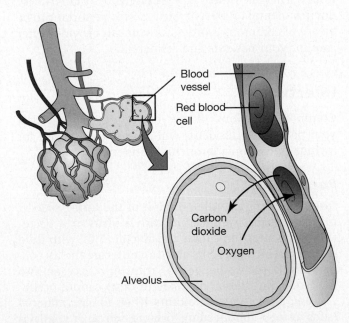

Figure 31-4 Gas exchange occurs in the alveoli. Oxygen moves from the alveolus into the blood vessel, and carbon dioxide moves from the blood vessel into the alveolus.

Because the concentration of oxygen is greater in the air than it is in the blood, the oxygen in the air moves (diffuses) across the wall of the alveolus into the blood vessel, oxygenating the blood. At the same time, carbon dioxide moves from the blood (where it is more concentrated) into the alveolus and is removed from the body when we exhale.

THE EFFECTS OF AGING ON THE RESPIRATORY SYSTEM

There is a good chance that many of the older people you will care for will have some type of respiratory problem. When the processes of aging are combined with chronic illness, immobility, or a lifetime of exposure to toxic chemicals (such as those in pollution and tobacco smoke), the respiratory system's ability to function properly is significantly reduced. For example, many people who are in their 60s, 70s, and 80s today began to smoke before anyone really knew the harmful effects. In addition, many older people worked before regulations such as those resulting from the Occupational Safety and Health Act were in place to keep them safe on the job. As a result, many were exposed to substances in the workplace that we now know are very harmful to the lungs, such as asbestos and coal dust. Due to these factors, respiratory disease is a leading cause of disability and of death in people over the age of 70.

When we inhale toxic substances (such as those in tobacco smoke and polluted air) day after day, the delicate membranes inside the lungs and airways become inflamed and stay that way. The chronic inflammation leads to scarring and may even cause changes that lead to cancer. In addition, chemicals in tobacco smoke paralyze the tiny cilia that line the trachea and bronchi. Recall that the purpose of the cilia is to sweep mucus upward, toward the pharynx, so that it can be eliminated from the respiratory tract. When the cilia are no longer able to perform this function because they have been paralyzed by tobacco smoke, the person must work harder to keep the airway and lungs clear of mucus. These attempts to keep the airway clear are what many of us know as a "smoker's cough." Fortunately, if a person is able to stop smoking, the cilia do regain their function and the tissues of the lungs will heal if the damage is not too severe.

Regular physical exercise and avoidance of tobacco smoke and other pollutants help to keep the respiratory system functioning properly well into old age (Fig. 31-5). However, as a person ages, there are three changes that are likely to occur to the respiratory system, even if the person is otherwise healthy. These changes include less efficient ventilation, decreased

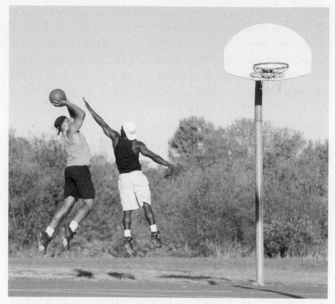

Figure 31-5 Exercise, especially when combined with avoidance of smoking and exposure to pollution, is a most effective way of keeping the respiratory system healthy for many years.

cough reflex, and an increased risk for respiratory tract infections.

Less Efficient Ventilation

As you have learned in other chapters, loss of tissue elasticity and loss of muscle mass occur as a person ages. In the respiratory system, these changes result in less efficient ventilation. The very elastic lung tissue loses some of its ability to expand and bounce back as a person breathes, which reduces the amount of air that is taken in and let out with each breath. The diaphragm and intercostal muscles become weaker, which means that the chest cavity may not expand as much with each breath, so the amount of air taken in will be smaller.

In healthy older people who do not smoke, these changes may not cause any problems. Often, the person will not be aware of any change, except possibly during exercise, when oxygen demands are significantly increased.

Decreased Cough Reflex

The cough reflex helps us to keep the airway clear of secretions. With age, the cough reflex decreases, affecting the older person's ability to keep the airway clear. As a result, the person may have a harder time eliminating microbes and secretions from the respiratory tract, putting the person at increased risk for respiratory tract infections and for choking on food or saliva.

Increased Risk of Respiratory Infections

The immune system becomes less efficient as a result of the aging process. This change in the immune system, combined with age-related changes to the respiratory system, makes older people more likely to get infections of the respiratory tract. In addition, a respiratory tract infection is likely to be more severe in an older person than it would be in a younger person. For example, what would have been a mild respiratory infection in a younger person can easily become a life-threatening respiratory infection in an older person.

Immobility also puts the older adult at higher risk for developing a severe respiratory infection. Many older people are less active because of changes in other body systems or because of chronic illness. In physically active people, the lungs are "exercised" along with the body, as they fully expand to meet the person's increased oxygen needs during exercise. But in a person who is confined to bed or a chair, the lungs do not get this "workout." A person who has become weak as a result of immobility may not be able to cough forcefully enough to clear the lungs of secretions. This can lead to the development of pneumonia, a serious lung infection.

DISORDERS OF THE RESPIRATORY SYSTEM

There is a wide range of disorders of the respiratory system. Some are caused by bacterial or viral infections, whereas others are strongly associated with environmental or lifestyle factors. It is important to be aware of common disorders so you can provide better care for your patients and residents.

Infections

Common infections of the respiratory system that your patients or residents will be at increased risk for include pneumonia, bronchitis, and influenza.

Pneumonia

Pneumonia is an inflammation of the lung tissue. It may be caused by infection with a virus or a bacterium. The infection causes the alveoli to fill with fluid and pus, which prevents air from entering the alveoli. As a result, gas exchange (the transfer of oxygen into the blood and carbon dioxide out of it) cannot occur.

Aspiration pneumonia occurs when foreign material (such as food, tube-feeding formula, saliva, or vomit) is inhaled into the lungs. The foreign material can damage the lung tissue, causing the alveoli to fill with fluid. The foreign material can also carry bacteria into the lungs, leading to bacterial pneumonia. Patients and residents who are receiving enteral nutrition (tube feedings) or who are unconscious are at increased risk for developing aspiration pneumonia because they are unable to protect their airway (by coughing or gagging).

Signs and symptoms of pneumonia include fever, pain when breathing, cyanosis (bluish skin as a result of decreased oxygen levels in the blood), and a productive cough. A productive cough is one in which a person coughs up sputum. **Sputum**, which is also known as "phlegm," consists of mucus and other respiratory secretions that are coughed up from the lungs, bronchi, and trachea. **Hemoptysis** is the coughing up of blood or blood-stained sputum (*heme-* means "blood," and *-ptysis* means "to spit"). Hemoptysis may be seen in pneumonia and can also occur with other respiratory disorders. In an older person, pneumonia may cause a fairly sudden change in mental status or delirium (see Chapter 9). The decreased oxygen levels in the blood impact the brain's ability to function and may result in increased confusion, behavioral changes, or both.

A vaccine is available to help prevent certain types of pneumonia and recommended for people 65 years or older.

Pneumonia is usually diagnosed with a chest x-ray and treated with antibiotics. Knowledge about which microbe is causing the pneumonia will allow the doctor to prescribe the most effective antibiotic therapy. You may be asked to assist by collecting a sputum specimen for analysis. Guidelines for collecting sputum specimens are given in Guidelines Box 31-1.

Pleurisy is an inflammation of the pleura, the membrane that lines the chest cavity and covers the lungs. Pleurisy often accompanies lower respiratory tract infections such as pneumonia. The inflammation of the pleura causes pain during breathing as the layers of the membrane rub against each other when the lungs expand and relax. Fluid may also collect in the pleural space between the chest wall and the lung. This build-up of fluid makes it difficult to breathe. The doctor may need to insert a needle into the chest cavity to drain the fluid.

Guidelines Box 31-1   Guidelines for Collecting a Sputum Specimen

WHAT YOU DO	WHY YOU DO IT
Explain to the person that the sputum for the specimen should be coughed up from deep down in the respiratory tract.	The sputum for analysis must come from the lungs because that is where most of the infection-causing microbes are located. Explaining this to the person helps to ensure that they produce a specimen that will result in an accurate diagnosis. If you do not explain this to the person, they may just cough up saliva, which will not result in an accurate diagnosis.
Provide privacy.	Having to spit mucus into a cup can be embarrassing and unpleasant for some people.
Have the person rinse their mouth with water before coughing up the specimen.	Rinsing with plain water helps to remove microbes that are normally present in the mouth, resulting in a "cleaner" specimen.
Do not have the person rinse with mouthwash before coughing up the specimen.	The antiseptic effects of the mouthwash might actually kill the microbes in the sputum specimen that are responsible for the infection, which will result in inaccurate test results.
Have the person spit the specimen directly into a sterile specimen container and close the lid.	Having the person spit directly into the sterile specimen container reduces the risk of contaminating the specimen and results in more accurate test results.
Make sure that the specimen container is labeled properly and that the information is correct.	Labeling errors can result in misdiagnosis or the need to repeat the test.
Take the specimen container to the laboratory immediately after collecting the specimen or ask the nurse how to store it.	Allowing a specimen to sit around or storing it the incorrect way can result in the need to repeat the test.

Bronchitis

Bronchitis is an inflammation of the bronchi. Like pneumonia, bronchitis can be caused by a viral or bacterial infection. Bronchitis may cause a dry, nonproductive cough that sounds like a "bark." But bronchitis can also cause a productive cough. Bacterial bronchitis is usually treated with antibiotics. Both bacterial and viral bronchitis can turn into pneumonia if the bronchial infection is not treated promptly.

Respiratory Viruses

Influenza, commonly referred to as the "flu," is an acute respiratory infection caused by the influenza virus. You are probably already familiar with symptoms of the flu: sore throat, dry cough, stuffy nose, headache, body aches, weakness, and fever. Influenza is different from the "common cold," which can be caused by many different types of viruses and usually only affects the upper respiratory tract.

Influenza season runs from November through April. The influenza virus is very contagious. Most people who get the flu will recover in about a week. However, older people, very young children, and people with chronic illnesses who get the flu are at risk for developing serious complications, such as an extremely severe form of pneumonia.

COVID-19 is caused by Severe Acute Respiratory Syndrome Coronavirus -2 (SARS-CoV-2). The symptoms of COVID-19 vary according to the strain and the person, but often include fever, cough, and tiredness. Some people lose their sense of taste and smell, which can impact their appetite. It can result in life-threatening pneumonia, especially in older individuals and those who did not receive a vaccine. As of 2022, the disease does not follow a seasonal pattern and is even more contagious than the influenza virus. Numerous vaccines exist that can limit the incidence and severity of the disease.

Residents of long-term care facilities are especially at risk for getting and spreading respiratory viruses to other residents and to the staff. An annual "flu shot" and frequent COVID-19 vaccine boosters for both staff members and residents are critical in reducing outbreaks of influenza and COVID-19 in long-term care facilities (Fig. 31-6).

Asthma

Asthma is a condition that affects the bronchi and bronchioles. In people with asthma, triggers (such as cold weather, allergies, respiratory infections, stress, smoke, and exercise) cause the bronchi and bronchioles to constrict (become narrower). This makes breathing difficult because air does not flow freely through the airways. An asthma attack can be very frightening for the person experiencing it because the airways can

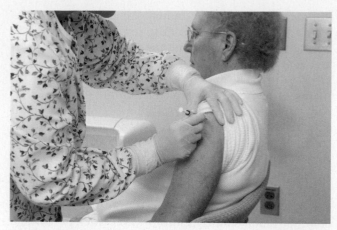

Figure 31-6 Flu shots are usually given to residents in the fall, before the start of flu season (November through April). Flu shots help to prevent infection with the influenza virus, which is very contagious and can cause serious complications in older adults, very young children, and people with chronic illnesses.

narrow to the point that breathing becomes almost impossible. If one of your patients or residents is having trouble breathing or is making wheezing sounds, you should call the nurse immediately.

An acute asthma attack is usually treated with inhaled medications called bronchodilators (Fig. 31-7). Bronchodilators stop the muscle spasms responsible for the constriction of the airways. People with chronic asthma may need to take medication on a regular basis to prevent attacks from occurring. These medications may be given orally, or they may be inhaled.

Chronic Obstructive Pulmonary Disease (COPD)

Chronic obstructive pulmonary disease (COPD) is a general term used to describe two related lung

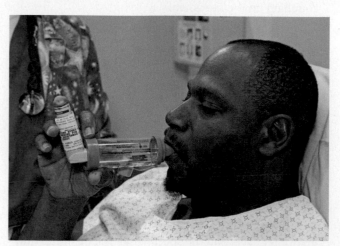

Figure 31-7 Asthma medications are often delivered through inhalers. (© *B. Proud.*)

disorders—emphysema and chronic bronchitis. These disorders often occur together in the same person, which is why some health care professionals prefer the more general term, COPD. The leading cause of COPD is smoking.

Emphysema

Emphysema is a form of COPD that involves damage to the alveoli. As you learned earlier, the walls of the alveoli are very thin and delicate. When a toxin, such as tobacco smoke, is inhaled, it damages the thin walls of the alveoli. Over time, the damage causes the fragile walls of the alveoli to break. Eventually, instead of having millions of tiny alveoli where gas exchange can take place, the person has fewer, large "merged" alveoli that are no longer effective for gas exchange (Fig. 31-8). Because the lung tissue is damaged, it is no longer "springy," and the air gets trapped in the large, damaged alveoli. The trapped air cannot be exhaled and exchanged for new oxygen-rich air, which limits the amount of oxygen that enters the blood by gas exchange. In addition, excess fluid can collect in the damaged alveoli, creating an excellent place for infection-causing microbes to collect and multiply.

A person with emphysema has trouble getting a "proper breath." The person's breathing is shallow and rapid, and they may have to stop to catch their breath quite frequently when talking or engaging in any type of physical activity. As the person's emphysema gets worse, they will need supplemental oxygen just to carry out even the simplest activities of daily living (ADLs). If you are caring for a person with emphysema, you may notice that their chest is enlarged and rounded. This finding is referred to as "barrel chest" and is caused by years of having extra air trapped in the lung tissue, which causes the chest cavity to enlarge over time.

Chronic Bronchitis

The other form of COPD is chronic bronchitis. **Chronic bronchitis** is caused by long-term irritation of the bronchi and bronchioles, such as that caused by inhaling tobacco smoke. The irritation leads to the production of thick mucus, which blocks the airways. Because the air cannot pass freely through the bronchi and bronchioles, breathing is impaired. In addition, infection-causing microbes can collect in the mucus and multiply, leading to infection.

A person with chronic bronchitis has a nagging, productive cough. They may complain of a "tightness" in their chest, or difficulty breathing. They are likely to have frequent respiratory tract infections. Like a person with emphysema, a person with chronic bronchitis will eventually need oxygen therapy.

Alveoli

Healthy alveoli   Emphysematous alveoli

Figure 31-8 Emphysema results from damage to the alveoli. The damage to the alveoli makes it difficult for the body to obtain oxygen and get rid of carbon dioxide. A healthy lung contains millions of tiny alveoli, where gas exchange takes place. In a person with emphysema, the walls of the alveoli break down, forming large areas where air can get trapped.

♥ Helping Hands and a Caring Heart

Focus on Humanistic Health Care

People who have chronic conditions of the respiratory system, such as asthma or COPD, may seem quite "needy." You may become frustrated with their frequent use of the call light control to ask for seemingly trivial things. Please stop for a moment and try to understand how frightening it would be to suddenly feel that you could not breathe! A person who is having an asthma attack or experiencing a flare-up of COPD feels that each breath might be their last. They might be afraid that in the event of another flare-up or attack, help will not arrive soon enough. Using the call light control frequently is the person's way of making sure that someone will actually come quickly if they are called. Instead of giving in to the desire to avoid a seemingly needy patient or resident, be patient and understanding of the underlying fears the person may have. Spend more time with the person and get into the habit of stopping by to check on them, even when they have not called you. By addressing the person's underlying need for safety and security, you will be providing truly humanistic care.

Cancer

In the United States, cancers involving the lungs and airway are the most common cause of cancer-related death. The types of cancers that affect the upper respiratory tract include tumors of the mouth, tongue, and vocal cords. Cancers of the lower respiratory tract can involve the lungs or the lining of the bronchi. People who smoke cigarettes are 10 times more likely to develop lung cancer than nonsmokers. In addition, some cancers that begin in other body parts, such as the breast or intestines, commonly spread to the lungs.

You may care for a person who is having diagnostic tests done to determine whether or not they have cancer of the lungs or airway. It is important for you to remember that the person and their family members may be worried about both the diagnostic test itself and the results of the test. You may notice that your patient or resident seems quiet or distracted, or that they are having trouble concentrating on tasks. Or, you might come into the room and find the person crying. Sometimes worrying makes a person angry, short-tempered, or agitated. Family members may show similar behaviors as they worry about their loved ones.

There are several different ways that the diagnosis of cancer can be made:

- **Radiologic studies**, such as chest x-rays, computed tomography (CT) scans, nuclear medicine scans (often called lung scans), and magnetic resonance imaging (MRI) scans, allow the doctor to see the tumor without actually entering the body.
- **Bronchoscopy** involves using a special instrument to look inside the airway and obtain tissue or fluids for analysis. The bronchoscope is passed through the mouth and pharynx and into the person's airway (Fig. 31-9). The person may have some discomfort during the procedure, as well as a scratchy throat afterward.
- **Surgery** may be necessary to obtain tissue for analysis. Of all of the diagnostic methods, surgery carries the most risk for the person and is associated with the most discomfort.

You may also care for people who are in a health care facility because they are receiving treatment for cancer of the respiratory system. There are many different ways of treating cancer, which are discussed in detail in Chapter 42. Treatment of cancer of the mouth, tongue, or vocal cords may involve surgery to remove the cancer and possibly some of the surrounding tissues as well. This type of surgery often changes the person's appearance, in very noticeable ways. For many people, coping with the change in their appearance as well as the diagnosis of cancer is very difficult. Treatment of lung cancer may involve surgical removal of all or part of the lung. A person who has had lung surgery will usually have drains inserted in the chest cavity for several days after the procedure to remove blood and fluid and to help keep the lungs expanded properly (Fig. 31-10). Make sure you have been shown how to care for a person with chest tubes if caring for a surgical patient is included in your responsibilities.

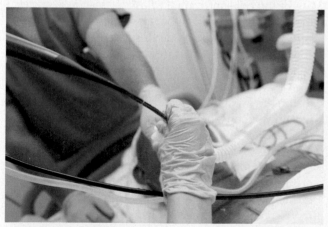

Figure 31-9 A doctor uses a flexible bronchoscope to examine a patient's airways. The bronchoscope is inserted into the patient's mouth, and an image of the trachea and bronchial tubes is displayed on a screen (*sfam_photo\Shutterstock.com*).

Helping Hands and a Caring Heart

Focus on Humanistic Health Care

When a person has a smoking-related illness, be careful not to be judgmental about the role the person's actions may have had in causing their disease. A person with a smoking-related illness, such as cancer or COPD, may choose to continue smoking, even though they know doing so may significantly shorten their life. Smoking is very physically addictive and quitting can be extremely difficult, especially when the person is trying to cope with the stress of having a chronic or terminal condition. Each of your patients or residents must be allowed to make decisions concerning their own quality of life. For some people, this may mean not giving up smoking, even when it would seem to be the best thing to do.

Pneumothorax and Hemothorax

Pneumothorax and hemothorax are often complications of chest trauma. **Pneumothorax** (sometimes called a "collapsed lung") occurs when air builds up

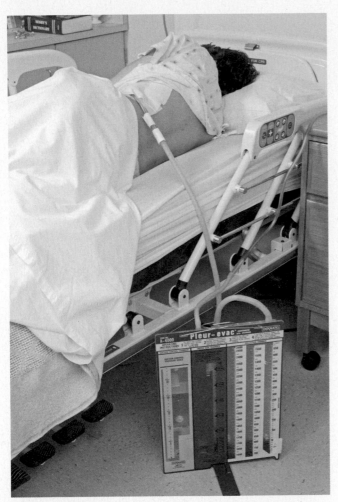

Figure 31-10 A chest tube drainage system is used to remove fluid (such as blood) or air that may build up in the chest cavity as a result of disease, injury, or surgery.

in the space between the lungs and the chest wall. For example, a penetrating chest wound, such as a stab wound to the chest, can lead to pneumothorax because the stab wound is a "sucking" wound. That means that because of the pressure difference between the inside and the outside of the body, air is drawn into the chest cavity through the wound. The air in the chest cavity prevents the lungs from expanding fully and makes it hard for the person to breathe. Pneumothorax can also be caused by small lesions that form on the surface of the lung and then rupture, releasing air from the lungs to the inside of the chest cavity. This condition is referred to as a *spontaneous pneumothorax*. Insertion of a chest tube to remove the air is usually necessary.

Hemothorax occurs when blood builds up in the space between the lungs and the chest wall. The bleeding can be caused by an injury to the chest or a rupture in the lung tissue. As with pneumothorax, the fluid build-up prevents the lungs from fully expanding and breathing becomes difficult. Sometimes surgery is

needed to stop the bleeding, and a chest tube is inserted to remove the blood.

RESPIRATORY THERAPY

Respiratory therapy is any treatment that is used to help a person achieve satisfactory respiration. Some of these treatments are relatively simple. For example, a humidifier may be used to add moisture to the air, helping to loosen secretions during a bout of bronchitis or pneumonia. Other treatments may be quite complex and involve the use of medications, such as oxygen, or mechanical ventilation.

Most health care facilities have a team of respiratory therapists who are specially trained to evaluate and treat problems of the respiratory system. The respiratory therapist listens to the person's breath sounds and looks at certain measurements to evaluate the person's respiratory function. For example, the respiratory therapist will measure the amount of air that is inhaled and exhaled, as well as the amount of oxygen in the person's blood. Next, the respiratory therapist helps to develop a treatment plan for the person. If you are caring for a patient or resident who is being cared for by a respiratory therapist, watch the therapist and ask questions about the types of treatments they are using. This knowledge will help you to better understand the specific needs of your patient or resident. The nurse or respiratory therapist can also alert you to signs or symptoms that you should watch for and report to the nurse immediately.

Oxygen Therapy

The air we breathe contains only about 20% oxygen. The rest is nitrogen and very small amounts of other gases. People with reduced lung function (for example, people with emphysema) may have trouble getting the oxygen their bodies need from inhaled air alone. For these people, the doctor might prescribe supplemental (extra) oxygen to increase the amount of oxygen that they take in with each breath. The supplemental oxygen is pure, 100% oxygen.

Some people who are receiving supplemental oxygen will only need it for a short time. Others will need it for the rest of their lives. Oxygen can be given continuously, or it can be given on an as-needed basis. Some people only need supplemental oxygen when they are physically active.

Oxygen is considered a medication and requires a doctor's order to be used. The doctor determines the rate at which the oxygen should be delivered, and how it should be given. Oxygen is usually delivered to the patient or resident at a rate of 2 to 15 liters of

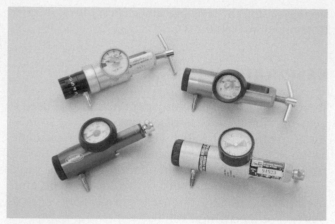

Figure 31-11 A flow meter controls the rate of oxygen flow to the patient or resident. Flow meters come in a variety of styles. You should learn how the flow meters used by your patients or residents work. This will allow you to check the flow meter to make sure that the person is receiving the ordered amount of oxygen.

oxygen per minute. The flow rate is set using a device called a **flow meter** (Fig. 31-11).

Many of the people you will care for will be receiving oxygen therapy. A nurse or respiratory therapist is responsible for setting up and adjusting the oxygen therapy. However, you need to understand how oxygen is given and what precautions are necessary while oxygen is being used. Some states and facilities do not allow nursing assistants to adjust or assist with the administration of oxygen, but others do.

Although you will not usually be responsible for adjusting the flow rate of oxygen, it is important for you to know what flow rate was ordered. You should check the flow meter frequently when you are caring for a person who is receiving oxygen therapy to make sure that the flow rate is set properly. A patient or resident (or a visitor) might accidentally change the setting on the flow meter. If you notice that the setting on the flow meter does not match the amount of oxygen that has been ordered, notify the nurse immediately. Receiving too much oxygen is just as dangerous as receiving too little oxygen.

Always make sure that you are familiar with your specific job responsibilities with regard to oxygen therapy. General guidelines for oxygen therapy are given in Guidelines Box 31-2. You should also review Chapter 13 for safety considerations related to oxygen therapy.

People who are receiving oxygen therapy may need to be monitored to make sure that enough oxygen is reaching the tissues. This monitoring may be constant for people who are critically ill. Other people will only require periodic monitoring. Monitoring of the oxygen content of the blood is done using a device called a *pulse oximeter*. The pulse oximeter has sensors that can be

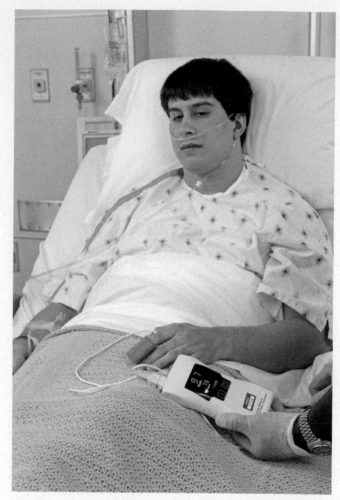

Figure 31-12 Pulse oximetry is used to monitor the amount of oxygen that is reaching a person's tissues.

used on a person's finger, toe, foot (for infants), earlobe, forehead, or bridge of the nose. It is important that you use the appropriate type of sensor for the body part (Fig. 31-12). Infrared light is passed through the tissue to a sensor on the other side of the device. The amount of light that reaches the sensor is translated into a measurement of how much oxygen the blood is actually carrying. A normal reading is between 95% and 100%. Readings below 90% indicate that the person's tissues are not receiving enough oxygen. An alarm will usually sound if the person's blood oxygen level is too low.

Because oxygen therapy can be very drying to a person's mouth or nose, moisture is often added to the supplemental oxygen using a humidifier bottle. The humidifier bottle is filled with distilled water. The oxygen passes through the water before it is delivered to the patient or resident. This increases the water content of the oxygen, making it less drying to the person's nose and mouth. As the oxygen flows through the water in the humidifier bottle, it creates bubbles. You should check the humidifier bottle frequently for bubbles, which indicate that the oxygen is flowing freely. You should also

Guidelines Box 31-2 Guidelines for Oxygen Therapy

WHAT YOU DO	WHY YOU DO IT
Avoid lighting matches or cigarette lighters in the person's room. Post a "No Smoking" sign, and remind the patient or resident and any visitors not to smoke when oxygen is in use.	Use of oxygen therapy can increase the oxygen content of linens and clothing in the immediate area. If burning ashes from a cigarette should happen to drop on the bed, a fire would be more likely to start and would burn much faster as a result of the added oxygen.
Make sure that all electrical equipment are in good working order and that cords are not frayed. Use a battery-operated razor or a blade razor when shaving a person who is receiving supplemental oxygen.	Electrical equipment that is not properly maintained can be the source of a spark, which could start a fire.
Make sure that the tubing through which the oxygen is delivered is free of kinks and that the person is not lying on it.	If the tubing is obstructed in any way, oxygen flow will be impaired and the person will not receive the correct amount.
Do not adjust the flow rate of oxygen.	Adjusting the flow rate of oxygen is out of the nursing assistant's scope of practice. Receiving too much oxygen can be as harmful to the patient or resident as receiving too little oxygen. The doctor decides how much oxygen the patient or resident should receive.
When you are caring for a person who is receiving supplemental oxygen, be aware of the ordered flow rate, and tell the nurse if the flow rate on the flow meter does not match the ordered flow rate.	The setting on the flow meter may get changed accidentally. Checking frequently to make sure that the ordered flow rate matches the flow rate on the person's medical chart helps to keep your patient or resident safe. Receiving too much oxygen can be as harmful to the patient or resident as receiving too little oxygen.
When providing personal care, do not remove a person's facemask or nasal cannula, unless you are specifically told to do so by the nurse.	Removing the facemask or nasal cannula will deprive the person of the supplemental oxygen. Some people may not be able to tolerate a decrease in the amount of oxygen they are receiving, even for just a few minutes.
Make sure that the water level in the humidifier bottle does not get too low.	Oxygen that is not humidified prior to delivery can be very drying to the mucous membrane lining of the person's nasal cavity and mouth. This dryness can be uncomfortable for the patient or resident.
Provide oral care frequently, as directed by the nurse.	Frequent oral care helps to relieve some of the dryness of the nose and mouth that occurs with supplemental oxygen therapy.
Watch for signs of skin irritation behind the person's ears, over their cheeks, or under their nose.	The pressure and friction from the tubing that holds the facemask or nasal cannula in place can cause skin breakdown.

check the water level often, to make sure that it does not drop too low. Your facility policy will specify how often the humidifier bottle should be changed.

Sources of Supplemental Oxygen

Supplemental oxygen can be supplied through a wall-mounted delivery system, in a pressurized tank, through an oxygen concentrator, or by small portable tanks containing liquid oxygen (Fig. 31-13).

Wall-Mounted Delivery Systems

In many facilities, the oxygen is piped into the patient's or resident's room from a central location. A special valve and flow meter device is inserted into the wall to

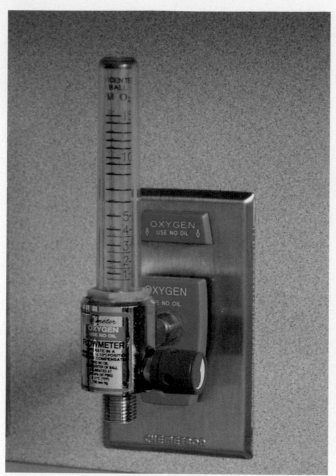

A. Wall-mounted delivery system

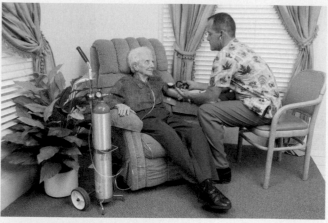

B. Pressurized tank

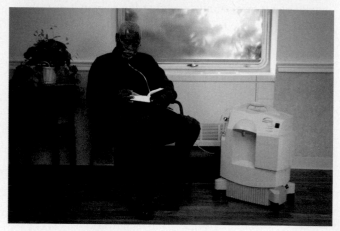

C. Oxygen concentrator

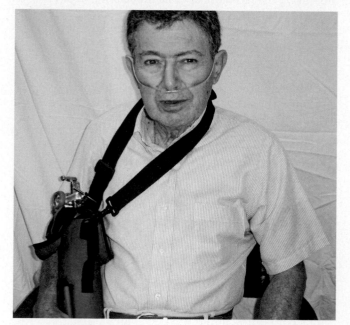

D. Liquid oxygen tank

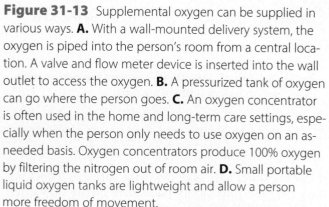

Figure 31-13 Supplemental oxygen can be supplied in various ways. **A.** With a wall-mounted delivery system, the oxygen is piped into the person's room from a central location. A valve and flow meter device is inserted into the wall outlet to access the oxygen. **B.** A pressurized tank of oxygen can go where the person goes. **C.** An oxygen concentrator is often used in the home and long-term care settings, especially when the person only needs to use oxygen on an as-needed basis. Oxygen concentrators produce 100% oxygen by filtering the nitrogen out of room air. **D.** Small portable liquid oxygen tanks are lightweight and allow a person more freedom of movement.

access the oxygen (see Fig. 31-13A). The nurse or respiratory therapist sets the flow meter so that the oxygen is administered to the person at the correct rate.

Pressurized Tank

These tanks, which are placed in the patient's or resident's room, contain oxygen under pressure. Some of these tanks are small enough to be carried or wheeled around with the person (see Fig. 31-13B). The nurse or respiratory therapist sets the flow meter on the tank so that the oxygen is administered to the person at the correct rate.

A gauge tracks the amount of oxygen remaining in the tank. You should note when the dial shows that the supply of oxygen is getting low. If you notice that the tank is nearly empty, tell the nurse or respiratory therapist so that they can exchange the nearly empty tank for a full one.

Because the portable oxygen tanks are pressurized, they should be moved with caution. If the tank is accidentally knocked over and the valve at the top breaks, the escaping gas in the tank could propel the tank across the room with quite a bit of force. If the tank hits someone, it could cause a serious injury.

Oxygen Concentrators

Oxygen concentrators are devices that take in room air and filter out the nitrogen, leaving behind pure oxygen (see Fig. 31-13C). The oxygen is then delivered to the person at the rate that has been programmed into the unit. Because the delivery amount is preset, the person (or caregiver) only has to turn the switch to "ON" when oxygen is needed. These units run on electricity and are often used in home and long-term care settings, especially if the person needs supplemental oxygen only once in a while.

Liquid Oxygen Tank

Oxygen becomes liquid when it is subjected to extremely cold temperatures. Liquid oxygen can be stored in a tank under pressure. When the oxygen is warmed, it returns to a gaseous state and can be delivered through a nasal cannula to a person who needs supplemental oxygen. Because these tanks are small and lightweight, they are easily carried in small packs or pouches (Fig. 31-13D). This gives a person who needs supplemental oxygen the ability to walk and go about their daily activities with much more freedom.

Due to the extreme cold temperature of the liquid nitrogen, a person should not allow the liquid to get on the skin.

Delivery of Supplemental Oxygen

A number of different devices are used to deliver oxygen to patients and residents. The type of delivery device used depends on several factors, including the amount of oxygen ordered, the condition being treated, and the overall physical condition of the patient or resident.

Nasal Cannulas

A nasal cannula is the most common method of administering oxygen. A **nasal cannula** is two prongs of soft plastic tubing, which are inserted into the nostrils (Fig. 31-14A). The tubing to the cannula is connected to an oxygen source with a humidifier bottle and a flow meter. A nasal cannula is easy to apply, it does not interfere with eating or talking, and it is less likely to create a feeling of suffocation. However, the nasal cannula can dry out the mucous membranes in the nasal cavity if the oxygen is delivered at a high flow rate. The tubing can irritate the skin around the nostrils and cheeks and behind the ears. Finally, a nasal cannula may not be suitable for use in a critically ill patient, or in a person who breathes through their mouth because the concentration of oxygen delivered may not be high enough.

Facemasks

Oxygen can also be delivered through a **facemask**. A facemask is made of soft, molded plastic material that fits over the nose and mouth (see Fig. 31-14B). A facemask may be a simple device that just delivers the oxygen to the mouth and nose, or it may be quite complex, with attachments (such as bags that act as a holding place for extra oxygen). A facemask can deliver oxygen at a higher concentration than a nasal cannula. In addition, a facemask is useful for a person who breathes through their mouth, instead of the nose. However, facemasks can make a person feel like they are suffocating (because they cover the person's nose and mouth), and they can interfere with the person's ability to eat, drink, and speak clearly. Sometimes a person is allowed to switch to a nasal cannula when it is time to eat or be shaved. Never remove a person's facemask without first asking the nurse. Removing the facemask, even briefly, can have serious consequences for the person.

Accessory Devices

There are some other devices that are often used in combination with nasal cannula or facemask oxygen delivery systems (Fig. 31-15). Sometimes a person is unconscious or has been sedated to the point that the muscles that keep the upper airway open relax. The lower jaw falls open and the tongue falls backward into the throat, blocking the passage of air into the body.

To prevent this from happening, a nasopharyngeal airway (nasal trumpet) may be used. A **nasopharyngeal airway** is a soft rubber tube that is inserted into

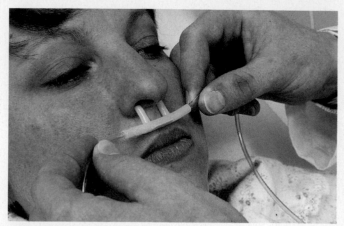

A. Nasal cannula

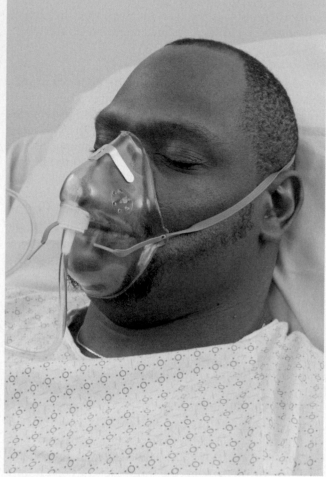

B. Facemask

Figure 31-14 Devices used for oxygen delivery. **A.** A nasal cannula is a two-pronged device that is inserted into the nostrils to deliver oxygen to the patient or resident. A person who has a nasal cannula in place is able to eat, drink, and speak normally. **B.** A facemask fits over the person's nose and mouth. A facemask may be used when a person requires a high level of supplemental oxygen. Facemasks come in a variety of styles.

the person's nose (see Fig. 31-15A). It extends back toward the throat, providing an opening that air can flow through. Another commonly used airway device is the oropharyngeal airway. An **oropharyngeal airway** is a hard plastic device that is inserted into the person's mouth (see Fig. 31-15B). The oropharyngeal airway stops the tongue from falling back into the throat, keeping the airway open. The oropharyngeal airway is used only for a person who is either heavily sedated or unconscious because it can cause gagging and choking in a conscious person.

Mechanical Ventilation

In **mechanical ventilation**, a machine called a *ventilator* breathes for a person who cannot breathe on their own (Fig. 31-16). There are many reasons that a person might need to be put on a ventilator. For example, a serious head injury, stroke, or drug overdose can affect the breathing control centers in the brain, which means that regular breathing will no longer occur automatically. In these situations, mechanical ventilation is needed. A spinal cord injury or a neurologic

disorder can interfere with the nerve impulses that cause the diaphragm to contract and relax automatically, resulting in the need for mechanical ventilation. Other conditions that may result in a person needing mechanical ventilation include acute respiratory infections and heart attacks. Mechanical ventilation is also often used both during and after surgery. Some people only need the ventilator for a short period of time, while others may need to be placed on a ventilator for the rest of their lives. Not all people who require mechanical ventilation are confined to bed. Some ventilators are portable (Fig. 31-17).

A ventilator works by forcing air into the person's lungs. The air is delivered through a tube that is inserted into the airway. Depending on the situation, an endotracheal tube or a tracheostomy tube may be used (Fig. 31-18).

Endotracheal Intubation

Many people who require mechanical ventilation for only a short time will have an endotracheal tube. The **endotracheal tube** is inserted into the person's nose or mouth. It extends to the trachea, where a balloon

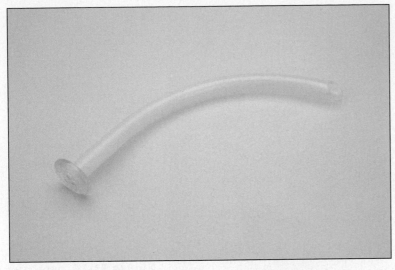
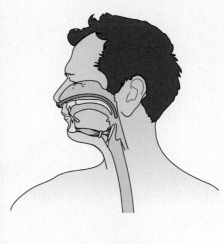

A. Nasopharyngeal airway

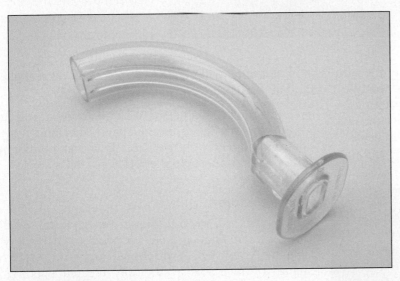
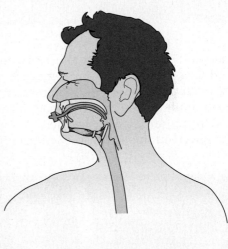

B. Oropharyngeal airway

Figure 31-15 An airway device may need to be used in a person who is unconscious or heavily sedated. The airway device keeps the airway open when the person cannot do this on their own. **A.** A nasopharyngeal airway is inserted into the person's nose. **B.** An oropharyngeal airway is inserted into the person's mouth.

cuff on the end holds it in place and prevents secretions that drain from the mouth from entering the respiratory tract (see Fig. 31-18A). Being intubated with an endotracheal tube can be very uncomfortable and frightening for the patient or resident.

- Because the endotracheal tube travels through the larynx (voice box), a person who has an endotracheal tube in place is unable to talk and will need to communicate using some other method, such as writing on a notepad. Imagine what it would be like to be dependent on a machine to breathe and unable to call out for help if you needed it. What would you do if

the machine stopped? This is something that a person on a ventilator might worry about. Making sure that the call light control is within easy reach and checking on the person frequently are things you can do to make an intubated person feel more secure.
- The endotracheal tube makes it impossible for the person to take food or fluids through the mouth. Frequent oral care can help to relieve some of the dryness and discomfort caused by having an endotracheal tube in place.
- Wrist restraints are often used for a person who is intubated, to keep the person from reaching up and removing the endotracheal tube from the

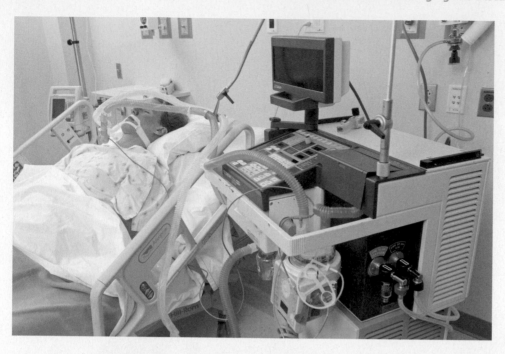

Figure 31-16 A mechanical ventilator performs the function of breathing for a person who cannot breathe on their own.

airway. The tube is uncomfortable, and it is natural for a person to try and remove it. Although the wrist restraints may be necessary, they can add to the person's anxiety. As is always the case when restraints are being used, you will need to check on the person very frequently, and the restraints will need to be removed and reapplied at regular intervals.

Ensuring that a person with an endotracheal tube is as comfortable as possible and checking on the person frequently will help to relieve some of the person's worries and help them to feel safe.

Tracheostomy

If a person will need to be on a mechanical ventilator for more than a week or so, a tracheostomy is usually performed. A **tracheostomy** (often referred to as a "trach") is a surgically created opening in the neck that opens into the trachea. A short tube, called a tracheostomy or "trach" tube, is inserted into the opening and attached to the ventilator tubing (see Fig. 31-18B). The tracheostomy tube is usually secured around the person's neck with ties or a special collar device (Fig. 31-19). If the tube is not secured, it could be coughed out very easily.

A tracheostomy tube is much more comfortable for the person than an endotracheal tube. The person is able to eat and drink normally. The tracheostomy and tubing require special care, which is performed by the nurse. You are responsible for making sure that the tubing stays connected at all times and for observing the person for any signs that they are having trouble breathing. Many people with a tracheostomy do not need a ventilator to help them breathe. They are able to breathe in and out through the trach.

Depending on the situation, a tracheostomy may be permanent or temporary. For example, a person who requires mechanical ventilation for several weeks will have a temporary tracheostomy that will

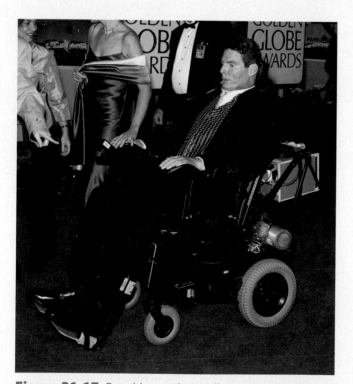

Figure 31-17 Portable ventilators allow some people with quadriplegia or other conditions that affect the muscles used for breathing to lead active lives. (*Featureflash Photo Agency\Shutterstock.com*)

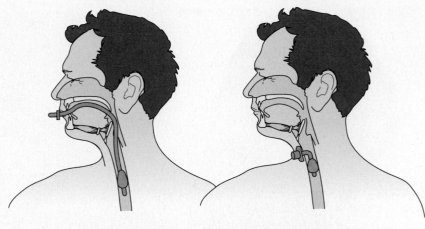

Figure 31-18 Mechanical ventilation requires the use of an endotracheal tube or a tracheostomy tube. **A.** An endotracheal tube is inserted into the person's nose or mouth and passed through the pharynx and larynx to the trachea. An inflatable balloon cuff at the end of the endotracheal tube holds it in place and helps to prevent secretions from passing into the lungs. **B.** A tracheostomy tube is inserted into a surgically created opening in the neck called a tracheostomy.

A. Endotracheal tube   **B.** Tracheostomy tube

be allowed to heal once the person no longer needs to be on the mechanical ventilator. However, a person who is paralyzed and will need to be on a ventilator for the rest of their life will have a permanent tracheostomy. A person who has had their larynx removed as a result of cancer will also have a permanent tracheostomy. The person breathes, talks, sneezes, and coughs through the tracheostomy because the airway between the pharynx and the trachea is no longer complete.

When caring for a patient or resident who has a tracheostomy, you will need to take special care not to allow anything to get into the opening because the person will "inhale" it into the lungs. Lint or small strings from dressing sponges can be easily inhaled through the opening in the trach. Many people wear a scarf or special cloth cover over their trach to protect from dust

and other particles. Be very careful when assisting the person with bathing and grooming to keep water or shaving cream from getting into the trach opening.

Suctioning

People with respiratory disorders often need help removing secretions from the airway. Conditions such as pneumonia or chronic bronchitis can cause the production of large amounts of sputum, which builds up in the lungs and bronchi and makes it difficult to breathe. Other conditions interfere with a person's ability to cough up secretions. For example, a person who is in a coma or heavily sedated may not have an intact cough reflex. Therefore, the person does not cough and the secretions continue to build up. **Suctioning** is the process of removing fluid and mucus from a person's airway.

Suctioning is done using various types of suction catheters. The suction catheter is attached to the tubing and a suction source, which works like a vacuum cleaner to remove the secretions from the airway. A Yankauer suction tip is used to remove secretions that collect in the back of the throat (Fig. 31-20). The Yankauer tip is placed in the person's mouth, and suction is applied. A long, thin, flexible catheter is used when it is necessary to suction the airways in the lower respiratory system. This soft catheter can be passed through the nose or mouth, or down an endotracheal or tracheostomy tube.

Because suctioning removes air along with the bothersome secretions, a person can easily become **hypoxic** (that is, deficient of oxygen) during the suctioning procedure. Nursing assistants are not responsible for suctioning patients and residents, but you will be responsible for letting the nurse know that suctioning may be needed and for assisting during the procedure. Usually it is quite obvious when a person needs to have their airway suctioned. The person's breathing becomes noisy, and they may keep trying to cough up secretions, with little success.

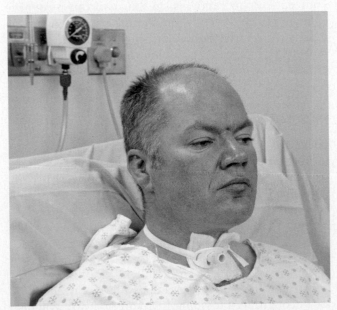

Figure 31-19 The tracheostomy tube is held in place with special ties or a collar.

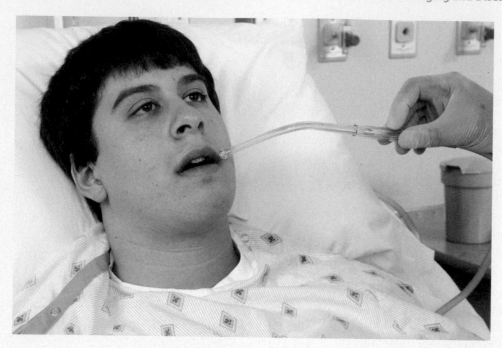

Figure 31-20 A Yankauer suction tip is used to remove secretions from the mouth and the back of the throat. You will be able to tell when a person needs to be suctioned. Always report this observation to the nurse so that they can perform the procedure.

GENERAL CARE MEASURES

Because there is little room for error when dealing with the respiratory system, many of the therapies that are used to help people with respiratory disorders can be carried out only by people who have received advanced training, such as nurses and respiratory therapists. However, many facilities and agencies offer additional training that will allow you to be more active in caring for people with special respiratory needs. For example, you may work in a facility that provides specialized care for people who depend on mechanical ventilators to breathe. In this case, your scope of practice may be widened to include procedures that are not normally part of a nursing assistant's responsibilities. Make sure that you have been adequately instructed in any special procedures that are required of you, and always be aware of what is and is not within your scope of practice, per your state's or facility's policy. No matter where you work, there are several general care measures related to the respiratory system that are within every nursing assistant's scope of practice.

Taking It to the Next Level:

Advanced Skills

More in-depth information related to advanced skills used when providing care for a person with respiratory disorders can be found in *Lippincott Acute Care Skills for Advanced Nursing Assistants*.

Visit thePoint at thepoint.lww.com for access to the ebook.

Observation

A nursing assistant's main responsibility in caring for any patient or resident with a respiratory problem is that of observation. Because you are the one who will spend the most time with your patients or residents, you will be the one who has the best opportunity to observe signs that a person may be having problems with ventilation or gas exchange. Some of your patients or residents who have chronic respiratory problems will always have difficulty breathing when they exert themselves. It is important for you to be able to recognize what is normal for each of your patients or residents, so that you can recognize changes if they occur. You should also be aware of a person's normal skin color, so that you are able to recognize changes that may indicate that their tissues are not receiving enough oxygen.

Promoting Comfort

There are many things that a nursing assistant can do to help a person with respiratory problems feel more comfortable. Positioning the person in the Fowler's or semi-Fowler's position is often helpful. Some people are more comfortable when they assume a forward-leaning position using pillows on the over-bed table (Fig. 31-21). If the doctor has not placed any restrictions on the person's fluid intake, encourage the patient or resident to drink plenty of fluids. Fluids help to thin respiratory secretions so that they are easier to cough up. Providing frequent oral care will also help keep the person comfortable and will reduce the number of microbes that are present in the mouth.

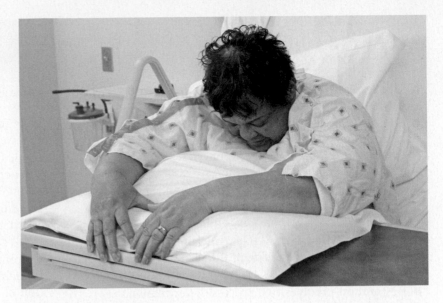

Figure 31-21 Certain positions make breathing easier for people with respiratory disorders. Many people find that leaning forward helps to make breathing easier.

Tell the Nurse!

Not receiving adequate oxygen, even for a very short time, places a person at risk for developing severe complications, or even dying. Tell the nurse immediately if you observe any of the following:

- A person experiences the sudden onset of chest pain or difficulty breathing

- A person develops noisy breathing (for example, wheezing, "barking," or "crowing")

- A person begins to make fluid-like, gurgling sounds (this is especially important to report if the person is very weak or comatose)

- The oxygen flow rate on the oxygen flow meter does not match the ordered amount of oxygen

- The gauge on a pressurized oxygen tank indicates that the oxygen level is low

- The screen on a pulse oximeter shows a reading of less than 90%

- A person's skin has a blue or gray tinge, either at rest or while exercising

- A person coughs up sputum that is discolored (green, frothy, brown, or red-streaked)

- A person's tracheostomy or endotracheal tube becomes dislodged

- A person becomes short of breath during a physical activity that they have performed without effort in the past

- A person's respirations become very slow and shallow, or they stop

SUMMARY

- The respiratory system provides the body with oxygen and rids the body of carbon dioxide.
- The respiratory system consists of the lungs and a group of structures known as the *airway*, which consists of the nasal cavities, pharynx, larynx, trachea, bronchi, and bronchioles.
  - The upper respiratory tract consists of those structures located outside of the chest cavity (the nasal cavity, pharynx, and larynx).
  - The lower respiratory tract consists of those structures located inside of the chest cavity (the trachea, bronchi, bronchioles, and lungs).
- Respiration involves two processes, ventilation and gas exchange. If one or the other of these processes is impaired, respiration will not be effective.
  - Ventilation is the process of physically moving air in and out of the lungs (breathing).
  - Gas exchange is the process of transferring oxygen from the air into the blood and transferring carbon dioxide from the blood into the air.
- Like all organ systems, the respiratory system is affected by aging.
  - Loss of elasticity in the lung tissue and weakening of the muscles of respiration make breathing less efficient because an older person is able to take in less air with each breath.
  - With aging, the cough reflex decreases.
  - The decreased ability of the immune system to fight infections may make an older person more at risk for pneumonia and other respiratory infections.
  - Chronic illness, immobility, or a lifetime of exposure to pollution, chemicals, or tobacco smoke can increase the effects of aging on the respiratory system.
  - Regular exercise combined with healthy habits helps keep the respiratory system healthy.
- Disorders of the respiratory system can make breathing very difficult.
  - Infections can be bacterial or viral and include pneumonia, bronchitis, COVID-19, and influenza.

- Asthma is a narrowing of the bronchioles in response to certain triggers, such as allergies, cold air, exercise, smoke, or stress. An asthma attack can be very frightening.
- Chronic obstructive pulmonary disease (COPD) is a general term for two smoking-related disorders.
  - In emphysema, the alveoli are destroyed. Trapping of air in the lungs results. Breathing is difficult and gas exchange is impaired.
  - Chronic bronchitis affects the bronchi and bronchioles. It is associated with the production of excessive amounts of secretions.
- Cancers of the lungs and airway are the most common cause of cancer-related deaths in the United States. People who smoke are 10 times more likely to develop lung cancer than non-smokers.
- Respiratory therapy is used to help improve a person's ventilation, gas exchange, or both.
  - Oxygen therapy is the administration of supplemental oxygen.
    - Oxygen is a medication and requires a doctor's order.
    - Oxygen may be supplied by way of a wall-mounted system, an individual pressurized tank, an oxygen concentrator, or a liquid oxygen tank.
    - Oxygen can be administered through a nasal cannula or facemask.
  - Mechanical ventilation is used for a person who cannot inhale and exhale on their own. A person who needs the assistance of a mechanical ventilator must be intubated with an endotracheal tube or a tracheostomy tube.
  - Suctioning is often necessary to remove excessive secretions from the respiratory tract.
- A nursing assistant's responsibilities when caring for a person with a respiratory disorder are mainly observation and the promotion of comfort. A nursing assistant also provides holistic care by helping the person feel safe and secure.

WHAT DID YOU LEARN?

Multiple Choice

Select the single best answer for each of the following questions.

1. Who has to write the order for oxygen to be used?
    a. The nurse
    b. The respiratory therapist
    c. The doctor
    d. No order is necessary

2. The nurse asks you to obtain a sputum specimen from Ms. Long, who has pneumonia. Which one of the following is correct to do when obtaining a sputum specimen?
    a. Have Ms. Long rinse her mouth with mouthwash before producing the specimen.
    b. Have Ms. Long cough the specimen into an emesis basin, and then transfer the specimen to the specimen container.
    c. Explain to Ms. Long that the specimen must come from deep within her chest.
    d. Put the specimen container in the refrigerator after you have collected the sputum specimen and labeled the container with Ms. Long's name and room number.

3. What color is a healthy lung?
    a. Blue
    b. Gray
    c. White
    d. Pink

4. Where does gas exchange take place?
    a. In the alveoli
    b. In the bronchioles
    c. In the pleura
    d. In the nasal cavity

5. Which of the following is true about a person who has an endotracheal tube in place?
    a. The person is able to eat and drink normally.
    b. The person is able to talk normally.
    c. The person will need frequent oral care.
    d. The person is unconscious.

6. You have been assigned to care for Mr. Fenley, who has chronic obstructive pulmonary disease (COPD). He is on continuous oxygen by a nasal cannula at a rate of 4 liters per minute. One morning, you enter Mr. Fenley's room to do your morning checks, and you notice that the flow rate on the flow meter is set at 8 liters per minute. What should you do?
    a. Call the nurse immediately.
    b. Decrease the flow rate back to the prescribed 4 liters per minute.
    c. Tell Mr. Fenley that it is very dangerous for him to make adjustments to the flow meter on his own.
    d. Nothing. A patient or resident can adjust the flow rate of oxygen to meet their own needs.

7. One of your responsibilities is to assist Mr. Tang with shaving. Mr. Tang is receiving continuous oxygen via a nasal cannula. What should you do when helping Mr. Tang to shave?
    a. Remove the nasal cannula before you begin the procedure.
    b. Use a battery-operated razor or a blade razor instead of an electrical razor.
    c. Increase the flow of oxygen during the procedure.
    d. Decrease the flow of oxygen during the procedure.

8. One of your newly admitted residents, Mr. Petersen, has emphysema. You are going to meet Mr. Petersen for the first time. Thinking back on what you learned during your nurse assistant training course about people with emphysema, which one of the following would you expect to be true of Mr. Petersen?
    a. His breathing will probably be shallow and rapid.
    b. He might need supplemental oxygen.
    c. He may have to catch his breath frequently while talking.
    d. All of the above.

Matching *Match each numbered item with its appropriate lettered description.*

_____ **1.** Respiration

_____ **2.** Lungs

_____ **3.** Nasopharyngeal airway

_____ **4.** Hemothorax

_____ **5.** Pharynx

_____ **6.** Trachea

_____ **7.** Pneumothorax

_____ **8.** Pleura

_____ **9.** Hypoxic

_____ **10.** Nasal cavity

a. Blood in the chest cavity

b. Also known as the "windpipe"; conducts air from the larynx to the bronchi

c. Membrane that covers the inside of the chest cavity and the outside of the lungs

d. Also known as the throat

e. A rubber tube that is inserted in a person's nose to keep the airway open

f. The process the body uses to obtain oxygen from the environment and remove carbon dioxide from the body

g. Primary organs of respiration

h. Space where air from the outside of the body is first warmed, humidified, and filtered

i. Air in the chest cavity

j. Deficiency of oxygen

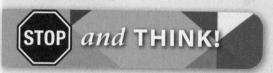

STOP *and* **THINK!**

- You have been assigned to care for Mrs. Nielsen, who has severe respiratory problems resulting from a long history of asthma. The light above Mrs. Nielsen's door is on, and you go to find out what she needs. When you enter the room, Mrs. Nielsen asks you if it is almost time for dinner and whether or not you think she will need to wear a sweater. You answer Mrs. Nielsen's questions, and then ask her if there is anything else she needs because surely there must be! She says, "no," she just wanted to ask you those questions. Do you think that Mrs. Nielsen has needs she may not be telling you about? What might you do for Mrs. Nielsen?

- Matthew is providing care for Mr. Tranh, who has smoked for more than 50 years. Mr. Tranh has advanced COPD and requires a lot of assistance with nearly everything (including smoking, which he continues to do). One day, you and Matthew are leaving work together and you see all of the "smokers" outside having their cigarettes, shivering because it is the middle of winter. Matthew tells you that he thinks smoking is a disgusting habit and that people who smoke are weak and lack willpower. How might Matthew's feelings about smoking affect his relationship with Mr. Tranh and other residents with smoking-related conditions?

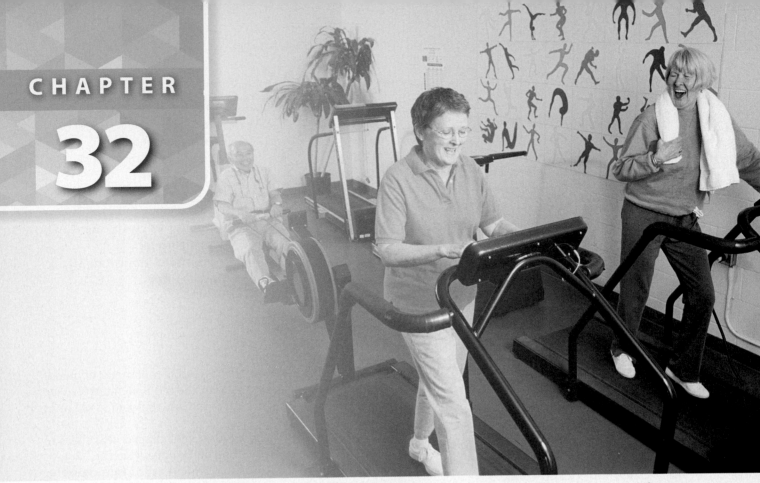

CHAPTER

32

Photo: Residents of a continuing care retirement community (CCRC) use the equipment at an on-site fitness center. Exercising regularly is one way to keep the cardiovascular system healthy.

The Cardiovascular System

 WHAT WILL YOU LEARN?

The heart and the other organs that make up the cardiovascular system are the subject of this chapter. According to the 2022 American Heart Association Statistical Update, about 127 million Americans lived with the effects of either heart disease or stroke (a neurologic problem caused by cardiovascular disease) between the years of 2015 and 2018. That's about 39% of the population! It is likely that some of the people you will care for daily will have some sort of a cardiovascular problem. Not only will an understanding of how the cardiovascular system works help you better serve your patients or residents, it will help you to keep your own cardiovascular system healthy! When you are finished with this chapter, you will be able to:

1. List and describe the major parts of the cardiovascular system.
2. Discuss the major functions of the cardiovascular system.
3. Describe how aging affects the cardiovascular system.
4. Explain how exercise and a healthy lifestyle can lessen the effects of aging on the cardiovascular system.
5. Discuss various disorders that affect the cardiovascular system.
6. List diagnostic tests that are often used to diagnose disorders of the cardiovascular system.

609

Vocabulary

Plasma	Lymph	Systole	Varicose veins
Erythrocytes	Lymph node	Diastole	Phlebitis
Hemoglobin	Endocardium	Cardiac cycle	Thrombophlebitis
Leukocytes	Myocardium	Anemia	Deep venous thrombosis
Thrombocytes	Epicardium	Leukemia	(DVT)
Coagulation	Pericardium	Thrombi	Pulmonary embolism
Hemostasis	Atria	Embolus	Venous (stasis) ulcers
Arteries	Ventricles	Atherosclerosis	Coronary artery disease (CAD)
Veins	Ischemia	Plaque	Angina pectoris
Arterioles	Circulation	Arteriosclerosis	Myocardial infarction (MI)
Capillary bed	Pulmonary circulation	Peripheral vascular	Heart failure
Venules	Systemic circulation	disease	

STRUCTURE OF THE CARDIOVASCULAR SYSTEM

The cardiovascular system, also known as the *circulatory system*, is made up of the blood, the blood vessels, and the heart. *Cardio-* means "heart," and *vascular* means "vessels." It is closely linked to the *lymphatic system*, which is also discussed in this chapter.

Blood

Blood is the life-giving fluid of our bodies. The blood has two main components, the plasma and the blood cells (Fig. 32-1A).

Plasma

More than half of the total blood volume is plasma. **Plasma** is the liquid part of the blood (see Fig. 32-1B). Plasma is about 90% water. The other 10% is made up of substances that are dissolved in the water (such as glucose, amino acids, fats, and salts) and proteins. Important plasma proteins include albumin, fibrinogen, and globulins. Albumin plays a role in driving fluid movement in and out of the bloodstream. Fibrinogen is used as part of the blood clotting process. Globulins known as *antibodies* help to fight infection.

Blood Cells

There are three main types of blood cells: red blood cells (erythrocytes), white blood cells (leukocytes), and platelets (thrombocytes).

Red Blood Cells (Erythrocytes)

Red blood cells, or **erythrocytes**, carry oxygen. The name *erythrocyte* comes from *eryth-*, which means "red," and *cyt*, which means "cell." There are approximately

5 million red blood cells per cubic millimeter of blood! Red blood cells are made in the red bone marrow (see Chapter 30) and are continuously replaced as old ones wear out.

Red blood cells are tiny, disc-shaped cells that are thinner in the center than at the edges (see Fig. 32-1A). Red blood cells contain a protein called **hemoglobin**. Oxygen molecules attach to the hemoglobin for transport to the tissues. When combined with oxygen, hemoglobin is bright red. This is what gives red blood cells their color and name.

The hemoglobin molecule on each red blood cell can carry many oxygen molecules. The hemoglobin on red blood cells that have just received a full load of oxygen from the lungs is filled almost to capacity with oxygen, and therefore, this blood is very bright red. As the blood circulates through the body, giving off oxygen and taking on carbon dioxide, the number of oxygen molecules on the hemoglobin molecule decreases, and the blood becomes darker red in color.

White Blood Cells (Leukocytes)

White blood cells, or **leukocytes**, fight infection. The name *leukocyte* comes from *leuk-*, which means "white" and *cyt*, which means "cell."

The blood of a healthy person contains 5,000 to 10,000 white blood cells per cubic millimeter. For comparison, a cubic millimeter of blood contains 4 to 6 million red blood cells. There are five different types of white blood cells (see Fig. 32-1A). Each type of white blood cell has a different function, related to fighting infection. Some destroy pathogens by surrounding them and "eating" them in a process called phagocytosis (see Chapter 10, Fig. 10-2). Others secrete substances that cause the pathogen to die. Still others make proteins called antibodies, which prevent us from getting some diseases twice.

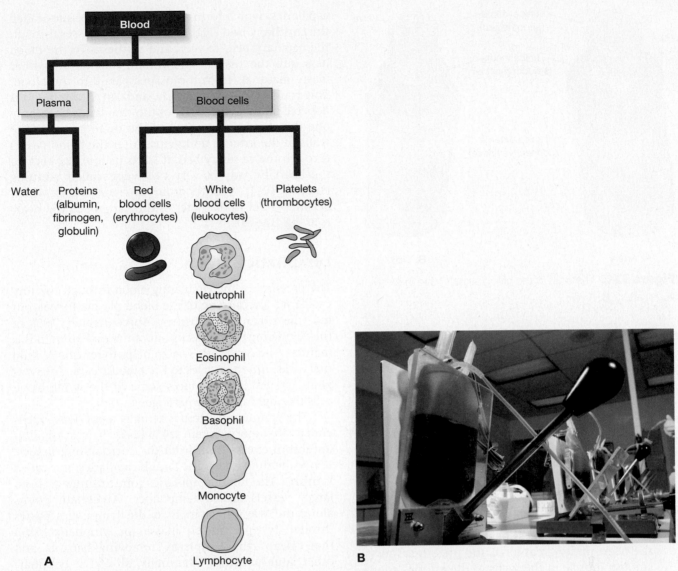

A

B

Figure 32-1   A. Blood consists of plasma and blood cells. **B.** When blood is put in a machine called a centrifuge and spun at high speeds, the blood cells sink to the bottom while the plasma rises to the top. Human blood is about 55% plasma. (*imging\Shutterstock.com*)

White blood cells are formed in the red bone marrow and the lymphatic system (discussed later in this chapter). An infection causes white blood cell production to increase, sending more "troops" into the bloodstream to battle the invading pathogen.

Platelets (Thrombocytes)

Platelets, or **thrombocytes**, are responsible for clotting (**coagulation**) of the blood. When an injury occurs, the platelets stick together to form a temporary plug over the site of injury. They also release chemicals that react with the plasma protein fibrinogen, causing a more permanent clot (or scab) to develop. This process, known as **hemostasis**, stops the loss of blood from the circulatory system (*heme-* = "blood," *stasis* = "stop").

Platelets are not actually whole cells (see Fig. 32-1A). They are pinched-off pieces of larger cells that are formed in the red bone marrow. There are about 150,000 to 450,000 platelets per cubic milliliter of circulating blood.

Blood Vessels

The blood vessels carry blood to and from all of the tissues in the body. The walls of the blood vessels have three layers (Fig. 32-2). The layer on the inside, the *tunica intima*, is a smooth lining that helps blood to flow smoothly through the vessel. The middle layer, the *tunica media*, is formed of smooth muscle tissue. The smooth muscle in the tunica media is what allows the blood vessels to constrict or dilate according to the body's needs. Constriction (narrowing) of the vessels

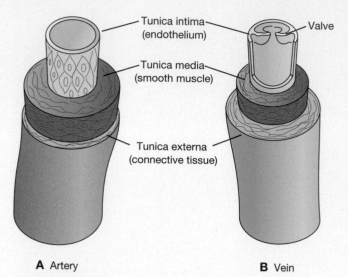

A Artery   **B** Vein

Figure 32-2 The walls of the blood vessels have three layers. **A.** An artery. **B.** A vein.

reduces the blood flow to the body region receiving blood from that vessel, while dilation (widening) of the vessels increases it. The outer layer of the vessel wall, the *tunica externa*, is a tough protective layer of connective tissue.

Arteries carry blood away from the heart, and **veins** carry blood to the heart. Looking at Figure 32-2, you can see that there are two major differences between the walls of the arteries and the walls of the veins:

- The walls of the arteries contain more smooth muscle than those of the veins because the arteries receive blood that is being pumped from the heart under great force and pressure. The smooth muscle in the walls of the arteries allows the arteries to handle the flow of blood from the heart. Smooth muscle in the walls of the smaller arteries also works to control the blood pressure. Constriction of the artery increases the blood pressure, while dilation of the artery will work to lower the blood pressure.
- The tunica intima of the veins contains valves, which help blood to flow back to the heart. This is especially important in the arms and the legs, where blood would tend to flow away from the heart, due to the effects of gravity. The valves are assisted by contraction of nearby skeletal muscles. For example, when we walk, contraction of the leg muscles compresses the veins, pushing blood toward the heart.

Arteries carry blood away from the heart. As the arteries get further away from the heart, they branch into a network, becoming smaller and smaller in diameter (Fig. 32-3A). The smallest arteries are called **arterioles**. Arterioles divide into branches called

capillaries, which form a network in the tissues called the **capillary bed** (Fig. 32-4). As blood passes through the capillary bed, oxygen and nutrients in the blood pass into the tissues, and carbon dioxide and other waste materials from the tissues pass into the blood. This transfer of substances in and out of the blood is possible because the walls of the capillaries have only one thin layer, as opposed to the three layers in the walls of the arteries and veins. After the blood passes through the capillary bed, it starts its journey back to the heart by way of very tiny veins called **venules** (see Fig. 32-4). Venules drain into small veins, which become larger in diameter as they approach the heart (see Fig. 32-3B).

Lymphatic System

The pressure of the circulating blood through the tiny capillaries forces some of the blood plasma to leak out into the surrounding tissues. Approximately 10% of the circulating plasma leaks out of the capillaries in this manner. The lymphatic system helps to return the fluid that leaks into the tissues to the bloodstream. The lymphatic system also produces some of the white blood cells that fight invading pathogens.

The lymphatic system is actually a one-way, open-ended circulatory system (Fig. 32-5). Lymph capillaries absorb excess fluid from the surrounding tissues. (Once the fluid enters the lymph capillaries, it is called **lymph**.) The lymph capillaries join together to form larger vessels, called lymphatics. At certain points along the way, the lymph in the lymphatics passes through **lymph nodes**, masses of lymphatic tissue that "clean" the lymph by removing bacteria and other large particles. Eventually, all of the lymphatics empty into the large veins in the shoulder region, returning the fluid to the general circulation.

Other parts of the lymphatic system include the thymus, which is located in the chest. The thymus helps produce certain white blood cells (T cells) in the event of an infection. (Recall from Chapter 11 that T cells are the cells that the human immunodeficiency virus [HIV] attacks.) The thymus atrophies (decreases in size) with age. Another organ, the spleen, located in the abdomen, helps to filter blood and break down worn-out red blood cells. The spleen also acts as a reservoir where extra blood is stored. The body draws on this "extra" blood supply during times of massive blood loss, for example, following a major injury. The tonsils are also part of the lymphatic system.

Heart

The heart is a hollow, muscular organ about the size of a fist that lies in the center of the chest, tilted a

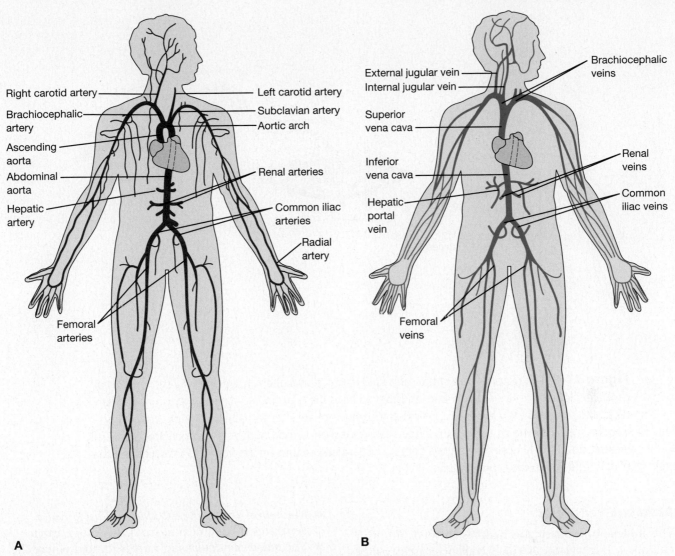

Right carotid artery
Brachiocephalic artery
Ascending aorta
Abdominal aorta
Hepatic artery
Left carotid artery
Subclavian artery
Aortic arch
Renal arteries
Common iliac arteries
Radial artery
Femoral arteries

External jugular vein
Internal jugular vein
Superior vena cava
Inferior vena cava
Hepatic portal vein
Brachiocephalic veins
Renal veins
Common iliac veins
Femoral veins

A

B

Figure 32-3 Blood vessels carry blood to every part of the body. **A.** The major arteries of the body. Arteries carry blood away from the heart. Note how the arteries get smaller in diameter the further away they get from the heart. **B.** The major veins of the body. Veins carry blood back to the heart. Note how the veins get larger in diameter the closer they get to the heart.

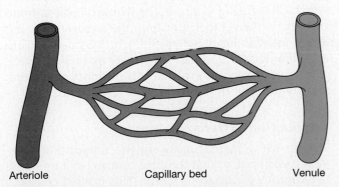

Arteriole   Capillary bed   Venule

Figure 32-4 The capillary bed is where the transfer of substances between the blood and the tissues occurs.

bit toward the left, behind the sternum (breastbone). Like the walls of the arteries and veins, the walls of the heart are made of three layers of tissue. The **endocardium** is the smooth inner layer of the heart. The **myocardium**, the middle layer, is formed of cardiac muscle. Coordinated contraction and relaxation of the myocardium is what causes the heart to pump. The **epicardium** is the smooth outermost layer of the heart. The epicardium forms part of the **pericardium**, a double-layered protective sac that surrounds the heart. A thin film of fluid between the epicardium and the outer layer of the pericardium allows the pericardial layers to slide smoothly against each other each time the heart pumps.

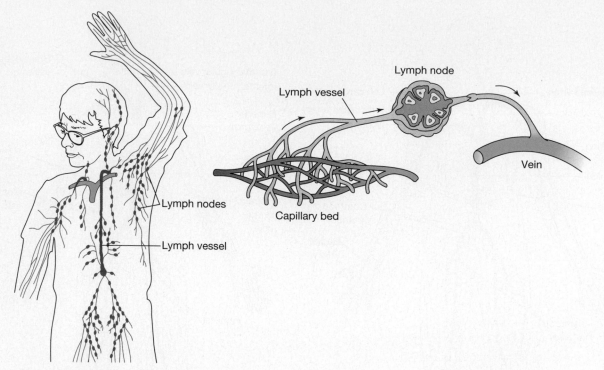

Figure 32-5 The lymphatic system returns fluid to the bloodstream. It is a one-way system. Lymph capillaries, located in the capillary bed, absorb fluid from the surrounding tissues. The lymph capillaries join together to form larger lymph vessels (called lymphatics). Eventually, the lymphatics empty into the subclavian veins, large veins in the shoulder region. Lymph nodes, masses of lymphatic tissue located along the lymphatics, remove bacteria and other foreign particles from the lymph before the fluid is returned to the bloodstream.

Atria and Ventricles

The hollow interior of the heart is divided into four chambers (Fig. 32-6). A thick wall of muscle, called the septum, separates the left side of the heart from the right side of the heart. Valves, flaps of tissue that help to ensure that blood flows only in one direction, separate the chambers on the top from the chambers on the bottom. The upper chambers are called the left atrium and right atrium, or the **atria**. The atria receive the blood that is being brought back to the heart from the body and send it into the lower chambers of the heart, called the **ventricles**. When the ventricles contract, they send blood from the heart to other parts of the body. Because the ventricles must send the blood much further with each contraction, they are larger than the atria and have thicker, more muscular walls.

Heart Valves

Blood can only flow through the heart in one direction. To keep blood flowing in the proper direction, the heart has four valves. Valves are flaps of tissue that snap shut after the blood passes through to prevent backflow.

- The *tricuspid (right atrioventricular) valve* separates the right atrium from the right ventricle.

- The *mitral (left atrioventricular or bicuspid) valve* separates the left atrium from the left ventricle.
- The *pulmonary (pulmonic) valve* is located where the pulmonary artery attaches to the right ventricle.
- The *aortic valve* is located where the aorta attaches to the left ventricle.

The four valves can be seen in Figure 32-6.

The valves of the heart may become diseased. For example, a type of infection called rheumatic fever can cause the valves to become thickened and scarred. Damaged valves are unable to create a seal when they close, which allows blood to flow in the wrong direction (from the atria to the ventricles, or from the aorta/pulmonary artery into the heart) when the ventricles pump. This condition is called *valvular insufficiency* or *valvular regurgitation*. A person with valvular insufficiency may need surgery to repair or replace the defective valve.

Conduction System

The muscle cells that make up the myocardium are very specialized, so that the atria contract as a unit and the ventricles contract as a unit. This unified contraction is what allows the heart to work efficiently as a pump, moving blood continuously through the body.

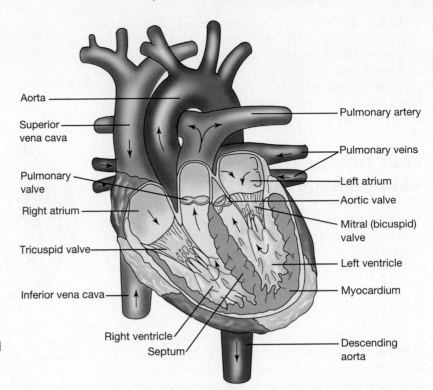

Figure 32-6 The heart has four chambers. The atria receive blood that is being returned to the heart from the veins. Blood leaves the heart after passing through the ventricles.

A small mass of special tissue in the heart, called the sinoatrial node (pacemaker), sets the pace for contraction by generating an electrical impulse. The electrical impulse travels through the myocardium via a special pathway called the conduction system. As it passes through, the electrical energy causes the cardiac muscle cells in the myocardium to contract. First the atria contract, there is a pause, and then the ventricles contract. The heart rests briefly and then the pacemaker generates another impulse, starting the cycle again.

Coronary Circulation

Like all organs, the heart needs oxygen and nutrients. In fact, the heart's demand for oxygen and nutrients is very high because it works continuously, without rest. Think about it—the normal resting heart rate of an adult is around 70 beats/min, or about 100,800 beats in a 24-hour period! The heart cannot stop to rest when it is tired; it has to continue pumping blood through the body. All of this hard work adds up to a very high, and constant, demand for oxygen and nutrients.

The coronary circulation meets this demand (Fig. 32-7). (*Coronary* is another word for "heart.") Many people think that the cells of the heart just absorb oxygen from the blood that is passing through the chambers, but this is not the case. The tissues of the heart have their own special network of arteries and veins, just like all of the other organs in the body.

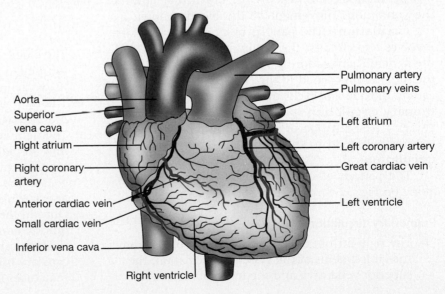

Figure 32-7 The heart has its own blood supply, called the coronary circulation.

Coronary arteries carry oxygen-rich blood into the heart tissue. Coronary veins remove carbon dioxide and other waste products. Any disruption in the flow of oxygen-rich blood to the tissues of the heart can cause **ischemia** (lack of oxygen to the tissues). Prolonged ischemia causes the tissue to die, resulting in permanent damage to the heart muscle.

FUNCTION OF THE CARDIOVASCULAR SYSTEM

The main function of the cardiovascular system is that of transport. However, the cardiovascular system also plays a role in regulating temperature and protecting the body from disease.

Transport

Bringing oxygen, nutrients, and other necessary substances (for example, hormones) to the cells and taking waste materials away from them is one of the most important functions of the cardiovascular system. Think of the cardiovascular system as a manufacturing company that serves customers across the nation. "Trucks" (red blood cells) are loaded up with merchandise at the "central warehouse" (the heart and lungs). The trucks set out on a huge network of "highways" (the blood vessels) to deliver their goods. When they reach their destinations, the ordered merchandise is unloaded, and the empty crates are put back on the trucks to be returned to the warehouse to receive another load.

Pulmonary and Systemic Circulation

While the blood is the vehicle that transports oxygen, nutrients, wastes, and other substances to their various destinations, the heart is the organ that powers the continuous movement of the blood (known as the **circulation**). The pattern of circulation actually involves two circuits, the pulmonary circulation and the systemic circulation (Fig. 32-8). The right side of the heart pumps blood to the lungs, where it releases carbon dioxide and picks up oxygen. This is the **pulmonary circulation** (*pulmonary* is another word for "lungs"). The left side of the heart pumps the newly oxygenated blood to the body. This is the **systemic circulation**.

The pattern of circulation goes like this (follow along on Fig. 32-8):

Pulmonary Circulation

■ The right atrium of the heart receives blood from the largest veins of the systemic circulation, the superior vena cava and the inferior vena cava.

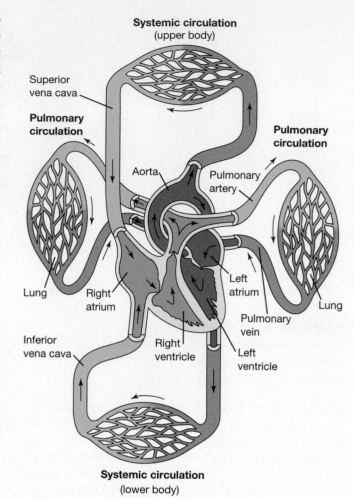

Figure 32-8 The pattern of circulation involves two circuits, the pulmonary circulation and the systemic circulation. In this diagram, *red* stands for oxygen-rich blood, and *blue* stands for oxygen-poor blood. Blood passes from the right ventricle into the pulmonary circulation. Once it is loaded up with oxygen, the blood returns to the left atrium, passes into the left ventricle, and is sent out to the rest of the body. This is the systemic circulation.

The blood in these veins is returning from its journey to the tissues, so it has given up most of its oxygen and taken on a load of carbon dioxide.
■ The right atrium pumps the oxygen-poor blood into the right ventricle.
■ The right ventricle pumps the oxygen-poor blood into the pulmonary artery. The pulmonary artery branches into the right pulmonary artery, which goes to the right lung, and the left pulmonary artery, which goes to the left lung.
■ Once in the lungs, the pulmonary arteries quickly branch into smaller arteries and arterioles to carry the oxygen-poor blood to the capillary beds surrounding the alveoli. As you remember from Chapter 31, gas exchange takes

place in the alveoli. The oxygen in the alveolus moves into the blood, and the carbon dioxide in the blood moves into the alveolus, to be exhaled from the body.

- The blood, which now contains fresh oxygen, is carried by the network of venules, then veins, to the pulmonary veins (right and left), which empty into the left atrium of the heart.

Systemic Circulation

- The left atrium pumps the oxygen-rich blood into the left ventricle.
- The left ventricle pumps the oxygen-rich blood into the largest artery of the body, the aorta.
- The aorta branches very quickly into the coronary arteries to carry oxygen-rich blood to the heart muscle, and then into large branches of arteries that carry oxygen-rich blood to the rest of the body.
- The arteries branch into arterioles and then into capillaries, which form a capillary bed. In the capillary bed, oxygen and nutrients move out of the blood and into the tissues, and carbon dioxide moves out of the tissues and into the blood.
- The blood, which now contains less oxygen, is carried by the network of venules, then veins, back to the right atrium, where the process begins again.

Cardiac Cycle

You may recall from Chapter 20 that the heart muscle contracts in two phases. During **systole**, or the active phase, the myocardium contracts, sending blood out of the heart. During **diastole**, or the resting phase, the myocardium relaxes, allowing the chambers to fill with blood. The atria are in systole when the ventricles are in diastole, and vice versa. The atria contract (atrial systole), sending the blood into the relaxed ventricles (ventricular diastole). Next, the atria relax (atrial diastole) while the ventricles contract (ventricular systole), sending the blood out to the body. Then there is a short period of complete diastole, during which both the atria and the ventricles are relaxed. This sequence is called the **cardiac cycle**.

The orderly sequence of systole and diastole is crucial for maximizing the amount of blood that is pumped throughout the body each time the heart contracts. During ventricular diastole, the ventricles are relaxed, which allows them to fill with blood. Without this rest period, the ventricles would never fill properly. Think about filing a plastic squirt bottle (the kind used for sauces like ketchup which squirts out sauce when it is squeezed) with water. If you fill the squirt bottle only partially with water, when you squeeze it, there is not enough force to push a large amount of water out. But, if you put as much water in the squirt bottle as it will hold and then squeeze, a small squeeze will cause a larger amount of water to squirt out with a lot more force. In other words, the heart is able to perform more efficiently when the ventricles are filled because less force is required to send the maximum amount of blood out to the body.

As you may recall from Chapter 20, there are two distinct sounds that you will hear with your stethoscope when you are taking an apical pulse. The first sound, "lubb," is the sound of the tricuspid and mitral valves (the valves that separate the atria from the ventricles) snapping shut during ventricular systole. The second sound, "dupp," is the sound of the pulmonary and aortic valves closing during ventricular diastole. The two sounds heard together ("lubb–dupp") is what we know as a heartbeat.

Regulation

Although transport is the cardiovascular system's major function, this system also plays a role in temperature regulation, as discussed in Chapter 29.

Protection

The cardiovascular system helps to protect the body in two major ways. First, white blood cells, which play an important role in helping us to fight off disease, are circulated throughout the body in the blood. Second, when injury to the body occurs, the blood has the ability to form a clot. The clot helps to protect us against excessive blood loss. It also helps to prevent microbes from gaining access to the body.

THE EFFECTS OF AGING ON THE CARDIOVASCULAR SYSTEM

Cardiovascular disorders are very common in the United States, especially among older people. Perhaps more than any other organ system, the cardiovascular system is affected by diet and lifestyle habits. For example, smoking, poor dietary habits, and a lack of exercise can all contribute to cardiovascular disease later in life. In addition, common medical problems, such as diabetes, obesity, and hypertension (high blood pressure) can cause the cardiovascular system to age faster.

Many national organizations, such as the American Heart Association, provide information and education about "healthy heart living." The American Heart Association recently embarked on an enhanced mission to stop heart disease before it's even started by sharing a message called "Life's Simple 7." The key components of "Life's Simple 7" are:

- Manage Blood Pressure: High blood pressure is a major risk factor for heart disease and stroke. Medication, exercise, a diet lower in sodium (salt), and weight control can help to keep blood pressure in a healthy range.
- Control Cholesterol: High cholesterol contributes to the formation of plaque, which can clog arteries and lead to heart disease. A healthy diet and medications (if needed) can help control cholesterol.
- Reduce Blood Sugar: Diets high in sugar and uncontrolled diabetes can lead to high blood sugar levels. Over time, this can cause damage to your heart, kidneys, eyes, and nerves.
- Get Active: Daily physical activity helps to keep the heart muscle strong, enhances the function of almost all body systems, and can increase your length and quality of life.
- Eat Better: A healthy diet that is low in saturated (unhealthy) fats is one of your best weapons for fighting cardiovascular disease (Fig. 32-9).
- Lose Weight: When you lose extra fat and unnecessary pounds, you reduce the workload placed on your heart, lungs, blood vessels, and skeleton. Losing weight can also help you reduce your chances of getting diabetes, or help control diabetes if you have it.
- Stop Smoking: Chemicals in tobacco smoke cause the arterioles and capillaries to constrict, depriving tissues of vital blood flow. Smoking should be avoided because it has a very negative impact on the heart, which requires a healthy supply of oxygen and nutrients to function properly.

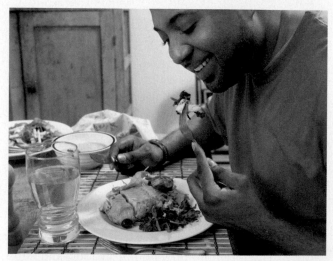

Figure 32-9 Regular exercise and a diet that is low in artery-clogging saturated fat are essential for maintaining a healthy heart throughout life.

In addition to preventing problems that affect the cardiovascular system directly, exercising, eating a healthy diet, and avoidance of tobacco smoke can help to prevent or control medical conditions that can contribute to cardiovascular disease, such as obesity, diabetes, and hypertension. By following the advice of these organizations, many people are able to maintain good cardiovascular function well into old age.

There are changes to the cardiovascular system that take place simply as a result of the aging process. In a healthy older person, these changes do not have a major impact on day-to-day life. However, when the processes of aging are combined with a chronic illness or a lifetime of unhealthy habits, the effect on cardiovascular function can be major. Age-related changes that occur include less efficient contraction of the heart, a loss of elasticity in the arteries and veins, and decreased numbers of blood cells.

Less Efficient Heart Contraction

Changes in the tissues of the heart, such as a loss of muscle tone and a loss of elasticity, affect the ability of the heart to contract forcefully, and it takes longer for the heart to complete the cycle of filling and emptying. A healthy older person might find that they tire faster while exercising because the heart is not able to deliver oxygen and nutrients to the body as efficiently as it once was, in times of increased demand. Medical conditions, such as obesity or hypertension, place additional strain on the heart muscle and make the effects of normal aging on the heart worse. The heart of an older person who is ill may barely be able to meet the body's needs for oxygen and nutrients when the person is at rest.

Decreased Elasticity of the Arteries and Veins

As we age, the walls of the blood vessels lose some of their elasticity. The loss of elasticity in the muscle layer of the arteries decreases the body's ability to control blood pressure and flow because the arteries are not able to expand and "bounce back" as easily. The "stretch" is gone from the vessel. The effects of this age-related change are especially noticeable when an older person with cardiovascular disease gets up quickly after lying down. Blood falls into the legs when we stand up, so blood pressure in the upper body decreases. Normally, the body senses low blood pressure and stimulates actions such as increased heart rate and vessel narrowing that increase blood pressure back to normal. However, the body can only sense the decrease in blood pressure if arteries are stretchy. If they are not, the body cannot react quickly enough to maintain adequate blood flow to the brain, and the person feels dizzy or lightheaded as a result. In other words, the person has orthostatic hypotension (see Chapter 20).

The loss of elasticity in the walls of the veins causes them to "stretch out," slowing the flow of blood back to the heart. The valves in the walls of the veins become less effective, which also slows the return of blood to the heart. Immobility and bed rest can worsen the effects of aging on the veins because the large muscles of the legs are not working to help move the blood back toward the heart.

Decreased Numbers of Blood Cells

The production of blood cells slows as a person ages. A decreased number of red blood cells affect the blood's ability to deliver oxygen to the tissues. A decreased number of white blood cells put the older person at higher risk for developing infections because the body's ability to fight them off is reduced.

DISORDERS OF THE CARDIOVASCULAR SYSTEM

Disorders of the cardiovascular system can involve the blood, the blood vessels, or the heart.

Disorders of the Blood

Blood disorders are often detected through laboratory analysis of the blood. Common blood disorders include anemia, leukemia, and clotting disorders.

Anemia

Anemia is a general term for a group of disorders affecting the red blood cells. Anemia decreases the blood's ability to transport oxygen to the cells. People who have anemia may become tired very easily. Their red blood cells simply are not able to transport the extra oxygen that is needed for exertion.

Anemia can result when the number of red blood cells is decreased, either because red blood cell production is impaired or the person is losing blood. For example, a disorder that affects the bone marrow, where blood cells are made, can cause a decrease in the number of circulating red blood cells, leading to anemia. Slow chronic blood loss (for example, from heavy menstrual periods or a stomach ulcer) can also cause anemia just by decreasing the amount of circulating blood.

Sometimes the number of red blood cells is adequate, but the red blood cells do not contain enough hemoglobin. Recall that hemoglobin is the molecule

Figure 32-10 In sickle cell anemia, the red blood cells are abnormally shaped. Here, normal red blood cells are shown alongside the crescent-shaped sickled red blood cells. (*extender_01\Shutterstock.com*)

that binds with oxygen, so if the red blood cells lack hemoglobin, then they are unable to carry as much oxygen, resulting in anemia. The body needs iron to make hemoglobin. Therefore, people who have diets that are low in iron or certain B vitamins (which help the body to absorb iron from the digestive tract) are at risk for anemia.

In sickle cell disease, red blood cells are produced, but they are abnormally shaped (sickled), which makes them unable to carry oxygen (Fig. 32-10). The abnormal shape of the sickled cells also causes them to get stuck in the tiny capillaries, obstructing the flow of blood and causing pain, swelling, and fevers. Sickle cell disease is an inherited disorder that is more common among people of African or Mediterranean heritage.

Leukemia

Leukemia is a cancer resulting in excessive production of white blood cells. The white blood cells are abnormal in structure and cannot perform their job of protecting the body from infection. Leukemia can be caused by cancer of the bone marrow or by cancer of the lymphatic tissue. Leukemia occurs in people of all ages and can cause death if treatment is started too late or is not effective. People who have leukemia are at higher risk for developing infections. They may also have bleeding disorders, which can cause them to bruise very easily or bleed from their gums during oral care.

Bleeding Disorders

There are two types of bleeding disorders. Either the blood clots too much, or not enough.

In some people, the blood clots too easily. Clots can form in the small blood vessels, blocking the flow of blood and depriving the tissues of oxygen and nutrients. The blood clots, called **thrombi**, can also break loose and travel to other parts of the body such as the brain, lungs, or heart. A blood clot that moves from one place to another is called an **embolus**. An embolus can be life-threatening. For example, the embolus may become stuck in the pulmonary artery, the artery that receives blood in need of oxygen from the heart. If blood cannot reach the lungs, then it cannot pick up the oxygen it needs for the rest of the body. People who have blood that clots too easily may need to take drugs called anticoagulants or "blood thinners" to help keep clots from forming where they are not needed.

Other people have the opposite problem—their blood does not form clots when it is supposed to (for example, after an injury). These people may lack one of many proteins that regulate clot formation. They may also lack fibrinogen, the blood protein that helps form the clot. Or, they may have a low platelet count. (Recall that platelets are the blood cells that participate in clot formation.) One type of leukemia affects the body's ability to form platelets. For these people, even a small bump can cause a large bruise, while a more severe injury can result in a fatal hemorrhage.

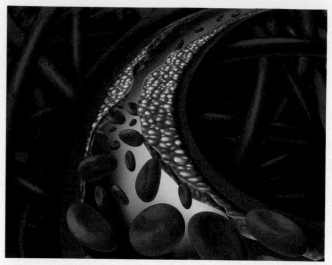

Figure 32-11 In atherosclerosis, fatty plaque builds up on the inside of the arteries, blocking the free flow of blood. This is particularly dangerous when the artery supplies a vital organ such as the heart, brain, or kidneys. (*Lightspring\Shutterstock.com*)

through the arteries because **plaque** (a fatty deposit) builds up on the inside of the vessel wall (Fig. 32-11). As a result, less oxygen and nutrients are delivered to the tissues of the body. In addition, plaque makes the normally smooth inner lining of the artery rough, which can cause blood clots to form. Sometimes the clots break off and become emboli. The plaque also weakens the vessel wall. The weakened vessel can burst, leading to hemorrhages (bleeding). Finally, the plaque interferes with the elasticity of the arterial walls, making them stiffer and less elastic. Atherosclerosis is a form of **arteriosclerosis,** which means "arterial hardening." This "hardening of the arteries" can lead to hemorrhages (bleeding) in the small vessels.

Depending on which arteries are affected, atherosclerosis can have serious consequences. The arteries that supply the brain, heart, kidneys, and legs are affected most often.

- Atherosclerosis of the arteries that supply the brain can cause a stroke. Strokes are discussed in detail in Chapter 33.
- Atherosclerosis of the arteries that supply the heart can cause myocardial infarction (MI) ("heart attack"). MI is discussed later in this chapter.
- Atherosclerosis of the arteries that supply the kidneys can cause renal failure, discussed in Chapter 37.
- Atherosclerosis of the arteries that supply the legs can cause **peripheral vascular disease (PVD)**. In peripheral vascular disease, decreased

Tell the Nurse!

People who are taking anticoagulant medications and those with disorders that affect the ability of the blood to form clots are at risk for bleeding, which can have serious consequences. Be sure to report any of the following observations to the nurse immediately:

- Any signs of bruising or bleeding under the skin
- Bleeding from any area of the body (such as the gums or nose)
- Blood in the urine or stool

Disorders of the Blood Vessels

In addition to disorders of the blood, it is also possible for people to develop disorders of the blood vessels themselves. Common disorders of the blood vessels include atherosclerosis and venous (vein-related) disorders.

Atherosclerosis

Atherosclerosis is a narrowing of the arteries that can result in blockage. Blood is unable to flow freely

blood flow to the leg muscles causes pain and cramping when the person walks. The pain and cramping, called *claudication*, occurs because the muscles are not receiving enough oxygen. In severe cases, the tissues in the leg die from lack of oxygen, and amputation may be necessary.

Although the exact cause of atherosclerosis is unknown, scientists now know that several factors contribute to the development of the disease. Diabetes, hypertension, and obesity are all medical conditions that have been associated with atherosclerosis. Heredity and stress may also play a role. Smoking, eating a diet high in cholesterol and saturated (unhealthy) fat, and a lack of physical activity can also increase a person's chances of developing atherosclerosis.

Venous Disorders

Loss of elasticity and decreased efficiency of the valves in the walls of the veins cause blood to "pool" in the legs, which can put the person at risk for several venous (vein-related) disorders:

- **Varicose veins.** In this condition, pooling of blood in the veins (especially the veins in the lower legs, causes the veins to become swollen and "knotty" in appearance (Fig. 32-12). A person with varicose veins may experience pain, aching, swelling, or a feeling of heaviness in the legs. Varicose veins also put the person at risk for

developing other venous disorders, such as phlebitis or venous (stasis) ulcers.

- **Phlebitis.** In this condition, pooling of blood in the vein causes the lining of the vein to become inflamed. The skin over the affected vein is reddened, and the area feels hard and hot to the touch. Phlebitis is often very painful.
- **Venous thrombosis.** In this disorder, blood clots (thrombi) form in the veins where the blood pools because the blood is moving so slowly. When the blood clots cause inflammation of the lining of the vein, you may hear this condition referred to as **thrombophlebitis**. Blood clots can form in the superficial veins or the deep veins. When the blood clots occur in the deep veins, the condition is called **deep venous thrombosis (DVT)**. Pain, redness, swelling, and warmth in the lower leg are all possible signs of DVT and should be reported to the nurse immediately. People with DVT are at high risk for **pulmonary embolism**, a life-threatening condition that occurs when an embolus becomes stuck in the pulmonary artery, the artery that carries oxygen-poor blood from the heart to the lungs. If blood cannot reach the lungs, then it cannot pick up the oxygen it needs for the rest of the body.
- **Venous (stasis) ulcers.** These ulcers are seen on the lower legs, usually in the ankle area. The pressure of the pooled blood in the veins forces

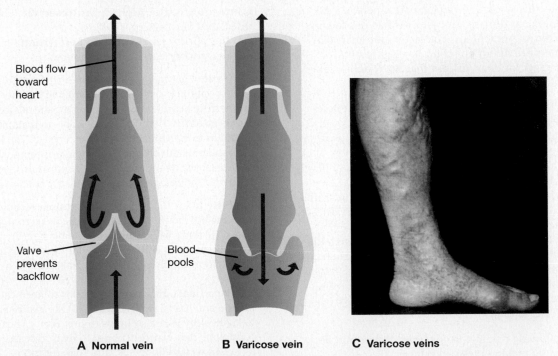

A Normal vein   **B** Varicose vein   **C** Varicose veins

Figure 32-12 Many older people, particularly females, have varicose veins. **A.** In a healthy vein, the valves help blood to flow back toward the heart and prevent it from pooling. **B.** In varicose veins, the valves no longer function properly, allowing the blood to pool. **C.** The pooling of blood in the veins causes them to become swollen and "knotty" in appearance.

plasma out of the blood vessels and into the surrounding tissues. Swelling occurs, and the skin becomes fragile and inflamed. Eventually, the skin breaks down, resulting in an open sore.

In general, people with venous disorders experience pain and have difficulty with mobility. The doctor may order the use of leg exercises, antiembolism (TED) stockings, or intermittent pneumatic compression (IPC) devices (see Chapter 43) to treat or prevent venous disorders.

Leg Exercises

Leg exercises help to move blood back to the heart and prevent the formation of clots. The doctor or physical therapist may order the leg exercises you learned as part of the range-of-motion exercises described in Chapter 30 (Procedure 30-1) to be carried out at routine times. Or, a specific exercise routine may be ordered. Always check with the nurse to see if there are any specific instructions or precautions for your patient or resident.

Antiembolism (TED) Stockings

TED stockings are made of a snug-fitting elastic fabric. The stockings, which may be knee-high or thigh-high, are specially fitted for the person by the nurse or the physical therapist. The elastic fabric applies pressure, compressing the veins and helping to return blood to the heart. This helps to prevent pooling of blood in the legs.

TED stockings are usually ordered to be applied before the person gets out of bed. Once the person stands up, gravity increases blood flow to the veins in the lower legs, causing the veins to widen and the blood to pool. The TED stockings are usually removed at bed time. Procedure 32-1 describes how to apply TED stockings.

Disorders of the Heart

Heart disorders affect children as well as adults. Most heart disorders in children are *congenital*, which means that they were "present at birth." Congenital heart disorders occur when the fetus's heart does not form correctly. Many babies who are born with congenital heart disorders grow up to live long and healthy lives following surgery to correct the heart defect.

Heart disorders are very common in the United States, especially among older people. Perhaps more than any other organ, the heart is affected by diet and lifestyle factors (Box 32-1). Common heart disorders in adults include coronary artery disease (CAD), heart failure, and dysrhythmias.

Box 32-1   Risk Factors for Heart Disease

Conditions that are known to increase a person's risk of developing heart disease are called cardiac risk factors. We can control some of our risk factors for heart disease. Others are out of our control.

Risk factors for heart disease that we cannot change include the following:

- **Age.** The risk of developing heart disease increases with age.
- **Sex.** Males are at greater risk of developing heart disease at an earlier age than females. However, after a female goes through menopause, their risk of developing heart disease is the same as a male's.
- **Heredity.** People who have parents or siblings with heart disease are more likely to develop heart disease themselves.
- **Body build.** Some people tend to accumulate fat in their abdominal cavity, resulting in an "apple"-shaped body profile, while others tend to accumulate fat just under the skin of the buttocks or thighs ("pears"). "Apple"-shaped people are more likely to develop heart disease than "pear"-shaped people.

The following risk factors for heart disease can be controlled by making lifestyle changes:

- **Smoking**
- **Being physically inactive**
- **Having a body mass index (BMI) above 25.0**

- **Consuming a diet high in saturated fat, cholesterol, and sodium**
- **Having poorly controlled hypertension**
- **Having poorly controlled diabetes**

Many national organizations, such as the American Heart Association, provide information and education about "healthy heart living." By following the advice of these organizations, many people are able to maintain good cardiovascular function well into old age. The keys to cardiovascular health are exercise; a diet that emphasizes fruits, vegetables, whole grains, and healthy fats (and is low in unhealthy saturated fats); and avoidance of smoking.

- **Exercise** helps to keep the heart muscle strong and working efficiently. Exercise also helps us to maintain a healthy body weight and is an important measure for preventing or controlling conditions that can contribute to heart disease, such as diabetes and hypertension.
- **Eating a heart-healthy diet** helps to keep the heart muscle and blood vessels healthy. Like exercise, a heart-healthy diet also helps to prevent or control conditions that can contribute to heart disease, such as excess weight, diabetes, and hypertension.
- **Avoiding smoking** is important because chemicals in tobacco smoke cause the blood vessels to constrict, depriving the heart of the oxygen and nutrients it needs to function properly.

Coronary Artery Disease

Coronary artery disease occurs when the coronary arteries narrow as a result of atherosclerosis. Recall that the coronary arteries supply the heart muscle with blood containing oxygen and nutrients. Initially, the heart muscle may receive enough oxygen to work properly when the body is at rest, but it may be unable to meet the increased needs brought on by activity. Eventually, one or more of the coronary arteries may become so narrow that no blood gets through, causing areas of the heart muscle to die.

Coronary artery disease (CAD) is treated in a number of ways. Medications are available that help to keep the arteries open, permitting maximum blood flow. Balloon angioplasty is a technique that involves inserting a catheter with a small balloon on the tip into the narrow part of the affected artery. The balloon is inflated, pressing the plaque against the arterial wall to create a larger opening for the blood to flow through. Then the balloon is deflated and the catheter is removed (Fig. 32-13A). Sometimes, balloon angioplasty is done along with placement of a small coiled wire called a *stent*. The stent supports the artery walls, helping to keep the artery open (see Fig. 32-13B). When the blockage is severe, surgery may be performed to bypass the blocked arteries and reestablish blood flow. The medical term for this type of surgery is coronary artery bypass graft (CABG) surgery. The acronym CABG is pronounced like "cabbage."

Conditions that are closely related to CAD include angina pectoris and MI.

Angina Pectoris

Angina pectoris is the classic chest pain that is felt as a result of the heart muscle being deprived of oxygen. Anginal pain varies among individuals. Some people

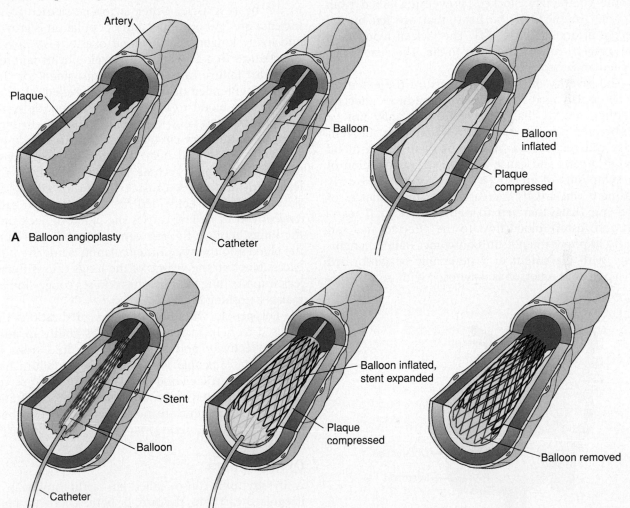

Figure 32-13 **A.** In balloon angioplasty, a catheter with a balloon on the tip is passed into the narrowed part of the artery. The balloon is expanded, pushing the plaque to the sides of the arterial wall and widening the artery. **B.** Sometimes, balloon angioplasty is done along with stent placement. The stent, a small wire cage, provides additional support to keep the artery open.

describe it as a pain in the center of the chest. Others experience pain that starts in the chest and extends to the arm or neck. A person who is experiencing angina may feel as though they are suffocating, and they may become very anxious.

Many people experience angina quite frequently and know what it is. These people often keep nitroglycerin pills on hand to relieve the pain when it occurs. Nitroglycerin widens the arteries, increasing the flow of blood. If you have been trained to help a person with their nitroglycerin, avoid handling the pills with your bare hands. The drug can be absorbed through the skin, which can cause a decrease in your blood pressure and a pounding headache.

Myocardial Infarction

A **myocardial infarction** is a "heart attack." An MI occurs when one or more of the coronary arteries become completely blocked, preventing blood from reaching the parts of the heart that are fed by the affected arteries (Fig. 32-14). The lack of blood (and vital oxygen) causes the tissue to die. The dead tissue is called an *infarct*.

The severity of the MI depends on the extent of the tissue damaged and the part of the heart affected. Although an MI that affects the atria may not be life-threatening, one that severely damages the ventricles can reduce the heart's ability to pump blood to vital organs and cause death. Early recognition of the symptoms of an MI (see Chapter 16) and early treatment can greatly increase a person's chances of surviving. Drugs that help to maintain a normal heartbeat and restore blood flow to the affected area can greatly improve the person's outcome. Balloon angioplasty with placement of a stent may be performed very soon after a person is diagnosed with an MI. This

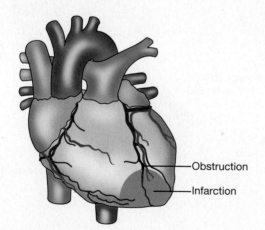

Figure 32-14 A heart attack occurs when one or more of the coronary arteries become blocked, preventing blood from reaching the myocardium. The lack of oxygen and nutrients causes the tissue that is supplied by the affected artery to die.

helps to restore blood flow and prevent further damage to the heart muscle.

Heart Failure

Heart failure occurs when the heart is unable to pump enough blood to meet the body's needs. Heart failure has many causes. For example, disorders that cause the ventricles to lose muscle tone and become large and flabby can cause heart failure. Heart failure can also occur as a result of an MI that leaves the ventricles unable to function properly.

At this time, the number of people in the United States who have heart failure is increasing and expected to rise to more than 8 million people affected by this disorder by 2030. One reason is related to advances in treatment for MI that are allowing more people to survive. This increases the risk that the person will later develop heart failure as a result of the initial damage to the heart muscle. Other factors attributed to this increase are that our older adult population is growing and living longer. Diabetes and obesity also increase the chances that a person will develop heart failure.

Heart failure can be either "right-sided" or "left-sided." Right-sided heart failure, also called *cor pulmonale*, causes blood to back up in the venous system because the right ventricle's ability to pump the blood into the pulmonary circulation is impaired. In a person with right-sided heart failure, the veins in the legs and abdomen become swollen, and fluid may leak into the tissues, causing significant edema and skin breakdown. Left-sided heart failure, also called *congestive heart failure*, causes the blood to back up in the lungs because the left ventricle's ability to pump the blood into the systemic circulation is impaired. The excess blood in the vessels of the lungs causes fluid to leak into the lung tissues, which causes congestion and makes breathing difficult.

For people with heart failure, medications may be used to help increase the heart's ability to pump more effectively and to pull excess fluid from the tissues. Many people with severe heart failure have their fluids restricted and their intake and output very carefully measured and monitored. When medication and other treatment are no longer effective, a heart transplant may be necessary.

Dysrhythmias

A dysrhythmia (also called an arrhythmia) is an irregular heart rate, rhythm, or both. There are many different types of dysrhythmias. Dysrhythmias can occur when the conduction system of the heart is not working properly. Dysrhythmias can cause a person to experience heart palpitations, fatigue, dizziness, or fainting. Dysrhythmias can also increase the person's risk for a heart attack or stroke. Many of your patients or residents will take medications to control a dysrhythmia.

Heart block is a common type of dysrhythmia. Heart block can result from an MI that damages the conduction pathway, or it may occur as part of the normal aging process. A heart block causes the heart to slow down significantly, leading to dizziness or fainting episodes.

Heart block is usually treated with a pacemaker, an electrical device that stimulates the heart to contract. The pacemaker consists of a small, battery-operated device implanted under the skin below the collarbone and two wires that connect to the right side of the heart (Fig. 32-15). When the person's heart rate drops below a programmed rate, the battery-operated device sends a small electrical impulse through the wires that stimulates the heart muscle to contract.

Taking It to the Next Level:

Advanced Skills

More in-depth information related to advanced skills used when providing care for a person with cardiovascular disorders can be found in *Lippincott Acute Care Skills for Advanced Nursing Assistants.*

Visit thePoint® at thepoint.lww.com for access to the ebook.

DIAGNOSIS OF CARDIOVASCULAR DISORDERS

Depending on where you work, you may be responsible for caring for people who are recovering from an acute cardiovascular disorder, such as a heart attack. Other people will be admitted to the hospital to have a

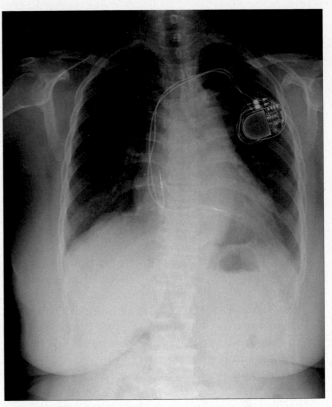

Figure 32-15 A pacemaker is a battery-operated device used to treat heart block. The pacemaker sends out an electrical signal that stimulates the heart to contract when the person's heart rate drops below a pre-programmed rate. In this x-ray, you can see the pacemaker (*in red*) above the person's ribcage. The wires, or leads, connect the pacemaker to the person's heart. (*Tridsanu Thopet\Shutterstock.com*)

procedure done to prevent a heart attack from occurring, such as balloon angioplasty. Often, people with cardiovascular disorders will have one or more tests done to help the doctor determine the extent of the

---

Tell the Nurse!

The routine taking of vital signs, especially the pulse and blood pressure, is one of the best ways to detect abnormalities in the functioning of the cardiovascular system at an early stage. In addition, there are many signs and symptoms you may observe that could indicate that a patient or resident is having a cardiovascular problem. Report any of the following observations to the nurse immediately:

- Complaints of chest pain or pressure
- Labored or difficult breathing
- A rapid or erratic pulse
- A slow, weak pulse
- A blood pressure reading that is either much higher or much lower than the person's usual reading
- Cyanosis of the face, lips, or fingers

- Decreased tolerance for usual exertion
- Red, painful, or swollen areas in the extremities, especially the calves of the legs
- Unusual swelling of the legs, especially if it is accompanied by red, shiny skin
- "Dusky" (blue or grayish) coloring of the legs, especially if it is accompanied by a diminished pulse and coldness of the skin

problem, plan a course of treatment, and monitor the person after the treatment. Tests you may hear mentioned include the following:

- **Electrocardiography.** In electrocardiography, sensors are attached to the person's chest. These sensors pick up the electrical activity of the heart and record it on a piece of paper. The tracing is called an *electrocardiogram* (EKG, ECG). An EKG shows abnormalities in the conduction system of the heart. Some people have an EKG done while they are exercising. This is called a stress test (Fig. 32-16).
- **Echocardiography.** In echocardiography, sound waves are bounced against the body to produce an image. A computer translates the sound waves into an image. Echocardiography can provide the doctor with much helpful information, including the size and shape of the heart, its pumping strength, and the location and extent of any damage to its tissues (especially the valves).
- **Doppler ultrasound.** In Doppler ultrasound, sound waves are used to check the blood flow in the large arteries and veins of the arms and legs.
- **Radiography.** Radiographs, commonly known as "x-rays," are often used in the diagnosis of cardiovascular disease. A chest x-ray can show

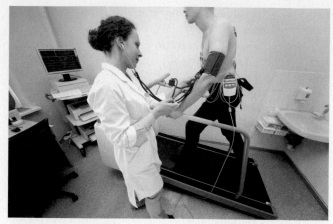

Figure 32-16 Electrocardiography is commonly used for diagnosis and monitoring of heart problems. This person is having a cardiac stress test. In a cardiac stress test, an electrocardiogram (EKG) is obtained while the person exercises. (*Pavel L Photo and Video\Shutterstock.com*)

enlargement of the ventricles. Sometimes, a special dye is injected into the veins and then an x-ray is taken. The dye allows the doctor to see any abnormalities in the vessels of the heart or other parts of the body.

SUMMARY

- The cardiovascular system, also known as the circulatory system, is made up of the blood, the blood vessels, and the heart. It is closely associated with the lymphatic system.
  - Blood consists of plasma and blood cells (red blood cells, white blood cells, and platelets).
  - Arteries carry blood away from the heart, and veins carry blood to the heart. The transfer of substances into and out of the blood occurs in the capillary bed.
  - The lymphatic system is a one-way system that returns fluid that leaks into the tissues to the bloodstream.
  - The heart is the muscular organ that powers circulation.
    - The heart has four chambers. The atria receive blood from the body, and the ventricles send blood to the body.
    - The heart valves make sure that blood flows through the heart in the proper direction.
    - The heart's conduction system makes and conducts the electrical impulses that cause the heart to contract regularly.

- The coronary circulation supplies the heart muscle with oxygen and nutrients.
- The main function of the cardiovascular system is to transport oxygen, nutrients, and other substances *to* the tissues, and to remove carbon dioxide and other wastes *from* the tissues.
  - The pattern of circulation involves two parallel circuits. The right side of the heart pumps blood into the lungs, where it picks up oxygen. The left side of the heart pumps the oxygenated blood to the rest of the body.
  - During systole, the heart contracts, sending blood out of the heart. During diastole, the heart relaxes, allowing the chambers to fill.
- When the effects of aging are combined with a lifetime of unhealthy habits or a chronic disease, the effect on cardiovascular function can be major.
  - Exercising, eating a diet low in saturated fat and cholesterol, and avoiding tobacco smoke help to keep the cardiovascular system healthy. Controlling chronic diseases such as diabetes and hypertension is also important.

- Risk factors for cardiovascular disease that cannot be changed include age, sex, heredity, and body build.
- Disorders of the cardiovascular system can affect the blood, the blood vessels, or the heart.
  - Disorders of the blood include anemia, leukemia, and bleeding disorders.
  - Disorders of the blood vessels include atherosclerosis, venous thrombosis, and venous (stasis) ulcers.
    - Atherosclerosis is narrowing of the arteries due to the buildup of plaque. Depending on which arteries are affected, atherosclerosis can lead to strokes, heart attacks, kidney failure, or peripheral vascular disease.
    - Disorders that affect the veins are usually caused by widening of the veins, which allows blood to pool in the legs. Venous disorders often cause pain and swelling and contribute to mobility problems.

- Disorders of the heart include coronary artery disease (CAD), heart failure, and dysrhythmias.
  - CAD is caused by a narrowing of the arteries that supply the heart muscle with oxygen and nutrients.
    - Angina pectoris is chest pain that results from the heart muscle being deprived of oxygen.
    - A myocardial infarction occurs when the blood supply to the heart muscle is completely obstructed.
  - Heart failure results from the heart's inability to pump blood in sufficient amounts to supply the body.
  - Dysrhythmias can occur when the conduction system of the heart is not working properly. A person with heart block, a type of dysrhythmia, may have a pacemaker implanted to stimulate regular contraction of the heart.

▶ **Procedure 32-1**

Applying Antiembolism (TED) Stockings

WHY YOU DO IT Use of TED stockings as ordered helps to prevent the formation of blood clots in the lower legs.

Getting Ready

1. Complete the "Getting Ready" steps.

Supplies

■ TED stockings in the correct size

Procedure

2. Make sure that the bed is positioned at a comfortable working height (to promote good body mechanics) and that the wheels are locked. If the side rails are in use, lower the side rail on the working side of the bed. The side rail on the opposite side of the bed should remain up.

3. Help the person into the supine position.

4. Fanfold the top linens to the foot of the bed. Adjust the person's hospital gown or pajama bottoms as necessary to expose one leg at a time.

5. Turn the stocking inside out down to the heel.

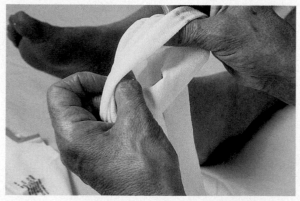

STEP 5 Turn the stocking inside out down to the heel.

6. Slip the foot of the stocking over the person's toes, foot, and heel. The stocking has an opening in the toe area, which allows the health care team to assess the person's toes to make sure they are receiving enough blood. Depending on the manufacturer, this opening may be on the top or on the bottom of the stocking.

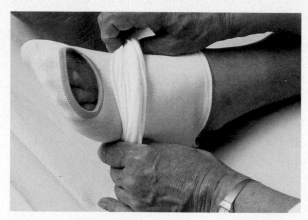

STEP 6 Slip the foot of the stocking over the person's toes, foot, and heel.

7. Grasp the top of the stocking and pull it up the person's leg. The stocking will turn itself right-side out as you pull it up the person's leg.

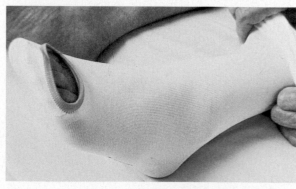

STEP 7 Grasp the top of the stocking and pull it up the person's leg.

8. Check to make sure that the stocking is not twisted and that it fits snugly against the person's leg, with no wrinkles. Also make sure that the stocking fits smoothly over the heel and that the opening in the toe area is correctly located in the toe region.

9. Cover that leg, expose the other leg, and repeat steps 5 through 8.

10. Help the person back into a comfortable position, straighten the bottom linens, and draw the top linens over the person. Raise the head of the bed as the person requests. Make sure that the bed is lowered to its lowest position and that the wheels are locked.

Finishing Up

11. Complete the "Finishing Up" steps.

What You Record

- Date and time
- Condition of person's skin on legs and feet. (Be especially observant of reddened, warm, or painful areas on the calves.)

WHAT DID YOU LEARN?

Multiple Choice

Select the single best answer for each of the following questions.

1. The formation of artery-clogging plaque on the inside of the arteries is called:
   a. Atherosclerosis
   b. Arterioles
   c. Anemia
   d. Myocardial infarction

2. What is the function of the cardiovascular system?
   a. Transport of substances throughout the body
   b. Regulation of body temperature
   c. Protection of the body from blood loss and infection
   d. All of the above

3. Which circulation supplies the tissues of the heart with oxygen and nutrients?
   a. Pulmonary circulation
   b. Cerebral circulation
   c. Coronary circulation
   d. Pericardial circulation

4. Which of the following is a risk factor for cardiovascular disease?
   a. Poorly controlled hypertension
   b. A diet high in cholesterol and saturated fats
   c. Lack of physical activity
   d. All of the above

Matching *Match each numbered item with its appropriate lettered description.*

_____ **1.** Red blood cells

_____ **2.** White blood cells (leukocytes)

_____ **3.** Ventricles

_____ **4.** Veins

_____ **5.** Atria

_____ **6.** Arteries

_____ **7.** Systole

_____ **8.** Pulmonary circulation

_____ **9.** Systemic circulation

_____ **10.** Diastole

a. Upper chambers of the heart, which receive blood from the body
b. Vessels that carry blood away from the heart
c. Active phase of the cardiac cycle
d. Blood cells that help the body to fight infection
e. Circuit that sends newly oxygenated blood to the body
f. Resting phase of the cardiac cycle
g. Blood cells that contain hemoglobin and carry oxygen
h. Lower chambers of the heart, which pump blood to the body
i. Circuit that sends oxygen-poor blood to the lungs to pick up oxygen
j. Vessels that return blood to the heart

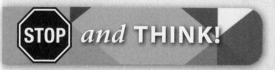

STOP *and* THINK!

You are caring for Mr. Becker, a 74-year-old man with a history of heart disease. Mr. Becker keeps nitroglycerin in his bedside table to use when he has an angina attack. As you are assisting Mr. Becker back into his room from the dining room, he starts to complain of a tightness in his chest and seems to be having difficulty breathing. His lips also look a little blue. He asks you to help him with his nitroglycerin pill. What safety precaution needs to be taken while handling nitroglycerin? What else should you do?

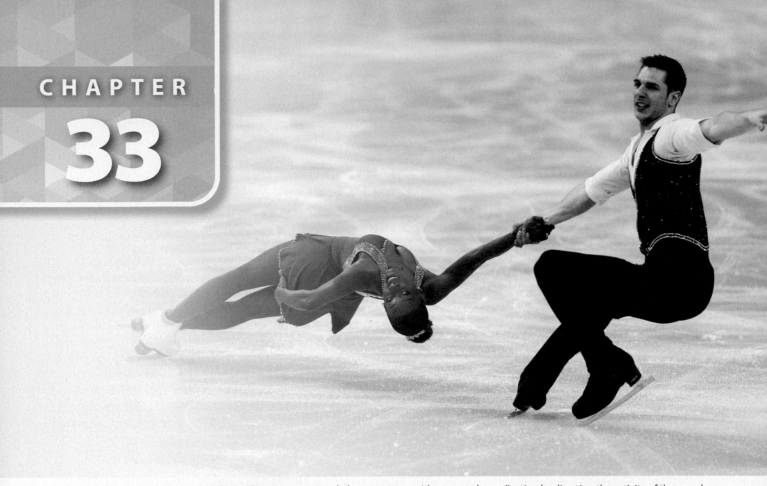

Photo: The nervous system helps us to move with grace and coordination by directing the activity of the muscles.
(Iurii Osadchi\Shutterstock.com)

The Nervous System

 WHAT WILL YOU LEARN?

The nervous system consists of the brain, the spinal cord, and the nerves. The nervous system receives information at a great rate, from both inside the body and outside of it. It then processes this information and issues instructions to other organ systems to carry out. "Command central" of the human body, the nervous system is the subject of this chapter. When you are finished with this chapter, you will be able to:

1. List and describe the structures that make up the two main divisions of the nervous system.
2. Discuss the main functions of the nervous system.
3. Describe how aging affects the nervous system.
4. Discuss various disorders that affect the nervous system.
5. List common diagnostic procedures that are used to help detect nervous system disorders.

Vocabulary

Neuron	Peripheral nervous	Transient ischemic attack	Coma
Dendrites	system (PNS)	(TIA)	Persistent vegetative
Axon	Meninges	Stroke	state
Synapse	Cerebrospinal fluid	Aphasia	
Myelin	(CSF)	Parkinson disease	
Central nervous system	Sensory nerves	Epilepsy	
(CNS)	Motor nerves	Multiple sclerosis (MS)	

STRUCTURE OF THE NERVOUS SYSTEM

Nervous tissue, which forms the organs of the nervous system, is made up of a special kind of cell called a neuron. A **neuron** is a cell that can send and receive information. A neuron consists of dendrites, a cell body, and an axon (Fig. 33-1). **Dendrites** are short extensions from the cell body that *receive* information. The **axon** is a long extension from the cell body that *sends* information. An electrical signal, called a nerve impulse, enters the neuron at the dendrites. It passes through the cell body and travels down the axon, and then on to the dendrites of the next neuron in line. The movement of the nerve impulse is called *conduction*. The axon of one neuron does not actually connect with the dendrites of the next (see Fig. 33-1). Instead, chemicals called neurotransmitters carry the nerve impulse across the gap between the axon of one neuron and the dendrites of the next. This gap is called a **synapse**. The axons of some neurons are wrapped in **myelin**, a fatty, white substance that protects the axon. Myelin also helps to speed the conduction of nerve impulses along the axon.

The nervous system has two main divisions, the central nervous system (CNS) and the peripheral nervous system (PNS) (Fig. 33-2). The **central nervous**

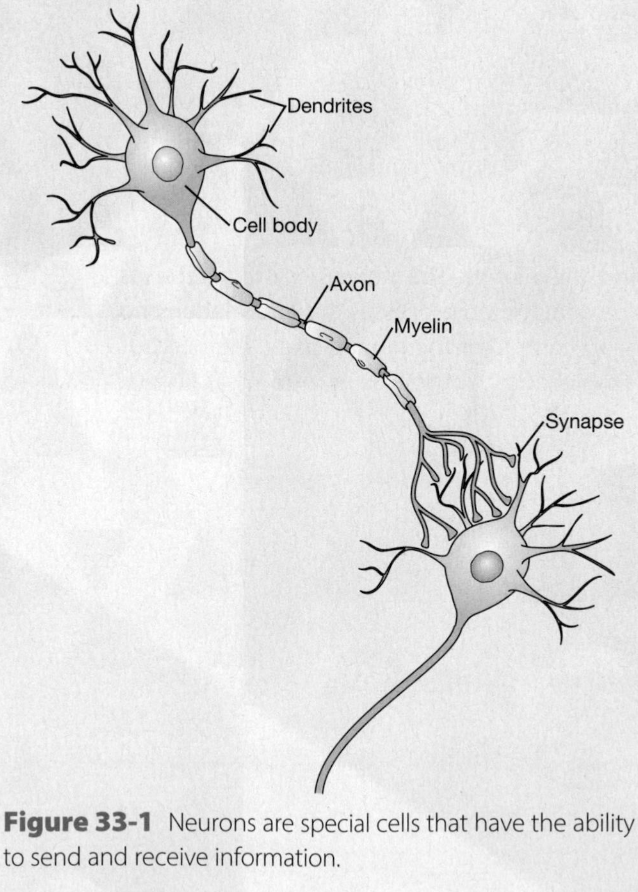

Figure 33-1 Neurons are special cells that have the ability to send and receive information.

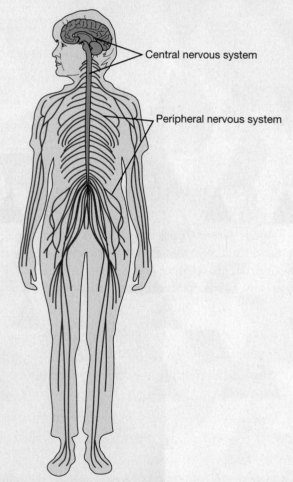

Figure 33-2 The nervous system has two main divisions, the central nervous system and the peripheral nervous system. "Peripheral" means "along the edge" or "away from the center."

system (CNS) consists of the brain and spinal cord. The CNS receives information, processes it, and issues instructions. The **peripheral nervous system (PNS)** consists of the nerves outside of the brain and spinal cord. A nerve is simply a bundle of axons, wrapped in a connective tissue sheath. The PNS receives information from the environment and carries commands from the brain and spinal cord to the other organs of the body, such as the muscles.

The Central Nervous System

Because it is so vital to the body's functioning, the central nervous system is well protected by three layers of connective tissue, called **meninges**, and the bony skull and vertebrae (Fig. 33-3). The three meninges are, from the inside out:

- The *pia mater*, a thin delicate layer of tissue rich in blood vessels that is attached to the surface of the brain and spinal cord
- The *arachnoid mater*, the web-like middle layer

- The *dura mater*, a thick, tough outer layer that is attached to the inside of the skull and the vertebrae

The space between the pia mater and the arachnoid mater contains **cerebrospinal fluid (CSF)**, a clear fluid that circulates around the brain and spinal cord and acts as an additional "shock absorber" to protect these structures.

The Brain

The brain, a large, soft mass of nervous tissue, is where information is processed and instructions are issued. The brain has four parts: the cerebrum, the diencephalon, the brain stem, and the cerebellum (see Fig. 33-3).

The Cerebrum

The cerebrum is the largest part of the brain, with the characteristic "folds" that you may picture when you think of a brain (see Fig. 33-3). The cerebrum:

- Controls the voluntary movement of muscles

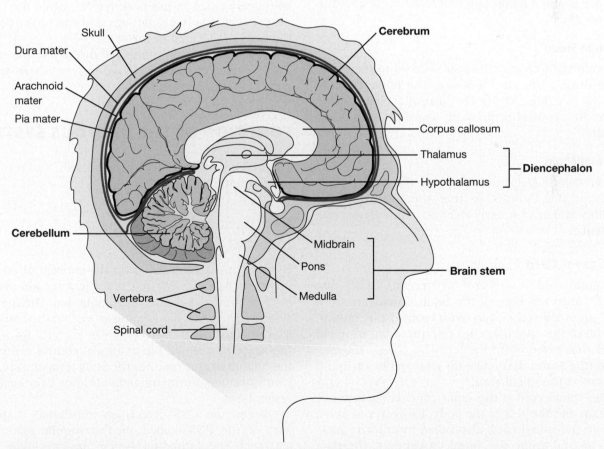

Figure 33-3 The brain and the spinal cord make up the CNS. The brain has four parts: the cerebrum, the diencephalon, the brain stem, and the cerebellum. Three layers of connective tissue, called the dura mater, the arachnoid mater, and the pia mater, help to cushion and protect the brain and spinal cord. Additional protection is provided by the bony skull and vertebrae.

- Gives meaning to information received from the eyes, ears, nose, taste buds, and sensory receptors in the skin
- Allows us to speak, remember, think, and feel emotions

A deep groove divides the cerebrum into two hemispheres, the left hemisphere (or "left brain") and the right hemisphere (or "right brain"). The right and left hemispheres communicate with each other and are connected by a structure called the *corpus callosum*. The right side of the brain controls the left side of the body, and vice versa. So, an injury to the tissues in the left side of the brain may result in loss of function on the right side of the body.

The Diencephalon

The diencephalon contains the thalamus and the hypothalamus (see Fig. 33-3). The thalamus sorts out the impulses that arrive via the spinal cord from other parts of the body and sends them to the correct part of the cerebrum. The hypothalamus controls body temperature, fluid balance, appetite, sleep cycles, and some of the emotions, and regulates the pituitary gland, a gland you will learn more about in Chapter 35.

The Brain Stem

The brain stem connects the spinal cord to the brain. It has three parts: the midbrain, the pons, and the medulla (see Fig. 33-3). The medulla contains the centers that control respiration, heartbeat, and blood pressure.

The Cerebellum

The cerebellum helps to coordinate the brain's commands to the muscles so that the muscles move smoothly and in an orderly fashion. It also plays a role in balance.

The Spinal Cord

The spinal cord is a "cord" of nervous tissue that extends from the base of the brain downward, to a point approximately even with your belly button. The end of the cord branches out into a fan of spinal nerves that extend into the legs and pelvis. The vertebrae (the bones that make up your spine) surround and protect the spinal cord.

The spinal cord is the main connection between the brain and the rest of the body. Pathways of nerve tissue in the spinal cord, also called *tracts*, carry messages to and from the brain. Ascending (heading upward) tracts carry information from the PNS to the brain. Descending (heading downward) tracts carry information from the brain to the PNS.

The Peripheral Nervous System

The PNS consists of the nerves, or the lines of communication between the central nervous system and the rest of the body. Every part of the body is innervated, or supplied, by nerves, which form a vast network throughout the body.

The nerves that form the PNS are either sensory nerves or motor nerves. **Sensory nerves** carry information from the "outside in." In other words, the sensory nerves carry information from the internal organs and the outside world to the spinal cord and up into the brain so that the brain can analyze the information. **Motor nerves** carry information from the "inside out." In other words, the motor nerves carry commands from the brain down the spinal cord and out to the muscles and organs of the body. Motor nerves allow the brain to control voluntary muscle movement and the involuntary functions of the internal organs.

Thirty-one pairs of nerves, called spinal nerves, connect to the spinal cord. Each spinal nerve contains both sensory and motor neurons. The spinal nerves that innervate the arms and the upper part of the body are located in the neck region, while the spinal nerves that innervate the legs and the lower part of the body are located in the back.

Some nerves are connected directly to the brain. These nerves are called cranial nerves. There are 12 pairs of cranial nerves.

FUNCTION OF THE NERVOUS SYSTEM

The nervous system receives, processes, and responds to information.

Regulation of the Internal Environment

By now, you are familiar with the concept of homeostasis, or balance. For the body to function well, a state of homeostasis must be maintained. The nervous system regulates what is going on within the body and makes adjustments as necessary to keep things within the range of normal. For example, control centers in the hypothalamus monitor the body temperature, and control centers in the medulla monitor heartbeat and respirations.

When the CNS detects an imbalance, a special part of the PNS, called the autonomic system, is activated. The autonomic system has two lower divisions, the sympathetic nervous system and the parasympathetic nervous system. Generally speaking, the sympathetic nervous system speeds things up, and the parasympathetic nervous system slows them back down. Perhaps you have heard of the "fight or flight" response. When we are put in a dangerous situation, our heart rate and breathing increase, and the adrenal glands release adrenaline, a chemical that helps us to cope with stress. These changes allow us to run faster or be stronger in a fight, and they are caused by activation of the sympathetic nervous system. Once the danger has passed, the parasympathetic nervous system slows things back down.

Interaction With the External Environment

The nervous system allows us to interact with the world around us. The special senses—touch, taste, smell, sight, and hearing—provide the brain with information about the outside world. The brain responds to this information. The ability to receive information about the outside world and respond to it not only makes life more pleasurable, it helps to protect us from harm. (The special senses are discussed in detail in Chapter 34.)

THE EFFECTS OF AGING ON THE NERVOUS SYSTEM

The cells of the CNS have a relatively low capacity for repair and replacement. As a result, the average person loses about 10% of their brain tissue between the ages of 50 and 90. Neurotransmitter levels are also slightly reduced. Nevertheless, healthy aging is associated with only minor changes in the functioning of the nervous system: slower reaction times, small attention deficits, and slight memory changes.

Slowed Reaction Times

You may notice that some of your older patients or residents are not as quick to react to things as they used to be. This is a normal age-related change that is caused by changes in the myelin sheath and the amount of neurotransmitters. As we age, the amount of myelin surrounding the axons decreases, reducing the speed of nerve conduction by approximately 10%. In addition, neurotransmitter imbalances can interfere with the ability of a nerve impulse to travel across a synapse, slowing conduction. These changes are a normal part of the aging process, and they occur gradually over time.

Slowed reaction times can increase an older person's risk for falling and other household accidents. For example, it will take an older person longer to regain balance if they start to fall, or to avoid an obstacle (such as a pet or small child) that suddenly darts into their path. For this reason, it is especially important to remember the general safety guidelines from Chapter 14 when caring for an older person. For example, when helping an older person to walk, you will want to make sure that the pathway is well-lit and clear, that the person's clothes and shoes fit properly, and, if the person wears glasses, that they are wearing them.

Memory and Attention Changes

Memory and thought processes usually remain intact with normal aging. It may take an older person slightly longer to remember names, dates, or other information from the past, but given enough time, the person will eventually remember. Many older people experience a mild loss of memory for recent events, while still having excellent long-term memory. There is also an age-related decline in a person's ability to pay attention without getting distracted. If you notice this change in your patients or residents, it can be helpful to repeat and even write down important information. Engaging in activities that stimulate the mind (such as reading, traveling, working crossword puzzles, and doing crafts and other handiwork) throughout life helps to keep thought processes sharp and active well into old age (Fig. 33-4). Physical exercise and social interactions have also been shown to promote brain health.

Dementia is a significant loss of mental capabilities. Dementia is a disorder, not a normal age-related change. If you work in a long-term care facility, it may seem to you that dementia is common because approximately 66% of the residents in long-term care facilities have some degree of dementia. However, in the United States, only about 15% of people 65 years or older have dementia, and of these 15%, only 5% have severe dementia. Dementia is discussed in detail in Chapter 9.

DISORDERS OF THE NERVOUS SYSTEM

There are many types of nervous system disorders. Some disorders affect a person's ability to control movement, or experience sensation. Other disorders may affect a person's ability to speak. Still other disorders affect a person's memory or behavior. Disorders can be the result of a disease process, such as Parkinson disease, or the result of an injury that damages the brain, spinal cord, or peripheral nerve pathways. Disorders of the nervous system are one

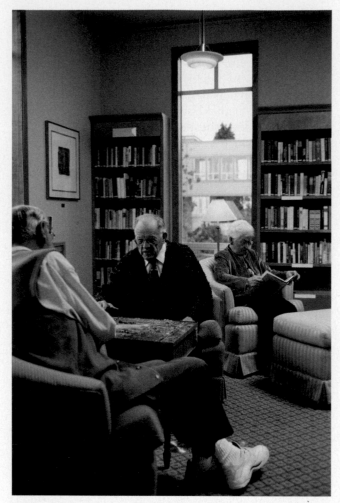

Figure 33-4 Use it or lose it! Studies have shown that actively exercising your mind throughout life helps to preserve mental function.

of the most common causes of disability among older adults. Approximately 50% of the disabilities seen in people older than 65 years are caused by a disorder of the nervous system.

Transient Ischemic Attacks (TIAs)

Ischemia is the decreased blood flow to the tissues. The tissue that is not getting enough blood is said to be *ischemic*. **Transient ischemic attacks (TIAs)** are temporary (transient) episodes of dysfunction that are caused by decreased blood flow (ischemia) to the brain. Any condition or situation that decreases blood flow to the brain can cause a TIA. For example, small blood clots can form in the heart or the arteries that supply the brain. These clots can break off and travel into the narrow arterioles of the brain, where they temporarily block the blood flow. Low blood pressure, certain medications, cigarette smoking, or standing up suddenly after lying down can also lead to a TIA.

Symptoms of a TIA vary according to the part of the brain affected by the decreased blood supply. Common symptoms may include dizziness, nausea, blurring or loss of vision, double vision, paralysis on one side of the body or face (with or without loss of sensation), or the inability to speak or swallow. The symptoms of a TIA may only last a few minutes, or they may last for several hours. The person usually recovers completely within 24 hours.

If you suspect that one of your patients or residents is having or has just had a TIA, please report this to the nurse immediately. TIAs are usually a warning that the person could have a stroke in the near future. A TIA may also be a sign of an underlying medical condition that needs to be addressed.

Stroke

A **stroke**, also known as a "brain attack" or cerebrovascular accident (CVA), occurs when blood flow to a part of the brain is completely blocked, causing the tissue to die. Unlike a TIA, a stroke causes permanent effects because the obstruction of blood flow lasts long enough for the brain tissue to die or become damaged. Stroke is the third leading cause of death in people older than 65 years. Even if death does not occur, the person may be left with significant disabilities following a stroke. A very high number of the residents in long-term care facilities are survivors of a stroke.

A stroke can occur suddenly in a person who was previously healthy. Signs and symptoms vary, depending on the area of the brain that is affected. Personality changes, drooping of the eyelid or corner of the mouth, slurring of speech, paralysis, severe headache, and loss of consciousness can all be signs of a stroke. If you notice a difference in a patient's or resident's usual behavior, appearance, or medical condition, report your observations to a nurse immediately (Fig. 33-5). The signs and symptoms of a stroke can be found in Chapter 16.

Causes of Stroke

The most common cause of a stroke is a blood clot that blocks the flow of blood to a part of the brain. Therefore, people who smoke, have atherosclerosis, have certain heart dysrhythmias, or have poorly controlled hypertension or diabetes are at high risk for having this type of stroke. Another, less common cause of a stroke is cerebral hemorrhage. A cerebral hemorrhage occurs when a small artery in the brain bursts. The bleeding into the surrounding brain tissue puts pressure on the delicate tissue, damaging it. A cerebral hemorrhage is more likely in people with chronic hypertension, arteriosclerosis ("hardening of

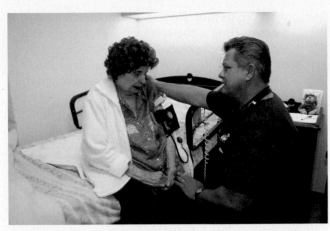

Figure 33-5 A severe headache, personality changes, slurring of speech, paralysis, or loss of consciousness may all signal the onset of a stroke.

the arteries"), or certain deformities of the blood vessels in the brain.

Effects of Stroke

The lasting effects of a stroke depend on the area of the brain that is affected and the amount of tissue that is damaged. For example, a stroke that affects the vital control centers of the brain stem will result in death, while a stroke that affects part of the cerebrum may result only in disability. The most common disabilities resulting from a stroke are hemiplegia and aphasia.

Hemiplegia, you will recall from Chapter 14, is paralysis on one side of the body. (Remember that the right side of the brain controls the left side of the body, and the left side of the brain controls the right side of the body—so, a stroke that damages the right side of the brain will affect the left side of the body, and vice versa.) Depending on the amount of tissue damage, the hemiplegia may be mild or severe. A person with mild hemiplegia may have slight muscle weakness or shaking on the affected side, while a person with severe hemiplegia may not be able to move or feel any type of sensation at all on that side of the body. A person with severe hemiplegia who has lost sensation on one side of the body will need frequent repositioning and positioning aids to prevent pressure ulcers from forming (Fig. 33-6). Care must also be taken to prevent other injuries, such as burns, because the person will not have the ability to detect extreme heat, cold, or pain on the affected side.

Aphasia is a general term for a group of disorders that affects the ability of the person to communicate with others.

■ *Expressive aphasia* is caused by damage to the motor centers of the brain that control the ability to speak or form sounds into meaningful words.

A person with expressive aphasia may also have trouble swallowing, increasing their risk of choking.

■ *Receptive aphasia* is caused by damage to the area of the brain that allows the person to understand words. The person can speak clearly, but they no longer know the meaning of the words. For example, a person with receptive aphasia may say "no" when they mean "yes." The person with receptive aphasia may not be able to follow your verbal instruction.

Treatment of Stroke

In the past, the treatment of stroke focused on stabilizing the person's medical condition and then using aggressive physical therapy to help retrain disabled muscles to perform simple tasks. However, now new treatments are available that can help to minimize the permanent damage caused by the stroke. For example, medications that dissolve blood clots are sometimes used to reestablish blood flow to the brain before permanent damage can occur. To work, these medications must be given very soon after the onset of the stroke.

Treatment immediately following a stroke depends on the severity of the damage to the brain, and on whether the person or family members want life-support measures to be taken. A person who has had a stroke may be very critically ill initially and need intensive nursing care. Respiratory support, oxygen, medications to support blood pressure, and continuous monitoring of vital signs may be necessary.

During this crisis period, the person's family members face uncertainty and difficult decisions. For

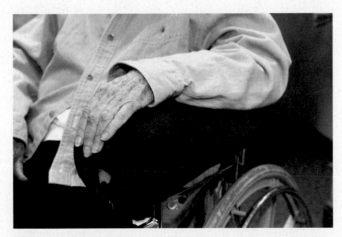

Figure 33-6 A person who has had a stroke may lose the ability to detect sensations on one side of the body. With these people, extra care must be taken to prevent pressure ulcers and other injuries because the person will be unable to sense warnings of impending injury, such as pain, cold, or heat.

example, they may need to decide whether or not to prolong life-support measures. If the person survives the stroke, family members may need to make some decisions about where the person will live in the future. For example, the person may need to move to a long-term care facility, or a home health care agency may need to be hired. During this difficult time, family members will appreciate a nursing assistant who demonstrates empathy, patience, and understanding.

A person who suddenly experiences a stroke and regains consciousness only to find that they are paralyzed or unable to communicate can be totally devastated. Rehabilitation, which is started as soon as the person's medical condition stabilizes, can be physically and emotionally difficult. Depression, frustration, anger, and major behavioral and personality changes can be expected. As a nursing assistant, you will be responsible for supporting the person both physically and emotionally during this difficult phase of their life.

Parkinson Disease

As you learned earlier, neurotransmitters are chemicals that carry nerve impulses across the gap between the axon of one neuron and the dendrites of the next. There are many different types of neurotransmitters. One neurotransmitter, called *dopamine*, is the neurotransmitter used by the neurons in an area of the brain called the *basal ganglia*, which works with other brain regions to plan and coordinate movements. In a person with **Parkinson disease**, dopamine is not produced in sufficient amounts, and signals between the basal ganglia and other brain regions are blocked because of the lack of dopamine. Because of this nervous system "short circuit," the brain loses its ability to properly control body movement.

Parkinson disease is a progressive disease, which means that it gets worse with time. The average age for the onset of Parkinson disease is 55 years. Males are affected more often than females. We do not know exactly what causes the neurons to stop producing dopamine.

Effects of Parkinson Disease

The effects of Parkinson disease can be easily remembered by thinking of the word **"TRAP"**:

T stands for *tremor*. Parkinson disease usually starts with a faint tremor that gets worse over a long period of time. The tremor is most apparent when the person is resting and decreases when the person attempts purposeful movement.

R stands for *rigidity*. The muscles become increasingly stiff. When rigidity is combined

with the tremor, there is a cogwheeling effect. Cogwheeling is the term used to describe the jerky, ratcheting feel to the movement.

A stands for *akinesia* (lack of movement). *Brady-kinesia*, or slowed movement, is also noted in Parkinson disease.

P stands for *postural instability*. The person's ability to maintain balance becomes increasingly worse, increasing the person's risk for falls.

As a result of these changes, the person has an abnormal gait. The person's steps are "shuffling," which means that their steps are short, there is a slight hesitation as the person tries to move the foot forward, and the foot barely comes off the floor. The person's posture is stooped forward, and they lose the natural arm swing that helps us maintain balance (Fig. 33-7). The person has difficulty initiating movement, but once the person gets going, the short, shuffling steps and forward posture make it difficult for them to control their speed and maintain balance. In addition, the person has difficulty turning. Instead of twisting the body and pivoting on the toes, a person

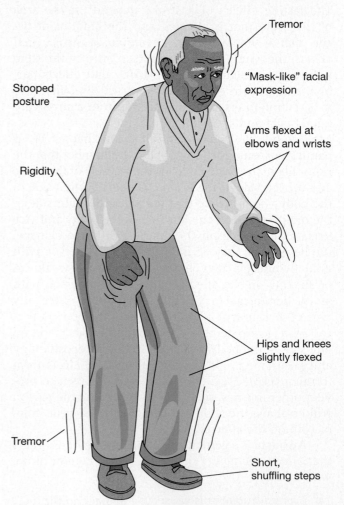

Tremor

"Mask-like" facial expression

Stooped posture

Arms flexed at elbows and wrists

Rigidity

Hips and knees slightly flexed

Tremor

Short, shuffling steps

Figure 33-7 People with Parkinson disease often develop a characteristic shuffling gait with a forward lean.

with Parkinson disease turns their whole body as one unit, taking many small steps to complete the turn. Because of these abnormal movements, the person with Parkinson disease is at very high risk for falling and significant injuries.

Difficulty controlling the muscles around the face and throat causes other symptoms that are characteristic of Parkinson disease. The person loses the ability to move the small muscles of the face that are responsible for facial expression, giving the face a "mask-like" appearance. Because the muscles used for swallowing are also affected, the person has trouble eating and is at high risk for choking and aspiration. Drooling is common.

The muscles used for speech are also affected. The person is unable to project their voice, so the volume is low and the speech pattern is monotone (that is, without variation). Sometimes the person's words come out very rapidly and are difficult to understand. Picture boards and asking simple questions that can be answered with a nod or shake of the head can help improve the person's ability to express themselves.

Other problems that are common with Parkinson disease include skin disorders, sleep disturbances, constipation, and as the disease progresses, incontinence. In the later stages of the disease, the person may develop dementia. In the end stage of Parkinson disease, the person becomes totally dependent on others for care and will be at risk for all of the complications of immobility.

Treatment of Parkinson Disease

Medications used in the treatment of Parkinson disease increase the concentration of dopamine in the brain. They are given on a set schedule to help maintain muscle control and coordination throughout the day. A person who is taking medications for Parkinson disease may seem to have "on" times and "off" times throughout the day. When the person is "on," the person's symptoms are well controlled by the medication and the person may be able to perform daily activities with minimal problems. During the "off" time, however, the medication dose is beginning to wear off, and the person's symptoms may reappear. Report your observations about the person's "on" and "off" times to the nurse. This information can help the nurse and the doctor schedule the person's doses of medication to achieve the best control of the person's symptoms. In addition, scheduling personal care and activities during the person's "on" times can help promote independence because the person functions better during these times. Other treatments for Parkinson disease may include speech therapy to help with swallowing problems and physical therapy to help with movement difficulties. Range-of-motion exercises, warm baths, and massage may help maintain and improve joint flexibility and use. Older people with Parkinson disease are at a very high risk for contracture development.

Epilepsy

Epilepsy is a disorder characterized by chronic seizure activity. Seizures are caused by interruptions of the normal electrical activity in the brain. A person with epilepsy experiences seizures periodically. The seizures may be grand mal (tonic–clonic) seizures, which are characterized by generalized and violent contraction and relaxation of the body's muscles, or they may be petit mal (absence) seizures, which can be very mild and hardly noticeable. Because the seizures often occur without any warning, a person with epilepsy may not be able to participate in certain activities, such as driving or swimming. Care for a person who is having a grand mal seizure is described in Chapter 16.

There are many possible causes of epilepsy. For example, a person may develop epilepsy following a head injury, brain infection, or stroke. A difficult delivery that results in the infant not getting enough oxygen during the birth process can also lead to epilepsy. Many times, the exact cause of a person's epilepsy is never determined.

Medications are available that help to reduce the frequency of seizures. For some people with epilepsy, these medications do not work, but for others, they are very successful. A person whose epilepsy can be well controlled with medications may have very few restrictions as far as activities are concerned.

Multiple Sclerosis (MS)

It is thought that **multiple sclerosis (MS)** is an autoimmune disorder—the immune system attacks and destroys the myelin sheaths that protect the nerves, resulting in faulty transmission of nerve impulses. MS usually affects the nerves in the hands, feet, and eyes first, and then moves inward toward the central nervous system. Muscle weakness, tingling sensations, twitching of the eyes, and visual disturbances may be early signs of MS.

MS usually strikes people early in life, between the ages of 20 and 40 years. The disorder progresses at different rates, depending on the individual. Some people may have a period of remission (mild or no symptoms) followed by a relapse (the symptoms return and are much worse). In the late stages of the disease, the person may become totally paralyzed. At this time, there is no cure for MS although some medications have been shown to slow the progression of the disease.

MS is one reason why a younger person may become a resident of a long-term care facility. Because a person with MS has difficulty controlling muscle movement, they are at increased risk for injury. It may be necessary to pad hard surfaces in the environment that could cause injury if the person accidentally bumps into them. Be aware of, and follow, any specific instructions for seating and positioning that are included on the person's care plan. Range-of-motion exercises may be ordered to help maintain muscle tone and prevent contractures. A person with MS often has difficulty with bowel and bladder elimination as a result of nerve damage. For example, the person may experience urinary retention, constipation, or incontinence. Be sure to communicate with the nurse about your patient's or resident's specific needs. Your attention to these needs is important to help minimize problems, promote comfort, and maintain the person's sense of dignity.

Amyotrophic Lateral Sclerosis (ALS, Lou Gehrig Disease)

Amyotrophic lateral sclerosis (ALS), like MS, is a nervous system disorder that causes progressive muscle weakness. In ALS, the neurons that transmit impulses between the spinal cord and the muscles are damaged and eventually die. People in the late stages of the disease have total paralysis, yet their minds remain sharp. Death occurs when a person loses the ability to breathe and swallow.

ALS usually affects people later in life, between the ages of 40 and 60 years. Males are affected more often than females. Most people who have ALS die within 10 years of the diagnosis.

Head Injuries

Head injuries leading to brain damage can be caused by falls, car and motorcycle accidents, bicycle accidents, and gunshot wounds (Fig. 33-8). Brain damage can also occur from events that cause a person to stop breathing for a long period of time, such as near-drowning, drug overdose, or choking.

Because neurons in the CNS do not easily repair themselves or "grow back," traumatic injuries to the brain often result in physical disability, loss of mental function, or both. The type of disability will depend on the area and extent of the brain tissue damaged. Some people with head injuries will have paralysis similar to that seen in people who have had a stroke. Others will develop epilepsy, memory problems, or behavioral problems. Still others will be comatose and will need ventilator assistance to live. The type of care and rehabilitation that a person with a head injury needs is very

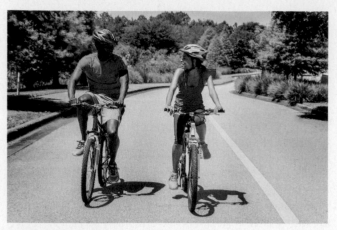

Figure 33-8 Taking standard safety precautions, such as wearing a helmet while riding a bike, can dramatically reduce the likelihood of a head injury should an accident occur. (*Spotmatik Ltd\Shutterstock.com*)

individualized, according to the person's specific needs. Many of the younger people who live in long-term care facilities are there because of a head injury that resulted in severe disability.

Altered States of Consciousness

A **coma** is a deep state of unconsciousness from which a person cannot be aroused. A coma can be caused by head injury, a tumor, a lack of oxygen, exposure to toxins, or illness. A person who is comatose is unaware of their environment and cannot deliberately respond to people or things in it. The person cannot move on their own, and they cannot talk or respond to commands.

Some people will come out of the coma and make a full recovery, or they will experience only some disability. If the coma persists longer than several weeks, the person is said to be in a **persistent vegetative state**. A person in a persistent vegetative state may have sleep–wake cycles and is able to breathe on their own. The person may even laugh, smile, or grimace. However, these are involuntary responses. The person is not actually deliberately responding to their environment. A person can live in a persistent vegetative state for years. It is generally believed that if a person remains in a persistent vegetative state for longer than 1 year, the condition is permanent.

A person who "awakens" from a coma or persistent vegetative state may be in a minimally conscious state, either temporarily or permanently. A person in this state appears to sleep most of the time but has episodes of awareness and responsiveness. For example, the person may open their eyes when someone is talking to them, and their eyes may even move toward the person who is speaking. Sometimes they will be able to hold an object or speak a few words. This state of consciousness may be temporary or permanent.

A person who is comatose or in a persistent vegetative state is totally dependent on others for care. Care measures are aimed at keeping the person physically healthy. For example, preventing infection and pressure ulcers is a primary concern. Nutritional support is provided by enteral nutrition.

Spinal Cord Injuries

Injuries to the spinal cord are usually caused by trauma, but they can also be caused by congenital deformities or tumors of the spine. Trauma can cause the vertebrae to break, and the sharp fragments of bone can cut the soft tissue of the spinal cord, causing damage. Permanent damage can also result from the swelling that occurs inside the spinal canal after an injury. Following an injury, the soft tissue of the spinal cord swells. The bones that surround the spinal cord do not "give." As a result, the spinal cord is squeezed, cutting off blood flow and resulting in tissue death from lack of oxygen.

The disability that results from a spinal cord injury depends on the severity of the injury and the level of the spine where the injury occurred. Remember that the spinal cord is the line of communication between the brain and the rest of the body. If this line is broken at any point, then nerve impulses cannot travel beyond the break in the line. So, an injury to the spinal cord in the neck area can result in quadriplegia, also known as tetraplegia (paralysis from the neck down) because nerve impulses are not able to travel past the neck. An injury further down the spinal cord may result in paraplegia (paralysis from the waist down). The paralysis may be partial or complete, depending on the severity of the injury.

As with other types of disorders of the nervous system, the care and rehabilitation needed by a person with a spinal cord injury will depend on the severity and extent of the injury. A person with quadriplegia will usually need total assistance with activities of daily living (ADLs), while a person with paraplegia may require little or no assistance following rehabilitation. For some people, the emotional effects of a spinal cord injury may be harder to overcome than the physical disabilities. Loss of control over one's body, and the accompanying loss of independence, can be very devastating. Some people may not be able to return to their jobs, which can cause financial problems. Others may never be able to enjoy a favorite hobby again. When you care for a person with a spinal cord injury, it is very important to encourage the person to do as much as possible for themselves. Doing so helps the person to maintain a sense of independence.

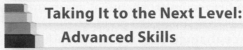

Taking It to the Next Level:

Advanced Skills

More in-depth information related to advanced skills used when providing care for a person with nervous system disorders can be found in *Lippincott Acute Care Skills for Advanced Nursing Assistants.*

Visit thePoint® at thepoint.lww.com for access to the ebook.

DIAGNOSIS OF NEUROLOGIC DISORDERS

When a person is showing signs or symptoms that suggest a neurologic disorder, the doctor may order one of several diagnostic tests to help determine the exact cause of the person's signs and symptoms. Improved diagnostic tools have led to the earlier detection of many neurologic disorders. Diagnostic tests that are often ordered for people with signs and symptoms of a neurologic disorder include the following:

■ **Imaging studies.** Tumors of the nervous system can occur in the brain, the spinal cord, or along the peripheral nerve tracts. Many of these tumors are not cancerous, but they may cause problems as they grow and press on healthy brain tissue or nerves. Imaging studies such as radiography ("x-rays"), computed tomography (CT), and magnetic resonance imaging (MRI) are used to help locate tumors of the brain, spinal cord, or surrounding bony structures (Fig. 33-9). Imaging studies are also useful for detecting fractures of the skull or vertebrae. When used with special dyes (injected into a vein), imaging

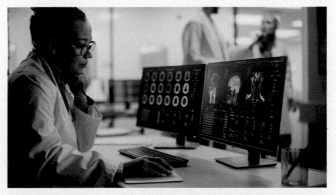

Figure 33-9 Imaging studies, such as CT scans, allow doctors to see physical abnormalities of the brain, spinal cord, and surrounding bony structures. Here, a doctor looks at a CT scan of a patient's brain. (*Gorodenkoff\Shutterstock.com*)

studies can help to reveal abnormalities in the blood vessels that supply the brain.

- **Electroencephalography.** An electroencephalogram (EEG) records the electrical activity of the brain. EEGs are used to pinpoint seizure activity within the brain. EEGs are also used to detect the presence or absence of brain activity following a severe brain injury.

SUMMARY

- Neurons are the basic cell of the nervous system.
  - A neuron can send and receive information.
  - Information, in the form of a nerve impulse, enters the neuron at the dendrites, travels through the cell body and down the axon, and then across the synapse and onto the dendrites of the next neuron in line.
- The nervous system consists of the central nervous system (CNS) and the peripheral nervous system (PNS).
  - The CNS consists of the brain and the spinal cord. The CNS receives information, processes it, and issues commands. The brain processes information and issues commands. The brain has four parts: the cerebrum, the diencephalon, the brain stem, and the cerebellum.
  - The spinal cord carries information to and from the brain.
- The PNS consists of the nerves. The nerves carry information to and from the CNS.
  - Sensory nerves carry information from the "outside in." Sensory nerves give the brain information about other organ systems or the outside world.
  - Motor nerves carry information from the "inside out." Motor nerves allow the brain to control the movement of muscles.
- The nervous system receives, processes, and responds to information.
  - The nervous system receives information from other organ systems and reacts to it, helping the body to maintain a state of homeostasis.
  - The nervous system allows us to experience the tastes, sounds, sights, and sensations of the world around us. The nervous system also enables us to move, think, and create.
- There are relatively few changes in the nervous system that result from normal aging.
  - Older people are not as quick to react to things as younger people, which increases the older person's risk for falling and other household accidents.
- Some older people find it harder to remember recent events, even though they remember events that happened long ago quite clearly. Extreme memory loss, such as that seen in people with dementia, is not a normal age-related change.
- Disorders of the nervous system can affect the brain, spinal cord, or nerves.
  - Transient ischemic attacks (TIAs) are caused by decreased blood flow to the brain. Once blood flow returns, the person's symptoms go away. Although the effects of a TIA are not lasting, a person who has had or is having a TIA needs medical attention because TIAs are often warnings that the person could have a stroke in the near future.
  - A stroke, also known as a cerebrovascular accident (CVA) or "brain attack," can be caused by a blood clot or hemorrhage that disrupts blood flow to the brain. The effects of a stroke may be permanent and can be mild or severe.
  - Parkinson disease affects the brain's ability to control movements because of a lack of the neurotransmitter dopamine.
  - Epilepsy is a seizure disorder caused by abnormal electrical activity in the brain.
  - Multiple sclerosis (MS) is a nervous system disorder that affects the motor neurons, resulting in muscle weakness that gets worse over time.
  - Head injuries that result in brain damage and spinal cord injuries are a major reason why many younger people come to live in long-term care facilities or require the services of a home health care agency.
  - A person who is in a coma or a persistent vegetative state requires total care to maintain physical health.
- Diagnostic procedures used to detect disorders of the nervous system include imaging studies—such as x-rays, computed tomography (CT) scans, and magnetic resonance imaging (MRI) scans—and electroencephalograms (EEGs).

WHAT DID YOU LEARN?

Multiple Choice

Select the single best answer for each of the following questions.

1. Any condition that temporarily decreases blood flow to the brain can cause what to occur?
   a. Multiple sclerosis
   b. A transient ischemic attack (TIA)
   c. A heart attack
   d. A cerebral hemorrhage

2. Ms. Ramirez has had a stroke and has a lot of trouble forming words. What term is used to describe Ms. Ramirez's difficulty with language?
   a. Aphasia
   b. Dysphasia
   c. Paraplegia
   d. Hemiplegia

3. Mr. Owens had a stroke that left the left side of his body paralyzed. Which one of the following statements is true?
   a. The stroke occurred in the left side of Mr. Owens' brain.
   b. The stroke occurred in the right side of Mr. Owens' brain.
   c. The stroke affected Mr. Owens' brain stem.
   d. Mr. Owens has paraplegia.

4. The effects of Parkinson disease can be easily remembered by thinking of the word _____.
   a. "TRIP"
   b. "TAPS"
   c. "TRAP"
   d. "TIPS"

5. Which of the following can increase a person's risk for a transient ischemic attack (TIA)?
   a. Low blood pressure
   b. Certain drugs
   c. Smoking
   d. All of the above

6. Which nervous system disorder is characterized by a lack of the neurotransmitter dopamine?
   a. Multiple sclerosis (MS)
   b. Epilepsy
   c. Parkinson disease
   d. Dementia

7. What neurologic disorder is characterized by chronic seizure activity?
   a. Multiple sclerosis (MS)
   b. Epilepsy
   c. Parkinson disease
   d. Stroke

8. What diagnostic test is used to monitor electrical activity of the brain?
   a. Electrocardiogram (EKG)
   b. Imaging studies, such as computed tomography (CT)
   c. Electroencephalogram (EEG)
   d. There is no test available to monitor the electrical activity of the brain

9. How does aging affect the nervous system?
   a. Older people usually become "senile" and forgetful.
   b. Older people lose the ability to form or understand words.
   c. Older people may take slightly longer to react to things.
   d. Aging does not affect the nervous system because old neurons are constantly replaced.

Matching *Match each numbered item with its appropriate lettered description.*

_____ **1.** Meninges

_____ **2.** Cerebrospinal fluid (CSF)

_____ **3.** Central nervous system

_____ **4.** Peripheral nervous system

_____ **5.** Axon

_____ **6.** Myelin

_____ **7.** Dendrite

_____ **8.** Neuron

_____ **9.** Synapse

a. The part of the neuron that sends information
b. Consists of the brain and spinal cord
c. Fatty white substance that speeds the conduction of nerve impulses
d. A cell that can send and receive information
e. The part of the neuron that receives information
f. The gap between the axon of one neuron and the dendrites of the next
g. Three layers of connective tissue that protect the brain and spinal cord
h. Consists of the nerves
i. Clear fluid that cushions the brain and spinal cord

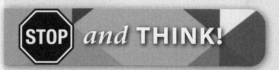

- You have been caring for Mr. Ishiguro, a resident in the long-term care facility where you work, for about 6 months now. Normally, you and Mr. Ishiguro have quite a lively chat while you help him get ready for breakfast in the mornings. However, this morning, while you are helping Mr. Ishiguro with his morning care, you notice that he seems to be slurring his speech and saying things that don't really make sense. What do you think might be going on? What should you do?

- Mr. Elba is a resident on your unit at the long-term care facility where you work. He has Parkinson disease and you have noticed a recent change in his facial expressions. When he tries to smile or laugh at something, his lips do not seem to be able to connect with his intention, creating a "mask-like" expression. Why do you think this is happening and what are some potential problems you should be watchful for?

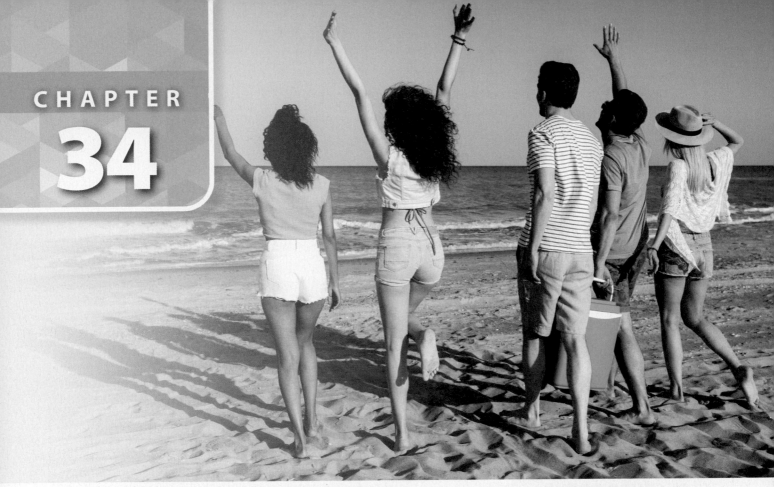

Photo: What would a day at the beach be like if you didn't have a sensory system? Would you miss the sound of the waves crashing on the beach, the seagulls squawking, and children laughing? The smell of the ocean? The taste of a treat from the boardwalk? The sight of the blue water? The feel of the hot sand between your toes? (Shift Drive\Shutterstock.com)

The Sensory System

 WHAT WILL YOU LEARN?

We rely on our special senses—sight, hearing, taste, smell, and touch—to understand and interact with the world around us. Our sensory system allows us to experience the beauty and joy of the world we live in. It also helps to protect us from harm. Many of the people you will care for will have disorders or disabilities involving the sensory system. In this chapter, you will learn how the sensory system works and about some of the disorders that can affect the sensory system. You will also learn how you can help to meet the needs of people who cannot see or hear well. When you are finished with this chapter, you will be able to:

1. List and describe the structures that make up the two main divisions of the sensory system.
2. Describe the body's general senses.
3. Describe how we experience taste and smell.
4. Discuss how aging affects a person's senses of taste and smell.
5. Describe how we experience sight.
6. Discuss the effects of aging on the eye.
7. List and describe disorders that can affect the eye.

8. Describe how to care for eyeglasses, contact lenses, and prosthetic (artificial) eyes.

9. Describe special considerations that are taken when caring for a person who is blind.

10. Describe how we experience sound.

11. Discuss the effects of aging on the ear.

12. List and describe disorders that can affect the ear.

13. Describe techniques for communicating with a person who has hearing loss.

14. Demonstrate proper technique for inserting and removing an in-the-ear hearing aid.

Vocabulary

Sensory receptors	Presbyopia	Cerumen	Conductive hearing
Sense organs	Conjunctivitis	Presbycusis	loss
Tactile receptors	Cataract	Cerumen impaction	Otosclerosis
Referred (radiating) pain	Glaucoma	Otitis media	Sensorineural hearing
Myopia	Diabetic retinopathy	Otitis externa	loss
Hyperopia	Macular degeneration	Vertigo	
Astigmatism	Braille	Tinnitus	

STRUCTURE OF THE SENSORY SYSTEM

The sensory system is part of the nervous system. The sensory system consists of **sensory receptors**, specialized cells or groups of cells associated with a sensory nerve. The sensory receptor picks up information, called a *stimulus*, and translates it into a nerve impulse, which is then sent via the sensory nerve to the brain for interpretation. Sensory receptors are found throughout the body. Some are found in the **sense organs**, which you probably can name already—the eyes, the ears, the nose, and the taste buds. Other sensory receptors are found throughout the skin and even in the tissues of internal organs.

The sensory system is sometimes divided into two major parts. This division is based on the location of the sensory receptors. The first part is called the *general senses*. The sensory receptors that are responsible for general senses are found everywhere throughout the body. The second part is called the *special senses*. The sensory receptors that are responsible for special senses are located in the specific sense organs (the eyes, the ears, the nose, and the taste buds).

GENERAL SENSES

The general senses allow us to detect touch, position, and pain.

Touch

Our sense of touch allows us to feel textures (such as the plush velvet of a party dress or the hot sand between our toes at the beach) and the shapes of objects. The sense of touch is made possible by tactile receptors found in the skin (Fig. 34-1). (*Tactile* is another word for "touch.") The **tactile receptors** are stimulated when something comes in contact with the surface of the body and presses on them, causing them to change shape. Some areas of the skin have more tactile receptors than others and are more sensitive to touch. For example, the tips of the fingers and toes and the lips contain many tactile receptors and are more sensitive to touch than other parts of the body.

Some of the tactile receptors in the skin allow us to sense pressure, also known as *deep touch*. Intolerance to prolonged pressure is what makes us shift our position when we have been sitting in one position for a long time. A person who is unable to sense pressure (for example, a person who is paralyzed) does not become uncomfortable from being in one position for a long time. Therefore, the person is not motivated to change positions. What effect do you think this has on the person's risk for developing skin breakdown and pressure ulcers?

Position

Position receptors, found in the muscles, tendons, and joints, keep the brain informed about the position of various body parts in relation to each other.

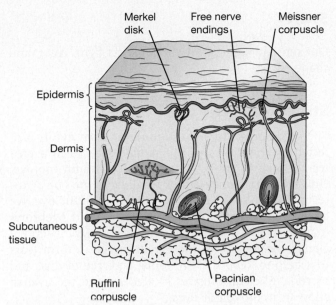

Figure 34-1 Tactile receptors and free nerve endings in the dermis of the skin allow us to feel things that come in contact with our bodies. There are four main types of tactile receptors: Ruffini corpuscles, Meissner corpuscles, Pacinian corpuscles, and Merkel disks.

For example, you can tell if your leg is bent or straight without actually looking down to check its position. These same receptors also relay information to the brain about the degree of muscle contraction, especially when the muscle is contracting against resistance (for example, when you are lifting weights). Position sense provides us with muscle tone and the ability to move our muscles in a smooth, coordinated way.

Pain

Pain is the body's distress signal. Pain tells us that we have been injured, that we have overworked a muscle group, that an organ is not working properly, or that we are ill.

Free nerve endings (dendrites) in the skin and the tissues of our internal organs allow us to detect pain. Your brain is usually pretty good at identifying what hurts when the cause of the pain is on the surface of your body (for example, when you burn your finger while removing a hot dish from the oven). But your brain may have more trouble pinpointing the exact location of pain that is coming from an internal organ. This results in the phenomenon known as **referred (radiating) pain**. For example, a person who is having a heart attack may complain of pain in the shoulder, neck, arm, or jaw. Gallbladder disease may cause pain in the back and shoulder on the person's right side. A back injury may cause pain to radiate down the leg and into a person's foot. Figure 34-2 shows

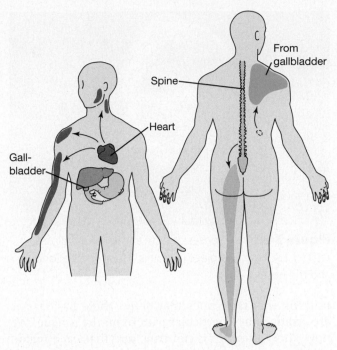

Figure 34-2 Pain may not always be felt at its exact source. Pain from the heart may be felt in the arm, shoulder, neck, or jaw (*red shading*). Pain from the gallbladder may be felt in the back and shoulder on the person's right side (*green shading*). A back injury can cause pain to radiate down the leg and into the foot (*yellow shading*).

how pain from certain internal organs can be referred to other areas of the body.

Many of the people you will care for will have some type of pain. The nursing assistant's role in caring for a person who experiences pain is described in Chapter 21.

TASTE AND SMELL

The sense organs of taste and smell are the taste buds and the roof of the nasal cavity, respectively. Special cells in these areas, called chemoreceptors, detect chemicals in the food we eat, the beverages we drink, and the air we breathe. The chemical signal is changed to an electric one and carried by sensory neurons to the brain, which tells us what we are tasting or smelling.

Taste buds cover the surface of the tongue. We have thousands of taste buds, and each taste bud consists of about 100 chemoreceptors, plus some supporting cells. The taste buds are bathed in fluid (either saliva or the liquids that we drink). The fluid contains dissolved chemicals, which stimulate the taste buds.

There are five basic tastes: sweet, salty, sour, bitter, and umami. Umami is the savory taste of cooked meats and some vegetables. Each of these tastes is detected by a different type of chemoreceptor. We used

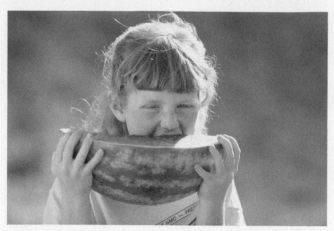

Figure 34-3 The senses of taste and smell are closely related. Eating a ripe piece of fruit is a treat for the tongue and the nose!

to think that taste buds that detect these basic tastes are arranged in a particular pattern on the tongue. We now know that this is not true, and that each region of the tongue can detect all five basic tastes.

The receptors that allow us to smell are located on the roof of the nasal cavity. Like the taste buds, these receptors are stimulated by chemicals that have been dissolved in fluid. However, in this case, the "fluid" is the moist mucous membrane lining of the nasal cavity. When exposed to the same chemical for a long period of time, the chemoreceptors stop sending signals to the brain. This explains why an odor that is very strong at first becomes less noticeable over time.

Together, taste and smell have a very powerful effect on the appetite (Fig. 34-3). Under normal circumstances, a person will not eat something that tastes or smells bad, even if they are hungry. But, how often have you found yourself eating too much of something just because it tastes or smells so good? Similarly, how often have you noticed that when you have a head cold and a stuffy nose, food seems to lose appeal? This happens in large part because you can't smell the food!

As we get older, the number of chemoreceptors on the tongue and on the roof of the nasal cavity decreases. In addition, we produce less saliva, which makes it harder to dissolve the chemicals that stimulate the taste buds. As a result of these changes, the senses of taste and smell become less intense, leading to an overall decrease in appetite. To make up for a diminished sense of taste and smell, older people often season their food more heavily than younger people.

There are many dangers associated with a diminished ability to taste or smell. For example, an older person may not be able to tell that food has spoiled and become ill from eating it. Or, they may not be able to detect the smell of smoke or a gas leak. It is surprising how much we rely on our senses of taste and smell to keep us safe.

SIGHT

Our sense of sight allows us to detect light, color, and shape.

Structure of the Eye

The sense organ of sight is the eye. Each eye is protected by the bones of the skull, which form a protective cavity ("orbit," "eye socket") around the eye. Only the very front of the eyeball lacks the bony protection of the skull. To protect the front of the eye, we have eyelids that close and eyelashes and eyebrows that serve as "dust catchers" (Fig. 34-4A). Lacrimal glands, located above the eye in the orbit, form tears that help to keep the eye moist and free of dust and bacteria. Skeletal muscles located around the eyeball allow us to move our eyes.

It may be helpful to look at Figure 34-4B as we go through the internal structure of the eyeball. The eyeball itself is made up of three layers of tissue—the sclera, the choroid, and the retina:

- The *sclera* is the tough outer layer. The sclera is made of connective tissue. Although most of the sclera is white (hence the term, "white of the eye"), the front of the sclera, which is called the *cornea*, is clear. Light passes through the cornea to the inside of the eye.

A. External structure of the eye

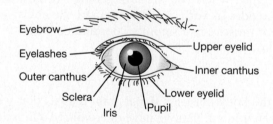

B. Internal structure of the eye

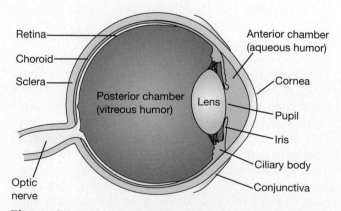

Figure 34-4 The eye. **A.** External view of the eye. **B.** Internal structures of the eye.

■ The *choroid* is the middle layer. This layer contains the blood vessels that supply the retina and other parts of the eye. At the front of the eye, the *choroid* also forms the ciliary body and the iris. The *ciliary body* is a muscular structure that attaches to the *lens*, a flexible, transparent, curved structure that adjusts to focus light rays onto the retina. The ciliary body changes the shape of the lens, allowing the eye to focus. The other structure formed by the choroid, the *iris*, is the colored part of the eye. The iris is actually a round muscle with an opening in the center (the *pupil*). The iris controls the amount of light that enters the eye through the pupil.

■ The *retina* is the innermost layer. The retina contains receptors, called *rods* and *cones*, which turn light into nerve impulses. The nerve impulses travel through the *optic nerve* to the brain for interpretation.

The eyeball also has two fluid-filled chambers (see Fig. 34-4B):

■ The *anterior chamber* is located between the cornea and the lens. Special cells in the ciliary body secrete *aqueous humor*, a watery fluid that fills the anterior chamber. The aqueous humor passes through the anterior chamber and is reabsorbed back into the bloodstream.

■ The posterior chamber is located between the lens and the retina. The posterior chamber is filled with *vitreous humor*, a jelly-like substance that gives the eyeball its shape.

Function of the Eye

Nowadays, we mostly use digital devices to capture pictures, but for a long time, film cameras were used. Think about how one of these cameras works. To take a picture, you need light and film. You also need a way of controlling the amount of light that enters the camera and adjusting the distance between the camera lens and the film. If the amount of light entering the camera is not sufficient, or if the distance between the lens and the film is not correct, the resulting photograph will be out of focus.

The human eye works much like a camera:

■ The retina is the "film."
■ The iris and pupil control the amount of light that enters the eye. In bright sunlight, the iris constricts, making the pupil smaller so that less light is allowed into the inner part of the eye. In low light, the iris dilates, making the pupil bigger so that more light can enter the eye.
■ The cornea and lens work to focus light rays onto the retina, resulting in a clear image. First, the curve of the cornea focuses the light rays as they enter the eye. Next, the light rays pass

through the lens, where the focus is refined (Fig. 34-5A). If the object the person is looking at is close, then the ciliary body contracts, causing the lens to become shorter and rounder. If the object is far away, then the ciliary body relaxes,

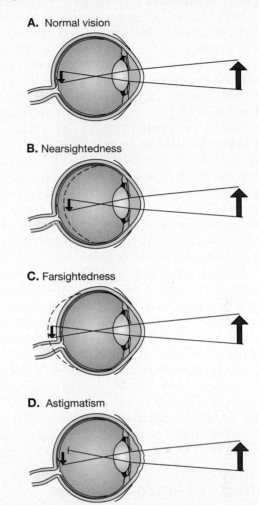

Figure 34-5 Many people need corrective lenses, such as glasses or contact lenses, to achieve clear vision. Three common problems that require the use of corrective lenses are nearsightedness (myopia), farsightedness (hyperopia), and astigmatism. **A.** Normal vision. Light rays pass through the cornea and the lens and are focused on the retina. **B.** Nearsightedness (myopia). The eyeball of a person who is nearsighted is more oval in shape than normal, which increases the distance between the lens and the retina. As a result, the image comes into focus before the retina. **C.** Farsightedness (hyperopia). The eyeball of a person who is farsighted is more round in shape than normal, which decreases the distance between the lens and the retina. As a result, the image is not yet focused when it hits the retina. **D.** Astigmatism. In astigmatism, the cornea is not uniformly curved. Some of the light rays that pass through the cornea are focused on the retina, but others are not, resulting in blurred vision.

causing the lens to become longer and flatter. The curved lens bends the light rays and brings them into focus on the retina, forming an image.

Clear, sharp vision is indeed a true gift. Many people need some help (in the form of corrective lenses, such as glasses or contact lenses) to see clearly. People who wear corrective lenses need help focusing the image properly on the retina. Some people need help focusing because of the shape of their eyeball. For example, the eyeball may be a little more oval than normal, causing the distance between the lens and the retina to be greater than usual. This results in nearsightedness, or **myopia** (Fig. 34-5B). People who are nearsighted are able to see fairly well close up, but they have trouble seeing images that are far away. This is because the distance between the person's lens and retina is longer than usual, which means that the image actually comes into focus before it hits the retina. This is a very common problem—20% of the people in the United States have some degree of nearsightedness!

Some people have the opposite problem, called farsightedness, or **hyperopia** (Fig. 34-5C). People who are farsighted are able to see objects in the distance fairly well, but they have trouble seeing objects that are close. In people who are farsighted, the eyeball is rounder than normal, causing the distance between the lens and the retina to be shorter than usual. Therefore, when the image hits the retina, it is not yet in focus.

Other people have trouble focusing images properly because the cornea is not perfectly curved. This condition is called **astigmatism** (Fig. 34-5D). The irregular curve of the cornea bends the light rays in such a way that it results in a blurred, distorted image.

The Effects of Aging on the Eye

As we age, many changes occur in the eye that can affect vision:

- The number of receptors in the retina decreases, and the lens becomes more opaque (cloudy). As a result, images are not focused as sharply as in younger days, and colors may not be as bright.
- The iris becomes more rigid, which means that it takes longer for an older person's eyes to adjust when they move from a bright area to a dim one, or vice versa.
- The lens becomes less flexible, which affects the older person's ability to focus on objects that are close, a condition known as **presbyopia**. Presbyopia is why many people start using reading glasses in their 40s (Fig. 34-6).
- There is a decrease in tear production, which leads to dryness and irritation of the eyes. Many older people use lubricating eye drops to help keep the eyes moist and comfortable.

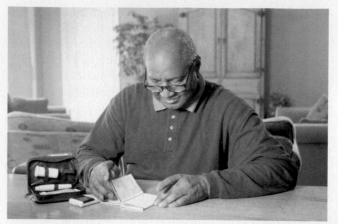

Figure 34-6 Presbyopia, which occurs when the lens becomes less elastic with age, is a common age-related change. People with presbyopia often need to use reading glasses to help them focus on things that are close.

Disorders of the Eye

There are several disorders of the eye that as a nursing assistant you should be aware may affect your patients or residents.

Conjunctivitis ("Pink Eye")

Conjunctivitis is an infection and inflammation of the conjunctiva, a clear membrane that lines the inside of the eyelids and covers most of the surface of the eye (see Fig. 34-4B). In conjunctivitis, the white of the eye appears red. The eye may itch or burn, and it tears excessively (Fig. 34-7). There may be a sticky white or yellow discharge.

There are many different causes of conjunctivitis. Microbes that cause colds and sinus infections can travel through the tear ducts and onto the surface of

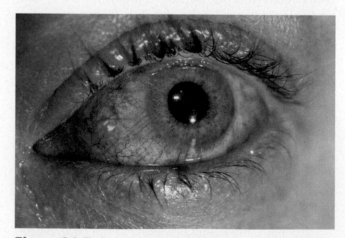

Figure 34-7 Conjunctivitis, or "pink eye," is a contagious infection of the conjunctiva, the clear membrane that covers most of the surface of the eye and lines the inside of the eyelids. The affected eye is red, itchy, and teary, and there may be a sticky white or yellow discharge. (*ARZTSAMUI\Shutterstock.com*)

the eye, causing an infection. Or, microbes from an infection somewhere else in the body can be transferred into the eye when the person touches the infected area and then rubs their eyes. For example, methicillin-resistant *Staphylococcus aureus* (MRSA) and herpes virus can cause conjunctivitis in this way.

Conjunctivitis is highly contagious. Rubbing the eyes and then touching something transfers the microbes to that surface, where they can easily be picked up by someone else. All that person has to do is touch their own eyes, and they could find themselves with their own case of conjunctivitis! Conjunctivitis is usually treated with eye drops or an eye ointment prescribed by a doctor.

Cataracts

Cataracts are very common in older people, but they can occur in younger people as well. Cataracts are the leading cause of low vision in older adults. It is thought that excessive exposure to sunlight increases a person's chances of developing cataracts. Diabetes, cigarette smoking, eye injury, and excessive alcohol consumption are also factors that can increase a person's chances of developing cataracts. A **cataract** is the gradual yellowing and hardening of the lens of the eye. The lens becomes opaque and eventually prevents light from passing through to the retina. The person's vision becomes more and more cloudy as the cataract worsens (Fig. 34-8). Total blindness can result as a cataract becomes more opaque.

Many people with cataracts have surgery to remove the opaque lens and replace it with an artificial one. Improvements in equipment and surgical techniques have made this procedure simple and routine. Surgery is usually performed on an outpatient basis using only a local anesthetic. The person can return home a few hours after the procedure. Cataract surgery enables people with cataracts to once again enjoy activities, such as needlework and reading, that would have been nearly impossible before.

Glaucoma

Glaucoma is a disorder of the eye that occurs when the pressure within the eye is increased to dangerous levels. This occurs when the aqueous humor in the anterior chamber is not reabsorbed into the bloodstream. As more and more aqueous humor is formed, it creates pressure, which builds up in the eye. The pressure squeezes the nerves and the blood vessels in the retina. Eventually, the nerves are destroyed and vision is lost.

People who are older than 40 years and have a family history of glaucoma are at high risk for developing glaucoma themselves. The most common type of glaucoma occurs gradually, over a period of time. However, in some people, the onset of glaucoma

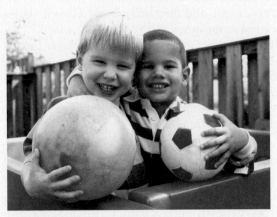

A. Normal vision

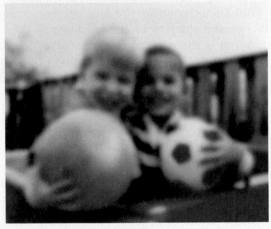

B. Cataract

Figure 34-8 Cataracts occur when the lens of the eye becomes yellow and hard over time, resulting in cloudy vision. This is what the world looks like to (**A**) a person with normal vision and (**B**) a person with cataracts. (*Courtesy of the National Eye Institute, National Institutes of Health.*)

happens suddenly and is accompanied by a great deal of pain. Both chronic and acute glaucoma can lead to blindness if left untreated. Glaucoma is the second leading cause of blindness in older people, making up 10% of all blindness in the United States.

Early detection and treatment of glaucoma can help to save the person's vision. This is why routine eye examinations are essential. If a person is found to have glaucoma, medicated eye drops are usually used to help control the pressure within the eye. Some people may need surgery if the eye drops are not effective.

Diabetic Retinopathy

Diabetic retinopathy is a complication of diabetes that can lead to blindness. In the early stages, the tiny blood vessels that supply the retina burst, leading to hemorrhages and damage the retina. As the retina tries to heal, new blood vessels start to grow along the retina and in the vitreous humor. These new vessels are very fragile and they often burst as well, damaging the retina even more.

The number of cases of blindness caused by diabetic retinopathy in the United States is rapidly increasing. Early detection during an eye examination is essential for preserving the person's vision. Laser treatment is often necessary to help seal off hemorrhages in the retina.

Macular Degeneration

The macula is the small area in the middle of the retina where images are sharpest. In **macular degeneration**, deposits build up under the macula (the dry form) or blood vessels develop over the macula (the wet form). The receptors in the area become damaged, and the person's ability to see is impaired. Macular degeneration is the most common cause of blindness in people over the age of 65. Factors that can increase a person's risk of developing macular degeneration are smoking, excessive exposure to sunlight, a diet high in cholesterol, and an inherited tendency for the disorder.

Blindness

Blindness has many different causes and takes many different forms. Many people are considered blind but have partial sight. Some people see nothing but darkness, but many others can see light, movement, shapes, and even colors, just not clearly enough to distinguish between them. Some people who are blind have been blind since birth and have never seen anything, while others may have lost their sight later in life. Most people who are blind adapt well and are very independent. People who have recently lost their sight, however, may be very frightened, especially of walking or moving around on their own.

Rehabilitation for a person who has recently lost their sight focuses on safety and the person's return to independence. Navigation skills are taught so that the blind person can be independent again. During rehabilitation, a blind person may learn to work with a companion animal that has been specially trained to guide the person as they walk (Fig. 34-9). The person may learn **Braille**, a system that uses letters made from combinations of raised dots (Fig. 34-10). The person runs their fingers over words written in Braille to read them. In addition, many books are available in the form of audio recordings for the person to listen to.

As a nursing assistant, treating a person who is blind with respect and allowing the person to be as independent as possible are the best things you can do to help the rehabilitation effort. Learn the techniques that your patient or resident is being taught and reinforce them by helping the person to practice them

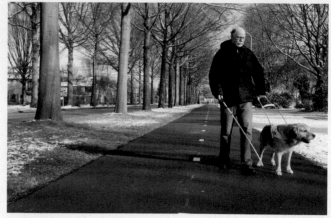

Figure 34-9 Many people who are blind have specially trained companion animals that help to keep them safe. For example, when preparing to cross a busy intersection, the blind person will listen to the traffic and tell the dog to move "forward" when they believe that the intersection is clear. If the dog judges that it is unsafe to move forward (for example, there is a car passing through the intersection that the person did not hear), the dog will refuse the command. This is called *intelligent disobedience*. Most companion animals require almost 2 years of training to learn how to do their jobs! (*Jeroen van den Broek\Shutterstock.com*)

continuously. Guidelines for caring for a person who is blind are given in Guidelines Box 34-1.

Caring for Eyeglasses, Contact Lenses, and Prosthetic Eyes

Many of your patients or residents will wear glasses or contact lenses. Some may even have a prosthetic (artificial) eye. Most people are able to care for their own vision accessories, but others may need your help.

Eyeglasses

Eyeglasses are commonly used to correct vision. Some people wear eyeglasses only for reading or close work,

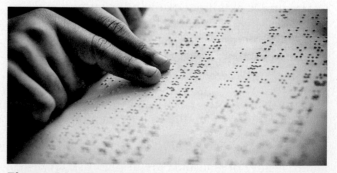

Figure 34-10 Braille uses a system of letters formed from raised dots to enable a blind person to read. (*vectorfusionart\Shutterstock.com*)

Guidelines Box 34-1 Guidelines for Caring for a Person Who Is Blind

WHAT YOU DO	WHY YOU DO IT
Speak in a normal tone of voice.	Unless the person is hearing impaired as well as blind, there is no need to raise your voice.
It is fine to use words such as "see," "look," and "watch." Be descriptive in the things you see around you. For example, tell the person that the sky is a beautiful shade of blue or that there are lovely yellow flowers blooming right outside the window.	There is no need to be self-conscious about your ability to see, as compared with the blind person's inability to see. Most people who are blind are comfortable with that fact. Many appreciate your ability to share what you see with them through your descriptions.
Ask the person about the extent of their blindness, and do not hesitate to ask the person what type of help they need from you.	Asking the person about their blindness will help you to better care for the person. You might be surprised at what the person is able to do for themselves, with little or no assistance from you!
When you enter the person's room, knock and tell the person who you are and why you are there. Similarly, when you leave, tell the person that you are leaving.	If you do not announce yourself when you enter the room, you could startle the person. Imagine how frightening it would be to hear someone walking around in your room and not know who they are or what they are doing! Similarly, if you do not tell the person that you are leaving, they may not be aware that you have left. How would you feel if you started talking to someone who was no longer in the room and were left to figure it out on your own that the other person had left?
Make sure you explain procedures completely and descriptively. Throughout the procedure, tell the person what type of equipment you are using, what you are doing, and what you are going to do next.	With all patients and residents, you should take care to explain procedures thoroughly. However, with a blind person, you may have to modify your approach a bit. For example, instead of just showing the person a piece of equipment, you will need to describe it to them, or let them touch it. Also, you should tell the person what is happening as it happens so that the person is not left wondering where you are in the procedure, or what is coming next.
Do not rearrange the furniture in the person's room, unless the person asks you to.	The person is used to moving around the room on their own. If you move the furniture, the person could injure themselves by running into something that has been moved and is now in an unfamiliar location.
Leave the door either completely open or completely closed.	If the door is partially open, the person may feel for the door, think that it is all the way open, and walk into the edge of the door.
When helping a blind person to walk, do not propel the person in front of you. Instead, let the person walk beside you and slightly behind you as they rest a hand on your elbow. Walk at a normal pace. Let the person know when you are about to turn a corner, or when a curb or step is approaching (and whether or not you will be stepping up or down).	In this way, you guide the person and reduce the risk of stumbles over unforeseen obstacles.

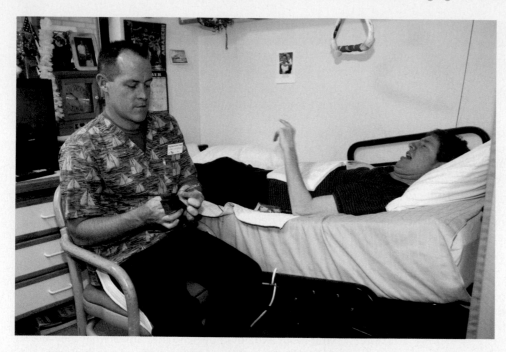

Figure 34-11 Take special care when handling a person's eyeglasses. They are expensive to replace.

while others may need to wear them all the time when they are awake. Always make sure that your patients or residents who need glasses wear them, especially if the person is confused or disoriented. Being unable to see clearly can make confusion and disorientation worse and adversely affects the person's quality of life.

Eyeglasses are very expensive to replace if broken or lost. As with all of your patients' or residents' personal belongings, you should be careful when handling a person's eyeglasses.

Clean eyeglasses with cloths or a special solution made specifically for that purpose, or with warm water (Fig. 34-11). If water or a special cleaning solution is used to clean the lenses, finish by drying them with a soft cloth or tissue. Paper towels or napkins may scratch the lenses and should not be used. When not in use, the person's eyeglasses should be stored in their case within easy reach.

Contact Lenses

Contact lenses are also commonly worn to help make vision sharp. Contact lenses are made of molded plastic and fit directly on the eyeball. Contacts may be soft or hard. Contact lenses are removed and cleaned daily. Many contact lenses are now disposable and are only worn for a specific length of time, for example a week or month, and then are thrown away and a new set is worn.

Contact lenses must be cared for carefully to prevent infection and irritation of the eyes (Fig. 34-12). Special cleaning and soaking solutions are used to clean and store the lenses. The types of solutions that are used vary according to the type of lens. Each lens

is kept in its own case ("left" and "right") because the correction and size for the left and right eyes may be different. If one of your patients or residents wears contact lenses, make sure you are familiar with the proper technique for helping the person to care for them. Report any complaints of eye irritation or discharge to the nurse immediately.

Prosthetic Eyes

Sometimes a person's eye must be surgically removed because of injury or disease. A person who has had an eye removed may choose to wear a patch to cover the missing eye, or they may wear a prosthetic (artificial) eye. Prosthetic eyes are made of ceramic or plastic and are usually designed to be very close in appearance to the person's own eye, in terms of color and shape

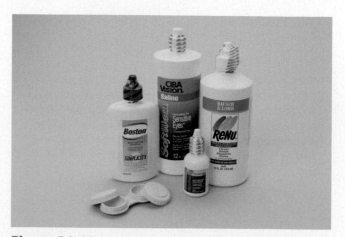

Figure 34-12 Contact lenses must be cleaned and stored properly to prevent infection and irritation of the eyes.

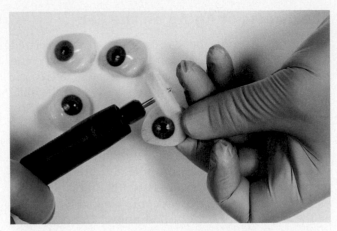

Figure 34-13 Artificial eyes are custom-made to look very similar to the person's other eye. *(Evil Khan\Shutterstock.com)*

(Fig. 34-13). When the person's natural eye is removed, a supporting structure is often inserted into the empty socket and the tissues inside the eyelids (the conjunctiva) are closed over it. Many times, the muscles that move the eyeball are attached to the supporting structure. This allows the prosthetic eye, if the person chooses to wear one, to move with the other eye.

A prosthetic eye is usually a curved disc (not a ball) that fits underneath the person's eyelids. Some prosthetic eyes are removable and others are permanent. If your patient's or resident's prosthetic eye is removable, you may need to help with cleaning and storing it. Like eyeglasses, a prosthetic eye is very expensive to replace and should be cared for carefully. Improper handling can cause scratches or nicks on the prosthetic eye that can injure or irritate the person's eyelids. Handling the prosthetic eye with dirty hands or not cleaning it properly can result in an infection.

If one of your patients or residents wears a prosthetic eye, make sure you have been instructed in the proper way to care for it.

HEARING AND BALANCE

The sense organ of hearing and balance is the ear.

Structure of the Ear

The ear has three main sections: the outer ear, the middle ear, and the inner ear (Fig. 34-14).

The Outer Ear

The outer ear consists of the part of the ear that you can see (called the *pinna* or the *auricle*), plus a short canal called the *external auditory canal* (see Fig. 34-14). The shape of the pinna allows it to collect sound waves and direct them down the external auditory canal toward the *tympanic membrane* (also called the eardrum). The external auditory canal is lined with small hairs and special glands that secrete **cerumen** (ear wax). Cerumen helps to protect the ear canal by trapping dirt and other particles.

The Middle Ear

The middle ear consists of an air space containing three very small bones (called *ossicles*) and the opening of the *eustachian tube*. The eustachian tube connects the middle ear to the pharynx (throat) and serves to equalize the pressure in the middle ear. If you have ever gone up or down a mountain or flown in an airplane, then you have probably felt your eustachian tube at work. As you change altitudes, your ears feel funny and you yawn to open them. The yawn allows

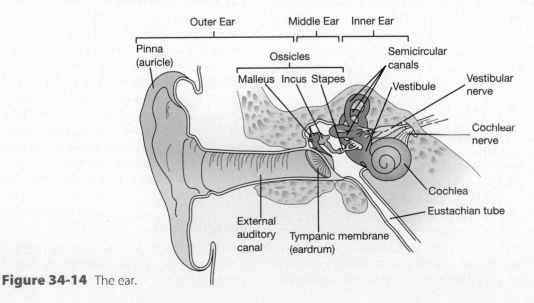

Figure 34-14 The ear.

air to travel through the eustachian tube, making the air pressure in the middle ear equal to the air pressure outside of your body. Equalizing the air pressures prevents the tympanic membrane from rupturing.

The three small bones (ossicles) in the middle ear are connected to the tympanic membrane. These bones, individually called the *malleus*, the *incus*, and the *stapes*, form a tiny bridge between the tympanic membrane and the inner ear (see Fig. 34-14).

The Inner Ear

The most complex part of the ear is the inner ear, which contains the receptors that make hearing and balance possible. The part of the inner ear that is responsible for hearing is called the *cochlea*. The cochlea looks like a snail's shell and is filled with fluid (see Fig. 34-14). Receptors for hearing are found within the cochlea.

The other part of the inner ear consists of two saclike structures, called the *vestibule*, and three *semicircular canals* (see Fig. 34-14). Like the cochlea, the semicircular canals are filled with fluid. The vestibule and the semicircular canals, which are referred to together as the *vestibular apparatus*, help us to keep our balance.

Function of the Ear

Hearing

Sounds travel in the form of sound waves. Sound waves are captured by the pinna and sent down the external auditory canal. As the sound waves travel down the external auditory canal, they come in contact with the tympanic membrane, causing it to vibrate. The tympanic membrane vibrations are then passed to the first bone of the middle ear, the malleus, which sends the vibrations to the second bone, the incus, and then to the last bone, the stapes. The stapes rests against the oval window, a membrane at the opening of the cochlea. When the stapes vibrates, it causes the oval window to vibrate, sending the vibrations through the fluid inside the cochlea. The moving fluid stimulates the receptors inside the cochlea, which then send nerve impulses via the cochlear nerve to the brain. The brain interprets these nerve impulses as sound.

Balance

When your body position changes, receptors in the vestibular apparatus are stimulated. These receptors then send nerve impulses via the vestibular nerve to the brain. These nerve impulses tell the brain what the body's position is, relative to the ground. Have you ever gotten sick on an amusement park ride, in a car, or on a boat? Motion sickness occurs when the messages your ears are sending to your brain about your body's position do not match the messages your eyes are sending to your brain about your body's position.

The Effects of Aging on the Ear

Like other organs, the ear is prone to age-related changes. The tympanic membrane and ossicles become stiffer, and the number of sensory receptors decreases. As a result, many older people gradually lose the ability to hear high-pitched sounds. This type of hearing loss is called **presbycusis**.

A person with presbycusis has trouble telling the difference between similar-sounding high-pitched sounds like *th* and *s*, which can lead to frequent misunderstandings. Conversations can be difficult to follow, especially when many people are talking at once or there is a lot of background noise. As a result, an older person with presbycusis may start to avoid social situations because they cannot hear well and are embarrassed to have to keep asking others to repeat themselves. Avoiding social gatherings can lead to a feeling of isolation and a decreased quality of life for the older person.

Many older people with presbycusis are mistakenly labeled "confused" or "disoriented" by family members, friends, or health care professionals. But think about it—how can a person answer a question correctly if they cannot hear it clearly in the first place? When speaking with an older person with presbycusis, it is helpful to speak slowly using a lower tone of voice. This may make it easier for the person to understand what you are saying.

Disorders of the Ear

There are several disorders of the ear that as a nursing assistant you should be aware may affect your patients or residents.

Cerumen Impaction

Cerumen impaction is a condition that occurs when ear wax (cerumen) builds up and becomes packed in the external auditory canal. In addition to decreased hearing, the person may experience a sense of fullness in the ear, ringing, itching, or pain. Routinely placing an object in the ear (such as a hearing aid or cotton swab) can cause cerumen impaction because the object pushes the cerumen deep into the external auditory canal. Treatment usually involves irrigating (flushing) the ear with a special solution to remove the wax. Some people have to use special ear drops on a routine basis to prevent this condition from occurring.

Ear Infections

Otitis media is an infection of the middle ear that is common in young children. It occurs when fluid builds up in the middle ear. Bacteria from the throat find their way into the middle ear through the eustachian tube. Once there, they start to grow and multiply in the trapped fluid.

Otitis media is usually accompanied by ear pain, fever, and difficulty hearing. If untreated, otitis media can cause scarring of the tympanic membrane and a permanent loss of hearing. If the infection is bacterial, antibiotics are usually given to treat it. Children who have frequent middle ear infections may need to have "tubes put in their ears." During this surgical procedure, called a *myringotomy*, the doctor makes a small slit in the eardrum and inserts a tube to equalize the pressure and prevent the build-up of fluid in the middle ear.

Another infection commonly seen in the ear involves the external auditory canal. **Otitis externa**, commonly referred to as "swimmer's ear," is an infection of the lining of the external auditory canal. Otitis externa is common in people who swim frequently or get the insides of their ears wet during showering or bathing. The ear becomes very painful to the touch. Antibiotic ear drops are usually needed to treat the infection.

Ménière Disease

Ménière disease, named after the French doctor who first described it, is a disease of the inner ear. The build-up of fluids interferes with the function of the receptors for hearing and balance. People with this disorder periodically experience episodes of dizziness **(vertigo)**, ringing in the ear **(tinnitus)**, temporary hearing loss, and a feeling of pressure or fullness in the ear. One or both ears may be affected, and with time, many people begin to experience permanent hearing loss in the affected ear or ears. There is usually no cure for this disorder.

Although Ménière disease is not fatal, it can be very difficult to live with. Each attack can last between 2 and 4 hours and is often accompanied by nausea, vomiting, or both. A person who is having an attack should lie down and keep their eyes fixed on an object that is not moving. This helps to reduce the nausea and lowers the risk of falling as a result of the dizziness. After a severe attack, the person may be very tired. A person with Ménière disease may need to take more time when getting up from a sitting or lying position, to prevent an attack from occurring.

Deafness

Like blindness, deafness has many different causes and takes many different forms. Some people have been deaf since birth, while others may have lost their hearing gradually later in life. Deafness can be partial or complete. The two main types of deafness are conductive hearing loss and sensorineural hearing loss:

- **Conductive hearing loss** occurs when something prevents sound waves from reaching the receptors in the cochlea. For example, the external auditory canal may be blocked by built-up cerumen, or by a tumor. The tympanic membrane may be damaged and not vibrate well, or the ossicles might not move freely. **Otosclerosis** is a disorder that causes a change in the stapes, preventing it from moving properly. Often, surgical removal and replacement of the stapes with a wire prosthesis can help to restore some hearing in people with otosclerosis.

- **Sensorineural hearing loss** occurs when the receptors are unable to receive stimuli or transmit nerve impulses. Presbycusis, or age-related hearing loss, is sensorineural. However, there are many other causes of sensorineural hearing loss that are not necessarily the result of aging. For example, prolonged exposure to loud noise (especially industrial noise), recurrent ear infections, trauma to the ear, and some types of medications can all cause sensorineural hearing loss.

A person with hearing loss may work with a speech therapist to learn how to speak more clearly. In addition, many adaptive devices are available to help a person with hearing loss maintain their independence. For example, telecommunications device for the deaf (TDD) systems can be used in combination with a standard phone to allow a person with hearing loss to communicate using the telephone. Television shows are available with "closed captioning," a system that prints the words that are being spoken at the bottom of the screen so that the person can read them. The person's doorbell, alarm clock, telephone, and smoke alarms may flash instead of ring. Like a person who is blind, a person who is deaf may have a companion animal that is trained to act as the person's "ears."

Communicating With a Person Who Has Hearing Loss

When caring for a person with hearing loss, there are a few easy things you can do to ensure good communication:

- **Face the person when you are speaking to them.** Many people who lose their hearing gradually develop the ability to partially lip-read what people are saying to them. You should always face the person as you speak so that the person has a clear view of your mouth (Fig. 34-15). Avoid chewing gum or speaking fast. Doing so can hinder the person's ability to lip-read.

- **Use a notepad to write down important questions or directions so that the person can read them.** This helps to eliminate misunderstandings. If the person cannot read or reads in a language that is unfamiliar to you, a picture

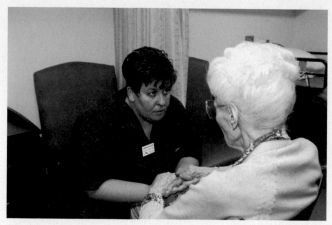

Figure 34-15 Always give a person who has a hearing deficit an unobstructed view of your mouth. This will help the person to lip-read.

board (see Chapter 5, Fig. 5-4) may be quite helpful.

■ **Make sure that the person fully understands what you said.** Some people, especially if the hearing loss is recent, hesitate to ask other people to repeat themselves. They may feel embarrassed by their hearing loss. When you are the "sender," you need to make sure that the person has gotten the message you were trying to send. If you are not sure that a person has understood what you have said to them, simply ask the person to repeat what you said back to you. For example, say, "If you could please repeat back to me what I said, I can make sure I told you everything I needed to." When the request is phrased in this way, the person feels as though they are helping you to do your job by repeating back the information. This helps to preserve the person's self-esteem and is a much better approach than just saying, "Now what did I say?"

■ **Let the person know if you cannot understand what they are saying to you.** Many people with hearing loss have difficulty speaking clearly. If you cannot understand what the person is saying to you, please do not pretend that you did to spare the person's feelings. The person may be trying to tell you something that is vitally important to their care or health. Tell the person that you did not understand and look for another way for them to get their message across. For example, you might offer them a notepad so they can write down what they need to tell you.

■ **Consider learning sign language.** Many people who have significant hearing loss use sign language to communicate (Fig. 34-16). Knowing how to communicate in this manner can be a very useful skill for a nursing assistant to have.

Hearing Aids

Many people who have hearing loss use a hearing aid. A hearing aid is a battery-powered device that amplifies sound (makes it louder) before it enters the external auditory canal. There are many different styles of hearing aids (Fig. 34-17). Some styles fit entirely within the external auditory canal. Others attach behind the ear or to the person's eyeglasses. Others take the form of a small box that the person carries in their pocket.

Not all people with hearing loss can benefit from the use of a hearing aid. It depends on the type of hearing loss the person has. An audiologist (ear specialist) evaluates the person's hearing deficit to determine whether a hearing aid will be useful and to determine what type of hearing aid should be used.

Hearing aids amplify all sounds, not just the voice of the person who is speaking. Noises from the environment, such as traffic noise or background music in a restaurant, are also amplified. This can be distracting to a person wearing a hearing aid, and as a result, the person may choose to keep the hearing aid turned off most of the time.

Hearing aids are expensive and must be cared for carefully. General guidelines for caring for hearing aids are given in Guidelines Box 34-2. If one of your patients or residents uses a hearing aid, make sure that you know how to care for it and operate it. If a person who uses a hearing aid seems unable to hear you, make sure the hearing aid is turned on, and that the volume is turned up high enough. If the hearing aid still does not seem to be working, check the batteries to see if they need to be replaced and make sure the sound passageway is not blocked with cerumen. As with eyeglasses, it may be your responsibility to make sure that your patients or residents have their hearing aids in place because they may forget them or be physically unable to put them in and turn them on. Procedure 34-1 explains how to help a person to insert and remove an in-the-ear hearing aid.

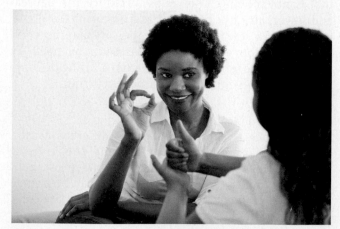

Figure 34-16 Some people who are deaf use sign language to communicate. (*Andrey_Popov\Shutterstock.com*)

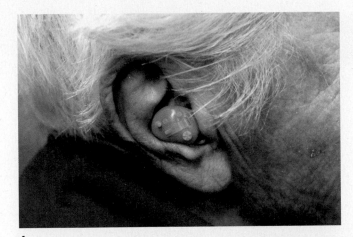

A

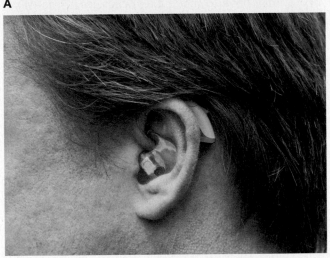

B

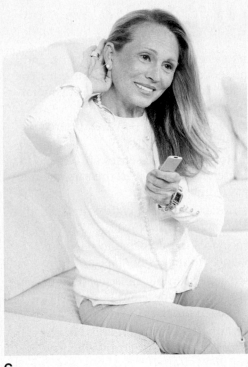

C

Figure 34-17 Hearing aids come in a variety of styles. **A.** This type of hearing aid fits entirely inside the external auditory canal. **B.** This type of hearing aid fits behind the person's ear. **C.** This type of hearing aid is carried in a pocket. (*B, andras_csontos\Shutterstock.com; C, Adam Gregor\Shutterstock.com*)

Guidelines Box 34-2   Guidelines for Caring for Hearing Aids

WHAT YOU DO	WHY YOU DO IT
Clean the hearing aid daily, according to the manufacturer's instructions.	If the hearing aid is not cleaned daily, the sound passages can become blocked with cerumen. The cerumen build-up can cause the hearing aid to stop working properly.
Make sure that the person has a spare set of batteries on hand at all times, and replace dead batteries immediately.	The hearing aid is battery-operated and will not work if the batteries are dead. It is very inconvenient for a person who uses a hearing aid to be without it for any length of time.
Keep hearing aids away from heat and moisture.	Heat and moisture can damage the plastic ear mold.
Do not use hairspray or other hair care products on a person who wears a hearing aid while the hearing aid is in place.	The chemicals in many hair care products can damage the plastic ear mold.
Store hearing aids at room temperature when they are not being worn.	Hearing aids are delicate instruments. Exposure to very hot or very cold temperatures is not good for them.
Keep replacement batteries and small hearing aids away from children and pets.	These small objects can pose a choking hazard to children and pets. In addition, hearing aids are expensive to replace.

SUMMARY

- Our sensory system protects us from harm and lets us experience the world that we live in. The sensory system has two main divisions: general senses and special senses.
    - The receptors for general senses are spread throughout the body.
    - The receptors for special senses are located in special sense organs (the eyes, the ears, the nose, and the taste buds).
- General senses are responsible for our sense of touch, position, and pain.
    - Tactile receptors in our skin allow us to feel textures and the shapes of objects.
    - Position receptors in our muscles, tendons, and joints let us know where our body parts are in relation to each other.
    - Pain receptors (free nerve endings) in our skin and internal organs let us know when we are injured or ill.
- Chemoreceptors in the taste buds and the roof of the nasal cavity give us our senses of taste and smell.
    - Together, taste and smell play a very large role in stimulating the appetite.
    - These senses also help to keep us safe by alerting us to signs of danger (such as spoiled food, a gas leak, or smoke from a fire).
- The eye is a complex organ that gives us our sense of sight.
    - Many people need corrective lenses (eyeglasses or contact lenses) to see clearly. Common problems with focusing include myopia (nearsightedness), hyperopia (farsightedness), and astigmatism.
    - Changes in the eye as a result of aging can lead to presbyopia (an inability to focus on objects that are close), cataracts, and dry eyes. Older people may also need more time to adjust when moving between brightly and dimly lit areas.
    - Some eye disorders, such as glaucoma and diabetic retinopathy, can lead to permanent vision loss if untreated.
    - There are many different degrees of blindness.
        - Most people who are blind manage well on their own.
        - When caring for a person who is blind, you may have to make a few changes in the way you normally do things.
    - Handle eyeglasses, contact lenses, and prosthetic (artificial) eyes with care. These are expensive and difficult to replace. Improper handling of contact lenses or prosthetic eyes can also lead to infection of the eye.
- The ear is responsible for our senses of hearing and balance.
    - Sensory receptors for sound are located in the cochlea.
        - Presbycusis is an age-related hearing loss caused by a gradual decrease in the number of sensory receptors for sound.
        - There are many different degrees of hearing loss. Hearing loss may be conductive or sensorineural in origin.
        - When talking to a person with hearing loss, be sure that the person can see your face, take care to speak clearly, and clarify information as necessary. It may be necessary to write information down or use a picture board to ensure understanding.
    - Sensory receptors for balance are located in the vestibular apparatus, which consists of the vestibule and the semicircular canals. These receptors tell the brain where the body is in relation to the ground.

Procedure 34-1

Assisting a Person With an In-the-Ear Hearing Aid

WHY YOU DO IT   Being able to hear clearly makes communication easier and enhances the person's quality of life.

Inserting an In-the-Ear Hearing Aid

Getting Ready

1. Complete the "Getting Ready" steps.

2. Check the hearing aid to make sure the volume is down and the hearing aid is turned off.

3. Help the person to a comfortable position, with their head turned so that the ear needing the hearing aid is closest to you.

4. Inspect the ear canal for excessive cerumen (ear wax). If you see excessive wax build-up in the ear canal, gently wipe the ear canal with a warm, moist washcloth.

5. Gently insert the tapered end of the hearing aid into the external auditory canal. Gently rotate the hearing aid so that it fits into the curve of the ear. With one hand, push up and in. Use your other hand to pull gently down on the person's earlobe. The hearing aid should fit snugly but comfortably, flush with the ear.

6. Turn on the control switch. Adjust the volume by talking to the person as you increase the volume. Stop increasing the volume when the person can hear you.

Finishing Up

7. Complete the "Finishing Up" steps.

Removing an In-the-Ear Hearing Aid

Getting Ready

1. Complete the "Getting Ready" steps.

2. Turn off the hearing aid.

3. Gently pull up on the person's ear. This will allow you to lift the hearing aid up and out of the person's ear.

4. Remove the batteries before storing the hearing aid in its case. Make sure the case is labeled with the person's name.

Finishing Up

5. Complete the "Finishing Up" steps.

WHAT DID YOU LEARN?

Multiple Choice

Select the single best answer for each of the following questions.

1. Where are sensory receptors that are responsible for the special senses located?
   a. In the muscles, tendons, and joints
   b. In the eyes, ears, nose, and taste buds
   c. In the brain and spinal cord
   d. In all of the organs of the body

2. Ms. Valencia is having a heart attack. She complains to the nurse of pain in her arm and jaw. What type of pain is Ms. Valencia experiencing?
   a. Chronic pain
   b. Referred (radiating) pain
   c. Imagined pain
   d. Musculoskeletal pain

3. One of the residents in the facility where you work, Mr. Hepberg, is 85 years old and in fairly good overall health. Mr. Hepberg always says to you, "Don't ever get old! When you get old, even the food doesn't taste good anymore." Why might Mr. Hepberg feel this way?
   a. The meals at the facility are very bland for dietetic reasons.
   b. Mr. Hepberg is depressed.
   c. As we get older, our sense of taste and smell decreases, making food less appealing.
   d. Mr. Hepberg has a head cold.

4. Which of the following are symptoms of conjunctivitis?
   a. Itching and burning of the eye
   b. Redness of the eye
   c. A sticky white or yellow discharge from the eye
   d. All of the above

5. Juanita is assigned to take care of Mr. Golden, who has recently become blind. What should Juanita remember when caring for Mr. Golden?
   a. Juanita should greet Mr. Golden and state her name when she enters his room.
   b. Juanita can help Mr. Golden to feel more secure when walking by walking a step or two ahead of Mr. Golden and letting Mr. Golden rest his hand lightly on her elbow.
   c. During procedures, Juanita should explain each step of the procedure to Mr. Golden as she does it so that he knows what is happening.
   d. All of the above

6. Which one of the following is true about cataracts?
   a. Many older people develop cataracts, but younger people can develop them too.
   b. Cataracts are very painful.
   c. There is no cure for cataracts.
   d. Cataracts are a complication of diabetes.

7. Matteo is taking care of Ms. Jordan, who has a hearing loss. Ms. Jordan is wearing her hearing aid, but it does not seem to be working. What should Matteo do first?
   a. They should raise their voice.
   b. They should make sure that the hearing aid is turned on, and that the volume is high enough.
   c. They should remove the hearing aid and replace its batteries.
   d. They should report the problem to the nurse immediately.

8. Mr. Campi, one of your older residents, has extensive hearing loss. What should you remember when you are talking to Mr. Campi?
   a. You should sit or stand so that Mr. Campi has a clear view of your face, and you should avoid chewing gum or speaking quickly.
   b. If you think that Mr. Campi has not completely understood what you are saying, you should demand that he repeat it back to you so that you can correct his mistakes.
   c. If you do not understand what Mr. Campi has said, you should just let it pass. Letting him know that you did not understand might embarrass or frustrate him.
   d. There is no point in talking to Mr. Campi. He cannot hear you anyway. It is better to just write everything down.

Matching *Match each numbered item with its appropriate lettered description.*

_____ **1.** Iris

_____ **2.** Cornea

_____ **3.** Lens

_____ **4.** Myopia

_____ **5.** Astigmatism

_____ **6.** Retina

_____ **7.** Hyperopia

_____ **8.** Pupil

_____ **9.** Vitreous humor

_____**10.** Ciliary body

a. Nearsightedness

b. Clear portion of the sclera, through which light passes to the inside of the eye

c. A round muscle; the colored portion of the eye

d. Farsightedness

e. A disorder of the cornea that results in blurred vision

f. The opening in the center of the iris

g. A flexible, transparent, curved structure that helps to focus images on the retina

h. Contains rods and cones, the sensory receptors responsible for vision

i. The jelly-like substance contained in the posterior chamber that helps to give the eyeball its shape

j. The muscle that allows the lens to either become shorter and rounder or longer and flatter

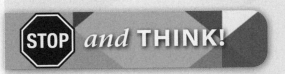

You work in an assisted-living facility and have known one of the residents, Mrs. Zinner, for almost 6 years now. Mrs. Zinner is in her 70s and enjoys very good health. In fact, her only disability seems to be related to macular degeneration, which is causing her to go blind. Mrs. Zinner's ability to see is now limited to being able to tell the difference between light and dark and make out the outlines of very large objects. What are some ways that you can help Mrs. Zinner adjust to her blindness physically? What are some things you can do that will help Mrs. Zinner adjust emotionally?

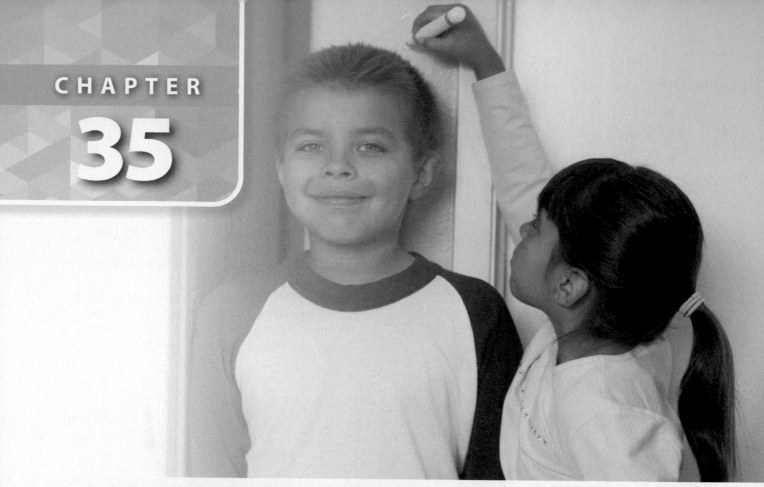

Photo: Hormones, which are produced by the endocrine system, set processes in motion. For example, hormones are what cause us to grow! (Blend Images\Shutterstock.com)

The Endocrine System

 WHAT WILL YOU LEARN?

The endocrine system produces hormones, chemicals that act on cells to produce a response. The word "hormone" comes from the Greek word *hormaein*, "to set in motion." This is, in fact, exactly what hormones do—set things in motion. Sometimes, the effects of the hormone occur over a long period of time. For example, hormones allow us to grow to our adult height, and they cause the physical changes that occur during puberty. Other times, the effects of hormones are more immediate. Hormones with short-term effects help the body to maintain homeostasis. For example, insulin is a hormone that regulates blood sugar levels.

The hormones produced by the endocrine system control many of the body's functions. In this chapter, you will learn about the glands of the endocrine system, some of the hormones they produce, and how these hormones act to "set things in motion." You will also learn about some of the disorders that occur when the body produces too much or too little of a certain hormone. When you are finished with this chapter, you will be able to:

1. List the glands that make up the endocrine system.
2. State the main function of the endocrine system.
3. Describe the feedback mechanism that controls the endocrine system.
4. List the hormones produced by the different glands of the endocrine system.

5. **Explain how the aging process affects the endocrine system.**

6. **Discuss various disorders that affect the endocrine system.**

7. **Discuss the special care needs of people who have endocrine system disorders.**

8. **Demonstrate the proper technique for monitoring a person's blood glucose level.**

Vocabulary

Hormones	Hyperthyroidism	Diabetes mellitus	Hypoglycemia
Goiter	(Graves disease)	Type 1 diabetes mellitus	Hyperglycemia
Tetany	Hypothyroidism	Type 2 diabetes mellitus	

STRUCTURE OF THE ENDOCRINE SYSTEM

A group of glands, called the endocrine glands, make up the endocrine system. Be careful not to confuse endocrine glands and exocrine glands! Endocrine glands produce hormones and release them into the bloodstream. Exocrine glands produce substances that are not hormones and release them into a hollow

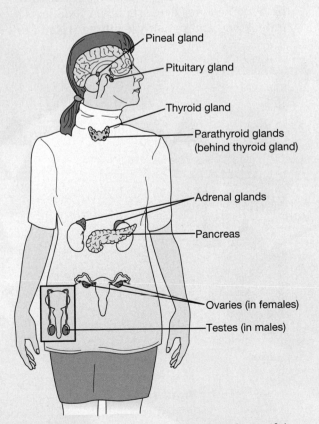

Figure 35-1 The endocrine system is made up of the endocrine glands, which are located throughout the body.

organ or onto a surface. Examples of exocrine glands include the salivary glands in the mouth, which produce saliva, and the sweat glands in the skin, which produce sweat. Exocrine glands are not part of the endocrine system.

The endocrine glands are located in specific places throughout the body (Fig. 35-1):

- The *pituitary gland* is about the size of a cherry and lies underneath the brain. It is connected by a stalk to the hypothalamus.
- The *pineal gland* is also located underneath the brain.
- The *thyroid gland* is located in the neck. It is butterfly-shaped, with two oval lobes located on either side of the larynx. The lobes are connected by a narrow band of tissue called the isthmus.
- The *parathyroid glands* are four tiny glands that are embedded in the back of the thyroid gland.
- The *adrenal glands* are located on top of the kidneys.
- The *pancreas* is located in the abdomen.
- The *sex glands (gonads)* are the ovaries in females and the testes in males. These glands are also considered part of the reproductive system and are discussed in detail in Chapter 38.

FUNCTION OF THE ENDOCRINE SYSTEM

The endocrine system controls many of the body's processes, such as growth and development, reproduction, and metabolism. It does this by producing **hormones**, chemicals that act on cells to produce a response. The hormones are released into the bloodstream, which means that they can affect cells far from the gland that produced them. A hormone travels in the blood until it reaches its target cell. Once there, it attaches to a special receptor in the cell's plasma membrane (or, more rarely, in the cell's nucleus). Just as turning a key in a lock causes a door to open, attaching a hormone to a receptor causes a specific reaction in the cell. Some hormones have receptors in all of the body's cells, while other hormones have receptors in only certain types of cells.

The release (secretion) of many hormones is regulated by a feedback system. In one type of endocrine feedback system, a specific change in the internal environment (the *stimulus*) causes a gland to increase production of its hormone (the *signal*). The hormone has an effect (the *response*) that corrects the change in the internal environment. Once the internal environment has returned to normal, the gland decreases production of the hormone. Other stimuli inhibit hormone production by the gland, and once the internal environment has returned to normal, hormone production increases.

The feedback system works very much like a central heating unit in a house. The thermostat is preset to keep the temperature inside the house within a certain range. When the thermostat detects that the temperature has dropped below this preset range (the stimulus), the thermostat signals the furnace to turn on to heat the air (the response). After the furnace creates heat and the temperature in the house rises to the desired range, the thermostat turns the furnace unit off. In this example, an electrical signal passes from the thermostat to the furnace. In the endocrine system, hormone signals pass from the gland to another organ.

In the rest of this section, we will explore the individual glands of the endocrine system, the hormones they secrete, and the effects of these hormones on the body.

Pituitary Gland

The pituitary gland, which is controlled by the hypothalamus, releases hormones that affect the function of other glands in the endocrine system. In this sense, the pituitary gland is like the "master gland." The pituitary gland has two parts, the posterior lobe and the anterior lobe.

Posterior Lobe Hormones

The posterior lobe of the pituitary gland stores and releases hormones that are produced by the hypothalamus. Two hormones are released by the posterior lobe (Fig. 35-2).

- *Antidiuretic hormone (ADH)* acts on the kidneys. ADH limits the amount of water that is lost from the body in the form of urine. When a person does not take in enough fluid or loses too much fluid through sweating, vomiting, or diarrhea, the hypothalamus detects a lower fluid level in the blood and signals the pituitary gland to

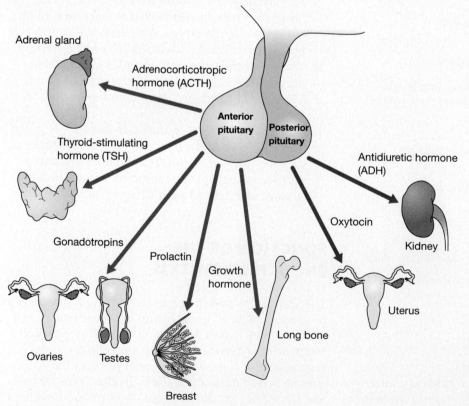

Figure 35-2 The pituitary gland, or "master gland," releases hormones that affect other glands in the endocrine system.

release more ADH. The ADH causes the kidneys to save body fluid by decreasing the amount of urine produced. Similarly, when the hypothalamus detects that fluid levels are too high, it signals the pituitary gland to secrete less ADH. The lack of ADH causes the kidneys to produce more urine, eliminating the excess fluid from the body.

- *Oxytocin* is the hormone that causes labor to begin and is responsible for the let-down of milk in the breasts of a nursing.

Anterior Lobe Hormones

The anterior lobe of the pituitary gland makes and releases several different hormones (see Fig. 35-2).

- *Growth hormone* is what causes our bodies to get bigger and taller as we move from infancy into adulthood. Growth hormone is usually released in greater amounts during short periods of time, resulting in a child's "growth spurts." Although the output of growth hormone is highest during childhood, the anterior lobe continues to release growth hormone long after the growing phase of development is finished. Cells need to be replaced throughout a person's lifetime, and growth hormone is necessary for that to occur.
- *Thyroid-stimulating hormone (TSH)* stimulates the thyroid gland to produce thyroid hormones, which affect the rate of metabolism in the body's tissues.
- *Adrenocorticotropic hormone (ACTH)* stimulates the adrenal glands to produce their hormones, which help the body to deal with stress.
- *Prolactin* stimulates the milk glands of the breast to produce milk when a baby is born.
- *Gonadotropins* regulate the functioning of the sex glands (gonads) in both males and females. There are two gonadotropins, *follicle-stimulating hormone (FSH)* and *luteinizing hormone (LH)*. The action of the gonadotropins is discussed in more detail in Chapter 38.

Pineal Gland

The pineal gland secretes *melatonin*, which helps to regulate the body's sleep–awake cycles. The pineal gland is stimulated by light and darkness and secretes melatonin during the dark part of the day.

Thyroid Gland

The thyroid gland produces *thyroxine*, which is often just called thyroid hormone. Thyroxine sets the rate of metabolism for the cells of the body. How quickly body cells and tissues use nutrients (especially protein) and produce energy is determined by the amount of thyroxine present in the bloodstream. If the thyroid gland releases more thyroxine, the metabolic rate of the cells increases, and if the thyroid gland releases less thyroxine, the metabolic rate of the cells decreases.

The thyroid gland needs iodine to produce thyroxine. Iodine is found naturally in fish and shellfish and is added to salt and other commercial products. When a person does not get enough iodine in their diet, the thyroid gland is not able to produce adequate amounts of thyroxine. The sensors in the hypothalamus and pituitary gland detect a decrease in the level of thyroxine in the bloodstream and release TSH to stimulate the thyroid gland to produce more. However, because the thyroid gland has no iodine, it cannot respond to the request for more thyroxine, and the cycle repeats itself. The constant stimulation of the thyroid gland causes it to enlarge. An enlargement of the thyroid gland is called a **goiter** (Fig. 35-3). Iodine deficiency is just one cause of goiter. Goiter can also occur when the thyroid gland does not produce enough hormone because of disease or tumors.

Parathyroid Glands

The parathyroid glands produce *parathyroid hormone (PTH)*, an important hormone for the regulation of blood calcium. Decreased blood levels of calcium stimulate PTH production. PTH causes calcium to be released from the bones into the bloodstream, increasing the amount of calcium in the bloodstream. In addition, PTH helps the kidneys to keep calcium by reducing how much is excreted in the urine.

PTH also stimulates the production of the active form of vitamin D, also known as *calcitriol*. Calcitriol

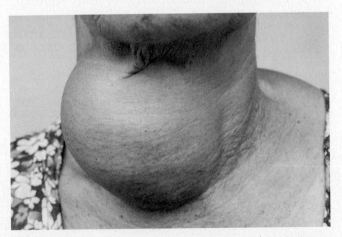

Figure 35-3 The swelling in this person's neck is a goiter, or an enlarged thyroid gland. Goiter can be caused by a lack of iodine in the diet or by a tumor or disease that affects the thyroid gland's ability to produce thyroid hormone. *(chatuphot\Shuttestock.com)*

helps to increase the absorption of calcium from the intestines, increasing blood calcium levels. As you learned in Chapter 30, a calcium-rich diet is important to build up stores of calcium in the bones. PTH and calcitriol working together is what allows us to draw on these stores later in life, when our bodies become less efficient at absorbing the calcium that we eat.

If the parathyroid glands are surgically removed or become damaged by disease, PTH is not produced in adequate amounts and the calcium levels may drop. The most common symptom of PTH deficiency is **tetany**, which is involuntary cramping of skeletal muscles. Some tumors of the parathyroid gland can cause an overproduction of PTH that results in too much calcium being removed from the bones. The bones then become very fragile and fracture easily. Because the kidneys are responsible for excreting the excess calcium, kidney stones are likely to form.

Adrenal Glands

Each adrenal gland has two separate parts: the *medulla*, or inner portion, and the *cortex*, or outer portion (Fig. 35-4). Each part secretes distinct hormones.

Medullary Hormones

The medulla of the adrenal glands secretes two hormones that are responsible for the "fight-or-flight" response of the body in emergency situations. Those hormones are *epinephrine* (also known as adrenaline) and *norepinephrine*. Epinephrine and norepinephrine help the heart and lungs deliver more oxygen and nutrients to the muscles, preparing the body to "stand up and fight or turn tail and run." A "side effect" of these hormones is the dry-mouthed, heart-pounding reaction that occurs when you are frightened!

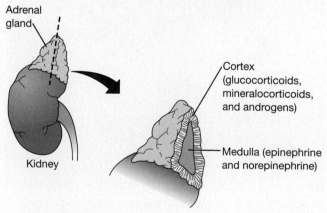

Adrenal gland

Kidney

Cortex (glucocorticoids, mineralocorticoids, and androgens)

Medulla (epinephrine and norepinephrine)

Figure 35-4 The adrenal gland consists of an inner part (the adrenal medulla) and an outer part (the adrenal cortex). Each part produces and secretes different hormones. Several of these hormones help us to deal with stressful situations.

Cortical Hormones

The outer portion of the adrenal glands secretes three main groups of hormones:

- *Glucocorticoids* play a role in the metabolism of fats and proteins and help the body to maintain a reserve of glucose (sugar) that can be used in times of stress. They are also able to suppress the body's inflammatory response. For this reason, glucocorticoids are often given in the form of medications for severe inflammatory disorders such as asthma, rheumatoid arthritis, or severe allergic reactions. Hydrocortisone is a common medication that is a glucocorticoid.
- *Mineralocorticoids* help to regulate the level of certain minerals in the body, particularly sodium and potassium. *Aldosterone* is the primary hormone in this group. Aldosterone helps the kidneys to reabsorb sodium and secrete potassium.
- *Androgens* are secreted in small amounts by the adrenal cortex. Androgens are converted by the body into the sex hormones *testosterone* and *estradiol*.

Pancreas

The pancreas is both an exocrine gland and an endocrine gland. It functions as an exocrine gland by producing and secreting into the small intestine enzymes that help to digest food. It functions as an endocrine gland by producing two hormones, *insulin* and *glucagon*.

Insulin

Special cells within the pancreas, called the *islets of Langerhans*, produce and secrete the hormone insulin. Insulin, which affects all of the body's cells, allows glucose (sugar) to be transported from the bloodstream into the individual cells, where it is used for energy. In this way, insulin lowers the blood glucose level.

When a person eats, food is digested and absorbed by the bloodstream in the form of glucose. The blood glucose levels determine how much insulin is released by the pancreas. After eating, a person's blood glucose is elevated, and the pancreas releases more insulin. The insulin causes the glucose to move from the bloodstream into the cells, where it can be used for energy. Any extra glucose is converted to glycogen. Glycogen is stored in the liver and muscle for later use, or it is converted to fat and deposited in various places on the body.

Glucagon

Glucagon has the opposite effect of insulin. While insulin is responsible for lowering blood glucose levels, glucagon is responsible for raising them. When the glucose levels in the bloodstream drop, as they normally do when a person has not eaten for some time, the pancreas secretes more glucagon. The glucagon stimulates the liver to release the glucose that has been stored as glycogen into the bloodstream, to supply the cells of the body with fuel for energy. Insulin and glucagon work together to keep the body's blood glucose levels stable.

Sex Glands

The sex glands (or gonads) secrete the hormones that result in the onset of puberty and that regulate reproduction. Because the ovaries and testes are also considered a part of the reproductive system, these glands are discussed in greater detail in Chapter 38.

THE EFFECTS OF AGING ON THE ENDOCRINE SYSTEM

The normal processes of aging decrease the amount of hormones produced and slow their secretion by the glands of the endocrine system. Many of the physical changes that are part of aging are directly related to the smaller amounts of hormone released. For example, decreases in growth hormone levels slow the rate at which the body's cells and tissues divide and replace themselves, and decreases in thyroid hormone levels slow the body's metabolism.

In females, menopause occurs as a result of decreased hormone production by the ovaries. In males, secretion of hormones by the testes decreases, affecting sexual drive and function.

DISORDERS OF THE ENDOCRINE SYSTEM

Disorders of the endocrine system occur when the body produces too much or too little of a certain hormone. Imbalances in hormone secretion can be caused by disorders of the hypothalamus, the pituitary gland, the specific endocrine gland responsible for the hormone, or as a result of poor nutrition. Corrective measures may be needed to restore the body's homeostasis and prevent the imbalances from causing health problems. There are many different types of endocrine disorders. Some of the ones you will be most likely to encounter in the health care setting are described here.

Pituitary Gland Disorders

The pituitary gland controls the function of the other endocrine glands and many other tissues and organs.

Because of this, disorders of the pituitary gland can affect numerous body systems in many different ways. Two well-known disorders are caused by abnormal secretion of growth hormone.

Growth Hormone Deficiency

Growth hormone deficiency during the growing years results in short stature. This condition is sometimes described as *pituitary dwarfism*. The body of a person with growth hormone deficiency during childhood is much smaller than average, but still well proportioned. If the condition is diagnosed while the person is still a child, growth hormone may be given to help stimulate growth.

Growth Hormone Excess

An excess in the amount of growth hormone secreted during the growing years results in a condition known as *pituitary gigantism* (Fig. 35-5). The body of a person with pituitary gigantism is much larger than average, but still well proportioned.

The secretion of too much growth hormone after a person has reached adulthood causes excessive

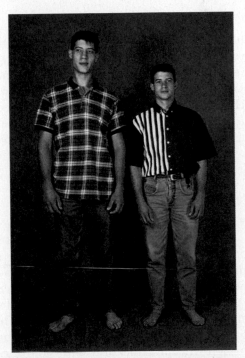

Figure 35-5 Pituitary gigantism occurs when the pituitary gland produces too much growth hormone during a person's growing years. These men are identical twins, but the man on the left is much taller than his average-sized brother because of the production of an excess amount of growth hormone. (From Gagel, R. F., & McCutcheon, I. E. Images in clinical medicine. Pituitary gigantism. *N Engl J Med.* 1999;350(7):524. Copyright © 1999 Massachusetts Medical Society. Reprinted with permission from Massachusetts Medical Society.)

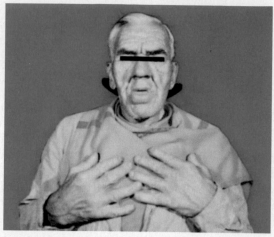

Figure 35-6 Secretion of too much growth hormone in an adult causes acromegaly, excessive growth of the bones of the hands, feet, and face.

growth of the bones of the hands, feet, and face. This condition is called acromegaly (Fig. 35-6). The person does not grow taller, but does have a disproportioned appearance, especially in the face and hands.

Thyroid Gland Disorders

Remember that the secretion of the thyroid hormones is controlled by the pituitary gland. Therefore, thyroid disorders can be caused by abnormalities of the pituitary gland or by abnormalities of the thyroid gland itself. Thyroid disorders can also result from nutrient deficiencies, such as a lack of iodine. A simple blood test can be used to detect imbalances in thyroid hormones. Once detected, these imbalances can usually be treated.

Hyperthyroidism

Hyperthyroidism is caused by the excessive secretion of thyroxine (*hyper* = "above"). The most common form, **Graves disease**, results from the body's own antibodies stimulating thyroid gland activity. In a person with hyperthyroidism, the metabolic rate of the body's cells is increased. Signs and symptoms of hyperthyroidism include increased hunger accompanied by weight loss, an irregular heartbeat, an inability to sleep, irritability, confusion, increased perspiration, and intolerance to heat. Hyperthyroidism may be treated by surgically removing part of the thyroid gland or by destroying part of the gland with radiation.

Hypothyroidism

Hypothyroidism results when thyroxine secretion is too low (*hypo* = "below"). Some babies are born with *congenital hypothyroidism* due to a failure of the thyroid gland to develop. Because thyroxine's control of the body's metabolism is essential for growth and development, congenital hypothyroidism is characterized by a lack of physical growth and mental development. However, if the hypothyroidism is detected and treated soon after birth, complications can be minimized. Hypothyroidism is treated by administering thyroxine in the form of a pill.

Most cases of hypothyroidism develop later in life, as a result of a disorder of the hypothalamus, pituitary gland, or thyroid gland. *Hashimoto thyroiditis* is the result of the body's own antibodies attacking and destroying thyroid tissue. In adults, hypothyroidism is more common among females and older adults. Hypothyroidism causes signs and symptoms that are opposite those of hyperthyroidism. Signs and symptoms of hypothyroidism include fatigue, weakness, depression, anorexia, weight gain, constipation, and intolerance to cold. The administration of oral thyroxine helps to restore the body's metabolism to a normal rate and relieves the signs and symptoms of hypothyroidism.

Adrenal Gland Disorders

Two of the most common adrenal gland disorders, Addison disease and Cushing syndrome, result from imbalances of the adrenal cortical hormones.

Addison Disease

In Addison disease, the adrenal cortex is not functioning normally, resulting in low levels of the adrenal cortical hormones. Because the glucocorticoids play a role in protein metabolism, a person with Addison disease develops muscle weakness and atrophy. Dark discoloration of the skin and disturbances in the body's salt and water balance are also seen. The person may have hypertension as a result of Addison disease. A person with Addison disease may need assistance with walking and range-of-motion exercises.

Cushing Syndrome

Cushing syndrome results from excessive secretion of glucocorticoids. Cushing syndrome can be caused by disorders of the pituitary gland that affect ACTH secretion or by disorders of the adrenal gland itself. Some people develop Cushing syndrome after taking high doses of steroid medications, such as hydrocortisone, for a long period of time. Because glucocorticoids help us to metabolize fat, people with Cushing syndrome tend to develop pockets of fat in the abdomen, on the back, and in the face. Increased facial hair is also common (Fig. 35-7). A person with Cushing syndrome will have high blood glucose levels because one of the effects of glucocorticoids is to decrease the

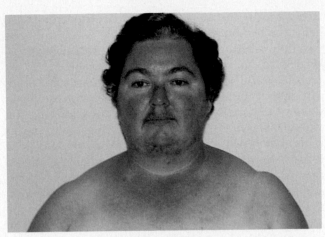

Figure 35-7 Cushing syndrome results from excessive amounts of the adrenal cortical hormones. The excessive secretion of androgens, which are converted into sex hormones, is what caused this female to develop facial hair. The accumulation of fat on the female's back and face is the result of excess glucocorticoids. (Reprinted with permission from Rubin, E., & Farber, J. L. [2005]. *Pathology* [4th ed., p. 1162]. Lippincott Williams & Wilkins.)

use of glucose by the tissues and stimulate glucose release from the liver. Easy bruising of the skin and muscle weakness is also seen.

Diabetes Mellitus

Diabetes mellitus results when the pancreas is unable to produce enough insulin, the body's cells are unable to properly use the insulin that is produced, or both. When there is not enough insulin in the body, or if the body's cells do not respond to the insulin that is produced, the body cannot use the glucose that enters the bloodstream. As a result, the amount of glucose in the bloodstream becomes very high. The high blood glucose levels may cause the person to experience symptoms such as fatigue, weakness, excessive thirst, excessive urination, blurry vision, and an increased number of infections. In an older adult, high blood glucose levels also increase the person's risk for dehydration and falling. Over time, if the blood glucose levels are not controlled, the person can develop serious complications, such as blindness, kidney failure, nerve damage, and cardiovascular disease.

Diabetes mellitus is the most common of all endocrine gland disorders and is a leading cause of death among older adults.

Types of Diabetes Mellitus

There are two types of diabetes mellitus, type 1 and type 2.

Type 1 Diabetes Mellitus

Type 1 diabetes mellitus, which accounts for 5% to 10% of all cases of diabetes, is caused by destruction of the insulin-producing cells of the pancreas. As a result, the body cannot produce its own insulin. A person with type 1 diabetes must receive regular injections of insulin to keep their blood glucose level within a normal range. Most people who have type 1 diabetes are diagnosed while they are children or young adults, which is why you may hear this type of diabetes referred to as "juvenile diabetes."

Type 2 Diabetes

Type 2 diabetes mellitus (also called "glucose intolerance"), which accounts for 90% to 95% of all cases of diabetes, occurs when the pancreas still produces some insulin, but the cells of the body are unable to respond to the insulin. This results in higher blood glucose levels because the body is unable to move the glucose out of the blood and into the cells. Risk factors for developing type 2 diabetes include increasing age and having a body mass index (BMI) that falls in the overweight or obese ranges. Because the number of people with a BMI in these ranges is increasing in the United States, we are seeing more and more cases of type 2 diabetes each year. And, while in the past type 2 diabetes was mostly considered a disease among older adults, now more people are developing type 2 diabetes at a younger age, even during childhood.

Some people, especially those whose BMI falls in the overweight or obese ranges, develop a condition known as "prediabetes." This means that their blood glucose level is higher than it should be but not as high as it would be in diabetes. Research has shown that people with "prediabetes" who make lifestyle changes (such as eating a healthy diet and exercising regularly) can often delay or prevent the onset of type 2 diabetes.

Management of Diabetes Mellitus

To keep blood glucose levels within the range of normal, three factors must be balanced: diet, exercise, and medication (Fig. 35-8). A change in any one of these factors can affect blood sugar control, resulting in **hypoglycemia** (a blood glucose level that is too low) or **hyperglycemia** (a blood glucose level that is too high). Box 35-1 reviews some of the causes and effects of hypoglycemia and hyperglycemia.

Diet

A person with diabetes needs to eat a well-balanced, nutritious diet, with limited sweets and fats. A diet that is high in fiber and complex carbohydrates helps to control the release of glucose into the bloodstream and works to prevent hypoglycemia and hyperglycemia. Following a proper diet helps to keep blood glucose

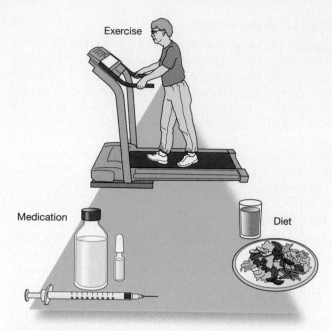

Figure 35-8 Diabetes mellitus is managed with diet, exercise, and medication. A change in any one of these three factors can affect the blood glucose level.

levels within the normal range. A proper diet also helps the person achieve or maintain a healthy body weight and reduces the person's risk for cardiovascular disease, which often accompanies diabetes.

Meals and snacks should be eaten at regular times throughout the day to help keep blood glucose levels steady. This is why, when you are caring for a person with diabetes, it is important to serve meals and snacks at the scheduled time (Fig. 35-9). You will also need to pay attention to how much and what the person eats. Specific amounts of carbohydrates, sugars, fats and proteins are needed to react with the medication the person takes for diabetes. If the person refuses the meal or snack, or only partially finishes it, their blood glucose level may become too low. Similarly, if the person eats more food than usual, or food with higher sugar content than usual, the amount of medication will not be sufficient and their blood glucose level may become too high.

Following a diabetic diet may be quite difficult, especially for a person who enjoys sweets. Lifelong eating habits can be hard to change. Sometimes special treats can be worked into the person's diet plan. However, some of your patients or residents may keep

---

Box 35-1 Hypoglycemia and Hyperglycemia

Hypoglycemia or hyperglycemia can result when diet, exercise, and medication are not in balance. A person's medication dose is planned to balance the person's usual food intake and amount of activity. A change in food intake or level of activity can lead to hypoglycemia or hyperglycemia if the person's medication dose is not adjusted accordingly. An older adult is more likely to experience hypoglycemia. Severe hypoglycemia is sometimes called "insulin shock" because it can result from taking too much insulin. The symptoms of hypoglycemia in an older person may be more subtle and present as confusion, abnormal behavior, altered sleep patterns, and slurred speech. Both hypoglycemia and hyperglycemia can have serious consequences, including death, if they are not treated.

Hypoglycemia (low blood glucose levels)

Causes
- Missing a meal or a snack
- A delayed meal or snack
- Eating too little food
- Vomiting
- NPO status
- Increased level of activity
- Too much medication

Effects
- Cool, clammy skin
- Sweating
- Feeling "shaky"
- Confusion or difficulty concentrating
- Rapid heart rate and rapid breathing
- Headache
- Blurry or "double" vision
- Restlessness and irritability
- Trembling
- A tingling sensation in the mouth or tongue
- Hunger
- Loss of consciousness

Hyperglycemia (high blood glucose levels)

Causes
- Eating too much food
- Decreased level of activity
- Too little medication
- Physical stress (illness or injury)
- Emotional stress
- Undiagnosed diabetes

Effects
- Excessive urination
- Excessive thirst
- Extreme hunger
- Unplanned weight loss
- Fatigue
- Blurry or "double" vision
- Headache
- Irritability
- Dry, flushed skin
- Sweet-smelling breath
- Dehydration
- Seizures
- Loss of consciousness (diabetic coma)

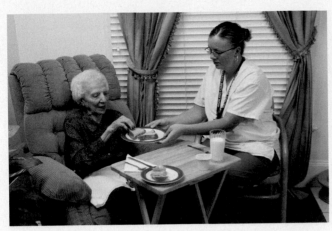

Figure 35-9 It is very important for a person with diabetes to eat regular, nutritionally sound meals and snacks. If one of your residents with diabetes refuses to eat or only eats part of a meal or snack, report this to a nurse immediately.

stashes of candy or other sweets in their rooms. If you notice that a person with diabetes is hoarding sweets, you should report this to the nurse.

Exercise

When we exercise, our muscles take up and use glucose for energy even in the absence of insulin. This helps to lower blood glucose levels. In addition, exercise plays an important role in achieving or maintaining a healthy body weight. An older person's ability to exercise may be limited by a chronic health condition or disability. You should encourage the person to participate in whatever level of exercise they can tolerate. Be sure you are aware of any specific instructions for exercise that are included in the person's care plan.

When you are caring for a person with diabetes, be aware that changes in the person's normal activity level could result in hypoglycemia or hyperglycemia. For example, a patient or a resident with diabetes who is beginning a new physical therapy program should be watched closely for signs and symptoms of hypoglycemia (see Box 35-1) because their activity level will be increased. Similarly, a decrease in the person's normal activity level could lead to hyperglycemia.

Medication

Medications used to treat diabetes include insulin and oral/injectable medications:

■ **Insulin.** All people with type 1 diabetes mellitus, and some people with type 2 diabetes mellitus, require insulin. Insulin can be administered using a needle and syringe, a special insulin "pen," or a pump (Fig. 35-10). Several types of insulin are available. The types of insulin differ in the speed at which they start working and how long they

last in the body. Many of your patients or residents who take insulin for the treatment of diabetes will receive multiple insulin injections each day.
■ **Oral/injectable medications.** Many people with type 2 diabetes mellitus take oral medications to help control their blood glucose levels. Other medications are being developed that are administered in injectable form. The different types of medications used to treat type 2 diabetes work in slightly different ways. Some stimulate the pancreas to produce more insulin, some act on the cells in the body to help them use the insulin that the body produces, and some decrease the amount of glucose that enters the bloodstream after eating.

Monitoring Blood Glucose Levels

As you have learned, diabetes control involves balancing diet, exercise, and medication. A person with diabetes needs to monitor their blood glucose levels regularly to make sure that their prescribed treatment is keeping their blood glucose level within the desired range. A *glucometer* (a type of blood glucose meter) is used to monitor blood glucose levels. Most blood glucose meters use a drop of blood obtained from the person's finger (Fig. 35-11). The "finger stick" method of monitoring blood glucose levels can be painful for the person and can also expose the health care worker to bloodborne diseases. If you are allowed to assist patients or residents with blood glucose monitoring using this method, make sure to wear gloves.

Many people with diabetes monitor their own glucose levels, but some patients or residents may need help with this. Different facilities will have different policies about who is responsible for blood glucose monitoring. You may work in a facility that allows nursing assistants to perform blood glucose monitoring. Make sure that you have been adequately trained in how to use the equipment and record your findings. A normal blood glucose level is between 70 and 120 mg/dL. A blood glucose level out of that range should be reported to the nurse immediately.

To obtain blood for use in the blood glucose meter, a *lancet* (a sharp instrument used to puncture the skin) is used to obtain a drop of blood from the patient's or resident's fingertip. The drop of blood is placed on a test strip, which is inserted into the blood glucose meter. The meter "reads" the amount of glucose in the blood. You may be required to document the reading in the person's medical record, or the blood glucose meter may send the reading directly to the facility's computer system. Blood glucose meters that communicate with the facility's computer system are often used in the health care setting.

Quality control (QC) tests are performed regularly on all blood glucose meters to ensure that the readings they give are accurate. Your facility will have a policy

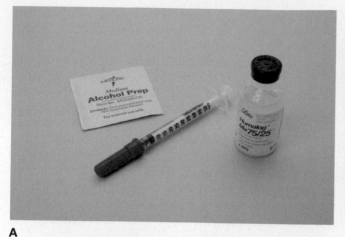

A

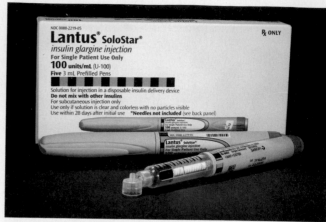

B

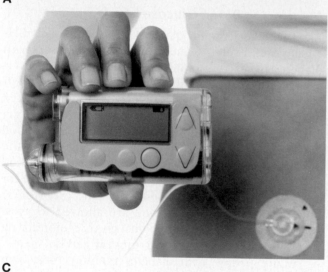

C

Figure 35-10 Insulin can be administered using (**A**) a needle and syringe, (**B**) an insulin pen, or (**C**) an insulin pump. (*B, Phil Lowe\Shutterstock.com; C, Click and Photo\ Shutterstock.com*)

stating how frequently QC tests should be performed (usually every 24 hours if the blood glucose meter is used daily). Some blood glucose meters do not permit you to perform a blood glucose check until the QC test is completed. Make sure that you are familiar with the particular QC test that is used with your facility's blood glucose monitors.

General guidelines for monitoring blood glucose levels are given in Guidelines Box 35-1. Procedure 35-1 gives step-by-step instructions for monitoring blood glucose levels.

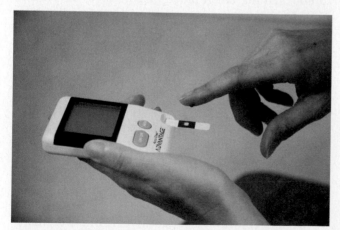

Figure 35-11 A glucometer is used to monitor blood glucose levels.

Tell the Nurse!

When caring for a person with diabetes, be sure to report any of the following observations to the nurse right away:

- The person has signs or symptoms of hypoglycemia or hyperglycemia (see Box 35-1)

- The person refuses a meal or snack, or only eats part of it

- The person has vomited

- The person has received gifts of food from visitors

- The person is taking food from others

- The person's activity level has changed significantly (either more active or less active than usual)

Guidelines Box 35-1 Guidelines for Monitoring Blood Glucose Levels

WHAT YOU DO	WHY YOU DO IT
Ensure that the blood glucose meter is properly calibrated (that is, it returns accurate readings for the testing solutions).	A blood glucose meter that is not properly calibrated will yield inaccurate results.
Use the testing strips specified by the manufacturer of the blood glucose meter.	The testing strips are specific to the blood glucose meter. Using the wrong kind of testing strips will yield inaccurate test results.
Remove the testing strip from the bottle right before you are going to use it. Replace the lid on the bottle of testing strips immediately after removing the testing strip you are going to use.	Testing strips are sensitive to light and humidity. Exposure to light and humidity affects their quality, which in turn affects the accuracy of the test results.
Note the expiration date on the bottle of testing strips. Do not use the testing strips past their expiration date.	Using expired testing strips will yield inaccurate test results.
When opening a new bottle of testing strips, write the date on the bottle.	The testing strips are only good for 3 to 4 months after opening the bottle. The manufacturer dictates how long an opened bottle of testing strips can be kept before it must be discarded. Using old testing strips may yield inaccurate test results.
Wear gloves when obtaining a blood glucose sample.	Blood puts you at risk for exposure to bloodborne pathogens.
Use a new lancet for each patient or resident.	The lancet comes in contact with the person's blood. Using the same lancet on multiple people could put your patients or residents at risk for bloodborne illnesses or other infections.
After use, dispose of the lancet in an approved sharps container.	Proper disposal of sharps (such as lancets) helps limit others' exposure to bloodborne pathogens.
Before obtaining the blood sample, have the patient or resident wash their hands with warm, soapy water.	Washing with warm soapy water helps remove pathogens that may be on the surface of the skin, lowering the person's risk of infection. Washing with warm, soapy water also removes any sugars that might be on the surface of the skin, preventing a false-high reading.
If using an alcohol swab to cleanse the skin, allow the skin to dry completely before using the lancet.	Alcohol can interfere with the accuracy of the test results, if not completely dried.
Insert the lancet on the side of the fingertip instead of in the center.	The center of the fingertip contains the highest number of nerve endings. If you obtain the blood sample from the side of the fingertip, the person will experience less pain.
If possible, avoid taking blood from the thumb or index finger.	The thumb and index finger are the fingers we use most frequently to perform day-to-day activities (for example, grasping small objects, buttoning a shirt). If these fingers are sore from blood glucose testing, the person will experience pain every time they try to use them.
Wipe away the first drop of blood with gauze or a cotton ball (if recommended by the manufacturer of the blood glucose meter or your facility policy).	Some manufacturers of blood glucose meters recommend discarding the first drop of blood because it may be mixed with serum or the cleansing agent, resulting in an inaccurate test result.
Apply the correct amount of blood to the testing strip. The manufacturer of the blood glucose meter will specify how much blood to apply to the testing strip.	Applying too much or not enough blood to the testing strip may result in inaccurate test results.

Complications of Diabetes

Many organ systems can be affected by uncontrolled diabetes mellitus of either type. Low insulin levels increase the release of lipids (fats) into the bloodstream. The lipids then build up in the linings of the arteries, damaging them. Atherosclerosis, high blood pressure, heart disease, kidney disease, and blindness (diabetic retinopathy; see Chapter 34) can result from the damaged blood vessels. In addition, peripheral nerve damage results from reduced blood flow to the neurons, causing diminished sensation in the arms and legs. Poor circulation to the feet and lower legs also increases the risk of infection and poor tissue healing in the event of injury.

Early detection of diabetes mellitus is essential for preventing complications. Once diabetes mellitus is diagnosed, there are many measures that can be taken to keep the disease under control and minimize the person's risk of developing complications. People whose BMI falls within the overweight range should try to lose the excess weight. In addition, exercising regularly, following the recommended diet closely, and taking prescribed medications correctly are also very important.

SUMMARY

- The endocrine system is made up of glands located in specific places throughout the body that produce hormones. Hormones are chemical messengers that allow the body to reproduce, grow, develop, metabolize energy, respond to stress and injury, and maintain homeostasis.
  - The pituitary gland is considered the master gland of the endocrine system because it secretes hormones that affect other glands. It is controlled by the hypothalamus.
    - The posterior lobe of the pituitary gland stores and releases antidiuretic hormone (ADH) and oxytocin.
    - The anterior lobe of the pituitary gland produces and releases growth hormone, thyroid-stimulating hormone (TSH), adrenocorticotropic hormone (ACTH), prolactin, and the gonadotropins (luteinizing hormone [LH] and follicle-stimulating hormone [FSH]).
  - The thyroid gland produces thyroxine, which helps to regulate metabolism.
  - The parathyroid glands secrete parathyroid hormone (PTH), which helps to move calcium from the bones into the bloodstream. PTH also stimulates the activation of vitamin D into calcitriol, which increases absorption of calcium from the intestines.
  - The adrenal glands produce hormones that help us to deal with stress.
    - The adrenal medulla secretes epinephrine and norepinephrine, which play a role in the "fight-or-flight" response.
    - The adrenal cortex secretes glucocorticoids, mineralocorticoids, and androgens.
  - The pancreas secretes insulin and glucagon, which play a role in regulating blood glucose (sugar) levels.

- Disorders of the endocrine system result from either too much or too little hormone.
  - Hypothyroidism (secretion of too little thyroid hormone) and hyperthyroidism (secretion of too much thyroid hormone) are common endocrine disorders. Thyroid hormone imbalances change the body's metabolic rate, causing many uncomfortable symptoms. Fortunately, hypothyroidism and hyperthyroidism can usually be treated.
- The most common of all endocrine disorders is diabetes mellitus.
  - There are two forms of diabetes mellitus:
    - Type 1 diabetes mellitus occurs when the insulin-producing cells of the pancreas are destroyed.
    - Type 2 diabetes mellitus occurs when the pancreas produces some insulin, but the cells of the body are unable to respond to the insulin that is produced.
  - Both types of diabetes mellitus are managed with diet, exercise, and medication.
  - A person with diabetes mellitus is prone to hyperglycemia (blood glucose levels that are too high) and hypoglycemia (blood glucose levels that are too low). Both hyperglycemia and hypoglycemia can cause complications, some of which are life-threatening.
  - Keeping blood glucose levels within the range of normal is very important to prevent long-term complications of diabetes, such as cardiovascular disease, stroke, nerve damage, kidney failure, blindness, and amputation.
  - A blood glucose meter is used to monitor blood glucose levels. If monitoring these levels is part of your job, make sure you have been trained in the proper use of the equipment at your facility and always follow standard precautions.

▶ **Procedure 35-1**

Monitoring the Blood Glucose Level

WHY YOU DO IT Blood glucose monitoring is necessary for people who are at risk of having blood glucose levels that are too high or too low.

Getting Ready

1. Complete the "Getting Ready" steps.

Supplies

- blood glucose meter
- nonsterile gloves
- sterile lancet
- testing strips
- cotton ball or gauze
- alcohol swab or
- wash basin and warm water
- soap
- washcloth and towel

Procedure

2. Perform hand hygiene and put on your gloves.

3. Help the person to wash their hands with soap and water. Dry the person's hands with a towel. If your facility policy requires, use a alcohol swab to cleanse the finger. Allow the skin to dry completely.

4. Turn the blood glucose meter on and wait until the "ready" sign appears on the display screen.

5. Remove a testing strip from the bottle. Immediately replace the cap on the bottle. Make sure that the code on the testing strip matches the code on the blood glucose meter. Depending on the type of blood glucose meter you are using, you may be required to insert the testing strip into the meter at this time.

6. Gently massage the side of the finger toward the intended puncture site to encourage blood to flow to the area.

7. Prepare the lancet by removing the safety cap. Grasp the person's finger and hold the lancet at a 90-degree angle to the skin. Press the lancet straight down to pierce the person's skin.

8. Wipe away the first drop of blood with gauze or a cotton ball (if recommended by the manufacturer or your facility's policy).

9. Lightly stroke the finger and/or lower the hand to encourage bleeding until a drop of blood forms. Do not squeeze the finger or touch the puncture site or blood drop with your gloved hands.

10. Transfer the drop of blood by touching it to the pad on the test strip without smearing it. Make sure to apply an adequate amount of blood to the test strip.

11. Press the test button on the blood glucose meter if directed by the manufacturer.

12. Apply pressure to the puncture site using gauze or a cotton ball.

13. When testing is completed, note the blood glucose results, remove the test strip and dispose of it in a facility-approved waste container. Dispose of the lancet in a sharps container.

14. Remove your gloves and perform hand hygiene.

15. Record the reading on the blood glucose meter. Turn off the meter if it does not automatically turn itself off.

Finishing Up

16. Complete the "Finishing Up" steps.

What You Document

- The date and time
- The person's blood glucose level

WHAT DID YOU LEARN?

Multiple Choice

Select the single best answer for each of the following questions.

1. Hormones are chemical messengers that allow the body to:
   a. Metabolize energy
   b. Grow
   c. Reproduce
   d. All of the above

2. Which endocrine disorder causes an increased metabolic rate, increased hunger, weight loss, an irregular heartbeat, an inability to sleep, irritability, and intolerance to heat?
   a. Hyperthyroidism
   b. Diabetes
   c. Acromegaly
   d. Pituitary gigantism

3. Mrs. Snow has type 1 diabetes mellitus. What special care considerations might a nursing assistant who is caring for Mrs. Snow need to keep in mind?
   a. Mrs. Snow will be unable to tolerate cold and therefore will often need a sweater.
   b. Mrs. Snow will need to eat meals and snacks on a regular schedule.
   c. Mrs. Snow may grow tired very easily.
   d. Mrs. Snow is likely to be irritable.

4. Why must a person with type 1 diabetes mellitus receive regular doses of insulin?
   a. The cells of the body do not respond to the insulin produced by the pancreas.
   b. The person's pancreas does not produce insulin on its own.
   c. The person's pancreas produces too much glucagon.
   d. People with type 1 diabetes do not need to take insulin; their disease can be controlled through diet, exercise, and oral medications.

5. Mr. Byron has type 2 diabetes mellitus. Although he knows that he should limit the amount of sweets that he eats, he has a real "sweet tooth" and often eats candy. In addition, he only monitors his blood glucose on days when he does not feel well. What complications is Mr. Byron at risk for developing if he does not make more of an effort to control his blood glucose levels?
   a. Kidney failure
   b. Blindness
   c. Heart disease
   d. All of the above

6. Ms. Banderes takes oral thyroxine to control her hypothyroidism. Without this medication, what sort of signs and symptoms do you think Ms. Banderes would have?
   a. Loss of appetite, weight gain, and constipation
   b. Frequent urination and excessive thirst
   c. Fat deposits on her back, abdomen, and face
   d. Excessive growth of the bones of the hands, feet, and face

Matching *Match each numbered item with its appropriate lettered description.*

_____ **1.** Parathyroid hormone (PTH)

_____ **2.** Antidiuretic hormone (ADH)

_____ **3.** Growth hormone

_____ **4.** Thyroid-stimulating hormone (TSH)

_____ **5.** Oxytocin

_____ **6.** Adrenocorticotropic hormone (ACTH)

_____ **7.** Thyroxine

_____ **8.** Norepinephrine and epinephrine

_____ **9.** Glucocorticoids

_____ **10.** Insulin

a. Secreted by the adrenal cortex; helps the body to deal with stress

b. Secreted by the posterior pituitary gland; acts on the kidneys to limit the amount of water lost in the urine

c. Secreted by the anterior pituitary gland; causes the body to get bigger and taller

d. Secreted by the pancreas; helps the body to manage blood glucose levels

e. Secreted by the posterior pituitary gland; stimulates milk release from the breasts

f. Secreted by the anterior pituitary gland; stimulates the adrenal glands to produce their hormones

g. Secreted by the thyroid gland; sets the metabolic rate for the cells of the body

h. Secreted by the parathyroid glands; stimulates the release of calcium from the bones into the bloodstream

i. Secreted by the anterior pituitary gland; stimulates the thyroid glands to produce their hormones

j. Secreted by the adrenal medulla; participates in the "fight-or-flight" response

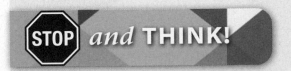

One of your residents, Mr. Singh, receives an insulin injection for his diabetes every morning. This morning, Mr. Singh had his injection and then ate most of his breakfast. About 30 minutes later, he vomited. Now Mr. Singh tells you that he feels shaky, and you can see that he is sweating. Why is it important for you to report these observations to the nurse immediately?

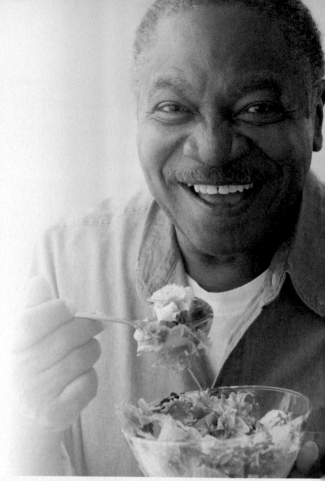

Photo: The digestive system processes the food that we eat.

The Digestive System

WHAT WILL YOU LEARN?

Did you know that over the course of a lifetime, you will eat about 50 *tons* (100,000 lb) of food? As you already know from Chapters 24 and 25, it is your digestive system's job to process that food so that your body can use it and to rid the body of the solid waste that is created as part of that process. In this chapter, you will learn more about the individual organs of the digestive system and how they work. You will also learn about some common disorders of the digestive system. When you are finished with this chapter, you will be able to:

1. List the organs that make up the digestive system.
2. Explain the function of the organs of the digestive system.
3. Discuss the effects of aging on the digestive system.
4. Discuss common digestive disorders and their symptoms.
5. Describe some of the tools used to diagnose digestive disorders.

Vocabulary

Esophagus
Stomach
Esophageal (cardiac)
   sphincter
Pyloric sphincter

Rugae
Salivary glands
Liver
Bile
Gallbladder

Pancreas
Mastication
Mechanical digestion
Enzymes
Chemical digestion

Villi
Hernia
Diverticulosis

STRUCTURE OF THE DIGESTIVE SYSTEM

The digestive system, also known as the gastrointestinal system, is a long tube, or *tract*, consisting of the mouth, pharynx, esophagus, stomach, small intestine, and large intestine (Fig. 36-1). In addition, several accessory organs (appendages) along the way assist in the process of breaking down food so that our bodies can use it. These accessory organs include the teeth, tongue, salivary glands, liver, gallbladder, and pancreas.

The Digestive Tract

The walls of the "tube" that forms the digestive tract are made up of four layers of tissue (Fig. 36-2). The layers are basically the same throughout the digestive tract although there is some variation from region to region. The four basic layers are the mucosa, the submucosa, the muscle layer, and the serosa:

■ The *mucosa*, a mucous membrane, lines the digestive tract. It is covered by a sticky fluid called mucus which helps to trap disease-causing

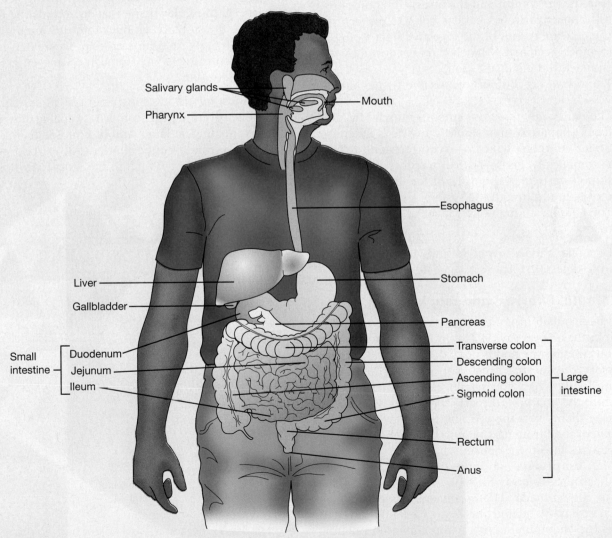

Figure 36-1 The digestive system breaks down food, absorbs nutrients, and gets rid of waste.

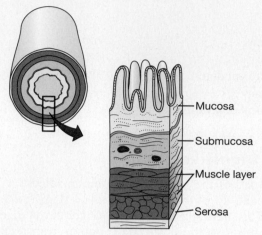

Figure 36-2 The walls of the digestive tract consist of four basic layers. This figure shows how these layers are arranged in the small intestine.

microbes. This is important because the digestive tract is open to the outside world at both ends (that is, the mouth and the anus). In addition to trapping microbes, mucus helps to protect the delicate tissues of the digestive tract from stomach acid, a very harsh fluid produced by the stomach to help digest food.

■ The *submucosa* contains connective tissue, blood vessels, and nerves.
■ The *muscle layer* contains smooth muscle. Recall from Chapter 28 that smooth muscle is not under voluntary control—it contracts and relaxes automatically. Peristalsis (contraction of the smooth muscle in the walls of the digestive tract) moves food through the system.
■ The *serosa* is a tough outer layer of connective tissue.

Let's take a look now at the individual organs that form the digestive tract.

The Mouth, Pharynx, and Esophagus

Food begins its journey through the digestive tract at the mouth, or oral cavity. The mouth is lined with a mucous membrane and houses the teeth and tongue, accessory organs that assist with chewing and swallowing food. When you swallow, the tongue pushes food into the pharynx (throat). The epiglottis (a flap of cartilage that covers the opening to the larynx) closes to prevent food from passing into the trachea. Instead, food moves into the esophagus.

The **esophagus**, a long narrow tube, serves mainly as a passageway for food to get from the pharynx to the stomach. The esophagus passes through the chest cavity, behind the heart (see Fig. 36-1). It enters the abdominal cavity at the *hiatus*, an opening in the diaphragm (the large, flat muscle that separates

the abdominal and chest cavities). After entering the abdominal cavity, the esophagus connects with the upper part of the stomach. The mucus secreted by the esophageal mucosa, as well as the action of the muscle layer, helps to move food downward and into the stomach.

The Stomach

The **stomach** is a hollow, muscular holding pouch for food. The stomach has three main regions (Fig. 36-3):

■ The *fundus* is the upper region.
■ The *body* is the main region. The esophagus enters the stomach here. The **esophageal (cardiac) sphincter**, a circle of muscular tissue, surrounds the place where the esophagus enters the stomach and keeps food from going back up the esophagus after it has entered the stomach. This sphincter is often called the *lower esophageal sphincter* or *LES* for short.
■ The *pylorus* is the bottom region. Food leaves the stomach through the **pyloric sphincter**, a circle of muscular tissue that surrounds the place where the stomach empties into the small intestine. The pyloric sphincter helps to prevent food from returning to the stomach once it enters the small intestine.

As most of us have experienced after eating a large holiday dinner, the stomach is capable of stretching and holding a large amount of food. Folds of the mucosa, called **rugae**, flatten out as food enters the stomach, almost doubling the stomach's holding capacity.

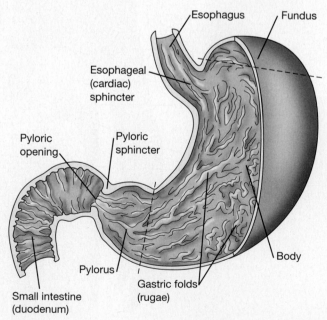

Figure 36-3 The stomach is a hollow holding pouch for food.

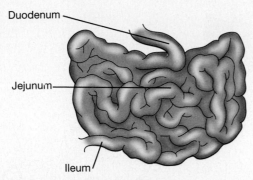

Figure 36-4 The small intestine has three regions: the duodenum, the jejunum, and the ileum.

The Small Intestine

The small intestine, which is about 20 feet long, is so named because its diameter is much smaller than that of the large intestine. The small intestine has three regions, called the *duodenum*, the *jejunum*, and the *ileum* (Fig. 36-4).

The Large Intestine

The large intestine (also called the *colon*) is approximately 4½ feet long and is much larger in diameter than the small intestine. Like the small intestine, the large intestine has several distinct regions (Fig. 36-5):

- The *cecum* is a small pouch below the *ileocecal valve*. Food passes through the ileocecal valve as it moves from the small intestine into the large intestine.
- The *ascending colon* travels upward from the cecum.

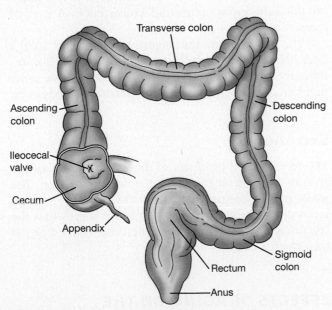

Figure 36-5 The large intestine has several regions: the cecum, the ascending colon, the transverse colon, the descending colon, the sigmoid colon, and the rectum. The appendix is a small pouch attached to the end of the cecum.

- The *transverse colon* travels across.
- The *descending colon* travels down.
- The *sigmoid colon* is an S-shaped curve at the end of the descending colon.
- The *rectum* is the last segment of the colon. The place where the rectum opens to the outside of the body is the *anus*.

The *appendix*, a tiny, closed pouch that dangles from the cecum, is thought to play a role in immunity. It also houses some of the resident bacteria that are necessary for good health. Inflammation or infection of the appendix causes *appendicitis*, a painful condition that is life-threatening if not treated. Treatment is surgical removal of the appendix.

The Accessory Organs

Several organs—the salivary glands, liver, gallbladder, and pancreas—play a role in digestion but are not actually part of the digestive tract (see Fig. 36-1).

- The **salivary glands** are located near the mouth. They produce and secrete saliva, a substance that helps with chewing and swallowing by moistening the food.
- The **liver** is a large organ located just underneath the diaphragm (see Fig. 36-1). The liver produces and secretes bile into the duodenum. **Bile** is a substance that helps with the digestion of fats. The liver has several other important functions that are not related to digestion. For example, it produces clotting factors (chemicals that help our blood to clot) and it helps to clear our blood of toxins, such as alcohol and drugs. The liver also stores sugar in the form of glycogen that can be converted into glucose and released into the bloodstream when the body needs extra energy or when we have not eaten in a while.
- The **gallbladder**, a small pouch that is attached to the liver, stores bile produced by the liver that is not secreted directly into the duodenum.
- The **pancreas** is located behind the stomach, in the curve of the duodenum (see Fig. 36-1). The pancreas produces substances that aid in digestion and secretes them into the duodenum. The pancreas also produces insulin and glucagon, hormones that are secreted into the bloodstream. (Recall from Chapter 35 that insulin and glucagon regulate glucose levels in the blood.)

FUNCTION OF THE DIGESTIVE SYSTEM

The digestive system breaks down the food we eat into nutrients, which are then absorbed into the bloodstream for use by the body's cells. In addition, the digestive system removes unusable digested food from the body, in the form of feces.

Digestion

Digestion, or the breaking down of food into simple elements (nutrients), begins in the mouth. First, we physically break the food into smaller pieces by chewing it. Another word for chewing is **mastication**. This physical breaking up of the food, such as occurs when we chew, is called **mechanical digestion**. Next, chemical substances in our saliva start to work on the smaller pieces of food, breaking them down even more by breaking the bonds that hold the food molecules together. Substances that have the ability to break chemical bonds are called **enzymes**. The human body produces many different types of enzymes, each with a specific function. The process of breaking down food through the use of chemical substances such as enzymes is called **chemical digestion**.

After passing through the esophagus, the food we eat stays in the stomach for 3 to 4 hours, where digestion continues to take place. Special glands in the stomach lining produce hydrochloric acid (sometimes called "stomach acid") and enzymes. The stomach acid and enzymes act on the pieces of food to break them down even further. The peristaltic action of the stomach helps to mix the food with the acid and enzymes, creating a liquid substance called *chyme.*

The chyme passes into the duodenum, the first segment of the small intestine. Once in the duodenum, the chyme mixes with bile (secreted by the liver) and digestive enzymes secreted by the pancreas. These substances cause further breakdown of the food. From the duodenum, the chyme passes into the jejunum.

Absorption

Once the chyme reaches the jejunum, absorption of nutrients begins. At this point, the food is fairly well digested. Now, it is time to start moving the nutrients from the digestive tract into the bloodstream. To reach the bloodstream, most nutrients pass through the mucosa and into the blood vessels in the next layer, the submucosa. Fats pass into lymphatic vessels, and then enter the circulation along with the lymph fluid (see Chapter 32). The mucosa of the small intestine has millions of tiny finger-like structures called **villi** (Fig. 36-6). The villi increase the small intestine's ability to absorb substances by increasing the surface area of the mucosa.

Although most of the absorption of nutrients, water, and minerals takes place in the small intestine,

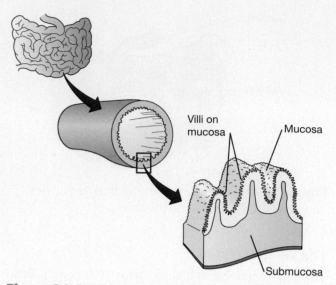

Figure 36-6 Villi are finger-like projections that increase the small intestine's ability to absorb nutrients.

the large intestine also plays a role in absorption. Bacteria that live in the large intestine act on the chyme to produce vitamin K and some B vitamins, which are absorbed by the body. The action of these bacteria on the chyme can also produce gas as a by-product, especially when high-fiber foods such as beans, onions, and broccoli are part of the diet. As the chyme passes slowly through the large intestine, water, vitamins, and other minerals called *electrolytes,* are absorbed into the bloodstream. By the time the chyme reaches the end of the long intestine, all nutrients and most of the water have been removed, and the chyme has taken on the soft, moist, semisolid consistency of normal feces.

The blood from the digestive tract goes to the liver before entering the general circulation. This preliminary "screening" allows the liver to remove some ingested toxins before they can affect other body cells.

Excretion

The feces (waste products of digestion) collect in the rectum, the last segment of the large intestine. The walls of the rectum gradually expand as the feces build up. At a certain point, the brain senses that the rectum is "full" and the urge to defecate (have a bowel movement) occurs.

EFFECTS OF AGING ON THE DIGESTIVE SYSTEM

Like all of the body's organ systems, the digestive system is affected by the aging process.

Less Efficient Chewing and Swallowing

In older people, the production of saliva decreases, which may make chewing and swallowing more difficult. In addition, many older people have dental problems, such as missing or painful teeth. An older person may choke as a result of trying to swallow food that has not been chewed properly. Remember this when you are helping an older person to eat. Create a relaxed, social environment for eating and help the person to cut food up into small, easy-to-chew pieces. Also, report complaints of poorly fitting dentures, sores in the mouth or on the tongue, or a toothache to the nurse immediately.

Less Efficient Digestion

Food is most easily digested when it has been thoroughly chewed. Mechanical digestion increases the effectiveness of chemical digestion by making the pieces of food smaller. In an older person, the production of saliva, stomach acid, and digestive enzymes slows, making chemical digestion less efficient. Digestion is less efficient because not only are fewer chemicals available for chemical digestion, but the pieces of food that the chemicals must work on may be larger, due to inefficient chewing.

Increased Risk for Constipation

In an older person, the movement of food through the digestive tract may be slower. This can put the older person at risk for constipation. The chyme spends more time in the large intestine, which allows more water to be reabsorbed into the bloodstream. As a result, by the time the chyme reaches the end of the large intestine, almost all of the water has been removed and the resulting feces are hard, dry, and difficult to pass. Certain medications (such as prescription pain relievers) and immobility can also increase a person's risk for constipation. Measures that you can take to help your patients and residents avoid constipation are described in Chapter 25.

DISORDERS OF THE DIGESTIVE SYSTEM

Many of the people you will care for will have a digestive disorder of some sort or will be recovering from one. Because the digestive system contains so many different organs, there are many different disorders that can occur. Five of the most common digestive disorders that you are likely to see in the health care setting are ulcers, hernias, gallbladder disorders, diverticulosis, and cancer.

Ulcers

Ulcers (sores caused by wearing away of the protective mucosa that lines the digestive tract) can occur anywhere along the digestive tract. The most common sites are the stomach (*gastric ulcer*) and the duodenum (*duodenal ulcer*). Ulcers are usually the result of infection with a bacterium called *Helicobacter pylori*. Factors that increase stomach acid production, such as smoking, frequent use of over-the-counter pain medications, and emotional stress can increase a person's chances of developing ulcers. In severe cases, the ulcer may affect all of the layers of the stomach or duodenum wall, not just the mucosa. This condition, called a *penetrating ulcer*, is life-threatening.

A person with an ulcer may feel uncomfortably full or nauseous after eating. Stomach pain is common, especially within 3 hours of eating (or when the person does not eat). Most ulcers are chronic. The person will have periods of feeling well, interrupted by flare-ups of symptoms.

Most ulcers can be treated with medication. For instance, antibiotics can eliminate the *H. pylori* bacteria. People with severe ulcers may need surgery.

Hernias

The abdominal cavity (the space in the body where most of the digestive organs are found) is bounded by muscular walls. The muscular walls of the abdominal cavity give structure to the body and help to keep the internal organs where they belong. A **hernia** occurs when an internal organ bulges through a weakness in the muscular wall of the abdominal cavity (Fig. 36-7). Sometimes the weakness occurs at the site of an old surgical incision. Other times, the muscle is just weak in certain areas. If there is a weak area in the muscular

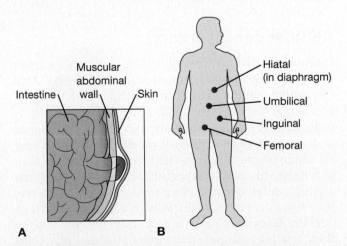

Figure 36-7 A. A hernia occurs when an internal organ bulges through a weakness in the abdominal wall. **B.** Hernias can occur in a number of different places.

wall, and the person does something that requires a lot of physical effort (such as lifting a heavy object), a hernia may occur. Hernias can occur in a number of different places:

- *Inguinal hernias* and *femoral hernias* occur from a weakness in abdominal wall in the groin area. Inguinal hernias are more common in males, and femoral hernias are more common in females. These types of hernias are repaired surgically.
- *Umbilical hernias* occur around the navel (belly button). If the umbilical hernia is very small, no treatment may be needed. However, surgery may be required to repair a larger umbilical hernia.
- *Hiatal hernias* occur when part of the stomach passes through the hiatus, the opening in the diaphragm that allows the esophagus to pass into the abdominal cavity. The chances of having a hiatal hernia increases with age and are greater in females than males. Approximately 50% of people in the United States over the age of 50 have a hiatal hernia. People with hiatal hernias often have heartburn because the stomach acid moves back up into the esophagus. This condition is known as *gastroesophageal reflux disease (GERD)* and the stomach acid can cause irritation and inflammation of the lining of the esophagus. A person with a hiatal hernia may find that eating small, frequent meals and sitting up for at least 2 hours after every meal helps to relieve the heartburn. Medication can also provide relief of symptoms. People with severe symptoms may need surgery to repair the hernia.

Complications occur if the weakened area of the muscle tightens around the tissue, such as a piece of intestine that has become trapped in the hernia, cutting off its blood supply. This situation, called a *strangulated hernia*, is a surgical emergency.

Gallbladder Disorders

Gallstones can form and block the flow of bile from the gallbladder into the duodenum (Fig. 36-8). This can lead to inflammation and infection of the gallbladder. A person with a gallbladder disorder has episodes of severe pain. The pain may stay in the upper abdominal region, or it may radiate to the back and shoulder on the person's right side. The person may also have indigestion, especially after eating foods that are high in fat. Because bile gives feces their characteristic brown color, in a person with a gallbladder disorder, the feces may be pale and "clay-colored" due to their low bile content. Remember also that bile helps the body to digest fat. Therefore, in a person with gallbladder disease, the feces may float because they contain a great deal of undigested fat.

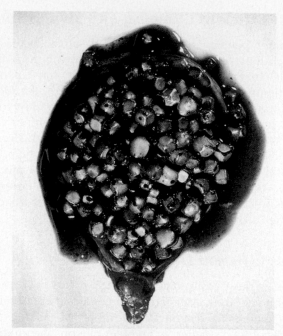

Figure 36-8 A gallbladder that has been removed and cut open to reveal the many gallstones inside. Gallstones can block the flow of bile into the duodenum, causing indigestion and severe pain. (Rubin, E., & Farber, J. L. [2005]. *Pathology* [4th ed., p. 803]. Lippincott Williams & Wilkins.)

Gallstones can also migrate into the *common bile duct* and block the flow of bile and other substances that are filtered from the liver into the duodenum. The backup of these substances into the liver can cause damage to the liver. A person with an obstructed common bile duct will become *jaundiced* (have yellowish skin and eyes) and will need acute medical, and possibly surgical, intervention to remove the obstruction. Inflammation or infection of the gallbladder due to gallstones is a common reason for a person to need a *cholecystectomy*, or surgical removal of their gallbladder.

Diverticulosis

Diverticulosis is a condition in which small pouches or sacs (called diverticula) form in the intestinal wall, usually the lower part of the colon (Fig. 36-9). These diverticula can become inflamed or infected, causing a condition known as *diverticulitis*. A person who has diverticulitis will have pain and tenderness, usually in their left lower quadrant, and may be febrile. Antibiotics are usually necessary to treat diverticulitis, although in severe cases, surgical removal of the affected section of colon may be necessary. If untreated, the diverticula can rupture causing a life-threatening emergency.

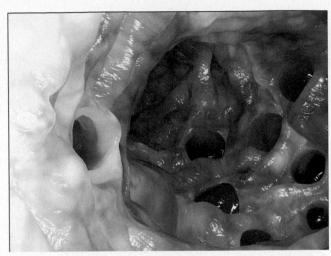

Figure 36-9 Diverticula are small sacs or pouches that can form in the intestines. (*Juan Gaertner\Shutterstock.com*)

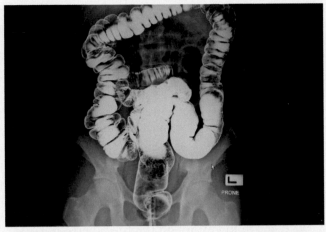

Figure 36-10 A person may be given a substance that coats the inside of the intestines prior to having an x-ray taken. This helps to enhance the x-ray image. This is a barium x-ray of a person's colon. (*Praisaeng\Shutterstock.com*)

Cancer

Any of the organs in the digestive system can be affected by cancer. Colorectal cancer is the second most common type of cancer in the United States. The person's signs and symptoms will vary, depending on the location of the tumor. A person with cancer involving the digestive system may have one or more of the following signs and symptoms: loss of appetite, indigestion, pain, vomiting, constipation, changes in bowel movements, or blood in the stool. Depending on the location and type of cancer, it may be treated with surgery, radiation, chemotherapy, or a combination of these. Many types of cancer affecting the digestive system can be easily cured if detected in the early stages. However, many people think that their symptoms are just related to aging or simple indigestion and do not seek professional treatment until the cancer has advanced.

DIAGNOSIS OF DIGESTIVE DISORDERS

Digestive complaints—such as heartburn, indigestion, nausea, vomiting, stomach ache, gas, diarrhea, and constipation—are common. Often, these symptoms are not a sign of anything serious. Sometimes, however, they may signal a serious disorder. Always report a new symptom, or a change in the person's symptoms, to the nurse immediately.

Sometimes, the doctor will order one or more tests to evaluate a person's symptoms. Some of these tests are simple, such as laboratory analysis of a stool sample. Others are more involved. Tests you may hear mentioned include the following:

- **Endoscopy** involves using a special instrument to look inside the digestive tract and obtain tissue or fluids for analysis. Endoscopy allows the doctor to look inside the digestive tract for tumors or other abnormal growths. The type of endoscope used depends on whether the instrument will be passed through the person's mouth (to view the upper digestive tract) or anus (to view the lower digestive tract).
- **Imaging studies**, such as x-rays, computed tomography (CT) scans, and magnetic resonance imaging (MRI) scans, allow the doctor to view the organs of the digestive system without actually entering the body. Sometimes, the person is asked to swallow a substance that will coat the inside of the digestive tract to help the structures in the intestines appear on x-ray, CT or MRI scans (Fig. 36-10).

You may find yourself caring for a person who is about to have one of these diagnostic procedures. The person may have a special diet in the days leading up to the procedure or be placed on NPO status (nothing to eat or drink). Sometimes, an enema or a type of cleansing laxative liquid is ordered to clean out the large intestine prior to the procedure. The nurse will let you know of any special care needs for a person who is having one of these procedures.

SUMMARY

- The digestive system consists of the digestive tract and several accessory organs.
  - The digestive tract consists of the mouth, pharynx, esophagus, stomach, small intestine, and large intestine.
    - The walls of the digestive tract are lined with a mucous membrane (mucosa).
    - The walls of the digestive tract contain smooth muscle, which contracts to help move food through the tube (peristalsis).
  - Accessory organs include the teeth, tongue, salivary glands, liver, gallbladder, and pancreas.
- The digestive system breaks down food into nutrients that can be used by cells. The digestive system also removes waste in the form of feces.
  - There are two types of digestion: mechanical and chemical.
    - Mechanical digestion is the physical breaking down of food (for example, chewing).
    - Chemical digestion is the breaking down of food through chemical means (such as digestive enzymes).
  - Absorption takes place in the small and large intestines.

- Most absorption of nutrients takes place in the jejunum and ileum, the last two segments of the small intestine.
- Additional water, electrolytes, and some vitamins are absorbed into the bloodstream as the chyme passes through the large intestine.
- Feces are what are left after all of the nutrients and most of the water are removed from the chyme during its passage through intestines. Feces collect in the rectum, the last segment of the large intestine, until the urge to defecate occurs.
- As a person ages, they may have more trouble chewing and swallowing. Digestion is less efficient, and the older person may be at higher risk for constipation.
- Common disorders of the digestive system include ulcers, hernias, gallbladder disorders, diverticulosis, and cancer. Always report a new gastrointestinal complaint, or a change in a person's usual symptoms, to the nurse immediately.
- A person who is about to have a diagnostic procedure to evaluate their digestive system may have special care needs prior to the test. The nurse will let you know of any instructions, which should be followed carefully.

WHAT DID YOU LEARN?

Multiple Choice

Select the single best answer for each of the following questions.

1. Where does the process of digestion begin?
   a. In the stomach
   b. In the large intestine
   c. In the mouth
   d. In the esophagus

2. What is the hollow, muscular pouch that holds food?
   a. The appendix
   b. The gallbladder
   c. The duodenum
   d. The stomach

3. What is another term for the large intestine?
   a. Stomach
   b. Duodenum
   c. Colon
   d. Appendix

4. Where does most absorption of nutrients take place?
   a. In the jejunum and ileum of the small intestine
   b. In the rectum of the large intestine
   c. In the stomach
   d. In the liver

5. Where is most of the water absorbed from the chyme, resulting in the formation of formed, semi-moist feces?
   a. In the large small intestine
   b. In the small intestine
   c. In the stomach
   d. In the gallbladder

6. Normal changes in the digestive system related to aging include:
   a. Less efficient chewing and swallowing
   b. Less efficient digestion
   c. Increased risk for constipation
   d. All of the above

7. You have been caring for Mrs. Zimmerman for several months. Mrs. Zimmerman has always had a "sensitive stomach." She often tells you that she is "queasy" or that something she ate "didn't agree with her." Although she always complains about the food at the facility, she usually cleans her plate. Today, however, you noticed that not only did Mrs. Zimmerman not eat her lunch, she has seemed particularly listless all afternoon. What should you do?
   a. Nothing; Mrs. Zimmerman always has "stomach issues"
   b. Record Mrs. Zimmerman's lack of appetite in her chart; the nurse will follow up later
   c. Report this change in Mrs. Zimmerman's behavior to the nurse immediately
   d. Wait and see if Mrs. Zimmerman has any appetite for dinner

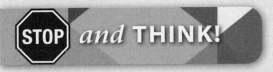

STOP *and* THINK!

■ Ms. Sanchez is a resident in the long-term care facility where you work. Although Ms. Sanchez has a partial disability from severe arthritis in her hips and knees, she remains active and positive. Ms. Sanchez has always told you that her favorite time of day is mealtime and she usually has a very good appetite, especially for foods a little on the fatty side. During the past few days, however, you have noticed a bit of a change in Ms. Sanchez's appetite. She has eaten very little of her favorite foods and has complained of some indigestion and bloating. You noticed that her bowel movement this morning had a peculiar "clay-colored" appearance, not the brown color you usually see, and it floated in the toilet bowl.

It is now about 2 hours after lunch and Ms. Sanchez calls you to her room. She is having pain in her abdomen and says that her back, especially up her right shoulder blade, also hurts. You take her vital signs and go to report your findings to the nurse. Using your knowledge of the digestive system, what would you think is happening to Ms. Sanchez?

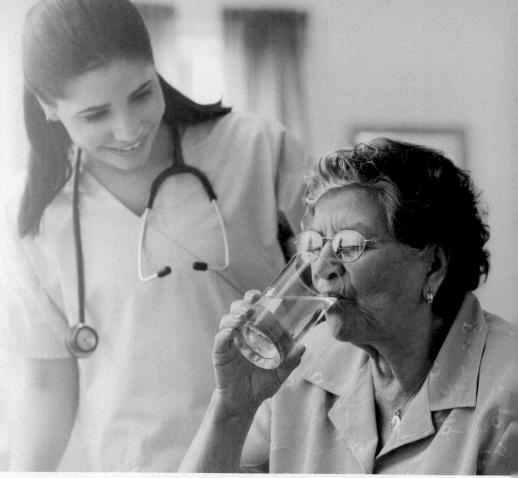

Photo: Drinking plenty of fluids helps to keep the urinary system healthy.

The Urinary System

 WHAT WILL YOU LEARN?

As you learned in Chapter 25, the urinary system rids the body of waste products that have been filtered from the bloodstream, along with excess fluid, in the form of urine. In Chapter 25, you also learned how to assist patients and residents with urinary elimination. In this chapter, you will learn a little bit more about the organs that make up the urinary system and how they work. As a nursing assistant, many of your daily responsibilities will allow you to observe changes in the functioning of a patient's or resident's urinary system that could indicate a serious problem. This is why it is important for you to know about the effects of aging on the urinary system and about some of the disorders that can affect this very important organ system. When you are finished with this chapter, you will be able to:

1. List the organs that make up the urinary system.
2. Describe the primary function of each organ of the urinary system.
3. Discuss the effects of aging on the urinary system.
4. Describe various disorders that can affect the urinary system.
5. Discuss the special care needs of people who have urinary system disorders.
6. List common diagnostic procedures that may be used to detect and diagnose urinary system disorders.

Vocabulary

Renal
Nephrons
Glomerulus
Filtrate

Urine
Urethritis
Cystitis
Pyelonephritis

Neurogenic bladder
Kidney stones
   (renal calculi)

Dialysis
Ureterostomy
Urostomy

STRUCTURE OF THE URINARY SYSTEM

The urinary system consists of the kidneys, the ureters, the urinary bladder, and the urethra (Fig. 37-1).

The Kidneys

We have two kidneys, which are like kidney beans in shape and color (only much larger!). The kidneys are located toward the back of the upper abdominal cavity, one on either side of the spinal column. The bottom of the rib cage and a layer of fat help to protect the kidneys.

Because the job of the kidneys is to filter the blood to remove waste products, the kidneys are supplied by two large arteries, called the left and the right renal arteries. (**Renal** is a word meaning "related to, involving, or located in the region of the kidneys.") The renal arteries are branches of the aorta, the largest artery in the body. The blood flow through the renal arteries is so efficient that the kidneys are able to filter all of the body's blood every half hour.

Inside each kidney are approximately 1 million tiny **nephrons**, the basic functional units of the kidney (Fig. 37-2). The nephrons are responsible for actually filtering the blood that passes through the kidney. Each nephron consists of a glomerulus and a tubule (see Fig. 37-2). The **glomerulus** is a capillary bed, enclosed within a structure called *Bowman capsule* that is the beginning of the tubule. The blood enters the kidneys through the renal arteries. Once inside the kidneys, the blood passes through a series of arteries that get smaller and smaller, until it reaches the capillary bed of the glomerulus. The blood enters the glomerulus through a vessel called the afferent arteriole (*afferent* means "cnter") and leaves the glomerulus through the efferent arteriole (*efferent* means "exit") (see Fig. 37-2). The efferent arteriole is smaller than the afferent arteriole, so the blood in the glomerulus is under a lot of pressure (think of what happens when you put your finger over the end of a garden hose). The walls of the capillaries in the glomerulus are semipermeable, which means that they have tiny openings in them. Because the blood is under a lot of pressure, some of the liquid in the blood squeezes through the walls, taking the wastes and nutrients

that are dissolved in it with it. This liquid, known as the **filtrate**, forms the basis of the urine. Next, two things happen (see Fig. 37-2B):

- The blood, minus the filtrate, leaves the glomerulus through the efferent arteriole. This arteriole branches into *peritubular capillaries* that surround each tubule (see Fig. 37-2). Eventually blood is returned to circulation through the renal veins, which empty into the inferior vena cava (the largest vein in the body).

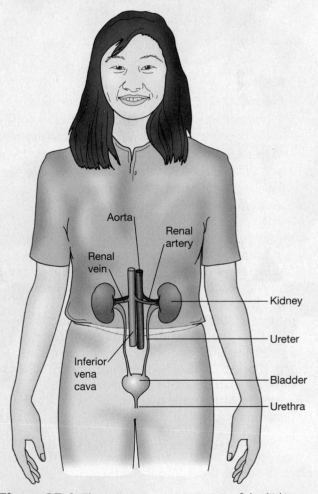

Aorta
Renal artery
Renal vein
Inferior vena cava
Kidney
Ureter
Bladder
Urethra

Figure 37-1 The urinary system consists of the kidneys, ureters, bladder, and urethra. Each kidney is supplied by a renal artery, which branches off of the aorta. After the kidneys filter the blood, the filtrate (urine) passes into the ureters and the blood passes into the renal veins, which empty into the inferior vena cava.

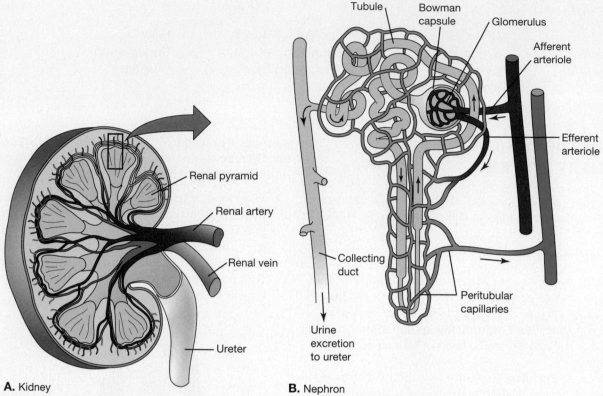

A. Kidney

B. Nephron

Figure 37-2 The kidney. **A.** If you were to cut open the kidney and look at the tissue through a microscope, you would see nephrons, the functional units where filtration actually takes place. Each kidney contains about 1 million nephrons, arranged in a radiating pattern. **B.** Each nephron consists of a glomerulus and a tubule. Blood (*red*) is filtered in the glomerulus, producing filtrate, the basis of urine (*yellow*). The portion of blood that does not enter the tubule (*purple*) leaves the glomerulus through the efferent arteriole and enters the peritubular capillaries. It is returned to the circulation through the renal veins.

■ Meanwhile, the filtrate enters Bowman capsule, and from there flows down the tubule that makes up the rest of the nephron. As the filtrate passes slowly through the tubule, the peritubular capillaries reabsorb useful substances such as water, nutrients, and minerals from the filtrate. By the time the filtrate reaches the end of the tubule, only excess fluid and waste substances remain. This is **urine**. The kidneys produce 160 to 180 liters of filtrate each day, but only about 1 to 1.5 liters are excreted from the body in the form of urine. (One liter is equal to about 1 quart.)

Urine from each nephron is emptied into a collecting area called the *renal pelvis*. From the renal pelvis, the urine flows into the ureters.

The Ureters

Two ureters, slender, muscular tubes approximately 10 to 13 inches (25 to 33 cm) long, carry urine from the kidneys to the bladder (see Fig. 37-1). The ureters are wider at the top where they connect to the renal pelvis, but they quickly become very narrow. Where the two ureters enter the bladder, a small triangular fold of tissue called the *trigone* keeps urine from flowing back into the ureters after it has emptied into the bladder.

The ureters are lined with a mucous membrane, which helps to protect against infection. Smooth muscle in the walls of the ureters contracts rhythmically, moving urine away from the kidney and toward the urinary bladder. The peristaltic movements that help move urine through the ureters are similar to the peristaltic movements that help move food through the digestive tract.

The Bladder

The bladder is a hollow sac that is a holding place (reservoir) for urine. Urine is constantly produced by the kidneys and transported through the ureters to the bladder, where it is stored until urination occurs. The bladder is very small when empty but can become quite large as it fills with urine. Like the ureters, the inside of the bladder is lined with a mucous membrane. The walls of the bladder contain three layers of smooth muscle. When the walls of the bladder contract, urination occurs. Where the bladder and the urethra join (the *bladder outlet*), the internal sphincter (a ring of involuntary muscle) keeps the bladder closed while it fills.

The Urethra

The urethra is a tube that carries urine from the bladder to the outside of the body. The urethra begins at the bladder outlet, just below the internal sphincter, and ends at the external urinary opening (called the *urinary meatus* or *urethral orifice*). Below the internal sphincter, the external urethral sphincter, a ring of voluntary muscle, relaxes to allow urine to pass during urination.

Male and female urethras are very different in size and function (Fig. 37-3). In females, the urethra measures about 1½ to 2½ inches and is used only as a

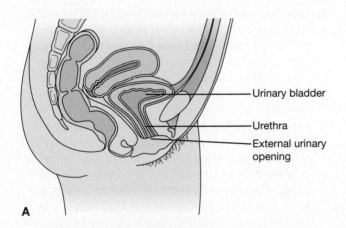

A

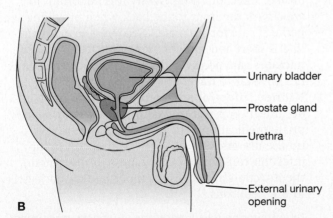

B

Figure 37-3 While the female urethra (**A**) is straight and only about 2 inches long, the male urethra (**B**) is curved in an "S" shape and is about 6 inches long. Because of the differences in anatomy, females are more prone to urinary tract infections than males, but males are harder to catheterize than females.

passageway for urine to leave the body. In males, the urethra measures about 6 to 8 inches and serves as a passageway for both urine and semen. In males, the urethra passes through the prostate gland soon after leaving the bladder outlet. The prostate gland produces seminal fluid, the fluid that, along with sperm cells, makes up semen.

FUNCTION OF THE URINARY SYSTEM

Removal of Liquid Wastes

The main function of the urinary system is to filter the blood and remove waste products and excess fluid from the body. A moderately full bladder usually contains about 1 pint (470 mL) of urine. When about 200 to 300 mL of urine collects in the bladder, the internal sphincter opens and allows urine to flood the upper segment of the urethra. At this point, the urge to urinate occurs. The person voluntarily relaxes the external urethral sphincter and the muscles of the bladder contract, allowing urine to pass out of the body through the urethra. Although it is possible to delay urination for some time, the bladder continues to fill with urine and eventually, the bladder will empty itself automatically.

Maintenance of Homeostasis

The urinary system plays several important roles in maintaining the body's homeostasis:

- The urinary system helps to keep fluid levels within the body constant. As the filtrate passes through the tubule in the nephrons, enough water is reabsorbed to maintain the body's fluid balance. Too much fluid in the blood can lead to fluid overload, causing swelling in parts of the body. Too little fluid can lead to dehydration.
- The urinary system regulates the levels of essential minerals—such as potassium, calcium, and sodium—by either saving them or releasing them through urine.
- The urinary system regulates the acidity of the blood. The pH scale, which you might remember from chemistry class, is used to rate the degree of acidity of a substance. Human blood is slightly above a 7 on the scale, which ranges from 1 to 14. Anything above 7 is said to be basic, or alkaline. Anything below 7 is acidic. Our blood cannot be either too acidic or too basic. When there is even a slight change in the blood's pH, damage to the cells can occur. Acid is a normal by-product of cellular metabolism. So, to maintain the blood at a constant pH level, the kidneys excrete the excess acids produced by cellular metabolism.

THE EFFECTS OF AGING ON THE URINARY SYSTEM

The normal processes of aging affect the urinary system:

- **Less efficient filtration.** After a person reaches 40 years of age or so, the number of functioning nephrons in the kidneys starts to decrease, decreasing the kidneys' ability to filter waste products from the bloodstream.
- **Decreased muscle tone.** Loss of muscle tone in the pelvic floor muscles and the urethral sphincter as a result of aging can contribute to stress incontinence. This type of urinary incontinence, which is most common in older females who have had children or are obese, can often be corrected with exercises or surgery.
- **Enlargement of the prostate gland (in males).** In older males, enlargement of the prostate gland is common. The enlargement may be benign (a normal effect of aging) or it may be due to cancer of the gland. As the prostate gland enlarges, it pushes against the urethra, causing it to narrow. Total emptying of the bladder of urine becomes difficult, and the person may experience episodes of overflow incontinence. As you recall from Chapter 25, overflow incontinence can occur when urine is retained in the bladder. Because the bladder does not empty completely when the person voids, it refills with urine quickly, and the urine simply overflows. As a result, the person may "dribble" urine in between visits to the bathroom. An enlarged prostate is treated with medications, surgery, or both.
- **Increased risk for urinary tract infections.** Older people are also more likely to get urinary tract infections. Incomplete emptying of the bladder can contribute to the development of infections, as can a decrease in immune system functioning.

Although it is important for everyone to drink plenty of water and other fluids, it is especially important for older people. Drinking plenty of fluids helps the kidneys to work properly, and regular urination flushes harmful bacteria from the bladder, helping to prevent urinary tract infections (Fig. 37-4).

DISORDERS OF THE URINARY SYSTEM

Illness or injury to any part of the urinary system affects the whole system and, eventually, the whole body. Common disorders of the urinary system include infections, neurogenic bladder, kidney stones, renal failure, and tumors.

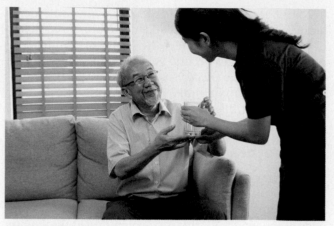

Figure 37-4 Encourage your patients or residents to drink plenty of fluids, unless a person has a medical condition that requires fluid restriction. (*ben Bryant\Shutterstock.com*)

Infections

Infections can affect any part of the urinary system:

- **Infection of the urethra (urethritis).** Urethritis is especially common in males because the urethra is longer and curved. Microbes responsible for sexually transmitted infections (STIs) such as gonorrhea, herpes, and chlamydia are common causes of urethritis in males. STIs are discussed in more detail in Chapter 38.
- **Infection of the bladder (cystitis).** Bladder infections are more common among females than males for two reasons. First, the urethral opening in females is located close to the anus. Because feces, which contain bacteria from the digestive tract, exit the body at the anus, this area is often contaminated with microbes that could cause a bladder infection. (This is why it is important to wipe from the front to the back when providing perineal care for a female.) Second, a female's urethra is short and straight, which means that once microbes gain access to the urinary tract, they do not have far to travel to infect the bladder.
- **Kidney infections (pyelonephritis).** If a bladder infection is not treated promptly with appropriate medications, the pathogens can travel up the ureters and infect the kidneys. A kidney infection can cause severe illness. If untreated, the infection might result in permanent damage to the nephrons.

In younger people, symptoms of urinary tract infections include urinary frequency, burning, and cramping. However, many older people do not have these symptoms. Urinary tract infections may also cause an older person to experience delirium. The nursing assistant may be the first to notice a change in the appearance or odor of the urine or a change in a person's voiding

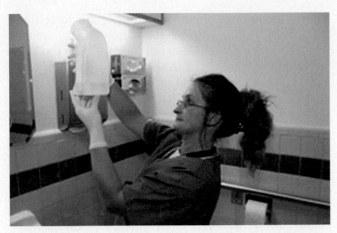

Figure 37-5 Urine that is cloudy, is an abnormal color, or has an abnormal odor may be a sign of a urinary tract infection. Always look at the urine before discarding it. If you notice anything unusual, get the nurse before discarding the urine.

habits or behavior that would indicate that a urinary tract infection may be present (Fig. 37-5).

Neurogenic Bladder

Neurogenic bladder is a condition caused by problems with the nerves that control the bladder. Neurogenic bladder can be caused by a spinal cord injury, a stroke, a tumor, or complications from diabetes. The bladder is either overactive or underactive:

- An overactive bladder is spastic or highly sensitive to stimulation. The person experiences bladder spasms (involuntary contractions of the smooth muscle in the walls of the bladder) that result in the frequent, uncontrolled release of small amounts of urine from the bladder (urge incontinence). In this condition, the amount of urine the bladder is able to hold (that is, the bladder's capacity) is reduced. There are medications that can be used to treat overactive bladder, but these medications are not often recommended for older people or for people with certain medical conditions because of their side effects. Treatment measures include carefully controlling fluid intake and emptying the bladder completely at regular intervals (for example, by applying pressure over the bladder to stimulate voiding). Sometimes catheterization with a straight catheter is ordered immediately following each attempt at voiding to check for residual urine (urine left in the bladder after voiding).
- An underactive bladder is flaccid or unable to contract forcefully. The smooth muscle that forms the walls of the bladder loses its tone, causing the bladder to "stretch out." As a result, the bladder's capacity is increased. Because of

nerve damage, the person may not be able to sense that the bladder is full, resulting in reflex incontinence (the bladder empties itself automatically when it becomes too full). Or, the muscular walls of the bladder may not be able to contract strongly enough to empty the bladder of all urine, leading to urinary retention and overflow incontinence. (Recall from Chapter 25 that overflow incontinence is characterized by dribbling of urine as the bladder overfills.) Treatment for an underactive bladder may include intermittent catheterization with a straight catheter or continuous catheterization with an indwelling urinary catheter to empty the bladder and prevent it from stretching, and careful monitoring of fluid intake and output.

Patients and residents with neurogenic bladder may be very self-conscious about the leakage of urine and the smell. Skin breakdown from urine may also occur. Your actions to help them with frequent hygiene to feel clean and fresh are very important.

Kidney Stones (Renal Calculi)

As you have learned, the main function of the kidney is to filter and remove waste products from the bloodstream. Many of these waste products are in the form of mineral salts, such as calcium salts and uric acid. If waste products become very concentrated, they can start to group together, forming tiny crystals that continue to grow in size as more of the mineral is deposited around them. These clumps of minerals are called **kidney stones (renal calculi)** (Fig. 37-6).

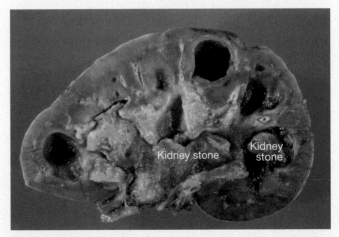

Figure 37-6 This kidney is cut open to reveal the kidney stones inside. Kidney stones can grow to be quite large, with sharp edges. They may cause obstruction of the ureters or urethra. Once the stone is passed, it is usually sent to the laboratory for analysis to determine which waste salt caused the stones to form. (© *Dr. E. Walker/Science Source*.)

Kidney stones are most common in middle-aged adults. Factors that may increase an older person's risk of developing kidney stones include immobility, not drinking enough fluids (which causes urine to become more concentrated with the waste salts), and infections of the urinary system.

Stones most often form in the collecting area (renal pelvis) of the kidney, but they can also form in the bladder. Kidney stones usually cause severe pain as they move downward through the ureter and then through the urethra. The rough edges of the stone can damage the mucosal lining of the ureter or urethra, causing it to bleed and resulting in hematuria (blood in the urine).

A person with a kidney stone usually needs to drink extra fluids to help flush the stone through the urinary tract. Medication may be necessary to help control the pain. You may be asked to collect all of the person's urine after each voiding and strain it to retrieve the stone. To strain the urine, place a piece of filter paper or a 4 × 4 gauze pad in a graduate, and then pour the urine into the graduate (Fig. 37-7). The urine will pass through the filter paper or gauze pad,

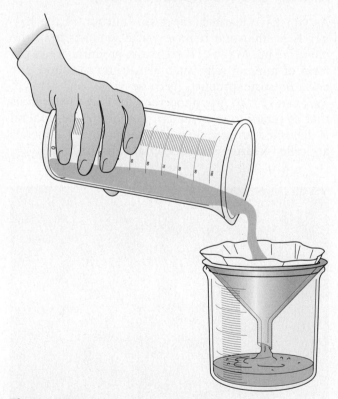

Figure 37-7 You may be asked to strain a person's urine to retrieve kidney stones. To strain urine, put a piece of filter paper or a 4 × 4 gauze pad in a graduate, and then pour the urine into the graduate. The urine will pass through the paper or gauze pad, leaving any stones behind. The stones are then transferred to a specimen container and sent to the laboratory for analysis.

leaving any stones behind. It is important to retrieve the kidney stones because then they can be sent to the laboratory for chemical analysis. Once the doctor knows which waste salt is causing the stones to form, they may be able to prevent future stones from developing.

If a stone becomes lodged in the narrow ureter, it can block the flow of urine to the bladder. The urine builds up, placing pressure on the delicate nephrons of the kidney. In this case, the person will need to have the stone removed surgically. Often, the stones are removed using a procedure called *lithotripsy*. In lithotripsy, high-frequency sound waves are directed at the stone, causing it to break into smaller pieces that can then be passed through the urinary tract. Sometimes, a surgical procedure will need to be done for stone removal.

Kidney (Renal) Failure

Kidney (renal) failure is the inability of the kidneys to filter blood effectively. As a result of kidney failure, waste products and fluid build up in the body, straining the heart and other organs. The person becomes very ill and can easily die if treatment is delayed.

Causes of Kidney Failure

Kidney failure can be either acute or chronic:

- Acute renal failure can result from a medical or surgical emergency that causes a decrease in the amount of blood flow through the kidneys. It can also be caused by poisoning, a severe infection, or a severe allergic reaction.
- Chronic renal failure results from a gradual loss of functioning nephrons. Because the kidneys gradually lose their ability to function, the person usually does not show signs of kidney failure until approximately 80% to 90% of kidney function is lost. The most common causes of chronic renal failure are hypertension and diabetes, chronic conditions that damage the blood vessels in the glomerulus. Other causes are related to chronic infections, blockage of the urinary system by stones or growths, and cancer.

Signs of Kidney Failure

Signs of renal failure may include:

- Dehydration from excessive loss of fluid (usually early in acute renal failure because the kidneys cannot reabsorb filtrate back into the bloodstream)
- Swelling from the build-up of fluid in the tissues of the body (later in chronic renal failure

when the kidneys are unable to eliminate excess fluid)

- Hypertension from fluid overload in the circulation
- Oliguria (scant amounts of urine, less than 400 mL in 24 hours), followed by anuria (the absence of urine)

Care of the Person With Kidney Failure

People with kidney failure often need to have dialysis. **Dialysis** does the job of the kidneys by removing waste products and fluids from the body. A person with acute renal failure may need dialysis treatment only for a short period of time, until kidney function returns. A person with chronic renal failure must remain on dialysis for the rest of their life, or until a donor kidney becomes available for transplant. There are two types of dialysis:

- In *hemodialysis,* the person's blood is drawn intravenously, passed through a machine with filters and solutions that clean the blood of waste, and then returned to the person's body through another vessel (Fig. 37-8A). A person who is receiving regular hemodialysis treatments will have surgery to create a *fistula* or *graft.* The fistula or graft provides access for the needles and

tubing used during the dialysis treatment. Sometimes, this access is provided through a temporary device called a *shunt.*

- In *peritoneal dialysis,* solutions that absorb waste products are instilled (placed) into a person's abdominal cavity through a tube that has been surgically inserted for this purpose (see Fig. 37-8B). The solution remains in the abdominal cavity for a specified period of time so that waste products can be absorbed into the solution through the membrane lining the abdominal cavity. The used solution is then drained into a collecting bag and is discarded according to facility policy.

Dialysis takes several hours and must be performed several times a week to keep the blood cleaned of waste products. Dialysis is performed by specially trained nurses. Most patients and residents who need dialysis travel to a health care center specifically designed to perform this service. Sometimes, a patient or resident is too ill to be taken to a dialysis center, so nurses and technicians may bring portable equipment to the facility where you work. You may be asked to monitor vital signs quite frequently after your patient or resident has had a dialysis treatment. Guidelines for caring for a person with kidney failure are given in Guidelines Box 37-1.

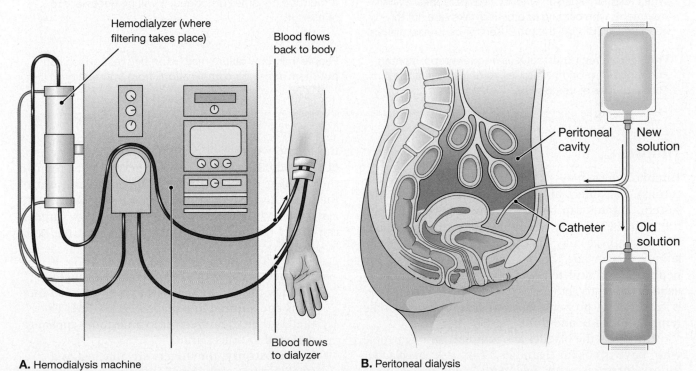

A. Hemodialysis machine   **B.** Peritoneal dialysis

Figure 37-8 Dialysis machines perform the job of the kidneys for people who have kidney failure.
A. Hemodialysis. The dialysis machine receives blood drawn from an artery in the person's arm. The blood is filtered and then returned to the body. **B.** Peritoneal dialysis. A special solution is placed in the person's abdominal cavity to absorb wastes, and then the solution is drained.

Guidelines Box 37-1   Guidelines for Caring for a Person With Kidney Failure

WHAT YOU DO	WHY YOU DO IT
Carefully measure the person's urine output and document the amounts accurately.	The doctor will use this information to monitor how well the person's kidneys are functioning.
Assist with obtaining urine samples as requested.	Testing the urine for waste products is another way of monitoring how well the person's kidneys are functioning.
Follow the person's care plan carefully with regard to food and fluid intake.	To reduce the amount of work the kidneys have to do, the person's fluid intake may be restricted and a special diet that is low in salt and protein may be ordered.
Monitor vital signs according to the person's care plan, and report any changes to the nurse immediately.	Changes in fluid balance, especially after dialysis, can significantly raise or lower a person's blood pressure.
If daily weights are ordered, make sure you weigh the person at the same time each day and with the same amount of clothing on.	Changes in a person's weight can indicate excess fluid that is being retained in the body.
When measuring the blood pressure of a person who receives hemodialysis treatments, avoid measuring the blood pressure in the arm in which the person's fistula, graft, or shunt is located.	Pressure can decrease blood flow through the fistula, graft, or shunt, which can lead to clots. Clots can make the fistula, graft, or shunt unusable for dialysis.
Provide frequent skin care.	Skin care helps prevent the skin irritation and itching that can be caused by kidney failure.
When assisting a person who receives peritoneal dialysis treatments with bathing or dressing, take care not to accidentally dislodge the tube used for peritoneal dialysis.	If the tube becomes dislodged, it will be necessary to reinsert it.
Provide care measures, such as frequent repositioning and range-of-motion exercises, to help prevent the complications of immobility.	People in kidney failure may be on bed rest, which can put them at risk for complications from immobility.

Tumors

Tumors, which may or may not be malignant (cancerous), can affect all of the organs of the urinary system. Tumors can block the flow of urine through the urinary system, resulting in kidney damage. Kidney damage may also result from tumors of the kidney that invade the healthy tissue, damaging the nephrons. Surgical removal of the affected kidney is usually necessary, but as long as the remaining kidney is functioning properly, it should be able to handle removal of waste and fluid.

Tumors of the bladder are common among people who have smoked cigarettes. The risk of bladder cancer increases with age, with older males twice as likely to develop bladder cancer as older females. Bladder tumors are usually malignant and may spread to other organs. Tumors may be treated with medication, radiation, or surgery, depending on the type of

tumor and whether or not it has spread to other parts of the body. In some cases, it is necessary to remove the bladder, disrupting normal flow of urine out of the body. Because the urine needs a new pathway to leave the body, a *urinary diversion* is created. A surgeon can divert (redirect) the urine's flow out of the body in several ways:

- In a **ureterostomy**, the ureters are brought through the abdominal wall by way of small incisions and sutured into place (Fig. 37-9A). The ureters then drain freely into an ostomy appliance designed to collect urine.
- In a **urostomy**, the ureters are attached to a small portion of the small intestine (usually the ileum) (see Fig. 37-9B). When the ileum is used, the person is said to have an *ileal conduit*. One end of the segment of intestine is sealed off, and the other end is brought through the abdominal

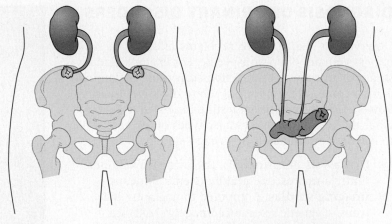

A. Ureterostomy   **B.** Urostomy (ileal conduit)

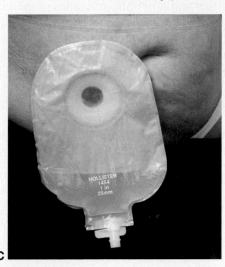

C

Figure 37-9 Urinary diversion procedures are necessary when part of the urinary system must be removed. **A.** In a ureterostomy, the ureters are brought through the abdominal wall and sutured into place. **B.** In a urostomy, the ureters are joined to a small segment of the small intestine, and then the intestine is brought to the surface of the body and sutured into place. **C.** An ostomy pouch is worn to collect the urine, in both cases. The person shown here had a urostomy following removal of their bladder to treat cancer. (C, *SPL\ScienceSource.*)

wall and sutured into place to create a stoma. The urine then drains freely into an ostomy appliance designed to collect urine (see Fig. 37-9C). For some patients, a surgeon is able to use the segment of intestine to form what is called a *neobladder*. This pouch of intestine collects the urine and holds it until the person inserts a small catheter into the stoma to drain it. With a neobladder, there is no need to wear an ostomy bag because it does not constantly drain urine.

Bladder cancer is a common reason for a person to have a ureterostomy or urostomy. However, injuries (for example, to the bladder or spinal cord) and congenital conditions (such as spina bifida) can also result in a person having a urinary diversion procedure done. Regardless of the reason for the procedure, good skin care around the ostomy site is essential. If urine is allowed to leak around the appliance, skin irritation and breakdown are very likely. The urostomy bags need to be emptied regularly and the urine may need to be measured and recorded. As always, the urine needs to be observed for any changes that might indicate infection or other urinary disorders.

Tell the Nurse!

Observations that may be a sign of a urinary system disorder and should be reported to the nurse immediately include:

- Complaints of sharp, sudden pain of the abdomen, side, or back
- Blood in the urine
- A significant increase or decrease in the amount of urine voided in a period of time
- Changes in a person's voiding habits, especially increased or decreased frequency, or a new onset of incontinence
- Pain or burning when urinating
- Urine that appears cloudy or has a strong ammonia smell
- Increased confusion, decreased alertness, or unusual behavior, especially in an older person

DIAGNOSIS OF URINARY DISORDERS

Observations that indicate problems affecting the urinary system are often nonspecific. For example, kidney stones or urinary tract infections can cause abdominal pain, a common symptom of many digestive disorders as well. Usually, additional testing is needed to find out what the real problem is. Many types of tests are used to diagnose disorders of the urinary system:

- **Urinalysis.** In urinalysis, the urine is examined under a microscope and by chemical means.
- **Imaging studies.** Computed tomography (CT) scans, magnetic resonance imaging (MRI) scans, and radiographs (x-rays) can allow a doctor to see tumors and other abnormalities of the urinary system. With x-rays, a special dye may be injected into the veins before the x-ray is taken to highlight the kidneys, ureters, and bladder (Fig. 37-10).
- **Ultrasound.** Ultrasound may be used to detect tumors of the urinary system.
- **Cytoscopy and ureteroscopy.** A small, lighted scope is inserted through the urethra and used to view the inside of the bladder (cytoscopy) or ureters (ureteroscopy).

You may be asked to collect and measure urine for testing or to help prepare a patient or resident for other diagnostic tests or procedures. Make sure that you are informed about any specific procedures that you will be responsible for, such as keeping the person on NPO status, restricting or encouraging fluids, or straining urine.

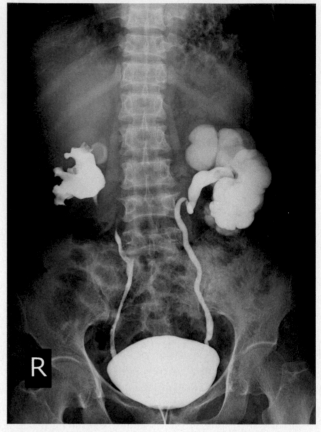

Figure 37-10 In intravenous pyelography (IVP), a type of radiographic (x-ray) procedure, a special dye is injected intravenously to allow visualization of the kidneys, ureter, and bladder. (*Jarva Jar\Shutterstock.com.*)

SUMMARY

- The organs of the urinary system are the kidneys, the ureters, the urinary bladder, and the urethra.
  - The two kidneys filter the blood to remove waste products and excess fluid.
  - The ureters carry urine from the kidneys to the bladder.
  - The bladder is a holding place for urine.
  - The urethra carries urine from the bladder to the outside of the body.
- The main function of the urinary system is to remove waste products and excess fluid from the body. The urinary system also plays a key role in homeostasis by maintaining fluid balance and regulating the pH of the blood.
- Aging affects the urinary system just as it affects the other organ systems.
  - In an older person, loss of muscle tone affects the bladder's ability to hold urine and empty properly.

- Older males may experience difficulty voiding as a result of an enlarged prostate gland.
- An older person is more likely to develop urinary tract infections because of decreased immune function and incomplete emptying of the bladder.
- As we age, the number of nephrons decreases, reducing the kidney's efficiency at filtering blood.
- Disorders of the urinary system include infections, neurogenic bladder, kidney stones (renal calculi), kidney (renal) failure, and tumors.
  - As a nursing assistant, you may be the first to notice signs and symptoms of a urinary problem that a patient or resident is having.
  - You may also be involved in helping a patient or resident to prepare for a diagnostic test used to evaluate the urinary system.

WHAT DID YOU LEARN?

Multiple Choice

Select the single best answer for each of the following questions.

1. Urine leaves the body through the:
   a. Nephrons
   b. Urethra
   c. Ureters
   d. Bladder

2. How does aging affect the urinary system?
   a. The number of nephrons is decreased, reducing the kidney's ability to filter blood efficiently.
   b. The ability to empty the bladder completely is decreased.
   c. Bladder capacity is decreased.
   d. All of the above

3. How much urine does an average adult pass each day?
   a. 200 mL
   b. 500 mL
   c. 1 to 1.5 liters
   d. 160 to 180 liters

4. Why are urinary tract infections more common in females than in males?
   a. A female's urethra is short, and the opening of the urethra is located close to the anus.
   b. A female's urethra is long and curved.
   c. Females tend to be more careless with perineal care.
   d. Females do not drink as much water as males.

5. Which of the following might be a sign of a urinary tract infection?
   a. Pain or burning while urinating
   b. Extreme thirst
   c. Anuria (absence of urine)
   d. Kidney failure

6. Which procedure uses high-frequency sound waves to break up kidney stones?
   a. Lithotripsy
   b. Dialysis
   c. Filtration
   d. Urostomy

7. How is the male urethra different from the female urethra?
   a. It is longer.
   b. It serves as a passageway for urine and for semen.
   c. The opening is further away from the anus.
   d. All of the above

8. Mr. Li has a urostomy, which was done to treat his bladder cancer. What do you need to remember when caring for Mr. Li?
   a. He may develop kidney failure at any time.
   b. He will require good skin care around the ostomy site to prevent skin irritation and breakdown.
   c. He is more at risk for kidney stones.
   d. He will not require any special care.

9. Usha is caring for Mrs. Brady, who has been going to the bathroom more frequently than usual. Now, Mrs. Brady is complaining of a burning sensation when she urinates. Why is it important for Usha to report what she has observed to the nurse?
   a. Mrs. Brady may be in kidney failure.
   b. Mrs. Brady may have a urinary tract infection.
   c. The nurse will assign another nursing assistant to help with Mrs. Brady's care.
   d. It is not necessary for Usha to report these observations to the nurse.

Matching *Match each numbered item with its appropriate lettered description.*

_____ **1.** Cystitis

_____ **2.** Renal calculi

_____ **3.** Pyelonephritis

_____ **4.** Glomerulus

_____ **5.** Neurogenic bladder

_____ **6.** Urethritis

a. Infection of the kidneys
b. Capillary bed in the nephron; surrounded by Bowman capsule
c. Infection of the urethra
d. Kidney stones
e. Infection of the bladder
f. Caused by problems with the nerves that control the bladder

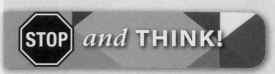

- Sunita works in a hospital and is assigned to care for Mr. Reyes, who is in the hospital because of kidney stones. This morning, while helping Mr. Reyes with his A.M. care, Sunita noticed that the urinal hanging on his side rail was full. Because Sunita knows that Mr. Reyes was admitted for kidney stones, what extra steps will she take when she empties his urinal?

- Jiayi has been assigned to care for Mrs. Rodriguez, who has a urostomy. She is unfamiliar with this term and doesn't know what to expect. If you were on Jiayi's team, what would you tell Jiayi to expect? What things would you tell Jiayi to look for in caring for Mrs. Rodriguez?

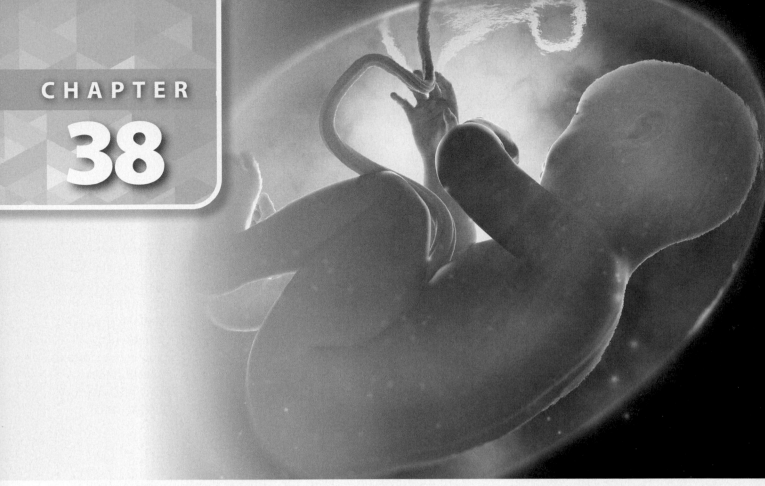

Photo: A fetus develops from a single fertilized egg. (Mopic\Shutterstock.com)

CHAPTER 38

The Reproductive System

 WHAT WILL YOU LEARN?

Of all of the systems that make up the human body, perhaps none is as fascinating and miraculous as the reproductive system. **Reproduction** is the process by which a living thing makes more living things like itself. Because all living things eventually die, the ability to reproduce is essential for the survival of any species. Without the ability to reproduce, the species would slowly die off and cease to exist.

In this chapter, you will learn about the male and female reproductive systems, which are very different from each other. You will learn about their structure and function, the effects of aging on each, and common disorders that can affect each. In addition, you will learn about sexually transmitted infections (STIs), which can affect both males and females. When you are finished with this chapter, you will be able to:

1. Describe the primary function of the reproductive system.
2. List the organs that make up the female reproductive system.
3. Discuss the normal function of the female reproductive system.
4. Explain the effects of aging on the female reproductive system.
5. Describe the disorders that may affect the female reproductive system.
6. List diagnostic tests commonly used to detect disorders of the female reproductive system.
7. List the organs that make up the male reproductive system.

8. Discuss the normal function of the male reproductive system.

9. Explain the effects of aging on the male reproductive system.

10. Describe the disorders that may affect the male reproductive system.

11. List diagnostic tests commonly used to detect disorders of the male reproductive system.

12. Discuss sexually transmitted infections (STIs) that may affect the male or female reproductive systems and ways to prevent them.

Vocabulary

Reproduction
Sex cell (gamete)
Sperm cell
Egg (ovum, ova)
Conception (fertilization)
Ovulation
Lactation
Menstrual period

Vaginitis
Amenorrhea
Dysmenorrhea
Menorrhagia
Infertility
Pelvic organ prolapse
Cystocele
Rectocele

Uterine prolapse
  (prolapsed uterus)
Pessary
Gynecologist
Postmenopausal
  bleeding
Mastectomy
Hysterectomy

Ejaculation
Erectile dysfunction
  (impotence)
Sexually transmitted
  infection (STI)
Pelvic inflammatory
  disease (PID)

Has anyone ever told you that you have "your mother's eyes" or "the family nose"? Do you look very much like your siblings, or not much like them at all? Each of us receives our genes, the bundles of DNA that determine how we develop and what we look like physically, from our parents. Each biologic parent gave you half of your genes to make a full set. This is why you may look a lot like either one of your biologic parents, or like a blend of the two. Or why you may look very much like one of your siblings and not much like another one. It all depends on the combination of genes that you received.

Each species has a set number of genes, or chromosomes. For example, human beings have 46 chromosomes. This means that to keep the number of chromosomes the same from generation to generation, the male parent contributes 23 chromosomes and the female parent contributes 23 chromosomes. The special cells contributed by each parent that contain half of the normal number of chromosomes are called **sex cells**, or **gametes**. The male sex cell is called a **sperm cell**. The female sex cell is called an **egg**, or **ovum** (*ova*, plural). When the sperm joins the egg, forming a cell that contains the complete number of chromosomes, **conception (fertilization)** occurs. During the 9 months leading up to the birth of a baby, the single original cell that formed at conception divides over and over again, forming all of the baby's tissues and organs.

One of the primary functions of the reproductive system in both males and females is to produce and transport sex cells. However, unlike other organ systems in the body, the organs that make up the reproductive system are very different in males and females. The male reproductive system is designed to produce sperm and deposit it inside the female's body. The female reproductive system is designed to produce eggs, receive sperm cells, contain and nourish a developing baby, give birth, and provide nourishment after the baby's birth by producing breast milk. Because of the physical and functional differences between the male and female reproductive systems, we will look at each system separately in the sections that follow.

THE FEMALE REPRODUCTIVE SYSTEM

Structure of the Female Reproductive System

The organs and structures of the female reproductive system are located both inside and outside of the body. The internal organs are the ovaries, fallopian tubes, uterus, and vagina (Fig. 38-1A). The outer structures are the labia, the clitoris, and the vaginal opening (see Fig. 38-1B). These outer structures are referred to collectively as the *vulva*. In addition, the breasts (mammary glands) are considered accessory

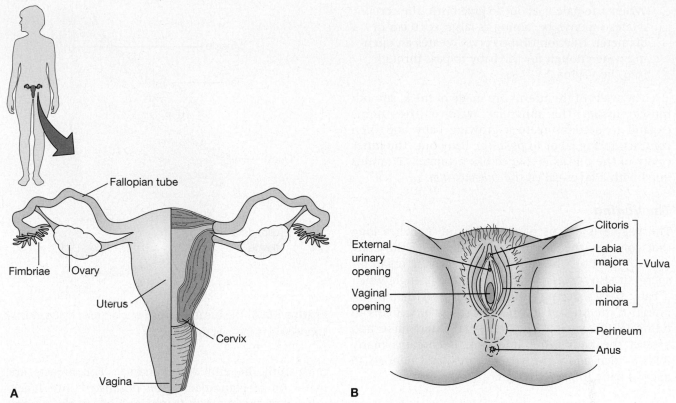

Figure 38-1 The female reproductive system. (**A**) Internal structures include the ovaries, fallopian tubes, uterus, and vagina. (**B**) External structures, collectively known as "the vulva," include the vaginal opening, labia, and clitoris.

organs of the female reproductive system because they play a role in nourishing a newborn baby.

The Ovaries

The ovaries are two small, almond-shaped organs located deep inside the abdomen on either side of the uterus (see Fig. 38-1A). The ovaries store the ova, or eggs. When a female baby is born, the ovaries contain all of the eggs that they will ever have. The stored eggs are kept in a "holding pattern" until they are needed. Once the child passes through puberty and reaches reproductive age, the ova begin to mature and ovulation begins. **Ovulation** is the release of a mature egg from the ovaries each month.

The Fallopian Tubes

The fallopian tubes, also called *uterine tubes* or *oviducts*, are slender tubes about 4 to 5 inches long that transport the egg from the ovary to the uterus. After leaving the ovary, the egg moves through the fluid in the abdomen to the entrance of the nearest fallopian tube. The open ends of the fallopian tubes nearest the ovaries have small, fringe-like projections called *fimbriae* (see Fig. 38-1A). The fimbriae beat in

a wave-like motion, helping to move the egg into the tube. Once in the fallopian tube, the egg moves toward the uterus, helped along by the peristaltic contractions of the smooth muscle layer in the walls of the fallopian tube and the tiny, hair-like cilia on the lining of the fallopian tube. Like the cilia in the airways of the lungs, the cilia in the fallopian tubes move gently back and forth, creating a sweeping motion that helps to move the egg along the length of the tube. Conception, if it occurs, occurs in the fallopian tubes.

The Uterus

The uterus, sometimes referred to as the *womb*, is a hollow, pear-shaped organ (see Fig. 38-1). The uterus has three sections:

- The *fundus* is the upper, rounded portion of the uterus.
- The *body* is the midportion of the uterus.
- The *cervix* is the lower, narrow portion of the uterus. Normally, the cervix is closed, except for a very tiny opening. This opening, which is no larger than a pinpoint, allows sperm to enter the uterus, and menstrual blood to pass out of it.

When a female is about to give birth, the cervix dilates (opens), becoming as large as 10 cm in diameter. Dilation of the cervix creates an opening wide enough for the baby to pass through into the vagina.

The walls of the uterus are made of thick, smooth muscle tissue. The muscular walls of the uterus expand to accommodate a growing baby and then contract during labor to push the baby out. The inner cavity of the uterus is shaped like a capital "T" and is lined with a layer called the *endometrium*.

The Vagina

The vagina is a muscular tube about 3 inches long that connects the uterus to the outside of the body (see Fig. 38-1A). The vagina is the receiving organ for sperm. It also serves as the birth canal, through which a baby passes during birth. The mucous membrane lining of the vagina secretes mucus, which helps to lubricate the vagina during sexual intercourse and protect the body from infection. It contains many folds, which allow the vagina to expand enough to allow a baby to pass through.

The Vulva

The vulva consists of the vaginal opening, the labia, and the clitoris (see Fig. 38-1B).

- The vaginal opening, also called the *vaginal orifice*, is where the vagina opens to the outside of the body. The vaginal opening is located between the external urinary opening (the urinary meatus or urethral orifice) and the anus. The area between the vaginal opening and the anus is often called the *obstetrical perineum*. However, the term *perineum* can also be used to describe the entire external genital area of both males and females.
- The labia, or "lips," are folds of tissue that surround the vaginal opening. The many folds of the external female reproductive system can create difficulties with hygiene, especially if the person is injured, ill, or otherwise unable to provide for their own cleanliness needs. Perineal care and hygiene assistance is discussed in Chapter 22.
- The clitoris is located at the upper folds of the internal labia. This tissue, which is very sensitive to touch, helps to initiate sexual arousal.

The Breasts (Mammary Glands)

In females, the breasts are considered accessory organs of the reproductive system because they play a role in nourishing the newborn. Although the female breasts develop during puberty, they do not start producing

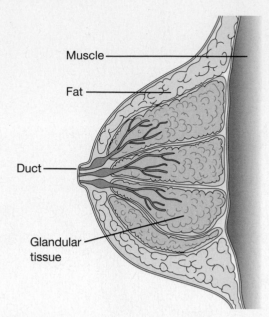

Figure 38-2 The breasts consist of glandular tissue, ducts, connective tissue, and fat.

milk until the end of pregnancy. The breasts are made up of glandular tissue organized into lobes, ducts that convey milk from the lobes to the nipple, and supporting fat and connective tissue (Fig. 38-2). When it is stimulated by the hormone prolactin (which is secreted by the pituitary gland in large amounts at the end of pregnancy), the glandular tissue of the breasts produces milk, a process known as **lactation**. In response to an infant's suckling, the pituitary gland releases the hormone oxytocin. This hormone stimulates the contraction of muscle cells in the duct walls, sending the milk through the ducts to the nipple.

Function of the Female Reproductive System

Each month during a female's reproductive years (from puberty to menopause), the body prepares for potential conception and pregnancy. If pregnancy does not occur, the person has a menstrual period, and the cycle begins again.

Each egg grows within its own "shell," called a follicle. The cycle begins when the pituitary gland releases more follicle-stimulating hormone (FSH), a hormone that stimulates the growth and maturation of multiple follicles (Fig. 38-3). FSH also stimulates the follicles to produce estrogen, another hormone. As the estrogen level increases, it inhibits FSH production. This feedback mechanism limits the number of follicles that mature each month. One egg-containing follicle continues to grow and mature, and the others die off.

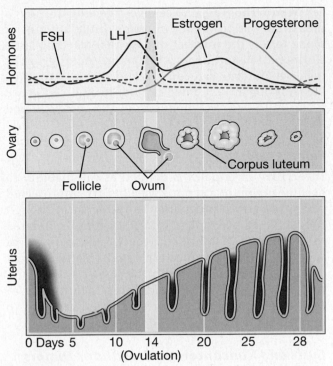

Figure 38-3 Each month during a female's reproductive years, the body prepares itself for a possible pregnancy. In response to hormones, a follicle fully develops and releases its ovum, and the lining of the uterus prepares itself to receive the fertilized ovum, should fertilization occur. If fertilization does not occur, the ovum and the lining of the uterus are shed during the female's menstrual period, and the cycle begins again.

When the follicle has matured, luteinizing hormone (LH), another hormone released by the pituitary gland, causes the follicle to burst, releasing the egg from the ovary (ovulation) (see Fig. 38-3). Following ovulation, the empty follicle becomes known as the *corpus luteum*. The corpus luteum continues to produce estrogen, and it also begins to produce progesterone. Estrogen and progesterone cause the uterus to begin to prepare itself to receive a fertilized egg.

In response to estrogen and progesterone, the lining of the uterus (the endometrium) thickens, creating a soft, nourishing environment for a fertilized egg, should one arrive (see Fig. 38-3). The fertilized egg attaches itself to the endometrium (a process called *implantation*). Even before the fertilized egg implants, it begins to divide, forming the cells and tissues that will eventually become a new human being. If fertilization does not occur, the egg passes into the uterus, where it usually dissolves. The levels of hormones decrease, causing the endometrial lining to break down and pass through the vagina as the **menstrual period**.

This cycle of hormone secretion and egg development occurs in a regular pattern throughout a female's reproductive years. The average cycle from the first day of one menstrual period until the start of another one is 28 days, but the cycle can be as short as 22 days or as long as 45 days.

The Effects of Aging on the Female Reproductive System

Unlike the age-related changes that affect other organ systems, the age-related changes that affect the female reproductive system are usually very noticeable.

Increased Difficulty Becoming Pregnant

Many females in their late 30s and early 40s have difficulty becoming pregnant. This is because each month, the number of healthy eggs remaining in the ovaries decreases. (Remember that at birth, the ovaries contain all of the eggs that they will ever have.) Becoming pregnant is often still possible at this age, just more difficult. Fertility treatments, such as the use of medications to cause more follicles to ripen each month or in-vitro fertilization (IVF), are often very helpful for people in this age group who wish to become pregnant.

Decreased Sex Hormone Production

As a female ages, the body produces lower amounts of sex hormones, especially estrogen and progesterone. Eventually, this decreased hormone production results in *menopause*. Menopause occurs in most females sometime between the ages of 45 and 55 years. Its symptoms result from the lack of estrogen and progesterone production by the ovary. People in menopause still have low levels of sex hormone production from the adrenal gland, as discussed in Chapter 35.

Menopause can cause many bothersome symptoms, including "hot flashes," irritability, a loss of energy, and an inability to sleep. Decreased production of estrogen and progesterone, which oppose the actions of androgens such as testosterone may also cause some females to develop facial hair and a coarse ("scratchy") voice. Some females experience vaginal dryness and irritation. When this is the case, use of a lubricant during sexual intercourse can be helpful. Vaginal dryness and irritation can also lead to **vaginitis** (inflammation of the vaginal tissues). Vaginitis can cause itching, burning, and a vaginal discharge, and it increases the risk of vaginal infections.

Many people who have gone through menopause choose to replace the hormones their bodies no longer produce by taking estrogen and progesterone orally or topically (applied to the skin or within the vagina). This is called menopausal hormone therapy (MHT), previously called hormone replacement therapy (HRT). MHT helps to minimize some of the more annoying "side effects" of menopause, such as hot flashes. In addition, some research shows that taking estrogen and progesterone after menopause can help keep bones strong and prevent heart disease and some types of dementia. However, MHT may increase a person's chances of developing certain types of cancer, especially if they are smokers or have a family history of these cancers. Each person must work with their health care provider to determine whether MHT is right for them, given their unique situation and health history.

Disorders of the Female Reproductive System

Many types of disorders can affect the female reproductive system. For example, many factors, such as hormone imbalances, can cause problems during the menstrual cycle. Cysts (fluid-filled sacs) and noncancerous tumors can interfere with the functioning of the reproductive system, or cause pain or excessive menstrual bleeding. Finally, cancer can occur in any organ of the female reproductive system.

Menstrual Disorders

A female may have problems during the menstrual cycle, such as irregular periods, excessive pain, or excessive bleeding. Common disorders associated with the menstrual cycle include the following:

- **Amenorrhea** is the absence of menstrual flow. Primary amenorrhea occurs when a female has not begun to menstruate by the age of 16 years. Abnormalities in the reproductive organs, a hormone disorder, or malnutrition may be the cause. Secondary amenorrhea is the absence of menstrual flow in a female who has had previous menstrual periods. Secondary amenorrhea can result from hormone imbalances or tumors; it is also usually the first sign of pregnancy.
- **Dysmenorrhea** is painful menstruation. Many females experience cramps in the lower abdomen during menstrual periods, but for some females the pain is severe enough to interfere with daily activities. Extremely painful periods that prevent a person from doing what they normally do should be brought to the attention of a health care provider. Severe dysmenorrhea may indicate a disorder called *endometriosis*, in which endometrial tissue develops on the outer surface of the reproductive organs.

Menorrhagia is excessive bleeding during a menstrual period, either in terms of the amount of blood lost or the number of days that bleeding lasts. Hormonal disturbances, infections, and growths inside the uterus can cause menorrhagia. Excessive bleeding for an extended period of time can cause a person to become anemic from the chronic blood loss.

Female Infertility

Infertility in females is defined as the inability to become pregnant after at least 1 year of unprotected sex or to carry a pregnancy to full term. Although the cause of a couple's infertility may be related to the male's inability to produce the amount of sperm needed to fertilize the egg, in many cases, it is related to a problem with the female's reproductive system. Hormone imbalances, deformities of the reproductive organs, or scar tissue can lead to infertility.

Cysts and Noncancerous Growths or Tumors

Many organs in the female reproductive system can be affected by cysts or other noncancerous growths. Although these cysts and growths are not cancerous, they can still cause problems.

- **Cysts** can form on the ovaries after ovulation, causing intense pain. Although not malignant, ovarian cysts may need to be surgically removed if they occur frequently and are painful. Cysts may also form in the lubricating glands located inside the vagina, creating a painful, infected lump that may have to be surgically drained.
- **Fibroids (myomas)** sometimes form in the muscle wall of the uterus. Fibroids can cause problems during pregnancy if they are large enough to crowd a developing baby inside the uterus. They may also cause severe menorrhagia if they grow toward the inside of the uterine cavity.

Pelvic Organ Prolapse

The female reproductive organs, the urinary bladder, and the rectum are supported in the pelvic cavity by connective tissue and muscles. Childbirth and the loss of estrogen that occurs with menopause, as well as obesity, can cause these supportive structures to weaken. As a result, a female may experience **pelvic organ prolapse**. In pelvic organ prolapse, the affected organ shifts downward from its normal position and may protrude into the vaginal wall through a weakness much like a hernia (Fig. 38-4):

- **Cystocele** occurs when the bladder shifts downward, pressing into the front (anterior) vaginal wall. Cystocele can contribute to incomplete

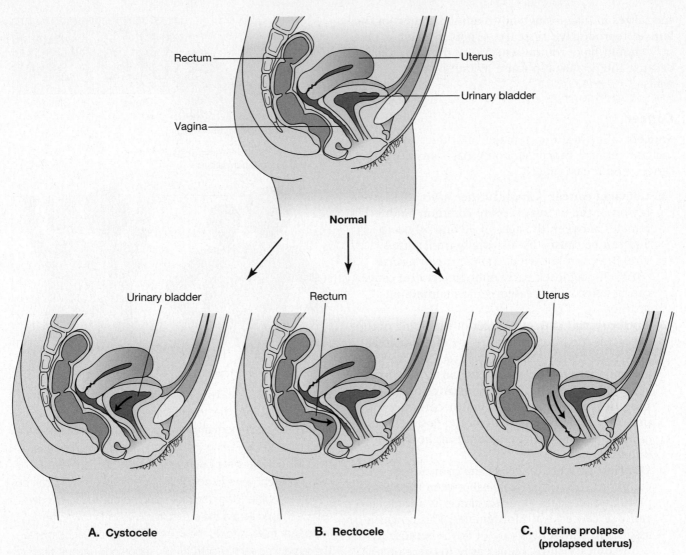

Rectum
Uterus
Urinary bladder
Vagina

Normal

Urinary bladder
Rectum
Uterus

A. Cystocele

B. Rectocele

**C. Uterine prolapse
(prolapsed uterus)**

Figure 38-4 Pelvic organ prolapse occurs in many females. (**A**) In cystocele, the bladder shifts downward, pressing into the front (anterior) wall of the vagina. (**B**) In rectocele, the front wall of the rectum shifts downward, pressing into the back (posterior) wall of the vagina. (**C**) In uterine prolapse (prolapsed uterus), the uterus slips downward, into the vagina.

emptying of the bladder and stress incontinence (see Chapter 25).

■ **Rectocele** occurs when the front wall of the rectum shifts downward, pushing into the back (posterior) vaginal wall. People with this condition may feel pressure in the rectal area, have difficulties having a bowel movement, or feel as if the rectum is not empty following a bowel movement.

■ **Uterine prolapse (prolapsed uterus)** occurs when the uterus shifts downward, into the vaginal canal. The uterus may slip only partway through the vagina, or it may pass all of the way through the vagina so that it is visible on the outside of the body. Symptoms of uterine prolapse can include a feeling of pelvic pressure or fullness,

low back pain, trouble having a bowel movement, leaking of urine, and urinary incontinence.

Treatment depends on the severity of the prolapse and the person's overall health. If the prolapse is mild, treatment may not be necessary, or estrogen may be administered (in the form of a cream that is applied to the mucous membrane lining of the vagina) to strengthen the supportive tissues and muscles. If the prolapse is more severe, surgery can be performed to remove the uterus and repair the weakened walls of the vagina. A nonsurgical option involves the use of a device called a **pessary** that is inserted into the vagina to support the prolapsed organ in the proper position. Pessaries come in a variety of styles and must be fitted by the doctor (usually a **gynecologist**, a doctor who specializes in diagnosing and treating disorders of the female reproductive system). A person using a pessary should have routine checks by the gynecologist because the pessary can cause irritation of the vaginal walls.

Cancer

Cancers affecting the female reproductive system include cervical cancer, endometrial cancer, ovarian cancer, and breast cancer.

- **Cervical cancer** (cancer of the cervix, the lower region of the uterus) is more common among females between the ages of 30 and 50 years and can be caused by a sexually transmitted viral infection known as *human papillomavirus (HPV)*. If diagnosed early enough, cervical cancer can be effectively treated while maintaining fertility.
- **Endometrial cancer** (cancer of the lining of the uterus) is the most common type of cancer that affects the female reproductive tract. It is most common in females after menopause. The first sign of this type of cancer is **postmenopausal bleeding**, uterine bleeding that occurs after a person has completed menopause. Postmenopausal bleeding can also result from hormone imbalances.
- **Ovarian cancer** (cancer of the ovary) most commonly occurs in females between the ages of 40 and 65 years. Ovarian cancer is a leading cause of cancer death for females. This cancer is associated with a high rate of death because it grows quickly and spreads easily to other organs. Early diagnosis and treatment can improve the chances of survival.
- **Breast cancer** is the most commonly occurring cancer in females. Breast cancer can develop in people with relatives with breast cancer, especially a female member of their immediate family. But it can also develop in people who have no family history of the disease. Females are encouraged to get into the habit of examining their breasts at the same time each month. During the breast self-exam (BSE), the person looks and feels for any changes in the breast tissue (Fig. 38-5). Monthly BSEs can help a person to become familiar with the way their breast tissue normally looks and feels. This knowledge may allow them to recognize lumps or other problems that need to be reported to the nurse or doctor for further evaluation. Many breast lumps are not cancer, but the only way to be sure is to have them checked. Early detection and new treatment methods for breast cancer allow many females to be completely cured of this disease.

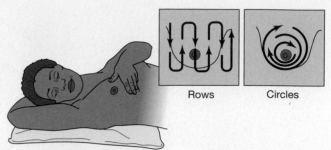

Rows   Circles

A. Feeling for abnormalities

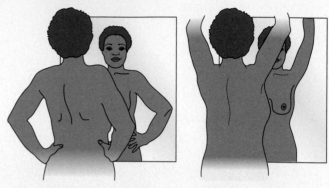

B. Looking for abnormalities

Figure 38-5 Females are encouraged to examine their breasts monthly so that they become familiar with the way their breast tissue normally looks and feels. A breast self-exam (BSE) involves (**A**) feeling the breasts for abnormalities and then (**B**) looking at the breasts for abnormalities. There are many different ways to do a BSE. For example, the BSE can be performed while lying down or standing up, and the fingers can be moved across the breast in circles or in rows. The important thing is to do the BSE the same way each time, at the same time each month, and to report any unusual findings to a health care provider immediately.

Common Diagnostic Procedures

As a nursing assistant, you may need to help prepare a female patient or resident for a procedure used to diagnose problems with the reproductive system. Many people are hesitant or embarrassed to discuss problems involving the reproductive organs. You must be especially careful to help maintain a person's modesty and privacy when they are being prepared for a diagnostic procedure involving the reproductive system. Make sure that the privacy curtains and the door are closed, and keep sensitive body parts (such as the breasts or vulva) covered as much as possible. Also be aware that your patient or resident may be fearful or anxious about the test results. Be careful not to give advice or tell the person what you would do if you were in their situation. Instead, listen, give competent and compassionate care, and report your observations to the nurse.

Tell the Nurse!

Your duties will include assisting your female patients or residents with their personal hygiene and toileting needs. Because of this, you may be the first to observe signs of a problem involving the reproductive organs. In addition, a female patient or resident may tell you about a problem that they are experiencing. Report any of the following observations or complaints to the nurse immediately:

- The person has an unusual vaginal discharge
- The person has vaginal bleeding, but they have already gone through menopause
- The person has very heavy vaginal bleeding during their menstrual period
- The person has pain or cramping in their lower abdomen
- The person complains of a feeling of pelvic pressure or fullness
- The person complains of problems emptying their bowel or bladder

- There is a protrusion from the vaginal opening
- The person reports itching or burning around the vulva
- The skin around the vulva is inflamed or irritated
- There are changes in skin coloring, sores that do not heal, lumps, unusual swelling, or thickened areas around the vulva
- There is a lump or thickened area in the breast
- There is a discharge from the nipples or puckering of the skin of the breasts

---

Routine physical examinations are very effective for detecting disorders of the female reproductive system while they are in the early stages and easier to treat. In addition to routine physical examinations, several diagnostic procedures are used to screen for female reproductive disorders:

- **Pap test.** A Pap test (named after the doctor who invented the test, George Papanicolaou) is routinely performed to detect changes in the cervix that may indicate early cervical cancer. The doctor uses a swab to gather a sample of cells from the cervix, and then the cells are examined under a microscope to make sure they are healthy.
- **Biopsy.** In a biopsy, a tissue sample is obtained and examined under a microscope for cancerous cells. A biopsy may be used to detect endometrial, cervical, or breast cancer.
- **Dilation and curettage (D&C).** A D&C is a surgical procedure. The cervix is dilated (made wider) and tissue is curetted (scraped) from the inside of the cervix and the uterus. This tissue is then examined to determine the cause of abnormal bleeding.
- **Imaging studies.** Radiographic imaging studies can allow a doctor to see tumors or scar tissue that may be blocking the fallopian tubes, a common cause of infertility.
- **Ultrasonography.** During an ultrasound study, sound waves are "bounced off" an organ and then translated into a three-dimensional image. Ultrasound can reveal tumors or cysts on the ovaries and in other structures of the female reproductive tract. Ultrasound can also be used to check breast cysts. In addition, ultrasound is used when a person is pregnant to check on the fetus and make sure that it is developing properly (Fig. 38-6).
- **Mammography.** A mammogram is an x-ray of breast tissue. Mammography can detect breast cancers at a very early stage, before they become large enough to be seen or felt. For this reason, it is recommended that females receive routine mammograms, in addition to performing monthly BSEs.

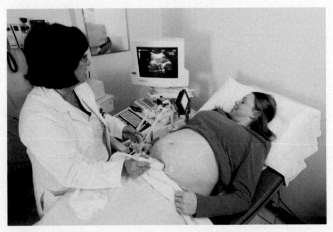

Figure 38-6 Ultrasound, a common diagnostic procedure, is used to view a developing baby inside the uterus. It can also be used to detect tumors or cysts on reproductive structures.

Common Surgical Procedures

Many of your patients or residents may be preparing for, or recovering from, surgery involving the reproductive organs. Common surgical procedures involving the female reproductive system include mastectomy and hysterectomy.

Mastectomy

A **mastectomy** (surgical removal of a breast) may be performed on a person who has been diagnosed with certain types of breast cancer. For some people with breast cancer, the cancer can be treated by removing only the cancerous lump and some of the surrounding tissue. This procedure is called a *lumpectomy*. But for many people, the entire breast must be removed to treat the cancer effectively. When this is the case, many people choose to follow the mastectomy with reconstructive surgery. A new breast is created either by inserting a prosthesis (implant) under the skin and muscle, or by grafting tissue from another part of the body. For many people, removal of a breast is very difficult to handle emotionally. This means that in addition to healing physically from the procedure, the person will need to heal emotionally.

Partial or reduction mastectomy procedures are often performed to reduce the size of breasts for people who have large breasts or who are having gender-affirming surgery. Breast enhancement procedures are performed to increase the size of the breasts.

Hysterectomy

A **hysterectomy** (surgical removal of the uterus) may be used to treat uterine cancer, excessive bleeding, or other disorders of the female reproductive tract. Removal of the uterus and ovaries is also performed for people desiring gender-affirming surgery. When a hysterectomy is performed through an incision in the abdomen, it is called a *total abdominal hysterectomy (TAH)*. When it is performed through the vagina by cutting around the cervix, it is called a *total vaginal hysterectomy (TVH)*. Many hysterectomy procedures are now performed using *minimally invasive surgery*, through a scope inserted into the abdomen or even by a robotic technique. The fallopian tubes and ovaries may or may not be removed, depending on the reason for the surgery. Invasive or widespread cancer of the uterus or ovaries may require surgical removal of other structures, such as the bladder or rectum, in order to remove all of the cancerous tissue.

THE MALE REPRODUCTIVE SYSTEM

Structure of the Male Reproductive System

The organs and structures of the male reproductive system include the testicles (testes), the epididymis, the vas deferens, and the penis (Fig. 38-7). Accessory

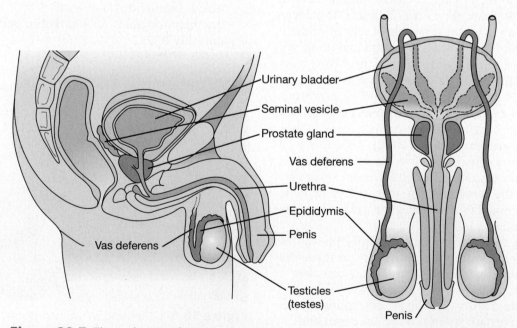

Figure 38-7 The male reproductive system consists of the testicles (testes), the epididymis, the vas deferens, and the penis. Accessory organs include the seminal vesicles and prostate gland.

organs include the seminal vesicles and prostate gland, which play a role in producing semen (the fluid that carries sperm cells out of the body).

The Testicles (Testes)

The testicles are two walnut-like organs located in the *scrotum*, a loose, bag-like sac that is suspended between the thighs. The testicles have two important functions: They secrete testosterone, the hormone that is responsible for the development of male secondary sex characteristics and for the proper functioning of the male reproductive system, and they produce sperm cells. The testicles are located outside of the torso because the temperature necessary for the proper development of sperm is lower than the temperature inside the torso.

The Epididymis

After the sperm cells leave the testes, they move into the epididymis, a series of coiled tubes where the sperm cells mature and gain the ability to "swim." A sperm cell's ability to swim comes from its flagellum, a whip-like "tail" (Fig. 38-8). The whip-like motion of the flagellum moves the sperm cell forward, allowing it to "swim" through the female reproductive tract in search of an egg to fertilize. The sperm cell is the only human body cell that has a flagellum.

The Vas Deferens

From the epididymis, the sperm cell moves into the vas deferens, a passageway that transports the sperm

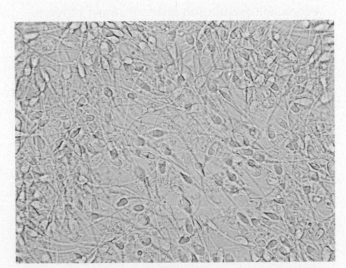

Figure 38-8 Each sperm cell has a whip-like "tail," called a flagellum, that allows it to move. The ability to move is important for sperm cells. This flagellum helps propel the sperm cell through the female's vagina, into the uterus, and then into the fallopian tube to meet the egg. (*Lukasz Pawel Szczepanski\Shutterstock.com*)

cell to the urethra (see Fig. 38-7). While in the vas deferens, the sperm cells are mixed with the secretions from the seminal vesicles and the prostate gland. These secretions, which nourish and protect the sperm cells, form the fluid portion of semen. In the prostate gland, the vas deferens joins with the urethra, which is the final passageway through which the sperm cells leave the body.

The Penis

The male urethra, described in Chapter 37, is contained in the penis. Semen leaves the body by way of the external urinary opening, which is located at the tip of the *glans penis,* the enlarged portion at the end of the penis. If a male has not been circumcised, a loose fold of skin called the *foreskin* covers the glans penis.

The urethra is surrounded by "spongy" tissue. Stimulation by the nervous system causes this spongy tissue to fill with blood. This in turn causes the penis to become hard and erect. For reproduction to occur, an erect penis is inserted into a female's vagina, allowing sperm cells to be deposited into the female's reproductive tract.

Function of the Male Reproductive System

The structures of the male reproductive system make sex hormones, produce and nourish male sex cells (sperm), and deliver these cells to the female reproductive system for fertilization to occur. While the mature female reproductive system usually produces only one egg each month, the mature male reproductive system produces sperm cells constantly. Many millions of sperm cells are needed to fertilize one egg because so many sperm cells die during their journey through the female reproductive tract. After puberty, sperm cells are produced in the testicles in response to the release of FSH by the pituitary gland. As in females, the pituitary gland also secretes LH, which stimulates the testicles to produce testosterone. Testosterone is needed for the continued development and growth of the sperm cells.

Sperm cells exit the body through the process of **ejaculation**. During sexual activity, stimulation of the erect penis causes the forceful release of semen from the body.

The Effects of Aging on the Male Reproductive System

Males do not go through menopause, because they continue to produce sperm cells and sex hormones throughout life. However, there are still age-related changes related to declining production of testosterone and enlargement of the prostate gland.

Decreased Frequency and Duration of Erections

Beginning at around the age of 20 years, production of testosterone and sperm begins to gradually decline. A male can remain fertile until late in life, even as late as 80 years of age, but most males find that as they get older, erections occur less frequently and last for shorter periods of time. This is a result of decreased production of testosterone. The ability to have and maintain an erection is also affected by the effects of aging on the cardiovascular system, which can result in decreased blood flow to the penis. Finally, medications taken for hypertension and other common disorders can also affect sexual abilities.

Enlargement of the Prostate Gland

As a male ages, the prostate gland tends to enlarge. Because the prostate gland surrounds the urethra, this enlargement can make urination difficult. Prostate problems associated with aging are discussed in Chapter 37.

Disorders of the Male Reproductive System

Common disorders of the male reproductive system include erectile dysfunction, infertility, and cancer.

Erectile Dysfunction

Erectile dysfunction (ED) (sometimes known as impotence) is the inability to achieve or maintain an erection long enough to engage in sexual activity. A patient or resident may experience erectile dysfunction for several reasons. Lowered levels of male hormones, circulatory problems that restrict blood flow to the penis, medications, or emotional disturbances can all affect the ability to have an erection, either temporarily or permanently. In many cultures, the ability to have an erection is often considered a mark of virility. Because of this, many males who have erectile dysfunction are embarrassed to tell a health care provider about this problem. However, once the cause has been discovered, many effective methods of treatment can allow the person to remain sexually active throughout the life span.

Male Infertility

Male infertility involves the inability to ejaculate enough functional sperm to fertilize an egg. As with females, hormone imbalances, deformities of the reproductive organs, or scar tissue resulting from infection can lead to male infertility.

Cancer

Cancers affecting the male reproductive system include testicular cancer, prostate cancer, and penile cancer. In addition, males may get breast cancer, although this cancer is much less common in males than in females.

- **Testicular cancer** usually affects young- to middle-aged adult males and can easily spread to other parts of the body through the lymphatic system before it is detected. Males of all ages are encouraged to examine their testicles regularly (Fig. 38-9). Testicular self-exam (TSE) can help detect lumps and other abnormalities at an early stage. Early detection and treatment of cancer leads to a better survival outcome.
- **Prostate cancer.** Cancer of the prostate gland most commonly occurs in males older than 50 years. Rectal examination, during which a doctor inserts a finger into the rectum to feel for enlargement of the gland, can lead to early detection. A blood test can also be used to screen for prostate cancer. Prostate cancer typically grows slowly and has a good cure rate with early detection.
- **Penile cancer.** Occasionally, lesions that appear on the penis may be cancerous. As always, it is important for you to report any changes in the skin of patients or residents on any part of the body.

Tell the Nurse!

A conscientious nursing assistant always observes a patient or resident for changes that indicate that something is "not quite right" and reports those observations to the nurse immediately. Listed below are some observations that may indicate disorders of the male reproductive system. Report any of the following observations or complaints to the nurse immediately:

- The person has an unusual discharge from the penis, especially if it contains blood or other discolored secretions
- The person has pain or burning when urinating
- There is a lump or thickened area in the testes
- There are changes in the skin surrounding the scrotum or penis
- There is reddened or irritated skin in the genital area
- The person complains of pain or aching in the scrotum or rectal area

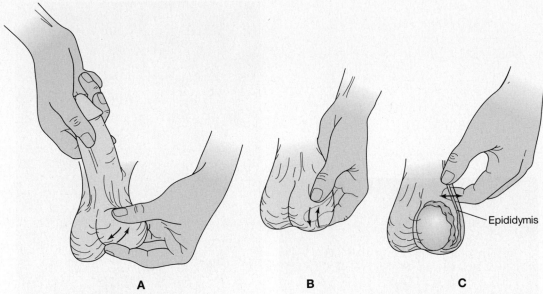

Epididymis

Figure 38-9 Males are encouraged to examine their testicles monthly. This is an effective and easy way to detect testicular cancer. To perform a testicular self-exam (TSE), first roll each testicle from side to side between the thumb and middle finger to feel for any lumps or abnormalities (**A**). Then repeat the procedure, except this time, roll the testicle between the fingers in an up-and-down direction (**B**). Finally, feel along the epididymis, the cord-like structure on the top and back of the testicle (**C**).

Common Diagnostic Procedures

Many of the diagnostic procedures that are used to detect disorders of the urinary system (see Chapter 37) are also used to detect disorders of the male reproductive system. You may care for a male patient or resident who is scheduled for one of the following tests:

■ **Blood work.** A blood sample can be used to determine hormone levels (for example, in a male with erectile dysfunction). A blood sample can also be analyzed for prostate-specific antigen (PSA), a substance that is found in the blood of people with prostate problems.

■ **Biopsy.** A biopsy may be necessary to test tissue for the presence of cancer in the prostate gland or the testes.

As always, be sensitive to how your patient or resident might be feeling. The person may be afraid of finding out that they have cancer or may be worried that problems with sexual functioning will be permanent.

SEXUALLY TRANSMITTED INFECTIONS

A **sexually transmitted infection (STI)** is an infection that is most often transmitted by sexual contact.

These infections, also known as sexually transmitted diseases (STDs), can be caused by bacteria or viruses. The pathogens are transmitted through semen and vaginal secretions. Infection of the organs of the reproductive system is most common, although the mucous membranes of the eyes, mouth, throat, or anus may also become infected following contact with infected semen or vaginal secretions. Some STIs, such as acquired immunodeficiency syndrome (AIDS), involve the entire body.

Types of Sexually Transmitted Infections

There are many different types of STIs. Some of the most common include the following:

■ **Herpes simplex** is a viral infection. There are two forms of herpes simplex. Herpes simplex type 1 causes the common "cold sore" or "fever blister" on the lip. Herpes simplex type 2, or genital herpes, causes painful blisters to form around the vaginal opening and perineum (in females) or the external urinary opening (in males) (Fig. 38-10). There is no cure for genital herpes, and the blisters may return over and over again throughout the lifetime of the person who is infected. Anti-viral medications can be used to decrease the severity of an infection and often delay recurrence.

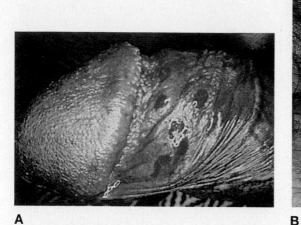

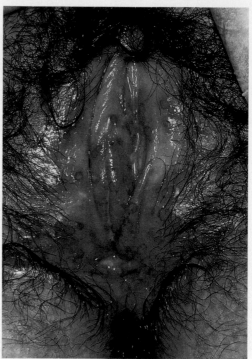

A   **B**

Figure 38-10 Genital herpes is a viral infection that causes blisters to form (**A**) on the penis (in males) and (**B**) on the vulva (in females). There is no cure for genital herpes. The sexual partner of a person with genital herpes is at risk for infection, even when blisters are not seen, if a condom is not used. (A, Used with permission from Goodheart, H. P. [2003]. *Goodheart's photoguide of common skin disorders. Diagnosis and management* [2nd ed., p. 284]. Lippincott Williams & Wilkins.) (B, Reprinted with permission from Beckmann, C. R., & Ling, F. W. [2015]. *Obstetricia y Ginecología* [7th ed.]. Lippincott Williams & Wilkins.)

■ **Gonorrhea** is a bacterial infection. In males, the bacterium that causes gonorrhea infects the urethra. The male may experience a burning sensation during urination and notice a greenish discharge from the urethra, or there may not be any symptoms. Females who are infected with the bacterium that causes gonorrhea also may not have any symptoms. Because the infection may not be detected and treated for some time, the bacterium can travel to the fallopian tubes and into the abdominal cavity, resulting in a condition called **pelvic inflammatory disease (PID)**. PID often results in severe pain and scar tissue that can lead to infertility. If detected, gonorrhea can be treated with antibiotics.

■ **Chlamydia,** the most commonly occurring STI, is caused by a type of bacteria. Like gonorrhea, chlamydia often is not associated with any noticeable symptoms. Chlamydia can cause infertility in both males and females and is treated with an antibiotic.

■ **Genital (venereal) warts** are caused by HPV. In males infected with the virus, small, wart-like growths may occur inside the urethra. In females, the warts may be seen around the vaginal opening, inside the vagina, or on the cervix. Infection with genital warts increases the risk of developing cervical cancer. Treatment may involve removal of the growths with a laser. Cancer of the tonsils and throat may occur in people infected by HPV. A vaccine is available that can help prevent infection from some types of HPV.

■ **Syphilis** is a bacterial infection. The signs and symptoms of syphilis occur in three stages. During the first stage, a painless lesion is seen on the genitals. This lesion heals, and 2 to 4 weeks later, the person develops a skin rash and a fever. This is the second stage. If not detected and treated, the infection becomes latent. This means that the pathogen that is causing the infection is still in the person's body, but it is not active. As many as 20 or more years later, the pathogen can become active again, resulting in the third stage. The third stage usually involves damage to the cardiovascular and nervous systems, which can result in confusion, dementia, and paralysis.

■ **AIDS** is caused by human immunodeficiency virus (HIV). HIV can be transmitted in semen, vaginal secretions, or blood. HIV infection used to be a terminal diagnosis, and many people have died of AIDS. However, thanks to modern treatments, many people infected with HIV will never develop AIDS. AIDS is discussed in detail in Chapter 11.

Prevention of Sexually Transmitted Infections

Although some STIs can be effectively treated and cured with antibiotics, the best treatment still remains prevention. The following methods are useful in the prevention of STIs.

■ When having sexual relations, use a barrier, such as a condom. Condoms help to prevent the transmission of infected secretions from one person to another. Some contraceptive creams, when used with a condom, help to increase the condom's effectiveness against both pregnancy and STIs.

■ If you or your partner has signs or symptoms of an STI, do not have sexual relations until treatment has been sought. Remember that you both must be treated. If you are not both treated, then reinfection can occur. After the course of treatment has been completed, it is important for both you and your partner to return to the health care provider for a follow-up examination to ensure that treatment was successful.

Knowing about STIs can help to keep you safe and healthy. In addition, this knowledge will help you to care for your patients or residents. Even if you work in a health care setting where you care mostly for older people, information about STIs is still useful. Some of the residents of long-term care facilities may continue to be sexually active and can still get an STI if they have relations with an infected partner. Also, symptoms of the third stage of syphilis may not appear until late in a person's life. To provide quality care to the people who depend on you for assistance, you need to be aware of the many different types of disorders that require the services of the health care industry.

SUMMARY

■ Reproduction is the process by which a living thing makes more living things like itself. Although in both males and females the reproductive system produces the cells and hormones that are necessary to create a new life, the organs that make up the reproductive system are very different in males and females.

■ The female reproductive system consists of internal structures (the ovaries, the fallopian tubes, the uterus, and the vagina), external structures (the labia, the clitoris, and the vaginal opening, referred to collectively as the vulva), and the accessory organs (the breasts).

■ The structures of the female reproductive system are capable of producing eggs and hormones, receiving sperm cells, containing and nourishing a developing baby, giving birth, and providing nourishment after the baby's birth by producing breast milk.

■ Each month during a female's reproductive years (from puberty to menopause), the body prepares for possible conception and pregnancy. If pregnancy does not occur, the female has a menstrual period, and the cycle begins again.

■ Aging affects the female reproductive system by causing a decline in the number of follicles that mature, and the amount of hormones produced.

■ Many disorders may affect a female's reproductive system throughout their lifetime, including menstrual disorders, pelvic organ prolapse, cancer, and infections. Female infertility can result from hormonal imbalances or structural abnormalities.

■ The male reproductive system consists of the testicles (testes), the epididymis, the vas deferens, and the penis. Accessory organs include the seminal vesicles and prostate gland, which play a role in producing semen (the fluid that carries sperm cells out of the body). Sperm cells leave the body through the urethra.

■ The structures of the male reproductive system are capable of producing sperm and sex hormones and delivering sperm outside the body.

■ After puberty, the male reproductive system continuously produces sperm cells, which are produced in the testes and mature in the epididymis.

■ As they get older, many males find that the frequency and duration of their erections decrease. Many males also develop enlargement of the prostate gland.

■ Disorders of the male reproductive system include erectile dysfunction, cancer, and infection. Male infertility may result from a lack of functional sperm production.

■ Sexually transmitted infections (STIs) are infections of the reproductive system that are commonly transmitted by sexual contact.

■ Some STIs do not cause signs or symptoms. Because they may not be diagnosed for a long time, the infected person can unknowingly spread the infection to sexual partners. In addition, the untreated infection can damage the passageways that carry the sperm or eggs, causing infertility.

■ Common STIs include herpes simplex, gonorrhea, chlamydia, HPV, syphilis, and HIV.

■ The best treatment for STIs is prevention. The risk of getting an STI can be lowered by using a barrier (such as a condom) when engaging in sexual activity and by avoiding sexual activity with infected partners.

WHAT DID YOU LEARN?

Multiple Choice

Select the single best answer for each of the following questions.

1. What occurs when a male sex cell joins the female sex cell, forming a cell that contains the complete number of chromosomes?
   a. Ovulation
   b. Menstruation
   c. Menopause
   d. Conception (fertilization)

2. Which one of the following is a sexually transmitted infection (STI)?
   a. Breast cancer
   b. Herpes
   c. Hepatitis A
   d. Tuberculosis (TB)

3. Which sexually transmitted infection (STI) is caused by a bacterium and may cause a male to have a burning sensation during urination and a greenish discharge from the urethra?
   a. Gonorrhea
   b. Syphilis
   c. Pelvic inflammatory disease (PID)
   d. HIV

4. Where does conception (fertilization) usually occur?
   a. In the uterus
   b. In the vagina
   c. In the fallopian tube
   d. In the vas deferens

Matching *Match each numbered item with its appropriate lettered description.*

_____ **1.** Sperm

_____ **2.** Estrogen and progesterone

_____ **3.** Amenorrhea

_____ **4.** Egg (ovum)

_____ **5.** Hysterectomy

_____ **6.** Menopause

_____ **7.** Menorrhagia

_____ **8.** Mastectomy

_____ **9.** Erectile dysfunction

_____ **10.** Infertility

a. Surgical removal of the uterus
b. Excessive menstrual bleeding
c. Male sex cell
d. Surgical removal of the breast
e. Female sex hormones
f. Absence of menstruation
g. The complete age-related ending of a female's menstrual cycles
h. Female sex cell
i. Inability to become pregnant or to carry a pregnancy to full term
j. Inability to achieve an erection

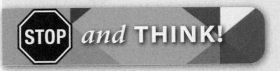

STOP *and* THINK!

You work in a busy health clinic that provides services for people with sexually transmitted infections (STIs). One day, one of your friends confides in you that they are afraid they might have an STI. Based on your knowledge of these infections, what advice can you offer your friend?

Respect

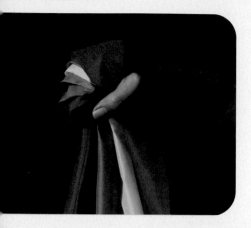

I am a nursing assistant who works in our local community hospital in the Gynecology/Surgical Unit. I also attend classes at the local college, working on my nursing degree. We are learning so much about how to care for different patients and how to be inclusive of all the differences among people in our society. We discuss topics including racial justice, cultural and religious diversity, and human sexuality. Between my classes where I learn so much, and my many friends from diverse racial and cultural backgrounds with different gender identities and sexual orientations, I've been thinking I understand a lot about what makes up a person's identity.

One day at the hospital, we were preparing to receive a patient following a hysterectomy to the unit. As part of the admission process, all patients are asked what their pronouns are, and this is entered on the electronic charting system along with the name they prefer to be called. As I opened the chart in anticipation of my patient's arrival, I was surprised to see that the name was Robert, and his pronouns were he/his. I thought someone must have made an entry error since I didn't think a man could have a hysterectomy.

As I set up the room, the Post-Anesthesia Care Unit nurse brought in our patient and introduced me to Robert, who said he really liked to be called Bob by his friends. As the PACU nurse gave the report to the receiving nurse, I set about trying to make our patient comfortable and welcome. Bob, who was assigned female at birth, is a transgender man; he was in the process of undergoing surgery so that his body's physical appearance and functions aligned with his gender. He had facial hair and a deeper voice from hormone therapy, and the surgical removal of his uterus and ovaries was part of the transition process.

During one of the several conversations that I had with Bob during his recovery, he looked at me and told me that he really appreciated how comfortable I had made him feel. He said that he felt like I just accepted him as Bob, with no judgments. He shared with me that his path in transitioning had been difficult because his religious upbringing didn't approve of LGBTQ+ individuals. However, he said that he was very lucky to have a supportive and loving family who helped him find gender-affirming care and mental health support.

He also said he felt the care he received by the health care team during his procedures was truly gender-affirming. From the medical guidance he received from the physician and nurses, to my warm and friendly welcome at the post-op unit, he felt truly respected for who he is. He wanted all transgender people to experience the same quality of care that honors their right to health and dignity.

I think this was one of the richest learning experiences I have had as a nursing assistant. I learned that people's gender identities don't always correspond to their sex assigned at birth, and respecting this difference is an important part of providing patients with holistic care. This lesson has certainly strengthened my view that respecting each patient as the unique individual they are is one of the greatest contributions nursing assistants can make.

(gnepphoto\Shutterstock.com)

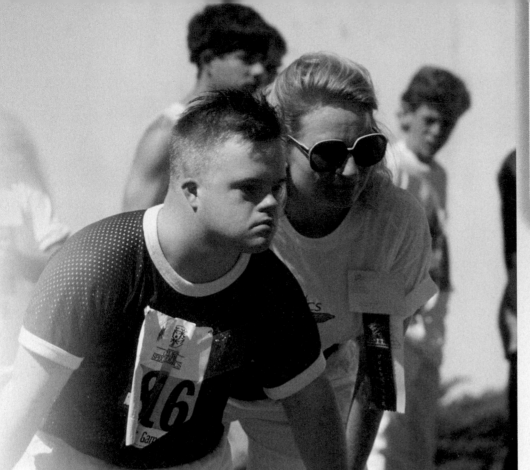

Special Care Concerns

BECAUSE NURSING ASSISTANTS ARE EMPLOYED IN SO MANY DIFFERENT HEALTH CARE settings, you may be involved with the care of patients, residents, or clients who are undergoing rehabilitation or who have developmental disabilities, mental illness, or cancer. Along with the normal assistance needed for feeding, bathing, and toileting, people in these groups have other unique needs. The purpose of this unit is to introduce you to these groups and help you to recognize and assist with meeting their special needs.

Photo: An athlete competes in the Special Olympics. (Joseph Sohm\Shutterstock.com)

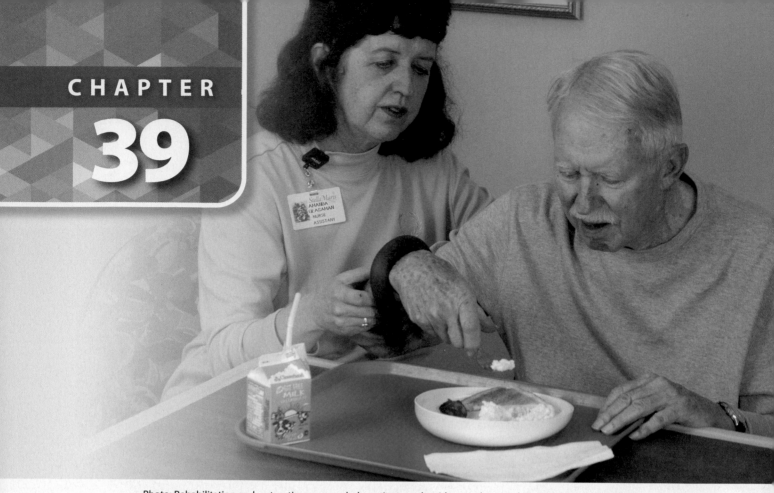

CHAPTER 39

Photo: Rehabilitation and restorative care can help patients and residents to be as independent as possible, for as long as possible. Here, a person uses an assistive device that enables them to eat independently.

Caring for People With Rehabilitation Needs

WHAT WILL YOU LEARN?

The word "rehabilitation" comes from the Latin word *habilitas*, "to make able." As you have learned, many of the patients or residents whom you will care for have some degree of disability or impaired function. As members of the health care team, we are responsible for helping each of our patients or residents reach or maintain their highest level of function. The ability to function is essential for maintaining or regaining independence and for ensuring the best quality of life. Rehabilitation services and restorative care are often needed to help people achieve their goal of reaching or maintaining their highest level of function. When you are finished with this chapter, you will be able to:

1. Define the terms rehabilitation and restorative care.
2. Explain why a person may require rehabilitation services, restorative care, or both.
3. Describe the major goals of rehabilitation and settings where it can take place.
4. List and define the three phases of the rehabilitation process.
5. Describe the responsibilities of key members of the rehabilitation team.

6. **Describe different types of rehabilitation that may be used in a rehabilitation program.**
7. **Identify factors that can affect the outcome of the rehabilitation effort.**
8. **Discuss the nursing assistant's role in rehabilitation and restorative care.**
9. **Describe how the concept of humanistic care applies to rehabilitation and restorative care.**
10. **Identify rehabilitation measures that are commonly used for different body systems.**

Vocabulary

Disability	Restorative care	Assistive devices	Frail
Rehabilitation	Supportive devices	Prosthetic devices	

REHABILITATION AND RESTORATIVE CARE

Many diseases and injuries may leave a person with a disability. The disability can be physical, emotional, or both. Like illnesses, some disabilities are acute whereas others are chronic. Some may be permanent (Fig. 39-1). A person with a disability may need minimal help with activities of daily living (ADLs) or total physical care, depending on how severe the disability is. One of the goals of the health care team is to help patients and residents learn to manage their disabilities and regain as much independence as possible.

Rehabilitation is the process of helping a person with a disability to return to their highest level of physical, emotional, or economic function. Rehabilitation involves treatment, education, and the prevention of

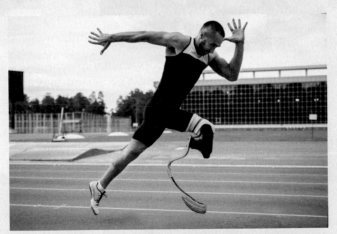

Figure 39-1 This young man has lost a leg, resulting in a permanent disability. However, he has adapted to the loss of the leg and is able to do everything that a person with two legs is able to do. Here, he is shown training to compete in the U.S. Paralympics. (*sportpoint\Shutterstock.com*)

further disability. **Restorative care** is the care provided by all of the members of the health care team that supports the rehabilitation effort and helps the person reach the goal of achieving or maintaining their highest level of function. Restorative care also focuses on helping prevent loss of function and independence, which is especially important for the older person. In most health care settings, the term "rehabilitation" usually refers to services provided by licensed therapists who specialize in various aspects of rehabilitation (such as physical therapists, occupational therapists, and speech–language pathologists), and the term "restorative care" usually refers to the actions taken by the nursing team to support the rehabilitation effort.

There are many reasons that a patient or a resident may need rehabilitation or restorative care. Injuries affecting bones and joints usually require physical therapy to retain function of the joints. In some instances, the therapy will last only for a week or two. In other instances, such as following an older person's hip fracture, the therapy may take much longer. Traumatic injuries that involve the brain and the spinal cord are very likely to cause permanent disability and require long-term, intensive therapy. Medical conditions, such as a heart attack or diabetes, require rehabilitation to help the person maintain strength and learn how to control the condition. Mental illness and substance and alcohol abuse are also disorders that may cause a person to need rehabilitation services.

Injuries sustained by people serving in the military require a combination of rehabilitation services. Missing limbs, head injuries, and the effects of *post-traumatic stress disorder* (discussed in Chapter 41) have placed a new emphasis on rehabilitation. Many of our armed service members receive rehabilitation care in VA care facilities where you may have the opportunity to work.

Settings for Rehabilitation

The rehabilitation effort focuses on the individual needs and capabilities of the patient or the resident. For example, following rehabilitation, some people will be able to leave the health care facility and live completely independently. Others will always be dependent to some degree on others for help with their ADLs, but following rehabilitation, they will be less dependent than they were before.

Rehabilitation services can be provided in a facility devoted exclusively to providing rehabilitation services or in specialized units within a hospital, subacute care facility, or long-term care facility. Some people receive rehabilitation services in their homes. Hospitals may offer a variety of rehabilitation services, from physical therapy to mental counseling. The Omnibus Budget Reconciliation Act (OBRA) requires long-term care facilities to provide rehabilitation services that meet the specific needs of the residents who live in the facility. Specialized rehabilitation centers provide rehabilitation services for people with specific rehabilitation needs. For example, one rehabilitation center may care only for people with brain and spinal cord injuries, and another may specialize in stroke rehabilitation. Burn injuries, acute mental illness, and substance use disorders are examples of other types of conditions a person may receive rehabilitation for in a specialized rehabilitation center.

The rehabilitation process can take varying amounts of time and often occurs in more than one setting. People who are expected to recover fairly quickly (for example, those who have had joint replacement surgery) may begin rehabilitation in the form of physical therapy while they are still in the hospital and may then continue rehabilitation on an outpatient basis. Some people are transferred to a subacute care unit or long-term care facility for additional rehabilitation before going home.

People with illnesses or injuries that are more severe (for example, brain or spinal cord injuries, strokes, myocardial infarction, burns) most likely will need long-term rehabilitation. Rehabilitation will begin in the hospital soon after the person's medical condition has stabilized. The person may then be transferred to a specialized rehabilitation center, a subacute care facility, or a long-term care facility for additional rehabilitation.

Phases of Rehabilitation

Rehabilitation takes place in three phases.

Acute Phase

For the first 24 hours after surgery, an injury, or a serious illness, the person is acutely ill and needs constant observation and care. The health care team's main focus during this phase is to keep the person alive, for example, by assisting with ventilation and helping the heart to function properly.

Subacute Phase

After 24 hours have passed, the person usually enters the subacute phase of rehabilitation. This phase usually lasts about 1 week. However, depending on the situation and the person's condition, active rehabilitation may actually begin right after the initial 24 hours. In the subacute phase, the health care team focuses on stabilizing the person's medical condition and preventing complications associated with immobility (for example, contractures, pressure ulcers, pneumonia, blood clots, bowel and bladder problems) so that the person's best rehabilitation potential is maintained. Proper nutrition, positioning, skin care, range-of-motion exercises, and urinary and bowel care (that is, measures taken to keep the urinary system and bowels functioning properly) are important. You may need to assist the person with eating, hygiene, and grooming tasks. Make sure to explain all procedures to the person and try to understand periods of anger, grief, and frustration. Many patients who have experienced an acute injury or illness are not used to being dependent on someone else for help with their ADLs.

Some patients and residents are able to begin taking fluids and food orally, start passive range-of-motion exercises, and progress to active range-of-motion exercises and ambulation during the subacute phase. Other people may still need ventilator support, intravenous fluids, and enteral feedings during the subacute phase. Many people who will be transferring to a specialized rehabilitation center transfer during the subacute phase.

Chronic Phase

During the chronic phase of rehabilitation, the work of intense rehabilitation begins. The person may still require medical support as they continue to recover from the injury or illness. In addition, the person will begin a rehabilitation and restorative care program designed to meet their special needs. Areas addressed as part of a rehabilitation program might include:

- Restoring or maintaining the person's ability to perform ADLs
- Restoring or maintaining the person's ability to move independently
- Restoring or maintaining the person's ability to communicate
- Restoring or maintaining the person's cognitive skills (such as problem solving, decision making, organizing, or concentrating)

TABLE 39-1 Health Care Workers Who Specialize in Rehabilitation

JOB TITLE	RESPONSIBILITIES
Rehabilitation physician (physiatrist)	• Works with the person's doctor to manage and direct the person's rehabilitation program
Rehabilitation nurse	• Develops a nursing care plan to maximize the person's functioning and quality of life • Provides patient/resident and family education • Helps the person practice skills learned in therapy • Takes measures to prevent complications and monitors for complications
Occupational therapist	• Helps the patient or the resident regain or maintain the ability to perform ADLs (for example, for eating, grooming, walking) • Teaches the person how to use assistive devices to carry out ADLs
Physical therapist	• Helps the person regain or maintain strength, endurance, coordination, posture, and flexibility
Speech–language pathologist (speech therapist)	• Helps the person regain or maintain the ability to communicate with others, chew, and swallow
Rehabilitation aide	• Assists the occupational therapist, physical therapist, and speech therapist with carrying out the rehabilitation program
Orthotist	• Fits the patient or the resident with supportive devices (such as braces or supports) to correct deformity, aid movement, and relieve discomfort
Prosthetist	• Fits the patient or the resident with prosthetic devices (such as an artificial arm or leg)
Neuropsychologist	• Helps the person regain or maintain cognitive skills

- Restoring or maintaining the person's mental health
- Restoring or maintaining the skills the person needs to return to work and achieve financial independence
- Educating the person and family members about the disorder or disability and about ways to prevent future complications

The Rehabilitation Team

The rehabilitation and restorative care program is designed and carried out by a team of health care workers. Just as with any health care team, the patient or the resident is always the focus of the rehabilitation team's efforts, and the goal of the rehabilitation team is to provide holistic care. Many jobs within the health care field have rehabilitation as their specific focus (Table 39-1). In addition to health care workers who specialize in various aspects of rehabilitation and restorative care, the rehabilitation team usually includes other health care team members, such as dieticians, social workers, and psychologists. The members of the rehabilitation team vary according to the patient's or the resident's specific needs.

TYPES OF REHABILITATION

There are many types of rehabilitation, and the one that a person receives depends on their specific disability and individual needs. In many cases, a person may need a combination of different types of rehabilitation. For example, imagine a patient named Mr. Hernandez. Mr. Hernandez was involved in a car accident that killed his wife and resulted in the loss of one of his legs. Mr. Hernandez now needs to learn to walk with a prosthetic leg. He also needs to overcome the emotional crisis associated with the loss of his wife. Depending on what sort of job Mr. Hernandez had before the accident, he may also need to learn new job skills so that he can work again. In this example, learning to walk with the prosthetic leg would be achieved through physical rehabilitation. Overcoming the grief and guilt caused by his wife's death would require emotional rehabilitation. Learning the skills needed to return to work would be achieved through vocational rehabilitation.

Physical Rehabilitation

Helping people to overcome physical disabilities is a common function of most health care facilities.

Physical Therapy

Physical therapy is used to help the person regain or maintain strength, endurance, coordination, balance, posture, and flexibility. Physical therapy is provided by, or under the supervision of, a licensed physical therapist. The primary goals of physical therapy are to improve or maintain a person's ability to move and to prevent complications that can result from the loss of function. These goals are achieved through a program of exercise, often combined with the use of supportive

SUPPORTIVE DEVICES

ASSISTIVE DEVICES

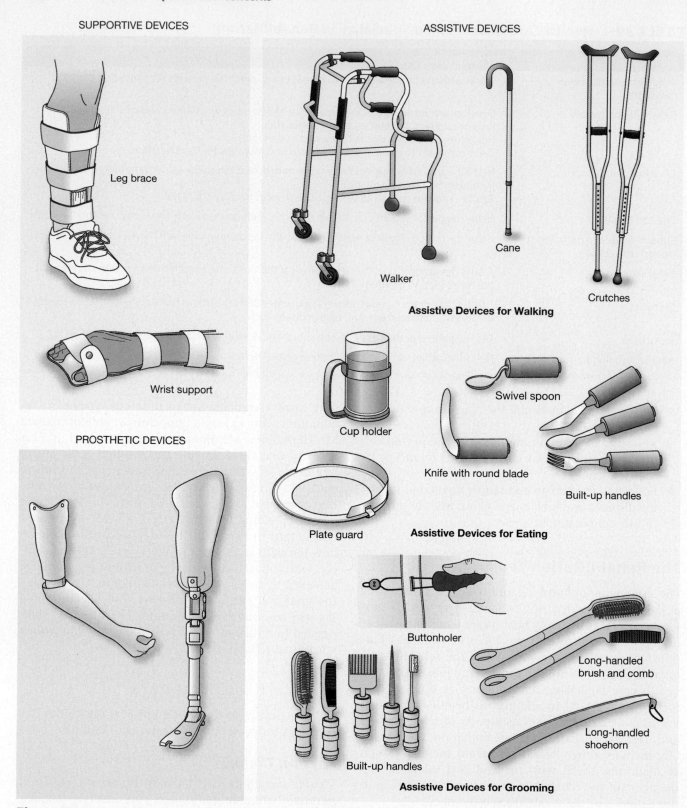

Leg brace

Wrist support

PROSTHETIC DEVICES

Walker

Cane

Crutches

Assistive Devices for Walking

Cup holder

Swivel spoon

Knife with round blade

Built-up handles

Plate guard

Assistive Devices for Eating

Buttonholer

Long-handled brush and comb

Long-handled shoehorn

Built-up handles

Assistive Devices for Grooming

Figure 39-2 Supportive devices, assistive devices, and prosthetic devices can help a person do certain tasks independently.

devices, assistive devices, prosthetic devices, or all three (Fig. 39-2):

- **Supportive devices**, such as splints and braces, help to stabilize a weak joint or limb.
- **Assistive devices** make certain tasks, such as transferring, walking, eating, or dressing easier. You have already learned about many assistive devices in previous chapters.
- **Prosthetic devices** are artificial replacements for legs, feet, arms, or other body parts.

Complications that can result from the loss of function include loss of strength and contractures. When a person does not use a part of the body for a long time, they lose muscle mass in that part. As the muscle mass is lost, so is the person's strength. For example, have you ever had a cast on an arm or a leg for a long period of time? When the cast finally came off, your arm or leg probably looked skinny and felt weak. That was because during the time your arm or leg was in the cast, you were not able to move it, and your muscle mass decreased or atrophied. After a period of being unable to use an arm or a leg, exercising the arm or leg helps to keep it working properly.

Occupational Therapy

Occupational therapy is a health care specialty that focuses on helping the person regain or maintain the skills needed for everyday life, including those related to ADLs. These ADLs include simple activities such as bathing and dressing; instrumental activities such as doing laundry and preparing food; and activities that the person engages in for personal enjoyment, such as a craft or hobby.

While physical therapy focuses on maintaining or improving the skills that involve bigger muscles and bigger movements, occupational therapy focuses more on maintaining or improving the skills that involve smaller muscles and smaller movements (Fig. 39-3). Like physical therapy, occupational therapy uses exercise combined with supportive devices, assistive devices, prosthetic devices, or all three to help the person regain function.

Speech–Language Pathology

Speech–language pathology is a health care specialty that focuses on helping the person regain or maintain the ability to communicate with others, chew, and swallow. Difficulty forming words, speaking, chewing, and swallowing can occur as a result of many different conditions, including disorders that affect the muscles of the mouth and throat (such as stroke), disorders that affect the brain (such as brain injury or dementia), and developmental disorders (such as cerebral palsy). A licensed speech–language pathologist

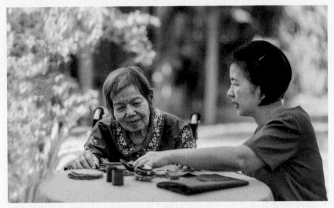

Figure 39-3 Occupational therapy helps a person regain skills needed for everyday life. Here, a patient performs an activity that helps to improve fine motor skills. Fine motor skills are needed for everyday activities such as using eating utensils, using a toothbrush, and writing. (*Toa55\Shutterstock.com*)

(sometimes called a speech therapist) works with the person to improve the person's ability to speak, chew, or swallow (Fig. 39-4).

Emotional Rehabilitation

The stresses that accompany disability can interfere with a person's ability to cope emotionally. Feelings of despair and a loss of self-esteem often accompany conditions that cause a disability. The loss of ability, the loss of a "normal" appearance, the loss of income, and the loss of independence will affect each person differently. You will see some people rally in the face of disability and actually find a new focus for their

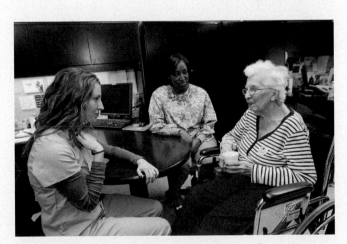

Figure 39-4 Speech–language pathology focuses on helping the person regain or maintain the ability to communicate with others, chew, and swallow. Here, a speech–language pathologist teaches a resident how to do a "chin tuck" when swallowing to help prevent choking.

life, whereas others withdraw emotionally and use the disability as a reason to not try to improve. Some people who have experienced a devastating illness or injury may even talk of suicide. If you think that one of your patients or residents is experiencing emotional distress, report your concerns to the nurse. The nurse will arrange for emotional counseling to help the person overcome their grief and learn to accept and work with their disability.

Vocational Rehabilitation

A *vocation* is a job. The goal of vocational rehabilitation is to return a person to gainful employment. Gainful employment is a job or career that will provide enough income for the person to live, without being dependent on financial assistance to survive. Vocational rehabilitation is used when a person's disability causes them to lose the skills they need to do the job they had prior to the disability. In some cases, the person may just need vocational rehabilitation to relearn the skills they had before. In other cases, the person will need to learn a completely new set of skills that will enable them to get another type of job (Fig. 39-5). Assistance

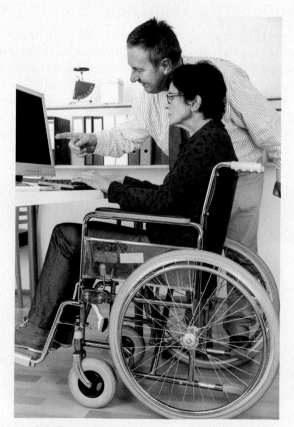

Figure 39-5 Vocational rehabilitation helps a person learn or relearn the skills they will need to return to work. (*Edler von Rabenstein\Shutterstock.com*)

may also be available to help the person locate a new job, new living arrangements, or a new mode of transportation that will allow them to become independent again.

FACTORS AFFECTING THE REHABILITATION EFFORT

Several factors can affect the outcome of the rehabilitation effort:

- **The person's attitude and coping skills.** For a person facing disability, the future can seem very difficult and frightening. The rehabilitation process requires a huge amount of effort and is often painful, and progress might be slow. The way a person responds to the challenges brought on by a disability is very personal and may be influenced by the person's upbringing, culture, values, beliefs, outlook on life, and experiences with life's challenges. A person with a positive attitude and good coping skills is more likely than a person with a negative attitude and poor coping skills to have a positive outcome.

- **The response of family members and caregivers to the person's disability.** Family members and caregivers who are doing everything for a person with a disability can actually do more harm than good. The person begins to believe that they cannot be independent and must rely on others to care for them. However, when family members and caregivers treat the person as a responsible, capable person, they build up the person's self-esteem, promote independence, and assist greatly in the rehabilitation process.

- **The person's overall health status.** In a person with a chronic illness or more than one illness, the rehabilitation process may take longer, and the person is at higher risk for developing complications. For example, chronic conditions that can result in poor blood flow to the tissues (such as diabetes) can increase the person's chances of developing pressure ulcers. Osteoporosis and arthritis may increase a person's risk of falling and fracturing bones. Complications such as these can delay the rehabilitation effort and might make full recovery of function impossible.

- **The person's age.** Normal age-related changes can make the rehabilitation process more difficult for an older person compared with a younger person. As we grow older, we tend to become **frail** (physically weak and fragile). We also have a greater chance of developing one or more chronic illnesses and of experiencing an acute illness or injury. Many older people undergo rehabilitation after an acute illness or injury. Some may begin a rehabilitation program when a combination of factors, such as normal age-related changes and a chronic medical condition, begin to affect the person's ability to perform ADLs and stay safe.

Concerns for Long-Term Care

Frailty is a special concern when caring for older adults. Age-related changes to skeletal muscles, combined with immobility or lack or exercise and poor nutrition, increases an older person's chances of being frail. A frail person usually has unplanned weight loss, walks slowly, is easily fatigued, and generally has a low level of activity. Older people who are frail are more likely to be at high risk for falls, disability, hospitalization, nursing home admission, and death. Rehabilitation and restorative care can help a frail person regain some strength and endurance and lower the risk of falling and other disability.

The Omnibus Budget Reconciliation Act (OBRA) requires nursing homes to provide each resident with the services the resident needs to reach and maintain their highest possible level of well-being and function. There are many specific OBRA requirements related to helping residents maintain or achieve their highest level of function. To be in compliance with OBRA, staff members must take steps to improve or maintain existing function, and to prevent the loss of function.

THE NURSING ASSISTANT'S ROLE IN REHABILITATION AND RESTORATIVE CARE

Nursing assistants play a key role in supporting the rehabilitation effort and providing restorative care. As a nursing assistant, you will be responsible for encouraging your patients and residents to practice the skills and techniques they are learning in rehabilitation. You will also be responsible for carrying out many of the actions specified in the person's care plan related to restorative care. Ask questions about rehabilitation or restorative care measures that have been planned for a person. Have the nurse

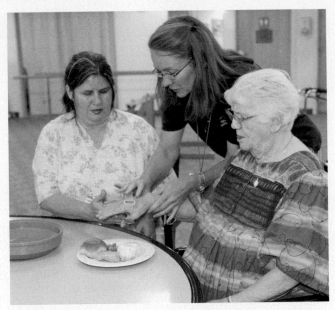

Figure 39-6 Ask the nurse or physical therapist to show you how to use assistive devices. This will allow you to help your patient or resident use the assistive device more effectively. Here, a physical therapist is showing a nursing assistant how to assist a resident with using a wrist supporter with a spoon attached.

or rehabilitation therapist explain how to use any special equipment and show you how to help your patient or resident to use it (Fig. 39-6). Also make an effort to learn about any specific techniques that the person should be practicing. Guidelines for assisting with rehabilitation and restorative care are given in Guidelines Box 39-1.

Because of the unique relationship that develops between nursing assistants and the patients and residents they care for, you will become the "eyes and ears" of the rehabilitation team. You will be able to observe the person for any changes, positive or negative, that are related to rehabilitation or restorative care. Make sure that you report your observations. If a rehabilitation or restorative care measure does not seem to be working for the person, perhaps a change is necessary. Your input can help initiate that change. Your daily care routines will also allow you to observe problems related to rehabilitation and restorative care measures (such as chafing or redness of the skin caused by a new splint or supportive device) that should be reported.

Rehabilitation is a continuous process that will change as the patient's or resident's needs and abilities change. It is always goal directed, with small accomplishments leading to greater ones. Rehabilitation requires active participation by the patient or resident.

Guidelines Box 39-1 Assisting With Rehabilitation and Restorative Care

WHAT YOU DO	WHY YOU DO IT
Ask questions about new rehabilitation measures that have been planned for a patient or a resident. Have the nurse or therapist explain to you how to use new equipment and show you how to help your resident to use it.	Knowing about the special techniques that are being used with the person will allow you to help the person to practice these techniques. Knowing how to use any special equipment will allow you to help the person to use the equipment properly.
Monitor the person's emotional status.	Working to regain or maintain function, or learning to adjust to a loss of function, can be a long, difficult, and painful process. It is very easy for residents to become frustrated and discouraged. Reporting your observations about the person's emotional status to the nurse ensures that steps are taken to get the person the help they need to manage these feelings.
Focus on the person's abilities, and celebrate all successes, no matter how small.	Achieving small goals gives the person an emotional boost and encourages them to keep working.
Encourage and reassure the person, but be realistic in your encouragement and be careful not to compare the person with someone else.	Each person will have individual responses to rehabilitation. Not all goals will be reached.
Give the person the time they need to complete a task independently. Offer assistance only as needed and only if the person seems overly frustrated.	Although it may be faster or easier to just complete the task for the person, it is important for the person's self-esteem to let the person do as much for themselves as possible.
Be empathetic, but do not pity the person.	When you pity someone, it means that you recognize their loss. When you empathize with someone, it means that you can imagine how the person feels about the loss. Empathy will help you deal more effectively with the person's anger and frustration.
If you find yourself feeling frustrated with a patient or a resident who is struggling with rehabilitation, talk to the nurse.	If you let the person's frustration and anger affect you, you may not be able to provide the person with the best care possible. You may need a break or a short reassignment from that person to continue to provide the best care possible.

Helping Hands and a Caring Heart

Focus on Humanistic Health Care

A person who is experiencing disability will have to face many losses. The loss of function, independence, and self-esteem can make the rehabilitation and restorative care effort seem futile. The person will need to grieve for these losses. Think for a moment how a disability might affect you. How would it feel to have to rely on someone else for help performing tasks you used to be able to do for yourself? People who experience disabilities often feel inadequate, helpless, or resentful of other "normal" people, especially at first. The rehabilitation and restorative care effort requires the person to work very hard, and the outcome of all of that hard work is uncertain. The person is likely to have good days and bad days. Be patient and empathetic. Focus on the person's abilities, rather than disabilities. Make an effort to learn what motivates the person—what are their goals and dreams? Offer realistic encouragement and reassurance, and celebrate every success, no matter how small. A holistic approach—considering the person's emotional needs, as well as physical ones—is essential for the rehabilitation and restorative care effort to be successful.

When a patient or a resident is receiving rehabilitation and restorative care, providing emotional and spiritual care is just as important as providing physical care. There are many things you can do to help meet the person's emotional needs. Focus on the person's abilities. Encourage and reassure the person, but remember to be realistic in your encouragement. For example, avoid saying things like, "Keep on working and you'll be back to normal in no time!" if it is unlikely that the person will ever return to the level of function they had before. Instead, say something like, "I am so impressed by your progress. You've gone so much further this week than you did last week!" Allow the person to hope for new treatments or advances in medical technology that can improve their quality of life. Finally, monitor the person's emotional status. Working to regain or maintain function, or learning to adjust to a loss of function, can be a long, difficult, and painful process. If you sense that your patient or resident is becoming depressed, angry, or frustrated, report this to the nurse. The nurse and the other members of the health care team will make sure that the person receives the help they need to work through these feelings.

Tell the Nurse!

When you are caring for a patient or a resident who is receiving rehabilitative therapy or restorative care, be sure to report the following observations to the nurse immediately:

- A supportive device or assistive device is broken or not working properly
- The person has a change in vital signs during or after the rehabilitation or restorative care activity
- The person has pain, swelling, redness, or signs of inflammation around supportive devices or prosthetic devices
- The person is showing signs of depression or excessive frustration, such as crying, withdrawal, anger, or talk of suicide
- The person is having excessive difficulty with a new rehabilitation technique or treatment

SPECIFIC REHABILITATION MEASURES

There are so many different situations that can make rehabilitation and restorative care necessary that it would be impossible to cover them all in this chapter. Some of the more common rehabilitation measures are described here, listed according to the related body system.

Integumentary System

Rehabilitation related to the integumentary system usually includes treatment for chronic wounds such as decubitus ulcers. The nursing assistant will be responsible for assisting with scheduled dressing changes, vacuum-assisted closure (VAC) therapy, and position changes. Burn injuries, depending on the severity, may require months of intensive rehabilitation that includes reconstructive surgery, physical therapy to prevent contractures, and emotional and vocational rehabilitation. Burn rehabilitation usually takes place at a specialized rehabilitation facility.

Musculoskeletal System

Many of your patients or residents will have some type of musculoskeletal disorder that will require rehabilitation and restorative care. Physical therapy is used to regain or maintain function of the joints and muscles and focuses on restoring mobility, flexibility, and balance. Physical therapy is also useful to help control the pain and stiffness that accompanies many musculoskeletal disorders or injuries. Assistive devices are used to help patients and residents ambulate and become more independent. Prosthetic devices will often be used to replace an amputated body part to assist with both function and appearance. Range-of-motion exercises and the use of heat and cold applications are common responsibilities of the nursing assistant.

Cardiovascular System

Cardiac rehabilitation is often necessary for a person who has had a heart attack or has had heart surgery. Cardiac rehabilitation focuses on helping a person regain strength and adopt habits that will help the cardiovascular system become healthier. A person who is in cardiac rehabilitation will begin an exercise program that is designed to strengthen the heart muscle and make it a more effective pump. As the person grows stronger, the therapist will work with the person to develop an exercise plan that will become a part of the person's daily routine. A dietitian will work with the person to teach them about dietary changes that are needed to help control obesity and blood cholesterol levels. Avoidance of unhealthy habits, such as smoking, may require the use of medications and supportive emotional therapy.

Nervous System

For people with neurologic disorders or injuries, rehabilitation is started as soon as possible after the person's medical condition stabilizes. One very important aspect of the rehabilitation effort is the prevention of complications of immobility, such as contractures, muscle atrophy, and pressure ulcers. These complications can lead to failure of the rehabilitation effort and permanent disability. The use of splints, supportive devices, and assistive devices can help prevent complications and promote independence. There are facilities that specialize in providing care and rehabilitation for people who are recovering from a brain or spinal cord injury.

For a person with a neurologic disorder, rehabilitation can be a very long, frustrating experience. Although the brain has an incredible capacity for relearning basic functions, this process can be very slow. Many injuries and disorders that affect the brain and the spinal cord result in permanent disability, leaving the person in need of emotional and vocational rehabilitation, as well as physical rehabilitation.

Endocrine System

The most common disorder affecting the endocrine system that requires rehabilitation is diabetes mellitus (Chapter 35). Education about the disorder and how to use diet management, weight loss, and exercise to control the symptoms make up the rehabilitation plan for diabetes.

Digestive, Urinary, and Reproductive Systems

Rehabilitation for these body systems involves measures such as bowel and bladder training programs (Chapter 25).

Taking It to the Next Level:
Advanced Skills

More in-depth information related to advanced skills used when caring for a person requiring rehabilitation can be found in *Lippincott Acute Care Skills for Advanced Nursing Assistants.*

Visit thePoint® at thepoint.lww.com for access to the ebook.

SUMMARY

- Many patients or residents will have some degree of disability.
  - Disability is impaired function and can be physical, mental, or emotional.
  - Disabilities can be short-term, long-term, or permanent.
- A primary goal of the health care team is to help a person learn to manage their disabilities and regain independence. Rehabilitation and restorative care can help achieve this goal.
  - Rehabilitation is the process of helping a person with a disability to return to their highest level of physical, emotional, or economic function and involves treatment, education, and the prevention of further disability.
  - Restorative care is the care provided by the health care team that supports the rehabilitation effort.
- Rehabilitation and restorative care services can be provided in specialized rehabilitation facilities, hospitals, subacute care facilities, long-term care facilities, and a person's home.

- The rehabilitation process takes place in three phases.
  - During the acute phase, the health care team focuses on keeping the person alive.
  - During the subacute phase, the health care team focuses on stabilizing the person's condition and preventing complications of immobility.
  - During the chronic phase, the health care team focuses on helping the person regain lost function.
- Rehabilitation involves a team working together to address the specific needs of the patient or the resident.
- Many types of rehabilitation are used to help a person with a disability regain function.
  - Physical rehabilitation focuses on regaining physical function and may involve specialized therapists.
    - Physical therapy focuses on helping the person regain or maintain strength, endurance, coordination, balance, posture, and flexibility.

- Occupational therapy focuses on helping the person regain or maintain the skills needed for everyday life, such as those related to self-care.
  - Speech–language pathology focuses on helping the person regain or maintain the ability to communicate with others, chew, and swallow.
- Emotional rehabilitation focuses on helping the person come to terms with the disability and cope with loss.
- Vocational rehabilitation focuses on providing the person with the skills they need to get a job and achieve financial independence.
- Many factors can affect the success of rehabilitation, including the attitude of the person and their family members and caregivers, the person's overall health, and the person's age.
- The nursing assistant plays a very important role in rehabilitation and restorative care.
  - Because of their unique relationship with their patients or residents, the nursing assistant becomes the "eyes and ears" of the rehabilitation team.
  - The nursing assistant is responsible for carrying out many of the actions in the person's care plan related to restorative care.
- Rehabilitation and restorative care is specific to different situations and affected body systems.

WHAT DID YOU LEARN?

Multiple Choice

Select the single best answer for each of the following questions.

1. The process that helps a person with a disability to return to their highest level of physical function and emotional well-being is called:
   a. Homeostasis
   b. Restoration
   c. Prosthetics
   d. Rehabilitation

2. Which of the following is a nursing assistant's responsibility that is related to the rehabilitation and restorative care effort?
   a. Encouraging the resident to use a trapeze to reposition themselves in bed, if this is part of the resident's care plan
   b. Taking the resident to the toilet every hour as part of normal care
   c. Teaching the resident techniques used for swallowing, such as the "chin tuck"
   d. All of the above

3. Someone who is *frail* is:
   a. Injured
   b. Old
   c. Feeble or weak
   d. Confused

4. A person who is having difficulty with balance when walking can benefit from which of the following?
   a. Emotional rehabilitation
   b. Occupational rehabilitation
   c. Physical rehabilitation
   d. Speech–language pathology

5. Mr. Dirkens has a history of stroke. He sometimes has difficulty keeping food in his mouth when chewing because he cannot close his lips all the way on the right side of his face. Which of the following might be of benefit to Mr. Dirkens?
   a. A visit to the dentist
   b. Speech–language pathology
   c. Occupational therapy
   d. Physical therapy

6. Mrs. Chao always liked to play cards. She is frustrated now because she is having difficulty holding her hand of cards. Which of the following statements is true?
   a. Occupational therapy could help Mrs. Chao regain her ability to play cards.
   b. Physical therapy could help Mrs. Chao regain fine motor control in her fingers.
   c. A restorative care program should be initiated to improve Mrs. Chao's card game.
   d. Mrs. Chao will need to find another pastime to enjoy because playing cards will not be possible for her anymore.

7. The rehabilitation process starts as soon as:
   a. The person's insurance approves of it
   b. The person is able to walk
   c. The person is medically stable
   d. The person is emotionally stable

8. The second phase of the rehabilitation process is called the:
a. Chronic phase
b. Subacute phase
c. Active phase
d. Acute phase

9. Devices used to stabilize a weak joint or limb, such as splints and braces, are known as:
a. Prosthetic devices
b. Assistive devices
c. ADL devices
d. Supportive devices

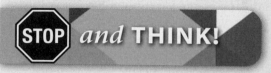

STOP *and* **THINK!**

- Jacob has been assigned to care for Mr. Huff, who has recently had his right leg amputated (removed) above the knee. Jacob is to assist Mr. Huff in his transfers until he is able to do them himself. Mr. Huff is to do all of his own ADLs, such as bathing, feeding, and dressing himself, with minimal help from Jacob. This morning when Jacob enters the room, he finds Mr. Huff on the floor between the bed and the wheelchair. Mr. Huff is struggling to climb into his wheelchair. When Jacob approaches him to help, Mr. Huff says angrily, "Leave me alone; I can do this. I'm OK, just leave me alone." What should Jacob do first? How might Jacob be able to help Mr. Huff maintain his independence and still be safe?

- Brylee is assigned to care for Mrs. Wong, who recently had a stroke. When the stroke occurred, Mrs. Wong had been preparing dinner at the stove. As a result, when she fell, she also suffered severe burns on her arms. Now Mrs. Wong is receiving rehabilitation therapy for her left-sided weakness, in addition to recovering from the skin grafts used to treat the burns on her arms. Mrs. Wong is a widow, and her children live out of state. She cries frequently because she believes there is no one to help her and she will probably end up staying in the nursing home for the rest of her life. Every time Brylee tries to get Mrs. Wong to participate in bathing and feeding herself, Mrs. Wong shakes her head and says, "I just don't feel up to the effort today." Mrs. Wong's grafts are healing well and she is doing great in therapy. Is there anything Brylee can do to help Mrs. Wong not feel so helpless?

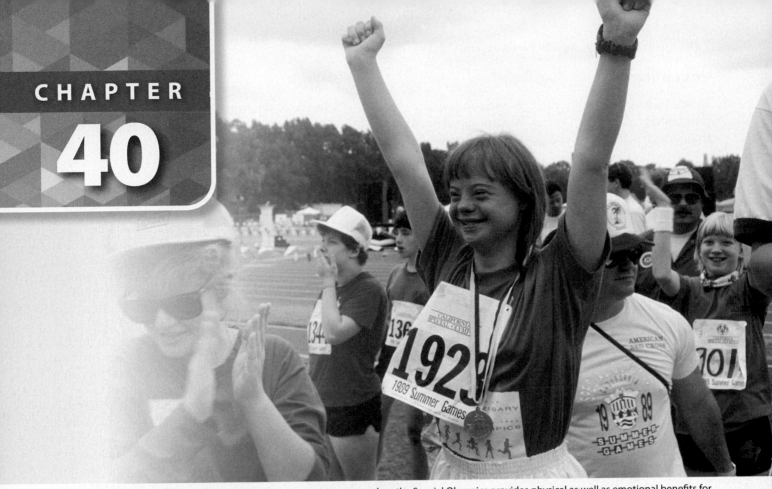

Photo: Participating in events such as the Special Olympics provides physical as well as emotional benefits for people with developmental disabilities. (Joseph Sohm\Shutterstock.com)

Caring for People With Developmental Disabilities

 WHAT WILL YOU LEARN?

In this chapter, you will learn about caring for people with developmental disabilities. Permanent disabilities that affect a person before adulthood are called *developmental disabilities* because they interfere with typical physical or intellectual development. As a nursing assistant, you will be primarily responsible for providing the assistance that people with developmental disabilities need to meet their physical and emotional needs on a daily basis. When you are finished with this chapter, you will be able to:

1. Define the term *developmental disabilities* and discuss various causes.
2. Describe the special needs of people who have developmental disabilities.
3. List common developmental disabilities and describe characteristics of each one.
4. Describe the nursing assistant's role in caring for a person who has a developmental disability.

Vocabulary

Developmental disability
Congenital
Intellectual disability

Down syndrome
Autism spectrum disorder
Cerebral palsy

Fragile X syndrome
Fetal alcohol spectrum
  disorder

Spina bifida
Hydrocephalus

WHAT IS A DEVELOPMENTAL DISABILITY?

A **developmental disability** is a permanent disability that affects a person before they reach adulthood (that is, before 19 to 22 years of age) and interferes with the person's ability to achieve developmental milestones. A developmental disability may be **congenital** (something a child is born with) or acquired (occurring after birth, as a result of trauma or illness). Common causes of developmental disabilities are shown in Box 40-1. A developmental disability may affect intellectual function, physical function, or both. Developmental disabilities vary in severity. Some people who have developmental disabilities are very independent while others require total care.

SPECIAL NEEDS OF PEOPLE WITH DEVELOPMENTAL DISABILITIES

People who have developmental disabilities have the same physical and emotional needs as everyone else, including good nutrition, plenty of exercise, and the sense of well-being that comes from feeling loved and cared for. However, many people with disabilities have additional special needs.

Special Education

Many children with developmental disabilities go to public school alongside friends and classmates who have no disabilities. This is called *mainstreaming.* Mainstreaming benefits children with developmental disabilities by making them feel less isolated. Children with disabilities who are "mainstreamed" often have higher self-esteem and better social skills (Fig. 40-1). Mainstreaming also benefits children who are not disabled by making them aware that people who have disabilities are just like they are, except that they may need extra help to do certain things.

Children who have developmental disabilities may also take part in special educational programs. Special educational programs are focused on the individual's needs and cover a wide range of topics, such as self-care skills (for example, eating or dressing), life skills (for example, counting money), and social skills (for example, understanding appropriate behavior and "limits"). Vocational training focuses on teaching work skills that help people with disabilities become less dependent on others for their care (Fig. 40-2).

Protection of Rights

Government agencies and organizations help protect the rights of people who have developmental disabilities. The Americans with Disabilities Act of 1990 ensures that people who have disabilities are treated

---

Box 40-1 Common Causes of Developmental Disabilities

Congenital (Present at Birth)
Genetic (inherited) disorders
Consumption of alcohol, drugs, or other toxic substances during pregnancy
Infections during pregnancy, such as rubella, Herpes virus, Cytomegalovirus (CMV), or Zika Virus
Poor nutrition during pregnancy
Conditions that deprive the baby of oxygen

Acquired (Occurring After Birth)
Birth trauma
Head injury
Near-drowning
Poisoning

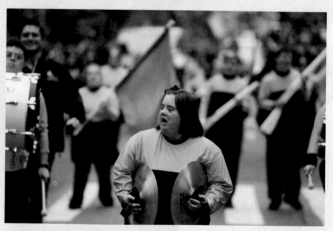

Figure 40-1 "Mainstreaming" benefits everyone. Here, a teenager with Down syndrome participates in marching band at their high school. (*a katz\Shutterstock.com*)

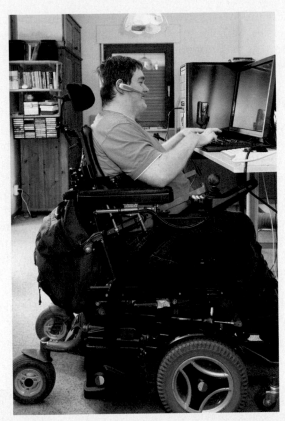

Figure 40-2 Vocational training helps to prepare people with disabilities for the work force. (*belushi\Shutterstock.com*)

the same as those without disabilities by guaranteeing people with disabilities access to public education; employment; and public places such as parks, restaurants, and transportation. The Arc of the United States is an organization that promotes the rights of people with intellectual disabilities, very similar to how the Omnibus Budget Reconciliation Act (OBRA) helps to protect the rights of older people.

Emotional and Social Needs

Reassurance, love, and acceptance are vital for everyone's well-being and especially for those who have disabilities that can make them appear or feel "different." Similarly, all people, even those with disabilities, have the need to interact with other people and participate in activities that they find enjoyable. One notable way in which people who have developmental disabilities can fulfill their emotional and social needs is through events like the Special Olympics. The Special Olympics is a sporting event established to promote the physical and emotional health of people with developmental disabilities. The participants are matched for their competitions according to their level of physical and intellectual ability. The athletes compete against their own personal best performance. The Special Olympics emphasizes the joy that comes with physical activity,

recognizing each athlete as a winner. Participating in events such as the Special Olympics benefits athletes with disabilities emotionally as well as physically.

TYPES OF DEVELOPMENTAL DISABILITIES

There are many different types of developmental disabilities. In general, developmental disabilities affect a person's physical and mental functioning, to different degrees. The following are common developmental disabilities you may encounter in the health care facility where you work.

Intellectual Disabilities

A person with an **intellectual disability** has certain limitations with intellectual functioning and adaptive skills. *Intellectual functioning* is the ability to reason, think, and understand. *Adaptive skills* are skills needed to live and work, such as communication skills, social skills, and self-care skills. A person may be identified as having an intellectual disability if they have an intelligence quotient (IQ) score of less than 70 points and limited adaptive skills in two or more areas.

An intellectual disability can be caused by abnormalities in the brain that are present at birth. It can also be caused by problems that interfere with oxygen getting to the brain before, during, or after birth. The severity of an intellectual disability, like that of other disabilities, varies from mild to profound:

- **Mild intellectual disability.** Most people with an intellectual disability fall into this category. Mild intellectual disability may go unnoticed until a child begins school and starts having trouble with reading or solving math problems. With special education, a person with a mild intellectual disability is usually able to achieve a third- to sixth-grade learning level and master the skills needed for socially appropriate behavior. Vocational (job) training is useful.
- **Moderate intellectual disability.** People with moderate intellectual disability have delays in both motor (manual) skills and speech development. With special education, a person with a moderate intellectual disability is usually able to learn self-care skills, communication skills, and safety habits. However, academically, they will probably not progress beyond a second-grade learning level. The person may also have trouble learning socially appropriate behavior.
- **Severe intellectual disability.** With special education, people with a severe intellectual disability are able to learn some communication

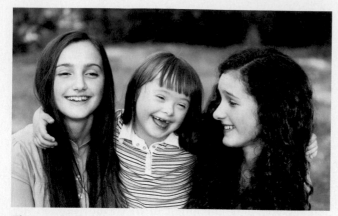

Figure 40-3 One of the great rewards that you will have as a nursing assistant is the satisfaction of helping a person with an intellectual disability to feel loved and allowing them to express love back to you. (*Denis Kuvaev\Shutterstock.com*)

and basic self-care skills, such as how to feed themselves. A person with a severe intellectual disability can usually learn to walk if they do not have other physical disabilities.

■ **Profound intellectual disability.** *Profound* means "deep." People with a profound intellectual disability have minimal function in all developmental areas, physical and mental. These people need complete assistance with their activities of daily living (ADLs) and constant supervision to provide for their safety.

One of the great rewards that you will experience as a nursing assistant is the satisfaction of helping a person with an intellectual disability to feel loved and allowing them to express love back to you (Fig. 40-3). Many people with intellectual disabilities need guidance with "appropriate" methods of displaying their love and affection to other people. In the same manner that a child learns that hugging a kitty too hard will lead to being scratched, people with intellectual disabilities may need gentle reminders that a hug may sometimes be too tight and that not everyone appreciates physical affection.

Adults with intellectual disabilities may function mentally at the level of a 7- or 8-year-old, with child-like curiosity and innocence. However, they are adults and will experience the same hormonal changes and sexual drives as everyone else. Because the person may not understand what is happening, these physical drives may be very confusing. Education and guidance from caregivers is very important to help a person with an intellectual disability learn about appropriate touch and sexual behavior. In addition, caregivers must protect the person from sexual abuse. Because people with an intellectual disability tend to be very trusting, and because they are not always able to understand what is happening to them, they are often targets of sexual abuse. As a nursing assistant, you must be especially observant for signs of sexual abuse when caring for a person with an intellectual disability. Any observations you make or suspicions that you have should be reported to the nurse immediately.

Down Syndrome

Down syndrome is a developmental disability that is the result of a genetic disorder. Typically, each of our body's cells contains 23 pairs of chromosomes, for a total of 46. A person with Down syndrome has one extra chromosome. Down syndrome is the most common chromosome-related disorder, affecting 1 in every 1,000 children born. Although the exact cause of Down syndrome is unknown, studies have shown that babies with Down syndrome are born more often to people who have children later in life.

People with Down syndrome have some degree of intellectual disability and muscle weakness. In addition, they may have certain physical features (Fig. 40-4):

■ Upward slanting eyelids
■ A large tongue and small mouth

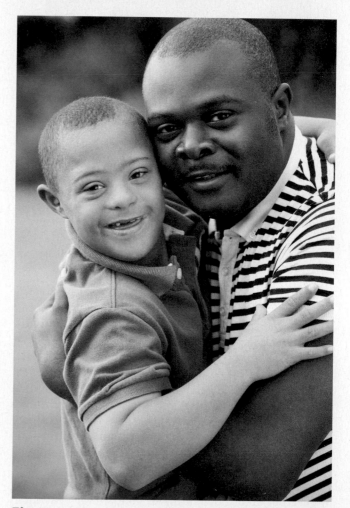

Figure 40-4 Certain physical characteristics are typical of Down syndrome. (*Monkey Business Images\Shutterstock.com*)

- Small hands and short fingers
- A small, wide nose and small ears
- Short stature and a wide, short neck

Some people who have Down syndrome are also born with heart defects that require corrective surgery or medication. Frequent respiratory tract infections are also common among people with Down syndrome, due to muscle weakness (which affects the muscles used for breathing) and a compromised immune system.

Many people with Down syndrome live independently and hold down jobs. Children with Down syndrome are usually raised in their own homes with their families. Once a person with Down syndrome reaches adulthood, the person may continue to live with family members, or they may choose to move to a group home. Group homes allow a person with Down syndrome to live independently within a supervised and supportive environment.

Autism Spectrum Disorder

A person with **autism spectrum disorder** has a condition related to brain development that affects how they understand and socialize with other people. It is called a *spectrum disorder* because there is a wide range of severity. People with autism spectrum disorder usually have difficulty communicating with and relating to other people and surroundings. Although the specific cause of autism spectrum disorder is unknown, experts suspect a genetic link. Like Down syndrome, autism spectrum disorder affects about 1 in every 1,000 children born. Male children are affected more often than female children, with signs of the disorder starting in early childhood, usually between 18 and 24 months of age.

Autism spectrum disorder affects a person's reasoning skills, language skills, ability to socialize, ability to perform self-care activities, and response to touch and pain. A person with autism may seem very withdrawn, like they are in their "own world" (*auto-* means "self"). The person may have lengthy or extreme tantrums or show aggressive or violent behavior that can result in self-injury. Other disorders, such as intellectual disabilities and seizure disorders, may accompany autism. At the same time, some people with autism spectrum disorder possess high levels of intellectual functioning. Therapy focusing on communication and social skills can be very useful for a person with autism spectrum disorder, especially when started at an early age.

Cerebral Palsy

Cerebral palsy is caused by damage to the cerebrum, the part of the brain involved with motor control. Cerebral palsy has many possible causes, including physical brain abnormality and conditions that

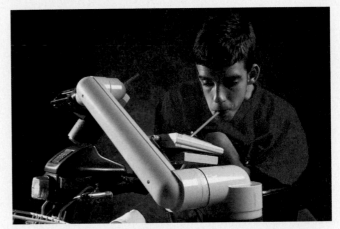

Figure 40-5 Cerebral palsy affects a person's motor function. Here, a child with cerebral palsy is using a pencil held in their mouth to operate a computer. (© *Richard T. Nowitz/Science Source.*)

interfere with the flow of oxygen to the baby's brain before, during, or shortly after birth. Babies who are born prematurely or have a low birth weight are at higher risk for cerebral palsy. Accidents in early childhood can also cause cerebral palsy. For example, head trauma that causes swelling or bleeding in the brain and events that interfere with the flow of oxygen to the brain (such as choking, near-drowning, or poisoning) can all cause this disability. The degree of disability depends on the extent of the damage to the brain.

The cerebrum plays a role in motor activity. This is why cerebral palsy typically affects the person's ability to voluntarily move parts of their body. Cerebral palsy can affect body movements in two different ways. One type of cerebral palsy causes spasms and shortening of the muscles. The affected joints may develop contractures. If the hands and arms are affected, the person may be unable to perform self-care skills such as feeding, bathing, or dressing. If the feet and legs are affected, the person may be unable to walk (Fig. 40-5). The second type of cerebral palsy causes involuntary movements of the arms, legs, and upper body. Facial and tongue muscles may also be involved, making the person frequently move around their lips and tongue. Varying degrees of intellectual disability may also accompany the physical disabilities associated with cerebral palsy.

Fragile X Syndrome

Fragile X syndrome is the most common inherited form of intellectual disability and is caused by a defect in the X chromosome. This defect in the chromosome prevents production of a particular protein needed for cell communication in the brain. Fragile X syndrome is more common and usually more severe in males than in females. People who have fragile X syndrome are usually moderately to severely intellectually disabled and may have physical characteristics such as large ears, a long face, flat feet, and soft skin. They usually have delayed speech and communication skills. They may be hyperactive and experience frequent changes in mood. Autism spectrum disorder may also accompany fragile X syndrome.

Special education helps people with fragile X syndrome learn self-care and behavior skills. A calm, structured environment that keeps distractions and disturbances to a minimum is useful when caring for a person with fragile X syndrome. Unfortunately, because the syndrome has only recently been identified as a developmental disorder, more research is still needed to determine the most effective methods of caring for people with this disability.

Fetal Alcohol Spectrum Disorder

Fetal alcohol spectrum disorder is a combination of physical and intellectual conditions that affect a child who was exposed to alcohol before birth. The degree of disability seems to depend on the amount and frequency of this exposure. Babies born with fetal alcohol spectrum disorder are usually smaller than average and have intellectual disabilities, behavioral problems, learning difficulties, and differences in the development of facial features.

The Arc states that alcohol is the leading preventable cause of intellectual disabilities. Although the disabilities caused by fetal alcohol spectrum disorder are permanent, special education and therapy can help to maximize the person's abilities.

Spina Bifida

Spina bifida is a congenital defect of the spinal column. Typically, the vertebrae enclose the spinal cord, protecting it from harm. In a person with spina bifida, the vertebrae do not close properly during development, leaving the spinal cord exposed. As with other developmental disabilities, spina bifida varies in severity. Some people with spina bifida have only a slight bone deformity that is not visible on the outside of the body, except for possibly a dimple or tuft of hair on the back. Other people have more severe deformities that result in the meninges, the spinal cord, or both bulging through a large opening on the back. In addition, the person may have weakness only in the legs, or they may have total paralysis below the waist (Fig. 40-6). Problems with bowel and bladder control are common. Sometimes, people with spina bifida also have intellectual disabilities.

Hydrocephalus

Hydrocephalus results from a build-up of cerebrospinal fluid (CSF) in the ventricles of the brain. Recall

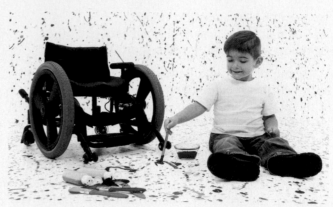

Figure 40-6 Spina bifida occurs when the vertebrae do not close properly during development. People with spina bifida have varying degrees of weakness or paralysis from the waist down, depending on the severity of the defect. (*Duplass\Shutterstock.com*)

from Chapter 33 that the ventricles of the brain constantly produce CSF, which circulates around the brain and spinal cord. Typically, the CSF is reabsorbed into the bloodstream after it circulates through the central nervous system (CNS). In hydrocephalus, either too much CSF is produced, or the CSF cannot drain properly. Eventually, the fluid builds up, placing pressure on the delicate tissues of the brain and putting the person at risk for permanent brain damage.

Many cases of hydrocephalus are congenital. For example, babies with spina bifida often have hydrocephalus as well. When hydrocephalus occurs in a child younger than 2 years, the child's head often enlarges because the bones of the skull have not yet fused together (Fig. 40-7A). Hydrocephalus may also occur later in life, as a result of a tumor, head trauma, or infection. Whether the hydrocephalus is congenital or acquired, it is often treated by surgically inserting a tube (called a *shunt*) that allows the fluid to drain from the brain to another part of the person's body (see Fig. 40-7B).

CARING FOR A PERSON WITH A DEVELOPMENTAL DISABILITY

During your career as a nursing assistant, you may have many opportunities to care for people who have developmental disabilities, in many different types of health care settings:

- **Hospitals.** If you work in a hospital, you may care for a person with a developmental disability while they are undergoing surgery or receiving treatment for an acute health problem, such as a heart problem, a respiratory tract infection, or a nutritional deficiency.
- **Home health care agencies.** Many parents who have children with disabilities choose to raise

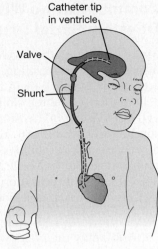

Catheter tip
in ventricle

Valve

Shunt

Figure 40-7 Hydrocephalus results from a build-up of cerebrospinal fluid (CSF). **A.** In children younger than 2 years, the accumulation of cerebrospinal fluid can cause the head to grow larger because the bones of the skull have not yet fused together. **B.** To prevent additional brain damage from occurring, a shunt is inserted to drain the cerebrospinal fluid. (*A, Angela kay Agnew\Shutterstock.com*)

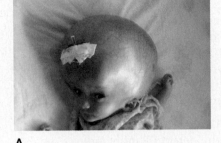

A

B

them at home instead of in a care facility. The parents of a child with severe disabilities may need the assistance of a home health care aide to provide the best care for the child at home.

- **Day care centers.** Some day care centers specialize in the care of people with developmental disabilities. Clients may be children with developmental disabilities or adults with developmental disabilities who live at home with their parents. These facilities provide care for the person while family members go to work. These facilities usually provide educational services and social activities for their clients.

- **Long-term care facilities.** People with developmental disabilities become residents of long-term care facilities for many reasons. A young person may become a resident of a long-term care facility because their disabilities are simply too difficult or too numerous for the family to manage at home. Older people with disabilities often become residents of long-term care facilities because their parents or other caregivers die or become unable to physically care for them.

Concerns for Long-Term Care

Today, because of improvements in medical care and nutrition, people who have developmental disabilities are living much longer than they used to. People with developmental disabilities experience the same changes that occur as a result of aging as everyone else. However, they usually experience these changes earlier, in middle age. In addition, many people with developmental disabilities are at risk for developing certain other health conditions as they age. As a result of these changes, a person with a developmental disability may require more care and assistance as they age. The aging parents

of an adult child with a developmental disability may find it difficult to provide that care for their child due to their own frailty or disability.

Moving to a long-term care facility can be difficult for the person, as well as their family. Having to leave home—where the person felt comfortable and safe—and move into a long-term care facility can be incredibly traumatic for a person with a developmental disability, just as it can be for any other resident. The person may feel angry, deserted, or alone, and will need your compassion and understanding to help become comfortable in their new surroundings.

Family members may have difficulty adjusting as well. A parent may have difficulty trusting the care of their child to someone else. In many cases, the parent has been the child's primary caregiver for the child's entire life. You can imagine how hard it would be to give up that role after 30, 40, or even 50 years! The parents may worry about how to afford their own care, as well as that of their child. In addition, they may worry about paying for the continued care that their child will need after their death.

Helping Hands and a Caring Heart

Focus on Humanistic Health Care

When working with a person who has a developmental disability, the care that you provide must be specific to the person's abilities and disabilities. Learn as much as you can about each person in your care. Focusing on each person's abilities will help you to provide the standard of care that each of your patients or residents needs from you.

Communicating With a Person With a Developmental Disability

Many people with developmental disabilities have difficulty communicating with other people. Some are unable to speak or to learn language skills due to a limitation of motor skills, intellectual functioning, or both. Vision or hearing problems can also make communication difficult. However, many people with developmental disabilities find other ways of communicating. For example, they may rely heavily on nonverbal communication techniques, such as facial expressions, nods, and body language. When caring for a person with a developmental disability:

■ Ask family members what communication techniques work best with the person. Family members are often happy to share with you what they have learned about which communication methods work best.

■ If the person has an intellectual disability, use simple words and short phrases. This allows the person to comprehend ideas or tasks one at a time.

■ Perhaps the most useful communication method is that of a touch, a smile, or a kind word, all of which transmit the message of your care and compassion for the person (Fig. 40-8).

Because many people with severe developmental disabilities have difficulty communicating, they may be unable to tell you if they are experiencing pain or discomfort. Learn to watch for small, subtle changes in your patients or residents, such as changes in behavior, eating habits, or sleeping habits. Changes like these may be a sign that the person is ill. Because you will most likely be the member of the health care team who spends the most time with the person, you will

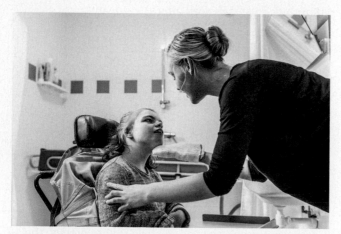

Figure 40-8 Good communication skills are especially important when working with people with developmental disabilities. (*martin bowra\Shutterstock.com*)

likely be the first to notice that "something is not quite right." Always be sure to report your observations to the nurse.

> ### Tell the Nurse!
>
> A person with a developmental disability may not be able to tell you when something is wrong. Use your observation skills and be sure to report any of the following to the nurse immediately:
>
> ● There is a change in the person's vital signs, especially body temperature or pulse rhythm
>
> ● There is a change in the person's appetite
>
> ● There is a change in the person's level of activity
>
> ● There is a change in the person's physical abilities (for example, a person who usually has no trouble walking starts having falls)
>
> ● There is a change in the person's level of intellectual functioning (for example, the person seems confused or disoriented)
>
> ● There is a change in the person's behavior (for example, a normally gentle person becomes aggressive)
>
> ● The person complains of pain or discomfort
>
> ● The person's skin is red or swollen in areas
>
> ● The person shows signs of physical, sexual, or emotional abuse

Meeting the Physical Needs of a Person With a Developmental Disability

A person with a developmental disability has the same physical needs as everyone else. Because of the person's disability, however, they may need some help in meeting those needs. As always, you will need to consider the specific needs of each person. Nursing assistants often are involved with assisting people with disabilities with their ADLs and with activities related to rehabilitation.

Assisting the Person With Activities of Daily Living

Depending on the severity and type of disability, the person may need assistance with ADLs. Some types of disability, such as cerebral palsy, can cause muscle weakness on one or both sides of the body, making dressing and grooming difficult. The short fingers of a person with Down syndrome may make it hard for the person to manage buttons or zippers on clothing. Assistive devices, many of which you have learned about in previous chapters, allow many people with physical disabilities to manage their ADLs independently or with minimal assistance. A person with intellectual disabilities may simply need supervision and reminders (for example, about which step comes next) to complete their ADLs. As with any patient or resident, helping a person achieve the greatest possible level of independence is the best type of assistance that you can give.

Assisting With Rehabilitation

Physical therapy or respiratory therapy may be needed to help the person maintain levels of function or to treat accompanying illnesses. For example, a person who has physical limitations may need assistance with passive range-of-motion exercises to keep the affected parts of their body functional. As a nursing assistant, you may play a very important role in helping the person with physical rehabilitation.

SUMMARY

- Permanent disabilities that affect a person before they become an adult are called *developmental disabilities* because they interfere with that person's physical or intellectual development.
    - Developmental disabilities can be due to congenital abnormalities, traumatic injury, infection, disease, deprivation of oxygen or nutrition, or the result of poisoning or drug use.
    - Developmental disabilities can affect a person physically or intellectually.
    - Special education, assistive devices, and rehabilitation can help a person with a developmental disability maximize their abilities and become more independent.
- Many people with developmental disabilities have special needs.
    - Educational opportunities designed specifically for people with developmental disabilities help teach self-care, communication, and social and vocational skills.
    - Legislation (such as the Americans with Disabilities Act of 1990) and organizations (such as The Arc of the United States) help to protect the rights of people with disabilities.
    - The Special Olympics was established to promote the physical and emotional health of people with developmental disabilities.
- There are many different types of developmental disabilities. The degree to which a person's abilities are affected varies considerably, even among people who have the same type of disability.
    - Intellectual disability affects a person's general intellectual functioning. A person with an intellectual disability has an IQ score of less than 70 and limited adaptive skills in two or more areas.
    - Down syndrome is a developmental disability that results from an extra chromosome. People with Down syndrome have some degree of

intellectual disability as well as certain physical characteristics.
- Autism spectrum disorder is a congenital disorder. People with autism spectrum disorder have difficulty communicating with and relating to other people and their surroundings.
- Cerebral palsy affects the motor region of the brain (the cerebrum) and causes varying degrees of paralysis. Some people with cerebral palsy also have some degree of intellectual disability.
- Fragile X syndrome is an inherited type of intellectual disability that is more common in males.
- Fetal alcohol spectrum disorder is a combination of physical and intellectual abnormalities that affect a child who was exposed to alcohol before birth.
- Spina bifida is a defect of the spinal column that can cause paralysis of the lower extremities.
- Hydrocephalus occurs when the ventricles of the brain produce too much cerebrospinal fluid (CSF), or when the fluid is not able to drain properly. Hydrocephalus can result in brain damage.
- Nursing assistants care for people with developmental disabilities in a variety of health care settings.
    - Because people with developmental disabilities may have trouble communicating with others, nursing assistants often must rely on their observation skills to tell when something is wrong.
    - Nursing assistants often must provide some or complete assistance with activities of daily living (ADLs). However, many people with developmental disabilities are able to manage their ADLs quite independently by using assistive devices.
    - Nursing assistants are often very involved in assisting people with developmental disabilities with tasks related to rehabilitation.

WHAT DID YOU LEARN?

Multiple Choice

Select the single best answer for each of the following questions.

1. Which of the following statements about intellectual disabilities is correct?
   a. It affects the motor region of the brain.
   b. It can occur before, during, or after birth.
   c. It is always severe.
   d. None of the above

2. What physical characteristics might a person with Down syndrome have?
   a. Large ears, a long face, flat feet, and soft skin
   b. Upward slanting eyes, small hands and short fingers, large tongue in a small mouth
   c. A large head
   d. Spinal abnormalities

3. A person with cerebral palsy may have difficulty with:
   a. Muscle control
   b. Social interactions
   c. Hearing and vision problems
   d. Certain heart conditions

4. Cerebral palsy can be caused by:
   a. Infection during pregnancy
   b. A lack of oxygen to the brain
   c. An extra chromosome
   d. Alcohol intake during pregnancy

5. A person with autism spectrum disorder may have:
   a. An extra chromosome
   b. Hearing and vision problems
   c. Problems with social relations
   d. Muscle weakness

6. A person with Down syndrome always has some degree of:
   a. Intellectual disability
   b. Spastic movements
   c. Cerebral palsy
   d. Autism

7. Which one of the following statements about fetal alcohol syndrome is correct?
   a. It occurs when a baby is exposed to cigarette use before birth.
   b. A newborn with fetal alcohol syndrome is larger than average.
   c. It occurs when a baby is exposed to alcohol before birth.
   d. It is caused by oxygen deprivation at birth.

8. What is spina bifida?
   a. A seizure disorder
   b. A defect of the spinal column
   c. A shunt
   d. Another name for fragile X syndrome

9. What is common in a person with spina bifida?
   a. Autism
   b. Bowel and bladder incontinence
   c. Drooling
   d. Seizures

10. Hydrocephalus occurs when:
    a. Cerebrospinal fluid (CSF) collects in the brain
    b. The person has a seizure
    c. A person is born with an extra chromosome
    d. A person has nerve damage

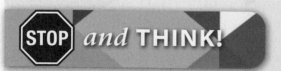

STOP *and* **THINK!**

Today a new resident has been admitted to the long-term care facility where you work. Mr. Siminski has severe cerebral palsy. He is an only child. His parents, who are in their 80s, are experiencing health problems of their own and are no longer able to provide the physical care that Mr. Siminski needs. Mr. Siminski is very upset. He is crying, and he keeps asking why his family doesn't want him anymore. What can you do in the coming days and weeks to help Mr. Siminski make the adjustment to his new home?

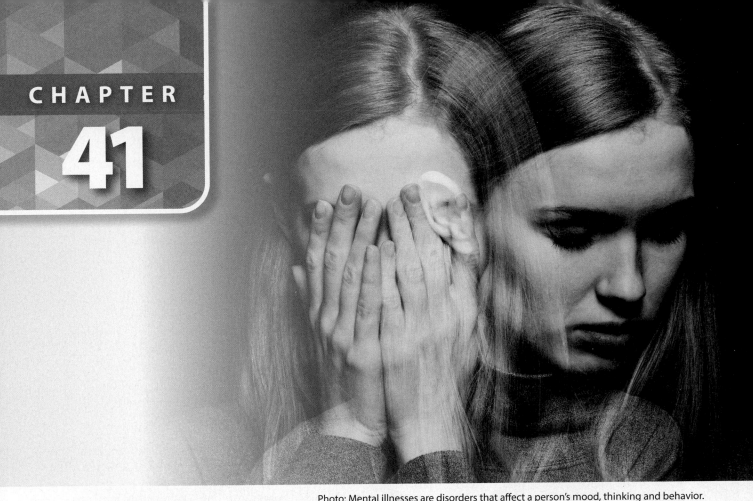

CHAPTER

41

Caring for People With Mental Illness

WHAT WILL YOU LEARN?

A **mental illness,** also known as a *mental health disorder*, refers to a wide range of mental health conditions. These disorders affect a person's mood, thinking, and behavior. (*Mental* means "mind.") In many societies and cultures, mental illness carries a stigma, meaning it is viewed negatively. The behavior of a person with mental illness may be perceived as frightening to those who do not understand it. In addition, movies, television, and books have contributed to many negative and often untrue images of mentally ill people as crazy, violent, and out of control. Although some people who are mentally ill may behave in violent or dangerous ways, most do not. There are many different types of mental illness, and mental illness varies in severity from person to person.

As a nursing assistant, you will care for many people with different types and degrees of mental illness. You may not feel comfortable about the idea of caring for a person with mental illness. Learning about common mental illnesses can help you to overcome this fear. In this chapter, you will learn about several common mental illnesses and how they affect the people who have been diagnosed with them. When you are finished with this chapter, you will be able to:

1. **Define the term *mental illness*.**
2. **Describe some of the qualities that define good mental health.**
3. **Discuss methods that people use to cope effectively with stress.**

745

4. List possible causes of mental illness.

5. Discuss the different treatments that are available for people who have mental health disorders.

6. Describe common mental illnesses that you may encounter in the health care setting.

7. Discuss special concerns related to the health care setting and aging that may affect a person's mental health.

8. Describe the responsibilities of the nursing assistant when caring for patients and residents who have a mental health disorder.

Vocabulary

Mental illness	Suicide	Post-traumatic stress disorder (PTSD)	Hallucinations
Stress	Anxiety	Depression	Substance use disorders
Coping mechanisms	Panic disorder	Bipolar disorder	Addiction
Defense mechanisms	Obsessive–compulsive disorder (OCD)	Schizophrenia	Withdrawal
Psychiatrist		Delusions	Anorexia nervosa
Psychologist	Phobia		Bulimia nervosa

MENTAL HEALTH

To better understand mental illness, it is often useful to start by understanding mental health. Simply put, mental health is the absence of mental illness. One of the main qualities of mental health is a state of emotional balance. In Unit 7, you learned how physical health is related to the body's ability to make adjustments to maintain a state of physical balance, or homeostasis. Similarly, mental health is characterized by a person's ability to make adjustments to maintain a state of emotional balance.

Stress, which can result from any change from the normal routine, affects a person's ability to maintain a state of balance. Changes that affect us physically, such as illness or disability, cause physical stress. Life events, such as getting married, getting divorced, starting a new job, having a baby, or losing a loved one cause a great deal of mental stress. For most of us, stress is a constant in our lives. Even day-to-day activities, such as reading about news and current events, raising children, or performing our jobs, are sources of stress (Fig. 41-1). Stress that is not managed properly can affect a person's physical health as well as their mental health. For example, not being able to manage stress can put a person at risk for cardiovascular problems, such as a heart attack, and digestive disorders, such as ulcers.

Each person has a limit to the amount of stress that they can deal with effectively at any given time. Fatigue, illness, and everyday stress sometimes affect our ability to cope well with change. Many times, stress does not come from a single source. For example,

a person may be able to cope fairly well with one type of stress, such as the loss of a job. But when other stresses, such as a sick child, are added, the person may reach their "breaking point." When this happens, the person may cry, sleep excessively, be unable to sleep, have difficulty concentrating, or feel depressed for a time. Most people with good mental health are able to eventually overcome these feelings and regain their emotional balance. People who are mentally ill cannot cope effectively with stress and may become unable to work, care for their children, make simple decisions, think clearly, or even provide their own self-care. A person with mental illness may need medication, counseling, or support groups to help regain emotional balance.

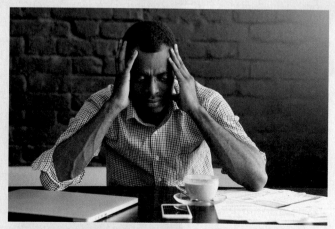

Figure 41-1 Stress is a constant in most people's lives. Work, family, and world events are common sources of stress. (*WAYHOME studio\Shutterstock.com*)

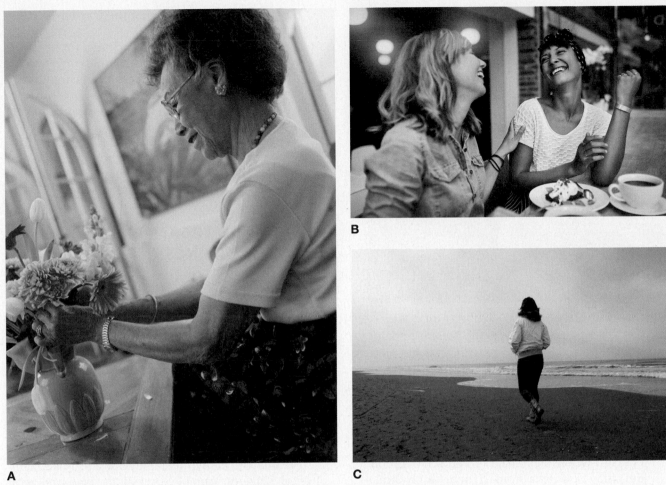

A   **C**

Figure 41-2 Our physical and mental health depend on our ability to manage everyday stress. Enjoying a hobby (**A**), laughing with friends (**B**), and taking a long walk (**C**) are just some of many positive approaches people take to relieve stress! (*B, Flamingo Images\Shutterstock.com; C, Thijs Schouten Fotografie\Shutterstock.com*)

Coping Mechanisms

What do you do when you start to feel overwhelmed or "stressed out"? Maybe you exercise, practice a hobby, get together with friends, meditate or pray, or just find a quiet place to relax (Fig. 41-2). Over time, many people come to know what they can do to make themselves feel better when they start to feel overwhelmed by life's pressures. These conscious and deliberate ways of dealing with stress are called **coping mechanisms**.

Many people rely on positive coping mechanisms, such as those mentioned above. Other people rely on less effective coping mechanisms that might provide short-term relief, such as nail biting, pacing, overeating or not eating enough, smoking, or abusing drugs or alcohol (Fig. 41-3). Initially, these behaviors may help the person to reduce stress. But over time, they place the person at risk for serious physical problems, mental problems, or both.

Defense Mechanisms

As you know, our bodies are "programmed" to try to return to a state of balance. Therefore, when a person is under stress, the mind may try to return the person to a state of emotional balance by using defense mechanisms. **Defense mechanisms** are methods of dealing with stress that "just happen." Usually the person is not even aware they are using them. Defense mechanisms help to protect us from emotionally traumatic events. The behaviors associated with defense mechanisms occur when the mind attempts to restore or maintain emotional balance in response to stress. Common defense mechanisms include the following:

- **Compensation** means to make up for a loss by "filling in" or "substituting" something else. For example, a person who feels lonely may eat too much. This person may be substituting food for affection.

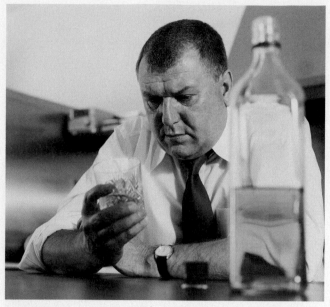

Figure 41-3 Many people drink alcohol excessively, use illegal ("street") drugs, or misuse legally prescribed drugs to deal with stress. This is called substance use disorder. Although substance use disorder may provide short-term relief from the pressures of daily life, in the long run it is not an effective coping mechanism.

- **Conversion** means "to change." For example, a person who is depressed (an emotional problem) may develop a stomach ache (a physical problem), and then use the physical problem as a reason to avoid participating in an activity.
- **Denial** is refusing to believe something that is true, especially if the truth is unpleasant. For example, a person who has been diagnosed with cancer may truly believe that the doctor has made the wrong diagnosis and that they do not have cancer.
- **Displacement** is shifting an emotion from one person to another who is less threatening. For example, a resident who is angry with their daughter for moving them to a long-term care facility—and who is afraid of expressing this anger because they fear the daughter will abandon them—may take their anger out on the nursing assistant instead.
- **Projection** is blaming someone else for your own uncomfortable or unacceptable actions or feelings. For example, a resident may accuse a nursing assistant of breaking a vase when in fact, the resident actually broke the treasured vase themselves.
- **Rationalization** is making excuses or creating acceptable reasons for poor behaviors or actions. For instance, a student who does not study for a test and then fails it may tell themself that

the reason they failed is that the teacher is "too hard."

- **Regression** means to turn back to a former or earlier state. For example, many older children who experience stress as a result of being hospitalized begin demonstrating behaviors from when they were younger, such as thumb-sucking or bed-wetting.
- **Repression (suppression)** is the refusal to remember or think about a frightening or painful memory. A person may repress memories of an automobile accident or childhood abuse.

CAUSES AND TREATMENT OF MENTAL ILLNESS

There are many different types of mental illness and many different causes. Some types of mental illness run in families (that is, they are inherited). Others result from chemical imbalances in the brain. For example, an imbalance in *neurotransmitters* (which you learned about in Chapter 33) can lead to some forms of mental illness. Finally, some mental illnesses may be influenced by a person's environment. For example, a person who is abused by a family member may develop ineffective coping or defense mechanisms that could contribute to a mental disorder.

Fortunately, many mental illnesses, just like many physical illnesses, can be successfully managed with medications, psychiatric counseling, or both. The word *psychiatric* comes from the Greek words *psyche* (the soul) and *iatreia* (healing). A **psychiatrist** is a medical doctor trained in diagnosing and treating mental illness. A psychiatrist is allowed to prescribe medications. A **psychologist**, while not a medical doctor, has education and training that allows them to provide counseling services to help people with mental illness. A psychologist is not allowed to prescribe medications. Depending on the person's situation, they may need the services of a psychiatrist, a psychologist, or both. With treatment, many people with mental illnesses are able to lead happy, productive lives. Because many people with mental illnesses are at risk for dying by **suicide** (taking their own lives, intentionally and voluntarily) or causing harm to other people, diagnosis and treatment of mental illness is very important.

Treatment for mental illness has changed dramatically over the last 50 years, because we know more about why mental illnesses occur and how they should be treated. For example, now that we know that moods and behaviors can be affected by chemical imbalances, we have developed new medications that help to restore the brain's chemical balance. And electroshock therapy, while still used in some cases, is used much more effectively.

TYPES OF MENTAL ILLNESS

Some of the more common mental illnesses include anxiety disorders, mood disorders, schizophrenia, substance use disorders, and eating disorders. In this chapter, you will receive only a brief overview of these disorders. As you care for patients or residents who have been diagnosed with these mental illnesses (or others not discussed here), make an effort to learn more about their disorders. Increasing your knowledge about your patients' or residents' specific disorders allows you to better understand and care for them. It is also important that you understand and remain aware that two people, both with the same type of mental illness, may have very different symptoms and very different methods of coping with their disorder. Do not make the mistake of assuming that every patient or resident with the same diagnosis will behave in the same way.

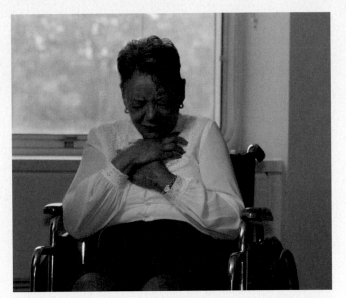

Figure 41-4 People with panic disorder suffer from "panic attacks," which are characterized by feelings of intense fear and anxiety, accompanied by physical signs and symptoms such as chest pain and a rapid heartbeat.

Anxiety Disorders

Anxiety is a feeling of uneasiness, dread, apprehension, or worry. Anxiety is a normal feeling that we have in response to situations that are threatening to our body, lifestyle, values, or loved ones. A certain level of anxiety is normal and may actually lead us to do something positive about a bad or potentially dangerous situation. But too much anxiety or prolonged periods of anxiety can make it hard for us to function or cope with everyday situations. Feelings of anxiety can cause many physical signs and symptoms, such as sleeplessness, restlessness, fatigue, changes in appetite, or increased heart rate and blood pressure. It is also common for an anxious person to be irritable and to have difficulty thinking clearly.

Although we all have periods of increased anxiety, some people have periods of anxiety that continue to build until they can no longer function. Anxiety is a typical symptom in many common mental health disorders. However, in some mental illnesses, overwhelming anxiety is the key feature of the disorder. These mental illnesses are grouped under the general term *anxiety disorders*. Common anxiety disorders include panic disorder, obsessive–compulsive disorder (OCD), phobias, and post-traumatic stress disorder (PTSD).

Panic Disorder

Panic is a sudden, overpowering fright. A person with a **panic disorder** has terrifying episodes or "panic attacks," during which they experience sudden increases in anxiety and feelings of intense fear. A person who is having a "panic attack" usually also has physical signs and symptoms, such as chest

or abdominal pain, a rapid heartbeat, shortness of breath, and dizziness (Fig. 41-4). These symptoms may be similar to those of a heart attack or other severe physical illness. Panic attacks can be brief, or they may last for some time. Some people will experience these attacks rarely while others will have them quite often. It is important to remember that even though the physical symptoms may not be a sign of a serious physical condition, they are no less real and frightening to the person who is experiencing them.

When speaking to a person who is having a panic attack, keep your voice low and calm. Ask the person to take a deep breath, and encourage them to focus on you. Reassure the person that they are safe and that you will help them. Remaining calm and speaking in a reassuring manner help to lower the person's anxiety level.

Obsessive–Compulsive Disorder

Obsessive–compulsive disorder (OCD) is an anxiety disorder that causes a person to experience intense and recurrent unwanted thoughts (*obsessions*). The obsessions are usually associated with rituals that the person cannot control (*compulsions*). The rituals may include actions such as handwashing, counting, or checking and are repeated over and over again in hopes that the obsessive thoughts will go away. Not performing the rituals increases a person's level of anxiety. When it is severe, OCD may cause a person to become unable to perform the tasks that are associated with normal daily activities because of the obsessions and compulsions.

Phobias

A **phobia** is an excessive, abnormal fear of an object or situation. A phobia can be incredibly disabling for the person affected by it. The person will do anything to avoid the thing they are afraid of, to the point where they may be unable to do something as simple as leaving the house. There are three main groups of phobias:

- *Simple phobias* are the most common type. A person with a simple phobia is abnormally afraid of a specific thing (for example, dogs, cats, insects, heights, water, or flying in an airplane).
- *Social phobias* involve a fear of being humiliated or embarrassed in front of other people. Social phobias may be related to feelings of inferiority and low self-esteem and may cause a person to drop out of school, avoid making friends, or remain unemployed.
- *Agoraphobia* is the fear of having a panic attack in a place from which there is no easy escape, or in a place where help is not available. For example, a person may be intensely afraid of having a panic attack in an elevator or on a crowded bus.

Post-Traumatic Stress Disorder

Post-traumatic stress disorder (PTSD) is an anxiety disorder that occurs after a person experiences an overwhelming traumatic event such as combat, natural disaster, serious injury, criminal assault, rape, or death of another person. PTSD can cause a person to have flashbacks (vivid memories of the event), panic attacks, nightmares, depression, and increased anxiety. In some cases, the symptoms can be so severe that the person becomes unable to function on a normal day-to-day basis. Substance use disorder can develop and is relatively common if PTSD is not treated. Medication and counseling are often necessary to help a person return to normal function. The use of *service animals* can help many people who suffer from PTSD remain focused and calm (Fig. 41-5). There are several organizations that train dogs to be companions to people, especially combat veterans, who suffer from the effects of PTSD.

Mood Disorders

Mood disorders affect how a person feels emotionally. Depression and bipolar disorder are two very common types of mood disorder.

Depression

Depression is a feeling of excessive sadness or hopelessness. Many events in life, such as the loss of a loved one, can cause temporary feelings of intense sadness and hopelessness. In a person with good mental

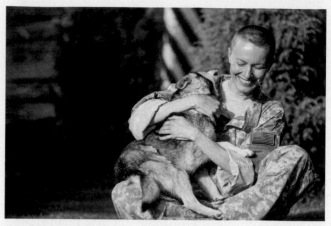

Figure 41-5 Many service animals are trained to help calm people who have PTSD. (*PEPPERSMINT\Shutterstock.com*)

health, the painful emotions of event-related depression decrease over time. Sometimes, short-term treatment with medication or counseling may be needed to help the person through the crisis.

Some people, however, experience intense feelings of sadness and hopelessness that do not decrease with time. These feelings may or may not be brought on by a sad event, such as the death of a loved one. When depression is severe and persistent, it is called *clinical depression*.

Clinical depression is one of the most common mental illnesses. It affects more than 19 million Americans each year. Some research indicates that a family history of clinical depression increases a person's risk of developing this mental illness. Females seem to experience clinical depression about twice as much as males do. Clinical depression is also the most frequently treated mental illness among older people (Fig. 41-6).

Several factors can lead to the development of clinical depression, including:

- Chemical imbalances in the brain
- Low self-esteem and poor coping skills
- Hormonal changes, such as those that affect people during pregnancy, menstruation, childbirth, and menopause
- Medications

A person who is depressed loses interest in activities that they usually find pleasurable or fulfilling, such as eating, working, socializing with friends, and pursuing hobbies. The person may feel sad or anxious and may cry frequently. Many people who are depressed have problems with sleeping. The person may sleep too much, or not enough. The person may be restless or irritable. Instead of being grateful when someone tries to help, the person may become angry and defensive. The person may have feelings of guilt and worthlessness and struggle with thoughts of death

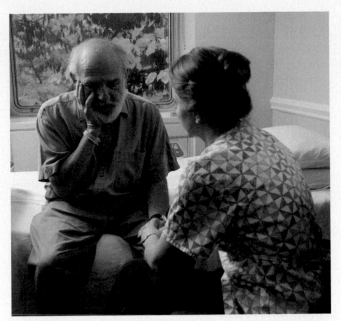

Figure 41-6 Depression is common among older people. If you think that one of your patients or residents is depressed, you should report your observations to the nurse.

or suicide. Physical complaints (for example, of pain or a digestive disorder) are also common among people who are depressed. Prompt treatment is needed to help a person with clinical depression return to an enjoyable, productive life.

The incidence of depression increases with age. Unfortunately, older people are less likely to seek treatment for this disorder. Many older people who are depressed feel that their depression is just part of getting older and must be accepted. If you will be working with older patients or residents, pay attention to changes in their behaviors or moods that may indicate clinical depression. By reporting these observations to the nurse, you play an important role in helping to ensure that the person receives treatment that will help them feel better.

Bipolar Disorder

Bipolar disorder is a mental health disorder that causes mood swings. Periods of excessive happiness and excitement that may cause the person to engage in impulsive or reckless behavior (*mania*) are followed by periods of excessive sadness and hopelessness (*depression*). Experts believe that bipolar disorder is caused by chemical imbalances in the brain that affect a person's moods.

A person with bipolar disorder may have mood swings several times a day, or less frequently, with days or even weeks passing between episodes. Between mood swings, a person with bipolar disorder may have periods of "normal" mood. Bipolar disorder can be difficult to recognize and properly diagnose.

Schizophrenia

Schizophrenia, although not as common as other mental health disorders, is a very disabling form of mental illness. It tends to run in families and may have a genetic basis. Symptoms of schizophrenia usually appear in people between the ages of 16 and 30. Rarely, children may also be diagnosed with schizophrenia. As with other mental illnesses, schizophrenia may be mild or severe. A person with severe schizophrenia that is untreated may be a danger to themselves or to others.

A person with schizophrenia has trouble determining what is real and what is imaginary. They may suffer from **delusions**, or false ideas. For example, the person may believe that they are someone famous or that someone is spying on them or trying to take their belongings. They may also experience **hallucinations**, or episodes where they see, feel, hear, smell, or taste something that does not really exist. For example, the person may hear voices in their head telling them to perform a certain act. The person's thinking and speech become disordered. They may switch from one topic to another during a conversation or may make up new words or patterns of speech. As a result of these symptoms, the person may say or do things that make it hard for them to function in a socially acceptable way in social situations. The behavior of a person who has schizophrenia may be frightening and confusing to others.

Substance Use Disorders and Addiction

Substance use disorders are disorders that involve the excessive or inappropriate use of drugs (prescription or illegal), alcohol, or inhalants. Some people misuse more than one substance. A person with a substance use disorder can develop a physical and emotional dependence on the substance. When this occurs, the person must have the substance in order to function. If they cannot get the substance, they may experience physical symptoms (such as tremors and delirium) and emotional symptoms (such as anxiety). **Addiction** is a physical need for a substance that results in withdrawal signs and symptoms if the substance is withheld. **Withdrawal** is an emotional and physical reaction that occurs when use of the addictive substance is discontinued. Withdrawal signs and symptoms depend on the type of substance that was used and on how frequently and how much the person was using.

Alcohol is the substance most often misused by older people. Many older people are able to hide their substance use, particularly if they are living alone and do not socialize with others on a regular basis. However, admission to a health care facility may trigger withdrawal signs and symptoms when the person no longer has access to the substance.

Patients and residents with substance use disorders may still try to seek out the substance, even after admission to a health care facility. A visitor may bring the desired substance to the person, or the person may seek a staff member's help in obtaining it. You should never agree to these types of requests, and you must report them to the nurse immediately. You should also report any suspicions you may have about a visitor supplying the substance to a patient or a resident. Be alert for signs that suggest that the person is continuing to engage in excessive substance use, such as changes in the person's behavior or mental status, or the smell of alcohol. Reporting your observations is important to help protect the patient or the resident, as well as others in the facility.

Eating Disorders

There are many different types of eating disorders. Two of the most common are anorexia nervosa and bulimia nervosa. No matter what the type, all eating disorders involve serious (and potentially fatal) changes in eating behavior, such as reducing the amount of food eaten to almost nothing, or severe overeating. Eating disorders cause many physical problems, including kidney failure and serious heart problems that can lead to death. Like people with other mental illnesses, people with eating disorders cannot voluntarily control their impulses, and they need treatment to help them recover from the disorder.

Eating disorders usually start during adolescence or early adulthood. Females are at higher risk than males for developing an eating disorder. Many people who suffer from depression or anxiety disorders also suffer from eating disorders.

Anorexia Nervosa

People with **anorexia nervosa** restrict food intake in an effort to lose weight, even though they may be excessively thin (Fig. 41-7). Anorexia (loss of appetite) is a key feature of this disorder. The person simply does not eat enough food. They will skip meals, take tiny portions at meal times, or make excuses for why they cannot eat. They may only allow themselves to eat small amounts of very "safe" low-calorie foods. Many people with anorexia nervosa exercise excessively in addition to severely reducing their food intake.

Bulimia Nervosa

A person with **bulimia nervosa** regularly eats excessive amounts of food (*binging*) and then induces vomiting or uses laxatives to rid the body of the food before it is digested (*purging*). A person with bulimia nervosa often is of average weight for their age and height. However, like a person with anorexia nervosa, a person with bulimia nervosa is extremely focused on their body weight and shape and believes that they are excessively overweight.

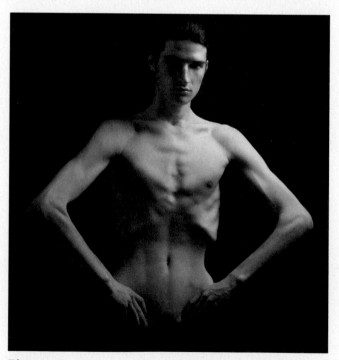

Figure 41-7 A person with anorexia nervosa has an intense and irrational fear of being overweight. Without treatment, many people with anorexia nervosa die. (*Africa Studio \Shutterstock.com*)

Binge-Eating Disorder

A person with a *binge-eating* disorder eats excessive amounts of food, but does not purge as a person with bulimia nervosa does. The need to continue eating is excessive, and the person may develop obesity. Weight-related health disorders, such as cardiovascular disease, diabetes, and hypertension, usually accompany the weight gain.

CARING FOR A PERSON WITH A MENTAL HEALTH DISORDER

You may choose to work in a facility that specializes in the care of people with mental health disorders. Treatment facilities for people with mental health disorders differ in purpose. Some facilities care for people with mental illnesses who cannot function on their own and need assistance with activities of daily living (ADLs) and safety. These facilities provide a form of long-term care specifically for people with mental illnesses. Other facilities specialize in acute care services. These facilities provide care to a person who is experiencing a mental crisis that may result in attempted suicide, drug overdose, or danger to others. After the crisis phase has passed, the person may be able to return home and receive treatment on an outpatient basis. Outpatient mental health clinics see people on a regular basis and offer services such as counseling, medication, and support groups. They may even help the person to obtain education, job training, or employment.

Even if you do not choose to work in a facility that specializes in the care of people with mental illnesses, it is likely that some of the patients or residents at the facility where you work will have or develop mental health disorders. The additional stress of illness or injury that brings a person to a health care facility could become the person's "breaking point," causing a mild mental health disorder to worsen. Remember all the new challenges that your patients or residents face when they enter a health care facility. They may have fears of disability or debilitation from illness or injury. The people you care for have been separated from loved ones and are now in unfamiliar surroundings. A lengthy illness can mean the loss of a job and income. Many people will have worries related to their current and future health. Any of these additional emotional stresses can become a contributing factor of mental illness if a person has poor or ineffective coping mechanisms.

In addition, many of the people cared for in health care facilities are older adults. Approximately 25% of older people in the United States have serious mental health problems. Of this 25%, approximately half are living in long-term care facilities, and approximately 10% have turned to excessive alcohol use as a way of dealing with their stress. Most older people have successfully lived through many struggles and stresses during their lives and have developed excellent abilities to cope. However, some of the unique losses and challenges that an older person faces may overwhelm the person emotionally and promote mental illness (Fig. 41-8). For example:

■ Older people face the loss of spouses, friends, and sometimes even adult children. Often, an older person has to face the death of several loved ones within a short period of time.

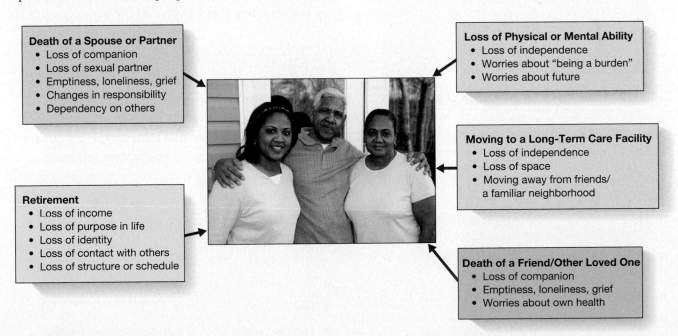

Death of a Spouse or Partner
- Loss of companion
- Loss of sexual partner
- Emptiness, loneliness, grief
- Changes in responsibility
- Dependency on others

Retirement
- Loss of income
- Loss of purpose in life
- Loss of identity
- Loss of contact with others
- Loss of structure or schedule

Loss of Physical or Mental Ability
- Loss of independence
- Worries about "being a burden"
- Worries about future

Moving to a Long-Term Care Facility
- Loss of independence
- Loss of space
- Moving away from friends/a familiar neighborhood

Death of a Friend/Other Loved One
- Loss of companion
- Emptiness, loneliness, grief
- Worries about own health

Figure 41-8 As we age, we face very challenging life events. These additional stresses can put an older person at risk for clinical depression and other mental illnesses. (*Rob Marmion\Shutterstock.com*)

■ Older people face retirement. Although many people view retiring from a job as an event to be celebrated, some people miss the structure, routine, and sense of identity that their jobs gave them. Retirement also means that a person's income becomes fixed, which can lead to money worries.

■ Older people face the loss of physical abilities and independence, either as a result of illness or the normal process of aging. As a result, many older people feel that they are a burden to their families. Others fear the need to move to a long-term care facility because of the associated loss of independence.

Listening and Observing

Listening and observation skills are very important when you care for a person with a mental health disorder. In some cases, your observations may lead to the diagnosis of a mental illness in one of your patients or residents. As noted earlier, the diagnosis and treatment of mental illness is very important. Not only might the person be suffering needlessly, they may be at high risk for dying by suicide. The rate of suicide increases as a person ages and is highest among older white males, especially those who have lost their spouses. Nearly 25% of all people who die by suicide are 65 years of age or older. As a nursing assistant, you may hear a person speak of "ending it all," or the person may wonder aloud "if anyone would miss me if I were gone." Take comments like these seriously and tell the nurse immediately.

Medications called *antipsychotics* are often used for the treatment of certain types of mental health disorders. These medications may make the person dizzy or drowsy and lethargic, putting the person at increased risk for accidents. Prolonged use of some types of antipsychotics can cause problems with movement, such as muscle rigidity or tremors, muscle spasms, or restlessness that results in an inability to keep still. These movement problems also increase the person's risk for accidents. Other types of antipsychotics can increase the person's risk for developing diabetes and high cholesterol, which can lead to significant medical problems. If you are caring for a patient or a resident who is taking an antipsychotic, you will need to be observant for side effects of the medication, as well as for signs that the medication is working (that is, reduced signs and symptoms of the person's mental illness). As a nursing assistant working closely with the person every day, you will be in an ideal position to help the nurse by making and reporting observations.

Patients and residents who have mental disorders that cause them to lose touch with reality (such as schizophrenia) can present a real challenge when providing care. You must understand that what the person thinks they see, hear, or feel is the person's reality. Listen very carefully to what the person is saying, and watch the person's facial expressions and other body language to try to understand what the person is experiencing. Then, respond to the mood or feeling that the person is conveying through their body language and tone of voice. As always, seek help from the nurse or your coworkers if you have difficulty understanding or caring for your patient or resident.

If you work in a facility that specializes in caring for people with mental illness, special methods of recording and reporting may be used. Know what is expected

---

Tell the Nurse!

There are many signs and symptoms of mental illness. Sometimes a physical problem or a medication will make a person show signs of mental illness. As a nursing assistant, you must know what types of behaviors and moods are "normal" for each patient or resident who is in your care. Watch for the subtle signs that something is not quite right and make sure to tell the nurse immediately if you notice any of the following in your patients or residents:

● Changes in appetite, such as eating too much or not eating enough

● Changes in sleep patterns, such as sleeping too much or not being able to sleep

● Restlessness, pacing, or unusual "handling" of objects such as bed linens

● Unusual movements of the mouth or eyes

● An inability to concentrate

● Crying frequently or for long periods of time

● Loss of interest in daily activities that were previously enjoyed

● Loss of interest in socializing with others

● An inability to focus during a conversation or an unwillingness to make conversation

● Unusual mood or behavioral changes

● Fatigue or irritability

● Expressions of feelings of hopelessness or helplessness

● Expressions of a desire to die

of you and how to report and record according to facility policy. When reporting and recording subjective information about patients and residents with mental illnesses, be very careful to use the person's own words, and avoid adding your own opinions or judgments. This is especially important when caring for a person with mental illness because certain phrases or words may have special meaning for the person. To accurately gauge the person's mental status, the health care team will need to know exactly what the person said.

Assisting With Activities of Daily Living

Mental illness may affect a person's ability to eat, sleep, rest, or manage routine grooming and hygiene. People with mental illnesses will need different levels of assistance with their ADLs, depending on the severity of their disorders. As always, help to promote the person's independence by allowing the person to provide as much of their self-care as possible. Because some mental health disorders affect a person's ability to think through the steps of routine care, you may need to gently remind the person of what step comes next. For instance, you may need to say, "OK, you're all dressed now . . . you just need to brush your teeth before we take our walk."

Concerns for Long-Term Care

Sometimes another medical problem can cause a person to appear to be mentally ill. This is especially common in older people. Nervous system disorders, kidney disorders, and the effects of other chronic illnesses such as hypertension and diabetes may cause a person to seem depressed or anxious. The symptoms that accompany hypothyroidism and anemia are often mistaken for clinical depression. Early signs of dementia (see Chapter 9) can also be very similar to some types of mental illness. Infections, dehydration, and the side effects of many medications can also affect an older person's behavior. When you notice a change in a patient's or resident's behavior or mental status and report this change to the nurse, you are taking the first step toward making sure the person gets the help they need. The health care team will work to determine the cause of the person's change in behavior, which will lead to prompt treatment. Never assume that your older patient or resident is just "entering their second childhood" or becoming senile. The person may have a serious mental or physical problem that needs to be treated.

SUMMARY

- One of the main qualities of mental health is a state of emotional balance.
  - Life causes stress, which can threaten our ability to maintain emotional balance.
  - People who are mentally healthy are able to manage stress effectively. People who are mentally ill have trouble coping effectively with stress.
  - Coping mechanisms and defense mechanisms help us to deal with stress.
- A mental illness, also called mental health disorder, is a disorder that affects a person's mood, thinking, and behavior.
  - Mental illnesses may be temporary or permanent, and of varying severity.
  - Mental illnesses may be related to genetics, chemical imbalances in the brain, or a person's environment.
  - Mental illnesses are typically treated using a combination of medication and psychiatric therapy.

- Mental illness places a person at risk for dying by suicide or possibly harming others. Diagnosis and treatment are extremely important.
- Common mental illnesses include anxiety disorders, mood disorders, schizophrenia, substance use disorders, and eating disorders.
  - Anxiety disorders are characterized by overwhelming feelings of uneasiness, dread, apprehension, or worry, and include panic disorder, obsessive–compulsive disorder (OCD), phobias, and post-traumatic stress disorder (PTSD).
  - Mood disorders affect how a person feels emotionally. Depression and bipolar disorder are two common mood disorders.
  - Schizophrenia causes a person to have trouble determining what is real and what is imaginary. The person may have delusions and hallucinations.
  - Substance use disorders involve the excessive or inappropriate use of drugs (legal or illegal),

alcohol, or inhalants. Substance misuse can lead to addiction, a physical need for a substance that results in withdrawal signs and symptoms if it is withheld.

■ Eating disorders such as anorexia nervosa and bulimia nervosa are characterized by serious (and potentially fatal) changes in eating behavior, such as severely restricting food or severely overeating.

■ Nursing assistants care for people with varying degrees of mental illness in all types of health care settings.

■ The additional stress of illness or injury that brings a person to a health care facility may trigger the onset of mental illness or make an existing one worse.

■ The unique losses and challenges that older persons face may trigger a mental illness.

■ By observing and listening, nursing assistants can give the health care team important information about changes in a person's behavior or mood and help ensure prompt treatment.

■ Learning more about specific mental illnesses and caring for people with them enables the nursing assistant to provide better care.

WHAT DID YOU LEARN?

Multiple Choice

Select the single best answer for each of the following questions.

1. Which physical sign or symptom can be caused by anxiety?
a. Sleeplessness
b. Fatigue
c. Increased heart rate and blood pressure
d. All of the above

2. What is depression?
a. An overwhelming feeling of uneasiness, dread, apprehension, or worry
b. An overwhelming feeling of sadness and hopelessness
c. A sudden, overpowering fright
d. Recurrent, unwanted thoughts

3. One of your residents insists that they are the Blessed Virgin Mary. What is your resident experiencing?
a. A manic episode
b. A hallucination
c. A delusion
d. A religious vision

4. You are caring for a resident who has schizophrenia. You know that when you are recording or reporting subjective information about this resident, you should:
a. Report or record what the resident has said, using their own exact words.
b. Report or record your interpretation of what the resident has said, since the resident often says things that do not make much sense.
c. Report or record your own opinion about what the resident has said, in addition

to reporting or recording the subjective information in the resident's own words.
d. Avoid reporting or recording any subjective information about this resident at all.

5. One of your older residents, Mrs. Sigfried, has been acting strangely the last few days. She is refusing to eat, and she insists on sleeping all of the time. Why is it important for you to report your observations to the nurse immediately?
a. Refusing to eat and extreme sleepiness are signs that death is approaching.
b. Mrs. Sigfried's change in behavior could be caused by a physical or mental problem, and sharing your observations with the nurse will help Mrs. Sigfried to get the help she needs, sooner.
c. Mrs. Sigfried is in violation of facility policy.
d. Mrs. Sigfried is a danger to the other residents.

6. One of your residents tells you that they hear voices inside their head telling them to contact aliens on another planet. What is this resident experiencing?
a. Paranoia
b. Hallucinations
c. Delusions
d. Mania

7. Which one of the following is a negative way to manage stress?
a. Drinking alcohol excessively
b. Taking an exercise class
c. Taking a bubble bath
d. Getting together with friends

Matching *Match each numbered item with its appropriate lettered description.*

_____ **1.** Panic disorder

_____ **2.** Phobia

_____ **3.** PTSD

_____ **4.** Obsessive–compulsive disorder

_____ **5.** Schizophrenia

_____ **6.** Bipolar disorder

_____ **7.** Anorexia nervosa

_____ **8.** Bulimia nervosa

_____ **9.** Substance use disorder

a. An eating disorder characterized by eating excessive amounts of food and then vomiting it up or taking laxatives to remove the food from the body before it can be digested

b. An anxiety disorder characterized by an extreme, abnormal fear of an object or situation

c. A mental illness characterized by an inability to tell what is real from what is imaginary

d. An anxiety disorder characterized by recurrent unwanted thoughts and rituals that the person cannot control

e. An anxiety disorder characterized by sudden increases in anxiety, often accompanied by physical signs and symptoms such as a rapid heartbeat and chest pain

f. An eating disorder characterized by an extremely reduced food intake

g. A mental illness characterized by mood swings from extreme highs to extreme lows

h. A disorder that involves the excessive use of drugs, alcohol, or inhalants

i. An anxiety disorder that occurs after a person experiences an overwhelming traumatic event

STOP *and* THINK!

- Think about an older person whom you know well. What major life events have this person experienced in recent years? How did these events affect the person? What coping mechanisms did the person use to deal with the stress caused by these life events?
- You work in a hospital. One patient on your floor is a 36-year-old woman named Evanka who is receiving treatment and evaluation following her second suicide attempt. In your opinion, Evanka has everything anyone could possibly want—a loving husband, two young children, and a comfortable lifestyle. You are finding it hard to understand why Evanka wants to kill herself, and as a result, you are having a hard time feeling empathetic toward her. What are you forgetting?

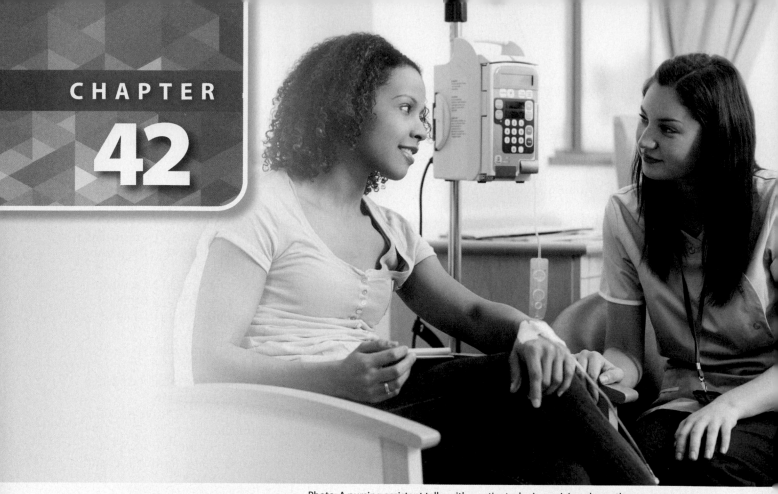

Photo: A nursing assistant talks with a patient who is receiving chemotherapy to treat cancer.
(Monkey Business Images\Shutterstock.com)

Caring for People With Cancer

 WHAT WILL YOU LEARN?

Cancer is the second leading cause of death in the United States. Only heart disease kills more people in this country each year. However, it is important to remember that many people who are diagnosed with cancer survive it, especially when the cancer is diagnosed and treated early. As a nursing assistant, you will play an important role in making sure that changes in a patient or resident that might be early signs of cancer are reported to the nurse promptly. In addition, you will care for people who have already been diagnosed with cancer and are receiving treatment for it, or who are waiting to find out if they have cancer. In this chapter, you will learn more about cancer, how it is diagnosed, and how it is treated. You will also learn about the special physical and emotional needs of people with cancer. When you are finished with this chapter, you will be able to:

1. Describe the difference between benign and malignant tumors.
2. List some common types of cancer.
3. List the common causes of cancer.
4. Describe the warning signs of cancer.
5. Describe how early detection and treatment affects the outcome of a cancer diagnosis.

6. **List and explain the types of treatment used for people with cancer.**

7. **Describe some of the side effects of cancer treatment and how a nursing assistant can help a person to manage them.**

8. **Discuss how cancer affects a person emotionally.**

Vocabulary

Tumor	Metastasis	Radiation therapy
Benign	Biopsy	Stomatitis
Malignant	Chemotherapy	Prognosis

WHAT IS CANCER?

The word *cancer* comes from the Greek word *karkinos*, or "crab." Indeed, cancers are "crab-like," with a central body and arms that reach out into the surrounding tissues (Fig. 42-1). The central body is a mass of abnormal cells, called a tumor. A **tumor** is simply an abnormal growth of tissue. All tumors are not necessarily cancer.

Tumors that are not cancerous are called benign. (*Benign* means "not harmful.") A **benign** tumor is made of abnormal cells that tend to stay together, without spreading into surrounding tissues. In addition, benign tumors tend to grow slowly because their cells do not divide rapidly. Many benign tumors are easily treated, simply by being removed surgically. However, an untreated benign tumor can enlarge and press on vital organs, which can cause serious problems (or even death), depending on the organs that are affected.

Cancerous tumors are called malignant. (*Malignant* means "evil.") A **malignant** tumor is made up of abnormal cells that do not function properly. Malignant cells divide rapidly and invade nearby healthy tissue. A cancer that stays in the organ where it originated is called *localized*. Malignant cells can also travel through the lymphatic system and bloodstream to other parts of the body, where they "take root" and start a new cancerous tumor. The process by which cancer cells spread from their original location in the body to a new location (which may be quite distant from the first) is called **metastasis** (Fig. 42-2). Death from cancer almost always results from metastasis. The cancer simply takes over the body.

Types of Cancer

It is estimated that 200 different types of cancer can affect the human body. All organ systems can be affected by cancer. Some cancers are very rare, while others are quite common. Common cancers that you may have heard of include skin cancer, lung cancer, breast cancer, brain cancer, colon cancer, ovarian cancer, prostate cancer, leukemia, and lymphoma. Cancer can occur at any age, but 67% of cancer deaths occur in people older than 65 years. The most common cancers seen in older people are breast, lung, prostate, and colon cancer.

Causes of Cancer

There has been much research into what causes cancer, and why some people get cancer and others do not. At present, the exact cause of cancer is still unknown. Currently, researchers believe that whether

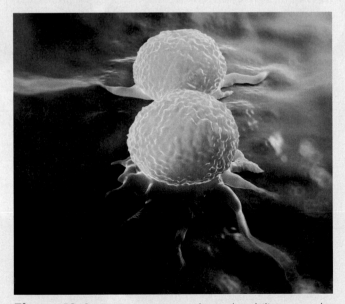

Figure 42-1 Cancerous tumors have the ability to send crab-like arms of cancerous cells into the surrounding tissue. This is an image of a dividing breast cancer cell. (*royaltystockphoto.com\Shutterstock.com*)

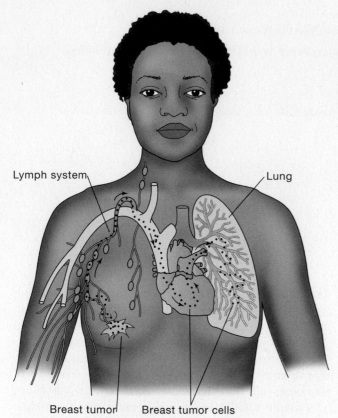

Lymph system

Lung

Breast tumor   Breast tumor cells

Figure 42-2 Metastasis is the process by which malignant cells spread to other parts of the body, or metastasize. A common example of metastasis is when a person with breast cancer also develops lung cancer. First, the malignant cells of the breast tissue gain access to the lymphatic system, which empties into the bloodstream. The malignant cells are pumped, along with the blood, through the right side of the heart. Some of the malignant cells are deposited in the tiny blood vessels in the lungs, where they begin to multiply and grow, forming a new tumor.

or not a person develops cancer may be related to a combination of many factors, including:

- **Inheritance.** Some cancers seem to "run in families." For example, a female with a close female relative who has breast or ovarian cancer is more likely to develop breast or ovarian cancer themselves. This suggests that genetics may play a role in whether or not a person develops cancer.
- **Environmental factors.** What we are exposed to on a daily basis also seems to play a role in the development of cancer. For example, a person who smokes or spends a lot of time around people who smoke is more likely to develop lung cancer than a person who is not exposed to tobacco smoke. Some people work in jobs or live in places that expose them to cancer-causing agents (*carcinogens*), such as radiation, asbestos, chemicals, and pollution.

- **Lifestyle.** Factors such as a person's diet and exercise habits have been shown to play a role in the person's risk for developing cancer. For example, diets that contain lots of fruit and vegetables are known to lower a person's risk for many cancers, while diets that are high in fat increase a person's risk for some cancers. Similarly, exercising on a regular basis can lower a person's risk for developing cancer, while not exercising can increase the person's cancer risk.
- **Age.** According to the National Cancer Institute, age is the single most important risk factor for cancer. Most new cancer cases are diagnosed in older adults, and cancer is the second leading cause of death in people who are 65 years old and older. Unfortunately, because older adults are less likely to receive early detection tests for cancer, their cancer is more likely to be in an advanced stage once it is diagnosed.

The American Cancer Society (ACS) reports that approximately one third of the deaths caused by cancer in the United States are the result of smoking, and another third are related to dietary habits. Eating a healthy diet, exercising, and avoiding smoking and job-related carcinogens are important steps that people can take to lower their risk of developing cancer.

DETECTION OF CANCER

Early detection of cancer can lead to early treatment, which greatly improves a person's chances of surviving the disease. Many cancers are caught in their early stages when a person notices signs and symptoms and reports them to a health care provider. For example, a person may feel an odd lump or notice blood in the stool. Other cancers are caught in their early stages through routine physical examinations and screening tests.

Warning Signs of Cancer

Our bodies are good at letting us know when something is not quite right. A person who has cancer may experience one or more of the following early warning signs. These warning signs can be remembered by thinking of the word *CAUTIONS*:

*C*hange in bowel or bladder habits. A person with colon cancer may have diarrhea or constipation, or may notice that their stool has become smaller in diameter. A person with bladder or kidney cancer may have urinary frequency and urgency.

A sore that does not heal. Small, scaly patches on the skin that bleed or do not heal may be

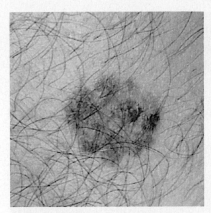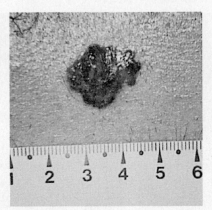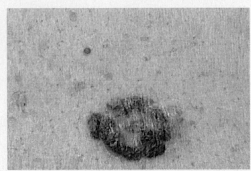

Figure 42-3 Moles that change in appearance or bleed, have jagged borders, display two or more colors (for example, brown, black, pink, gray, or white), or are larger than a pencil eraser may be malignant melanoma. Malignant melanoma is the most lethal type of skin cancer, accounting for 4% of deaths from cancer overall. (Photographs courtesy of Goodheart, H. P. [2003]. *Goodheart's photoguide of common skin disorders: Diagnosis and management* [pp. 325, 354]. Lippincott Williams & Wilkins.)

a sign of skin cancer. A sore in the mouth that does not heal can indicate oral cancer.

- *Unusual bleeding or discharge.* Blood in the stool is often the first sign of colon cancer. Similarly, blood in the urine is usually the first sign of bladder or kidney cancer. Postmenopausal bleeding (bleeding after menopause) may be a sign of uterine cancer.
- *Thickenings or lumps.* Enlargement of the lymph nodes or glands (such as the thyroid gland) can be an early sign of cancer. Breast and testicular cancers may also present as a lump.
- *Indigestion or difficulty in swallowing.* Cancers of the digestive system, including those of the esophagus, stomach, pancreas, and biliary system, may cause indigestion, heartburn, or difficulty swallowing.
- *Obvious change in a wart or mole.* Moles or other skin lesions that change in shape, size, or color should be reported (Fig. 42-3).
- *Nagging or persistent cough or hoarseness.* Cancers of the respiratory tract, including lung cancer and laryngeal cancer, may cause a cough that does not go away or a hoarse (rough) voice.
- *Sudden, unexplained weight loss.* Loss of a significant amount of weight (for example, about 10 pounds) without trying may be an early sign of cancer.

Unfortunately, many people recognize these early warning signs of cancer but put off making an appointment with a health care provider because they are embarrassed or scared. As a nursing assistant, you may be the first to notice that a patient or resident has an early warning sign of cancer. Reporting your concerns to the nurse immediately can lead to early detection and treatment.

Routine Physical Examinations and Screening Tests

Many cancers are detected during routine physical examinations or by screening tests that are done on a regular basis. Examples of screening tests include mammograms (used to detect breast cancer), Pap smears (used to detect cervical cancer), and colonoscopies (used to detect colon cancer). Some cancers are detected by using blood tests. These tests can help to detect cancer long before the person develops noticeable signs or symptoms of the disease. The early detection of cancer allows the tumor to be removed before it has time to spread (metastasize) to nearby tissues or other organs.

If physical examination or screening tests reveal that a person might have cancer, the doctor may order additional studies or exploratory surgery (surgery that is performed when a person is thought to have a significant medical problem but the doctor does not know the extent of the problem or what is causing it). As a nursing assistant, you may need to help prepare a patient or resident for surgery or other diagnostic tests that will be performed to determine if cancer is present. Examples of additional studies that may be ordered for a person who might have cancer include the following (Fig. 42-4):

- **Imaging studies,** such as x-rays, computed tomography (CT) scans, and magnetic resonance imaging (MRI) scans, allow the doctor to see the tumor without actually entering the body (see Fig. 42-4A).
- **Endoscopic studies** involve using a special lighted instrument to look inside the body and obtain tissue or fluids for analysis (see Fig. 42-4B). Examples of endoscopic studies that you read about in Unit 7 include bronchoscopy (when a scope is passed into the lungs through the

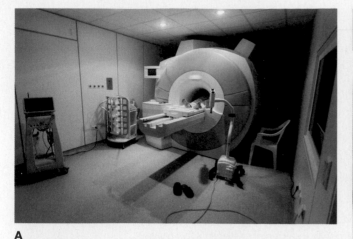

A

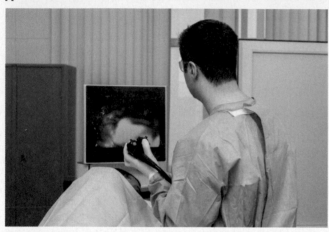

B

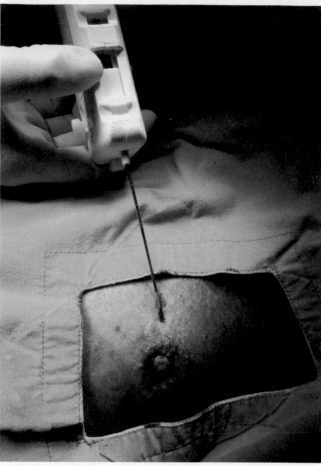

C

Figure 42-4 As a nursing assistant, you may need to help prepare a patient or resident for studies that are done to diagnose cancer. **A.** Radiologic imaging studies, such as magnetic resonance imaging (MRI) scans, allow the doctor to see the tumor without actually entering the person's body. **B.** Endoscopic studies, such as gastroscopy, involve passing a lighted instrument through an opening in the body to view the inside of a structure. **C.** In a needle biopsy, cells are removed from the body so that they can be examined under a microscope for abnormalities. Here, a surgeon is performing a core needle biopsy to check for breast cancer in a patient. (*A, zlikovec\Shutterstock.com; B, Beloborod\ Shutterstock.com; C, Pthawatc\Shutterstock.com*)

mouth), gastroscopy (when a scope is passed into the stomach through the mouth), and colonoscopy (when a scope is passed into the large intestine through the anus).

■ **Biopsy** is the surgical removal of cells or a small piece of tissue for microscopic examination (see Fig. 42-4C). Biopsy is done to determine if cells are cancerous and to determine exactly what type of cancer is present.

TREATMENT OF CANCER

There are three main approaches to treating cancer (Fig. 42-5). The approach used depends on the type of cancer and the extent to which the cancer has spread to other tissues and organs. Treatment methods may be used alone or in combination with each other, depending on the type and extent of the cancer.

■ **Surgery** involves cutting away the tumor and surrounding tissue to remove the cancer and stop the spread of the disease (see Fig. 42-5A). Many cancer surgeries change the person's physical appearance significantly. For example, a person with breast cancer may lose one or both breasts. A person with bone cancer may lose all or part of an arm or leg. A person with colon cancer may need to use an ostomy appliance for the rest of their life. Although it is a relief to have the cancer gone, the person must still deal emotionally with the change in their appearance.

■ **Chemotherapy** involves the use of medications (chemical agents) to destroy the cancer cells (see

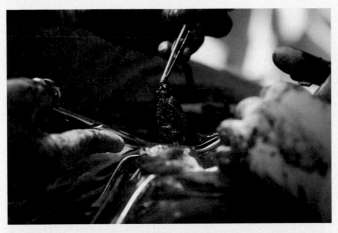

A

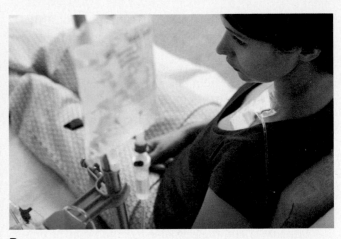

B

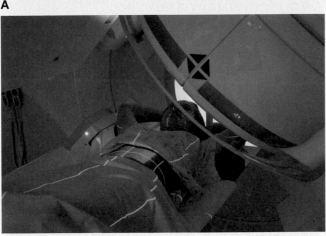

C

Figure 42-5 The three main approaches to treating cancer are (**A**) surgery, (**B**) chemotherapy, and (**C**) radiation therapy. Doctors may choose to use these methods alone or in combination, depending on the type and extent of the cancer. (*A, vz maze\Shutterstock.com; B, Image Point Fr\ Shutterstock.com; C, Mark_Kostich\Shutterstock.com*)

Fig. 42-5B). There are many different chemotherapy drugs available now, each for specific types of cancer. Chemotherapy is often used in combination with surgery to help destroy any malignant cells that the surgery may not have removed completely. Alopecia (the loss of hair) may accompany chemotherapy. Chemotherapy works by killing cells that divide rapidly, such as cancer cells. Unfortunately, some types of normal cells in the body also divide rapidly, such as the cells in the hair follicles. This is why people who are receiving chemotherapy often lose their hair. Many people may be very self-conscious about their hair loss. These people may find that wearing a wig, hat, or scarf helps them to feel more confident about their appearance (Fig. 42-6).

■ **Radiation therapy** involves the use of powerful x-ray beams or implanted radioactive materials to destroy the cancer cells (see Fig. 42-5C). The radiation is directed at the tumor to destroy the cells. Sometimes tiny pellets that contain radiation are placed inside the tumor so that the cells are destroyed from the inside. This is a common method of treating prostate cancer—radioactive pellets are placed inside the prostate

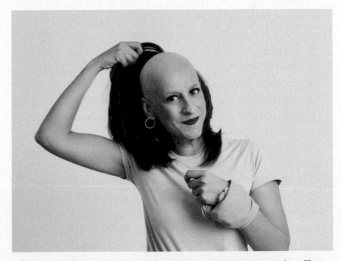

Figure 42-6 Hair loss (alopecia) is a common side effect of cancer chemotherapy. Many people who have lost their hair temporarily as a result of chemotherapy find that wearing a wig, hat, or scarf helps them to feel more confident about their appearance. (*Retamosa\Shutterstock.com*)

gland with a needle-like instrument to destroy the cancerous cells. Patients or residents who have recently received radioactive implants for cancer treatment may be placed under special precautions to help keep visitors and health care workers from being exposed to the low levels of radiation that will be given off for a while. Visitors and health care workers who are pregnant or younger than 18 years should not be in close contact with the patient. Be sure that you have been properly trained according to your facility's policies when caring for a person who is being treated with radioactive implants.

Surgery, chemotherapy, and radiation may be either *curative* or *palliative*. When a treatment is performed with the goal of curing the person of cancer by completely removing or destroying the cancerous cells, the treatment is said to be *curative*. However, sometimes the cancer cannot be cured. When this is the case, the goal of treatment is to make the person as comfortable as possible until death occurs. This sort of treatment is referred to as *palliative* (see Chapter 26). Examples of palliative cancer treatments include surgery to bypass an obstruction caused by a tumor and chemotherapy or radiation to shrink a large tumor that is pressing on an organ and causing pain.

Helping Hands and a Caring Heart

Focus on Humanistic Health Care

A person who has cancer may need to decide among several different treatment options. Sometimes, the person will have to decide whether they even want to go ahead with treatment. Some people may choose to have every type of treatment available. Others may choose to skip treatment, even if it means giving up the chance for longer survival. You must always remember that each patient or resident has the right to choose. The reasons behind treatment choices are unique and specific for each individual person. Although one choice may be right for one person, a different choice will be the right one for another. To truly provide humanistic care to a person with cancer, you must respect the person's decisions concerning treatment. Use your listening skills to show the person that you care. Allow the person to verbalize their fears and feelings without adding your own opinion as to whether you think the person is doing the right thing or not. When you respect the decisions of the people you provide care for and support them emotionally, you demonstrate true compassion and caring.

Biologic Therapy

Biologic therapy is often used in addition to the more conventional types of cancer treatment or for specific types of cancer that do not respond to surgery, chemotherapy, or radiation. Biologic therapy, also called "immunotherapy," involves the use of living organisms (such as bacteria), substances produced by living organisms, or similar substances that can be produced in the laboratory (such as vaccines or antibodies). These substances either treat the cancer or the side effects of other cancer treatments. They can either boost a person's immune system to act against cancer cells or prevent infections from other organisms.

Complementary and Alternative Medicine

Many people who have cancer choose to use *complementary and alternative medicine (CAM) therapies*. Complementary therapies are used with standard treatment, such as chemotherapy and radiation, and include techniques such as special diets, massage and therapeutic touch, acupuncture, special herbs, and meditation. Alternative medicine is used instead of standard treatment and may also include many of the healing approaches used with complementary therapies. Both types of therapy focus on the holistic approach to the person's treatment.

CARING FOR A PERSON WITH CANCER

Many of us know someone who has had cancer. In fact, the experience of losing someone to cancer, or of witnessing someone's recovery from cancer, may be what inspired you to become a nursing assistant in the first place. Like all patients and residents, those with cancer have special physical and emotional needs that must be met.

Meeting the Physical Needs of a Person With Cancer

People with cancer have special physical needs that are directly related to the cancer, the treatment, or both. Cancer can be very painful. The pain may be temporary, related to surgery or radiation treatment. Or it may be chronic, related to the cancer itself. In addition, many of the treatments used for cancer have unpleasant side effects. As a nursing assistant, you will play an important role in helping your patients or residents who have cancer to manage their pain and deal with the unpleasant side effects of treatment.

Managing Pain

Pain control is an essential part of the treatment for a person with cancer. Advanced cancerous tumors often cause severe pain that can only be relieved by the regular use of strong pain medications. Report any observations that suggest that a patient or resident is in pain, or any complaints that the person may have of pain, to a nurse promptly. (See Chapter 21 for a complete discussion of pain and the nursing assistant's role in detecting it and helping to control it.) As a nursing assistant, you will also need to be aware of and look for side effects of pain medication, such as constipation. The discomfort from the constipation alone may be as bad as the tumor pain. Recall what you learned in Chapter 25 about the measures you can take to help prevent your patients or residents from becoming constipated. If one of your patients or residents does become constipated, please report this to the nurse immediately.

Managing Side Effects of Treatment

The treatments used for cancer, especially chemotherapy and radiation therapy, may have severe side effects:

- **Digestive problems.** Nausea, vomiting, anorexia (loss of appetite), and diarrhea are common with chemotherapy and radiation treatments. Patients or residents who are having digestive problems as a result of cancer treatment will appreciate frequent mouth care. In addition, you can offer ice chips to prevent the person from becoming dehydrated. Many people are able to tolerate ice chips when nothing else will stay down. If a person is able to tolerate some foods or liquids and has an appetite for something special, try to accommodate the person's request. Medication may be used to help control the nausea and vomiting.
- **Skin problems.** People who are receiving radiation therapy may develop irritation and burning where the skin is exposed to the treatment rays. Skin breakdown can be prevented with gentle, thorough skin care. Special creams and lotions may be used to help soothe irritated skin.
- **Mouth problems.** People who are having chemotherapy may develop **stomatitis** (inflammation of the mouth). Sores in the mouth may be very painful and cause discomfort during eating. Offering the person drinks that are blended with ice, ice cream, yogurt, and fruit may be very soothing and provide much needed nutrition at the same time. Frequent, gentle oral care is necessary to prevent infection. A special mouthwash or spray may be used to numb the inside of the person's mouth before providing oral care.
- **Fatigue.** People who are receiving cancer treatment may be very tired, all of the time. Mild exercise combined with periods of rest is necessary to maintain muscle strength.

- **Increased risk for infection.** Some cancer treatments temporarily interfere with the body's ability to fight off infections. People who are having these treatments will be at high risk for getting contagious illnesses, such as colds or the flu. In addition, if they do get a cold or the flu, it could turn into something more serious, such as pneumonia. For this reason, you must be very careful to protect patients or residents with lowered immunity from contact with other people who have a contagious illness.

Tell the Nurse!

When caring for a person who has cancer, be sure to report any of the following observations to the nurse immediately:

- The person has severe nausea, vomiting, or both
- The person has pain or sores in the mouth
- The person's skin is red or irritated in areas
- The person has an unusual discharge or bleeding from the vagina, urethra, or rectum
- The person complains of pain or shows body language that suggests they are in pain
- The person has diarrhea or is constipated
- The person has redness, swelling, or pain around an intravenous (IV) or venous access site
- The person has a fever or other signs of infection

Meeting the Emotional Needs of a Person With Cancer

A person who is awaiting test results or who has just been diagnosed with cancer will have many emotional needs. The word *cancer* is very frightening to many people because the disease is so often associated with death. However, a diagnosis of cancer is not necessarily a "death sentence." Many types of cancer can be successfully treated. Still, many people are very anxious about their prognosis, especially right after the cancer is diagnosed. A **prognosis** is the doctor's prediction of the course of a disease, and their estimation of the person's chances of recovering from it.

A person who has cancer may have many other fears as well. For example, the person may fear the side effects of treatment. Or they may worry about how their body will look during treatment or following surgery. The person may be afraid of experiencing a great deal of pain as a result of the cancer or treatment.

The person may worry that even if the cancer is treated successfully now, it may return later in life.

If one of your patients or residents has been diagnosed with cancer, be sure to check in on the person as often as you check in on your other patients or residents. Spend time with the person. Many nursing assistants are uncomfortable with the subject of cancer and as a result may avoid a person with cancer without even being aware that they are doing so. You might be afraid that you "won't know what to say." Remember, caring for a person with cancer does not require you to say anything—the person will be comforted just by the fact that you are there and willing to listen.

Often, people with cancer find comfort in their spiritual beliefs and practices. The person may request visits from religious or spiritual leaders. Time spent praying, reading religious texts, meditating, or listening to spiritual music may be comforting to the person. Provide privacy for the person during these times, and make sure you relay any requests for visits from religious leaders to the nurse so that the appropriate calls can be made according to facility policy.

Concerns for Long-Term Care

Many of your older residents with cancer will receive palliative treatment or no treatment at all. Because of advanced age, a chronic health condition, or both, the person may be too frail to tolerate aggressive treatment of the cancer. For example, a resident with heart disease may not be able to tolerate the recommended chemotherapy because the medications used are potentially toxic to the heart. Another resident may not be able to have surgery because their chronic respiratory disorder makes anesthesia too risky. A resident with dementia may not be able to lie still through radiation treatments. In cases like this, the treatment may be harder on the person than the cancer itself. As a result, the person (or their health care agent) and the doctor may agree not to screen for common cancers (or not to do further testing for cancer even if the person has symptoms that suggest cancer). Instead, palliative care is provided to minimize symptoms and keep the person as comfortable as possible.

SUMMARY

- A tumor, or mass of abnormal cells, may be *malignant* or *benign*. The cells that make up malignant tumors divide rapidly and spread into nearby tissues. They can also enter the lymphatic system and bloodstream and spread to distant organs, a process called *metastasis*.

- Early detection of cancer can lead to early treatment, which greatly improves a person's chances of surviving the disease.

  - The nature of your duties as a nursing assistant will put you in an ideal position to observe changes in a patient or resident that may be early warning signs of cancer.

  - Many cancers are detected at an early stage through routine physical examinations or screening tests. If the doctor suspects cancer, they may recommend follow-up tests (such as radiologic studies, endoscopic studies, or biopsy).

- The three main approaches to treating cancer are surgery, chemotherapy, and radiation therapy.

  - These approaches may be used alone or in combination, depending on the type of cancer and whether it has spread.

  - Treatment may be curative or palliative. The goal of curative treatment is to rid the body of

the disease. The goal of palliative treatment is to keep the person comfortable when the disease cannot be cured.

- Cancer treatment can be associated with unpleasant side effects, including hair loss, nausea, vomiting, diarrhea, loss of appetite, mouth sores, skin breakdown, lowered immunity, and fatigue.

- A person with cancer often faces many treatment choices, including the choice of not having treatment at all.

- An older person may not be a good candidate for cancer treatment because of advanced age, the effects of chronic disease, or both.

- A patient or resident with cancer requires humanistic care, just as any other patient or resident does.

  - A person with cancer has many physical needs that are directly related to the cancer or to its treatment. Nursing assistants play an important role in helping the person with cancer to manage pain and deal with unpleasant side effects of cancer therapy.

  - A person with cancer will need assistance to meet emotional and spiritual needs as well.

WHAT DID YOU LEARN?

Multiple Choice

Select the single best answer for each of the following questions.

1. Which one of the following statements best describes a malignant tumor?
   a. It consists of abnormal cells that divide rapidly and are capable of spreading to nearby tissues and distant organs.
   b. It consists of abnormal cells that divide slowly and tend to stay together.
   c. All tumors are malignant.
   d. All malignant tumors are fatal.

2. Which of the following factors may play a role in whether or not a person develops cancer?
   a. Inheritance (genes)
   b. Lifestyle factors, such as diet and exercise
   c. Environment
   d. All of the above

3. Mrs. Worthington is receiving chemotherapy following surgery to remove a malignant tumor. Following each treatment, she is nauseous, and often she vomits. What could you do to help Mrs. Worthington feel better?
   a. Offer her strong pain medications
   b. Offer her ice chips, and report her nausea to the nurse
   c. Enter her room only when necessary to avoid disturbing her
   d. Serve her meal tray as usual, in hopes that the smell of the food will increase her appetite

Matching   *Match each numbered item with its appropriate lettered description.*

_____ **1.** Alopecia

_____ **2.** Stomatitis

_____ **3.** Biopsy

_____ **4.** Metastasis

_____ **5.** Palliative

_____ **6.** Tumor

_____ **7.** Prognosis

a. Surgical removal of cells or tissue for examination under a microscope
b. Treatment done with the goal of reducing pain and discomfort, not curing the disease
c. Loss of hair
d. The doctor's prediction of the course of a person's disease and the person's chance of recovering from it
e. Inflammation of the mouth
f. The spread of malignant cells to other parts of the body
g. Abnormal growth of tissue

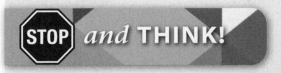

You are caring for Mr. Bengali, a resident who was recently diagnosed with cancer. The doctors have presented Mr. Bengali and his family with a number of different treatment options, and for the last few days, Mr. Bengali has been weighing the pros and cons of each. In addition, he is still trying to adjust to the diagnosis he has just been given, and what it means for his future. One morning, while you are making Mr. Bengali's bed, he starts to talk to you about his father, who died of cancer after going through several months of agonizing treatments. He tells you that he is scared that he, too, will go through the treatments and in the end, all of his suffering might be for nothing. "Maybe it would just be easier to give up now and die peacefully," he says. How would you react to what Mr. Bengali is telling you? Is there anything you can do or say that might help Mr. Bengali with the difficult choices he needs to make?

Respect

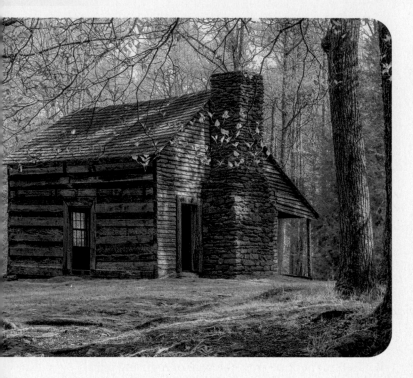

I am a nursing assistant who has been working in a long-term care facility in Eastern Tennessee for about 10 years. The majority of our residents have lived in this part of the country for all of their lives. I really enjoy getting to know each of them and hearing about their lives.

One of our residents, Mrs. Clemens, has quite an interesting and long life full of lessons. She was a high school science teacher for many years. Apparently, she inspired many students to go on to college and become nurses, doctors, and scientists. One day, I started asking her about her students and what she loved about teaching them. Her answer surprised me.

She said that she loved science and how it could be used to prove theories and ideas, but what she really loved was nature. She said that she always introduced her students to a series of books known as *The Foxfire Books*. These books were about the ways of the people who had first settled in Appalachia, in this part of the country. The books covered everything about the lives of the people: how they hunted and cooked, how they farmed, how they made wine, and especially how they practiced "healing."

Healing practices in those early days in Appalachia were very different from modern medicine. People generally relied on herbs from surrounding forests and remedies that had been handed down through the generations. Mrs. Clemens said that people used willow bark tea to treat pain and fever and that it naturally contains the ingredient now found in aspirin. She told me that a plant called foxglove could be used for heart problems because it contains digitalis. She said that faith healing was also a common practice in those times.

Mrs. Clemens said that her purpose in exposing her students to this local history of medicine was to help them realize that "doctoring folks" was not just about modern medications and technology, but it had so much to do with what folks believed would heal them. She said that to be an effective healer, a person had to learn to listen to their patients and ask them what they thought would help them get well. Then perhaps, the modern healer would add a little of their modern medicine to what the person was already doing.

I think that Mrs. Clemens taught me the most important lessons about caring for people in the health care setting during those conversations. Of course, I had to read *The Firefox Books* for myself and learn about the histories of the residents in our facility! Now that I am back in college with the goal of becoming a family doctor, I know that I will always hear Mrs. Clemens' voice telling me to remember how to "doctor folks." You have to be able to respect different ways of healing.

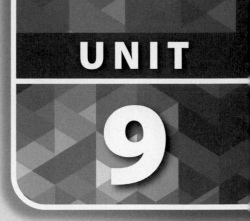

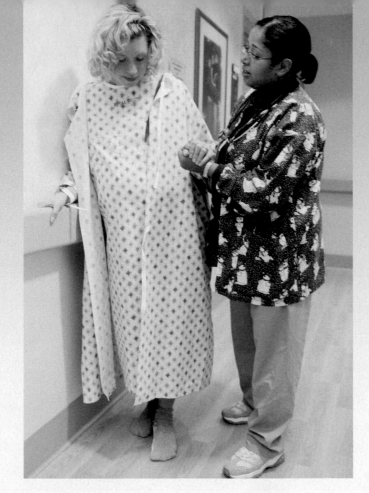

Acute Care

THE ACUTE CARE SETTING CAN BE AN EXCITING PLACE TO WORK. If you choose to work in an acute care setting, such as a hospital, you will have the opportunity to meet and care for many different people. In this unit, you will learn about how to care for three special groups of patients who often receive treatment in hospitals: surgical patients; patients who are about to deliver, or have just delivered, babies; and children.

Photo: The acute care setting offers the opportunity to work with many different types of patients. Here, a nursing assistant helps a patient who is in labor.

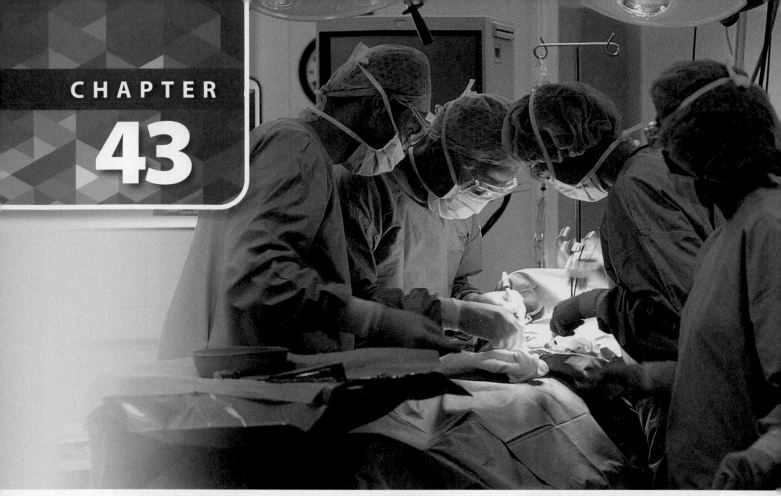

Photo: A surgical team performs an operation.

Caring for Surgical Patients

 WHAT WILL YOU LEARN?

Surgery is a branch of medicine that involves treating diseases and disorders by entering the body and physically removing or repairing damaged organs or tissues. Advances in surgical instruments and techniques have made surgeries safer and opened up treatment options for many diseases and disorders that were considered fatal in the past. Surgeries that once made headlines, such as kidney transplants, are now done fairly routinely.

The longer a person lives, the greater the chance the person will need surgery sometime during their lifetime, simply because the person will have more of a chance to develop a disease or disorder that is treated surgically. As a nursing assistant, you may have many opportunities to help prepare people for surgery and care for them afterward. When you are finished with this chapter, you will be able to:

1. Explain the various reasons surgery is done and the preparations for it.
2. Define the term *anesthesia* and describe the three main types of anesthesia.
3. Understand the fears and concerns of a preoperative patient and describe actions the nursing assistant can take to help relieve some of them.
4. Describe physical preparations required for a person before surgery and explain the nursing assistant's role in these preparations.

5. Describe potential complications of surgery and the measures taken to prevent them.
6. Discuss observations that are important to report to the nurse when caring for a patient who is recovering from surgery.

Vocabulary

Exploratory surgery	Emergent	Preoperative phase	Preoperative teaching
Definitive surgery	General anesthesia	Intraoperative phase	Postanesthesia care unit
Elective	Regional anesthesia	Postoperative phase	(PACU)
Urgent	Local anesthesia	Perioperative period	Atelectasis

INTRODUCTION TO CARING FOR SURGICAL PATIENTS

A person may need surgery for many different reasons. **Exploratory surgery**, also known as *diagnostic surgery*, may be performed when a person has a significant medical problem but the doctors do not know how bad the problem is or exactly what is causing it. For example, doctors might want to do exploratory surgery following an accident when the extent of the damage to the person's internal organs is unknown, or when cancer is suspected but cannot be confirmed by other means. Often, the problem is discovered and solved during the same surgery.

Definitive surgery is performed when the person's medical problem is known and the best way to address it is through surgery. For example, surgeries are performed to repair organ defects or injuries, as in a hernia repair or surgical repair of a fractured bone. Surgeries are also performed to remove diseased body parts, as when the cancerous part of the colon is removed as treatment for colon cancer. Definitive procedures are usually considered to be *curative*. However, some surgical procedures are only *palliative procedures*. Remember that Chapter 26 describes palliative care as care that focuses on relieving uncomfortable symptoms, not curing the illness.

Surgeries may be elective, urgent, or emergent. Surgeries are performed on an **elective** basis when the procedure is planned for and scheduled ahead of time. An example of an elective procedure would be cataract surgery or a plastic surgery procedure, such as a face-lift. **Urgent** surgeries are planned and scheduled ahead of time, but usually an effort is made to schedule the procedure as soon as possible to prevent the person's condition from getting worse. Examples of urgent procedures would include a mastectomy (in a person with breast cancer) or removal

of a gallbladder (in a person who has gallstones). An **emergent** or emergency surgery is one that must be performed immediately to prevent the person from dying or becoming disabled. Emergent surgeries are unplanned and unscheduled and are usually the result of an acute illness or injury, such as a ruptured appendix.

Most patients who are having elective or urgent surgery will have any necessary lab work or other diagnostic testing done in the surgeon's office or on an outpatient basis in the days leading up to the surgery. The person remains home until the morning of surgery and goes to the hospital or surgical center an hour or two before the surgery is scheduled. Hair is removed from the surgical site and the skin is cleaned in the operating room or in a preparation area next to the operating room just prior to the procedure. As a nursing assistant, you may be involved in assisting a patient or resident with some of these preparations for surgery.

Most surgical procedures are done under anesthesia. Anesthesia prevents the person from feeling pain during the surgery and is accomplished through the use of medications. Depending on the situation, the doctor may choose to use a general anesthetic, a regional anesthetic, a local/topical anesthetic, or a combination of these:

- **General anesthesia** causes a loss of consciousness. Usually, a combination of inhaled medications (in the form of a gas) and injected medications is given to cause general anesthesia. The person is "put to sleep" for the duration of the surgical procedure. When the procedure is completed, the medications are stopped and the person "wakes up." The person will be sleepy for several hours after the procedure and may experience some nausea or vomiting during the recovery period.

■ **Regional anesthesia** causes a loss of sensation in part, but not all, of the body. The person remains conscious throughout the procedure. A sedative may be given in addition to the anesthetic to help the person relax. The anesthetic is injected near a nerve pathway, causing the part of the body beyond the injection site to become numb. After surgery, the sensation returns gradually. The person may experience temporary paralysis and weakness of the anesthetized body part until the anesthetic has worn completely off. An example of regional anesthesia is an epidural block, which numbs the body from the waist down and is often given to patients during childbirth.

■ **Local** (and topical) **anesthesia** causes a loss of sensation in only a very small part of the body (the surgical site). As with regional anesthesia, the medication is injected near a nerve pathway, the person remains conscious throughout the procedure, and a sedative may be given to help the person relax. Topical medications are applied to mucous membranes to numb them. Eye drops, nasal sprays, or oral sprays are examples of topical anesthetics. The surgical site remains without sensation until the local anesthetic wears off. Eye surgeries, breast biopsies, and hernia repairs are examples of surgeries that are often performed under local and/or topical anesthesia.

Combinations of these anesthetic approaches are now frequently used to improve comfort after surgery. For example, it is common practice to inject a long-lasting local anesthetic around an incision site during surgery even if the patient has a general anesthetic. This allows the person to wake up relatively pain-free. Regional blocks are also used for postoperative pain control and may be injected either before the person is put to sleep with a general anesthesia or afterward.

After the surgery, the person is often discharged from the hospital within a few hours to recover at home, in an extended care facility, or in a long-term care facility. Even though surgery is performed in a hospital or surgical center, as a nursing assistant, you can expect to care for people who are either preparing for surgery or recovering from it, no matter where you work.

There are three phases of care for the person having surgery (Fig. 43-1). These phases are:

■ The **preoperative phase**, or before surgery
■ The **intraoperative phase**, or during surgery
■ The **postoperative phase**, or after surgery

The term **perioperative period** is used to describe all three phases of the surgical process as a whole.

CARE OF THE PREOPERATIVE PATIENT

The preoperative phase begins when the person is first informed about the need for surgery and ends when the person actually enters the operating room. The preoperative phase can be as long as several weeks (for an elective, scheduled procedure) or as short as a few minutes (for an emergent procedure). During the preoperative phase, the person who is having surgery is prepared both emotionally and physically for the procedure.

Emotional Preparation

A person facing surgery usually has many fears, concerns, and worries. For example, the person may be afraid of not waking up from the anesthesia, dying as

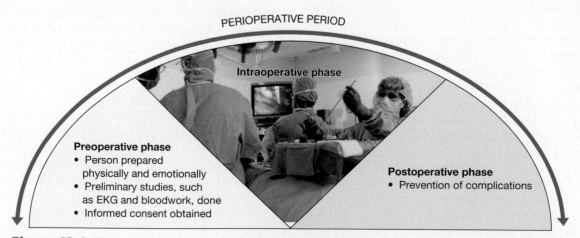

Figure 43-1 There are three phases of care for the person having surgery. As a nursing assistant, you will provide care during the preoperative and postoperative phases.

a result of the surgery, or experiencing pain during or after the procedure. If the person is having exploratory surgery, the person may be worried about what the doctor will find (for example, a malignant tumor). Many people worry about how long it will take to recover from the surgery and what this will mean in terms of time missed from work and lost income needed to support a family.

To help reduce a person's anxiety about the upcoming surgery, the health care team spends time talking with the person and family members about the procedure, its benefits and possible risks, and what can be expected during the postoperative recovery phase. These conversations are commonly called **preoperative teaching**. Preoperative teaching begins with the doctor's explanation of why they feel the procedure is the best treatment option for the person. The doctor tells the person what complications can occur as a result of the procedure, what will actually occur during the procedure, and what other treatment options, if any, are available (Fig. 43-2).

The doctor must explain these things in a way that is understandable to the person, so that the person can make an informed decision about whether they want to have the surgery. To go ahead with the procedure, informed consent must be given by the person and documented in the person's medical record. If the person is not able to make an informed decision on their own, informed consent must be obtained from the person's family members or legal representative. The nurse is responsible for making sure that informed consent has been obtained and that the person signs a form giving permission for the procedure to take place. As a nursing assistant, you will not be responsible for either explaining the procedure to the person or obtaining the person's signed consent for it.

Once informed consent for the procedure is obtained, the nurse continues the preoperative teaching by explaining the preoperative procedures that are done to physically prepare the person for surgery, as well as the purpose of any medications or tests that are required during the preoperative phase. The nurse also explains what will happen during the postoperative phase and teaches the person how to do any exercises that may be necessary to prevent complications following the surgery.

Although as a nursing assistant you will not participate directly in preoperative teaching, you will still play a very important supporting role. You will reinforce what the nurse has told the person, and keep the nurse informed of any questions the person may ask you about the procedure. Anxiety can make the person forget to ask important questions when the doctor or nurse is explaining the surgery. Often, the person will remember questions they wanted to ask later, when the doctor or nurse is no longer in the room. The person may ask you the questions instead. If the question is about an aspect of preoperative or postoperative care that you are directly involved with, such as the reason for the NPO status prior to the procedure or the purpose of taking vital signs frequently after the procedure, you can answer the question yourself. But if you do not know the answer to the person's question, or if the question is about the surgical procedure itself, please tell the nurse immediately that the person has a question. The nurse will see to it that the person's question is answered.

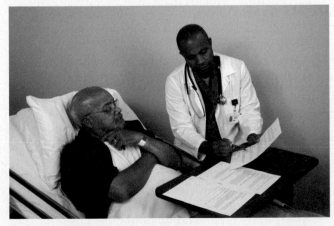

Figure 43-2 During the preoperative phase, the doctor tells the person why the surgery is the best treatment option, explains the surgical procedure and any associated risks to the person, and obtains informed consent to perform the surgery.

Helping Hands and a Caring Heart

Focus on Humanistic Health Care

It is very easy to tell a person that a procedure is "minor" or "just routine." Many surgical procedures are, indeed, relatively low risk and considered "routine" by health care professionals, who see these procedures done every day. But no matter how simple or low-risk a surgical procedure is, there is nothing minor or routine about it to the person who is having it! Recognizing the person's fears, listening to their questions and concerns, and taking action to get those questions or concerns addressed are all very important things that you can do to help a person to prepare emotionally for the upcoming surgery.

Physical Preparation

Several things are done to physically prepare the person for surgery.

In the Days Leading Up to the Surgery

Typically, a person who is having surgery will need to have several tests done before the surgery to assess their level of health. Tests to assess the functioning of the person's cardiovascular, respiratory, and urinary systems are typically done. In addition, the doctor may request blood work.

The Evening Before Surgery

A person who is scheduled for surgery will usually be on NPO status for 6 to 8 hours before surgery (Fig. 43-3). This is necessary to ensure that the person's stomach is empty during and after the procedure. For some procedures, clear liquids are allowed up to 4 hours before the surgery is scheduled. Sometimes, a person who is having surgery under a general anesthesia may vomit as the anesthesia is given or starts to wear off. Vomiting while in a semiconscious state puts the person at risk for aspiration (the inhalation of foreign material into the lungs). Aspiration puts the person at risk for developing pneumonia. Going into the procedure with an empty stomach helps to reduce the risk of aspiration and pneumonia.

You will need to tell the person, as well as any visitors, that NPO means that the person may not have anything by mouth, including water, ice, gum, and mints. It can be difficult for a person who is on NPO status to be around other people who are eating and drinking. For this reason, it may be helpful to show visitors to an area outside of the person's room where

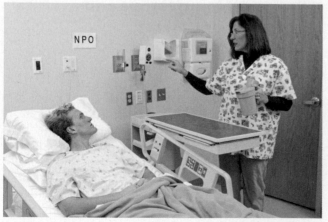

Figure 43-3 Many people will not be allowed to have anything by mouth for 6 to 8 hours before the surgery. When a person is on NPO status, the water pitcher and drinking glass are removed from the person's room.

they can enjoy their snacks and beverages, away from the person who is on NPO status. Remember to remove the water pitcher and the drinking glass from the bedside table. Frequent mouth care helps to keep the person on NPO status comfortable. The person is usually allowed to brush their teeth as long as no water is swallowed.

The Morning of Surgery

Many things are done the day of surgery to prepare the patient. You should arrange your schedule as necessary, allowing enough time to help the person get ready for surgery. This is especially important if you work in a long-term care facility or for a home health care agency, to ensure that the person arrives at the hospital or surgical center at the appointed time. The nurse will tell you what you need to do to help to prepare the person for surgery. Tasks that you may be involved with include the following:

- **Bowel prep.** Unlike surgeries in the past, a routine enema before surgery is not necessary. However, some abdominal procedures may require that the person completes a total bowel prep. The bowel prep consists of a liquid that the person drinks the day prior to surgery. The liquid acts similar to a laxative and clears any fecal material from the intestines. In some instances, the bowel prep may be followed by an enema. For example, an enema and/or a bowel prep may be given if the person is scheduled for intestinal surgery to prevent feces from contaminating the abdominal cavity during the surgery.
- **Bathing.** You may need to help the person to bathe and wash their hair prior to the surgery. Bathing and shampooing reduce the number of microbes on the skin. In some cases, the doctor may order a special antimicrobial soap to be used.
- **Grooming.** Make-up should be removed before surgery, especially if the procedure is on the face or neck. Prosthetic devices, glasses, contact lenses, hearing aids, dentures, wigs, jewelry, and hair accessories may also be removed prior to the surgery. Although the person may want or need to wear some of these items up until the very last minute, you should let the person know about these restrictions and encourage them to leave all but the most necessary items at home.
- **Dressing.** If the person will be going to the hospital or surgical center the day of the surgery, have them wear clothing that is loose and comfortable. This will make changing into a hospital gown before the procedure easier, and it will

also ensure that when the person goes home, the clothing will fit over any bulky dressings or casts that may have been applied during the procedure.

Immediately Before the Surgery

There are a few additional steps taken immediately before surgery for both outpatients and inpatients that are important to be aware of as a nursing assistant.

Outpatients

Once the person arrives at the hospital or surgical center, they will go to a preparation area next to the operating room. The person will be shown to a private area and asked to undress and put on a clean hospital gown and surgical cap.

A nurse will check that all paperwork has been properly completed and will answer any questions that the person has. Vital signs will be taken and documented, and the person will be asked about any medication allergies. The person will then be asked to void and may be given a sedative (to help relieve anxiety). After giving the sedative, which can make the person drowsy and weak, the side rails must remain up on the bed or stretcher and the person must not get up without assistance (Fig. 43-4). Make sure the call-light control is within easy reach and that the person is comfortable and warm.

If the surgery will be performed under general anesthesia, the person's glasses or contact lenses, hearing aids, dentures, prosthetic devices, jewelry, and hair accessories may be removed at this time. If the surgery will be performed under regional or local

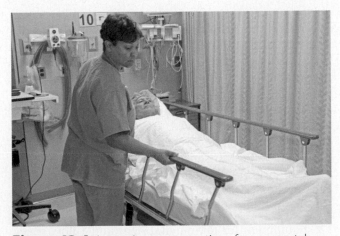

Figure 43-4 Last-minute preparations for surgery take place in the preparation area near the operating room. Once medications have been given to prevent nausea and reduce anxiety, the person must remain in bed with the side rails up to reduce the risk of falling.

anesthesia, the doctor may request that the person wear hearing aids or dentures during the surgery, to make communication easier. Items that are removed from the person are documented and given to the person's family.

The surgical site may be prepared at this time, or this may be done in the operating room. The surgical site is the area of the body that will be operated on. Preparation of the surgical site may or may not involve removal of body hair. If hair removal is ordered, an electric clipper with a disposable head will most likely be used. Current practice now usually involves removing hair only along the incision line. If one of your duties is to perform preoperative hair removal, make sure you have been instructed in the proper technique.

Last, a preoperative checklist is completed (Fig. 43-5). The checklist is used to confirm that all preoperative tests and procedures have been completed. The nursing assistant is often responsible for completing and recording many of the tasks on the checklist.

Inpatients

If the person was admitted to the hospital prior to the surgery, the tasks that are completed immediately before the surgery may be completed in the person's room, before taking them to the operating room. Let the person's family members know where they can wait while the person is in surgery. Some facilities have surgical waiting rooms while others allow the family to wait in the person's room. Please remember that family members are often anxious and nervous about the surgery. Refer any questions family members may have about the procedure or the person's condition to the nurse.

CARE OF THE POSTOPERATIVE PATIENT

Immediately after surgery, the person is taken to the **postanesthesia care unit (PACU),** also known as the recovery room (Fig. 43-6). While in the PACU, the person is closely monitored by the health care team to make sure that they are recovering without complications from the surgery or the anesthesia. The person is usually groggy but can be awakened. Once awake, the person will usually be oriented to person and place. The person will remain in the PACU until their condition is stable. While in the PACU, the person usually receives supplemental oxygen. Suctioning is also available, in case the person vomits or has secretions that interfere with breathing.

1. Patient's name: _____ Date: _____ Height: _____ Weight: _____
   Identification band present: _____
2. Informed consent signed:: _____ Special permits signed: _____
3. Surgical site: _____ (Ex: Sterilization)
4. History & physical examination report present: _____ Date: _____
5. Laboratory records present:_____
   CBC: _____ Hgb: _____ Urinalysis: _____ Hct: _____

6.	Item	Present	Removed
	a. Natural teeth		
	Dentures; upper, lower, partial	_____	_____
	Bridge, fixed; crown	_____	_____
	b. Contact lenses	_____	_____
	c. Other prostheses—type: _____	_____	_____
	d. Jewelry:		
	Wedding band (taped/tied)	_____	_____
	Rings	_____	_____
	Earrings: pierced, clip-on	_____	_____
	Neck chains	_____	_____
	Any other body piercings	_____	_____
	e. Make-up	_____	_____
	Nail polish	_____	_____
7.	Clothing		
	a. Clean patient gown	_____	_____
	b. Cap	_____	_____
	c. Sanitary pad, etc.	_____	_____

8. Family instructed where to wait? _____
9. Valuables secured? _____
10. Blood available? _____ Ordered? _____ Where? _____
11. Preanesthetic medication given: _____
    Type: _____ Time: _____
12. Voided: _____ Amount: _____ Time: _____ Catheter: _____
    Mouth care given: _____
13. Vital signs: Temperature: _____ Pulse: _____ Resp: _____ Blood Pressure: _____
14. Special problems/precautions: (Allergies, deafness, *etc.*): _____
15. Area of skin preparation: _____
16. _____ Date: _____ Time:_____
    Signature: Nurse releasing patient

Figure 43-5 A preoperative checklist documents that all of the tasks that must be completed during the preoperative period have been completed. The preoperative checklist goes in the person's medical record and must be completed before the person goes into surgery.

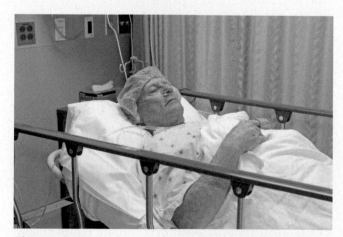

Figure 43-6 Following surgery, the person is taken to a postanesthesia care unit (PACU), also known as a recovery room. The person remains here and is monitored closely until their condition is stable.

While the person is in surgery, you will most likely be responsible for preparing the person's room for their postoperative arrival (Fig. 43-7). The bed linens are usually changed and a surgical bed is prepared (see Chapter 19). The bed is raised to make transferring the person from the stretcher to the bed easier. Furniture is moved, if necessary, to ensure a clear pathway for the stretcher. In many facilities, the patient may be transferred to their bed immediately after surgery. Finally, items that may be needed at the time of the person's arrival are gathered and placed in the room. Items that may be needed include:

- Equipment for taking vital signs and a flow sheet or electronic chart for recording the vital signs
- An intravenous (IV) pole
- A towel and washcloth
- An emesis basin
- A bed protector

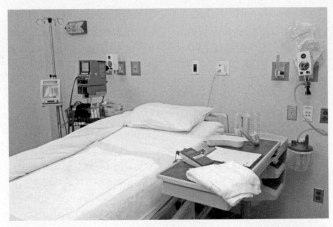

Figure 43-7 The nursing assistant prepares the person's room for their return while the person is in surgery. The linens are changed and a surgical bed is made. The bed is raised to a height that will make transferring the person from the stretcher to the bed easier. The equipment that may be needed during the postoperative phase is gathered and placed in the room. Before the occupant of this room arrives, the over-bed table will need to be moved out of the way to ensure a clear pathway from the door to the bed.

- Suction to connect to drainage devices
- Supplemental oxygen
- Pillows or other positioning aids to elevate the extremities
- Warmed blankets

When the person is returned to their room, you will need to assist in transferring the person from the stretcher to the bed, unless they arrive already in their hospital bed. The nurse assesses the person's overall condition, checks for blood on the dressing and for the presence of drains and catheters, and adjusts the IV flow rate. While the nurse is doing this, you may be asked to take the person's vital signs. Vital signs are taken as ordered and recorded in the person's chart. Postoperatively, routine vital sign measurements, including temperature, are usually taken every 15 minutes for the first hour, every 30 minutes for the next 1 to 2 hours, every hour for the next 4 hours, and then every 4 hours as ordered (Fig. 43-8). As always, any changes in vital signs must be reported to the nurse immediately. In a person who is recovering from surgery, a change in a vital sign could be the first sign that the person is developing a postoperative complication.

The person may need to be positioned in a particular way postoperatively. Children may be positioned laterally or in the Sim position to help prevent aspiration in the event of vomiting. If the person had surgery on an arm or leg, the arm or leg is usually elevated on a pillow or folded blanket to help prevent swelling and pain. Make sure you check with the nurse for any specific instructions or restrictions

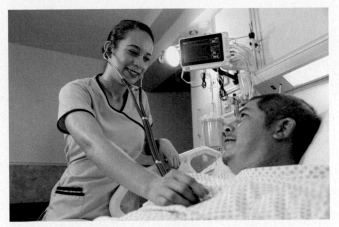

Figure 43-8 Vital signs are taken frequently during the immediate postoperative phase because a change in vital signs could signal a complication of the surgery or the anesthesia. (*FERNANDO MACIAS ROMO\Shutterstock.com*)

regarding the person's position. In all cases, the person should be positioned comfortably and in a way that will prevent stress on the surgical incision.

In the hours and days that follow surgery, the health care team focuses on preventing complications and assisting the person with routine tasks, such as grooming and elimination, as necessary. As a nursing assistant, you will play an important role in helping the person to make a good recovery.

Taking It to the Next Level:
Advanced Skills

More in-depth information related to advanced skills when caring for a person having surgery can be found in *Lippincott Acute Care Skills for Advanced Nursing Assistants*. Visit the Point® at thepoint.lww.com for access to the ebook.

Preventing Complications

People who have had surgery are at risk for developing complications, especially related to breathing and circulation. In addition, the surgical site may become infected or the wound may not stay closed. As a nursing assistant, there are several things that you will do to prevent complications from developing. Also, if one of your patients develops a complication from surgery, you may be the first one to notice. Reporting your observations to the nurse promptly helps to ensure that action will be taken quickly to prevent the person's condition from getting worse.

Respiratory Complications

The combined effects of general anesthesia, the medications given to relieve postoperative pain, and a painful incision make it difficult for a person who is recovering from surgery to clear the lungs and airways of fluid and mucus. The person is drowsy from the anesthesia and pain medication, and it hurts to cough! If the person also has a chronic respiratory disorder, such as asthma or chronic obstructive pulmonary disease (COPD), or if the person smokes, then their risk of developing a respiratory complication increases even more.

Common respiratory complications of surgery include pneumonia (fluid fills the alveoli) and **atelectasis** (the alveoli collapse). Both atelectasis and pneumonia make it difficult for oxygen to pass into the blood and carbon dioxide to pass out of it.

To prevent fluid and mucus from collecting in the person's lungs, you may need to assist the person with frequent repositioning and with performing respiratory exercises. Commonly used respiratory exercises include coughing and deep breathing, and incentive spirometry (Fig. 43-9).

- **Coughing and deep breathing.** The person is helped into a comfortable position and then instructed to take a few deep breaths and cough forcefully. If the person has had abdominal or chest surgery, you may need to support the incision site with a small pillow or folded towel while the person coughs (see Fig. 43-9A). Supporting the incision site helps to minimize pain.
- **Incentive spirometry.** The person forcefully inhales through a special device called an incentive spirometer (see Fig. 43-9B). The device consists of a tube and a chamber that contains balls. The goal is for the person to inhale hard enough through the tube to raise the balls in the chamber.

If your patient has orders to perform respiratory exercises, these exercises will need to be done every few hours or as directed. Elevating the head of the bed while the person is supine will also make it easier for the person to breathe.

Cardiovascular Complications

Anesthetic agents, pain medications, and general immobility after surgery can cause the body's circulation to slow down, leading to pooling of the blood in the legs. When blood flow slows and blood pools, a thrombus, or blood clot, may form. Surgical patients who are older or have a history of circulatory problems are at the most risk for developing thrombi. Certain conditions (such as fractures of the femur, or thigh bone) and certain surgeries (such as joint replacement surgery) also carry a high risk of thrombus formation.

A thrombus in one of the veins of the legs causes inflammation and pain, a condition known as *thrombophlebitis* (Chapter 32). Sometimes the blood clot will break loose and travel through the bloodstream. A blood clot that breaks loose and moves through the bloodstream is known as an *embolus*. The embolus can travel to the brain and get stuck in one of the blood vessels there, causing a stroke. Or, the embolus can travel to the pulmonary artery, the artery that carries blood from the heart to the lungs so that it can receive oxygen. Blocking of the pulmonary artery by an embolus is called a *pulmonary embolism* (Chapter 32) and it can be fatal. Restlessness and shortness of breath may be signs of pulmonary embolism and should be reported to the nurse immediately.

A number of different measures are taken to lower the person's risk of cardiovascular complications.

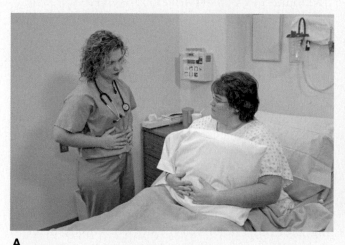

A

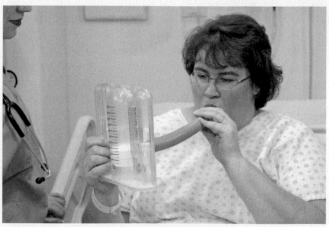

B

Figure 43-9 Respiratory exercises may be ordered during the postoperative phase to prevent the person from developing respiratory complications such as pneumonia and atelectasis. **A.** Coughing and deep breathing exercises. The person takes a few deep breaths and then coughs forcefully. **B.** Incentive spirometry. The person inhales through an incentive spirometer with the goal of causing the balls to rise in the chamber.

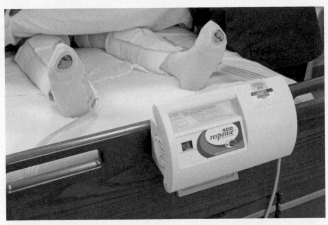

Figure 43-10 Intermittent pneumatic compression (IPC) devices help to prevent pooling of blood in the lower extremities. The plastic sleeves around the person's lower legs contain multiple chambers, which alternatively inflate and deflate, pushing blood through the veins.

Intermittent Pneumatic Compression (IPC) Devices

Intermittent pneumatic compression (IPC) devices (known as sequential compression devices in the past) are applied to the calves to help prevent pooling of blood in the lower legs (Fig. 43-10). Disposable plastic sleeves are wrapped around the person's lower legs. The sleeves, which have several different compartments, are connected to an air pump via tubing. Air is pumped into the first compartment (the one closest to the foot) to inflate it. Then the next compartment inflates, then the next, helping to move the blood from the lower legs toward the heart. When the topmost compartment has been inflated, all the compartments deflate and the cycle begins again at the bottom. The inflating and deflating action massages the veins, pushing the blood through the veins and back to the heart. Many of your patients will return from the PACU with these devices in place.

Antiembolism (TED) Stockings

Antiembolism (TED) stockings are made of a tight-fitting elastic fabric. The stockings, which may be knee-high or thigh-high, are specially fitted for the person by the nurse or the physical therapist. The elastic fabric applies pressure, compressing the veins and helping to return blood to the heart. This helps to prevent pooling of blood in the legs.

TED stockings may be applied before surgery, or ordered afterward. If the stockings are allowed to be removed at night, they should be reapplied before the person gets out of bed for the day. Once the person stands up, gravity increases blood flow to the veins in the lower legs, causing the veins to widen and the blood to pool. You will find the procedure for how to properly apply TED stockings in Chapter 32.

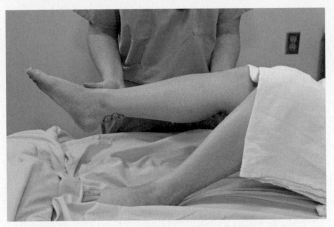

Figure 43-11 If your patient is weak or unconscious, you may have to help them to perform leg exercises. Leg exercises help to prevent blood from pooling in the veins of the legs.

Leg Exercises

The doctor may also order leg exercises for the person following surgery to help reduce the risk of embolism. If the person is weak or unconscious, you may need to help them with these exercises (Fig. 43-11). The person usually must do these exercises every 1 to 2 hours while awake.

Tell the Nurse!

During the postoperative phase, you may be the first person to notice signs of a postoperative complication. Report any of the following observations to the nurse immediately:

- There is an increased amount of bright red drainage (blood) on the person's wound dressing or in the drainage device
- There is a significant change in the person's vital signs (blood pressure, pulse, respirations, temperature)
- The person is having trouble breathing, experiencing chest pain, or is making wheezing or gurgling sounds
- The person is restless, confused, or disoriented
- The person's lips or nail beds are very pale or have a bluish tinge
- The person's skin is cool and clammy
- The person complains of increased pain, tingling, or numbness of an extremity with a cast or bandage
- The person complains of pain or swelling at the IV site, or the IV is not dripping
- The person complains of abdominal pain, nausea, or vomiting

The exercises are done while the person is in the supine position. One leg is exercised at a time. The person rotates the ankle, flexes and points the foot, flexes and extends the knee, and finishes by raising the leg off the bed and lowering it again. Each movement is repeated five times, and then the movements are repeated with the other leg, unless the person had leg surgery. In this case, the exercises might only be done on the "well" leg. A doctor's order is required to exercise the leg that was operated on. Always check with the nurse to see if there are any specific instructions for your patient.

Assisting With Positioning

During the postoperative phase, most people will need assistance with repositioning themselves every 1 to 2 hours. Frequent repositioning is necessary for the person's comfort. In addition, it helps to prevent the postoperative complications of pneumonia and embolism. Depending on where the incision is, moving may be very painful for the person. Use a lift sheet to help reposition the person, and move them gently and slowly.

Assisting With Nutrition

A person who is recovering from surgery usually needs intravenous (IV) therapy until they are able to take fluids orally and are no longer nauseated. If the person has had surgery involving the digestive system, they may have a nasogastric tube. The nasogastric tube is connected to suction to keep the stomach empty. These patients will be NPO and may need to remain on IV fluids for several days.

Once the person is able to take fluids orally and is no longer nauseated, they will usually be started on a clear liquid diet. The diet is progressed as the person's condition improves. From a clear liquid diet, the person usually progresses to a full liquid diet and then gradually to a regular diet. Good hydration and a proper diet help with the healing process.

Assisting With Elimination

Following surgery, the person may have difficulties related to elimination. Some people may need to use a bedpan or a urinal after surgery. The person's NPO status, pain medications, and immobility can lead to constipation. A full bladder can increase pain from an abdominal incision, making voiding difficult. As a result, some people may need to be catheterized. Other patients will return from surgery with an indwelling urinary catheter already in place. Your responsibilities will include reporting the person's first voiding after surgery. Often, you will also need to measure and record the person's intake and output (I&O) for a period of time following surgery as well.

Assisting With Hygiene

People who are recovering from surgery may need help with personal hygiene. Assisting with frequent oral care, helping the person to wash their face and hands, and changing soiled gowns promptly are all things you can do to help promote comfort. Many people will not be able to take a bath or a shower for a few days following surgery because the incision cannot get wet. These people will need your help in the form of either partial or complete bed baths.

Assisting With Walking (Ambulation)

Early and frequent ambulation is helpful in preventing many of the complications that can result from surgery. Many times, a person who has had surgery is able to get out of bed within a few hours of returning to their room. Because the person will be weak and unsteady, they will need your help when ambulating. Allow the person time to sit on the edge of the bed ("dangle") before getting out of bed. If the person complains of feeling dizzy or lightheaded while dangling, help the person to lie back down and call the nurse. Otherwise, check the person's pulse and blood pressure and then help the person to stand. Usually, you and the person will walk only a short distance to begin with. As the person's strength returns, you can go for longer walks.

Concerns for Long-Term Care

Many older people who are residents in a long-term care facility will need surgery at some point. If you work in this type of health care setting, you will have many responsibilities related to preparing your residents for their surgical procedures and then caring for them after they return to the facility after surgery. Many people, especially older people, may need to go to a long-term care facility for a short period of time after having surgery. There they can continue to recover and receive any necessary therapy until they are strong enough to return to their own homes.

An older person is more likely to suffer complications related to surgery than a younger person. Many older people have other chronic health conditions not directly related to the reason they are having surgery. It takes an older person longer to wake up completely from sedation or general anesthesia. As a result, you will need to monitor their respirations and level of consciousness closely. An older person is more likely to become dizzy and fall when trying to get out of bed and walk after surgery. The use of side rails to help prevent falling out of bed and reminding the person to call for assistance may be necessary for a while.

Respiratory complications are more likely to occur in an older person after surgery. Confusion and restlessness may be an indication of decreased oxygenation and not pain. Some types of sedation and pain medication can cause temporary delirium in older people. Make sure you observe your residents closely as they recover from surgery, and report anything that does not seem quite normal to the nurse immediately.

SUMMARY

- Surgery involves treating diseases and disorders by removing or repairing damaged organs or tissues.
  - Surgery may be exploratory or definitive. It may be elective, urgent, or emergent.
  - Surgery is performed under general, regional, or local/topical anesthesia. Many instances involve a combination of anesthetics.
  - Because many surgeries are now done on an outpatient basis, you may be responsible for helping a person to prepare for and recover from surgery, even if you do not work in a hospital or other acute care setting.

- There are three phases of care for a person who is having surgery. The term *perioperative period* is used to describe all three phases of the surgical process as a whole.
  - During the preoperative phase, the patient is prepared emotionally and physically for the procedure.
  - During the intraoperative phase, surgery is performed.
  - During the postoperative phase, the nursing team's efforts focus on preventing complications and helping the person to recover.

WHAT DID YOU LEARN?

Multiple Choice

Select the single best answer for each of the following questions.

1. Mrs. Wong is recovering from surgery. How often will she need assistance with repositioning?
   a. Every shift
   b. Every 1 to 2 hours
   c. Every 3 to 4 hours
   d. Every 15 minutes

2. Which one of the following patients is at high risk for an embolism?
   a. Mr. Solis, who is 75 years old and has just had cardiac bypass surgery
   b. Mrs. Greene, who is 60 years old and has just had a hip joint replaced
   c. Ms. Kirkpatrick, who is 40 years old and has just had surgery to repair a fractured leg
   d. All of the above

3. Which one of the following may be a sign of pulmonary embolism?
   a. Fever
   b. Fatigue
   c. Profuse sweating
   d. Restlessness and shortness of breath

4. The nurse asks you to help Mr. Huang in Room 340 with coughing and deep breathing exercises. What is the purpose of these exercises?
   a. To help Mr. Huang build up his strength following the surgery
   b. To lower Mr. Huang's risk of pulmonary embolism
   c. To lower Mr. Huang's risk of pneumonia or atelectasis
   d. All of the above

5. In which case might emergent surgery be necessary?

   a. The person has been in a car accident and is bleeding internally

   b. The person needs to have a cataract removed

   c. The person needs to have a hip joint replaced

   d. The person needs to have a tumor in the breast removed

6. During which type of anesthesia is the person unconscious?

   a. Regional anesthesia

   b. Local anesthesia

   c. General anesthesia

   d. All of the above

7. Which one of the following activities takes place before surgery?

   a. Frequent ambulation

   b. Completion of the preoperative checklist

   c. Performance of coughing and deep breathing exercises

   d. Careful monitoring in the postanesthesia care unit (PACU)

8. Why must a person who is having surgery avoid taking food or fluids by mouth for 6 to 8 hours before the surgery?

   a. If the person vomits as a result of the anesthesia, they could be at risk for aspiration.

   b. An empty stomach is necessary to prevent infection of the abdominal cavity.

   c. The anesthesia is more effective if the person's stomach is empty.

   d. An empty stomach helps to prevent problems with elimination after the surgery.

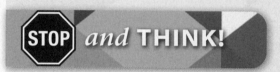

STOP *and* **THINK!**

■ You are a nursing assistant in an assisted living facility. One of your residents, Mrs. Sanchez, is scheduled to have a surgical procedure done on an outpatient basis at the local hospital. Mrs. Sanchez is a very stylish woman who takes a lot of pride in her appearance. Her nails are always done, she always accessorizes her outfits, and she always makes sure to apply a fresh coat of lipstick before leaving her room. Mrs. Sanchez knows that she is not permitted to wear make-up during the surgery, but when you arrive in her room to help her get ready the day of the surgery, you find that she is looking like her usual self—nails done, jewelry on, lipstick applied. What would you do, and why?

■ You work as a nursing assistant in a hospital. One of your patients, Mr. Newman, is scheduled for exploratory surgery to determine whether a tumor in his brain is cancerous. Mr. Newman is married, with three children ranging in age from 8 to 14 years. He has a very large extended family, many of whom have been staying at the hospital day and night since Mr. Newman was admitted. How might Mr. Newman and his family members be feeling right now? Is there anything you could do to help them?

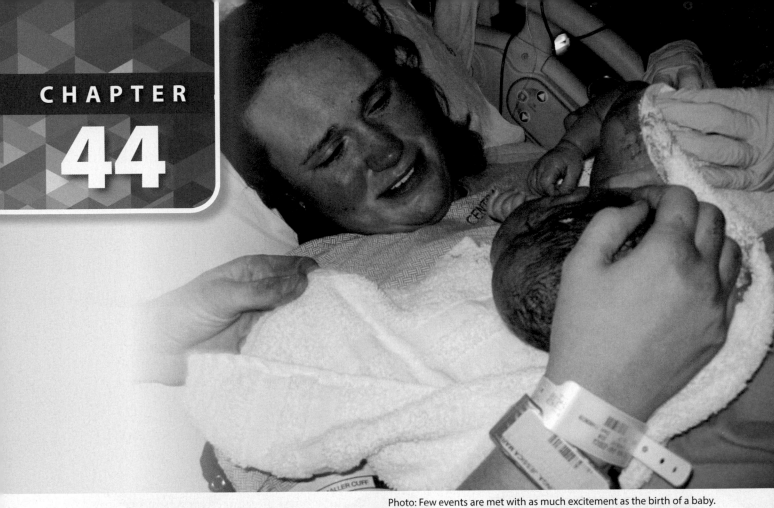

Photo: Few events are met with as much excitement as the birth of a baby.

Caring for Birthing Parents and Newborns

 WHAT WILL YOU LEARN?

In this chapter, you will learn how to care for a newborn baby. You will also learn about the care required by a patient during pregnancy in the months leading up to birth, during birth, and following birth. Although many states and health care facilities do not allow nursing assistants to participate in the care of a pregnant patient or a newborn, others do. You may work in a hospital, providing care for birthing parents and newborns before, during, and after delivery. Or you may be employed by a home health care agency that provides home care to patients during pregnancy as well as after delivery, to both them and their newborns. When you are finished with this chapter, you will be able to:

1. Describe physical changes that occur in the female reproductive system during pregnancy.
2. Define *prenatal care* and give examples of advice given during the prenatal period.
3. List reasons that home care or hospitalization may be required during pregnancy.
4. Describe the nursing assistant's responsibilities for meeting a person's physical and emotional needs during pregnancy.

5. Describe the two ways of delivering a baby.

6. Describe the nursing assistant's responsibilities when caring for a person who has just given birth.

7. List observations you might make while caring for a person who has just given birth that should be reported immediately to the nurse.

8. Discuss important security and safety issues related to caring for a newborn.

9. Explain how to care for the umbilical cord stump.

10. Explain how to care for a baby who has been circumcised.

11. Explain how to bottle-feed a baby.

12. Explain how to bathe a baby.

Vocabulary

Antepartum (prenatal) period
Placenta
Prenatal care
Preterm labor

Pregnancy-induced hypertension (PIH)
Eclampsia
Labor
Cesarean section

Epidural block
Vernix
Bonding period
Postpartum period
Lochia

Episiotomy
Sitz bath
Colostrum
Umbilical cord

THE ANTEPARTUM (PRENATAL) PERIOD

During pregnancy, the period of time from conception until the baby is born is called the **antepartum (prenatal) period**. (The prefixes *ante-* and *pre-* both mean "before," and the roots *partum* and *natal* both mean "birth.") The antepartum period lasts approximately 9 months and is divided into three trimesters of 3 months each.

Physical Changes in Pregnancy

Very soon after conception, the body undergoes dramatic changes that allow for the growth and development of the new life carried inside. The changes are the result of hormones secreted by the pituitary gland and the **placenta**, the structure that develops on the inside lining of the uterus during pregnancy and participates in the exchange of gas and nutrients between the pregnant person and the developing baby (called a *fetus*). Prolactin, a hormone secreted by the pituitary gland, causes the breasts to enlarge and prepare for the production of milk to nourish the baby after birth. The uterus enlarges to make room for the growing fetus. More blood is formed to manage the extra demand created by the fetus's need for oxygen and nutrients. The extra blood also helps to remove the extra waste products created by the fetus.

These physical changes can result in many "signs and symptoms" of pregnancy. For example, changes in hormone levels may be responsible for the morning sickness that many have during the first trimester of pregnancy. In a pregnancy that is progressing normally, certain "signs and symptoms" are expected at certain times (Fig. 44-1).

Routine Prenatal Care

Prenatal care, or the health care provided during the pregnancy in the months leading up to birth, helps to ensure the health of both the pregnant parent and the fetus. Routine prenatal care involves screening tests and regular check-ups. The pregnant person is also given advice about how to care for themselves and the developing fetus:

- **Nutrition.** During pregnancy, a person should eat a healthy diet containing a variety of nutritious foods. Because a pregnant person must meet their own body's nutritional needs, plus those of the developing fetus, nutritional needs are increased. For example, because of an increased need for calcium, a pregnant person should consume 3 to 4 servings of dairy foods each day (versus 2 to 3 servings for a person who is not pregnant). Most doctors also suggest that a special prenatal vitamin supplement be taken daily to ensure that nutritional needs are met.

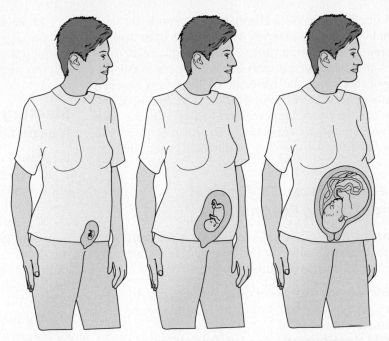

First trimester
- First missed menstrual period
- Morning sickness
- Swollen, tender breasts

Second trimester
- Visibly enlarged uterus
- Weight gain
- Breast enlargement
- Will feel baby move

Third trimester
- Indigestion and shortness of breath (caused by enlarged uterus pressing on stomach and lungs)
- Difficulty sleeping
- Swollen ankles

Figure 44-1 The antepartum period is divided into three trimesters. In a pregnancy that is progressing normally, certain signs and symptoms are expected at certain times.

■ **Avoidance of toxins.** A pregnant person should avoid smoking, drinking alcohol, or taking any medications that have not been specifically approved by their doctor. Many of these substances are known to harm the growth and development of the fetus.

■ **Exercise.** Moderate exercise throughout pregnancy has been shown to have benefits for both the pregnant parent and the fetus. If a pregnant person is interested in either starting an exercise program or continuing one during pregnancy, the health care team will provide information about how to safely do this.

Helping Hands and a Caring Heart

Focus on Humanistic Health Care

When caring for a person who is pregnant, be aware that their feelings may differ from what you consider "normal." Some have mixed emotions when they find out that they are pregnant. The pregnancy may be unplanned, or another child may cause financial hardship for the family. Sometimes there are health concerns associated with the pregnancy. All of these are reasons that an expectant parent may not behave in a "typical" way. It is important to respect your patient's feelings, even if they differ from what yours would be in a similar situation. Also, avoid being judgmental about the relationship status of a pregnant person or other lifestyle choices. Remember that not all pregnant people have (or necessarily want) partners.

Complications During Pregnancy

Prenatal care helps to prevent complications from developing during the pregnancy. It also helps to detect complications at an early stage, should any develop. If a complication develops, the pregnant person may be hospitalized or placed on partial or complete bed rest at home for the rest of the pregnancy to help protect their own health, as well as that of the fetus. Examples of complications that can develop during pregnancy include **preterm labor** (labor begins too early, before the fetus can survive on its own) and **pregnancy-induced hypertension (PIH)**, sometimes called *pre-eclampsia* (when dangerously high blood pressure develops). PIH may lead to **eclampsia** if untreated and cause serious complications or death for both the baby and the pregnant parent. Some pregnancies are "high risk" right from the start—for example, the person has had trouble carrying a baby to term in the past, is carrying more than one baby, or has a chronic health condition such as diabetes. Hospitalization or bed rest may also be ordered at some point during these pregnancies.

A pregnant person who is having, or is at risk for, complications may be hospitalized for weeks or even months prior to the birth of the baby. Depending on the situation, they may be permitted to stay at home with extreme limitations on activity. In this case, they will often need the services of a home health care aide.

Meeting a Person's Physical Needs During Pregnancy

A nursing assistant who is caring for a pregnant person in the hospital or home health care setting may have the following responsibilities:

- **Measuring and recording vital signs.** Any change in vital signs must be reported to the nurse immediately.
- **Obtaining urine samples.** Depending on the situation, the urine samples may need to be provided on a regular basis. The urine is tested for glucose and protein. You may be responsible for obtaining these samples.
- **Helping with personal care.** Many pregnant people who are on bed rest are allowed to get up to go to the bathroom, but they will need assistance with bathing in bed and grooming. If the patient is not allowed to get out of bed at all, then they will also need assistance with toileting.

Tell the Nurse!

Complications during a pregnancy can endanger the life of both the pregnant person and the baby if they are not reported promptly. When caring for a pregnant person, report the following observations to the nurse immediately:

- There is a change in vital signs (especially an elevated blood pressure or body temperature)
- The person complains of a headache or of seeing "spots" or "bright flashes" in front of their eyes
- The person faints or is dizzy
- The person has nausea, vomiting, or diarrhea
- The person complains of abdominal pain
- The person is experiencing uterine contractions that are frequent or severe and are not relieved by resting
- The person has vaginal bleeding or there is fluid leaking from the vagina

Make sure you follow all directions that are given to you regarding the care required, and ask the nurse for help if you are unsure about how to complete any of your assigned duties.

Meeting a Person's Emotional Needs During Pregnancy

Pregnancy can be a time of great joy and anticipation. It can also be a time of great stress, especially if complications develop that jeopardize the person's health and that of the baby.

A pregnant person who is experiencing complications and has been placed on partial or complete bed rest prior to the birth of the child may have many emotional needs. They may feel lonely and bored—imagine what it would be like to be stuck in the same bed, in the same room, for weeks, or even months. Making pleasant conversation as you complete your duties can help to ease this loneliness. The person may also have lots of worries. They may be worried about their own health and that of their unborn child. They may worry about children they already have and how they are being cared for in their absence. They may worry about how they will pay for bills during the time that they cannot work. Taking the time to listen to these concerns and reporting them to the nurse is important (Fig. 44-2).

Sometimes pregnancy does not end with the birth of a healthy baby. Many pregnancies result in miscarriage. Some babies are born too early to survive on their own, and they die. Some babies are stillborn (born dead). The loss of a child is an emotional time for the family. Loss affects each person differently. Be respectful of the family's feelings. Acknowledge the loss, and simply say "I'm sorry."

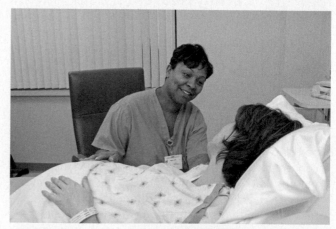

Figure 44-2 A pregnant person who is having complications is likely to be lonely, bored, scared, or all three. Making yourself available to listen is part of providing humanistic care.

LABOR AND DELIVERY

Labor

When it is time for a baby to be born, the pituitary gland releases oxytocin, a hormone that stimulates the uterus to contract. The contractions of the uterus squeeze the baby downward, forcing the head against the cervix so that it opens, or *dilates*. This process is known as **labor**. The length of time labor occurs varies greatly from person to person. Some people have very short labors, while other labors may last as long as 36 hours or so. When caring for a person who is in labor, your responsibilities will be defined by facility policy. In many cases, your only responsibility will be to measure and record vital signs and other observations. However, some facilities or birth centers provide additional training, which will allow you to perform more specialized tasks when assisting during labor.

Taking It to the Next Level:

Advanced Skills

More in-depth information related to advanced skills when caring for a person having a baby can be found in *Lippincott Acute Care Skills for Advanced Nursing Assistants*.

Visit thePoint® at thepoint.lww.com for access to the ebook.

Delivery

A person may deliver (give birth to) the baby vaginally or by cesarean section (Fig. 44-3). Delivery of the baby through the vagina (a vaginal delivery) is usually preferred, unless there are complications. A **cesarean section** (delivery of the baby through a surgical incision made in the abdomen) is done when a vaginal delivery is not possible or safe for the parent or baby. For example, many doctors choose to do a cesarean section when labor has gone on for too long, when the baby is not positioned correctly for a vaginal delivery, or when the birthing parent has a serious health problem (such as heart disease) that would make a prolonged labor dangerous. Because a cesarean section is a surgical procedure, the recovery time following a cesarean delivery is generally longer than the recovery time following a vaginal delivery.

Women who give birth vaginally may choose to deliver with or without pain medications. Many women choose to have an **epidural block**, which is anesthesia given through a catheter that is placed in the spinal canal. The catheter is placed in the lower back, so that the anesthetic affects only the pelvis and legs. This allows the person to be awake and participate fully in the birth of the child while numbing the pain of labor.

A person who gives birth by cesarean section is having major abdominal surgery and therefore requires an anesthetic of some sort. The person may be given an epidural block or, in some cases, general anesthesia. An incision is then made in the abdomen, and the baby is lifted out of the uterus. After delivery, the incision is closed, and the birthing parent recovers in the same manner as with any other type of operation (see Chapter 43).

Immediately Following Delivery

Immediately following the birth of the baby, if the baby is breathing well and otherwise stable, they may be handed directly to their parent for a few moments.

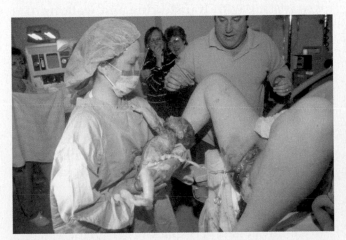

A. Vaginal delivery

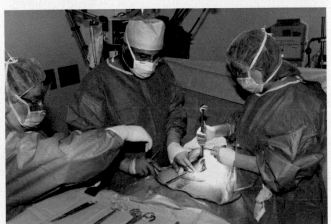

B. Cesarean delivery

Figure 44-3 A baby may be delivered (**A**) vaginally or (**B**) by cesarean section. (*A*, © *B. Proud.*)

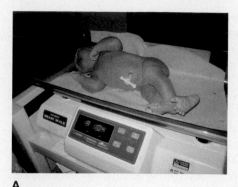

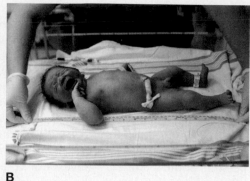

A   **B**

Figure 44-4 The baby is (**A**) weighed and (**B**) measured.

Then, the baby is weighed and measured and evaluated by the nurse or doctor (Fig. 44-4). The baby's footprints are taken, and identification bracelets are applied to their wrists and ankles. Because it takes a while for a newborn's body to adjust to life outside of the womb, the baby may be placed for a short period of time in a special bed to help keep them warm. A temperature monitor may be taped to the baby's skin, or you may need to measure the baby's axillary temperature as often as ordered or until the baby's temperature has stabilized. Once the baby's temperature has stabilized, they will be given a bath to remove blood and **vernix**, a protective, cheese-like substance that is present on the skin of newborns. Finally, the baby is wrapped snugly in a blanket; a soft, stretchy cap is put on the baby's head to prevent heat loss; and the baby is placed in the waiting arms of their parents.

The first hour or two immediately following delivery is important for parent–infant bonding. This **bonding period** helps to develop emotional and physical attachment. It is important to remember the importance of the bonding process for the non-birthing parent, as well (Fig. 44-5).

THE POSTPARTUM PERIOD

During the **postpartum period** (the 6-week period of time following the birth), you may be involved in the care of both the parent who has just given birth and the new baby.

Care of the Birthing Parent

Birth is a stressful, difficult activity affecting the entire body. After delivery, the birthing parent will likely be tired, hungry, and thirsty. They may want to sleep, especially if the labor was long and difficult. They may only want privacy, to cuddle and get to know their new baby.

When caring for a person who has just delivered a baby, you will have several general responsibilities, including:

- **Taking vital signs as ordered.** You will need to take the person's vital signs as often as ordered. As always, any change in vital signs should be reported immediately.
- **Assisting with transferring and walking.** If the person has had an epidural block, they may be unsteady on their feet for some time after delivery and will need help with transferring and walking.
- **Assisting with toileting.** Assist the new parent to the bathroom, or provide a bedpan if needed. Measure and record the amount of urine voided. Many people experience swelling after delivery and may not be able to void. If this is the case with your patient, tell the nurse. The patient may need to be catheterized.
- **Observing.** A complication that develops during the immediate postpartum period can become life-threatening very quickly. Being observant can make the difference between life and death for the new parent.

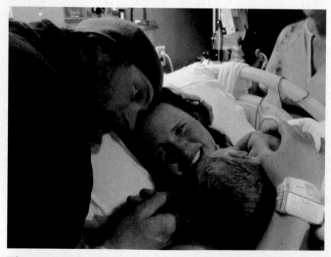

Figure 44-5 The first 1 to 2 hours following birth is a critical time for parents to bond with their newborn, and vice versa.

You may also have additional responsibilities, as described in the sections that follow.

Managing Vaginal Discharge

Vaginal discharge occurs following delivery. This discharge, called **lochia**, changes over the days and weeks following delivery:

■ *Lochia rubra.* Initially, the discharge is bright red and is called *lochia rubra* (*rubra* means "red"). Special pads may be worn to collect this flow, which may last for 2 to 3 days. If a person is recovering from a cesarean section or is on bed rest for other reasons, you may have to assist with changing these pads. Note the amount and color of the discharge and report your observations to the nurse. Remember that vaginal secretions should be handled according to standard precautions. Always wear gloves any time you might come into contact with soiled pads, bed linens, or bed protectors.

■ *Lochia serosa* follows for approximately 3 to 10 days longer. Serosa is a pink- or brown-tinged fluid. Any large clots are abnormal and should be reported immediately.

■ *Lochia alba* follows for another week or two and is mostly creamy white to yellowish in color (*alba* means "white").

Assisting With Perineal Care

If the person delivered their baby vaginally, they may have perineal tears caused by the baby's head as it exited the birth canal. Sometimes, doctors perform an episiotomy to prevent the perineum from tearing so much. An **episiotomy** is an incision made in the perineum to enlarge the vaginal opening, making delivery of the baby's head easier. If the perineum was torn during the delivery, or if an episiotomy was done, the perineum will be sore and tender for several days and the new parent may find sitting uncomfortable.

Ice may be applied to the perineum for a period of time immediately following delivery to help prevent swelling. Afterward, the use of sitz baths may help ease the discomfort. A **sitz bath** is a warm water soak for the perineal area. The basin, which usually fits over the toilet seat, is filled with warm water (105° to 110°F [40.5° to 43.4°C]) and the person sits in it for the prescribed amount of time. Be sure to follow the nursing care plan; the maximum amount of time allowed is 20 minutes. After the sitz bath, help the person to stand up. They may be dizzy because the warm water causes the blood vessels to dilate. Depending on facility policy, birthing parents may also be instructed to cleanse the perineal area after each trip to the bathroom by spraying warm water over the area using a small plastic sprayer. Increased pain, swelling, or drainage from the episiotomy site could indicate an infection and should be reported immediately to the nurse.

Assisting With Breastfeeding

Many people choose to breastfeed their babies. Immediately following delivery of the baby, the breasts produce **colostrum**, a thin yellowish fluid that contains extra calories and protein, as well as important antibodies. Colostrum is usually secreted for 2 to 3 days after birth and is then replaced by breast milk. Breastfeeding requires that extra calories and fluids be consumed. Therefore, you should offer fresh water frequently, as directed by the nurse.

Breasts may become swollen and painful when the milk comes in. Frequent nursing of the infant will help to ease the discomfort, which usually only lasts for a couple of days. The appearance of a painful lump, reddened areas, or an elevated temperature could indicate a breast infection and should be reported immediately to the nurse.

If a person chooses to breastfeed their baby, the nurse will teach them how. You may need to help them get in a comfortable position, especially if they have had a cesarean section or an episiotomy. Help to first wash their hands and then gently clean the nipple of the breast with warm water. Next, hand the baby to them. There are several different ways to hold a baby during breastfeeding. With time, a parent will usually find the way of holding the baby that works best for them. Have the parent stroke the baby's cheek with their nipple to stimulate the baby's rooting reflex. The baby will turn their head toward the breast and open their mouth. All

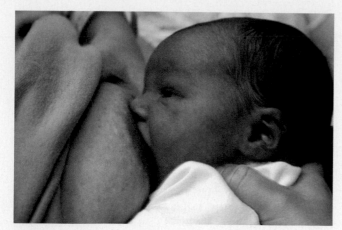

Figure 44-6 When breastfeeding, the baby's mouth covers both the nipple and the areola.

of the nipple and part of the *areola* (the colored portion of the breast surrounding the nipple) need to be placed into the baby's mouth (Fig. 44-6). As the baby sucks on the breast, the parent may experience cramping pains in the lower abdomen. This is normal. After the baby has finished feeding from the first breast, have the parent insert their finger gently into the baby's mouth to break the suction before they remove them from the breast. After burping the baby, the process is repeated with the other breast.

After the baby has finished nursing, have the parent allow their nipples to air-dry. Any colostrum or breast milk remaining on the nipples will help protect the nipples from drying and cracking. Soap should not be used because it can cause dryness or irritation of the nipples. Some people use special creams or ointments when they first start breastfeeding to help keep the nipples from cracking and becoming sore. Some find that a supportive nursing bra is more comfortable than a regular bra, while others do not.

Care of the Baby

A newborn is considered a neonate for the first 28 days of their life. You may help to care for a neonate in the hospital or birth center, or in the home as a home health aide. You may also find yourself caring for older babies, especially if you work in the home health care setting or in the pediatrics unit of a hospital.

Taking Vital Signs

You may be responsible for taking vital signs on the newborn infant. If the baby is in the room with the parents, make sure you explain what you are going to do before beginning.

■ A newborn's temperature may be measured either by the axillary or temporal method (Fig. 44-7).

> ## Tell the Nurse!
>
> A baby can become very sick very quickly. When caring for an infant, report any of the following observations to the nurse immediately:
>
> ● The baby appears weak or "floppy"
>
> ● The baby is pale
>
> ● The baby cries, and nothing you try makes them stop
>
> ● The baby's temperature is abnormal (either high or low)
>
> ● The baby's heart rate is abnormal (either fast or slow)
>
> ● The baby is breathing rapidly and shallowly
>
> ● The baby cannot be wakened
>
> ● The baby has a rash
>
> ● The baby will not eat
>
> ● The baby's eyes are red or discolored
>
> ● The baby has vomited

Rectal temperatures are not routinely taken on newborns. The range of normal is 97.6° to 98.6°F (36.6° to 37°C).

■ A newborn's apical pulse is taken for a full minute by listening (auscultating) with a stethoscope over the heart. The normal heart rate in a newborn is 110 to 160 beats/minute. A newborn's respirations are also counted for a full minute by watching the abdomen rise and fall. The normal respiratory rate in a newborn is 30 to 60 breaths/minute. Vital signs taken on a crying baby are not going to be accurate, so it is best to measure

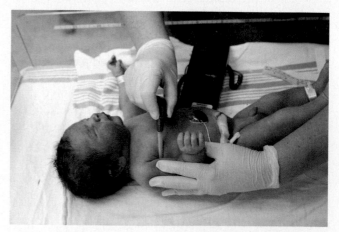

Figure 44-7 A newborn's temperature is measured using either the axillary or temporal method. The axillary method is shown here.

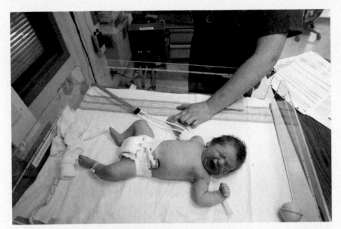

Figure 44-8 A newborn's blood pressure may be measured manually or using an electronic measuring device. Here, an electronic measuring device is being used. Note the very small cuff, which is sized according to the baby's weight.

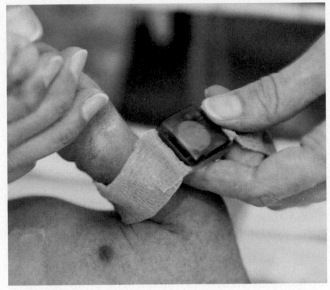

Figure 44-9 Protecting the security of the newborn is very important. Many facilities attach a sensor device to the newborn's arm (shown here) or umbilical cord stump (see Fig. 44-10). If someone tries to remove the baby from the unit, the device sounds an alarm.

the baby's pulse and respirations while the baby is sleeping, if possible.

■ A newborn's blood pressure is measured in the baby's arm using a cuff specifically sized according to the babys weight (Fig. 44-8). Most facilities use electronic blood pressure devices for taking a newborn's blood pressure. These devices inflate the cuff and measure the blood pressure automatically. The range of normal for a newborn is 50 to 80 mm Hg systolic, 30 to 50 mm Hg diastolic.

Ensuring Security

If you work in the postpartum unit of a hospital or in a birthing center, there will be many policies and procedures in place to ensure the security of the newborn (Fig. 44-9). These security measures are taken to prevent newborns from being kidnapped from the facility by people posing as relatives or health care workers. Always follow the security procedures in place at your facility. These procedures usually require visitors to sign in. The baby is brought from and returned to the nursery by a member of the health care team. Finally, the identification bands on the baby's wrist and ankle are always checked against the parent's identification band before the baby is handed to the parent. The identification bands cannot be removed until after the baby goes home with their parents.

Caring for the Umbilical Cord Stump

The **umbilical cord** carries oxygen and nutrients from the placenta to the growing fetus. When the baby is born, the umbilical cord is clamped and cut. Eventually, the "stump" (the part of the cord that remains) dries up and falls off, leaving behind the navel (or belly button). Until the stump dries up and falls off, it must be cared for properly to prevent

infection (Fig. 44-10). Make sure you perform proper hand hygiene and wear gloves before touching the area around the stump. If necessary, clean the skin surrounding the stump with a mild baby soap and warm water. Keep the area dry. Fold the diaper down in front so that it does not cover the stump. If the stump or surrounding area is red, bleeding, or has any drainage, tell the nurse. The baby should not be given a complete bath (in a bath basin) until the umbilical

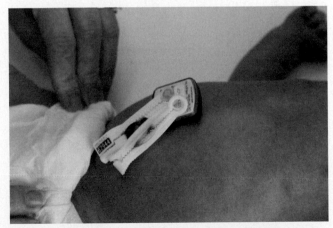

Figure 44-10 Proper care of the umbilical cord stump is necessary to prevent infection. At each diaper change, the umbilical cord stump and surrounding skin is observed for drainage and redness, and the diaper is folded down so that it does not cover the stump. The stump will dry up and fall off in about 10 days.

cord stump has dried up and fallen off. This usually occurs within about 10 days of the birth.

Providing Circumcision Care

Circumcision is the surgical removal of the foreskin from the head of the penis. Many studies have been done regarding the long-term benefits and risks associated with circumcision. To date, whether to circumcise or not remains largely a matter of parental choice. Circumcision is also a rite of some religious faiths.

The circumcision is done using local anesthetic. The procedure can be performed at the hospital before the baby is discharged home, or it may be done at the doctor's office. Following circumcision, the penis should be kept clean and dry. A petrolatum dressing may be applied to keep the penis from sticking to the diaper. Depending on the technique used for the circumcision, petroleum jelly or an ointment may be applied around the circumcision site at each diaper change for the first 24 to 48 hours. Be sure to follow any specific instructions that are given to you regarding care of the circumcision.

The baby's penis will be red and sore (Fig. 44-11). If you notice bleeding, drainage, or odor when you are changing the baby's diaper, tell the nurse. The circumcision should heal within 10 to 14 days. After the circumcision has healed, the baby can be given a complete bath in a bath basin.

Feeding

Babies who are not being breastfed are fed with a bottle. The bottle may contain breast milk or a prepared formula. Infants who are younger than 1 year should not be fed cow's milk, as it can cause the baby to develop food allergies. In addition, it does not contain many of the nutrients that are essential for the baby's growth.

Many commercial formula preparations are available. Some formulas come prepared and ready to feed to the baby, while others are in the form of a powder or a concentrated liquid that must be mixed with water prior to feeding (Fig. 44-12A). Make sure you follow the instructions on the label carefully

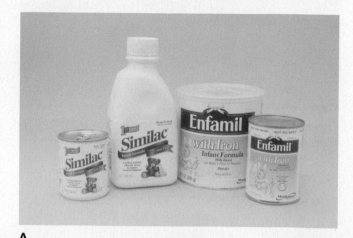

A

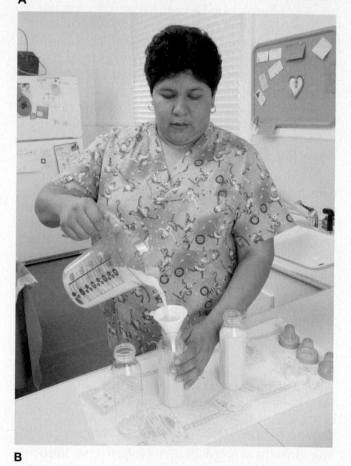

B

Figure 44-12 Babies who are not breastfed are bottle fed. **A.** Many types of prepared formulas for bottle feeding are available. **B.** When preparing bottles, always be sure to mix the formula according to the label instructions if the formula is not "ready-to-feed."

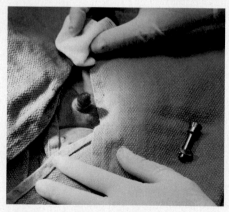

Figure 44-11 Following circumcision, the penis will be red and sore, but there should not be any bleeding, discharge, or odor. Report any of these observations to the nurse immediately.

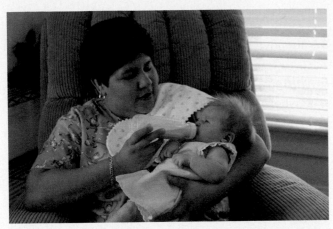

Figure 44-13 Always hold a baby upright to feed them.

movement. Disposable diapers are very absorbent, allowing the baby to urinate several times before a change is necessary. An infant usually urinates six to ten times each day. The frequency of bowel movements depends on whether the baby is fed breast milk or formula.

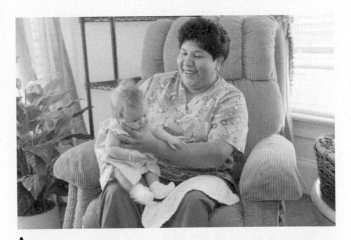

A

when preparing infant formula, so that the prepared formula is neither too strong nor too weak. Often, several bottles are prepared at once and stored in the refrigerator (see Fig. 44-12B). Before preparing a bottle, wash your hands thoroughly.

Prepared bottles that have been stored in the refrigerator will need to be brought to room temperature before feeding the baby. To warm the bottle, place the prepared bottle in a container of warm water. Check the temperature of the bottle by shaking a few drops of the formula onto your wrist before feeding the baby. Never use a microwave to warm the bottle. Microwaving can cause the formula inside the bottle to become very hot in some spots while remaining cool in others. When you test the formula on your wrist, the "hot spots" might go undetected. The hot formula will then burn the baby's mouth when they swallow it.

Hold the baby upright during bottle feeding (Fig. 44-13). Never prop the bottle up during feeding, or lay the baby down to take the bottle. After every few ounces of formula, stop feeding the baby so that they can burp. Burping gets rid of the excess air that is swallowed during feeding. The baby can be burped in several ways (Fig. 44-14). Hold the baby upright on your knee, or place the baby over your shoulder, and gently rub or pat their back. Be patient—some infants burp easily, while others may need more time.

Bottles, nipples, and rings should be cleaned in the dishwasher. They can also be washed by hand in hot, soapy water and rinsed well. Bottles do not need to be boiled for sterility, unless the doctor specifies that this should be done. In a hospital setting, disposable bottles are usually used.

Diapering

Infants are diapered using disposable or cloth diapers. To prevent diaper rash and skin breakdown, change the baby's diaper every time the baby has a bowel

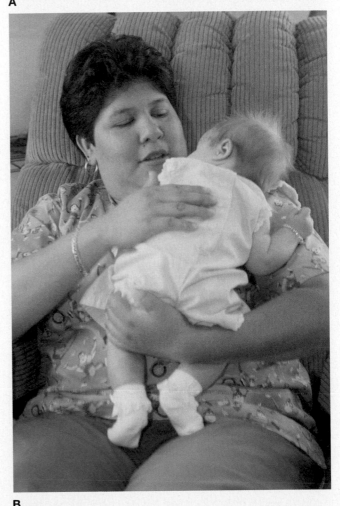

B

Figure 44-14 To burp the baby, (**A**) hold them upright on your knee, or (**B**) place them over your shoulder.

To change a diaper:

1. Perform hand hygiene and gather your supplies. It is important to gather all of your supplies first because you must never leave a baby alone, even for a moment. Even very young infants can easily roll off the changing table or other surface, leading to serious injury.

2. Put on gloves, and remove the soiled diaper. Clean the perineal area, wiping from front to back if the baby is female. The perineal area can be cleansed with baby wipes (soft disposable wet cloths that contain a cleansing agent) or with a warm, wet washcloth. A mild baby soap may be used in addition to a warm, wet washcloth if the baby had a bowel movement. Be sure to rinse and dry the area thoroughly. Apply diaper rash ointment or a light dusting of cornstarch powder, if used. Remove your soiled gloves and put on a clean pair.

3. Position the clean diaper, fastening it with the provided tabs. Place the baby in an infant carrier or some other secure place.

4. Dispose of the soiled diaper in an appropriate waste container. Before placing a cloth diaper that is soiled with stool in the diaper pail, rinse it in cool water to prevent the stool from drying in the diaper.

5. Remove your gloves and perform hand hygiene.

Bathing

A newborn infant is given a complete bath at birth. Once the umbilical cord stump has fallen off and the circumcision has healed (if the baby was circumcised), the baby may be given a complete bath in a bath basin on a routine basis. It is usually not necessary to fully bathe the baby every day. Until that time, partial baths (sponge baths) are given as needed.

To bathe a baby in a bath basin:

1. Perform hand hygiene and gather all of your supplies. It is important to gather all of your supplies first because you must never leave a baby alone in a bath or on a surface.

2. Fill the bath basin with only 1 to 2 inches of warm water. Check the water temperature with a bath thermometer or the inside of your wrist before putting the baby in the bath basin (Fig. 44-15A). The temperature should be between 100° and 105°F (37.8° and 40.5°C).

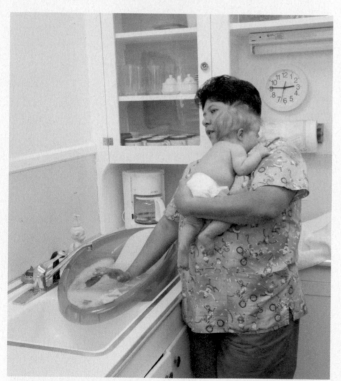

A. Check the water temperature.

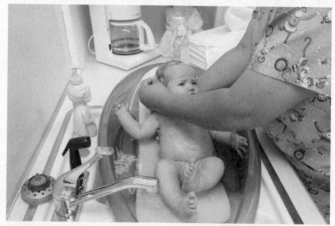

B. Wash the baby's hair.

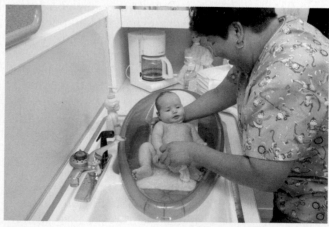

C. Wash the baby's body.

Figure 44-15 Bathing a baby. **A.** The bath basin is only filled to a depth of 1 to 2 inches. Always check the temperature of the bath water before you put the baby in it. **B.** Wash the baby's hair first. **C.** Then wash the baby's body.

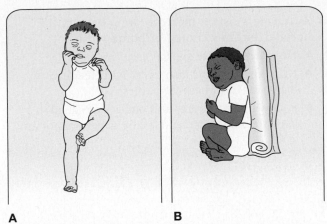

A   **B**

Figure 44-16 A baby is placed on their back or side to sleep, never on their abdomen. **A.** Positioning on the back. **B.** Positioning on the side. Note the rolled receiving blanket bolstering the baby's back.

3. Place the baby in the bath basin. Lather the baby's hair with a baby shampoo and rinse well (see Fig. 44-15B). Next, use a washcloth and soap formulated for infant skin. Wash the baby's face first. Then move on to the rest of the body, making sure to rinse all soap from the skin (see Fig. 44-15C). Keep a firm grip on the baby at all times and work quickly to avoid chilling the baby.

4. After the bath, dry the baby thoroughly. Baby lotion may be applied as desired.

Putting a Baby Down to Sleep

A baby should be placed on their back or side to sleep. Research has shown that positioning babies on their backs or sides is safer than positioning them on their abdomen (Fig. 44-16). When placing a baby on their side to sleep, roll a receiving blanket or towel and tuck it securely next to the baby's back. This will help the baby to stay in the side-lying position. Remove all blankets, pillows, and toys from the sleeping area. These items pose a suffocation risk (the baby may get tangled in them and not be able to breathe). Instead of using blankets, place the baby in a blanket sleeper to keep them warm.

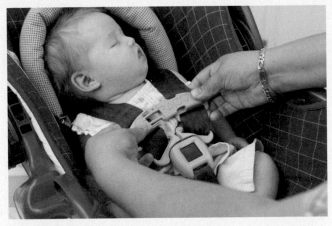

Figure 44-17 A baby may also sleep in a carrier. Always make sure to secure the baby in the carrier.

A baby can also be placed in an infant carrier to sleep. After putting the baby in the carrier, make sure that the carrier straps are properly secured (Fig. 44-17). Place the carrier on a low, level surface (such as the floor) so that it does not tip. Make sure that the carrier is out of the reach of pets or other small children who could accidentally knock the carrier over. Never place an infant carrier on a table or counter.

Transporting a Baby

A baby's first ride in a car seat occurs when the parents leave the hospital or birthing center. In all states, it is against the law to transport a baby in a car without first properly securing them in a car seat. You may need to help the parents install the car seat correctly, and show them how to place the baby in it. Written instructions for installation are provided with the car seat packaging. Instructions for installation can also be found on many manufacturers' websites.

An infant car seat is placed in the back seat. The baby faces the back of the car, not the front. This is safer in the event of an accident. An infant car seat is required until the child reaches the age of 1 year and weighs more than 20 pounds. The use of car seats for older babies and children is discussed in Chapter 45.

SUMMARY

- Nursing assistants often are involved in the care of pregnant people, people who are in labor or have just given birth, and newborns.
  - Complications during pregnancy can require complete or partial bed rest, either at home

or in the hospital, for weeks or even months before delivery.

- When assisting a person who is in labor, the nursing assistant is usually only responsible for measuring and recording vital signs and other observations, unless they have received advanced training from the facility.

- Following delivery, the nursing assistant cares for both the birthing parent and the baby.
- During the postpartum period, the nursing assistant helps the birthing parent recover.

- A nursing assistant may care for a baby in the hospital, birthing center, or home setting.
  - Neonates require special care.
  - Nursing assistants also assist with feeding, diapering, and bathing babies.
  - Following procedures and policies designed to keep the infant safe and secure is very important.

WHAT DID YOU LEARN?

Multiple Choice

Select the single best answer for each of the following questions.

1. Mrs. Gutierrez had an episiotomy during the birth of her baby. What might the nursing assistant do to help relieve the soreness and tenderness at the episiotomy site?
   a. Apply triple antibiotic ointment to the perineum
   b. Give Mrs. Gutierrez a bed bath
   c. Assist Mrs. Gutierrez with a sitz bath
   d. Avoid washing the area until the episiotomy has healed

2. What is the period of time after delivery during which the parents and the new baby develop an emotional and physical attachment called?
   a. The epidural period
   b. The prenatal period
   c. The bonding period
   d. The antepartum period

3. You are caring for Ms. Bergen, who just had a baby. Which of the following observations should you report immediately to the nurse?
   a. Ms. Bergen has what you think is an abnormal amount of vaginal discharge
   b. Ms. Bergen's pulse rate is elevated
   c. Ms. Bergen's blood pressure is low
   d. All of the above

4. Mrs. Ling has just delivered a baby by cesarean section. You are helping her to breastfeed her baby, and she complains of cramping in her lower abdomen while the baby nurses. What is this a sign of?
   a. Mrs. Ling may be hemorrhaging
   b. The baby is kicking her in the stomach
   c. Cramping in the abdomen is a normal response during breastfeeding
   d. Mrs. Ling is not holding the baby correctly for breastfeeding

5. In what position should an infant be placed to sleep?
   a. On their back
   b. On their abdomen
   c. On their side
   d. Either on the back or side

6. Which of the following observations would be a cause for alarm when caring for a baby?
   a. The baby is pale
   b. The baby cries all the time, no matter what you do
   c. The baby will not eat
   d. All of the above

7. A couple is going home from the hospital today with their new baby. How should the car seat be placed?
   a. In the front seat, facing the back of the car
   b. In the back seat, facing the back of the car
   c. In the back seat, facing the front of the car
   d. It makes no difference, as long as the baby is secure

8. You are checking vital signs on a newborn. Which one of the following measurements would you report to the nurse immediately?
   a. Heart rate 80 beats/minute, respiratory rate 20 breaths/minute
   b. Heart rate 160 beats/minute, respiratory rate 34 breaths/minute
   c. Heart rate 152 beats/minute, respiratory rate 58 breaths/minute
   d. None of the above

Matching *Match each numbered item with its appropriate lettered description.*

_____ **1.** Lochia

_____ **2.** Colostrum

_____ **3.** Vernix

a. Whitish, cheese-like protective coating on the skin of newborns

b. Vaginal discharge following the birth of a baby

c. Thin, yellowish fluid produced by the breasts before the milk comes in; rich in calories, protein, and antibodies

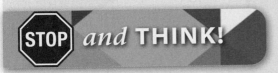

- You work in the newborn nursery at your local hospital. The other nursing assistant who works in the nursery with you, Shelly, has just left to take a baby to their parent for the noon feeding. You are attending to the other babies, when a pleasant-looking woman approaches and asks to see the new Sitko baby. She explains that she is the baby's grandmother, and she has just arrived from out of town to visit her son, daughter-in-law, and new grandchild. How would you respond to this request?

- Donna is a home health care aide who has been assigned to care for Mrs. Upchurch and her new baby, David. David was born very prematurely and spent several months in the hospital, but now the doctors have allowed him to come home. David still has numerous problems related to his premature birth, but coming home is a big milestone. Donna cannot help but notice that Mrs. Upchurch does not seem to be as thrilled about David's homecoming as Donna herself would be. Mrs. Upchurch seems very high-strung and almost frightened of the baby. In addition, she cries frequently. Why might Mrs. Upchurch be feeling this way? If you were Donna, how would you behave around Mrs. Upchurch?

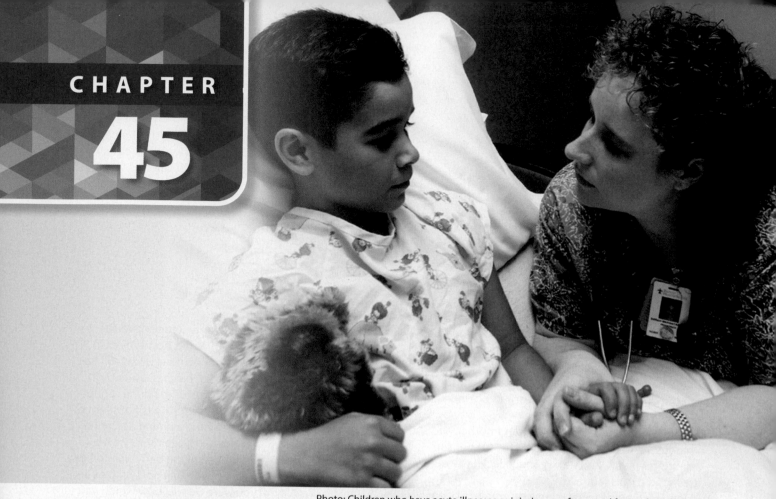

Photo: Children who have acute illnesses or injuries are often cared for in a hospital setting.

Caring for Pediatric Patients

 WHAT WILL YOU LEARN?

Children receive health care in many different types of health care settings. For example, children who have acute illnesses or injuries are often cared for in a hospital setting. Children who need regular therapy or medical treatment for congenital or chronic health conditions may receive this care in a hospital, clinic, or home health care setting. Other children are residents of long-term care facilities because of developmental disabilities, injuries, or illnesses. Although many of the procedures used to provide physical care to a child are very similar to those used with adults, it is very important to remember that children are not simply "little adults." In this chapter, you will learn about the unique physical and emotional needs of children of different ages. You will also learn about your role in reporting suspected cases of child abuse. When you have finished with this chapter, you will be able to:

1. **Understand how the stages of development affect the emotional needs of children in health care settings.**
2. **Discuss the specific physical needs that children in health care settings have, including infants, toddlers, preschoolers, school-aged children, and adolescents.**

3. Describe measures that the nursing assistant can use to help meet the physical and emotional needs of infants, toddlers, preschoolers, school-aged children, and adolescents in a health care setting.

4. List safety considerations that are specific for infants, toddlers, preschoolers, school-aged children, and adolescents.

5. Discuss signs of child abuse and the nursing assistant's role in reporting suspected abuse.

Vocabulary

Failure to thrive   Magical thinking   Shaken baby syndrome
Regress   Egocentric   Munchausen syndrome by proxy

INTRODUCTION TO CARING FOR PEDIATRIC PATIENTS

In Chapter 6, you learned about the stages of growth and development that we all pass through as we live our lives. An understanding of the basic stages of growth and development will better prepare you to provide the type of care that each child requires.

Remember that childhood is a time of rapid growth and development. A child's physical and emotional needs change constantly as they grow. Although only a few years separate a 3-year-old from an 8-year-old, there is a huge difference between these two age groups in terms of growth and development. Think about what a frightening place a health care setting must be to a child. A child's ability to understand and cooperate with the health care team depends on their particular stage of development. A child, especially a very young child, does not understand illness and pain.

Think also about the effect a child's illness has on the family as a whole. If the child's injury or illness is severe or acute, family members may wonder whether the child will survive the event and, if they do, what effect the illness or injury will have on their future growth and development. Sometimes, a child's illness requires one family member to travel to a distant health care facility to be with the child, while the rest of the family stays at home. Families may worry about how they will pay for the health care that the child is receiving. The other children in the family may feel "left out" while most of the family's attention is focused on the child who is sick or injured. Including the child's family members in their care whenever possible is one thing you can do to help the family better cope with a child's illness (Fig. 45-1). The family members will feel like they are actively doing something to help the child, and the child will be happier being cared for by familiar people.

When working with children and families, remember that families come in all different shapes and sizes. Many families are "traditional," in the sense that they consist of two parents and one or more children. However, many families consist of only one parent and the children. Children may also be raised by grandparents, guardians, foster parents, or other caregivers. Regardless of the family structure, the effects of a child's illness on the people who care about the child are the same.

Taking It to the Next Level:
Advanced Skills

More in-depth information related to advanced skills when caring for children can be found in *Lippincott Acute Care Skills for Advanced Nursing Assistants*.

Visit thePoint® at thepoint.lww.com for access to the ebook.

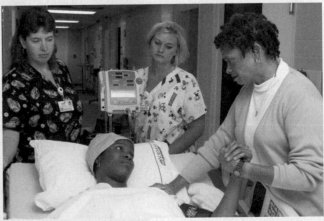

Figure 45-1 A child's illness can be very stressful for the family.

CARING FOR INFANTS

Infancy is the period of time from a child's birth to their first birthday. Infants grow and develop very rapidly during the first year of life. They progress from being totally helpless—unable to roll over, sit up, or move about without help—to being able to crawl, walk, and feed themselves small pieces of food by the time they reach the age of 1 year.

Meeting the Infant's Physical Needs

An infant is totally dependent on their caregiver to help them meet their most basic physical needs. The procedures for feeding, diapering, bathing, and positioning a newborn that you learned in Chapter 44 apply for older infants as well. In addition, you may be responsible for monitoring food and fluid intake and output, and for monitoring the infant's temperature:

- **Monitoring food and fluid intake and output.** An infant who is ill or unable to drink or eat properly can quickly become dehydrated. An infant who is receiving adequate food and fluid will urinate regularly and have regular bowel movements. Since it is not possible to know exactly how much breast milk a nursing infant is taking at each feeding, keeping track of the number of wet diapers or weighing the wet diapers may be necessary to ensure that the baby is not dehydrated. Observing and recording the number, consistency, and amount of bowel movements may also be one of your responsibilities.
- **Monitoring body temperature.** An infant, especially one who is ill or very young, must be kept warm. A very small infant can be swaddled securely in a blanket. An older, more mobile infant can be clothed in snuggly one-piece pajamas if the weather is cold. A change in body temperature (either above or below the normal range) is cause for concern and should be reported immediately.

Because an infant's medical condition can change very quickly, you must report any unusual signs or symptoms (see Chapter 44) to the nurse immediately.

Meeting the Infant's Emotional Needs

Aside from being clean, warm, and fed, an infant's greatest need is to feel secure. Infants need to be spoken to or sung to softly (Fig. 45-2). They need to be rocked gently, touched, and held. Human contact is essential for an infant to develop physically and emotionally. Many studies have shown that infants, even those who are well cared for physically, fail to grow

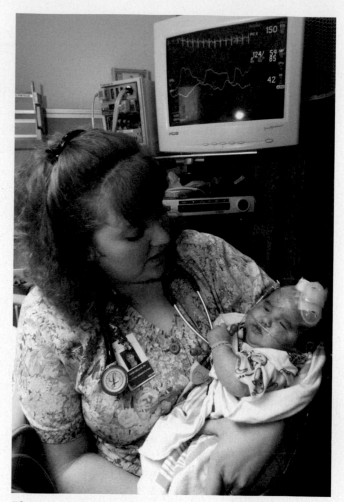

Figure 45-2 The infant's greatest emotional need is to feel safe and secure. Infants need to be held, cuddled, rocked, and spoken or sung to.

and develop both physically and emotionally if they are not held and talked to. This is called **failure to thrive**.

To help meet an infant's emotional needs, you must take the time to touch, cuddle, stroke, and talk soothingly to them. Encourage family members to hold the baby if the baby's condition allows. The nurse can show family members how to hold the baby without disturbing medical devices, such as monitors and tubes. Provide music and infant-appropriate toys. If possible, position the infant's bed so that they can watch activity through a window or a doorway.

Meeting the Infant's Need for Safety

Safety and the prevention of accidents are essential for children of all ages, but especially for the youngest. As helpless as they may seem, infants can wriggle, roll, and twist themselves into dangerous situations very quickly.

- Never leave an infant on a surface unattended, even for a moment. Even very young infants can easily roll off of a bed, changing table, or examination table. An infant who falls to the floor could receive severe or fatal head injuries. If you are changing diapers, taking vital signs, or bathing an infant, keep one hand on the child at all times to prevent a fall.

■ As the infant grows and is placed in an infant carrier, swing, or high chair, make sure that safety straps are securely fastened both across the infant's chest and shoulders and between their legs to prevent them from falling out of or sliding down in the carrier, swing, or chair.

■ Infants should sleep on their backs in a safety-approved crib. Do not place bumper pads, blankets, pillows, or stuffed toys in the bed with the baby. According to the CDC, nearly 1,000 infants die each year from accidental suffocation.

■ Always secure the infant in a car seat when traveling in a car or other vehicle. An infant car seat is placed in the back seat. The baby faces the back of the car, not the front.

■ An infant explores the world by placing everything they can get their hands on in their mouth. Make sure that toys are age-appropriate and that they have no small, removable parts that the infant could choke on. Clean the toys by washing them frequently in warm, soapy water and rinsing them thoroughly. As the infant learns to crawl and move about, make sure that the floor or play area is free of small objects or plants that the infant could place in their mouth.

■ Keep plastic bags and balloons away from infants. A young infant could roll over and become tangled in a plastic bag. An older infant could put the bag over their head. The infant is unable to breathe through the plastic, and suffocates. Balloons are also a suffocation risk. The infant may put the balloon (or a piece of a broken balloon) in their mouth. When the infant inhales, the rubber balloon gets sucked into the airway, blocking air flow and leading to suffocation.

■ Do not leave an infant unattended, even for a moment, in water of any depth. Babies who can stand up have drowned in a mop bucket.

■ Make sure that electrical cords and window blind cords are out of the reach of the infant. The infant could become tangled in the cord and strangle themself. Or, they could put the electrical cord in their mouth, which could result in electrocution.

These are just a few of the many safety concerns that you must be aware of when caring for very small children. A primary rule of thumb is that if a child can reach an object, they will grab it and try to put it in their mouth. Child-proofing everything, whether in the home or the health care setting, is critical for the safety of the infant.

CARING FOR TODDLERS

A toddler is a child between the ages of 1 and 3 years. Toddlers are mobile, curious, and independent. They explore everything. Toddlers can feed themselves and are busy learning how to communicate, how to use the potty, and how to dress themselves. Because of their new independence, toddlers may not cooperate with the efforts of health care workers.

Toddlers who need health care services are also likely to be very frightened. It is common for a child of this age to **regress**, or return to an earlier stage of development. For instance, a child who has been potty-trained for some time may suddenly start wetting their pants, or they may ask for a bottle or pacifier after being previously weaned from these items. While frustrating, especially for the child's caregivers, regression is just a normal way for a young child to cope with stress. A toddler is still too young to talk about their fears or even understand what exactly they are afraid of, so they just return to an earlier, more comfortable stage of development temporarily until the stress passes. When caring for a toddler, it is important to recognize regression for what it is and ignore it.

Meeting the Toddler's Physical Needs

A toddler will need your help to meet many of their physical needs. Ask the toddler's regular caregiver how much help the child usually needs with eating, toileting, and dressing. Find out what words the child uses for urination and bowel movements. It is important for you to allow the toddler to remain as independent as possible. One way to do this is to offer choices that are realistic. For example, instead of asking the child what they want to wear, limit their choices to those that are actually possible ("Do you want to wear your red pajamas, or your blue ones?").

Because a toddler's physical growth slows during this stage, their appetite may also be small. Being scared can also affect the toddler's appetite. Ask the child's caregiver what the child prefers to eat and drink. Many children in this age group have very clear and very limited food preferences. Most toddlers enjoy finger foods such as crackers, fruit cut into small pieces, and dry cereal. They can drink from a cup and may enjoy a variety of juices and milk. Toddlers are usually on an "eat and run" type of dietary schedule and need to have small amounts of food provided throughout the day. You may be responsible for monitoring and recording the toddler's food and fluid intake. If the toddler's fluid intake is low, try offering foods such as popsicles, ice cream, or gelatin. These foods count toward the fluid intake and may be more enticing than a cup of water.

Older toddlers who sleep in a regular bed at home may be offered a small adjustable bed in the health care facility if their condition allows. However, a toddler who is at risk for falling out of bed may need a crib with side rails and a top cover. The use of restraints is common among children in this age group because toddlers are simply too young to understand that intravenous lines, drains, catheters, and other medical devices are a necessary part of their treatment and should not be pulled out. If restraints are being used, be sure to check on the toddler very frequently (at least every 10 minutes). The best alternative to using a restraint is to keep the toddler occupied by offering distracting activities and toys and by having someone stay with the toddler at all times.

Meeting the Toddler's Emotional Needs

Most toddlers are afraid of strangers and prefer to be with their usual caregivers. Remember that you are a stranger to the toddler. Speak softly and get down on the toddler's level when you are talking with them. That way you will not appear quite so tall and scary. Many toddlers are more cooperative during procedures if they are allowed to sit in their usual caregiver's lap. They also like to touch any equipment that is being used in the procedure (Fig. 45-3). Allow the child to handle your stethoscope and blood pressure cuff before attempting to measure vital signs.

Toddlers love to play with brightly colored toys such as blocks, simple puzzles, and stuffed toys. They also love to clap, move, and sing along with children's songs. Because their attention spans are very short, toddlers become bored and fretful very quickly. Make sure that the toddler has access to activities that can help keep them entertained. Toddlers also may need to nap in the middle of the day, especially if they are sick or injured. Provide quiet time, soothing music, and a comforting touch to help the child fall asleep.

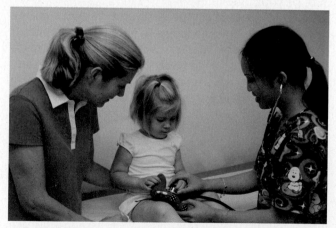

Figure 45-3 Most toddlers enjoy handling the equipment that will be used in a procedure. Procedures will usually go more smoothly if it is possible for the toddler's usual caretaker to be present.

Meeting the Toddler's Need for Safety

Toddlers are sometimes referred to as "tornadoes in training pants" because of their boundless energy, mobility, and natural curiosity. They learn to open locked doors quickly and can wander away from the facility or home. They run, climb, and reach for things without any thought to safety. They love to explore cabinets and will taste the contents of any containers they find there. As a result, accidental poisonings are very common among this age group. Toddlers must be observed at all times to help prevent accidents, and safety locks on doors, cabinets, and drawers are essential.

Toddlers should be placed in a size-appropriate, government safety–approved car seat with a 5-point harness. It is recommended that babies and toddlers remain rear-facing in the back seat for as long as possible. That can mean up to 35 or 40 pounds in most car seats, unless they outgrow it by height first. At that time, toddlers should be placed in a forward-facing car seat in the back seat of the vehicle. As with infants, it is illegal in all states to transport a toddler in a car without first properly securing them in a car seat.

CARING FOR PRESCHOOLERS

Preschoolers are children between the ages of 3 and 5 years. Like toddlers, preschoolers are very physically active and love to run, jump, ride on toys, and swing. Because the preschooler enjoys being physically active, being confined to bed or indoors because of an injury or illness can lead to boredom. Art supplies, games, computer tablets, movies, and television can be good entertainment for a child of this age (Fig. 45-4). Preschoolers also love to have stories read to them, and many are learning to read simple books on their own.

Meeting the Preschooler's Physical Needs

At this age, a child has developed most of their self-care skills. A healthy preschooler can dress themselves, go to the bathroom unassisted, and brush their own teeth. However, a sick or injured preschooler may need help with these daily tasks.

Most preschoolers are picky eaters and eat only a small variety of foods in small amounts. You may find it frustrating when your attempts to get a preschooler to eat nutritious foods fail. A preschooler who is not feeling well is even less likely to have an appetite for foods that are "good for them." Offering a variety of nutritious foods in small amounts throughout the day is often more effective than insisting that the preschooler eat regular meals.

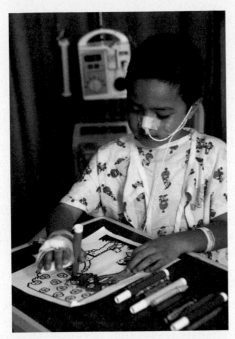

Figure 45-4 Art projects, books, games, movies, and television can be good entertainment for the preschooler who is injured or ill.

Obesity in children has become a major issue and a significant health risk in the United States. According to the CDC, in the past 30 years the rate of obesity in children has doubled. Currently, over one third of children have a body mass index (BMI) that falls into the overweight or obese ranges. Health problems related to obesity, such as cardiovascular disease and type 2 diabetes, are occurring more often in children at younger ages. Promoting healthy eating and lifestyle habits is very important throughout the child's life.

You may be required to help hold or restrain a preschooler during a procedure. Make sure you plan ahead and have been shown how to hold a child gently but securely, so that the procedure can be performed as efficiently as possible. A frightened child can be very strong and may kick, pinch, hit, or bite to get away. You will have to protect both the child and yourself from injury in this situation.

Meeting the Preschooler's Emotional Needs

Preschoolers have vivid imaginations and enjoy pretend play. As a result, preschoolers may have a lot of anxiety about being in a health care facility. A young preschooler may fear that a procedure will involve "cutting off" body parts or other drastic measures. An older preschooler has begun to understand the concept of death and may think that the hospital is "where people go to die." Because children of this age are learning to understand that discipline or punishment is the consequence of bad behavior, they may think that the reason they have to have a painful treatment or stay in bed is because they were "bad."

"Magical thinking" is a thought process that is common among preschoolers. Preschoolers believe that if they wish for something hard enough, it will happen. As a result, a preschooler may think that because they wished for something bad to happen to a parent or a sibling, their current medical condition is punishment for having those bad thoughts. Or they may think that their bad thoughts actually made something bad happen (for example, if several members of a family are now hospitalized because of an accident).

Preschoolers need their questions answered simply and honestly. They are very interested in whether a procedure will "hurt." If the procedure will cause discomfort, be truthful and describe what the procedure will feel like in words that the child can understand. For example, you might tell the child that the procedure will "pinch," "squeeze," or "pull." Not being honest about the procedure and what it will feel like will destroy the child's ability to trust you and the other members of the health care team.

Using a stuffed animal or doll to demonstrate the procedure helps the child to understand what is expected of them and will help to relieve the child's fears. For example, you could use a doll to demonstrate how you do range-of-motion exercises. Similarly, the preschooler will enjoy being able to listen to their own heart through the stethoscope, or seeing a demonstration of how the blood pressure cuff "squeezes the arm to check their muscles."

Meeting the Preschooler's Needs for Safety

A preschooler is beginning to learn the difference between right and wrong behavior. As a result, they are more able to follow the rules of safety, if these rules are explained in a way that they understand. Some preschoolers are still likely to place items in their mouths and are therefore at risk for choking. As in younger children, balloons pose a choking risk and should be used with caution. Scissors used for craft projects should be blunt-tipped, and markers, crayons, glue, and other art supplies should be nontoxic and approved for use for children between the ages of 3 and 5 years.

The toddler car seat is used until the child weighs 40 pounds. At that point, the child will have outgrown the toddler car seat and will need a larger booster seat. Many child automobile seats are convertible, allowing it to be adjusted as the child grows. Head and back supports, combined with an adjustable 5-point harness, can accommodate children up to 100 pounds.

The booster seat is placed in the back seat of the car, facing forward. Children should continue to ride in a booster seat until they are 4 feet 9 inches tall, usually between 8 and 12 years of age. As with younger children, it is illegal to drive with a child in the car who is not properly restrained.

CARING FOR SCHOOL-AGE CHILDREN

School-age children are children between the ages of 5 and 12 years. School-age children are developing many interests outside of their own families. They are learning to socialize and spend a lot of time playing with their friends. They enjoy physical activities, such as riding bicycles, swimming, skating, skiing, and climbing. Unfortunately, these activities often result in injury and the need for health care. "Fitting in" socially is very important to the school-age child, and children who have physical or intellectual disabilities may be excluded from play or teased by their peers.

Caring for a child of this age in a health care setting involves answering lots of questions. School-age children are typically very cooperative if their questions are answered in a manner that they can understand. These children like to be included as active participants in their own care and are very good at following directions.

Meeting the School-Age Child's Physical Needs

School-age children are very independent and are quite proud that they no longer have to rely on anyone else for self-care, although they do need to be reminded that the purpose of a bath or shower is to clean their bodies. If a child is not able to bathe, dress, or go to the bathroom by themself as a result of injury or illness, they will need the assistance of others, and this is likely to make them very unhappy. Allow the child to do as much as they are able to by themself. Sometimes, taking the approach that the child is helping you because you simply cannot do the task without their assistance is helpful.

When caring for a school-age child, you must check on them frequently. Although the child may be badly injured and in pain, they may not pay attention to your directions to call for help if they need to get out of bed. A reward system for following the rules may be necessary. For example, you might tell the child that if they use the call light control to ask for your assistance each time they need to get out of bed, then you will allow them to choose a small treat or privilege. Rewards and praise work very well for children of this age.

Meeting the School-Age Child's Emotional Needs

School-age children expect to receive direct, simple answers to their questions. If a school-age child asks you a question that you cannot answer, be sure to relay the question to the nurse so that they can answer it for the child. Never make promises or assurances about a school-age child's condition or treatment that are not certain. Children of this age are usually aware of when they are being told the truth and when they are not. A school-age child usually has developed a strong moral conscience and feels very strongly about what is right and what is wrong.

A school-age child will enjoy reading, doing arts and crafts projects, playing video games, and talking with caregivers. If possible, allow the child to accompany you throughout the health care facility in a wheelchair for company, or take them to a common area where there may be other children their age to socialize or play games with. For a child of this age who is confined due to accident or illness, staying in touch with friends is a huge emotional boost. Texts and video calls, internet access for e-mail, visits (if possible), and cards from friends and classmates are thoroughly enjoyed (Fig. 45-5). Make sure you help the child to place cards and notes safely on a table or bulletin board so they can be looked at often.

Meeting the School-Age Child's Need for Safety

The school-age child is less vulnerable to certain dangers than younger children are. For example, school-age children generally know not to drink poisonous

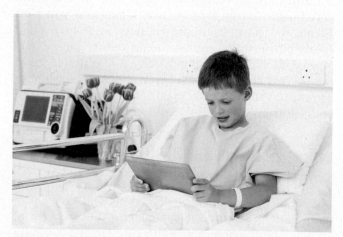

Figure 45-5 School-age children who must be confined to bed due to injury or illness will miss socializing with their friends. Email messages, phone calls, or video calls with friends and family members are thoroughly enjoyed. (*wavebreakmedia\Shutterstock.com*)

liquids or stick objects into an electrical outlet. However, their curiosity and habit of pushing their physical abilities to the limit bring new dangers. School-age children are often interested in fire. They may dart into the path of oncoming traffic on bicycles and skateboards or when chasing a ball. They climb trees and buildings and then fall. Burns, broken bones, and head injuries are the reason many children in this age group require hospitalization and rehabilitation.

When transporting a school-age child in a car, use a booster seat until the lap and shoulder restraints of the car's seatbelts fit the child properly. This usually occurs when the child reaches a height of 4 feet 9 inches, and a weight of about 80 pounds. Children should continue to ride in the backseat until the age of 12 years.

CARING FOR ADOLESCENTS

Adolescents are children between the ages of 12 and 20 years. Adolescence is a time of tremendous growth and development. We enter adolescence as children and exit as young adults. During adolescence, logical thinking skills develop. Adolescents have the ability to understand possibilities and make judgments. As a result, it is essential that children of this age be included in plans and decisions regarding their medical care.

Meeting the Adolescent's Physical Needs

Allow the child to be as independent as possible with their daily care. An adolescent may hesitate to ask for help or for pain medication if they are trying to seem "tough," mature, or grown-up. They may act angry or aloof when in reality they are frightened. Adolescence is a difficult time of life to require health care. The physical changes that occur during adolescence can make adolescents self-conscious about their bodies. As a result, they are often very embarrassed by care or treatments that expose their bodies to others. Remember this when caring for an adolescent and make a special effort to provide privacy. Also be aware that an adolescent who is menstruating may need your assistance with obtaining or changing sanitary napkins or tampons, if they are too ill to manage this task on their own. Be sensitive to the embarrassment they may feel at having to ask for your help.

To help adolescents meet their nutritional needs, offer the types of foods that they like to eat. A teenager may totally refuse the types of meals served in a health care facility but will eat pizza, milkshakes, or other nutritional alternatives. Because of the increased need for extra calories during periods of growth spurts, an adolescent may need nutritious snacks in between meals. Peanut butter and crackers, cheese, fruit, yogurt, and ice cream are good nutritious alternatives for chips and soda and should be readily available for the teenager if their dietary orders allow.

Meeting the Adolescent's Emotional Needs

Psychologically, the period of adolescence is stormy. Adolescents are **egocentric**, meaning that they place themselves at the center of the world and often overestimate their importance to others. They begin to question the moral teachings of authority figures and parents. As a result, experimentation with alcohol, drugs, and sex may occur during this stage. Many adolescents begin to question their own sexual orientation. They may fear being "different" or being shamed or outcast from their own families if they have same-sex attractions. Many adolescents also find themselves questioning their own gender identity.

Adolescents are torn between wanting to be treated as grown-ups and being afraid to make their own decisions. They need adults to respect their individuality. When caring for an adolescent, listen to what they are saying. Try not to lecture them on morals or proper behavior. Include the adolescent in discussions and decisions regarding their care and treatment. Adolescents need to feel that their opinions count (Fig. 45-6).

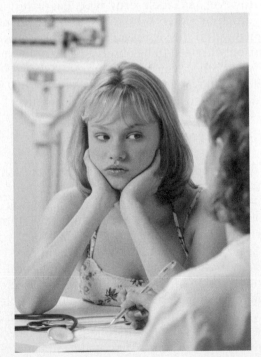

Figure 45-6 Adolescents need to be included in plans and decisions regarding their medical care. It is important to listen to what the adolescent is telling you. Avoid lecturing them on morals or proper behavior.

Many adolescents require care in a health care facility because of complications related to mental health issues, such as depression, attempted suicide, or eating disorders. Attempted suicide is more prevalent in this age group than any other. In fact, suicide is the third leading cause of death in people 15 to 24 years of age.

Other adolescents may have had accidents related to drug or alcohol use. An adolescent may need health care as a result of a pregnancy, which may not be planned or wanted. Sexually transmitted infections (STIs) are common among people in this age group. Many adolescents have become victims of sexual abuse. All of these situations require tact and sensitivity on the part of caregivers. Be very observant for any changes in the adolescent's emotional behavior or mood and report anything unusual to the nurse immediately.

Most adolescents have mobile phones and are constantly communicating with their friends via social media. They may like to take photos of themselves and their environment to post. Make sure that your young patients are aware that taking photos of other patients or making comments about other people's health status or condition violates their rights of confidentiality and should not be done.

Meeting the Adolescent's Need for Safety

In the health care setting, most adolescents are fairly safe. However, an adolescent who has a history of using drugs or other substances may try to obtain pain medication that is not needed. Adolescents with depression will need to be observed closely for suicide attempts or other types of self-injury. Make sure that the adolescent knows you are available if they need assistance, and answer the call light promptly.

Concerns for Long-Term Care

As you will recall from Chapter 8, there are some instances where a resident of a long-term care facility will be a child. Intellectual and physical disabilities may require that the child have round-the-clock skilled nursing care. The challenge when caring for young people in the long-term care setting is that most often their level of physical development and their level of emotional/intellectual development do not match. For example, a 15-year-old resident may have total paralysis from an accident but will be emotionally and intellectually a typical adolescent. They will need conversation and interaction that can meet their emotional needs while still needing complete care from others to meet their physical needs. Another resident may physically be a typical teenager, with

normal bodily functions and drives. However, they may intellectually be at the developmental level of a 6-year-old child. You will need to always remember to adjust the emotional and physical care you give younger residents as needed.

CHILD ABUSE

Children, like older adults, are often targets of abuse.

Forms of Abuse

Like elder abuse, child abuse (also known as *child maltreatment*) can be physical, psychological (emotional), or sexual in nature.

Physical Abuse

Neglect is the most common form of physical abuse in children. The child's caregiver simply fails to provide for the child's basic physical needs. For example, the child may be malnourished from lack of nutritious food, dirty from lack of proper hygiene, or ill from a lack of medical care.

Physical abuse can also take the form of striking, biting, slapping, shaking, or handling a child roughly. Some children are punished by placing them in water that is too hot. Scald burns and sometimes cigarette burns may be present. Violently shaking an infant or toddler can cause the child's brain to hit the inside of the skull repeatedly, leading to severe brain damage or death. This is called **shaken baby syndrome**. Shaken baby syndrome is most often seen in children younger than 1 year. About 25% of children with shaken baby syndrome die, and the rest suffer from permanent disabilities. Many cases of shaken baby syndrome occur accidentally, when a frustrated caregiver shakes a child to get them to stop crying. Because of the risk of head injury, it is never acceptable to shake an infant or toddler.

In **Munchausen syndrome by proxy**, another form of physical abuse seen in children, the child's caregiver deliberately does things to make the child appear ill. For example, the caregiver may feed the child soap or other substances to make them vomit. Or they might smother the child for a period of time to deprive them of oxygen, leading to neurologic symptoms. Often, the child is forced to have painful diagnostic procedures or surgery as health care providers try to discover the cause of the child's strange signs and symptoms. Munchausen syndrome by proxy is often difficult to detect and to prove because nearly constant observation is needed to determine the cause of the child's health problems. In some cases, it becomes necessary to conceal a camera in the child's hospital room to observe what happens when the caregiver is alone with the child.

Psychological (Emotional) Abuse

A caregiver can inflict psychological (emotional) abuse on a child in many ways. A caregiver might make a child fearful by threatening them with physical harm or abandonment. Or they might say cruel things to the child, such as "You're no good," "You're stupid," or "I wish you had never been born." Isolating a child by preventing them from seeing friends or other family members (an act called *involuntary seclusion*) is another form of psychological abuse. Involuntary seclusion can involve keeping a child in a room alone with the door closed. In extreme cases, it may involve locking a child in a closet or attic for years. Children who are the victims of psychological abuse can struggle for the rest of their lives with emotional pain, depression, thoughts of suicide, and lack of self-esteem.

Sexual Abuse

Sexual abuse occurs when a parent or caregiver:

- Touches or fondles a child's sexual organs
- Shows their sexual organs to a child or asks the child to touch or otherwise stimulate them
- Forces a child to have sexual intercourse with them (rape)
- Forces a child to engage in a sexual act and then films or photographs it (pornography)
- Forces a child to engage in a sexual act for money, often with many different people (prostitution)

When a stranger sexually abuses a child, it is called *sexual assault.*

Risk Factors for Child Abuse

Child abuse can occur in all levels of society and in all ethnic groups. However, there are certain situations that seem to increase the risk that abuse will occur. Risk factors for child abuse include the following:

- Caregivers who are very stressed by situations such as unemployment, depression, marital or relationship problems, substance use, or health problems of their own
- Caregivers who are very young, lack parenting skills, or lack knowledge about the normal behaviors and developmental stages of children
- Caregivers who have no family or social support and feel "trapped" by their parenting responsibilities
- Children who are "difficult" to care for, such as those who cry frequently, do not sleep well, are hyperactive or aggressive, wet the bed, or have physical or intellectual disabilities

Role of the Nursing Assistant in Reporting Abuse

As a nursing assistant, you may suspect that one of your pediatric patients is being abused (Box 45-1). You may see physical signs that suggest abuse, or the child's behavior or play-acting may raise your suspicions. In some cases, the child might tell you something that makes you suspicious. Make sure to listen carefully to what the child is telling you. Report the child's words exactly as you heard them. Be very careful not to influence the child's ideas or "put words in their mouth." In the event of an abuse investigation, a young child may repeat what they have been told, rather than describe what actually happened. If you are suspicious about something a child has told you, do not question the child further yourself. Report your suspicions to the nurse and allow a person who has experience and training in detecting child abuse to continue the questioning.

It may be difficult to work with parents or caregivers if you suspect that they have abused their child. You may feel angry toward the parents or caregivers or disgusted by their behavior. Remember that

---

Box 45-1 Signs of Child Abuse

- Unclean or unsafe living conditions, as evidenced by rotting food, unchanged sheets, or a lack of heat or water services
- Poor personal hygiene, as evidenced by an unclean body, clothes, or both; uncombed hair; skin irritation (from wearing urine-soaked undergarments for long periods of time); dried stool on buttocks; or a lack of oral hygiene
- Loss of weight or dehydration
- Multiple unexplained fractures or bruises in various stages of healing; explanations of injuries that are not consistent with the location of the injury
- Burn marks (for example, from cigarettes or stove burners) or scalds (for example, from having a hand or foot held in hot water)

- Abrasions from ropes or other bindings
- Patches of missing hair
- Vaginal bleeding or discharge; urinary tract infection; or pain, itching, redness, or bruising around the genitals or anus
- Excessive sexual curiosity or play
- Sleeping problems or nightmares
- An anxious, fearful or withdrawn demeanor, especially in the presence of the abuser
- Uncontrolled medical conditions (possibly the result of a lack of prescribed medication or treatment)
- A history of requiring health care for similar injuries

it is not your place to pass judgment on a parent or caregiver. Your responsibility is to simply report your suspicions and to let the state agencies that handle abuse reports determine if abuse has occurred and, if so, who did it. The agencies will also determine how the child will be protected going forward. Your top priority is to meet the child's physical and emotional needs as best you can while the child is in your care. If you feel that your emotions about a particular situation may affect your ability to provide care, talk with your supervisor and ask for help or to be assigned to another area.

SUMMARY

- Children receive health care in many different types of health care settings for many different reasons. Understanding the basic stages of growth and development will better prepare you to provide the type of care that each child requires.
- Pediatric patients range in age from newborn through 20 years.
  - Infants are children younger than 1 year. Infants are totally dependent on others for their physical care. Their greatest emotional need is to feel secure and to develop trust.
  - A toddler is a child between the ages of 1 and 3 years. Toddlers may have a fear of strangers that could affect their response to health care providers. They commonly regress to an earlier stage of development in response to the stress of a health care setting.
  - Preschoolers are children between the ages of 3 and 5 years. Preschoolers have vivid imaginations and enjoy pretend play. Preschoolers may indulge in magical thinking. The preschooler's questions must be answered simply and honestly.

- School-age children are children between the ages of 5 and 12 years. School-age children like to be included as active participants in their own care and are very good at following directions. However, they may resist asking for help when they need it.
- Adolescents are children between the ages of 12 and 20 years. Adolescents have a great need for privacy and for control over what is happening to them.
- Children are frequently the targets of many types of abuse. All members of the health care team are legally obligated to report any type of suspected abuse.
  - Physical abuse can take the form of neglect or deliberate injury.
  - Psychological (emotional) abuse can involve threatening a child, saying demeaning or cruel things to a child, or isolating the child from others.
  - Sexual abuse occurs when an adult touches a child inappropriately or forces the child to perform sexual acts.

WHAT DID YOU LEARN?

Multiple Choice

Select the single best answer for each of the following questions.

1. A pediatric patient is most likely to cooperate with the health care team when:
   a. Members of the health care team treat them like a "little adult"
   b. Members of the health care team recognize the child's particular stage of development and provide age-appropriate care
   c. Members of the health care team always give the child what they want
   d. The child is restrained

2. To help determine whether a breast-fed infant is receiving an adequate amount of milk, the nursing assistant may need to:
   a. Supplement the breastfeeding with extra formula
   b. Monitor the baby's intravenous (IV) line
   c. Have the parent pump their breasts and measure the amount of milk produced
   d. Weigh the infant's wet diapers

3. A behavior that could indicate regression in a toddler might be:
a. Asking for a bottle or pacifier
b. Becoming potty-trained
c. Feeding themselves
d. Fearing strangers

4. Which one of the following is an example of magical thinking?
a. Believing in Santa Claus
b. Fearing strangers
c. Thinking that an accident occurred because you were mad at your sibling
d. Pretending to be a princess

Matching *Match each numbered item with its appropriate lettered description.*

_____ **1.** Infant

_____ **2.** Toddler

_____ **3.** Preschooler

_____ **4.** School-age child

_____ **5.** Adolescent

a. This child has developed a very strong moral conscience and will expect truthful answers to their many questions.

b. This child may be very self-conscious and become embarrassed if they are exposed during a medical procedure.

c. This child needs to be touched, cuddled, stroked, and spoken to soothingly to thrive.

d. This child has a vivid imagination and may fear monsters under the bed and doctors who will "cut off" body parts.

e. This child is at the highest risk for accidental poisoning.

STOP *and* **THINK!**

- You are the nursing assistant on a pediatric floor of a hospital. One of your small patients, Saryah, is 5. As you walk into her room, you notice that she is playing with a doll and a teddy bear. As you listen, you hear her talking to the toys. Saryah is pretending that the bear is asking the doll to touch him between the legs. When the doll refuses, the bear becomes very angry and demands that the doll touch him. What is happening in this room? What should be your response?

- You are caring for a 2-year-old child who has a fractured arm. You notice that the parent seems very fearful of talking about what happened and their version of the story changes frequently. As you are helping to bathe the child you notice small burn marks on his buttocks and some bruises on his back. What do you report and to whom?

Respect

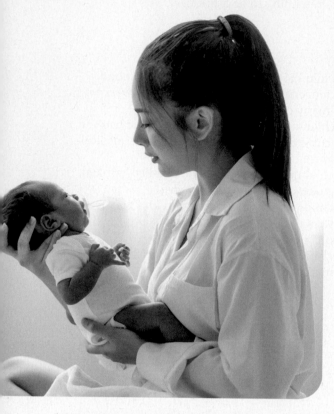

I have been a nursing assistant for many years now and currently work in the maternity unit of a small city hospital. I love caring for new parents and their babies. Getting to experience new life and the joy of those young families is so rewarding. It reminds me of my own children coming into this world.

We recently had a young mother, Julia, who needed to be hospitalized for pre-term labor a couple of weeks before her baby was born. Because she was with us for an extended period of time, I got to know her better than most of our patients. She was only 17, and I noticed that she didn't have any family or friends who would visit her. Julia seemed very quiet and sad but expressed a lot of concern for her unborn baby. As she learned to trust me and the rest of the nursing staff caring for her, she would tell us a little about herself.

When Julia found out she was pregnant, she was unhoused. She sought help through the local Planned Parenthood office and through them was able to find temporary housing. They also put her in contact with the local technical college where she was able to finish her high school diploma and start some career training. Julia shared that she had an interest in pursuing a career in the health care field, and she had many questions for us about our jobs.

Soon enough, Julia went into hard labor and delivered a beautiful little boy. She was holding him gently and talking to him when we were notified that a social worker had arrived. Julia was placing her baby for adoption, and the social worker had brought the adoptive parents to receive Julia's little boy. Julia asked the social worker if she could please meet the adoptive parents.

I watched with my eyes full of tears as Julia told her son that she loved him so much but that she would not be able to care for him as he deserved. She told him that hopefully one day when he was grown up, he would understand. And, if he chose to find her, that she would have grown into someone he would be proud to know as his birth mother. She then kissed him tenderly and placed him in the waiting arms of his new parents, Angela and Susanna. I think everyone in the room was crying as Angela and Susanna welcomed the child they felt made their little family complete. They told Julia that when the child was older, they would tell their son about the remarkable person that his birth mother was and how brave she was to make sure he had a loving family to raise him.

I learned so much about love and families that day. I saw a very young mother's love for a child, so deep and pure, and how she was brave enough to give her child a life she did not believe she could provide. I have learned more respect for people and families facing situations I have not faced.

(SritanaN\Shutterstock.com)

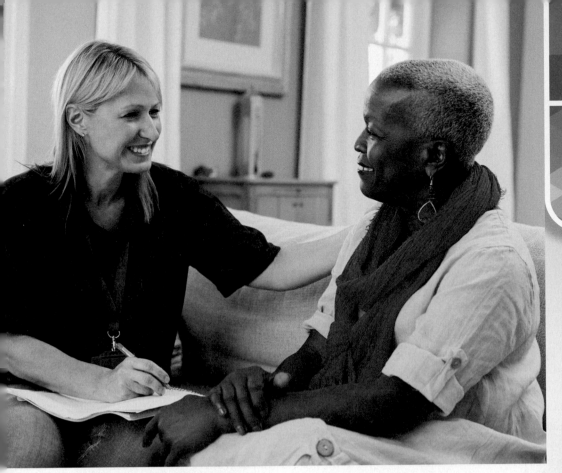

Home Health Care

46 Introduction to Home Health Care

47 Safety and Infection Control in the Home Health Care Setting

HOME HEALTH CARE—SKILLED NURSING CARE that is provided to a person in their home—is a rapidly growing part of the health care industry. Currently, more than 15 million Americans use the services of more than 35,000 home health care agencies. The purpose of this unit is to introduce you to the home health care setting.

Photo: Home health aides care for clients in their homes. (Monkey Business Images\Shutterstock.com)

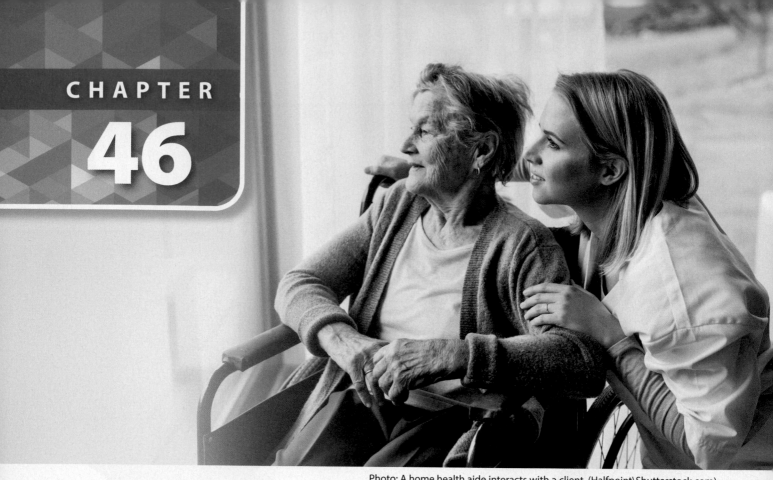

Photo: A home health aide interacts with a client. (Halfpoint\Shutterstock.com)

CHAPTER 46

Introduction to Home Health Care

 ## WHAT WILL YOU LEARN?

Many nursing assistants choose to work in home health care. A nursing assistant who works in home health care is often called a **home health aide**. Perhaps becoming a home health aide is something you have thought about. The basic skills and concepts that you have learned will apply no matter where you decide to work. But some aspects of providing care to a person in their own home are unique. In this chapter, you will learn about why a person might need the services of a home health care agency and how these services are paid for. You will also learn about some of the key responsibilities you will have if you decide to work in the home health care setting. Finally, we will discuss the personal qualities that a person must have to succeed as a home health aide. When you are finished with this chapter, you will be able to:

1. Describe why a person might need home health care.
2. Discuss how home health care is paid for.
3. List some of the members of the home health care team.
4. Describe how the home health care team works together to provide client care.
5. Describe the primary duties of a home health aide.
6. List personal qualities that a home health aide must have to be successful.

Vocabulary

Home health aide   Respite care   Homebound   Case manager

WHAT IS HOME HEALTH CARE?

If you were ill, where would you rather be? In your own home, surrounded by the people, pets, and things that you love? Or in a hospital or long-term care facility? Given a choice, most people would prefer to stay in the comfort of their own home when they are sick. Home health care, also known as *home care*, makes it possible for people who are not critically ill to receive health care in the comfort of their own home. A person who is receiving the services of a home health care agency is called a *client*, instead of a "patient" or a "resident." People of all ages may need the services of home health care, but the majority are 65 years of age or older. There are many reasons why a person might become a client of a home health care agency:

- **The person may have just been discharged from the hospital following surgery or an acute illness or injury.** The care provided in a hospital is costly, and a person's health insurance or Medicare will only cover admission for a limited number of days. For these reasons, a person may be discharged from the hospital as soon as their condition is stable but before they are fully recovered. Many of these people will continue to need IV antibiotics or other medications, wound care, or physical therapy before they fully recover. In this situation, a home health aide may be needed to help care for the person at home until they have made a full recovery.
- **The person may have a chronic illness or disability that makes it hard for them to manage some tasks independently.** For example, a person who is paralyzed might need a home health aide to help get them out of bed and ready for work each morning.
- **The person may have a condition, such as dementia, that makes it dangerous for the person to be left alone in the house.** In this case, a home health aide might come to the home on a regular basis to provide care and companionship for the person and to relieve the primary caregiver. Care that allows the primary caregiver to rest or leave the house for a short period of time is called **respite care** (Fig. 46-1). Being able to "take a break" and leave the house is critical for managing the stress that can be caused by providing constant care for a family member who is ill.
- **The person may be terminally ill.** Hospice care is often provided in the person's home. A home health aide who works for a hospice agency will receive special training in providing end-of-life care.

Home health care can also be given to a person who lives in an assisted living facility. Most assisted living facilities do not provide skilled nursing services, and a resident may need skilled care for a short period of time (for example, following hip replacement surgery). This way, the person is able to remain in their "home" and receive the necessary care.

Paying for Home Health Care

Home health care is paid for in many different ways. A client may pay for home health care entirely from their own income or savings. Or, they may have insurance coverage that covers all or part of the costs. Insurance coverage is provided by insurance companies and by government agencies, such as Medicare or state Medicaid. Medicare is the most common method of reimbursement for home health care.

Home health care services are usually divided into two different categories. *Skilled home care* services are meant to be short term and are usually paid for by Medicare and other health insurance programs. In

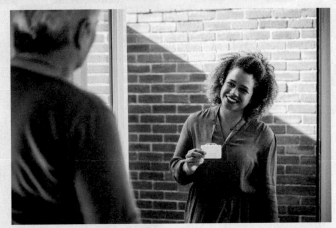

Figure 46-1 Part of a home health aide's duties may be to provide respite care. Respite care allows the family member who has primary responsibility for caring for the client to have time to themselves. (*DGLimages\Shutterstock.com*)

order to qualify for skilled home care, a client must meet all of the following criteria:

- The person must be **homebound**
- The services must be ordered by the person's primary care doctor or nurse practitioner
- There must be a need for skilled nursing or rehabilitative care
- The person must require intermittent (several times a day or week), but not full-time, care

After meeting the criteria, Medicare will pay for home health services for a period of 60 days. The goal of skilled home care services is to help the client return to optimal health. At the end of the 60-day period, the client's condition is reevaluated and if necessary, the services can be extended for an additional 60 days. If the client needs home health care services after a hospitalization, Medicare will pay the cost of up to 100 home visits.

Insurance companies and government agencies may also control the length of each visit and the number of visits a person may have each week. For example, a client who needs minimal assistance with bathing may be allowed three visits per week, while a client who cannot get out of bed and is at risk for developing pressure ulcers may be allowed two visits each day. One client may be allowed a 1-hour visit, while another client is allowed a 2-hour visit. Proper documentation (recording) of the care provided to the client during each visit is necessary to justify continued payment for home care services and to determine the frequency and length of future visits.

Long-term home care services (also referred to as home health sitting services) are available for many older people who need home care but do not meet the criteria for skilled home care. Long-term care services are usually made up of nonskilled duties, such as meal preparation, light housekeeping, assistance with personal care, grocery shopping, and other errands. This type of home care service is usually paid for by the individual or their family members. Some services may be offered as part of a community outreach project.

Box 46-1	**Members of the Home Health Care Team**
Doctor or Nurse Practitioner	The doctor or nurse practitioner usually initiates the order for the client to receive home health care services. The doctor is responsible for writing orders for the treatment, therapy, special diets, and medications that the client will receive.
Case manager	The clinical case manager, usually a registered nurse (RN), is responsible for overseeing all of the client's care, from admission to discharge. The case manager assesses the client and works with the client and their family to create the care plan. They will also coordinate the client's care and make assignments to the home health care aide and other members of the care team. The case manager receives input from other team members and is responsible for reevaluating the client's care needs should their condition decline or improve.
Registered Nurse (RN) and Licensed Practical Nurse (LPN)	RNs and LPNs visit the client and provide skilled nursing care that may be needed. For example, the nurses will provide wound care, intravenous medications, specialized procedures, and client/family teaching about the client's condition or care measures.
Home Health Aide	The home health aide follows the care plan set up by the case manager and provides personal care for the client. Home health aides assist clients with hygiene and grooming needs, toileting, positioning and transferring, monitoring vital signs, observing and reporting any changes in the client's condition, and other duties required to ensure the client's safety and comfort. The home health aide may visit a client two times a week or up to twice a day, each day of the week, depending on the client's needs and the care plan.
Physical Therapist	Physical therapists provide exercises geared toward helping clients gain strength, balance, mobility, movement, and gait.
Occupational Therapist	Occupational therapy assists clients to relearn and gain the ability to perform ADLs. The occupational therapist makes recommendations for home safety modifications or adaptive equipment that will improve the client's level of independence.
Speech Therapist	Speech therapy helps clients improve their ability to speak and communicate more clearly, especially after an accident or stroke that causes aphasia. Speech therapists also assist clients who have eating and swallowing difficulties.
Registered Dietician	Registered dieticians provide consultation and teaching on diet and nutrition choices and concerns, especially for clients with a medically prescribed diet.
Social Services/Social Worker	Social workers provide assistance to clients and their families with needs such as financial issues, meal assistance, or obtaining medical or assistive devices (for example, hospital beds, bedside commodes, ambulation devices). Some social workers provide counseling services; advance directives; and ongoing support in the home, such as respite care.

The Health Care Team

Just as in any other health care setting, health care that is provided in the home is provided by a health care team. The health care team consists of the client, the client's family members, the home health aide, and other specialized members. Box 46-1 lists the members of the home health care team and gives a brief description of each member's primary role. As always, the client is the focus of the health care team's efforts, and the goal of the health care team is to provide holistic care. Each team member provides a specific aspect of care for the client. For example, the home health aide may be responsible for monitoring vital signs and helping the client with routine activities of daily living (ADLs), while the nurse may be responsible for giving medications or providing wound care (Fig. 46-2). The health care team provides care in the home as directed by the client's care plan. The care plan is a set of instructions for the client's care, created by the case manager with input from all members of the health care team. The **case manager**, usually a registered nurse, is responsible for overseeing all of the client's care, from admission through discharge.

The home health aide is a very important member of the health care team. Because the home health aide is often scheduled to visit the client on a frequent, routine basis, they have the best chance to observe changes that could indicate a change in the client's health. In addition, the client may feel most comfortable with the home health aide and, as a result, may tell them things they may not share with other members of the health care team. By communicating their observations to the rest of the health care team, the home health aide becomes the "eyes and ears" of the members of the team who do not see the client as frequently. For this reason, communicating with the case manager and other members of the health care team is an essential part of the home health aide's responsibilities.

In the hospital and long-term care settings, team members often have the chance to communicate face-to-face because everyone is together in the same building. This is not true in the home health care setting. Team members travel to the client's home according to their own individual schedules. As a result, they may rarely see each other. In the home health care setting, most communication among team members takes place through documentation. As always, you must accurately document the care you provide on the appropriate forms, including the date, time, and duration of the visit. As in most other health care settings, electronic methods of documentation are used for recording care given in the home. Proper documentation is necessary to ensure that all members of the home health care team are kept "in-the-know."

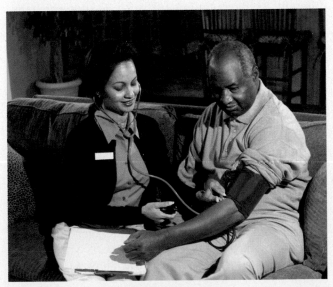

Figure 46-2 Home health aides are often responsible for monitoring the vital signs of their clients.

Tell the Nurse!

As a home health aide, you will play an important role in reporting changes in a client's medical condition that could indicate a serious problem. Your agency will have specific guidelines about observations that should be reported. Make sure you are familiar with these guidelines, and if you are ever in doubt about whether an observation should be immediately reported to the case manager, choose to err on the side of safety and report it. Make sure you report any of the following observations to the case manager immediately:

- One or more of the client's vital signs is above or below the standards set by the agency
- The client has a fever or other signs of infection
- There is a change in the client's mental alertness or orientation
- The client has signs of skin breakdown or pressure sores
- The client has signs or symptoms that could indicate a medical emergency
- You suspect that the client is being abused (physically, sexually, or emotionally)
- There are unsafe or unsanitary conditions in the home

RESPONSIBILITIES OF THE HOME HEALTH AIDE

The home health aide usually assists clients with tasks related to personal care. Depending on the client's needs, the home health aide may also be assigned light housekeeping duties, such as cleaning, preparing meals, and doing laundry. The home health aide's responsibilities are clearly outlined in the client's care plan. You must follow the care plan exactly. Any changes to the care plan must first be approved by the case manager.

In addition to documenting the care that you provide to the client, you may be required to keep a daily record of your activities. For example, you might be asked to keep a *time and travel log*, which details how much time you spent at each client's house, how much time you spent traveling between houses, and your mileage for the day. Always record information in a timely manner. If you must wait until the end of the day to record something, keep accurate notes so that the information you record will be accurate.

You will most likely provide care for many clients who live in very different types of homes. One client may live in a single-family house in a quiet neighborhood. Another client may live in an inner-city apartment building. Some clients may be well-off and have beautiful homes with modern accommodations. Others may live on very limited funds and have a house or apartment that is old and in need of repair. Some clients may not even have modern plumbing and a bathtub or shower. Regardless of the setting, you are responsible for providing the same quality of care for each of your clients. Each home, and each family, is different. Remember that you are a guest in the client's home. You must be careful not to allow your opinions about how a person lives affect the care that you provide. If you feel that something about a client's home environment puts the client at risk for injury (such as extremely dirty conditions, an abusive relationship with a family member, or a potential fire hazard), report your concerns to the case manager.

Personal Care

As a home health aide, many of your responsibilities will be related to helping your clients with activities such as bathing, eating, getting dressed, exercising, toileting, repositioning, and transferring (Fig. 46-3). As always, the amount of help you will need to provide will vary from client to client, and you should encourage the client to do as much as possible for themselves.

The skills you will use to assist with personal care are the same no matter where you work. However,

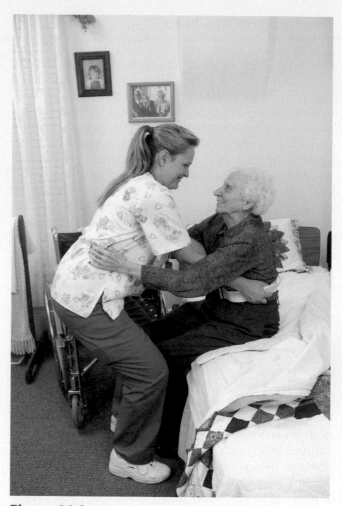

Figure 46-3 Home health aides assist with all types of personal care. Here, a home health aide helps a client to transfer out of bed.

in the home setting, some of the equipment may be different. Medical equipment, such as shower chairs, bedside commodes, or adjustable beds, can be purchased or rented from a medical supply store for use in the home, but this can be expensive. Many clients will not be able to afford this expense. Therefore, many times you must be resourceful and use items that are readily available in the home. For example, if the person's bed is not adjustable, you can use extra pillows or a back rest to position the person in Fowler's position. A sturdy webbed or plastic lawn chair may substitute for a shower chair (Fig. 46-4). However, as with the use of any type of equipment, safety is a top priority. If you think that a client is at risk for injury because they do not have a certain piece of medical equipment, ask the case manager for advice. The case manager may be able to work with outside resources to get the equipment the client needs at low cost or no cost.

If a client starts to decline your assistance with ordered tasks that are listed on the person's care plan,

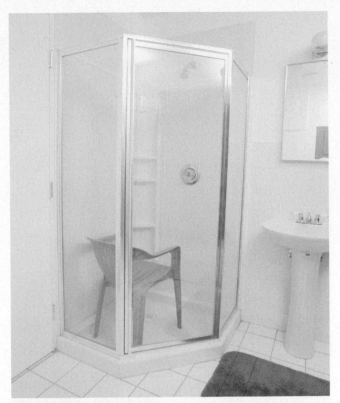

Figure 46-4 Sometimes common household items can be used in place of expensive medical equipment. Here, a plastic lawn chair is used as a shower chair.

it may indicate the need to reevaluate the care plan or the need for continuing care. Make sure you report this to your case manager.

Homemaking

Depending on the client's needs, part of your responsibilities as a home health aide may include preparing and serving meals, cleaning, and doing laundry. Homemaking duties are outlined on the client's care plan. You will document the homemaking duties that you perform on a *homemaker flow sheet*, according to your agency's policies. The homemaker flow sheet becomes part of the client's medical record. As always, you must accurately document your work.

Meal Preparation

Preparing meals is a duty frequently assigned to the home health aide (Fig. 46-5). Some states require home health aides who will be preparing and serving food to have a food handler's permit. Because requirements may differ from state to state, it is important for you to know your agency's policies and to check with the nurse aide registry in the state where you work.

When preparing a meal, consider the special needs and individual preferences of the client. The

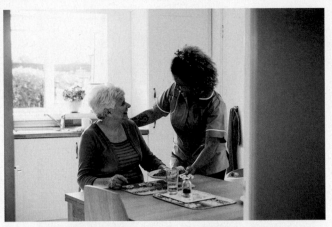

Figure 46-5 Meal preparation is often part of the home health aide's routine duties. *(DGLimages\Shutterstock.com)*

meal should be nutritious. If the person is on a special diet, such as a restricted sodium diet, then you must make sure that the meal you prepare meets the diet's requirements. For some clients, you may have to cut the food into very small pieces or puree it in a blender before serving it.

Serve the meal or snack at the time specified in the care plan. As always, make an effort to make meal time as pleasant as possible. Present the meal in an attractive way, and sit down and talk with the person as they are eating. The amount of assistance with eating that your client will need will vary. For example, some clients will be able to feed themselves if you assist with opening cartons or peeling a piece of fruit. Others will need more help. Involve the person in the process of eating by allowing them to do as much as possible for themselves.

Housekeeping

Many times, the home health aide is also responsible for providing some light cleaning services (Fig. 46-6). These tasks may be done on a weekly basis or as scheduled on the care plan. Depending on the client's needs, you may be responsible for:

- Dusting
- Vacuuming carpets
- Mopping floors
- Disinfecting kitchen and bathroom surfaces
- Changing the client's bed linens
- Washing and drying the client's bed linens and clothing

When providing housekeeping services, care for the client's home as if it were your own. Be careful not to damage decorative items on tables and shelves. Pay attention to details. For example, when vacuuming a room, be thorough. Don't just vacuum the center of the room—make sure the edges and baseboards

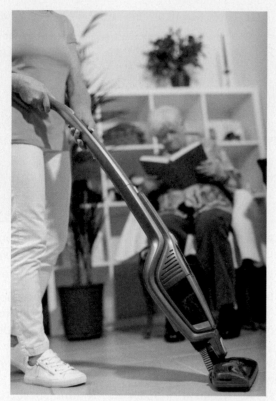

Figure 46-6 Light housekeeping might also be part of the home health aide's responsibilities. (*thodonal88\ Shutterstock.com*)

are clean too. When using cleaning solutions, make sure that the product you are using is approved for use on the surface you are cleaning, to avoid causing permanent damage (Fig. 46-7). It is important to be respectful of the client's home and its contents. When you show respect for a client's home and personal belongings, you are letting the person know that you truly care for them.

QUALITIES OF THE SUCCESSFUL HOME HEALTH AIDE

So maybe you are thinking that you would like to work in the home health setting. Of course, just as in any health care setting, a strong work ethic is important. For example, being honest, compassionate, courteous, conscientious, and reliable will serve you well, no matter where you work. However, the people who make the best home health aides also have other qualities that help them to succeed in the home health care setting. The most successful home health aides:

- Enjoy working independently and are self-motivated
- Are organized and able to manage their time well

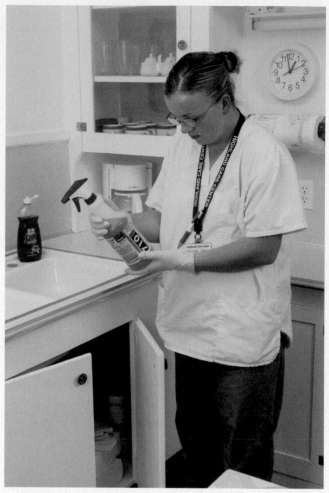

Figure 46-7 When using cleaning solutions, make sure the product you are using is approved for use on the surface you are cleaning. Cleaning solutions should always be kept in properly labeled containers.

- Are reliable
- Are able to set and maintain professional boundaries
- Have good communication skills
- Look and act professional

Let's look at each of these qualities in more detail.

Ability to Work Independently

As a home health aide, you will be working in a client's home without direct supervision most of the time. If you like a lot of feedback and guidance as you complete your assignments, then working in the home health care setting might not be right for you. To work in the home health care setting, you need to be very comfortable with your own caregiving and problem-solving skills. You also need to be self-motivated. No one will be there to help you or to tell you what to do next.

Ability to Be Organized and Manage Time

Because you will be working independently, you will be responsible for making sure that you complete your assigned duties as scheduled. You will be given a list of the clients you must care for each day, and you will be told the length of each client visit. However, it will be up to you to determine how to best provide the required care, complete the necessary documentation, and travel between clients during the workday. You must work efficiently and safely.

Organization is one key to working efficiently and safely. When preparing to visit a client's home, gather all of the supplies you will need before you enter the person's home. Having the necessary supplies on hand allows you to work more efficiently because you will not have to interrupt care to search for something you need. Many items that you will use to provide personal care for your clients may be stored in the client's home in a designated place (Fig. 46-8). Other needed supplies may need to be taken to the client's home each time you visit. Supplies specific for each client are usually filled by your agency from a central area and placed in delivery bags. This helps to ensure that you have the necessary supplies available for each of your clients and helps prevent the transmission of infection because you are not taking container bags from one client's house to another. It also helps to control costs.

Only take supplies specific to that client into the house. Unused supplies are not to be returned to the agency after being taken into the home. This practice is for infection control in addition to cost management.

Equipment that is used with each client, such as for measuring vital signs, is carried in a small tote bag

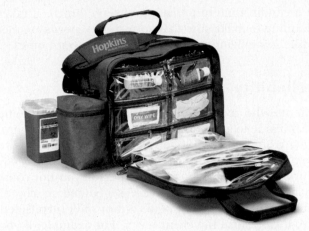

Figure 46-9 A small tote bag is used to carry supplies that will be used with every client, such as equipment for taking vital signs and personal protective equipment. The many compartments help you to keep the bag organized and clean. (Courtesy of Hopkins Medical Products, Baltimore, MD/(800)835-1995, www.hmponline.com)

(Fig. 46-9). Other things that you may carry in your tote bag include:

- Forms needed for documentation and a pen or an electronic device (if used by your agency)
- Personal protective equipment (PPE)
- Supplies for cleaning your equipment
- Alcohol-based hand rub
- Storage bags to enclose any specimens or small equipment that is to be returned to the agency
- Barrier to place tote bag on (disposable waterproof sheets of paper)

Your tote bag has many compartments, which makes it easy for you to organize and find your supplies and equipment. Keeping each item in a special place makes it easy for you to see if you need to restock your tote bag. It also makes it easy for you to check that you have everything you need before you leave for the day. Planning is the other key to working efficiently and safely. If possible, you should plan your day so that you visit clients in an order that allows for the most efficient use of travel time. For example, it would not be the best use of your time to spend all day traveling back and forth across town, when you could see all of your clients on the east side in the morning and all of your clients on the west side in the afternoon. When planning your day's work, map out your clients' addresses and try to limit your travel time as much as possible. However, keep in mind that your clients' preferences and needs must also be taken into account when arranging care schedules. For example, a client with paraplegia may need your help to get ready for work in the morning, while another client with diabetes might need you at their house

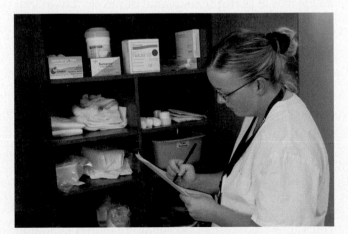

Figure 46-8 Many of the supplies and equipment you will need to care for your client may be kept in a special place in the client's home. Here, a home health aide is checking to see if any of the supplies are getting low.

at a certain time to prepare and serve lunch. It takes planning to make sure that your clients' needs are met while minimizing your travel time between homes.

Reliability

Clients who receive home care depend on the home health aide to arrive and provide the appropriate care. How would you feel if you depended on someone to help you get out of bed, shower, and get ready for work in the morning, and that person did not come to help you when they were scheduled to come? Failing to keep appointments is not only inconsiderate, it can cause the client harm. For example, if you are responsible for preparing lunch for a client with diabetes, then you must do that at the scheduled time, or else the person is at risk for an adverse insulin reaction due to low blood glucose levels. Being reliable is a critical quality for a home health aide to have.

The term *abandonment* means to withdraw one's support or help from another person, in spite of duty or responsibility. A home health aide who fails to show up at a client's home to provide scheduled care is guilty of abandonment (Fig. 46-10). Similarly, a home health aide who leaves a client's home without completing the scheduled tasks may also be guilty of abandonment. As with any job, there may be situations beyond your control that will cause you to be unable to keep your appointments. If you are running late, it is your responsibility to notify the home health care agency. You must also try to contact the clients who are expecting you and let them know that you will be late. If you are unable to report to work at all, you must notify the home health care agency so that another aide can be sent to care for your scheduled

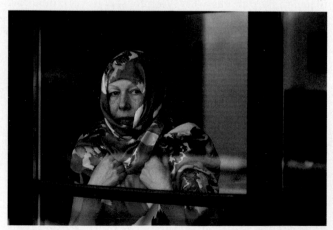

Figure 46-10   Your clients depend on you to arrive and provide the appropriate care, as scheduled. Leaving a client alone and without proper assistance is called *abandonment.* (*Zelma Brezinska\Shutterstock.com*)

clients. Also make sure you notify your agency if a personal emergency arises during your work day that would make it necessary for you to leave before completing your scheduled visits and care duties. Follow your agency's policies regarding situations of this nature so that the care needed by your clients is provided without delay.

Ability to Set Professional Boundaries

Many of your clients and their family members will come to regard you as a friend, or maybe even part of the family. You may also become close to clients and their family members. As a result, the line between your professional life and your personal life might become blurry. To succeed as a home health aide, you must be able to maintain a professional relationship with both clients and their family members at all times. Although it may be tempting to "drop in" on a client, or to go to the client's home after working hours to visit socially, this is not appropriate. Also, you should refuse any gift (including gifts of food or money) that may be offered to you by a client or family member. Your employer will have very specific policies regarding personal relationships between health care professionals and clients and the acceptance of gifts. Make sure that you always follow these policies, and if you are in doubt about any type of relationship or gift, ask your supervisor for clarification.

Professional boundaries are also necessary to prevent clients or their family members from taking advantage of you. You will have a helping relationship with the client and family members that can easily be taken advantage of in many different ways. For example, a family member might ask you to provide care that has not been listed in the care plan. If you ever have any question about whether or not it is acceptable to perform additional duties or "favors" for a client or family member, make sure you ask your supervisor first.

Good Communication Skills

Clear communication with the other members of the home health care team has already been discussed. You will also need to remember the communication skills you learned in Chapter 5 when working with your clients and their family members. Because you may be the team member who is working with the client most frequently, the client and their family will come to view you as the agency's representative. They may tell you important information about the client's condition or abilities that they "forgot" to mention to the nurse or the case manager. Be sure to listen carefully to what the client and family members share with you and to report promptly to your case manager any information that may affect the client's care or condition. Your client or their family may also ask you additional questions about the client's condition or care. If possible, and if the client is able, refer any questions by family members or neighbors to the client directly. Confidentiality when caring for a person in their home is very important. Make sure that you know with whom the client has agreed to share information about their condition. You should also refer any questions to the nurse or the case manager.

Look and Act Professional

Dress and personal hygiene are very important. Dress according to your agency's policy and always wear proper identification. Since mishaps can occur, either while providing care in a client's home or while traveling between visits, that can cause your clothing to become soiled, it is a good idea to carry an additional set of clothing. That way, you can always look clean and neat for every client.

SUMMARY

- Home health care is skilled nursing care that is given to a person in their home.
  - People of all ages and with all types of illnesses and disabilities use home health care services. Home care may be needed for a short time to help a person recover from an acute illness or injury, or it may be needed for the rest of the person's life.
  - Home health care can be paid for privately by the client, by insurance, or by Medicaid or Medicare.
  - Home health care is provided by a health care team consisting, at a minimum, of a client, their family members, the home health aide, a nurse, a doctor, and a case manager. Other specialists may be included depending on the client's needs.
    - The home health aide is the "eyes and ears" of the health care team. Most communication with other health care team members takes place through documentation.
    - The home health aide's major responsibilities include tasks related to personal care and light housekeeping.
- To succeed, a home health aide must be:
  - Resourceful, since not all of the standard equipment that is available in other health care settings may be available in a person's home.
  - Able to work independently, without a lot of supervision or help from others.
  - Organized, with good time management skills.
  - Reliable, because leaving a client alone and without proper assistance is abandonment.
  - Able to set appropriate professional boundaries with the client and family.
  - A good communicator who always looks and acts professional.

WHAT DID YOU LEARN?

Multiple Choice

Select the single best answer for each of the following questions.

1. Which one of the following may be a routine responsibility of a home health aide?
   a. Providing assistance with a client's ADLs
   b. Picking up a client's prescription at the drug store
   c. Grocery shopping for the family
   d. Washing the windows of the home

2. One of your clients is turning 90 next week, and their family has invited you to attend the birthday party. What should you do?
   a. Accept the invitation, and take a card or a gift to the party
   b. Decline the invitation, but give the client a card or gift during your next scheduled visit
   c. Decline the invitation after thanking the family for inviting you
   d. Accept the invitation, but avoid bringing a card or a gift to the party

3. You are scheduled to work today, but the weather is beautiful and your best friend is begging you to take the day off and go to the beach. What should you do?

    a. Ask your friend if they would be willing to go with you in the afternoon. You will rush to take care of all of your scheduled clients in the morning, and then you will be free to go.

    b. Call the case manager on your way to the beach and tell them that you will not be able to visit your clients today. This will allow the case manager to find another aide to cover for you.

    c. Tell your friend that you are sorry, but you cannot go to the beach today.

    d. Call each of the clients who you are scheduled to visit and ask them if it would be okay if you came tomorrow instead.

4. Why is documentation a very important responsibility of the home health aide?

    a. Documentation is the main way that the members of the home health care team communicate with each other about the care given to the client and the client's condition, and the home health aide has the most frequent contact with the client.

    b. Documentation provides information that is used to determine if a client's condition is improving, or getting worse.

    c. Documentation of all care provided is needed to justify continued payment for home care services.

    d. All of the above.

5. Vamika is a home health aide. Today, while Vamika is helping a client, her son's teacher calls her on her phone to tell her that her son has had an accident on the playground, and he needs to be picked up. What should Vamika do?

    a. Tell the client that she has a family emergency and she has to leave

    b. Tell the teacher that she will be there to pick up her son after her shift ends, in another 2 hours

    c. Call her supervisor and ask if there is another aide who could cover for her while she goes to pick up her son at school

    d. Take the client in the car with her to pick up her son

6. Elizabeth has been caring for Mrs. Ricardo for several months and has become friendly with her son Jose, who is single. One day, Jose asks Elizabeth out for a cup of coffee after she is finished working. What should Elizabeth do?

    a. Decline Jose's invitation because dating family members of clients is against the home health care agency's policy

    b. Accept Jose's invitation—after all, she is single too and she likes to date

    c. Ask Mrs. Ricardo if it is all right if she dates her son

    d. Ask Jose if he would be willing to go for a cup of coffee on a day when she is not scheduled to work

Matching *Match each numbered item with its appropriate lettered description.*

_____ **1.** Case manager

_____ **2.** Care plan

_____ **3.** Respite care

_____ **4.** Hospice care

_____ **5.** Time and travel log

_____ **6.** Homemaker flow sheet

a. End-of-life care provided to a person who is terminally ill

b. Member of the health care team responsible for overseeing a client's care, from admission through discharge

c. Form the home health aide uses to record how much time is spent at each client's house, how much time is spent traveling between houses, and mileage for the day

d. Form used to document housework that is done

e. A set of instructions for the client's care

f. Care that allows the primary caregiver to rest or leave the house for a short period of time

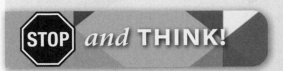

■ You are thinking about becoming a home health aide, and you decide to talk to your friend Tanzi, who has worked in both the long-term care setting and as a home health aide. What do you think Tanzi will tell you is different about working in the home health care setting? What will she tell you is the same?

■ You work for the Home-Aid Home Health Care Agency, which is located in a city called Evergreen. You have received your assignments for the day and are trying to plan your day's work. Look at the assignment list and the map of Evergreen below, and decide how you will organize your day. You know that it will take you 15 minutes to travel between each client's home.

CLIENT	ASSIGNMENT	LENGTH OF VISIT	ADDRESS
Mr. Diaz, a 93-year-old man who is confined to bed	Assist client with toileting and repositioning	45 minutes, twice daily	13th & Chestnut
Miss Louise, an 84-year-old woman who is blind and has diabetes	Assist client with eating snack, change bed linens	45 minutes	7th & Spruce
Ms. Lindgren, a 65-year-old woman with advanced dementia	Assist client with activities of daily living (ADLs) and provide respite care for client's daughter	3 hours	16th & Walnut
Ms. Chang, a 26-year-old woman with paraplegia	Assist client with morning care and breakfast so that she can leave for work by 8:30 AM	90 minutes	14th & Arch

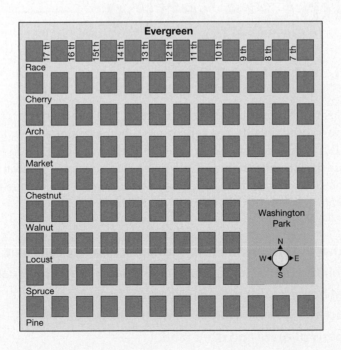

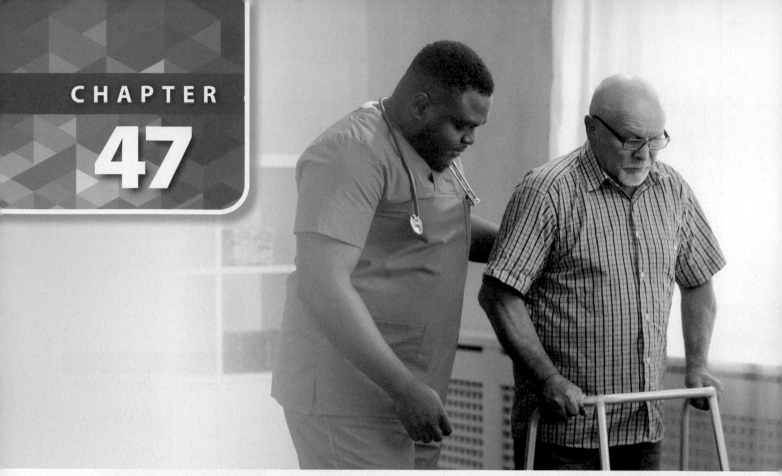

Photo: A home health aide checks to make sure a client is comfortable using their walker. This is just one of many ways that home health aides help to keep their clients safe. (*Maksim Shmeljov\Shutterstock.com*)

Safety and Infection Control in the Home Health Care Setting

 WHAT WILL YOU LEARN?

Keeping yourself and your clients safe from both physical hazards and infection is a priority in the home health care setting, just as it is in other health care settings. As a home health aide, you must be aware of unsafe situations that could put your client at risk for injury in their own home. In addition, working as a home health aide poses unique risks to your safety and well-being. In this chapter, you will learn how to adapt the principles of safety and infection control that you learned earlier to meet the unique needs of the home health care setting. When you are finished with this chapter, you will be able to:

1. List safety concerns that are unique to the home health care environment.
2. Discuss the responsibilities of the home health aide in an emergency situation.
3. Understand ways that home health aides can spread infection.
4. Identify ways to reduce the spread of infection within the home.
5. Identify ways to properly prepare and store food.
6. Describe measures that the home health aide should take to help ensure their own personal safety.

Vocabulary

Bag technique

WORKPLACE SAFETY

Many of us consider our homes places of safety and security. However, the home environment can actually be quite dangerous. As a home health aide, you need to be aware of conditions in the home that put the client at risk. You also need to know how to react in the event of an emergency.

Accidents and Medical Emergencies

Health care settings, such as long-term care facilities and hospitals, are built with safety in mind. The hallways are wide and well lit; there are no throw rugs to trip over; and the bathrooms come equipped with handrails and other safety devices. A person's private home is a different story, however.

Falls

Many factors in the home can put a person at risk for falling, especially if the person has limited mobility or poor eyesight:

- Many homes are older, with worn carpets or uneven floors.
- Hallways, rooms, and staircases may be dimly lit, or not at all.
- The bathroom may be small, or not located in a place that is easy for a person with poor mobility to reach.
- The bathroom may not be equipped with handrails to assist a person with poor mobility to get on and off the toilet or in and out of the bathtub.
- The home may be filled with a lifetime of collected objects and furniture, which can lead to crowding and clutter.
- Many people have pets, which can run underfoot.

Remember from Chapter 14 that falling is the most common type of accident that occurs in the health care setting, and the number one cause of accidental death among older people.

Fire

Fire is also a concern in the home:

- The wiring in the house may be old.
- Outlets may be overloaded. Overload can be caused by plugging too many cords into a single outlet, or by using extension cords.
- Electrical cords may be covered by rugs. This is a fire hazard as well as a tripping hazard.
- The family may rely on space heaters, wood burning stoves, or fireplaces to provide heat.
- Many people do not have functioning smoke detectors in their homes.

Guidelines for helping to maintain a safe home environment are given in Guidelines Box 47-1. It is not your responsibility to change the client's home to ensure safe conditions. However, your observations about the overall safety of the home are important and should be reported to the case manager. For example, based on your observations, the case manager might decide that the client needs better lighting and a smoke detector installed in the hallway, handrails installed on the staircase, and grab bars installed in the bathroom. The client may also need assistive devices, such as an elevated toilet seat or a bedside commode (to make toileting easier) or a stand-assist device (for help with getting into and out of bed). The case manager will arrange for the necessary modifications and equipment. Your job is to make the case manager aware of the client's needs. It is important to remember that you are a guest in the client's home. You are not allowed to make changes or rearrange furniture without the client's or the family's permission.

It is quite possible that despite your efforts to maintain a safe home environment, an accident, fire, or medical emergency will occur. For example, you may arrive at the home to find that your client has fallen and hurt themselves. You may smell smoke or gas when you enter the client's home. The client may have a medical emergency such as a heart attack or stroke while you are there, or they may choke on food. Remember what you learned in Chapters 13 and 16 about reacting to fire and medical emergencies. Remain calm, and use good judgment. Call the fire department or activate the emergency response system by calling 911 or the emergency telephone number specified by your agency. Then provide appropriate care until help arrives. After the situation has been resolved, you will need to report and record according to your agency's policy. For example, if an accident occurred while you were working, most agencies will require you to complete an incident (occurrence) report (see Chapter 14).

Guidelines Box 47-1 Guidelines for Maintaining a Safe Home Environment

WHAT YOU DO	WHY YOU DO IT
Make sure that the furniture is arranged to allow for wide walkways. Chairs and small tables should be placed around the edges of the room rather than in the center.	A cluttered, narrow walkway increases a person's risk of tripping and falling.
Remove any clutter or obstacles from indoor and outdoor walkways and steps. Provide adequate lighting.	Proper lighting enhances the ability to see, which helps to prevent falls. Removing obstacles and clutter that a person could trip over helps to prevent falls as well.
Place a small lamp and a telephone on the person's bedside table.	Having these items close at hand can help to prevent falls. If the phone rings, the person can answer it without getting out of bed. If the person needs to get out of bed in the middle of the night, they can turn on the light first. The ability to see helps to prevent falls.
Install night-lights as needed.	Some people may hesitate to turn on the light when they get up in the middle of the night. Night-lights can help the person to see the route to the bathroom or kitchen without turning on the lights in the room or hallway. The ability to see helps to prevent falls.
Avoid running electrical cords across walkways. Instead, move the furniture so that the electrical cords for lamps and other appliances are close to the outlet.	A person could trip over a cord that is placed across a room or walkway.
In wintry climates, make arrangements for snow and ice to be removed from outdoor walkways and steps.	A person could easily slip and fall on icy or snowy walkways and steps.
Clean up spills on the bathroom or kitchen floor promptly.	Tile or linoleum floors become very slippery when wet, increasing the person's risk of falling.
Use a non-slip rubber bath mat on the floor of the bathtub.	A non-slip rubber bath mat helps to provide traction, reducing the person's risk of falling while getting into or out of the bathtub.
Provide a bath bench or a shower chair for the person to use while showering.	An unsteady person will be more stable and at less risk for falling if they can sit down during the shower.
Be aware of potential fire hazards (for example, frayed wires and overloaded outlets) and report these immediately.	A house fire can have tragic consequences, especially when the people who live in the home are relatively unable to help themselves should a fire break out.
Keep chemicals, cleaning solutions, and other poisonous substances in a secure storage area.	Poor eyesight, confusion, or a decreased sense of taste or smell can cause an older person to eat or drink something that will cause them harm. Children are also at risk for accidental poisoning because they are curious.
Program emergency telephone numbers into the telephone (for example, for the person's doctor, a family member, and emergency services), or keep a written list next to the telephone.	Having emergency phone numbers handy will make it easier for the person to call for help in the event of an emergency.

Abusive Situations

In Chapter 4, you learned about abuse. Abuse can be physical, psychological (emotional), financial, or sexual. Anyone can be a target for abuse. Families are complex, and many things go on "behind closed doors." As a home health aide, you may witness some of these things. For example, one of the family members may be the target of abuse, either by another family member or a friend of the family. An older person or a person with a disability is more likely to be abused in the privacy of their own home because the abuser may feel that the abuse will go undiscovered. Children are also often targets of abuse.

As a home health aide, you may find yourself in a situation where you suspect that one of your clients is being abused (see Chapter 4, Table 4-1). Laws require that any health care worker who suspects the abuse of a child or vulnerable adult must report their suspicions to the proper authorities. Your agency will have specific policies regarding the chain of reporting. It is not your responsibility to investigate whether or not abuse has actually occurred or who has caused it. The state agencies that handle abuse reports will proceed through the proper channels. Your responsibility is simply to report your suspicions.

If a family situation turns violent while you are in the client's home, and you feel unsafe, you should leave the home after doing your best to make sure that the client is also safe. Please do not try to intervene if the situation is turning violent or you may become a victim yourself. Activate the emergency response system by calling 911 or the emergency telephone number specified by your agency if you feel that someone in the house is in immediate danger, and then report the situation to the case manager.

INFECTION CONTROL

Just as in any other health care setting, infection control is a top priority. Many of the people you will care for as a home health aide will have risk factors for infection. Your clients will be sick, be recovering from surgery, be older or have a chronic illness or conditions that will increase their risk of getting an infectious disease. One of your major responsibilities is to protect the people you care for from infection.

As a home health aide, you will visit several clients' homes each day. Improper or careless use of infection control methods can result in pathogens being carried from the home of one client to the home of another one. You can transmit pathogens via your hands, respiratory tract, clothes, or equipment. By maintaining a sanitary environment and using standard precautions, you can protect your clients and yourself from communicable disease.

Maintaining a Sanitary Environment

No matter where you work, you will do many things to help maintain a sanitary work environment (see Chapter 12, Guidelines Box 12-1). When working in a client's home, you will have additional responsibilities related to maintaining a sanitary environment and preventing the spread of infection.

Using Proper Bag Technique

Bag technique is a procedure that is used to keep your tote bag free from contamination. Using proper bag technique helps to prevent the transmission of microbes from one client's home to another client's home or to your car. To practice proper bag technique:

1. When you arrive at the client's home, place your tote bag on a clean surface, such as the kitchen table, after laying down a clean barrier. Placing a barrier between your tote bag and the surface helps to prevent contamination of the bag.

2. After performing hand hygiene, remove the equipment you will need from your tote bag.

3. After you use the equipment, clean it and disinfect it according to agency policy and return it to its proper location in your tote bag (Fig. 47-1). Equipment that is used with all clients, such as your stethoscope, should not be returned to your tote bag until it has been properly cleaned and disinfected. Equipment that has been cleaned and disinfected is stored in the "clean" area of the tote bag.

4. Some items that are used for a client's care must be returned to the agency for proper cleaning and disinfection before they are used again. You may also be required to transport specimens, such as urine or sputum samples, to the agency or laboratory. Used equipment and specimens

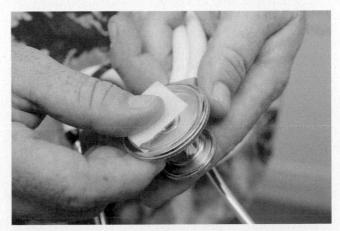

Figure 47-1 Equipment that is used for each client, such as equipment for measuring vital signs, is cleaned after each use and before placing it back in the tote bag.

are considered contaminated and should be contained in a sealed plastic bag for transport back to the agency. When placing the sealed plastic bag into your car, do not place it near clean supply bags that are to be used for other clients. Have a separate area to keep those supplies.

Cleaning Equipment and Household Surfaces

You will use many pieces of equipment as you care for your clients. Some of this equipment will be kept in the client's home, such as a bedside commode or equipment used for bathing. As always, this equipment must be properly cleaned and disinfected after each use. Many people like to use a mixture of vinegar and water for cleaning their homes. However, according to the Centers for Disease Control and Prevention (CDC), vinegar is not effective as a disinfectant and should not be used for that purpose. A commercial disinfectant solution or a solution of bleach and water mixed 1:10 (1 cup of bleach to 10 cups of water) may be used, according to your agency's policy. Wear gloves when cleaning any equipment.

Many of your duties as a home health aide will be related to keeping clean areas where food is prepared or personal care is given. A disinfectant solution is used to clean floors, kitchen counters, bathroom fixtures (including the toilet, bathtub, sink, and counters), and surfaces that are frequently touched by many people (such as doorknobs, telephone receivers, and refrigerator handles). These areas should be cleaned according to agency policy to decrease the spread of pathogens in the home. When cleaning floors and other household surfaces, remember the following:

- Empty dirty mop water into the toilet, *not* into sinks where food will be prepared.
- Disinfect mop heads and sponges after use by soaking them in a 1:10 bleach and water solution. Removable mop heads may be placed in the washing machine and laundered on the hottest setting.
- Clean up blood or body fluid spills immediately. Wearing gloves, use paper towels to soak up as much fluid as possible. Place the soiled towels in a plastic bag and seal it. Then place that plastic bag in a second plastic bag. Seal the second bag, write "biohazard" on the outside of it, and dispose of it in the trash, or according to your agency's policies. Then clean the area where the spill occurred with a disinfectant solution.
- People who are pregnant and people who have weak immune systems should not clean litter boxes, bird cages, or other pet-related items. Cat feces, bird droppings, and other animal wastes can contain microbes that can cause harm to a developing fetus or to a person with a weak immune system.

Handling Food Properly

Depending on a client's care plan, you may be responsible for preparing simple meals or snacks. Before preparing any food, always wash your hands using proper handwashing technique, and make sure that the surface where you will be preparing the food is clean. When preparing foods, remember to:

- Take note of expiration dates on packaged foods
- Avoid using eggs that are cracked
- Thoroughly wash and dry fresh fruits and vegetables before serving them
- Wash your hands after handling raw meat or poultry and before touching anything else
- Wash cutting boards, utensils, and dishes used to prepare raw meat or poultry in hot, soapy water immediately after use
- Cook meat and poultry thoroughly, according to the U.S. Department of Agriculture (USDA) safe food-handling labels that are attached to all supermarket meat packages
- Use a clean spoon each time if you must taste the food to check the seasoning
- Prepare food according to the client's dietary orders (see Special Diets in Chapter 24)

Raw or cooked food that is not stored properly can easily spoil and cause foodborne illnesses. Leftovers should be placed in appropriate sealed containers, labeled with the date and contents, and refrigerated (Fig. 47-2). Food in the refrigerator should be inspected and disposed of before it is outdated or spoiled. The refrigerator itself should be cleaned with hot, soapy water periodically.

After each use, clean kitchen counters and stovetops with a disinfectant solution. If the house has a dishwasher, rinse the dishes and utensils and place them in the dishwasher. When the dishwasher is full, run it using the hot water cycle and dishwasher detergent. Items that are not dishwasher safe should be washed by hand using hot, soapy water. If possible, allow these items to air dry in a rack. Otherwise, use a clean dish towel or paper towels to dry them. If no dishwasher is available, the dishes and utensils will need to be washed by hand and dried. Be sure to wear household gloves when washing dishes.

Assisting Clients With Personal Hygiene

Helping your clients to maintain good personal hygiene is essential to maintaining a sanitary environment. Bathing, washing hair, brushing teeth, and wearing clean clothing are all practices that help prevent the spread of infection. Change the client's bed linens frequently, and encourage the client to wear clean clothing each day. (As always, soiled bed linens

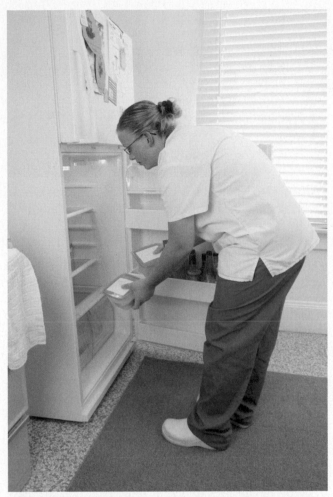

Figure 47-2 Leftovers should be placed in appropriate sealed containers, labeled (contents and date), and stored in the refrigerator.

and clothing should be changed immediately.) Wash soiled linens and clothing in the washing machine, using the warmest water temperature available. Use a lengthy wash cycle and laundry detergent. Make sure to follow laundering directions found on a garment's tag so that you do not damage it. Dry the laundry on the appropriate heat setting in a dryer. If a dryer is unavailable, hang laundry in the sun to dry.

Using Standard Precautions

Maintaining a sanitary workplace is one important way to limit the spread of pathogens. In addition, you must always use standard precautions when providing client care. Standard precautions, covered in detail in Chapter 11, are used to reduce your risk of getting a communicable disease from a client. Proper use of standard precautions also helps to prevent the transmission of an infection to family members or other clients.

Tell the Nurse!

As a home health aide, you will have the unique opportunity to observe the home for conditions and situations that may increase a client's risk of spreading or getting an infection. You must be very diligent about observing your client for signs or symptoms of a developing infection. You must also be aware of practices of the client or family members that may spread an infection. Report any of the following observations to the case manager immediately:

- The client has signs of an infection, such as fever, pain, reddened skin, coughing, a thick nasal discharge, vomiting, or diarrhea

- A family member has signs of infection, especially if the client is at high risk for catching a communicable infection because of a weakened immune system

- Members of the household have poor sanitation practices (for example, there is spoiled food, accumulated trash, or soiled linens lying around the house)

- The house lacks running water or toilet facilities

- The house is infested with insects or rodents (mice or rats)

Hand Hygiene

Proper hand hygiene is the single most important method of preventing the spread of infection in any type of health care setting (see Chapter 12). Always perform proper hand hygiene:

- When you first arrive at a client's home
- Whenever your hands become visibly soiled with blood or other body fluids or substances
- Whenever you remove your gloves
- After each task or procedure that you perform
- Before you leave the client's home

Wash your hands with soap and warm water, using the technique you learned in Chapter 12 (Fig. 47-3). If paper towels are not available, use a *clean* cloth towel to dry your hands.

If handwashing facilities are not available or are inadequate, and your hands are not visibly soiled with dirt, blood, or other body fluids or substances, you can use an alcohol-based hand rub to decontaminate your hands (Fig. 47-4). If your hands are visibly soiled, then you should seek proper handwashing facilities as soon as possible.

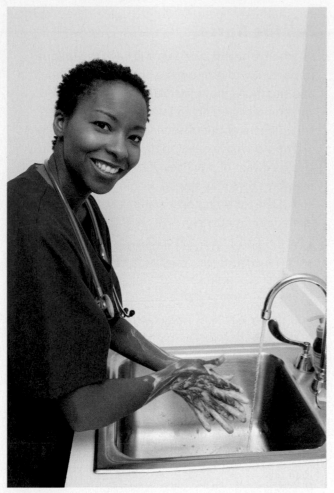

Figure 47-3 Proper hand hygiene is the single most important method of preventing the spread of infection, no matter where you work. Here, a home health aide washes their hands at the kitchen sink. (*sirtravelalot\Shutterstock.com*)

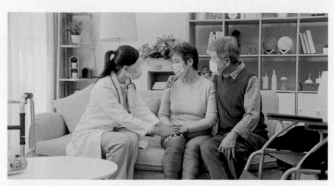

Figure 47-5 It may be necessary for both the home health aide and their clients to wear masks during a visit. (*aslysun\Shutterstock.com*)

Using Personal Protective Equipment (PPE)

As in other health care settings, gloves, gowns, masks, and goggles are worn as necessary to control the spread of pathogens. Your agency is required by the Occupational Safety and Health Administration (OSHA) to provide you with adequate personal protective equipment (PPE). You may carry PPE in your tote bag, or it may be included in the client's supply bag or stored in the home. It is your responsibility to make sure that you have the PPE that you need before you leave for work and to use the PPE consistently, conscientiously, and correctly (see Chapter 12). Eye protection that is not disposable must be cleaned and disinfected after each use.

Due to the prevalence of infections that are easily spread through airborne and droplet transmission, such as influenza and COVID-19, you may need to wear a mask and gloves when visiting your clients (Fig. 47-5). This is especially important during "flu

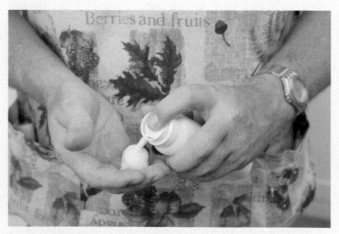

A

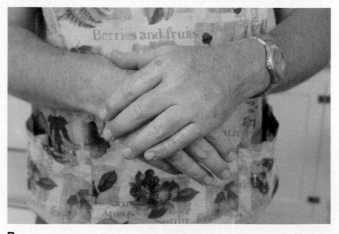

B

Figure 47-4 An alcohol-based hand rub can be used for routine hand hygiene. Alcohol-based hand rubs are easy to use. **A.** Apply the recommended amount of product to one of your palms. **B.** Rub your hands together, covering your hands and fingers (front and back) with the product. Keep rubbing your hands together until your skin is dry.

season." It may be necessary to remind your clients and their family members to wear a mask also. Please remember to wear your mask properly and change it frequently according to your agency's policies.

Disposing of Sharps

Many clients will use needles, lancets, or other sharp instruments or devices on a routine basis. For example, a client who has diabetes may routinely prick their finger with a lancet to check their blood sugar, and then use a syringe and needle to inject their daily doses of insulin. Clients who routinely use needles and lancets will be taught by the nurse how to properly dispose of these items safely. You may use disposable razors when providing care to your clients. These razors should also be disposed of safely. Clients may be provided with an OSHA-approved sharps disposal container by the home health care agency. One of your duties may be to close and dispose of the sharps containers as they become full. Follow your agency's policy on proper sharps disposal measures.

PERSONAL SAFETY

As a home health aide, you will use standard methods to keep yourself safe on the job. For example, you will use proper body mechanics to minimize your risk of physical injury when lifting or transferring clients, and you will use infection control methods to protect yourself from infection. But some aspects of the home health

aide's job pose unique safety risks. Instead of working in one building, you will be required to travel from one client's home to another. This puts you at increased risk for traffic accidents, flat tires, and other driving hazards. In addition, some of your clients may live in unsafe neighborhoods, which could put you at risk for being attacked. Protecting yourself while traveling to and from your clients' homes is a top priority. Box 47-1 describes some things you can do to keep yourself safe while traveling between clients' homes.

Other Safety Concerns

The home health care setting presents some safety concerns that are unique to that environment. Many of your clients may have pets in the home. Dogs, either large or small, that are normally friendly may become protective of an owner who is ill. A dog may think you are a threat to its owner, especially when you are touching or moving a client while providing personal care. The dog may become nervous and protective, resulting in bites or scratches to the home health aide. It is a good idea to call the client before entering the home and request that the dog be confined to another room or area while you are providing care.

Many people have multiple pets in their homes. If a client or family members are unable to care for multiple pets, you may notice unsanitary conditions involving pet waste, food, or other issues. You may also notice conditions in which there are insect, mouse, or rat infestations in a client's home. Any of these situations can

---

Box 47-1   Personal Safety Suggestions

- Keep your car in good repair, and always start out with a full tank of fuel.
- Choose the safest route of travel. Avoid driving or walking through unknown areas and alleys.
- Take a defensive driving course.
- Keep an emergency kit in the trunk of your car. Include flares, a blanket, a shovel, food, drinking water, a flashlight and batteries, jumper cables, and a tire jack.
- Be aware of the dangers of driving in ice and snow. When the weather is bad, be prepared with snow tires, a bag of sand or kitty litter (for weight and traction), and windshield washer fluid.
- Always keep your car doors locked and stay alert for strangers who may wish to cause you harm.
- Leave personal items (such as jewelry or electronics) at home. Do not leave items in plain view on the car seat. Instead, take them with you or put them in the trunk or under the seat before leaving the car. Always lock your car.
- Visit clients who live in unsafe neighborhoods during the day, preferably during the morning hours. Or

- speak with the case manager about arranging an escort to help ensure your safety.
- Park your car in a safe, well-lit area as close to the client's home as possible.
- Choose the safest walking route to reach the home. When walking between your car and the client's home, be aware of other people, animals, and your surroundings in general.
- Wear a name badge identifying yourself as a home health care provider according to your agency policy. If you are attacked, let the attacker know that you do not carry syringes, needles, or medication.
- Consider taking a self-defense course. If you are attacked, use your bag, arms, and hands to protect your face, neck, and throat. Kick the attacker with your legs. Use your car keys to slash the attacker's face. Scream or yell loudly to attract attention.
- Make sure that someone else (your case manager, a friend, or family member) knows your planned schedule. Follow your schedule and check in with the office frequently.
- Carry a fully charged phone with you at all times.

create a health concern and should be reported to the case manager.

Depending on where you live, inclement weather can also create safety concerns, both for the client and the home health aide. Snow and ice can make steps and sidewalks treacherous and lead to falls. Heavy rains that can lead to floods and storms can cause structural damage to a person's home. Weather conditions can make it difficult for you to even reach a client's home.

SUMMARY

- Home health aides are responsible for protecting themselves and those in their care from physical harm and infection.

- The home environment poses many safety risks. Home health aides are responsible for noting dangerous situations and reporting their observations to the case manager and for knowing how to react should an emergency occur.
  - Worn carpets or uneven floors, poor lighting, and clutter increase a person's risk of falling, especially if they have poor mobility or eyesight.
  - Fire is always a risk in the home.
  - Abuse can take place in the home.

- Infection control is a priority in the home health care setting, just as in any other health care setting. The home health aide helps to prevent the spread of infection by maintaining a sanitary environment and using good infection control practices.

- Using proper bag technique helps to prevent the spread of microbes from one client's home to another's.

- Disinfecting household surfaces, especially those where food is prepared or personal care is given, is essential to maintaining a sanitary environment.

- Handling and storing food properly are important for preventing foodborne illnesses.

- Practicing good personal hygiene and helping clients to do the same are important parts of infection control.

- Home health aides must keep themselves safe while traveling between clients' houses. Keeping your car in good repair, being prepared for roadside and weather emergencies, using common sense, and being aware of your surroundings are important safety measures.

WHAT DID YOU LEARN?

Multiple Choice

Select the single best answer for each of the following questions.

1. You have just entered a client's home and are preparing to wash your hands at the kitchen sink when you notice that there is no soap. How else could you accomplish the task of decontaminating your hands?
   a. Wipe your hands with moisturizing hand lotion and a tissue
   b. Use an alcohol-based hand rub
   c. Run your hands under hot water and dry them with a dish towel
   d. Skip washing your hands at this time because you have just arrived in the home, and you have not done anything yet

2. Where should laboratory specimens be stored for transport?
   a. In a sealed plastic bag placed separately from the clean supply bags in your car
   b. Next to the clean supply bags in your car
   c. In the home health aide's uniform pocket
   d. In a cooler on the front seat of the car

3. You have just finished mopping a client's kitchen floor. Where do you dispose of the dirty water?
   a. Out the back door
   b. Down the kitchen sink
   c. Down the toilet
   d. Down the bathroom sink

4. You arrive at a client's home and find the client tied down in bed. The client's daughter tells you that her mother keeps falling out of bed, so she has tied her to the bed for her own protection. What should you do about this situation?
   a. Ignore it. The client's daughter obviously knows what is best for her mother.
   b. Report your observations to the case manager immediately.
   c. Call the police.
   d. Untie the client and tell the daughter that she is guilty of abusing her mother.

5. You are caring for Mrs. DiTomo, who has advanced emphysema. Suddenly, Mr. DiTomo, who also has health problems, complains of chest pain and slumps to the floor. What should you do first?
   a. Call the case manager.
   b. Dial 911 to activate the emergency response system.
   c. Call the DiTomos' daughter and ask her to come over right away.
   d. Put Mr. DiTomo to bed and leave for your next assignment. You owe it to your next client to be on time.

6. Which one of the following observations about a client's home should be reported to the client's case manager?
   a. The client has all of the most modern kitchen appliances.
   b. The client has newspapers and magazines stacked 3 feet high lining both sides of a hallway.
   c. The client has a large collection of dishes stored in a sideboard in the dining room.
   d. The client has very poor taste in decorating.

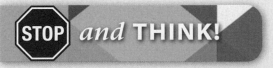

STOP *and* THINK!

■ Juanita has been assigned a new client, Mrs. Pascal. Mrs. Pascal is a widow who lives alone in a small home on a limited income. She is recovering from a stroke, so her ability to get around independently is limited. Juanita is expected to assist Mrs. Pascal with her activities of daily living (ADLs) and to do some light housekeeping. When Juanita arrives at Mrs. Pascal's home for her first visit, she notices the garbage cans outside of the house are overflowing, and there are a lot of flies. On entering the kitchen she notices the kitchen sink is full of dirty dishes, there are dirty dishes all over the counter, and there is a strange odor coming from the refrigerator. After Juanita finishes helping Mrs. Pascal to bathe and she has cleaned up the bathroom, she starts to wonder what to do about Mrs. Pascal's breakfast. Mrs. Pascal needs breakfast, but the kitchen is too filthy to do any cooking. In addition, Juanita only has another half hour before she must leave for her next appointment. If you were Juanita, what would you do?

■ You have been assigned to provide home health care for Mrs. Abrams. Mrs. Abrams is pregnant with her third child and on complete bed rest because of pregnancy-related complications. During your visits, you are assigned to help Mrs. Abrams with personal care and to look after her twin 2-year-old boys, Sammy and Alex. When you arrive at the Abrams home today, you learn that both Sammy and Alex have had diarrhea and have been vomiting since the middle of the night as the result of a virus. You really do not want to take this virus home to your own kids, or get it yourself. Nor do you want Mrs. Abrams to get it since being sick will only make her more uncomfortable than she already is. And you definitely do not want the client you will be visiting next, Mrs. Jefferson, to get it. Mrs. Jefferson has been receiving chemotherapy as part of her treatment for cancer and as a result, her immune system is weak. What measures will you take to try to contain the virus and prevent anyone else from getting it?

Respect

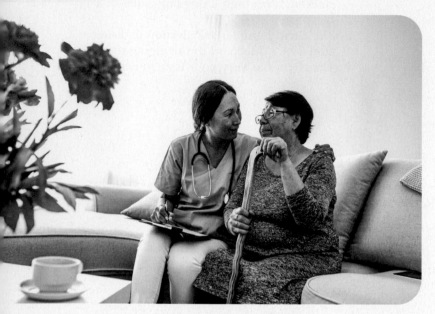

My name is Selina and I am a home health care nurse. I began my career as a nursing assistant and fell in love with home health care. I love visiting clients in their homes and helping them so that they can stay at home, where they feel safe.

One Monday, a few months ago, I received notice that I had a new client. She was an older patient who had just come home from the hospital following knee replacement surgery. I briefly noticed that her name seemed familiar, but it was also a common name in this community. After arriving at her home, her sister answered the door and led me in to meet my new client, Mrs. Santiago. Much to my surprise, my client was none other than my nursing assisting instructor from 15 years ago!

Mrs. Santiago immediately recognized me and started asking me about my journey to become a nurse. As I cared for her, we chatted happily and I told her about the places I had worked and about going to nursing school. I told her that it had been tough to do because at the time I was a single mother to two young boys. I reminded her that she had always told us during our nursing assisting training that we would face challenges in life, both personal and professional, and that we had to believe in our ability to succeed. In fact, Mrs. Santiago and her continuous support of her students had inspired many of us to pursue our careers in nursing.

I continued to care for Mrs. Santiago for the next few weeks as she recovered from her surgery. On the last day of the scheduled visits, she took my hand in hers and asked me to sit down beside her on the sofa. She told me that she was so proud of me and the career I had worked so hard for. She said that one of the reasons she had loved to teach nursing assistants was to help us become confident in our abilities and pursue our dreams. She said that she had always had the utmost respect for her students and it filled her heart with joy to see them overcome obstacles and succeed. As I hugged her goodbye, I promised to stay in touch. Soon, I will let her know that she has inspired my next career objective. I have decided I want to become a teacher of nursing assistants myself and hopefully inspire the next generation of health care professionals like Mrs. Santiago inspired me.

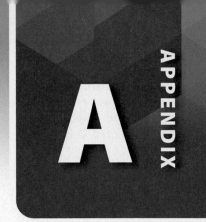

Answers to the
What Did You Learn? Exercises

Chapter 1: The Health Care System
Matching: 1-a, 2-c, 3-d, 4-b, 5-e, 6-g, 7-f, 8-i, 9-j, 10-h

Chapter 2: The Nursing Assistant
Multiple choice: 1-c, 2-b, 3-c, 4-b, 5-b, 6-d

Chapter 3: Professionalism and Job-Seeking Skills
Multiple choice: 1-b, 2-c, 3-b, 4-d, 5-a, 6-d, 7-b, 8-c, 9-c, 10-d, 11-a, 12-b, 13-c

Chapter 4: Legal and Ethical Issues
Multiple choice: 1-b, 2-a, 3-b, 4-b, 5-d, 6-d, 7-c, 8-a, 9-b, 10-a, 11-d, 12-a
Matching: 1-e, 2-a, 3-d, 4-b, 5-c

Chapter 5: Communication Skills
Multiple choice: 1-b, 2-a, 3-d, 4-b, 5-c, 6-a, 7-b, 8-c, 9-b, 10-b
Matching: 1-e, 2-a, 3-d, 4-c, 5-b

Chapter 6: Those We Care For
Multiple choice: 1-d, 2-a, 3-a, 4-b, 5-b, 6-a, 7-d, 8-b
Matching: 1-d, 2-c, 3-f, 4-g, 5-a, 6-b, 7-e

Chapter 7: Overview of Long-Term Care
Multiple choice: 1-a, 2-a, 3-c, 4-b, 5-c
Matching: 1-i, 2-b, 3-a, 4-c, 5-h, 6-g, 7-j, 8-f, 9-e, 10-d

Chapter 8: The Long-Term Care Resident
Multiple choice: 1-d, 2-b, 3-d, 4-d, 5-a, 6-d, 7-a, 8-d, 9-d, 10-d
Matching: 1-g, 2-e, 3-b, 4-c, 5-f, 6-d, 7-a

Chapter 9: Caring for People With Dementia
Multiple choice: 1-d, 2-a, 3-b, 4-c, 5-d, 6-d, 7-a, 8-b, 9-a, 10-d

Chapter 10: Communicable Disease
Multiple choice: 1-d, 2-d, 3-a, 4-c, 5-b, 6-a
Matching: 1-c, 2-d, 3-f, 4-g, 5-e, 6-a, 7-h, 8-i, 9-j, 10-b

Chapter 11: Common Communicable Diseases and Transmission in the Health Care Setting
Multiple choice: 1-d, 2-d, 3-d, 4-b, 5-d, 6-d, 7-c

Chapter 12: Infection Control Measures
Multiple choice: 1-d, 2-b, 3-b, 4-a, 5-d, 6-c, 7-d, 8-b, 9-b, 10-c

Chapter 13: Workplace Safety
Multiple choice: 1-a, 2-b, 3-d, 4-a, 5-c, 6-c, 7-c, 8-a, 9-a, 10-c, 11-b, 12-b, 13-b, 14-d, 15-b

Chapter 14: Patient Safety and Restraint Alternatives
Multiple choice: 1-d, 2-b, 3-c, 4-b, 5-b, 6-c, 7-c, 8-b, 9-c, 10-d

Chapter 15: Positioning, Lifting, and Transferring Patients and Residents
Multiple choice: 1-a, 2-a, 3-d, 4-c, 5-d, 6-d, 7-d, 8-c, 9-b, 10-c, 11-d, 12-b, 13-d, 14-c, 15-d, 16-a

Chapter 16: Basic First Aid and Emergency Care
Multiple choice: 1-d, 2-b, 3-c, 4-c, 5-b, 6-d, 7-d, 8-d
Matching: 1-g, 2-f, 3-i, 4-b, 5-c, 6-e, 7-j, 8-h, 9-d, 10-a

Chapter 17: The Patient or Resident Environment
Multiple choice: 1-c, 2-d, 3-c, 4-b, 5-a, 6-c, 7-d
Matching: 1-e, 2-d, 3-a, 4-b, 5-c

Chapter 18: Admissions, Transfers, and Discharges
Multiple choice: 1-c, 2-b, 3-a, 4-d, 5-b, 6-c, 7-c, 8-c, 9-c

Chapter 19: Bedmaking
Multiple choice: 1-b, 2-d, 3-c, 4-b, 5-c, 6-c, 7-a, 8-d

Chapter 20: Vital Signs, Height, and Weight
Multiple choice: 1-c, 2-a, 3-b, 4-c, 5-d, 6-d, 7-a, 8-c, 9-d, 10-d, 11-b, 12-c

Chapter 21: Comfort and Rest
Multiple choice: 1-d, 2-c, 3-d, 4-c, 5-b, 6-a, 7-c, 8-b, 9-b, 10-c
Matching: 1-f, 2-h, 3-g, 4-a, 5-e, 6-b, 7-c, 8-d

Chapter 22: Cleanliness and Hygiene
Multiple choice: 1-a, 2-c, 3-d, 4-d, 5-c, 6-d, 7-b, 8-a, 9-d, 10-d, 11-d, 12-c
Matching: 1-g, 2-b, 3-f, 4-d, 5-c, 6-e, 7-a

Chapter 23: Grooming
Multiple choice: 1-c, 2-a, 3-a, 4-c, 5-b, 6-d, 7-d, 8-c, 9-d, 10-c, 11-a, 12-d
Matching: 1-d, 2-b, 3-e, 4-c, 5-a

Chapter 24: Basic Nutrition
Multiple choice: 1-c, 2-b, 3-c, 4-b, 5-b, 6-a, 7-c, 8-c, 9-b, 10-c, 11-b, 12-d, 13-d
Matching: 1-c, 2-f, 3-a, 4-e, 5-d, 6-b

Chapter 25: Assisting With Urinary and Bowel Elimination
Multiple choice: 1-b, 2-a, 3-a, 4-a, 5-c, 6-d, 7-b, 8-d, 9-a, 10-c, 11-a, 12-b
Matching: 1-i, 2-j, 3-e, 4-f, 5-b, 6-c, 7-g, 8-d, 9-h, 10-a

Chapter 26: Caring for People Who Are Terminally Ill
Multiple choice: 1-d, 2-d, 3-d, 4-a, 5-c

Chapter 27: Caring for People Who Are Dying
Multiple choice: 1-c, 2-c, 3-b, 4-b, 5-a, 6-d, 7-b, 8-a
Matching: 1-d, 2-e, 3-b, 4-c, 5-a

Chapter 28: Basic Body Structure and Function
Multiple choice: 1-d, 2-c, 3-d, 4-b
Matching: 1-c, 2-g, 3-b, 4-h, 5-a, 6-e, 7-d, 8-f

Chapter 29: The Integumentary System
Multiple choice: 1-d, 2-c, 3-a, 4-d, 5-b, 6-d, 7-b, 8-a, 9-c
Matching: 1-g, 2-j, 3-i, 4-f, 5-a, 6-h, 7-e, 8-d, 9-c, 10-b

Chapter 30: The Musculoskeletal System
Multiple choice: 1-b, 2-b, 3-d, 4-b, 5-d, 6-b, 7-d, 8-c, 9-b, 10-b
Matching: 1-f, 2-c, 3-d, 4-e, 5-b, 6-a

Chapter 31: The Respiratory System
Multiple choice: 1-c, 2-c, 3-d, 4-a, 5-c, 6-a, 7-b, 8-d
Matching: 1-f, 2-g, 3-e, 4-a, 5-d, 6-b, 7-i, 8-c, 9-j, 10-h

Chapter 32: The Cardiovascular System
Multiple choice: 1-a, 2-d, 3-c, 4-d
Matching: 1-g, 2-d, 3-h, 4-j, 5-a, 6-b, 7-c, 8-i, 9-e, 10-f

Chapter 33: The Nervous System
Multiple choice: 1-b, 2-a, 3-b, 4-c, 5-d, 6-c, 7-b, 8-c, 9-c
Matching: 1-g, 2-i, 3-b, 4-h, 5-a, 6-c, 7-e, 8-d, 9-f

Chapter 34: The Sensory System
Multiple choice: 1-b, 2-b, 3-c, 4-d, 5-d, 6-a, 7-b, 8-a
Matching: 1-c, 2-b, 3-g, 4-a, 5-e, 6-h, 7-d, 8-f, 9-i, 10-j

Chapter 35: The Endocrine System
Multiple choice: 1-d, 2-a, 3-b, 4-b, 5-d, 6-a
Matching: 1-h, 2-b, 3-c, 4-i, 5-e, 6-f, 7-g, 8-j, 9-a, 10-d

Chapter 36: The Digestive System
Multiple choice: 1-c, 2-d, 3-c, 4-a, 5-a, 6-d, 7-c

Chapter 37: The Urinary System
Multiple choice: 1-b, 2-d, 3-c, 4-a, 5-a, 6-a, 7-d, 8-b, 9-b
Matching: 1-e, 2-d, 3-a, 4-b, 5-f, 6-c

Chapter 38: The Reproductive System
Multiple choice: 1-d, 2-b, 3-a, 4-c
Matching: 1-c, 2-e, 3-f, 4-h, 5-a, 6-g, 7-b, 8-d, 9-j, 10-i

Chapter 39: Caring for People With Rehabilitation Needs
Multiple choice: 1-d, 2-a, 3-c, 4-c, 5-b, 6-a, 7-c, 8-b, 9-d

Chapter 40: Caring for People With Developmental Disabilities
Multiple choice: 1-b, 2-b, 3-a, 4-b, 5-c, 6-a, 7-c, 8-b, 9-b, 10-a

Chapter 41: Caring for People With Mental Illness
Multiple choice: 1-d, 2-b, 3-c, 4-a, 5-b, 6-b, 7-a
Matching: 1-e, 2-b, 3-i, 4-d, 5-c, 6-g, 7-f, 8-a, 9-h

Chapter 42: Caring for People With Cancer
Multiple choice: 1-a, 2-d, 3-b
Matching: 1-c, 2-e, 3-a, 4-f, 5-b, 6-g, 7-d

Chapter 43: Caring for Surgical Patients
Multiple choice: 1-b, 2-d, 3-d, 4-c, 5-a, 6-c, 7-b, 8-a

Chapter 44: Caring for Birthing Parents and Newborns
Multiple choice: 1-c, 2-c, 3-d, 4-c, 5-d, 6-d, 7-b, 8-a
Matching: 1-b, 2-c, 3-a

Chapter 45: Caring for Pediatric Patients
Multiple choice: 1-b, 2-d, 3-a, 4-c
Matching: 1-c, 2-e, 3-d, 4-a, 5-b

Chapter 46: Introduction to Home Health Care
Multiple choice: 1-a, 2-c, 3-c, 4-d, 5-c, 6-a
Matching: 1-b, 2-e, 3-f, 4-a, 5-c, 6-d

Chapter 47: Safety and Infection Control in the Home Health Care Setting
Multiple choice: 1-b, 2-a, 3-c, 4-b, 5-b, 6-b

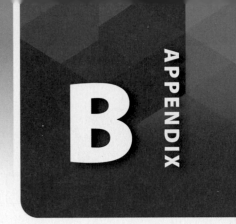
Introduction to the Language of Health Care

All professions have their own sets of words and abbreviations that are used to describe objects and situations that are specific to that particular profession. The health care profession is no different. In fact, the health care profession has so many unique words and abbreviations, you might think that health care professionals are speaking a different language from everyone else!

Understanding the words and abbreviations that are unique to the health care profession is essential if you expect to be able to communicate effectively with the other members of the health care team. Not knowing these words and abbreviations will make it difficult for you to read and follow orders for patient or resident care. In addition, you will need to know these words and abbreviations to accurately record and report.

In this appendix, you will learn some tricks that will allow you to figure out the meaning of many unfamiliar words you may hear or read. We will also introduce you to some commonly used medical words and abbreviations. Finally, you should always make it a point to look up new words or abbreviations in a medical dictionary as soon as you hear or read them. Or, you can ask the nurse to explain the meaning of the word or abbreviation to you. Before long, you will become very comfortable using and understanding the language of the health care profession!

MEDICAL TERMINOLOGY

Although the strange-sounding language of the health care profession may seem overwhelming at first, it is really quite easy to pick up. Some medical words come from the names of people (for example, Down syndrome, Alzheimer disease, Parkinson disease, Papanicolaou smear). Other words come from Greek or Latin words, just as many everyday English, Spanish, French, and Italian words do. For example, you know what a rhinoceros looks like, right? A rhinoceros is a large animal with a huge horn growing out of its nose (Fig. B-1). *Rhin-* comes from the Greek word for "nose," and *-ceros* comes from the Greek word *keras,* or "horn." Now where else might you find the Greek word *rhin-*? Well, if the mucous membranes on the inside of your nose are inflamed because you have a cold or allergies, the doctor might say that you have *rhinitis* (*rhin-,* nose + *itis,* inflammation). If a person has had a "nose job," then their medical record will say they had a *rhinoplasty,* the medical term for a nose job (*rhin-,* nose + *-plasty,* surgical repair).

Perhaps you have noticed a pattern here. Big words can be broken down into smaller parts, and if you know the meaning of the individual parts, you can figure out the meaning of the entire word. There are four types of word parts (Fig. B-2):

- **Roots** contain the essential, basic meaning of the word. For example, *cardi-* means "heart." Common roots are listed in Table B-1, at the end of this appendix.
- **Suffixes** are attached to the end of a root to make the root more specific. For example, *carditis* is "inflammation of the heart" (*cardi-,* heart + *-itis,* inflammation). Common suffixes are listed in Table B-2, at the end of this appendix.
- **Prefixes** are attached to the beginning of a root to make the root more specific. For example, *pericarditis* is "inflammation of the sac that surrounds the heart" (*peri-,* around + *cardi-,* heart + *-itis,* inflammation). Common prefixes are listed in Table B-3, at the end of this appendix.
- **Combining vowels** are often added in between the root and the suffix to make the new word easier to pronounce. When a word has more than one root, combining vowels may also be used between the roots. For example, *cardiomyopathy* is "disease of the heart muscle" (*cardi-,* heart + *o* + *my-,* muscle + *o* + *-pathy,* disease). The combining vowel is usually "o," but "a" or "i" may

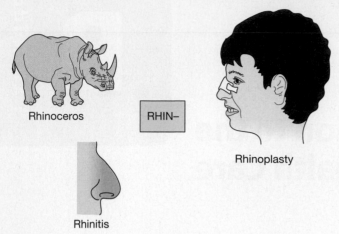

Rhinoceros

RHIN–

Rhinoplasty

Rhinitis

Figure B-1 Many of the words you use in everyday conversation have the same Greek or Latin origins as medical words that you may be less familiar with. For example, the Greek word *rhin-* means "nose." You see *rhin-* in words such as *rhinoceros, rhinitis,* and *rhinoplasty.* When you are trying to figure out the meaning of a new medical word, think about similar-sounding words that you may already know!

also be used. The combining vowel that is used most often with each root is listed in Table B-1.

You will come across many medical words as you study each chapter in this textbook. When you come across a term in your reading that is new to you, try using what you have learned about the different word parts to guess at the word's meaning. Then look up the word in the glossary and see how well you did!

ANATOMICAL TERMS

Anatomy is the study of the structure of the body. To describe the location of one body part in relation to

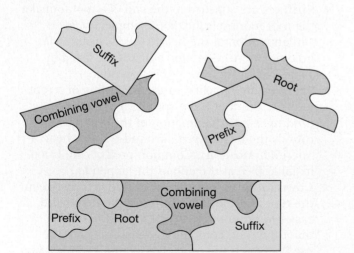

Figure B-2 Big words can be broken down into smaller parts, and if you know the meaning of the individual parts, then you can figure out the meaning of the entire word.

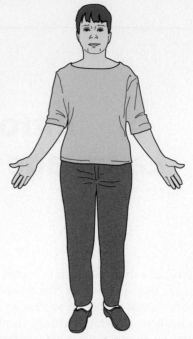

Figure B-3 When describing the location of one part of the body in relation to another, we imagine the body to be in normal anatomical position. In normal anatomical position, the person is standing upright, facing forward, with the legs slightly apart and the arms at the sides, with the palms facing forward.

another, health care professionals use specific terms. To ensure that these terms always have the same meaning to everyone, we always imagine the body to be in *normal anatomical position* when we describe it. A person who is in normal anatomical position is standing upright and facing forward, with their feet slightly spread apart, with arms to the sides and palms facing forward (Fig. B-3). *Anatomical planes* are used as standard points of reference when describing the body. A *plane* is a flat surface, like a pane of glass. Health care professionals use three main imaginary planes to divide the body (Fig. B-4):

■ The **sagittal plane** is a vertical plane that divides the body into right and left sides. A sagittal plane that divides the body into exact right and left halves is sometimes called the *mid-sagittal plane*.
■ The **transverse plane** is a horizontal plane that divides the body into upper and lower segments.
■ The **frontal (coronal)** plane is a vertical plane that divides the body into front and back segments.

Directional Terms

When describing the body, health care professionals often need to describe something that is above, under, to the side of, or further away from something else. To do this, they use standard directional terms.

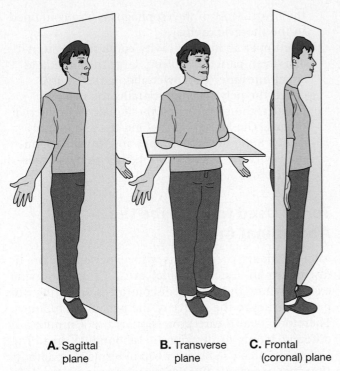

A. Sagittal plane   **B.** Transverse plane   **C.** Frontal (coronal) plane

Figure B-4 The body is divided into imaginary planes, which are used as points of reference when describing the location of one body part with relation to another. **A.** The sagittal plane is a vertical plane that divides the body into right and left segments. Shown here is the mid-sagittal plane, which divides the body into equal right and left halves. **B.** The transverse plane is a horizontal plane that divides the body into upper and lower segments. **C.** The frontal (coronal) plane is a vertical plane that divides the body into front and back segments.

Directional terms are used to describe the location of one body part in relation to another. When we use directional terms, we need a point of reference that stays the same. If not, just changing a person's body position would change a directional reference. This is where normal anatomical position and the anatomical planes come in.

Using the anatomical planes as reference points gives us the following directional terms (Fig. B-5):

- **Medial:** closer to the mid-sagittal plane of the body (toward the inner side or middle). For example, the nose is medial to the eyes.
- **Lateral:** further away from the mid-sagittal plane of the body (toward the outer side). For example, the ears are lateral to the nose.
- **Superior:** closer to the top of the body (closer to the head). For example, the chin is superior to the breast.
- **Inferior:** further away from the top of the body (closer to the feet). For example, the belly button is inferior to the breast.
- **Anterior:** toward the front, or *ventral surface*, of the body. For example, the abdomen is anterior to the buttocks.
- **Posterior:** toward the back, or *dorsal surface*, of the body. For example, the buttocks are posterior to the abdomen.

Two other directional terms are used to describe the location of one body part in relation to another. These terms describe the relationship between parts of the extremities (the arms and legs) and their points

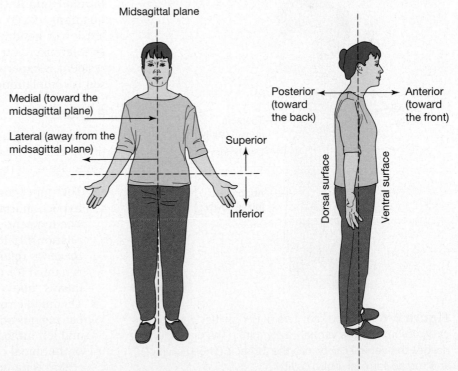

Figure B-5 Directional terms are used to describe the location of one body part in relation to another.

of attachment to the body (the shoulders and hips). These two terms are also used to describe locations on tubular structures, such as the gastrointestinal tract:

- **Proximal:** closer to the point of origin in relation to something else (for example, the elbow is proximal to the wrist)
- **Distal:** further away from the point of origin in relation to something else (for example, the wrist is distal to the elbow)

Like other words used in the health care profession, many of these directional terms have similar meanings to words you use every day. For example, *distal* sounds like *distant*, or "further away." Similarly, *proximal* sounds like *proximity*, which means "close by." If you find the terms *ventral* and *dorsal* hard to remember, just think of a shark swimming close to the surface of the water. The shark's dorsal fin, the fin located on the shark's back, is usually visible above the water.

Terms Used to Describe Body Cavities

A *cavity* is a hollow space. In the body, cavities contain organs. There are two major cavities inside the body. The *dorsal cavity,* which contains the brain and spinal cord, is toward the back of the body. The *ventral cavity* is toward the front of the body (Fig. B-6). The ventral cavity is divided by the diaphragm into the *thoracic (chest) cavity* and the *abdominal (belly) cavity.*

- The thoracic cavity contains the lungs, the heart, and the large blood vessels that enter and leave

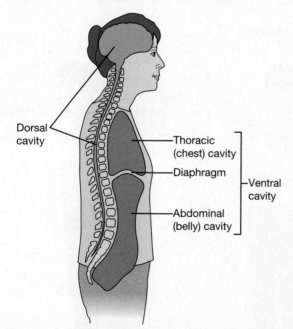

Figure B-6 The body has two major cavities, the dorsal cavity (blue) and the ventral cavity (pink). The diaphragm divides the ventral cavity into the thoracic (chest) cavity and the abdominal (belly) cavity.

the heart. Most of the esophagus is also contained in the thoracic cavity.

- The upper abdominal cavity contains the stomach, liver, pancreas, spleen, large intestine, and small intestine. The lower abdominal cavity, called the pelvic cavity, contains the urinary bladder, the rectum, and the female reproductive organs. The kidneys lie behind the abdominal cavity. Sometimes the upper and lower abdominal cavity are referred to together as the *abdominopelvic cavity.*

Terms Used to Describe the Abdominal Area

Many patients or residents will experience pain or discomfort in the abdominal area. Often, knowing exactly where the pain or discomfort is occurring can provide clues to the source of the person's symptoms. Therefore, health care professionals use a number of different words to describe the abdominal area. The abdominal area can be described in terms of quadrants (fourths) or regions (Fig. B-7). Quadrants are typically used to describe general information, such as where a person is experiencing pain. Regions are used when it is necessary to be very specific (for example, when describing where an incision is located).

Quadrants

Quad means "four." The simplest way to describe the abdominal area is to divide it into fourths, or quadrants. The quadrants are named according to their location: right upper quadrant (RUQ), left upper quadrant (LUQ), right lower quadrant (RLQ), and left lower quadrant (LLQ). By using these quadrants as reference, you can describe where your patient or resident is experiencing pain by saying, "Mrs. Johansen is complaining of a sharp pain in her RUQ."

Regions

The abdomen can also be divided into smaller sections, called *regions,* for the purpose of description. There are nine regions (three rows of three):

- The upper row consists of the right and left hypochondriac regions and the epigastric region. The hypochondriac regions are named for their relationship to the ribs: *hypo-* means "below" and *chondr/o-* refers to the ribs. The epigastric region is named for its relation to the stomach: *epi-* means "above" and *gastric* means "stomach."
- The middle row consists of the right and left lumbar regions and the umbilical region. The right and left lumbar regions are named for the region of the spinal column in that area. The umbilical region is named for the umbilicus, or belly button.

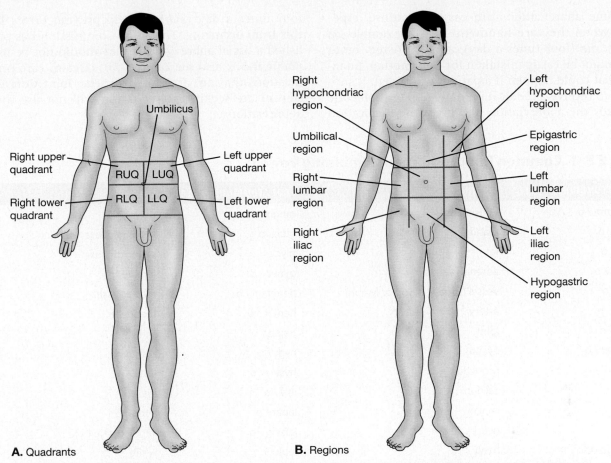

A. Quadrants

B. Regions

Figure B-7   The abdominal area can be described in terms of (**A**) quadrants or (**B**) regions. (Remember that when you are using the terms *right* and *left*, these terms are used in relation to the patient's or resident's right or left, not your right or left.)

■ The lower row consists of the right and left iliac regions and the hypogastric region. The iliac regions are named after the iliac crest, the bone that forms the hip bones. The iliac regions are also sometimes called the inguinal (groin) regions. The hypogastric region is named for its relation to the stomach: *hypo-* means "below" and *gastric* means "stomach."

ABBREVIATIONS

Abbreviations are shortened versions of words or phrases. Health care professionals use abbreviations to make recording more efficient. Some abbreviations come from English words. For example, you just learned that *RUQ* means "right upper quadrant." Other abbreviations come from Latin or Greek words, and therefore may seem foreign at first. For example, *bid* is the abbreviation for "twice daily," from the Latin words *bis* (twice) *in* (a) *die* (day). And *NPO*, which means "nothing by mouth," comes from the Latin

words *nils* (nothing) *per* (by) *os* (mouth). As with other terms used in health care, you can often remember the meaning of a new abbreviation by relating it to an everyday word that you already know. For example, *bid*, *tid*, and *qid* are abbreviations that describe how many times a day an action is to be carried out. The abbreviation *bid* means "twice daily." Now think of how many wheels a *bi*cycle has: two, right? Similarly, the abbreviation *tid* means "three times daily." How many wheels does a *tri*cycle have?

Abbreviations that are commonly used in health care settings are listed in Table B-4, at the end of this appendix. Although abbreviations can help us save time and space when recording, it is very important to use only abbreviations that are approved for use in your facility. Otherwise, other members of the health care team may be confused by your meaning. In addition, if you are unsure of the meaning of an abbreviation that you read in a patient's or resident's care plan, please either look the abbreviation up or ask the nurse to explain it to you. It is important not to just guess at the meaning, because guessing could cause harm to the patient or resident.

Some abbreviations are easy to confuse, especially when they are handwritten. For example, *qd* (daily), *qid* (four times a day), and *qod* (every other day) might be easily mistaken for one another. Imagine what could happen if a patient or resident is supposed to receive a medication daily (*qd*) but someone misreads the abbreviation and gives the medication four times a day (*qid*)! To help prevent errors like this from occurring, The Joint Commission has published a list of abbreviations that should not be used (Table B-5A; also see Table B-5B). Health care organizations that are accredited by The Joint Commission or are seeking accreditation will not use these abbreviations.

TABLE B-1 Common Roots and Their Combining Vowels

ROOT / COMBINING VOWEL	MEANING	ROOT / COMBINING VOWEL	MEANING
abdomin / o	abdomen	gingiv / o	gum
aden / o	gland	gluc / o	sugar, glucose
adip / o	fat	glyc / o	sugar, glucose
adren / o	adrenal glands	gynec / o	female
angi / o	vessel (usually blood or lymph)	hemangi / o	blood vessel
arteri / o	artery	hemat / o	blood
arthr / o	joint	hepat / o	liver
blephar / o	eyelid	hydr / o	water
bronchi / o	bronchus	hyster / o	uterus
calc / o	calcium	irid / o	iris
carcin / o	cancer	lapar / o	abdomen
cardi / o	heart	laryng / o	larynx (voice box)
cephal / o	head	leuk / o	white
cerebr / o	cerebrum (brain)	lingu / o	tongue
chol / e	bile, gall	lip / o	fat
cholecyst / o	gallbladder	lith / o	stone, calculus
choledoch / o	bile duct	lumb / o	lower back
chondr / o	rib or cartilage	lymphangi / o	lymph vessel
col / o	colon	lymph / o	lymph
cost / o	ribs	mamm / o	breast
crani / o	cranium (skull)	mast / o	breast
cutane / o	skin	megal / o	enlargement
cyan / o	blue	melan / o	black
cyst / o	bladder	mening / o	meninges
dent / o	teeth	men / o	menses, menstruation
dermat / o	skin	muc / o	mucus
dipl / o	double	myel / o	spinal cord, bone marrow
electr / o	electric	my / o	muscle
encephal / o	brain	myring / o	tympanic membrane (eardrum)
enter / o	intestine (usually the small intestine)	nas / o	nose
		necr / o	death
erythr / o	red	nephr / o	kidney
esophag / o	esophagus	neur / o	nerve
femor / o	femur (thigh bone)	noct / o	night
gastr / o	stomach		

TABLE B-1 Common Roots and Their Combining Vowels *(Continued)*

ROOT / COMBINING VOWEL	MEANING	ROOT / COMBINING VOWEL	MEANING
odont / o	teeth	spin / o	spine
oophor / o	ovary	spondyl / o	vertebra (backbone)
ophthalm / o	eye	stern / o	sternum (breastbone)
orchi / o	testis	stomat / o	mouth
os / o	mouth	tend / o	tendon
oste / o	bone	therm / o	heat
ot / o	ear	thorac / o	chest
pancreat / o	pancreas	thromb / o	blood clot
pelv / i / o	pelvis	thyr / o	thyroid gland
pharyng / o	pharynx (throat)	toxic, tox / o	poison
phleb / o	vein	trache / o	trachea (windpipe)
pleur / o	pleura	tympan / o	tympanic membrane (eardrum)
pneum / o	lung, air	ureter / o	ureter
proct / o	anus, rectum	urethr / o	urethra
pyel / o	renal pelvis	ur / o	urine
radi / o	x-rays, radiation	uter / o	uterus
ren / o	kidney	vagin / o	vagina
retin / o	retina	vascul / o	blood vessel
rhin / o	nose	vas / o	vas deferens, vessel
salping / o	fallopian tube	ven / o	vein
scler / o	hardening, sclera (white of the eye)	ventricul / o	ventricle (of brain or heart)
sigmoid / o	sigmoid colon	vesic / o	bladder
spermat / o	sperm	vertebr / o	vertebra (backbone)

TABLE B-2 Common Suffixes

SUFFIX	MEANING	SUFFIX	MEANING
-al	pertaining to	-graphy	process of recording
-algia	pain	-ia	condition
-ar, -ary	pertaining to	-ic	pertaining to
-cele	hernia, swelling	-ism	condition
-centesis	surgical puncture	-ist	specialist
-cyte	cell	-itis	inflammation
-derma	skin	-lith	stone, calculus
-dipsia	thirst	-logist	specialist in the study of
-ectomy	excision, removal of	-logy	study of
-edema	swelling	-lysis	separation, destruction, loosening
-emesis	vomiting	-malacia	softening
-emia	blood	-megaly	enlargement
-gram	record	-meter	measure, instrument for measuring

(continued)

TABLE B-2 Common Suffixes *(Continued)*

SUFFIX	MEANING	SUFFIX	MEANING
-oid	resembling	-plegia	paralysis
-oma	tumor	-pnea	breathing
-opia	vision	-rrhaphy	suture
-osis	abnormal condition	-rrhea	flow, discharge
-pathy	disease	-scope	instrument to view
-pause	cessation	-scopy	visual examination
-penia	decrease	-stenosis	structure, narrowing
-pepsia	digestion	-stomy	forming a new opening
-pexy	fixation	-therapy	treatment
-phagia	swallow, eat	-tome	instrument to cut
-phasia	speech	-tomy	incision, cut into
-phobia	fear	-tripsy	crushing
-plasty	surgical repair	-uria	urine, urination

TABLE B-3 Common Prefixes

PREFIX	MEANING	PREFIX	MEANING
a-, an-	without, not, absent	macro-	large
Ab	away from	micro-	small
amb-, ambi-	both, on two sides	neo-	new
auto-	self	para-	near, beside, around
bi-	two, double	peri-	around
brady-	slow	poly-	many, much
dys-	bad, painful, difficult	post-	after, behind
epi-	above, upon	pre-	before
hemi-	half, partly	quadri-	four
hyper-	excessive	sub-	under, below
hypo-	under, below	supra-	above
inter-	between	tachy-	rapid
intra-	within	tri-	three

TABLE B-4 Common Medical Abbreviations

ABBREVIATION	MEANING	ABBREVIATION	MEANING
abd	abdomen	CMS	Centers for Medicare & Medicaid Services
ac	before a meal	CNA	certified nursing assistant
AD	Alzheimer disease	CNS	central nervous system
ADA	Americans with Disabilities Act of 1990	c/o	complains of
ADL	activities of daily living	COPD	chronic obstructive pulmonary disease
ad lib	as desired	CP	cerebral palsy
Adm (adm)	admitted or admission	CPR	cardiopulmonary resuscitation
AED	automated external defibrillator	CVA	cerebrovascular accident (stroke)
AIDS	acquired immunodeficiency syndrome	dc (d/c)	discontinue
AIIR	airborne infection isolation room	DD	developmental disability
AKA	above-the-knee amputation	disch	discharge
ALS	amyotrophic lateral sclerosis	DJD	degenerative joint disease
AM (am)	morning	DNR	do not resuscitate
amb	ambulate, ambulatory	DOA	dead on arrival
amt	amount	DOB	date of birth
ap	apical	DON	director of nursing
approx	approximately	drsg	dressing
ASAP	as soon as possible	DS	Down syndrome
as tol	as tolerated	DV	Daily Value
ax	axillary	Dx	diagnosis
bid	twice a day	ECG (EKG)	electrocardiogram
BKA	below-the-knee amputation	EEG	electroencephalogram
BLS	basic life support	EMS	emergency medical services
BM (bm)	bowel movement	ePHI	electronic protected health information
BP, B/P	blood pressure	ER	emergency room
B.R.	bed rest	F	Fahrenheit
BRP	bathroom privileges	FBAO	foreign-body airway obstruction
BSC	bedside commode	FBS	fasting blood sugar
C	centigrade, Celsius	FF	force fluids
c̄	with	fl (fld)	fluid
CA	cancer	ft	foot or feet
CAD	coronary artery disease	Fx	fracture
cath	catheter, catheterize	gal	gallon
CBC	complete blood count	GB	gallbladder
CBR	complete bed rest	GERD	gastroesophageal reflux disease
CCRC	continuing care retirement community	GI	gastrointestinal
CCU	coronary care unit	GSW	gunshot wound
CDC	Centers for Disease Control and Prevention	gtt	drops
CHD	coronary heart disease	GU	genitourinary
CHF	congestive heart failure	h (hr)	hour
cl liq	clear liquids	HAI	health care–associated infection

(continued)

TABLE B-4 Common Medical Abbreviations *(Continued)*

ABBREVIATION	MEANING	ABBREVIATION	MEANING
H$_2$O	water	NG	nasogastric
HBV	hepatitis B virus	NIDDM	noninsulin–dependent diabetes mellitus
Hg	mercury	nil	none
HIPAA	Health Insurance Portability and Accountability Act of 1996	no	number
		noc, noct	night
HIV	human immunodeficiency virus	NPO (npo)	nothing per mouth (nils per os)
HOB	head of bed	N&V	nausea and vomiting
HS (hs)	hour of sleep (bedtime)	O$_2$	oxygen
ht	height	OB	obstetrics
HTN	hypertension	OCD	obsessive–compulsive disorder
ICU	intensive care unit	OJ	orange juice
ID	identification	OOB	out of bed
IDDM	insulin-dependent diabetes mellitus	O	oral
in	inch	OR	operating room
I&O	intake and output	OSHA	Occupational Safety and Health Administration
IV	intravenous		
IQ	intelligence quotient	OT	occupational therapy
L	left, liter	oz (Oz)	ounce
lab	laboratory	PACU	post anesthesia care unit
lb	pound	pc	after a meal
lg	large	Peds	pediatrics
liq	liquid	PEG	percutaneous endoscopic gastrostomy
LLQ	left lower quadrant	PHI	protected health information
LMP	last menstrual period	per	by, through
LPN	licensed practical nurse	PM (pm)	afternoon or evening
lt	left	PPE	personal protective equipment
LVN	licensed vocational nurse	po (per os)	by mouth
LUQ	left upper quadrant	post op	postoperative
MDRO	multidrug-resistant organism	pre op	preoperative
MDS	Minimum Data Set	prep	preparation
meds	medications	prn	as necessary
mg	milligram	Pt (pt)	patient
MI	myocardial infarction (heart attack)	PT	physical therapy
min	minute	PTSD	posttraumatic stress disorder
mL	milliliter	PVS	persistent vegetative state
mm	millimeter	q	every
MRSA	Methicillin-resistant *Staphylococcus aureus*	qd	every day
		qh	every hour
MS	multiple sclerosis	q2h, q3h, q4h, etc.	every 2 hours, every 3 hours, every 4 hours, etc.
MSD	musculoskeletal disorder		
NA	nursing assistant	qhs	every night at bedtime
NB	newborn	qid	four times a day
neg	negative	qod	every other day

TABLE B-4 Common Medical Abbreviations *(Continued)*

ABBREVIATION	MEANING	ABBREVIATION	MEANING
qs	sufficient quantity	Sx	symptoms
qt	quiet	TB	tuberculosis
R	rectal	TBI	traumatic brain injury
RA	rheumatoid arthritis	tbsp	tablespoon
RBC	red blood cell, red blood cell count	tid	three times a day
rehab	rehabilitation	TIA	transient ischemic attack
resp	respiration	TJC	The Joint Commission
RLQ	right lower quadrant	TLC	tender loving care
RN	registered nurse	TPN	total parenteral nutrition
ROM	range of motion	TPR	temperature, pulse, and respirations
rt (R)	right	tsp	teaspoon
RT	respiratory therapy	Tx	treatment
RUQ	right upper quadrant	Ty	tympanic
Rx	treatment	UA (u/a)	urinalysis
s̄	without	UK	unknown
s̄s̄	half	URI	upper respiratory infection
SCD	sequential compression device	UTI	urinary tract infection
SNF	skilled nursing facility	VRE	Vancomycin-resistant Enterococci
SOB	shortness of breath	VS (vs)	vital signs
Spec (spec)	specimen	WA	while awake
SSE	soapsuds enema	WBC	white blood cell, white blood cell count
ST	speech therapy	w/c	wheelchair
STAT, stat	at once, immediately	WNL	within normal limits
STI	sexually transmitted infection	wt	weight
Surg	surgery		

TABLE B-5A The Joint Commission Official "Do Not Use" List

DO NOT USE	POTENTIAL PROBLEM	USE INSTEAD
U, u (unit)	Mistaken for "0" (zero), the number "4" (four), or "cc"	Write "unit"
IU (International Unit)	Mistaken for IV (intravenous) or the number 10 (ten)	Write "International Unit"
Q.D., QD, q.d., qd (daily)	Mistaken for each other	Write "daily"
Q.O.D., QOD, q.o.d, qod (every other day)	Period after the Q mistaken for "I" and the "O" mistaken for "I"	Write "every other day"
Trailing zero (X.0 mg)[a]	Decimal point is missed	Write X mg
Lack of leading zero (.X mg)		Write 0.X mg
MS	Can mean morphine sulfate or magnesium sulfate	Write "morphine sulfate"
MSO_4 and $MgSO_4$	Confused for one another	Write "magnesium sulfate"

This list applies to all orders and all medication-related documentation that is handwritten (including free-text computer entry) or on pre-printed forms.
[a]**Exception:** A "trailing zero" may be used only where required to demonstrate the level of precision of the value being reported, such as for laboratory results, imaging studies of lesions, or catheter/tube sizes. It may not be used in medication orders or other medication-related documentation.
© Joint Commission Resources: "Do Not Use" List of Abbreviations. Oakbrook Terrace, IL: Joint Commission on Accreditation of Healthcare Organizations, 2018. Reprinted with permission.

TABLE B-5B Additional Abbreviations, Acronyms, and Symbols for Possible Future Inclusion in the Official "Do Not Use" List

DO NOT USE	POTENTIAL PROBLEM	USE INSTEAD
> (greater than) < (less than)	Misinterpreted as the number "7" (seven) or the letter "L" Confused for one another	Write "greater than" Write "less than"
Abbreviations for drug names	Misinterpreted due to similar abbreviations for multiple drugs	Write drug names in full
Apothecary units	Unfamiliar to many practitioners Confused with metric units	Use metric units
@	Mistaken for the number "2" (two)	Write "at"
Cc	Mistaken for U (units) when poorly written	Write "mL" or "milliliters"
Mg	Mistaken for mg (milligrams), resulting in one thousand-fold overdose	Write "mcg" or "micrograms"

© Joint Commission Resources: "Do Not Use" List of Abbreviations. Oakbrook Terrace, IL: Joint Commission on Accreditation of Healthcare Organizations, 2018. Reprinted with permission.

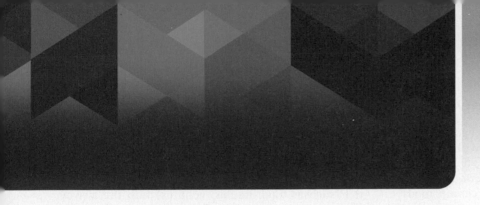

Glossary

A

Abandonment: the act of withdrawing support or help from another person, in spite of duty or responsibility (4)

Absorption: transfer of nutrients from the digestive tract into the bloodstream (24)

Abuse: intentional act that causes harm to another person (4)

Acceptance: one of the stages of grief; the person comes to terms with the reality of their own impending death, and is finally at peace with this knowledge (26)

Accident: an unexpected, unintended event that has the potential to cause bodily injury (14)

Accreditation: official recognition that an organization meets certain standards of quality (1)

Acquired immunodeficiency syndrome (AIDS): a disease caused by human immunodeficiency virus (HIV), a bloodborne virus that attacks the body's immune system; death results when the body becomes unable to recognize and fight off infections (11)

Activities of daily living (ADLs): routine tasks of daily life, such as bathing, eating, and grooming (compare with instrumental activities of daily living) (8)

Acute care setting: a place where health care is provided for people who require a high level of care; patients usually have severe illnesses, or are medically unstable, and length of stay in the facility is typically short (compare with post-acute care setting and long-term care setting) (1)

Acute illness: an illness with a rapid onset and a relatively short recovery time, usually unexpected (6)

Acute pain: sharp, sudden pain, typically produced by a sudden injury or illness (21)

Addiction: a physical need for a substance that results in withdrawal signs and symptoms if the substance is withheld (41)

ADLs: see activities of daily living

Admission: official entry of a person into a health care setting (18)

Advance directive: a document that allows a person to make their wishes regarding health care known to family members and health care workers, in case the time comes when they are no longer able to make those wishes known themselves; examples include living wills and durable powers of attorney for health care (4)

Aerobic: an adjective used to describe bacteria that need oxygen in order to live (compare with anaerobic) (10)

Afterlife: a state of being where the dead meet again with loved ones who have passed on before them (27)

Afternoon care: care that is provided before and after lunch and dinner (22)

Against medical advice (AMA): term used to describe a person's actions when a person leaves a health care facility without a doctor's order (18)

Agnosia: difficulty recognizing sensory input; one of the "4 As" of dementia (9)

AIDS: see acquired immunodeficiency syndrome

Airborne infection isolation room (AIIR): single-occupancy patient-care room with special ventilation and filtration systems used to isolate persons with an airborne infectious disease (12)

Airborne pathogen: pathogens that can be transmitted through the air (11)

Airborne precautions: used when caring for people infected with pathogens that can be transmitted through the air; include placing the patient or resident in a private room with the door closed, wearing a mask when caring for the person, and minimizing the amount of time the person spends out of their private room (12)

Alignment: good posture; the "A" in the ABCs of good body mechanics (13)

Alopecia: baldness, loss of hair (23)

Alveoli (singular, alveolus): grape-like clusters of tiny air sacs in the lungs, where gas exchange takes place (31)

Alzheimer disease: the most common type of dementia; characterized by the permanent and progressive loss of the ability to think and remember caused by damage to the brain (9)

Ambulate: to walk (15)

Amenorrhea: absence of menstrual flow (38)

Amino acids: molecules that are the building blocks of the body's cells; found in proteins (24)

Amnesia: memory loss; one of the "4 As" of dementia (9)

Amputation: the surgical removal of all or part of an extremity (30)

Anaerobic: an adjective used to describe bacteria that can survive without oxygen (compare with aerobic) (10)

Anaphylactic shock: shock caused by a serious allergic reaction to a medication, bee sting, or certain foods (16)

Anatomy: the study of what body parts look like, where they are located, how big they are, and how they connect to other body parts (28)

Anemia: a general term for a group of disorders that affect the ability of the red blood cells to carry oxygen to the cells and tissues of the body (32)

Anger: one of the stages of grief; the person realizes that they are actually going to die as a result of their illness and has feelings of rage, which may be directed toward themselves or others (26)

Angina pectoris: the classic chest pain that is felt as a result of the heart muscle being deprived of oxygen (32)

Anorexia: loss of appetite (24)

Anorexia nervosa: an eating disorder characterized by an intense fear of gaining weight or becoming obese; people with this disorder cannot maintain a healthy body weight because they engage in activities such as extreme dieting, excessive exercising, or both (41)

Antepartum (prenatal) period: the period of time from conception until the baby is born (44)

Antibodies: specialized proteins produced by the immune system that help our bodies to fight off specific microbes, preventing infection (10)

Antiperspirant: a grooming product that contains ingredients to stop or slow the production of sweat (22)

Antisepsis: practices that kill microbes or stop them from growing; one of the techniques of medical asepsis (compare with sanitization, disinfection, and sterilization) (12)

Anuria: the state of voiding less than 100 mL of urine over the course of 24 hours (25)

Anxiety: feeling of uneasiness, dread, apprehension, or worry (41)

Aphasia: a general term for a group of disorders that affect a person's ability to communicate with others; may be expressive (an inability to form words) or receptive (an inability to understand words); often occurs following a stroke; one of the "4 As" of dementia (9, 33)

Appetite: the desire for food (compare with anorexia) (24)

Apraxia: difficulty coordinating the steps to complete a task; one of the "4 As" of dementia (9)

Arteries: vessels that carry blood away from the heart (32)

Arterioles: the smallest arteries (32)

Arteriosclerosis: "hardening of the arteries"; occurs when atherosclerotic plaque interferes with the elasticity of the arterial walls, making them brittle and prone to breaking (32)

Arthritis: inflammation of joints, usually associated with pain and stiffness (30)

Aspiration: the accidental inhalation of foreign material (such as food, liquids, vomitus) into the airway (16)

Assault: threatening or attempting to touch a person without the person's consent (4)

Assisted-living facility: type of long-term care facility that provides residents with limited assistance with tasks such as medication administration, transportation, meals, and housekeeping (1)

Assistive devices: devices that make certain tasks (such as walking, eating, or dressing) easier for a person with a disability (39)

Asthma: a condition that affects the bronchi and bronchioles of the lungs; triggers (such as cold weather, allergies, respiratory infections, stress, smoke, and exercise) cause the bronchi and bronchioles to become narrower, making breathing difficult (31)

Astigmatism: an inability to focus images properly because the cornea of the eye is not perfectly curved (34)

Atelectasis: collapse of the alveoli of the lungs; a common respiratory complication following surgery (43)

Atherosclerosis: blocking of the arteries, caused by the build-up of fatty deposits called plaque on the inside of the vessel wall (32)

Atria (singular, atrium): the upper chambers of the heart (32)

Atrophy: the loss of muscle size and strength (30)

Attitude: the side of ourselves that we display to the world, communicating outwardly how we feel about things (3)

Autism spectrum disorder: a condition related to brain development characterized by difficulty communicating and relating to other people and surroundings (40)

Automated external defibrillator (AED): a small, portable device that automatically detects a person's heart rhythm and delivers and electrical shock to the heart to stop fast, abnormal heartbeats and restore the heart's normal rhythm (16)

Autopsy: examination of a person's organs and tissues after the person has died, done to confirm or identify the cause of the person's death (27)

Axon: a long extension from the body of a neuron that sends information to other neurons (compare with dendrites) (33)

B

Bag technique: an infection control procedure used in the home health care setting to keep the tote bag free from contamination (47)

Balance: stability produced by the even distribution of weight; the "B" in the ABCs of good body mechanics (13)

Bargaining: one of the stages of grief; the person wants to "make a deal" with someone they feel has control over their fate, such as God or a health care provider (26)

Basic life support (BLS): basic emergency care techniques, such as rescue breathing and cardiopulmonary resuscitation (CPR) (16)

Bath blanket: a lightweight cotton blanket used to cover a person during a bed bath or linen change to help provide modesty and warmth (19)

Battery: touching a person without their consent (4)

Bed cradle: a metal frame that is placed between the bottom and top sheets to keep the top sheet, the blanket, and the bedspread away from the person's feet; used when pressure on the person's feet could result in pain or skin breakdown (19)

Bedpan: a device used for elimination when a person is unable to get out of bed; females use a bedpan for both urination and bowel movements; males use a bedpan for bowel movements only (25)

Bed protector: a square of quilted absorbent fabric backed with waterproof material that measures approximately 3 feet by 3 feet; used to prevent soiling of the bottom linens; sometimes called an incontinence pad or a soaker pad (19)

Bedside commode: a device used for elimination when a person is able to get out of bed, but unable to walk to the bathroom; it consists of a chair-like frame with a toilet seat and a removable collection bucket (25)

Bell: the small, rounded surface on a stethoscope that is used to pick up faint sounds; commonly used to listen to the apical pulse in infants and small children (20)

Benefit period: a unit of time used by the Medicare program to track how many days of skilled health care services a person uses, and how many are still available; begins with hospitalization and ends when a person has not received any skilled health care services, either in the hospital or nursing home, for 60 days (7)

Benign: adjective used to describe a noncancerous tumor (that is, a tumor that does not progress or invade other tissues) (compare with malignant) (42)

Bile: a substance produced by the liver that helps with the digestion of fats (36)

Biopsy: a diagnostic procedure that involves obtaining a tissue sample and examining it under a microscope for cancerous cells (42)

Bipolar disorder: a mental health disorder characterized by mood swings; people with this disorder experience excessively "high" or happy periods, followed by excessively "low" or depressed periods (41)

Bisexual: a person who is sexually attracted to members of both sexes (6)

Bloodborne pathogen: a disease-producing microbe that is transmitted to another person through blood or other body fluids (11)

Blood pressure: the force that the blood exerts against the arterial walls; one of the vital signs (20)

BLS: see basic life support

Body alignment: positioning of the body so that the spine is not twisted or crooked (15)

Body fluids: liquid or semi-liquid substances produced by the body, such as blood, urine, feces, vomitus, saliva, drainage from wounds, sweat, semen, vaginal secretions, tears, cerebrospinal fluid, amniotic fluid, and breast milk (11)

Body mechanics: the efficient and safe use of the body (13)

Body temperature: how hot the body is; one of the vital signs (20)

Bonding period: the first hour or two immediately following delivery of a baby, during which emotional and physical attachments between the parents and the infant develop (44)

Bony prominences: parts of the body where there is very little fat between the bone and the skin, such as the ankles, heels, hips, and elbows (29)

Bradycardia: a heart rate that is slower than normal (less than 60 beats/min in an adult) (20)

Bradypnea: a respiratory rate that is lower than normal (less than 10 breaths/min in an adult) (20)

Braille: a system that uses letters made from combinations of raised dots that allows a person who has a visual impairment to read (34)

Breakthrough pain: pain that occurs before a person's next regularly scheduled dose of pain medication (21)

Bronchi (singular, bronchus): passageways that carry air from the trachea ("windpipe") to the lungs, one bronchus goes to the right lung and the other goes to the left (31)

Bronchioles: the smallest branches of the bronchi (31)

Bronchitis: inflammation of the bronchi (31)

Bulimia nervosa: an eating disorder characterized by an intense fear of gaining weight or becoming obese; people with this disorder cannot maintain a healthy body weight because they engage in activities such as binging (eating large amounts of food in one sitting) and purging (vomiting the food back up) (41)

C

Call light system: a system that allows a patient or resident to call for help; usually consists of a call light control, a light in the hall, and a panel of lights at the nurses' station or some other central location (17)

Calories: the unit of measure used to describe the energy content of food (24)

Capillary bed: the network of tiny vessels in the tissues where the oxygen and nutrients in the blood pass into the tissues, and carbon dioxide and other waste materials from the tissues pass into the blood (32)

Cardiac arrest: the condition that is said to occur when the heart stops beating (16)

Cardiac cycle: the pumping action of the heart in an organized pattern (all of the events associated with one heartbeat) (32)

Cardiac rehabilitation: therapy that helps a person regain strength and adopt habits that will help the cardiovascular system become healthier (39)

Cardiogenic shock: shock that occurs when the heart is unable to pump enough blood throughout the body to meet the tissues' need for oxygen (16)

Cardiopulmonary resuscitation (CPR): a technique used to sustain breathing and circulation for a person who has gone into respiratory or cardiac arrest (16)

Carrier: a person who is infected with a virus but never develops symptoms of the disease; the virus lives in the person's body and can be transmitted to another person (11)

Cartilage: a tough, fibrous substance found in joints and other parts of the body; in slightly movable joints, the cartilage acts as a "shock absorber"; in freely movable joints, the cartilage provides a smooth surface for the bones of the joint to move against (30)

Case manager: in the home health care setting, the member of the health care team who is responsible for overseeing the client's total care, from admission through discharge (46)

Cataract: the gradual yellowing and hardening of the lens of the eye (34)

Catastrophic reaction: an extreme reaction to a situation that would normally cause minimal or no stress; often seen in people with dementia (9)

Catheter: a tube that is inserted into the body for the purpose of administering or removing fluids (25)

Catheter care: thorough cleaning of the perineal area (especially around the urethra) and the catheter tubing that extends outside of the body, to prevent infection (25)

CDC: see Centers for Disease Control and Prevention

Cell: the basic unit of life (28)

Centers for Disease Control and Prevention (CDC): a federal agency based in Atlanta, Georgia, that is dedicated to protecting the health and safety of people in the United States (11)

Centers for Medicare and Medicaid Services (CMS): the government agency that provides oversight of government-funded insurance programs and is responsible for monitoring nursing homes to ensure compliance with Omnibus Budget Reconciliation Act (OBRA) regulations; under the umbrella of the United States Department of Health and Human Services (DHHS) (7)

Central nervous system (CNS): the brain and spinal cord; responsible for receiving information, processing it, and issuing instructions (compare with peripheral nervous system) (33)

Cerebral palsy: a developmental disability caused by damage to the cerebrum, the part of the brain involved with motor control (40)

Cerebrospinal fluid (CSF): a clear fluid that circulates around the brain and spinal cord and acts as a "shock absorber" to protect these structures (33)

Cerumen: a waxy substance that helps to protect the external auditory canal by trapping dirt and other particles; commonly referred to as "earwax" (34)

Cerumen impaction: a condition that occurs when ear wax builds up and becomes packed in the external auditory canal (34)

Cesarean section: delivery of a baby through a surgical incision made in the pregnant person's abdomen (44)

Chain facility: a facility that is owned and operated by a corporation that owns multiple, similar facilities (compare with free-standing facility) (7)

Chain of infection: the six key conditions that must be met for a person to get a communicable infection (pathogen, reservoir, portal of exit, method of transmission, portal of entry, and susceptible host) (10)

Chain of survival: the series of events that must take place in an emergency situation to increase the person's ability to survive the emergency without any permanent damage (16)

Charge nurse: a registered nurse (RN) or licensed practical nurse/licensed vocational nurse (LPN/LVN) who supervises the other nurses for a particular shift (2)

Chemical digestion: the process of breaking down food through the use of chemical substances such as enzymes (compare with mechanical digestion) (36)

Chemical restraint: any medication that alters a person's mood or behavior, such as a sedative or tranquilizer (compare with physical restraint) (14)

Chemotherapy: the use of medications to destroy malignant cancer cells (42)

Cheyne–Stokes respiration: very irregular, shallow breaths, in an alternating fast–slow pattern; often seen in people who are dying (27)

Chronic bronchitis: a disorder caused by long-term irritation of the bronchi and bronchioles, such as that caused by inhaling tobacco smoke; one of two forms of chronic obstructive pulmonary disease (COPD) (31)

Chronic condition: a condition that is ongoing and often needs to be controlled through continuous medication or treatment (8)

Chronic illness: an illness that is ongoing and often needs to be controlled through continuous medication or treatment (6)

Chronic obstructive pulmonary disease (COPD): a general term used to describe two related lung disorders, emphysema and chronic bronchitis; the leading cause of COPD is smoking (31)

Chronic pain: slow, diffuse, constant pain (21)

Chyme: the liquid substance produced by the digestion of food in the stomach (25)

Circulation: the continuous movement of the blood through the blood vessels; powered by the pumping action of the heart (32)

Circumcision: a procedure involving the removal of the foreskin, the fold of loose skin that covers the head of the penis; often performed on male infants for religious or cultural reasons (22)

Civil laws: laws concerned with relationships between individuals (4)

Client: a person who is receiving the services of a home health care agency (1)

Closed bed: an empty, made bed (19)

CNS: see central nervous system

Coagulation: clotting of the blood (32)

Coexistent medical conditions: more than one medical condition at the same time in the same person (8)

Cognitive impairment: problems processing, learning, or remembering information (8)

Coitus: sexual intercourse (6)

Collagen: a protein that supports connective tissue, such as that found in the dermis; loss of collagen contributes to the formation of wrinkles (29)

Colonies: groups of bacteria (10)

Colostomy: an alternative way of eliminating feces from the body; done when only part of the large intestine must be removed due to disease; after removing the diseased part of a person's large intestine, an artificial opening, called a stoma, is made in the abdominal wall and the remaining portion of the large intestine is connected to it (compare with ileostomy) (25)

Colostrum: a thin yellowish fluid that contains extra calories and proteins as well as antibodies and is produced by the breasts immediately following delivery of the baby; after 2 to 3 days, colostrum is replaced by breast milk (44)

Coma: a state of unconsciousness from which a person cannot be aroused (33)

Comatose: the state of being in a coma, a state of unconsciousness from which a person cannot be aroused (14)

Communicable disease: a disease that can be transmitted from one person to another (10)

Communication: the exchange of information (5)

Competency evaluation: an exam consisting of a written portion and a skills portion that must be passed at the end of the nursing assistant training course to obtain certification (2)

Conception (fertilization): occurs when the male and female sex cells join, forming a cell that contains the complete number of chromosomes (38)

Condom catheter: a device used to manage urinary incontinence in males; it consists of a soft plastic or rubber sheath, tubing, and a collection bag for the urine (25)

Conduction disorders: conditions that affect the pathway that the heart uses to transmit the electrical impulses that cause contraction (32)

Conductive hearing loss: hearing loss that results when something prevents sound waves from reaching the receptors in the cochlea of the ear; compare with sensorineural hearing loss (34)

Confidentiality: keeping personal information that someone shares with you to yourself (4)

Conflict: discord resulting from differences between people; can occur when one person is unable to understand or accept another's ideas or beliefs (5)

Congenital: adjective used to describe a disorder that a person is born with (40)

Conjunctivitis ("pink eye"): infection and inflammation of the conjunctiva, a clear membrane that lines the inside of the eyelids and covers most of the surface of the eye; characterized by redness, swelling, itching, burning and excessive tearing (34)

Constipation: a condition that occurs when the feces remain in the intestines for too long, resulting in hard, dry feces that are difficult to pass (25)

Contact precautions: used when caring for people infected with pathogens that can be transmitted directly (by touching the person), or indirectly (by touching fomites); include using barrier methods whenever contact with the infected person or items contaminated with wound drainage or body substances is necessary (12)

Contaminated: adjective used to describe an object that is soiled by pathogens (10)

Continuing Care Accreditation Commission (CCAC): an independent, non-profit organization that sets national standards for continuing care retirement communities (CCRCs), as well as for some other types of organizations that provide long-term care services (such as adult day care centers), and officially recognizes (accredits) organizations that meet these standards (7)

Continuing Care Retirement Community (CCRC): a type of long-term care setting that provides many different levels of care (for example, independent living, assisted living, and nursing home care) and multiple services on the same campus (7)

Continuous positive airway pressure (CPAP) therapy: a treatment that involves forcing air into the airway to keep it open; used in the treatment of sleep apnea (21)

Continuum of care: the delivery of health care over time as a person moves from being independent to needing assistance with personal care, medical care, or both (7)

Contractures: a condition that occurs when a joint is held in the same position for too long a time; the tendons shorten and become stiff, possibly causing permanent loss of motion in the joint (15)

Coordinated body movement: using the weight of the body to help with movement; the "C" in the ABCs of good body mechanics (13)

COPD: see chronic obstructive pulmonary disease

Coping mechanisms: conscious and deliberate ways of dealing with stress (compare with defense mechanisms) (41)

Coronary artery disease: a disorder that occurs when the arteries that supply the heart (the coronary arteries) narrow as a result of atherosclerosis, preventing adequate blood flow to the heart muscle (32)

CPR: see cardiopulmonary resuscitation

Cradle cap: see seborrheic dermatitis

Criminal laws: laws concerned with the relationship between the individual and society (4)

CSF: see cerebrospinal fluid

Culture: the beliefs (including religious or spiritual beliefs), values, and traditions that are customary to a group of people; a view of the world that is handed down from generation to generation (6)

Cuticle: the skin along the edges of the nail (23)

Cyanotic: adjective used to describe skin, lips, or nail beds that have a blue or gray tinge (27)

Cyanosis: blue or gray discoloration of the skin, lips, and nail beds; develops when the skin does not receive enough oxygen and is a sign of a respiratory or circulatory disorder (29)

Cystitis: infection of the bladder (37)

Cystocele: a condition that occurs when the bladder shifts downward, pressing into the front (anterior) vaginal wall (38)

Cytoplasm: the jelly-like substance within a cell within which the organelles float (28)

D

Dandruff: excessive itching and flaking of the scalp (23)

Decision-making capacity: the ability to make a thoughtful decision based on an understanding of the potential risks and benefits of taking a certain course of action (4)

Deep venous thrombosis (DVT): a condition where blood clots form in the deep veins, usually in the legs (32)

Defamation: the act of making untrue statements that hurt another person's reputation (4)

Defecate: to have a bowel movement (25)

Defense mechanisms: unconscious ways of dealing with stress (compare with coping mechanisms) (41)

Definitive surgery: surgery that is done when the person's medical problem is known and the best way to address it is through surgery (43)

Degenerative condition: a condition that gets progressively worse over time (8)

Dehydration: too little fluid in the tissues of the body (compare with edema) (24)

Delegate: to authorize another person to perform a task on your behalf (2)

Delirium: a temporary state of confusion (9)

Delusions: false ideas or beliefs, especially about oneself (41)

Dementia: the permanent and progressive loss of the ability to think and remember (9)

Dendrites: short extensions from the body of a neuron that receive information from other neurons (compare with axon) (33)

Denial: one of the stages of grief; the person refuses to accept the diagnosis or feels that a mistake has been made (26)

Dental caries: dental cavities or tooth decay, caused by poor oral hygiene (22)

Deodorant: a grooming product that covers or masks odor (22)

Depression: (1) an alteration in a person's mood that causes them to lose pleasure or interest in all usually pleasurable activities such as eating, working, or socializing; a feeling of hopelessness (41); (2) one of the stages of grief; the person fully realizes that death will be the end result of the illness and experiences sadness and regret (26)

Dermatitis: a general term for inflammation of the skin (29)

Dermis: the deepest layer of skin, where sensory receptors, blood vessels, nerves, glands, and hair follicles are found (29)

Depth of respiration: the quality of each breath (20)

Development: changes that occur psychologically or socially as a person passes through life (6)

Developmental disability: a permanent disability that affects a person before they reach adulthood (that is, before 19 to 22 years of age) and interferes with the person's ability to achieve developmental milestones (40)

Diabetes mellitus: an endocrine disorder that results when the pancreas is unable to produce enough insulin (35)

Diabetic retinopathy: a complication of diabetes that can lead to blindness (34)

Dialysis: a procedure that is done to remove waste products and fluids from the body when a person's kidneys fail and can no longer perform this task (37)

Diaphoretic: excessive sweating (22)

Diaphragm: (1) the large flat surface of the stethoscope that is used to hear loud, harsh sounds (20); (2) the strong, dome-shaped muscle that separates the chest cavity from the abdominal cavity and assists in breathing (31)

Diarrhea: the passage of liquid, unformed stool (25)

Diastole: the resting (relaxation) phase of the cardiac cycle; during which the myocardium relaxes, allowing the chambers to fill with blood (compare with systole) (32)

Diastolic pressure: the pressure that the blood exerts against the arterial walls when the heart muscle relaxes; the second blood pressure measurement that is recorded (compare with systolic pressure) (20)

Dietitian: a person who has a degree in nutrition (24)

Digestion: the process of breaking food down into simple elements (nutrients) (24)

Digital examination: examination that is done when a person is thought to have a fecal impaction; a finger is inserted into the person's rectum to feel for the impacted mass (25)

Director of Nursing (DON): the registered nurse who directs all of the nursing care within a facility (2)

Disability: impaired physical or emotional function (39)

Disaster: a sudden, unexpected event that causes injury to many people, major damage to property, or both (13)

Discharge: the official release of a patient or a resident from a health care facility to their home (18)

Discharge planning: the process used by the members of the health care team to help prepare a patient or resident to leave the facility; helps to make sure that the person continues to receive quality care, either from a home health care agency or from family members, after the discharge (18)

Disease: a condition that occurs when the structure or function of an organ or an organ system is abnormal (28)

Disinfection: the use of strong chemicals to kill pathogens on non-living objects that come in contact with body fluids or substances, such as bedpans, urinals, and over-bed tables; one of the techniques of medical asepsis (compare with antisepsis, sanitization, and sterilization) (12)

Disoriented: the state of being unable to answer basic questions about person, place, or time; a state of confusion (compare with oriented to person, place, and time) (16)

Diuresis: excessive urine output of urine; also called polyuria (25)

Diverticulosis: a condition in which small pouches form in the wall of the intestine, usually the lower colon (36)

DNR: see do not resuscitate order

Do not resuscitate (DNR) order: an order written on a person's chart specifying the person's wishes that the usual efforts to save their life will not be made; also called a no-code order (26)

Down syndrome: a developmental disability that is the result of having 47 chromosomes instead of 46; people with this disorder have some degree of intellectual disability and certain key physical features, such as upward slanted eyes and small hands with short fingers (40)

Draw sheet: a small, flat sheet that is placed over the middle of the bottom sheet, covering the area of the bed from above the person's shoulders to below the buttocks; see also lift sheet (19)

Droplet precautions: used when caring for people infected with pathogens that can be transmitted by direct exposure to droplets released from the mouth or nose (for example, when the person coughs, sneezes, or talks) (12)

Durable power of attorney for health care: a type of advance directive that transfers the responsibility for making medical decisions on the person's behalf to a family member, friend, or other trusted individual, in the event that the person is no longer able to make these decisions on their own behalf (4)

Dysmenorrhea: painful menstruation (38)

Dysphagia: difficulty swallowing (24)

Dyspnea: labored or difficult breathing (20)

Dysrhythmia: an irregular pulse rhythm (20)

Dysuria: painful or difficult urination (25)

E

Early morning care: care provided after a person wakes up to prepare them for breakfast or early testing or treatment (22)

Eclampsia: a severe hypertensive disorder of pregnancy which can cause convulsions and coma (44)

Eczema: a type of chronic dermatitis that is usually accompanied by severe itching, scaling, and crusting of the surface of the skin (29)

Edema: too much fluid in the tissues of the body (compare with dehydration); swelling (24)

Edentulous: without teeth (22)

EEOC: see Equal Employment Opportunity Commission

Egg (ovum, ova): female sex cell (38)

Egocentric: an adjective used to describe someone who places themselves at the center of the world and often overestimates their importance to others; a common character trait during adolescence (45)

Ejaculation: the forceful release of semen from the body; method by which sperm cells leave the male's body through the penis (38)

Elder abuse: physical, emotional, or sexual abuse of an older person (4)

Elective: adjective used to describe a surgical procedure that is planned for and scheduled ahead of time (43)

Embolus: a blood clot in a vessel that breaks off and moves from one place to another (32)

Emergency: a condition that requires immediate medical or surgical evaluation or treatment to prevent the person from dying or having a permanent disability (16)

Emergency response system: a network of resources (including people, equipment, and facilities) that is organized to respond to an emergency (16)

Emergent: adjective used to describe surgery that must be performed immediately to prevent the person from dying or becoming disabled (43)

Empathy: the ability to imagine what it would feel like to be in another person's situation (3)

Emphysema: a disorder caused by long-term exposure of the alveoli to toxins, such as tobacco smoke; one of two forms of chronic obstructive pulmonary disease (COPD) (31)

Endemic: describing a disease that is constantly or continuously present in a specific area (12)

Endocardium: the smooth inner lining of the heart wall (32)

Endotracheal tube: a device that is inserted into a person's nose or mouth and extends to the trachea; used when a person must receive mechanical ventilation for a short time (31)

Enema: the introduction of fluid into the large intestine by way of the anus for the purpose of removing stool from the rectum (25)

Enteral nutrition: placing food directly into a person's stomach or intestines, using a nasogastric tube, nasointestinal tube, gastrostomy tube, jejunostomy tube, or percutaneous endoscopic gastrostomy (PEG) tube; also called a "tube feeding" (24)

Entrapment: occurs when a person becomes trapped in the side rail, or between the side rail and the mattress (14)

Enzymes: substances that have the ability to break chemical bonds (36)

Epicardium: the smooth outermost layer of the heart wall (32)

Epidemic: an outbreak of a disease that suddenly affects a large group of people in a specific geographic area (12)

Epidermis: the outer layer of the skin (29)

Epidural block: anesthesia given through a catheter that is placed in the spinal canal (44)

Epilepsy: a disorder characterized by chronic seizure activity (33)

Episiotomy: an incision made in the perineum to enlarge the vaginal opening, making delivery of the baby's head easier (44)

Equal Employment Opportunity Commission (EEOC): a government agency that says it is illegal during the hiring process for an employer to ask a candidate questions related to age, marital status, weight, religion, sexual preference, and plans to have children at any time (3)

Erectile dysfunction (ED): the inability to achieve or maintain an erection long enough to engage in sexual activity (38)

Ergonomics: the practice of designing equipment and work tasks to conform to the capability of the worker (13)

Erythema: redness of the skin (29)

Erythrocytes: red blood cells; responsible for carrying oxygen to all of the tissues of the body (32)

Esophageal (cardiac) sphincter: a circle of muscular tissue that surrounds the place where the esophagus enters the stomach and keeps food from going back up the esophagus after it has entered the stomach (36)

Esophagus: a long narrow tube that serves mainly as a passageway for food to get from the pharynx to the stomach (36)

Ethics: moral principles or standards that govern conduct (4)

Eupnea: a normal respiratory rate (20)

Evening (hour of sleep, hs) care: care provided in preparation for sleep (22)

Excoriation: an abrasion, or a scraping away of the surface of the skin; can be caused by trauma, chemicals, or burns (29)

Exhalation (expiration): the phase of respiration during which carbon dioxide is transported out of the lungs (compare with inhalation [inspiration]) (20)

Exploratory surgery: surgery that is performed when a person has a significant medical problem but the doctors do not know exactly how bad the problem is or exactly what is causing it (43)

Exposure control plan: a plan that states what actions must be taken if an employee is exposed to blood or other body fluids while on the job (11)

F

Facemask: a device used for delivering oxygen that is made of soft, molded plastic material that fits over the nose and mouth (31)

Failure to thrive: failure of an infant to grow and develop both physically and emotionally, as a result of not being held and talked to (45)

False imprisonment: confining another person against their will (4)

Fanfolded: adjective used to describe the top sheet, blanket, and bedspread of a closed bed when they have been turned back (toward the foot of the bed) (19)

Fat-soluble: adjective used to describe a substance that dissolves in fat (for example, certain vitamins) (24)

Febrile: adjective used to describe the state of having a fever, or increased body temperature (20)

Fecal impaction: a condition that occurs when constipation is not relieved (25)

Fecal (bowel) incontinence: the inability to hold one's feces, or the involuntary loss of feces from the bowel (25)

Feces: the semi-solid waste product of digestion; stool (25)

Fetal alcohol spectrum disorder: a group of physical and intellectual conditions that affect children who were exposed to alcohol before birth (40)

Fiber supplement: a tablet or drink additive that is used to add bulk to the feces, causing them to hold fluid, and preventing constipation (25)

Filtrate: the liquid that forms the basis for urine (37)

First aid: the care given to an injured or sick person while waiting for more advanced help to arrive (16)

Fissure: a crack in the skin (29)

Five rights of delegation: a set of guidelines that help nurses to make good decisions about which tasks to delegate and to whom (2)

Fixation: the process of holding a broken bone in one position until the fracture heals; may be external (accomplished through the use of a cast) or internal (accomplished through the use of metal plates, screws, rods, pins, or wires attached to the bone) (30)

Flatulence: the presence of excessive amounts of flatus (gas) in the intestines, causing abdominal distension (swelling) and discomfort (25)

Flatus: gas that is formed as part of the digestion process (25)

Flow meter: a device used to set the rate at which oxygen is delivered to a patient or resident who is receiving oxygen therapy (31)

Fluid balance: a state where the amount of fluid taken into the body equals the amount of fluid that leaves the body (24)

Flushing: redness of the skin (29)

Fomite: a non-living object that has been contaminated (soiled) by pathogens (10)

Footboard: a padded board that is placed upright at the foot of the bed; used to keep the person's feet in proper alignment (19)

Foreskin: the fold of loose skin that covers the head of the penis (22)

For-profit facility: a facility that is owned and operated by a company or organization with the intention of making money (compare with non-profit [not-for-profit] facility) (7)

Fowler's position: one of the basic positions in which the head of the bed is elevated to between 45 and 60 degrees; variations include semi-Fowler's (low-Fowler's) position and high-Fowler's position (15)

Fracture: a broken bone (30)

Fracture pan: a wedge-shaped bedpan that is used when a person has an injury or disability that makes it too uncomfortable or dangerous to use a regular bedpan (25)

Fragile X syndrome: an inherited type of intellectual disability caused by a defect in the X chromosome (40)

Frail: physically weak and fragile (39)

Fraud: deception that could cause harm to another person (4)

Free-standing facility: a facility that is independently owned and operated (compare with chain facility) (7)

Frequency: the term used to describe voiding that occurs more often than usual (25)

Friction: a term used to describe the force created when two surfaces (such as a sheet and a person's skin) rub against each other; can lead to skin breakdown (15)

Frontotemporal dementia: a disorder characterized by damage to the areas of the brain that are responsible for personality, behavior and language; in addition to a progressive decline in mental abilities, people with frontotemporal dementia have extreme changes in behavior and personality, difficulties with language, or both (9)

G

Gallbladder: a small pouch-like organ that is attached to the liver; it stores bile produced by the liver that is not secreted directly into the duodenum (36)

Gas exchange: the transfer of oxygen into the blood, and carbon dioxide out of it (31)

Gastrostomy tube: a tube used for enteral nutrition that is inserted into the stomach through a surgical incision in the abdomen (24)

Gatches: the joints at the hips and knees of the mattresses of most adjustable beds that allow the mattress to "break" so that the person's head can be elevated or their knees bent (17)

Gay: a term used to describe a man who is attracted to other men (6)

General anesthesia: a loss of consciousness brought on by the administration of a combination of inhaled and injected drugs (compare with local anesthesia and regional anesthesia) (43)

General lighting: lighting that supplies overall illumination (light), allowing a person to see and move about safely (compare with task lighting) (17)

Gingivitis: inflammation of the gums (22)

Glaucoma: a disorder of the eye that occurs when the pressure within the eye is increased to dangerous levels (34)

Glomerulus: part of the nephron, the functional unit of the kidney where blood is filtered to form urine (37)

Glucose: the body's most basic type of fuel; supplied by carbohydrates and sometimes referred to as "blood sugar" (24)

Goals: descriptions of what nursing interventions (nursing actions that are taken to help a patient or resident) are meant to achieve (5)

Goiter: enlargement of the thyroid gland (35)

Graduate: a measuring device used to measure fluids (24)

Grand mal (tonic–clonic) seizure: a seizure characterized by generalized and violent contraction and relaxation of the body's muscles (compare with petit mal [absence] seizure) (16)

Grief: mental anguish, specifically associated with loss (26)

Grooming: activities related to maintaining a neat and attractive appearance, such as shampooing and styling the hair, shaving, and applying make-up (23)

Grounded: an adjective used to describe electrical equipment that has a way of returning stray electrical current to the outlet so that the risk of electrical shock is reduced (13)

Growth: changes that occur physically as a person passes through life (6)

Gynecologist: a doctor who specializes in diagnosing and treating disorders of the female reproductive system (38)

H

Halitosis: bad breath that does not go away (22)

Hallucinations: episodes when a person sees, feels, hears, or tastes something that does not really exist (41)

Hangnails: broken pieces of cuticle (23)

HAV: see hepatitis A virus

HBV: see hepatitis B virus

HCV: see hepatitis C virus

HDV: see hepatitis D virus

Head nurse: a registered nurse (RN) who is in charge of a department or section (2)

Health care agent: the person who is responsible for making decisions on the person's behalf (4)

Health care–associated infections (HAIs): infections that patients or residents get while receiving treatment in a hospital or other health care facility, or that health care workers get while performing their duties within a health care setting (12)

Health care team: group of people with different types of knowledge and skill levels who work together to provide holistic care to the patient or resident (1)

Health Insurance Portability and Accountability Act (HIPAA): a federal privacy regulation that helps to keep personal information about patients and residents private (4)

Heart failure: a condition that occurs when the heart is unable to pump enough blood to meet the body's needs (32)

Hematuria: blood in the urine (25)

Hemiplegia: paralysis on one side of the body (compare with paraplegia and quadriplegia) (14)

Hemoglobin: a protein found in red blood cells that combines with oxygen to carry it to the tissues of the body (32)

Hemoptysis: the coughing up of blood or blood-stained sputum (31)

Hemorrhage: severe bleeding (16)

Hemorrhagic shock: shock that results from massive blood loss (16)

Hemostasis: the process of stopping blood loss from the circulatory system (32)

Hemothorax: a condition that occurs when blood collects in the space between the lungs and the chest wall (31)

Hepatitis: inflammation of the liver (11)

Hepatitis A virus (HAV): a virus that is transmitted through the oral–fecal route and causes a form of acute hepatitis (11)

Hepatitis B virus (HBV): a bloodborne virus that causes a form of hepatitis that is acute in most people but may become chronic; a serious health threat for the health care worker (11)

Hepatitis C virus (HCV): a bloodborne virus that causes a form of chronic hepatitis that can eventually lead to end-stage cirrhosis (a fatal liver disease), liver failure, or liver cancer (11)

Hepatitis D virus (HDV): a bloodborne virus that is found only in people who are already infected with hepatitis B virus (HBV) (11)

Hepatitis E virus (HEV): a virus that is transmitted through the oral–fecal route and causes a form of hepatitis (11)

Hernia: a disorder that occurs when an internal organ bulges through a weakness in the muscular wall of the abdominal cavity (36)

Heterosexual: a term used to describe women with an attraction to men and men with an attraction to women (6)

HEV: see hepatitis E virus (11)

High-Fowler's position: one of the basic positions in which the head of the bed is elevated to between 60 and 90 degrees (15)

HIPAA: see Health Insurance Portability and Accountability Act

HIV: see human immunodeficiency virus

HIV positive: the state of being infected with human immunodeficiency virus (HIV) (11)

Holistic: an adjective used to describe care of the whole person, physically and emotionally (1)

Homebound: adjective used to describe a person who cannot leave the house without a lot of help from another person (46)

Home health aide: a nursing assistant who provides skilled care in the home (46)

Home health care agency: an agency that provides skilled care in a person's home (1)

Homeostasis: a state of balance (28)

Hopper: a sink-like fixture that empties into a sewer line and is used for tasks such as cleaning bedpans or rinsing soiled linens or clothing (17)

Hormones: chemicals that act on cells to produce a response (35)

Hospice organization: a health care organization that provides care for people who are dying, and their families (1)

Hospital: a health care facility that provides treatment for people with acute medical or surgical conditions (1)

Human immunodeficiency virus (HIV): a virus transmitted in blood and other body fluids (such as semen) that targets the T cells of the immune system; some people infected with HIV go on to develop acquired immunodeficiency syndrome (AIDS), a fatal illness (11)

Human resources (HR) department (personnel): the department within an organization that is concerned with matters related to employees; often responsible for hiring new employees (3)

Hydrocephalus: a condition that results from the build-up of cerebrospinal fluid (CSF) in the ventricles of the brain (40)

Hygiene: personal cleanliness (3)

Hyperalimentation: see total parenteral nutrition

Hyperglycemia: a state of having too much glucose in the bloodstream (35)

Hyperopia: farsightedness; trouble seeing objects that are close (compare with myopia) (34)

Hypertension: high blood pressure; a blood pressure that is consistently greater than 140 mm Hg (systolic) and/or 90 mm Hg (diastolic) (20)

Hyperthyroidism: a condition caused by the excessive secretion of thyroxine, one of the thyroid hormones; characterized by increased hunger accompanied by weight loss, an irregular heartbeat, an inability to sleep, irritability, confusion, increased perspiration, and intolerance to heat (35)

Hyperventilation: increased rate and depth of breathing (20)

Hypoglycemia: a dangerous drop in blood glucose levels (35)

Hypotension: low blood pressure; a blood pressure that is consistently lower than 90 mm Hg (systolic) and/or 60 mm Hg (diastolic) (20)

Hypothyroidism: a condition caused by the low secretion of thyroxine, one of the thyroid hormones; characterized by fatigue, weakness, depression, anorexia, weight gain, constipation, and intolerance to cold (35)

Hypoventilation: decreased rate and depth of breathing (20)

Hypoxic: the state of being deficient of oxygen (31)

Hysterectomy: surgical removal of the uterus (38)

I

Ileostomy: an alternative way of eliminating feces from the body; done when the entire large intestine must be removed due to disease; after removing the person's diseased large intestine, an artificial opening, called a stoma, is made in the abdominal wall and the end of the small intestine is connected to it (compare with colostomy) (25)

Incident: an occurrence that is considered unusual, undesired, or out of the ordinary, and that disrupts the normal routine for the patient or resident, the health care facility, or both (14)

Incident (occurrence) report: a preprinted document that is completed following an accident or incidence involving a patient or resident (14)

Indwelling catheter: a urinary catheter that is left inside the bladder to provide continuous urine drainage; also known as a retention catheter or a Foley catheter (25)

Infection: disease caused by pathogenic microbes (10)

Infection control: basic practices designed to decrease the chance that an infection will spread from one person to another in a health care setting (12)

Infertility: the inability to become pregnant or to carry a pregnancy to full term (38)

Influenza: an acute respiratory infection caused by the influenza virus; characterized by a sore throat, dry cough, stuffy nose, headache, body aches, weakness, and fever; commonly known as "the flu" (31)

Informed consent: permission granted by a patient or resident to begin treatment or perform a procedure after receiving a full explanation of the treatment or procedure from the health care provider (4)

Ingestion: the intake of food or fluids (24)

Inhalation (inspiration): the phase of respiration during which oxygen is taken into the lungs (compare with exhalation [expiration]) (20)

Insomnia: a disorder characterized by an inability to fall asleep, or to stay asleep (21)

Intermittent pneumatic compression (IPC) devices: a device that is applied to the calves to help prevent pooling of blood in the lower legs; often used following surgery to prevent cardiovascular complications (43)

Instrumental activities of daily living (IADLs): more complex tasks that a person must be able to do in order to continue to live independently, such as using the telephone or handling money (compare with activities of daily living) (8)

Intake and output (I&O) flow sheet: a document used for recording measurements of all of the fluids that enter and leave the body (24)

Intellectual disability: the state of having certain limitations with intellectual functioning (that is, ability to reason, think, and understand) and with adaptive skills (that is, skills needed to live and work, such as communication skills, social skills, and self-care skills) (40)

Intentional tort: a violation of civil law committed by a person with the intent to do harm (4)

Intentional wound: a wound that is the result of a planned surgical or medical intervention (compare with unintentional wound) (29)

Interdisciplinary care plan: a specific plan of care for each patient or resident developed with input from all members of the health care team (5)

Interventions: actions that are taken by the nursing team to help the patient or resident (5)

Interview: a meeting between an employer and a potential employee, during which information is exchanged regarding the organization, the job, and the potential employee's qualifications for the job (3)

Intimacy: a feeling of emotional closeness to another human being (6)

Intraoperative phase: one of three phases of care for a person who is having surgery; the phase during which the surgery is actually performed (compare with preoperative phase and postoperative phase) (43)

Intravenous (IV) therapy: an alternative method of providing fluids and nutrition; fluids are given through a small catheter (tube) that is inserted into a vein (24)

Invasion of privacy: the act of violating another person's right to keep certain information and aspects of themselves away from the examination of others (4)

Ischemia: the state that occurs when the flow of oxygen-rich blood to the tissues is interrupted, leading to an oxygen deficiency in the tissues (32)

Isolation precautions: guidelines, based on a pathogen's method of transmission, that health care workers follow to contain the pathogen and limit others' exposure to it as much as possible (12)

J

Jaundice: a yellow discoloration of the skin and the whites of the eyes; usually associated with liver disorders (29)

Jejunostomy tube: a tube used for enteral nutrition that is inserted into the jejunum (part of the small intestine) through a surgical incision in the abdomen (24)

Joint: the area where two bones join together (30)

K

Kardex: a card or electronic file that contains condensed versions of each patient's or resident's medical record (5)

Keratin: a substance that causes mature skin cells to thicken and become resistant to water (29)

Kidney stones (renal calculi): a painful disorder characterized by the formation of clumps of minerals ("stones") in the kidney and bladder (37)

Korotkoff sounds: sounds that are heard while taking a person's blood pressure (20)

L

Labor: the process of giving birth to a baby, during which the uterus contracts to push the baby out (44)

Lactation: the process by which the glandular tissue of the female breast produces milk (38)

Larceny: the act of stealing another person's property (4)

Laryngitis: inflammation of the larynx (the "voice box") (31)

Larynx: part of the respiratory airway; also known as the "voice box" (31)

Lateral position: one of the basic positions in which the person lies on their side (15)

Laws: rules that are made by a controlling authority, such as the state or federal government, with the intent of preserving basic human rights (4)

Laxative: a medication that chemically stimulates the bowels to move; a treatment for constipation (25)

Lesbian: a term used to describe a woman who is attracted to other women (6)

Lesion: a general term used to describe any break in the skin (29)

Leukemia: a general term for a cancer resulting in the excessive production of white blood cells that are abnormal in structure (32)

Leukocyte: white blood cell (32)

Lewy body dementia: a disorder characterized by the build-up of abnormal protein deposits (called Lewy bodies) in areas of the brain that are responsible for thinking and movement; in addition to a progressive decline in mental abilities, people with Lewy body dementia have problems controlling body movement similar to those seen in people with Parkinson disease, visual hallucinations, and distinct changes in mental alertness (9)

Libel: written statements that injure someone's reputation; a form of defamation (4)

Licensed practical nurse (LPN): a specially trained person who is licensed by a state to provide routine care for the sick under the supervision of a registered nurse (RN); completes a 1- to 2-year program in a vocational school, community college, or hospital (2)

Licensed vocational nurse (LVN): another term for licensed practical nurse (2)

Life-sustaining treatment: treatments that will prolong life, such as mechanical ventilation, cardiopulmonary resuscitation (CPR), and the placement of a feeding tube or intravenous (IV) line for the provision of nutrition (26)

Lift sheet: a draw sheet that is used to help lift or reposition a person who needs assistance with moving in bed (19)

Ligaments: very strong bands of fibrous tissue that cross over the joint capsule, attaching one bone to another and stabilizing the joint (30)

Liver: an organ that performs several important functions in the body, including the secretion of bile (a substance needed for digestion of fats), the production of clotting factors (chemicals that help our blood to clot), and the clearance of toxins (such as alcohol and drugs) from the body (36)

Living will: a type of advance directive that allows the person to give instructions about what medical treatments they would or would not want done in an effort to save their life (4)

Local anesthesia: a loss of sensation in only a very small part of the body brought on by the injection of drugs (compare with general anesthesia and regional anesthesia) (43)

Lochia: vaginal discharge following the birth of a baby (44)

Logrolling: a technique for turning a person in which the person's body is moved in one fluid motion to keep the spine in alignment (15)

Long-term care facility: a health care facility that provides care for people who are unable to care for themselves at home, yet do not need to be hospitalized; sometimes referred to as a "nursing home" (1)

Long-term care insurance: a private insurance policy that can be purchased by an individual to help pay for long-term care in the future, should it be needed (7)

LPN: see licensed practical nurse

Lungs: the primary organs for respiration, the process the body uses to obtain oxygen from the environment and remove carbon dioxide (a waste gas) from the body (31)

LVN: see licensed vocational nurse

Lymph: fluid in the lymph vessels (vessels that return the fluid that leaks into the tissues to the bloodstream) (32)

Lymph nodes: masses of lymphatic tissue that "clean" the lymph by removing bacteria and other large particles before returning the fluid to the bloodstream (32)

M

Macular degeneration: a vision disorder that results from the build-up of deposits in the macula (part of the retina) and can eventually lead to blindness (34)

Macule: a small, flat, reddened skin lesion (29)

Magical thinking: a thought process that is common among preschoolers; the child believes that if they wish for something hard enough, it will happen (45)

Malignant: adjective used to describe a cancerous tumor (that is, a tumor that has the ability to progress or invade other tissues) (compare with benign) (42)

Malpractice: negligence committed by people who hold licenses to practice their profession, such as doctors, nurses, lawyers, dentists, and pharmacists (4)

Managed care system: a system designed to control health care costs by delivering health care to people who need it by arranging contacts with various health care providers; examples include preferred provider organizations (PPOs) and health maintenance organizations (HMOs) (1)

Mastectomy: surgical removal of a breast (38)

Mastication: chewing (36)

Masturbation: stimulation of the genitals for sexual pleasure or release, by a means other than sexual intercourse (6)

Mechanical digestion: the process of breaking down food through the use of physical means, such as chewing (compare with chemical digestion) (36)

Mechanical ventilation: a life-sustaining treatment in which a machine breathes for a person who cannot breathe on their own (31)

Medicaid: a federally funded and state-regulated plan designed to help people with low incomes to pay for health care (1)

Medical asepsis: techniques that are used to physically remove or kill pathogens (see also sanitization, antisepsis, disinfection, and sterilization) (12)

Medical record: a legal document where information about a patient's or resident's current condition, the measures that have been taken by the medical and nursing staff to diagnose and treat the condition, and the patient's or resident's response to the treatment and care provided are recorded; also called a "medical chart" (5)

Medicare: a type of insurance plan that is federally funded by Social Security and which all people 65 years and older, and some younger people with disabilities, are eligible to participate in (1)

Melanin: a dark pigment that gives our skin, hair, and eyes color (29)

Menarche: the onset of the first menstrual period (6)

Meninges: the three layers of connective tissue that cover and protect the brain and spinal cord (33)

Menopause: the cessation of menstruation and fertility that females typically experienced in their early 50s (6)

Menorrhagia: excessive bleeding during a menstrual period, either in terms of the amount of blood lost or the number of days that bleeding lasts (38)

Menstrual period: the monthly loss of blood through the vagina that occurs in the absence of pregnancy (38)

Mental illness: also known as a mental health disorder, refers to a wide range of mental health conditions that affect a person's mood, thinking and behavior (41)

Metabolism: the word used to describe the physical and chemical changes that occur when the cells of the body change the food that we eat into energy (20)

Metastasis: the process by which cancer cells spread from their original location in the body to a new location, which may be quite distant from the first (42)

Methicillin-resistant *Staphylococcus aureus* **(MRSA):** a type of bacteria that has become resistant to methicillin, a powerful antibiotic (10)

Microbe (microorganism): a living thing that cannot be seen with the naked eye; examples include bacteria and viruses (10)

Micturition: the process of passing urine from the body; also known as urination and voiding (25)

Midstream ("clean catch") urine specimen: a method of collecting urine that prevents contamination of the urine by the bacteria that normally exist in and around the urethra (25)

Minimum Data Set (MDS): a report that focuses on the degree of assistance or skilled care that each resident of a long-term care facility needs (1)

Mission: the officially stated purpose of a health care facility or organization (1)

Mitered corner: a corner that is made by folding and tucking the sheet so that it lies flat and neat against the mattress (19)

Morning (AM) care: care provided in the morning, to ready the person for the day, such as completion of personal hygiene and grooming activities, and bed-making (22)

Motor nerves: nerves that carry commands from the brain down the spinal cord and out to the muscles and organs of the body (33)

MRSA: see methicillin-resistant Staphylococcus aureus

MS: see multiple sclerosis

Mucous membrane: a sheet of epithelial tissue that lines many of the organ systems in the body and is coated with mucus (31)

Mucus: a slippery, sticky substance that is secreted by special cells and serves to keep the surfaces of mucous membranes moist (31)

Multidrug-resistant organisms (MDROs): bacteria that are resistant to one or more classes of antimicrobial agents (10)

Multiple sclerosis (MS): a disorder of the nervous system in which the myelin sheaths that cover the nerves are damaged, resulting in faulty transmission of nerve impulses (33)

Munchausen syndrome by proxy: a form of physical abuse seen in children; the child's caregiver deliberately does things to make the child appear ill (45)

Muscle tone: the steady contraction of the skeletal muscles that helps us to maintain an upright posture, such as sitting or standing (30)

Muscular dystrophy: a general term for a group of disorders that cause the skeletal muscles to become more and more weak over time (30)

Myelin: a fatty, white substance that protects the axon and helps to speed the conduction of nerve impulses along the axon (33)

Myocardial infarction: a "heart attack"; occurs when one or more of the coronary arteries become completely blocked, preventing blood from reaching the parts of the heart that are fed by the affected arteries (32)

Myocardium: the thick, muscular middle layer of the heart wall; responsible for the pumping action of the heart (32)

Myopia: nearsightedness; trouble seeing objects that are far away (compare with hyperopia) (34)

N

Nasal cannula: a device used to deliver oxygen to a patient or resident; consists of two prongs of soft plastic tubing that are inserted into the nostrils (31)

Nasal cavity: the inside of the nose (31)

Nasogastric tube: a tube used for enteral nutrition that is inserted through the nose, down the throat, and into the stomach (24)

Nasointestinal tube: a tube used for enteral nutrition that is inserted through the nose, down the throat, and into the small intestine (24)

Nasopharyngeal airway: a soft rubber tube that is inserted into a person's nose and extends back toward the throat to create an opening that air can flow through (31)

Necrosis: tissue death as a result of a lack of oxygen (29)

Need: something that is essential for a person's physical and mental health (6)

Neglect: the failure to provide for a dependent person's basic physical needs; a form of physical abuse (4)

Negligent: adjective used to describe a person who fails to do what a "careful and reasonable" person would do in any given situation (4)

Neonate: a newborn infant, 28 days or younger (6)

Nephron: the basic functional unit of the kidney; consists of a glomerulus and a tubule (37)

Neurogenic bladder: a condition caused by problems with the nerves that control the bladder (37)

Neuron: a cell that can send and receive information (33)

Nits: the eggs of head lice, seen on the hair, near the scalp, in people with pediculosis capitis (head lice infestation) (23)

No-code order: an order written on a person's chart specifying the person's wishes that the usual efforts to save their life will not be made; see also do not resuscitate (DNR) order (26)

Nocturia: the need to get up more than once or twice during the night to urinate, to the point where sleep is disrupted (25)

Nocturnal emission: the harmless involuntary discharge of semen during sleep; commonly called a "wet dream" (6)

Non-profit (not-for-profit) facility: a facility that is owned and operated by a service organization (such as a church or charitable group) with the intention of fulfilling a need in the community (compare with for-profit facility) (7)

Nonverbal communication: a way of communicating that uses facial expressions, gestures, and body language, instead of written or spoken language (5)

Normal (resident) flora: the harmless microbes that live in and on the body and help it to function properly (compare with transient flora) (10)

Nosocomial infections: infections that patients or residents get while receiving treatment in a hospital or other health care facility; a type of health care–associated infection (HAI) (12)

NPO status: a doctor's order specifying that a patient or resident is to have "nils per os" (nothing by mouth) (24)

Nucleus: the cell's "brain"; it contains all of the information the cell needs in order to do its job, grow, and reproduce (28)

Nursing care plan: a specific plan of care for each patient or resident developed by the nursing team (5)

Nursing diagnosis: a statement that describes a problem the person is having that can be identified and treated by the nursing staff independently (5)

Nursing history: a report that is completed by the nurse when a patient or resident is admitted to a health care facility that gathers information about the person's preferences, abilities, disabilities, and habits (18)

Nursing process: a process that allows members of the nursing team to communicate with each other regarding the patient's or resident's specific needs (in regard to nursing care), what steps will be taken to meet those needs, and whether the steps were effective in meeting the person's needs; consists of five parts: assessment, diagnosis, planning, implementation, and evaluation (5)

Nutrients: substances in foods and fluids that the body uses to grow, to repair itself, and to carry out processes essential for living (24)

Nutrition: the process of taking in and using food (24)

Nutritional supplement: a flavored shake or drink that is used to supply extra calories or protein; often served with meals or as a snack in between meals (24)

O

Obese: having a BMI of 30.0 or higher (24)

Objective data: information that is obtained directly, through measurements or by using one of the five senses (sight, smell, taste, hearing, touch) (5)

OBRA: see Omnibus Budget Reconciliation Act of 1987

Observation: something that you notice about the patient or resident, typically related to a change in the person's physical or mental condition (5)

Obsessive–compulsive disorder (OCD): an anxiety disorder that causes a person to suffer intensely from recurrent unwanted thoughts (obsessions) that are usually associated with rituals the person feels obligated to complete constantly (compulsions) (41)

Occult: adjective used to describe something that is hidden or cannot be seen with the naked eye; often used in reference to blood in a urine or stool sample (25)

Occupational Safety and Health Administration (OSHA): an agency within the Department of Labor that establishes safety and health standards for the workplace, to protect the safety and health of employees (1)

Occupied bed: a bed with a person in it (19)

OCD: see obsessive–compulsive disorder

Oliguria: the state of voiding a very small amount of urine over a given period of time (25)

Omnibus Budget Reconciliation Act of 1987 (OBRA): an act passed in 1987 to improve the quality of life for people who live in long-term care facilities by making sure that residents receive a certain standard of care (1)

Open bed: a bed with the top covers folded down that is ready to receive a patient or resident (19)

Opportunistic microbes: microbes that are considered normal (resident) flora when they are in or on one part of the body, but can cause infection if they move out of that area and into or onto another part of the body (10)

Oral–fecal route: a method of transmitting an infection; occurs when feces containing a pathogen contaminate food or water, which is then consumed by another person (11)

Organ: a group of tissues functioning together for a similar purpose (28)

Organelles: structures inside of the cell that help the cell to make the energy it needs to stay alive and to rid itself of waste products (28)

Organism: a living thing, such as an animal or a plant (28)

Organ system: a group of organs that work together to perform a specific function for the body (28)

Oriented to person, place, and time: the state of being able to answer basic questions about person, place, or time; alert (compare with disoriented) (16)

Oropharyngeal airway: a hard plastic device that is inserted into a person's mouth to stop the tongue from falling back into the throat; used to keep the airway open (31)

Orthostatic hypotension: a sudden decrease in blood pressure that occurs when a person stands up from a sitting or lying position (20)

OSHA: see Occupational Safety and Health Administration

OSHA Bloodborne Pathogens Standards: standards created by the Occupational Safety and Health Administration that all employers must follow to help protect employees from exposure to bloodborne pathogens (11)

Osteoporosis: a disorder characterized by the excessive loss of bone tissue (30)

Ostomy: a surgically created opening between an internal structure and the skin, usually located on the abdomen (see also ileostomy and colostomy) (25)

Otitis externa: an infection of the lining of the external auditory canal; commonly referred to as "swimmer's ear" (34)

Otitis media: an infection of the middle ear that is common in young children (34)

Otosclerosis: a condition caused by fixation of the small bones in the inner ear that can result in hearing loss (34)

Over-bed table: a table that fits over a bed or a chair and can be raised or lowered as needed (17)

Ovulation: the release of a ripe, mature egg from the ovaries each month (38)

P

PACU: see post anesthesia care unit

Pain: an unpleasant sensation that can range from mild discomfort to intense suffering (21)

Pain scale: a tool or guide that helps to translate a person's subjective rating of their pain into an objective measurement (21)

Pain threshold: the point at which a person becomes aware of pain (21)

Pain tolerance: the level of pain that a person can endure before taking action to seek relief (21)

Palliative care: care that focuses on relieving uncomfortable symptoms, not on curing the problem that is causing the symptoms (26)

Pallor: paleness of the skin (29)

Pancreas: an organ that produces enzymes that aid in digestion, as well as the hormones insulin and glucagon (36)

Pandemic: a disease or outbreak that affects large populations throughout the world; an exceptionally widespread epidemic (12)

Panic disorder: a mental health disorder in which a person experiences episodes of sudden, overpowering fright (panic) and anxiety, usually accompanied by chest or abdominal pain, a rapid heart rate, shortness of breath, and/or dizziness (41)

Papule: a small, raised, firm skin lesion that can be easily felt by passing your fingers lightly over the affected area (29)

Paraplegia: paralysis from the waist down (compare with quadriplegia and hemiplegia) (14)

Parkinson disease: a progressive neurologic disorder that is characterized by tremor and weakness in the muscles and a shuffling gait (33)

Pathogen: a microbe that can cause illness; commonly referred to as a "germ" (10)

Patient: a person who is receiving health care in a hospital, clinic, or extended-care facility (1)

Patient-centered or patient-focused care: cross-functional teams consisting of groups of professional and assistive personnel that work together as a unit-based team to provide care to a given group of patients (2)

Patient Self-Determination Act of 1990: an act passed to ensure that the wishes patients and patients' family members have regarding measures to be taken on their own behalf (or on the behalf of their loved one) are followed (4)

Pediculosis capitis: head lice (23)

Pelvic inflammatory disease (PID): infection of the fallopian tubes and abdominal cavity that can lead to infertility (38)

Pelvic organ prolapse: a condition that occurs when a pelvic organ shifts downward from its normal position (38)

Percutaneous endoscopic gastrostomy (PEG) tube: a special type of gastrostomy tube that is inserted into the stomach with the aid of an endoscope (24)

Pericardium: a double-layered protective sac that surrounds the heart (32)

Perineal care (peri-care): cleaning the perineum and anus, as well as the vulva (in females) and the penis (in males) (22)

Perineum: the area from the bottom of the vagina to the anus (in females) or the area from the root of the penis to the anus (in males) (22)

Periodontitis: infection and inflammation of the soft tissue and bones that support the teeth; can lead to tooth loss (22)

Perioperative period: the term used to describe all three phases of the surgical process as a whole—the preoperative, intraoperative, and postoperative phases (43)

Peripheral nervous system (PNS): the nerves outside of the brain and spinal cord; receives information from the environment, and carries commands from the brain and spinal cord to the other organs of the body, such as the muscles (compare with central nervous system) (33)

Peripheral vascular disease: a disorder characterized by pain and cramping in the legs, caused by atherosclerosis of the arteries that supply the legs (32)

Peristalsis: involuntary wave-like muscular movements, such as those that occur in the digestive system to move chyme (partially digested food) through the intestines (25)

Perseveration: the inappropriate and constant repetition of a phrase or act; often seen in people with dementia (9)

Persistent vegetative state: a state of altered consciousness in which the person appears to be awake, but cannot respond in a deliberate or meaningful way to the environment (33)

Personal protective equipment (PPE): barriers that are worn to physically prevent microbes from reaching a health care provider's skin or mucous membranes, such as gloves, gowns, masks, and protective eyewear (12)

Pessary: a device that is inserted into the vagina to support a prolapsed organ in the proper position (38)

Petit mal (absence) seizure: a seizure characterized by a sudden, brief break in consciousness or activity (compare with grand mal seizure) (16)

Phantom pain: the feeling that a body part is still present, after it has been surgically removed (amputated) (30)

Pharyngitis: inflammation of the throat (pharynx) (31)

Pharynx: throat region (31)

Phlebitis: inflammation of a vein (32)

Phobia: an excessive, abnormal fear of an object or situation (41)

Physical abuse: the repetitive and deliberate infliction of physical injury on another person, such as that caused by striking, biting, slapping, shaking, or failing to meet a dependent person's physical needs (for example, for food, water, and cleanliness) (compare with psychological [emotional] abuse and sexual abuse) (4)

Physical restraint: a device that is attached to or near a person's body to limit a person's freedom of movement or access to their body (compare with chemical restraint) (14)

Physiology: the study of how the body parts work (28)

Placenta: the structure that develops from the inside lining of the uterus during pregnancy and participates in the exchange of gases and nutrients between the parent and the fetus (44)

Plaque: a fatty deposit that builds up on the inside of the artery wall, blocking blood flow to the tissues and making the artery wall brittle and prone to breaking (32)

Plasma: the liquid part of the blood (32)

Plasma membrane: a membrane that surrounds the cytoplasm and gives the cell its shape (28)

Pleura: the membrane that lines the chest cavity and covers the outside of the lungs (31)

Pleurisy: inflammation of the pleura, the membrane that lines the chest cavity and covers the lungs (31)

Pneumonia: inflammation of the lung tissue, caused by infection with a virus or a bacterium, and resulting in impaired gas exchange (31)

Pneumothorax: the build-up of air in the space between the lungs and the chest wall (31)

PNS: see peripheral nervous system

Podiatrist: a doctor who specializes in the care of the feet (23)

Polyuria: excessive urine output; see also diuresis (25)

Postanesthesia care unit (PACU): the recovery room where patients are taken following surgery so that they can be closely monitored by the health care team to make sure that they are recovering without complications from the surgery or the anesthesia (43)

Postmenopausal bleeding: uterine bleeding after menopause (38)

Postmortem care: the care of a person's body after the person's death (27)

Postoperative phase: one of three phases of care for a person who is having surgery; the phase after the surgery is actually performed (compare with preoperative phase and intraoperative phase) (43)

Postpartum period: the 6-week period of time following the birth of a baby (44)

Post-procedure actions: steps that are routinely performed at the end of each patient or resident care procedure, called "Finishing Up" actions in this book (compare with pre-procedure actions) (13)

Post-traumatic stress disorder (PTSD): an anxiety disorder that occurs after a person experiences an overwhelming traumatic event such as combat, natural disaster, serious injury, criminal assault, rape, or death of another person (41)

PPE: see personal protective equipment

Pregnancy-induced hypertension (PIH): dangerously high blood pressure in a pregnant person (44)

Prenatal care: the health care given to a pregnant person in the months leading up to the birth of a baby (44)

Preoperative phase: one of three phases of care for a person who is having surgery; the phase before the surgery is actually performed (compare with intraoperative phase and postoperative phase) (43)

Preoperative teaching: teaching done by members of the health care team to prepare a person and their family members for surgery; during preoperative teaching, the person learns about the surgical procedure, its benefits and possible risks, and what can be expected during the postoperative recovery period (43)

Pre-procedure actions: steps that are routinely performed before each patient or resident care procedure; called "Getting Ready" actions in this book (compare with post-procedure actions) (13)

Presbycusis: age-related hearing loss (34)

Presbyopia: age-related loss of the eye's ability to focus on objects that are close (34)

Preschooler: a person between the ages of 3 and 6 years (43)

Pressure points: bony areas where pressure ulcers are most likely to form; include the heels, ankles, knees, hips, toes, elbows, shoulder blades, ears, the back of the head, and along the spine (29)

Pressure-relieving mattress: a mattress that is placed on top of the regular mattress to help prevent skin breakdown in patients and residents who must stay in bed for long periods of time (19)

Pressure ulcer: a difficult-to-heal (and possibly even fatal) sore that forms when part of the body presses against a surface (such as a mattress or chair) for a long period of time; also known as pressure sores and decubitus ulcers (15)

Preterm labor: labor that begins too early, before the fetus can survive on its own (44)

Private pay: adjective used to describe and expense that is paid "out-of-pocket," using one's own money (7)

Procedure: a series of steps followed in a particular order when providing care to a patient or resident that helps to ensure that the care provided is safe and correct (13)

PRN (as-needed) care: personal hygiene care that is provided whenever a patient or resident needs it, throughout the day or night (22)

Professional: a person who has credentials, obtained through education and training, that enable them to become licensed or certified to practice a certain profession; also, a person who demonstrates a professional attitude (3)

Professionalism: the attitude of being a professional, characterized by a positive outlook and a commitment to doing one's best at all times (3)

Prognosis: a doctor's prediction of the course of a person's disease, and their estimation of the person's chances for recovery (42)

Prone position: one of the basic positions in which the person lies on their abdomen with their head turned to one side (15)

Prosthetic devices: artificial replacements for legs, feet, arms, or other body parts (39)

Psychiatrist: a doctor who specializes in the diagnosis and treatment of mental illness (41)

Psychological (emotional) abuse: the repetitive and deliberate infliction of emotional injury on another person, such as that caused by threatening a person with physical harm or abandonment, teasing a person in a cruel way, or preventing a person from interacting with others (compare with physical abuse and sexual abuse) (4)

Psychologist: a health care professional who is trained to provide counseling services for people with mental illness (41)

Puberty: the period during which the secondary sex characteristics appear and the reproductive organs begin to function (6)

Pulmonary circulation: the pattern of circulation that takes blood from the heart to the lungs to pick up oxygen and release carbon dioxide (compare with systemic circulation) (32)

Pulmonary embolism: a life-threatening condition that occurs when an embolus becomes stuck in the pulmonary artery, the artery that carries un-oxygenated blood from the heart to the lungs (32, 43)

Pulse: the wave of blood sent through the arteries each time the heart beats (20)

Pulse amplitude: the force or quality of the pulse (20)

Pulse deficit: the difference between the apical pulse rate (the pulse that is measured by listening over the apex of the heart with a stethoscope) and the radial pulse rate (the pulse that is measured by placing the middle two or three fingers over the radial artery, located on the inside of the wrist) (20)

Pulse points: the points where the large arteries run close enough to the surface of the skin to be felt as a pulse (16)

Pulse pressure: the difference between the systolic and diastolic pressures (20)

Pulse rate: the number of pulsations that can be felt over an artery in 1 minute; an indication of the heart rate (one of the vital signs) (20)

Pulse rhythm: the pattern of the pulsations and the pauses between them (20)

Pustule: a small, blister-like skin lesion that contains pus, a thick, yellowish fluid that is a sign of infection (29)

Pyelonephritis: a kidney infection (37)

Pyloric sphincter: a circle of muscular tissue that surrounds the place where the stomach empties into the small intestine and helps to prevent food from returning to the stomach once it enters the small intestine (36)

R

Race: physical differences that groups and cultures consider socially significant (6)

RACE fire response plan: the general actions that are taken in the event of a fire emergency (rescue/remove to safety, activate the alarm, contain the fire, extinguish or evacuate) (13)

Radiation therapy: a type of therapy that uses energy transmitted by x-ray beams or implanted radioactive material to destroy cancer cells (42)

Radiating pain: pain that travels from one area to another (21)

Range of motion: the complete extent of movement that a joint is normally capable of without causing pain (30)

Rash: a group of skin lesions (29)

Reciprocity: the principle by which one state recognizes the validity of a license or certification granted by another state (2)

Recording: communicating information about a patient or resident to other health care team members in written form; sometimes called charting (5)

Rectocele: a condition that occurs when the front wall of the rectum shifts downward, pushing into the back (posterior) vaginal wall (38)

Reduction: the word used to describe the process of bringing the ends of a broken bone into alignment (30)

Reference list: a list of three or four people who would be willing to talk to a potential employer about a job candidate's abilities (3)

Referred (radiating) pain: pain that is felt somewhere other than where it originated (21)

Regional anesthesia: a loss of sensation in part, but not all, of the body brought on by the injection of medications (compare with general anesthesia and local anesthesia) (43)

Registered nurse (RN): a specially trained person who is licensed by a state to develop nursing care plans and coordinate all aspects of patient or resident care, as well as to provide that care; holds a baccalaureate degree from a liberal arts college or university (4 years) or an associate degree from a junior or community college (2 years) (2)

Registry: an official record maintained by the state of the people who have successfully completed the nursing assistant training program (2)

Regress: to return to an earlier stage of development, as when a child who is experiencing stress as a result of being hospitalized begins demonstrating behaviors from when they were younger, such as thumb-sucking or bedwetting (45)

Rehabilitation: the process of helping a person with a disability to return to their highest level of physical, emotional, or economic function (39)

Reincarnation: the idea that a person's spirit or soul will live again on Earth in the form of an animal or human being yet to be born (27)

Religion: a person's spiritual beliefs (6)

Reminiscence therapy: a technique used for interacting with people who have dementia, in which the person with dementia is encouraged to remember and share experiences from their past with others (9)

Renal: related to, involving, or located in the region of the kidneys (37)

Renal calculi: kidney stones (37)

Reporting: the spoken exchange of information between health care team members (5)

Reproduction: the process by which a living thing makes more living things like itself (38)

Rescue breathing: a basic life support (BLS) technique in which the rescuer blows air into the victim's mouth to perform the function of breathing for the victim until the victim begins breathing again on their own (16)

Resident: a person who is living in a long-term care facility or assisted-living facility (1)

Resident inventory sheet: a document that lists and briefly describes all of the resident's personal belongings; completed when a resident is admitted to a long-term care facility (18)

Respiration: the process the body uses to obtain oxygen from the environment and remove carbon dioxide (a waste gas) from the body (31)

Respiratory arrest: the condition where breathing has stopped (16)

Respiratory rate: the number of times a person breathes in 1 minute (one breath is both an inhalation and an exhalation); one of the vital signs (20)

Respiratory rhythm: the regularity with which a person breathes (20)

Respiratory therapy: any treatment that is used to help a person achieve satisfactory respiration (31)

Respite care: home care that gives the primary caregiver an opportunity to rest or leave the home for a short period of time (46)

Restorative care: measures that health care workers take to help a person regain health, strength, and function; the means by which rehabilitation is achieved (39)

Restraint alternatives: measures taken to avoid the use of chemical or physical restraints (14)

Résumé: a brief document that gives a possible employer general information about a job candidate's education and work experience (3)

Reverse Trendelenburg position: one of the basic positions in which the head of the mattress is raised so the person's head is higher than their feet (compare with Trendelenburg position) (17)

Rigor mortis: the stiffening of the muscles that usually develops within 2 to 4 hours of death (27)

Rugae: folds in the lining of the stomach (36)

S

Safety Data Sheets (SDS): a document that summarizes key information about a chemical, such as its composition, which exposures may be dangerous, what to do if an exposure should occur, and how to clean up spills (13)

Salivary glands: glands located near the mouth that produce and secrete saliva, a substance that helps with chewing and swallowing by moistening the food (36)

Sanitization: practices associated with basic cleanliness, such as handwashing, cleansing of eating utensils and other surfaces with soap and water, and providing clean linens and clothing; one of the techniques of medical asepsis (compare with antisepsis, disinfection, and sterilization) (12)

Schizophrenia: a mental health disorder that affects how a person thinks, feels and acts; the person has difficulty determining what is real from what is imaginary (41)

Scope of practice: the range of tasks that a nursing assistant is legally permitted to do (2)

Seborrheic dermatitis ("cradle cap"): severe scaling of the scalp with thick, yellow, crusty patches (23)

Sebum: an oily substance secreted by glands in the skin that lubricates the skin and helps to prevent it from drying out (29)

Semi-Fowler's (low-Fowler's) position: one of the basic positions in which the head of the bed is elevated approximately 30 to 45 degrees (15)

Sense organs: a general term used to describe the eyes, the ears, the nose, and the taste buds (34)

Sensorineural hearing loss: hearing loss that occurs when the receptors in the ear are unable to receive stimuli or transmit nerve impulses (compare with conductive hearing loss) (34)

Sensory nerves: nerves that carry information from the internal organs and the outside world to the spinal cord and up into the brain so that the brain can analyze the information (33)

Sensory receptors: specialized cells or groups of cells associated with a sensory nerve (34)

Septic shock: shock caused by a severe bacterial infection that involves the entire body (16)

Sex: the physical activity one engages in to obtain sexual pleasure and reproduce (6)

Sex cell (gamete): special cells contributed by each parent that contain half of the normal number of chromosomes (38)

Sexual abuse: forcing another person to engage in sexual activity (compare with psychological [emotional] abuse and physical abuse) (4)

Sexuality: a broad concept that includes our sexual feelings and behaviors, including how a person perceives of their gender and sexual identity (6)

Sexually transmitted infection (STI): an infection that is most commonly transmitted by sexual contact; also known as venereal disease (38)

Shaken baby syndrome: severe brain damage or death in an infant or toddler resulting from violent shaking that causes the child's brain to hit the inside of the skull repeatedly (45)

Shearing: a term used to describe the force created when something or someone is pulled across a surface that offers resistance; can lead to skin breakdown (15)

Shingles (herpes zoster): a disorder, caused by the same virus that causes chickenpox, that is most frequently seen in people older than 65 years and is characterized by a blistering, painful rash that typically follows the pathway of a nerve (29)

Shock: the condition that results when the organs and tissues of the body do not receive enough oxygen-rich blood; see also cardiogenic shock, hemorrhagic shock, anaphylactic shock, and septic shock (16)

Shroud: a covering used to wrap the body of a person who has died (27)

Signs: objective observations (that is, observations based on information that is obtained directly, through measurements or by using one of the five senses) (compare with symptoms) (5)

Sims' position: one of the basic positions in which the person lies on their side with their head turned to one side and their knee sharply bent and supported by a pillow; the corresponding arm is bent at the elbow with the hand in front of the face, palm down, resting on a pillow; the lower leg is straight and the lower arm extends out from the side with the hand down near the hips and the palm turned upward (15)

Sitz bath: a warm water soak for the perineal area (44)

Skeleton: the framework for the body formed by the bones (30)

Slander: spoken statements that injure someone's reputation; a form of defamation (4)

Sleep apnea: a disorder that causes the person to stop breathing for varying periods of time during sleep (21)

Sperm cell: male sex cell (38)

Sphygmomanometer: a device used to measure blood pressure (20)

Spina bifida: a congenital defect of the spinal column that occurs when the vertebrae do not close properly during development, leaving the spinal cord exposed (40)

Sputum: mucus and other respiratory secretions that are coughed up from the lungs, bronchi, and trachea; also known as phlegm (31)

Standard precautions: precautions that a health care worker takes with each patient or resident to prevent contact with bloodborne pathogens; includes the use of barrier methods (such as gloves) as well as certain environmental control methods (12)

Sterilization: the process of completely eliminating microbes from the surface of an object using an autoclave or chemicals; one of the techniques of medical asepsis (compare with antisepsis, disinfection, and sanitization) (12)

Stethoscope: a device that amplifies sound and transfers it to the listener's ears (20)

STI: see sexually transmitted infection

Stomach: a hollow, muscular pouch for holding food (36)

Stomatitis: inflammation of the mouth, often seen in people who are receiving chemotherapy (42)

Stool: a term used to refer to fecal material after it has left the body (25)

Stool softener: a medication that helps to prevent constipation by keeping fluid in the feces (25)

Straight catheter: a urinary catheter that is inserted and then removed immediately, after the urine in the bladder has drained out (25)

Stress: a physical or emotional factor that changes the body's normal balance or equilibrium (41)

Stroke: a disorder that occurs when blood flow to a part of the brain is completely blocked, causing the tissue to die; also known as a "brain attack" or cerebrovascular accident (CVA) (33)

Stump: the end of an amputated limb that is left after surgery (30)

Sub-acute care unit (skilled nursing unit, skilled nursing facility): a unit within a hospital or a long-term care facility, or a separate facility, that provides care focused on rehabilitation and helping the patient to move from hospital care to home care (1)

Subcutaneous tissue: the layer of fat that supports the dermis (the deepest layer of the skin) (29)

Subjective data: information that cannot be objectively measured or assessed (5)

Substance use disorder: disorders that involve the excessive or inappropriate use of drugs (prescription or illegal), alcohol, or inhalants (41)

Suicide: the act of taking one's own life intentionally and voluntarily (41)

Suctioning: the process of removing fluid and mucus from a person's airway (31)

Sundowning: the worsening of behavioral symptoms in the late afternoon and evening (as the sun goes down) of a person with dementia (9)

Supine (dorsal recumbent) position: one of the basic positions in which the person lies on their back, with the bed flat and the head supported by a pillow (15)

Supportive care: treatments that will not prolong life, but will make a person more comfortable, such as oxygen therapy, nutritional supplementation, pain medication, range-of-motion exercises, grooming and hygiene, and positioning assistance (26)

Supportive devices: (1) devices used when positioning a person to help the person maintain proper body alignment, such as pillows or rolled sheets, towels, or blankets (15); (2) devices that help to stabilize a weak joint or limb; used in physical therapy to help a person with a disability regain function (39)

Suprapubic catheter: a urinary catheter that is inserted into the bladder through a surgical incision made in the abdominal wall, right above the pubic bone (25)

Surgical bed: a closed bed that has been opened to receive a patient or resident who will be arriving by stretcher; the top sheet, blanket, and bedspread are folded toward the side of the bed, leaving one side open and ready to receive the person (19)

Survey: an inspection of a nursing home carried out by the government to ensure that care is being provided according to standards and regulations (1)

Symptoms: subjective observations (that is, observations that are based on information that cannot be measured or observed first-hand, such as a patient's or resident's complaint of pain) (compare with signs) (5)

Synapse: the gap between the axon of one neuron and the dendrites of the next (33)

Syncope: fainting (16)

Systemic circulation: the pattern of circulation that takes blood from the lungs to the rest of the body to release oxygen and pick up carbon dioxide (compare with pulmonary circulation) (32)

Systole: the active (contracting) phase of the cardiac cycle, during which the myocardium contracts, sending blood out of the heart (compare with diastole) (32)

Systolic pressure: the pressure that the blood exerts against the arterial walls when the heart muscle contracts; the first blood pressure measurement that is recorded (compare with diastolic pressure) (20)

T

Tachycardia: a heart rate that is faster than normal (more than 100 beats/minute in an adult) (20)

Tachypnea: a respiratory rate that is higher than normal (more than 24 breaths/minute in an adult) (20)

Tactile receptors: receptors found in the skin that are stimulated when something comes in contact with the surface of the body and presses on them, causing them to change shape (34)

Task lighting: bright light directed toward a specific area, used for activities that require good lighting to prevent eyestrain (compare with general lighting) (17)

Tasks: growth and development milestones that must be completed before a person can move on to the next stage of growth and development (6)

TB: see tuberculosis

T cells: special white blood cells (leukocytes) that play a role in the immune response to invading pathogens; the main target of the human immunodeficiency virus (HIV) (11)

Team nursing: a model for organizing the nursing team's efforts in which a team leader (a registered nurse) determines all of the nursing needs for the patients or residents assigned to the team, and assigns tasks according to each team member's skills and level of responsibility (2)

Tendons: bands of connective tissue that attach the skeletal muscles to the bones (30)

Terminal illness: an illness or condition from which recovery is not expected (6)

Tetany: a condition that occurs when the body's calcium level drops too low; characterized by cramping of the skeletal muscles and an irregular heartbeat (35)

Tetraplegia (quadriplegia): paralysis from the neck down; compare with paraplegia and hemiplegia (14)

Thrombi (singular, thrombus): blood clots that form in the small blood vessels, blocking the flow of blood and depriving the tissues of oxygen and nutrients (32)

Thrombocytes: pinched-off pieces of larger cells that are found in the red bone marrow and are responsible for clotting of the blood; also called platelets (32)

Thrombophlebitis: inflammation of the lining of a vein caused by a blood clot (32)

TIA: see transient ischemic attack

Tinea capitis: a fungal infection of the scalp (23)

Tinea pedis: a fungal infection of the skin and nails, commonly known as "athlete's foot" (23)

Tinnitus: ringing in the ear (34)

Tissue: a group of cells similar in structure and specialized to perform a specific function (28)

Toddler: a person between the ages of 1 and 3 years (45)

Toe pleat: loosening of the top linens over a person's feet to relieve pressure and promote comfort (19)

Tort: a violation of civil law (4)

Total parenteral nutrition (TPN, hyperalimentation): an alternative method of providing fluid and nutrition; nourishment is delivered directly into the bloodstream through a large catheter (tube) inserted into a large vein near the heart (24)

TPN: see total parenteral nutrition

Trachea: the passage that carries air from the larynx down into the chest toward the lungs; commonly known as the "windpipe" (31)

Tracheostomy: a surgically created opening in the neck that opens into the trachea; often used with a tracheostomy tube (instead of an endotracheal tube) when a person must be on a mechanical ventilator for more than a week or so (31)

Traction: a treatment for fracture in which the ends of the broken bone are placed in the proper alignment and then weight is applied to exert a constant pull and keep the bone in alignment (30)

Transfer: (1) to move a person from one place to another, for example, from the bed to a wheelchair (15); (2) to move a patient or resident within or between health care settings (18)

Transfer belt (gait belt): a webbed or woven belt with a buckle that is used to assist a weak or unsteady person with standing, walking, or transferring; called a gait belt when used to help a person walk (15)

Transgender: a term used to describe an individual whose gender identity is not what they were assigned at birth (6)

Transient flora: microbes that are picked up by touching contaminated objects or people who have an infectious disease (compare with normal [resident] flora) (12)

Transient ischemic attack (TIA): a temporary (transient) episode of dysfunction caused by decreased blood flow to the brain (33)

Transmission-based precautions: precautions that a health care worker takes when a person is known to have a disease that is transmitted in a certain way; include airborne precautions, droplet precautions, and contact precautions (12)

Trapeze bar: a device that is attached to the overhead frame of a person's bed; used to assist with movement (30)

Trendelenburg position: one of the basic positions in which the foot of the mattress is raised so that the person's head is lower than their feet (compare with reverse Trendelenburg position) (17)

Tuberculosis (TB): an airborne infection caused by a bacterium that usually infects the lungs (11)

Tumor: an abnormal growth of tissue; the cells that form the tumor may be benign or malignant (42)

Type 1 diabetes mellitus: a type of diabetes caused by destruction of the insulin-producing cells of the pancreas (35)

Type 2 diabetes mellitus: a type of diabetes caused by the inability of the cells of the body to respond to insulin; the pancreas still produces some insulin (35)

U

Ulcer: a shallow crater on the surface of the skin that is formed when the tissue dies and is shed (29)

Umbilical cord: a cord that supplies the growing fetus with nutrients and oxygen, and removes waste (44)

Unintentional tort: a violation of civil law that occurs when someone causes harm or injury to another person or that person's property without the intent to cause harm (4)

Unintentional wound: an unexpected injury that usually results from some type of trauma (compare with intentional wound) (29)

Unit: a patient's or resident's room (17)

United States Department of Health and Human Services (DHHS): the primary government agency responsible for protecting this nation's health; includes organizations such as the Food and Drug Administration (FDA), the Centers for Disease Control and Prevention (CDC), the National Institutes of Health (NIH), and the Centers for Medicare and Medicaid Services (CMS) (1)

Unresponsive: adjective used to describe a person who is unconscious and cannot be aroused, or conscious but not responsive when spoken to or touched (16)

Ureterostomy: an alternative way of eliminating urine from the body; a surgical procedure in which the ureters are brought through the abdominal wall by way of small incisions and sutured in place (37)

Urethritis: infection of the urethra, the passageway that carries urine from the bladder to the outside of the body (37)

Urgency: a need to urinate immediately (25)

Urgent: adjective used to describe surgery that is planned and scheduled ahead of time, but must be done as soon as possible to prevent the person's condition from getting worse (43)

Urinal: a device used for urination when a male is unable to get out of bed (25)

Urinalysis: examination of the urine under a microscope and by chemical means (25)

Urinary incontinence: the inability to hold one's urine, or the involuntary loss of urine from the bladder (25)

Urinary retention: the inability of the bladder to empty either completely during urination, or at all (25)

Urination: the process of passing urine from the body; also known as micturition and voiding (25)

Urine: formed by the kidneys; consists of waste products that have been filtered from the bloodstream, along with excess fluid (37)

Urostomy: an alternative way of eliminating urine from the body; a surgical procedure in which the ureters are attached to a small portion of the small intestine, one end of the segment of intestine is sealed off, and the other end is brought through the abdominal wall and sutured into place to create a stoma (37)

Uterine prolapse (prolapsed uterus): a condition that occurs when the uterus shifts downward, into the vaginal canal (38)

V

Vaginitis: inflammation of the vaginal tissues (38)

Validation therapy: a technique used for interacting with people who have dementia, in which the caregiver acknowledges the person's reality; rather than correcting the person, the caregiver attempts to distract the person and redirect the conversation whenever possible (9)

Value: a cherished belief or principle (4)

Vancomycin-resistant enterococcus (VRE): a type of bacteria that has become resistant to vancomycin, a powerful antibiotic (10)

Varicose veins: a condition that results from pooling of blood in the veins, especially those in the lower legs, causing them to become swollen and "knotty" in appearance (32)

Vascular (multi-infarct) dementia: a type of dementia caused by the loss of function in multiple areas of the brain due to tissue death caused by a lack of adequate oxygen and nutrients (9)

Vector: a living creature, such as an insect, that can transmit disease (10)

Veins: vessels that return blood to the heart (32)

Venous thrombosis: the formation of blood clots (thrombi) in the veins as a result of pooling of the blood (32)

Venous (stasis) ulcers: open sores that occur on the lower legs, usually in the ankle area, as a result of pooling of blood in the veins (32)

Ventilation system: a system that provides fresh air and keeps air circulating throughout a building (17)

Ventricles: the lower chambers of the heart (32)

Venules: the smallest veins (32)

Verbal communication: a way of communicating that uses written or spoken language (5)

Vernix: a protective, cheese-like substance that is present on the skin of newborns (44)

Vertigo: dizziness (34)

Vesicle: a small, blister-like skin lesion that contains fluid (29)

Villi (singular, villus): tiny, finger-like structures on the lining of the small intestine that increase the small intestine's ability to absorb nutrients (36)

Virulence: the strength or disease-producing potential of a pathogen (10)

Vital signs: certain key measurements that provide essential information about a person's health (20)

Voiding: the process of passing urine from the body; also known as urination and micturition (25)

VRE: see vancomycin-resistant enterococcus

Vulnerable adult: a person who is 18 years of age or older who may be in need of community care services because they have an intellectual or other disability, an illness, or is at an age (older adult) that causes them to be unable to care for or protect themselves against significant harm or exploitation (4)

W

Water-soluble: adjective used to describe a substance that dissolves in water (for example, certain vitamins) (24)

Weight bearing: a term used to refer to a person's ability to stand on one or both legs (15)

Will: a legal statement that expresses a person's wishes for the management of their affairs after death (26)

Work ethic: a person's attitude toward their work (3)

Workplace violence: violent acts (including physical assaults and threats of assaults) directed persons at work or on duty (13)

Wound: an injury that results in a break in the skin (and usually the underlying tissues as well) (29)

Note: Page number followed by b, f, t indicates text in box, figure, table respectively.